Blood Pressure and Arterial Wall Mechanics in Cardiovascular Diseases

Michel E. Safar • Michael F. O'Rourke
Edward D. Frohlich
Editors

Blood Pressure and Arterial Wall Mechanics in Cardiovascular Diseases

Springer

Editors
Michel E. Safar, MD
Hôtel-Dieu Hospital Diagnosis
and Therapeutics Center
Paris Descartes University
Paris
France

Edward D. Frohlich, MD, MACP, FACC
Department of Cardiology
Ochsner Clinic Foundation
New Orleans, LA
USA

Michael F. O'Rourke, MD, DSc
St Vincent Clinic and Hospital
University of New South Wales
Victor Chang Cardiac Research Institute
Darlinghurst, Sydney
New South Wales
Australia

ISBN 978-1-4471-7216-1 ISBN 978-1-4471-5198-2 (eBook)
DOI 10.1007/978-1-4471-5198-2
Springer London Heidelberg New York Dordrecht

Printed on acid-free paper

Springer is part of Springer Science+Business Media (www.springer.com)

Contents

Part V Stratifications of Cardiovascular Risk and Therapeutic Consequences on Arterial Stiffness and Wave Reflections

Contributors

Davide Agnoletti, MD, PhD Diagnosis and Therapeutics Center, Hôtel-Dieu Hospital, Assistance Publique des Hôpitaux de Paris, Paris Descartes University, Paris, France

Majd AlGhatrif, MD Human Cardiovascular Studies Unit, Laboratory of Cardiovascular Science, National Institute on Aging, National Institutes of Health, Baltimore, MD, USA

Department of Medicine, Johns Hopkins School of Medicine, Baltimore, MD, USA

Sola Aoun Bahous, MD, PhD Division of Nephrology, Department of Medicine, University Medical Center–Rizk Hospital, Ashrafieh, Beirut, Lebanon

Lucas S. Aparicio, MD, DDS Internal Medicine – Hypertension Section, Hospital Italiano De Buenos Aires, Buenos Aires, Argentina

Annayya R. Aroor, MD, PhD Research Service Harry S Truman Memorial Veterans Hospital, Columbia, MO, USA

Division of Endocrinology and Metabolism, Department of Medicine, University of Missouri School of Medicine, Columbia, MO, USA

Kei Asayama, MD, PhD Studies Coordinating Centre, Division of Hypertension and Cardiovascular Rehabilitation, Department of Cardiovascular Sciences, University of Leuven, Leuven, Belgium

Department of Planning for Drug Development and Clinical Evaluation, Tohoku University Graduate School of Pharmaceutical Sciences, Sendai, Japan

Department of Hygiene and Public Health, Teikyo University School of Medicine, Tokyo, Japan

Jeffrey Atkinson, BA, MA, PhD Cardiovascular Pharmacology Laboratory, Pharmacy Faculty, Lorraine University, Nancy University, Nancy, France

Abraham Aviv, MD, PhD Center of Human Development and Aging Rutgers, The State University of New Jersey, New Jersey Medical School, Newark, NJ, USA

Alberto P. Avolio, PhD, BE The Australian School of Advanced Medicine, 2 Technology Place, Macquarie University, North Ryde, Sydney, NSW, Australia

Tine De Backer, MD, PhD Clinical Pharmacology, Heymans Institute of Pharmacology, University Hospital Ghent, Ghent, Belgium

Cardiovascular Diseases, University Hospital Ghent, Ghent, Belgium

Hélène Beaussier Clinical Research Unit and Pharmacy, Fondation Hôpital Saint Joseph, Paris, France

Hopital Europeen Georges Pompidou, Assistance Publique Hôpitaux de Paris, Université Paris Descartes, Paris, France

Jérémy Bellien, PharmD, PhD Department of Pharmacology, Rouen University Hospital, Rouen, France

Athanase Benetos, MD, PhD Department of Geriatrics, University Hospital of Nancy, Universite De Lorraine, Vandoeuvre Les Nancy, France

INSERM U1116, Université de Lorraine, Nancy, France

Yvonnick Bezie, PharmD, PhD Pharmacy Department, Groupe Hospitalier Paris Saint – Joseph, Paris, France

Jacques Blacher, MD, PhD Department of Medicine, Diagnosis and Therapeutics Center, Hôtel-Dieu Hospital, Assistance Publique des Hôpitaux de Paris, Paris Descartes University, Paris, France

José Boggia, MD, PhD Centro de Nefrología and Departamento de Fisiopatología, Hospital de Clínicas, Montevideo, Uruguay

Luc M. Van Bortel, MD, PhD Clinical Pharmacology, Heymans Institute of Pharmacology, Ghent University, Ghent, Belgium

Pierre Boutouyrie, MD, PhD Department of Pharmacology and Institut National de la Santé et de la Recherche Médicale U970(Eq7)-PARCC, Hôpital Européen Georges Pompidou, Assistance Publique-Hôpitaux de Paris, Université Paris-Descartes, Paris, France

Marie Briet, MD, PhD Department of Pharmacology, Centre Hospitalo-Universitaire d'Angers, Université d'Angers, Angers, France

Lady Davis Institute for Medical Research, McGill University, Montreal, QC, Canada

Mark Butlin, PhD, BE The Australian School of Advanced Medicine, 2 Technology Drive, Macquarie University, North Ryde, Sydney, NSW, Australia

Julio A. Chirinos, MD, PhD Philadelphia Veterans Affairs Medical Center, University of Pennsylvania School of Medicine, Philadelphia, PA, USA

John R. Cockcroft, FRCP, FESC Department of Cardiology, Wales Heart Research Institute, University Hospital, Cardiff University, Cardiff, UK

Julia L. Cook, PhD Research Division, Ochsner Health System, New Orleans, LA, USA

Yazan Daaboul, MSc Department of Medicine, Gilbert and Rose Marie Chagoury School of Medicine, University Medical Center – Rizk Hospital, Ashrafieh, Beirut, Lebanon

Michel Delahousse, MD, PhD Department of Nephrology and Transplantation, Foch Hospital, Suresnes, France

Richard B. Devereux, MD Greenberg Division of Cardiology, New York Presbyterian Hospital, Weill Cornell Medical College, New York, NY, USA

Javier Diez, MD, PhD Program of Cardiovascular Diseases, Centre for Applied Medical Research, Pamplona, Spain

Department of Cardiology and Cardiac Surgery, School of Medicine, University Clinic, University of Navarra, Pamplona, Spain

Feng-Hua Ding, MD, PhD Centre for Epidemiological Studies and Clinical Trials, The Shanghai Institute of Hypertension, Ruijin Hospital, Shanghai Jiaotong University School of Medicine, Shanghai, China

Department of Cardiology, Ruijin Hospital, Shanghai Jiatong University School of Medicine, Shanghai, China

Isabel Ferreira, PhD Department of Internal Medicine, Maastricht University Medical Centre, Maasricht, The Netherlands

Stanley S. Franklin, MD, FACO, FAHA, FASN Preventive Cardiology Program, Division of Cardiology, Department of Medicine, C240 Medical Sciences, University of California, Irvine, CA, USA

Edward D. Frohlich, MD, MACP, FACC Department of Cardiology, Ochsner Clinic Foundation, New Orleans, LA, USA

Sylvie Gautier, MD Department of Geriatrics, University Hospital of Nancy, Universite De Lorraine, Vandoeuvre Les Nancy, France

Yumei Gu, MD, PhD Studies Coordinating Centre, Division of Hypertension and Cardiovascular Rehabilitation, Department of Cardiovascular Sciences, University of Leuven, Leuven, Belgium

Tine W. Hansen, MD, PhD Department of Complications, Steno Diabetes Center, Gentofte, Denmark

David G. Harrison, MD Division of Clinical Pharmacology, Departments of Medicine and Pharmacology, Vanderbilt University, Nashville, TN, USA

Scott L. Hummel, MD, MS Division of Cardiovascular Medicine, Department of Internal Medicine, University of Michigan, Ann Arbor, MI, USA

Piotr Jankowski, MD, PhD I Department of Cardiology and Hypertension, Institute of Cardiology, Jagiellonian University Medical College, Krakow, Poland

Guanghong Jia, PhD Research Service Harry S Truman Memorial Veterans Hospital,Columbia, MO, USA

Division of Endocrinology and Metabolism, Department of Medicine, University of Missouri School of Medicine, Columbia, MO, USA

Xiongjing J. Jiang, MD Department of Cardiology, Hypertension Centre, Fuwai Hospital, Cardiovascular Institute, Chinese Academy of Medical Sciences, National Centre for Cardiovascular Diseases, Peking Union Medical College, Beijing, China

Robinson Joannidès, MD, PhD Department of Pharmacology, INSERM U1096 Institute for Research and Innovation in Biomedicine, Rouen, France

Bronwyn A. Kingwell, PhD Metabolic and Vascular Physiology, Baker IDI Heart and Diabetes Institute, Melbourne, VIC, Australia

Serge Korjian, MSc Department of Medicine, Gilbert and Rose Marie Chagoury School of Medicine, University Medical Center – Rizk Hospital, Ashafieh, Beirut, Lebanon

Roel J.J. van de Laar, MD, PhD Department of Internal Medicine, Maastricht University Medical Centre, Maastricht, The Netherlands

Patrick Lacolley Faculte de Medecine, Unité INSERM UL U1116, Vandoeuvre Les Nancy, France

INSERM U1116, Université de Lorraine, Nancy, France

Edward G. Lakatta, MD Laboratory of Cardiovascular Science, Biomedical Research Center, Baltimore, MD, USA

Laboratory of Cardiovascular Science, IRP, National Institute on Aging, National Institutes of Health, Baltimore, MD, USA

Stéphane Laurent, MD, PhD Department of Pharmacology and Institut National de la Santé et de la Recherche Médicale U970(Eq7)-PARCC, Hôpital Européen Georges Pompidou, Assistance Publique-Hôpitaux de Paris, Université Paris-Descartes, Paris, France

Stephanie Lehoux, PhD Department of Medicine, Lady Davis Institute for Medical Research, Sir Mortimer B. Davis-Jewish General Hospital, McGill University, Montreal, Canada

Bernard I. Lévy, MD, PhD Cardiovascular Research Center- Inserm UMRS 970, Paris, France

Blood and Vessel Institute, Paris, France

Yan Li, MD, PhD Centre for Epidemiological Studies and Clinical Trials, The Shanghai Institute of Hypertension, Ruijin Hospital, Shanghai Jiaotong University School of Medicine, Shanghai, China

Li-Hua Li, MD Centre for Epidemiological Studies and Clinical Trials, The Shanghai Institute of Hypertension, Ruijin Hospital, Shanghai Jiaotong University School of Medicine, Shanghai, China

Yanping Liu, MD, PhD Studies Coordinating Centre, Division of Hypertension and Cardiovascular Rehabilitation, Department of Cardiovascular Sciences, University of Leuven, Leuven, Belgium

Gérard London, MD Department of Nephrology, Hopital Manhes, Fleury-Mérogis, France

Laurent Macron, MD, PhD Radiology, HEGP, APHP, Inserm U970 Eq7, Université Paris Descartes, Paris, France

RadiologyHopital Europeen Georges Pompidou, Paris, France

Kaisa M. Mäki-Petäjä, PhD, BSc Clinical Pharmacology Unit, University of Cambridge, Addenbrooke's Hospital, Cambridge, UK

Yoshio Matsui, MD, PhD Division of Cardiovascular Medicine, Department of Medicine, Jichi Medical University School of Medicine, Shimotsuke, Tochigi, Japan

Department of Internal Medicine, Iwakuni Medical Center, Iwakuni, Yamaguchi, Japan

Carmel M. McEniery, PhD Clinical Pharmacology Unit, University of Cambridge, Addensbrooke's Hospital, Cambridge, UK

Gerald A. Meininger, PhD Dalton Cardiovascular Research Center, University of Missouri School of Medicine, Columbia, MO, USA

Department of Medical Pharmacology and Physiology, University of Missouri School of Medicine, Columbia, MO, USA

Jean-Jacques Mourad, MD, PhD Department of Internal Medicine and Arterial Hypertension, Avicenne University Hospital – APHP, Bobigny, France

Elie Mousseaux, MD, PhD Radiology, HEGP, APHP, Inserm U970 Eq7, Université Paris Descartes, Paris, France

RadiologyHopital Euopeen Georges Pompidou, Paris, France

Teemu J. Niiranen, MD, PhD Department of Chronic Disease Prevention, National Institute for Health and Welfare, Turku, Finland

Department of Medicine, Turku University Hospital, Turku, Finland

Caroline O'Brien, PhD Harvard-MIT Biomedical Engineering Center, Institute for Medical Engineering and Science, Massachusetts Institute of Technology, Cambridge, MA, USA

Michael F. O'Rourke, MD, DSc Department of Cardiovascular and Hypertension, St. Vincent's Clinic, University of New South Wales, Victor Chang Cardiac Research Institute, Darlinghurst, Sydney, NSW, Australia

Augustine Nonso Odili, MD Department of Internal Medicine, Faculty of Clinical Sciences, College of Health Sciences, University of Abuja, University of Abuja Teaching Hospital, Abuja, Nigeria

Division of Hypertension and Cardiovascular Rehabilitation, Department of Cardiovascular Sciences, Studies Coordinating Centre, University of Leuven, Leuven, Belgium

Bruno Pannier, MD Service de Medecine Interne-Cardiologie, Centre Hospitalier F.H. Manhes, Fleury Merogis, France

Gianfranco Parati, MD Department of Health Sciences, University of Milano- Bicocca, Milan, Italy

Marc A. Pfeffer, MD, PhD Division of Cardiovascular, Department of Medicine, Brigham and Women's Hospital, Harvard Medical School, Boston, MA, USA

Gerard E. Plante Institut de Pharmacologie, Universitye de Sherbrooke, Sherbrooke, QC, Canada

Athanase D. Protogerou, MD, PhD Cardiovascular Research Laboratory and Hypertension Center, First Department of Propedeutic and Internal Medicine, "Laiko" Hospital, Medical School, National and Kapodistrian University of Athens, Athens, Greece

Francesco Mattace Raso, MD, PhD Department of Internal Medicine, Erasmus MC, University Medical Center, Rotterdam, The Netherlands

Richard N. Re, MD Research Division, Ochsner Health System, New Orleans, LA, USA

Véronique Regnault Department of Geriatrics, Université De Lorraine, Vandoeuvre Les Nancy, France

Unité INSERM, U1116, Vandoeuvre Les Nancy, France

Mary J. Roman, MD Greenberg Division of Cardiology, New York Presbyterian Hospital, Weill Cornell Medical College, New York, NY, USA

Julian W. Sacre, BScApp, PhD Metabolic and Vascular Physiology, Baker IDI Heart and Diabetes Institute, Melbourne, VIC, Australia

Michel E. Safar, MD Department of Medicine, Diagnosis and Therapeutics Center, Hôtel-Dieu Hospital, Assistance Publique des Hôpitaux de Paris, Paris Descartes University, Paris, France

Paolo Salvi, MD, PhD Department of Cardiology, S. Luca Hospital, IRCCS Istituto Auxologico Italiano, Milano, Italy

Department of Geriatrics, University Hospital of Nancy, Universite De Lorraine, Vandoeuvre Les Nancy, France

INSERM U1116, Université de Lorraine, Nancy, France

Ernesto L. Schiffrin, MD, PhD Department of Medicine, Lady Davis Institute for Medical Research, Sir Mortimer B. Davis-Jewish General Hospital, McGill University, Montreal, QC, Canada

Angelo Scuteri, MD, PhD School of Geriatrics – Faculty of Medicine, University of Rome Tor Vergata, Rome, Italy

Patrick Segers, PhD Institute Biomedical Technology (IBiTech), iMinds Medical IT, Ghent University, Campus Heymans- Blok B, Ghent, Belgium

Jean-Sébastien Silvestre, PhD Cardiovascular Research Center- Inserm UMRS 970, Paris, France

Harold Smulyan, MD Cardiology Division, Department of Medicine, Upstate Medical University, Syracuse, NY, USA

James R. Sowers, MD Division of Endocrinology and Metabolism, Department of Medicine, University of Missouri School of Medicine, Columbia, MO, USA

Research Service Harry S Truman Memorial Veterans Hospital, Columbia, MO, USA

Department of Medical Pharmacology and Physiology, University of Missouri School of Medicine, Columbia, MO, USA

Dalton Cardiovascular Research Center, University of Missouri School of Medicine, Columbia, MO, USA

Jan A. Staessen, MD, PhD Department of Cardiovascular Sciences, UZ Leuven Campus Sint Rafael, University of Leuven, Leuven, Belgium

Department of Epidemiology, Maastricht University, Maastricht, The Netherlands

Research Unit Hypertension and Cardiovascular Epidemiology, Department of Cardiovascular Sciences, Studies Coordinating Centre, University of Leuven, Leuven, Belgium

Division of Hypertension and Cardiovascular Rehabilitation, Department of Cardiovascular Sciences, Studies Coordinating Centre, University of Leuven, Leuven, Belgium

Christodoulos Stefanadis, MD, PhD Hypertension and Peripheral Vessels Units, 1st Department of Cardiology, Athens Medical School, Hippokration Hospital, Athens, Greece

Coen D.A. Stehouwer, MD, PhD Department of Internal Medicine, Maastricht University Medical Center, Maastricht, The Netherlands

Jonathan Stone, BSc (Med), PhD, DSc Department of Physiology, Bosch Institute, University of Sydney F 13, Sydney, NSW, Australia

Harry A.J. Struijker-Boudier, PhD Department of Pharmacology, CARIM, Maastricht University, Maastricht, The Netherlands

Kenji Takazawa, MD, PhD Department of Cardiology, Hachioji Medical Center, Tokyo Medical University, Hachioji City, Tokyo, Japan

Isabella Tan, BE The Australian School of Advanced Medicine, 2 Technology Drive, Macquarie University, North Ryde, Sydney, NSW, Australia

Alain Tedgui, PhD Institut National de la Santé et de la Recherche Médicale (Inserm), Unité 970, Paris Cardiovascular Research Center, Université Paris-Descartes, Paris, France

Dimitrios Terentes-Printzios, MD Hypertension and Peripheral Vessels Units, 1st Department of Cardiology, Athens Medical School, Hippokration Hospital, Athens, Greece

Lutgarde Thijs, MSc Studies Coordinating Centre, Division of Hypertension and Cardiovascular Rehabilitation, Department of Cardiovascular Sciences, University of Leuven, Leuven, Belgium

Simon N. Thornton, PhD Faculté de Médecine, Unité INSERM UL U1116, Nancy, France

Christian Thuillez, MD, PhD Department of Pharmacology, INSERM U1096, Institute for Research and Innovation in Biomedicine, Rouen, France

Charalambos Vlachopoulos, MD, PhD Hypertension and Peripheral Vessels Units, 1st Department of Cardiology, Athens Medical School, Hippokration Hospital, Athens, Greece

Ji-Guang Wang, MD, PhD Centre for Epidemiological Studies and Clinical Trials, The Shanghai Institute of Hypetension, Ruijin Hospital, Shanghai Jiaotong, University School of Medicine, Shanghai, China

Ghassan Watfa, MD, PhD Department of Geriatrics, University Hospital Of Nancy, Universite De Lorraine, Vandoeuvre Les Nancy, France

INSERM U1116, Université de Lorraine, Nancy, France

Thomas Weber, MD Department of Cardiology, Kinikum Wels-Grieskirchen, Wels, Austria

Paracelsus Medical University, Salzburg, Austria

Ian B. Wilkinson, FRCP, DM, BM BCh Clinical Pharmacology Unit, University of Cambridge, Addenbrooke's Hospital, Cambridge, UK

Jing Wu Division of Clinical Pharmacology, Departments of Medicine and Pharmacology, Vanderbilt University School of Medicine, Nashville, TN, USA

Alexandra Yannoutsos, MD Diagnosis and Therapeutics Center, Hôtel-Dieu Hospital, Assistance Publique des Hôpitaux de Paris, Paris Descartes University, Paris, France

Yi Zhang, MD, PhD Department of Cardiology, Shanghai Tenth People's Hospital, Tongji University School of Medicine, Shanghai, China

Introduction

Three colleagues whose background in medicine arose from their similar interests in cardiovascular research, although they never worked at the same institution, conceived the concept of this textbook. Further, even more unique, they lived throughout their professional careers in three disparate continents and countries: France, Australia, and the United States. Each of them conducted their clinical investigation in cardiovascular medicine. Initially, Professors Safar and Frohlich were interested primarily in a developing area concerned with the hemodynamics of hypertension. They first met in 1962 when Ed Frohlich was on staff of the Research Division of the Cleveland Clinic in Ohio. Michel Safar visited the Cleveland group at that time to exchange thoughts on a now-forgotten topic concerning the underlying mechanisms of "labile" hypertension. Michel was on the Faculty of Medicine at the Broussais Hospital in Paris. They both shared similar thinking about one aspect in the pathogenesis of hypertensive disease: an initial increased cardiac output, which was produced by total body venoconstriction resulting in increased venous return associated with an "inappropriately normal" total peripheral resistance. Ed continued his work with the role of the heart in hypertension and the underlying mechanisms which may explain its increased risk for morbidity and mortality associated with left ventricular hypertrophy. This, of course, stimulated further interest in left ventricular hypertrophy and its interaction with antihypertensive therapy and its impact on cardiac risk. Other factors confounded that risk including the effects of long-term dietary sodium excess on the cardiovascular and renal inter-relationships. Thus, Michel and Ed continued to remain closely related personally and academically in their clinical investigative interests.

During these years, Michel Safar focused his efforts on the pathophysiological mechanisms responsible for the role of the large arteries in hypertension and its consequences in patients with essential hypertension. He and his team of investigators made their major impact on the development of a new area of clinical research responsible for the increasing interest in systolic hypertension in the elderly and the field of "stiffness" of the large arteries. This, of course, brought Michel Safar into the third relationship with Michael O'Rourke whose fundamental research on large arteries in Australia involved work with a physiological pioneer, Michael Taylor, on comparative physiology and computer modeling of arterial networks. This led to clinical studies on ventricular/vascular interactions, intra-aortic balloon counterpulsation, cardiac transplantation and mechanical heart assist devices. His studies promoted interests in the aging process, which develops slowly from early adulthood and involves stiffening and dilation of the aortic wall. These hemodynamic interests led to the collaborative efforts of Michael and Michel in the fields of pulsatile arterial parameters and aortic rigidity. They now consider the possibility that small vessel disease in the brain, causing dementia, is another consequence of aortic stiffening and early wave reflection, which may be prevented or delayed by measures which reduce effects of aortic stiffening. The immediate result of their relationship was Michel's establishment of a regular series of international workshops in Paris on this new area of research resulting in a remarkably increased pursuit of scholarly activity in both the fundamental and clinical investigative aspects in this area.

Contemporaneously, during these years, Ed Frohlich assumed editorial responsibility for the American Heart Association's journal *Hypertension*, and was delighted to join "forces" with Michel and Michael to publish the periodic proceedings of the workshop in that journal. This is the story of our personal collaborations and continuing research, based on long-standing friendship and the influence of Michel Safar in the three of us joining together our mutual interest. This now has resulted in publication of this volume involving similarly committed colleagues from the world-wide academic community. Indeed, it explains our joint conception of the title and content of this work of long-standing friends and academic co-workers and the large co-authorship of its contributors.

Basic Concepts of the Book

Our most common and classical knowledge on blood pressure and hypertension has been primarily influenced by three key-points. First, the hemodynamic mechanisms of hypertension have been primarily associated with an increase in total peripheral resistance, pointing to a major contribution of the role of small arteries. Second, the respective contributions of the heart, vessels, and kidneys involve major interactions affecting particularly the renin-angiotensin-aldosterone system. Finally, drug treatment modifies substantially cardiovascular morbidity and mortality through the dominant role of blood pressure reduction.

The development of hypertension has considerably matured over the years for two reasons. Firstly, hypertension was no longer considered as a single homogeneous disease, but rather as a mosaic of interacting mechanisms associated with many other interrelated cardiovascular risk factors. Secondly, the primary objectives of study were no longer limited to a discussion of only control of arterial pressure. Primary objectives were focused on the means to diminish the underlying risk of cardiovascular stiffness and its consequences on morbidity and mortality. This goal was considered and pursued through numerous therapeutic trials designed to intervene on those pathophysiological mechanisms and the interrelationships that are involved with the development of injury and disease outcomes of these target organs.

Parts I and II of this book are related to blood pressure involving two different and complementary aspects: the role of arterial wall mechanics and the underlying mechanisms of risk involving left ventricular hypertrophy and the role of dietary salt excess on the development of cardiac and renal failure through structural and functional impairment.

In Part I, the role of blood pressure in hypertension and cardiovascular diseases was no longer limited to the role of brachial artery BP measurements, frequently explored in the past but extended to the overall remaining portions of circulation, mainly located at the origin of the aorta. Thus, the concept of central blood pressure was introduced for those organs most related to the presence of cardiovascular risk (i.e., the heart, the brain and kidneys). Pressure measurements were associated to evaluations of flow, impedance to pulsatile flow, arterial stiffness, and other critical parameters as pulse amplification. An important aspect of Part I was the difference noted between steady and pulsatile arterial hemodynamics, two parameters highly and differently related to cardiovascular risk. As noted by Michael O'Rourke, most of these parameters refer to the approach suggested in the past by the principal pioneers of pulsatile arterial hemodynamics, McDonald, Womersley and Taylor. One important aspect is the concept of heart-vessel coupling and its consequences on cardiac structure and function.

Part II refers to the relation between blood pressure, the heart and kidneys. The role of vasoactive interactions are not primarily focused in this discussion but involve primarily the role of the underlying mechanisms of risk in left ventricular hypertrophy, heart failure, oxidative stress and nitric oxide, in relation with mainly dietary salt excess in the heart and kidney. Also investigated are details of the value of multicenter trials of pharmacological therapy on cardiovascular and renal function in hypertension and heart failure.

As a consequence, Part III summarizes the principal findings characterizing hypertension and cardiovascular diseases and the disturbed arterial wall mechanics and sodium balance within the cardiovascular system. Such modifications are studied successively in terms of brachial and central BP measurements and take into account both steady and pulsatile arterial hemodynamics, particularly the role of heart rate and pulse pressure amplification. In addition, organ damages are described extensively in Part III, evaluating the particular and specific roles of the heart, the brain and the kidneys.

Parts IV and V are focused on the different aspects of the clinical involvement necessary for evaluation of the cardiovascular system. First, the role of age, sex, metabolic and inflammatory factors is considered in detail. Second, a description of risk stratification is given, primarily affecting arterial stiffness and pulse pressure. The major role of ethnicity is particularly taken into account. Finally, among the various cardiovascular medications associated to treatment, the antihypertensive agents are mainly (but not exclusively) taken into account, studying in particular their impact on arterial stiffness and wave reflections. Each of these considerations are presented in terms of large vessels, based on the privilege of knowledge and not necessarily the evidence of recommendations frequently difficult to demonstrate.

Finally, this book has developed new conceptual approaches of hypertension and cardiovascular risk, taking into account three major points. First, hypertension should involve in its definition not only vascular resistance but also arterial stiffness, wave reflections and vascular rarefaction. Second, hypertension does not reflect a simple linear relationship between blood pressure and target organ damage but is more complex – and not necessarily linearly affecting mechanical factors and different complications individually associated with the heart, brain and kidneys. Finally, the aim of treatment is no longer limited to a decrease in blood pressure but, rather, a reduction of cardiovascular risk and, in the long term, of residual risk. In this context, it is important that, whereas increased stiffness and early wave reflections caused by aging magnify cardiovascular risk (studies in Part I), the improvement of cardiac function by drug treatment (studies in Part II) may actually exacerbate the adverse effect of increased stiffness and wave reflections when these arterial parameters remain untreated, thereby further increasing cardiovascular risk. Again, it is evident that treatment must verify in the long term the major role of heart-vessel coupling. Modern concepts must include arterial properties as well as peripheral resistance and cardiac function.

Content of the Book

This book is published at the peak of a special evolution during which new concepts and knowledge on blood pressure and cardiovascular risk have been developed over recent years, which is associated with continued exciting aspects of disease and its treatment. First, studies have recognized that the duration of life has increased considerably in recent years promoting research into novel aspects of therapeutic interventions. Second, current investigations on the interactions between genetics and environment still remain difficult to delineate clearly in our patients. These difficulties explain the necessity to obtain numerous contributors participating in all five sections of this volume. Each section is composed of several chapters, each detailed by their respective authors. Importantly, their specific contributions and responsibility, and reflecting any changes by the co-editors. Due to the complexity of the subject, repetitions within this book have not been completely excluded from the studied description by the authors, other than in editorial context to facilitate reading.

Michel E. Safar — Paris, France
Michael F. O'Rourke — Sydney, NSW, Australia
Edward D. Frohlich — Orleans, LA, USA

Part I

Blood Pressure: Basic Concepts of Steady and Pulsatile Arterial Hemodynamics

1 Arterial Stiffness, Wave Reflection, Wave Amplification: Basic Concepts, Principles of Measurement and Analysis in Humans

Michael F. O'Rourke, Caroline O'Brien, and Thomas Weber

Abstract

The arterial system has two functions – as a conduit to deliver blood at high pressure to the organs and tissues of the body according to need, and as a cushion, to reduce pulsations generated by the intermittently-pumping left ventricle, so that blood flow through peripheral high and low resistance vascular beds is steady with little residual pulsation (O'Rourke, Chapter 1: Principles and definitions of arterial stiffness, wave reflections and pulse pressure amplification. In: Safar ME, O'Rourke MF (eds) Arterial stiffness in hypertension. Handbook of hypertension, vol 23. Elsevier, Amsterdam, 2006; Nichols et al., McDonald's blood flow in arteries, 6th edn. Arnold Hodder, London, 2011). The arterial system in man is beautifully suited to serve these functions, at least through childhood, adolescence and young adulthood (Taylor, Gastroenterology 52:358–363, 1967). By mid-life, effects of pulsatile strain on non-living elastic fibres in the highly pulsatile aorta lead to their fracture and to progressive passive aortic dilation, with transfer of stress to more rigid collagen fibres in the media (Nichols et al., McDonald's blood flow in arteries, 6th edn. Arnold Hodder, London, 2011). Such changes have adverse effects on arterial function and ideal timing of vascular/ventricular interaction (O'Rourke and Nichols, Hypertension 45:652–658, 2005; Laurent et al., Eur Heart J 27:2588–2605, 2006; O'Rourke and Hashimoto, J Am

M.F. O'Rourke, MD, DSc (✉)
Department of Cardiovascular and Hypertension,
St Vincent's Clinic, University of New South Wales,
Victor Chang Cardiac Research Institute,
Suite 810 St Vincent Clinic, 438 Victoria Street,
Darlinghurst, Sydney, NSW 2010, Australia
e-mail: m.orourke@unsw.edu.au

C. O'Brien, PhD
Harvard-MIT Biomedical Engineering Center,
Institute for Medical Engineering and Science,
Massachusetts Institute of Technology,
77 Massachusetts Ave, Cambridge, MA 02139, USA
e-mail: ccob@mit.edu

T. Weber, MD
Department of Cardiology, Klinikum Wels-Grieskirchen,
Grieskirchnerstrasse 42, Wels 4600, Austria

Paracelsus Medical University, Salzburg, Austria
e-mail: thomas.weber3@liwest.at

M.E. Safar et al. (eds.), *Blood Pressure and Arterial Wall Mechanics in Cardiovascular Diseases*,
DOI 10.1007/978-1-4471-5198-2_1, © Springer-Verlag London 2014

Coll Cardiol 50:1–13, 2007). As later years pass, impaired arterial function plays an important role in morbidity and mortality, becoming a key factor in development of Isolated Systolic Hypertension of the Elderly (ISHE), and cardiac failure (Chirinos et al. 2012; Weber et al. 2013) and of cerebral micro-infarcts and hemorrhage with cognitive impairment and dementia (O'Rourke and Safar ME, Hypertension 46:200–204, 2005; Stone, Med Hypotheses 71:347–359, 2008; Gorelick, Stroke 42:2672–2713, 2011). This introductory chapter discusses mechanisms and introduces strategies for treatment and prevention.

Keywords

Arterial stiffness • Wave reflection • Pressure amplification • Aging • Pulse wave velocity • Impedance

Concepts

Arterial stiffness and distensibility (Table 1.1) are difficult to measure directly in the human arterial system. Normally up to young adulthood, distensibility is high (stiffness is low) in the proximal thoracic aorta and distensibility is less (stiffness greater) in the abdominal aorta and peripheral arteries [1, 2]. This is the pattern seen in most other mammals throughout life; benefits resulting have been set out by Taylor [3]. Distensibility measured in one arterial segment is not necessarily the same as distensibility at another segment [2]. Further, pressure pulsation is not the same in all arteries and diameter change is small – (2–16 %), and hard to measure accurately [1–6]. The arterial wall is not homogeneous, and stresses are controlled by the medial, not intimal elements. Stiffness and distensibility are not only difficult to measure, but measures are bound to be inaccurate, and they have not always been shown of value in predicting cardiovascular events [1, 5, 8]. However, indirect measures of arterial stiffness have proved useful, and are widely used now to predict cardiovascular events [1, 5]. Such indices are directly (pulse wave velocity [1, 2]), or indirectly, related to arterial stiffness (aortic augmentation index), and amplification of the arterial pressure wave between aorta and radial artery (to be later discussed).

Table 1.1 Indices of arterial stiffness

Elastic modulus	The pressure step required for (theoretic) 100 % stretch from resting diameter at fixed vessel length, $(\Delta P \cdot D) \div \Delta D$ (mmHg)
Arterial distensibility	Relative diameter change for a pressure increment; the inverse of elastic modulus, $\Delta D \div (\Delta P \cdot D)$ (mmHg^{-1})
Arterial compliance	Absolute diameter; change for a given pressure step, $\Delta D \div \Delta P$ (cm·mmHg^{-1})
Volume elastic modulus	Pressure step required for (theoretic) 100 % increase in volume $\Delta P \div (\Delta V \div V)$ (mmHg) $= \Delta P \div (\Delta A \div A)$ (mmHg) (where there is no change in length)
Volume compliance	Absolute volume change for a given pressure step or an arterial segment $\Delta V \div \Delta P$ (cm^3·mmHg^{-1}) or $\Delta A \div \Delta P$ (cm^2·mmHg^{-1}), if there is no change in length
Young's modulus	Elastic modulus per unit area; the pressure step per square centimetre required for (theoretic) 100 % stretch from resting length $(\Delta P \cdot D) \div (\Delta D \cdot h)$ (mmHg·cm^{-1})
Pulse wave velocity	Speed of travel of the pulse along an arterial segment, distance $\div \Delta t$ (cm·s^{-1})
Characteristic impedance	Relationship between pressure change and flow velocity in the absence of wave reflections $(\Delta P \div \Delta V)$ (mmHg. cm^{-1}.s)
Stiffness index	Ratio of logarithm (systolic/diastolic pressures) to (relative change in diameter) $\beta = \ln(P_s \div P_d) \div [(D_s - D_d) \div D_d]$ (nondimensional)

Distensibility (and stiffness) are useful and necessary concepts, and had been used in the past to characterise properties of the arterial tree. The whole arterial tree was likened by Stephen Hales (the first to actually measure blood pressure [12]), to the inverted air-filled dome ("Windkessel" in the German translation) of contemporary (circa 1770) hand-pumped fire engines. The problem with this model was its inability to explain pressure wave contour under different physiological or pathophysiological conditions. In such a model, pressure is everywhere the same – there is no wave travel, no wave reflection, no augmentation and no amplification of the pulse in peripheral arteries. Readers will find support for Windkessel models in other chapters of this book, usually by non-clinicians. Clinicians who see a future for analysis of pulse waveforms require comprehensive realistic models for use in situations such as intensive care where a wide range of blood pressure, heart rate, age and disease exist. Here, the model of transmission line is necessary for realistic monitoring, analysis and diagnosis.

The best and the only comprehensive model of the arterial tree is a simple tube (Fig. 1.1) [1, 2], open at one end to receive blood in spurts from the left ventricle, and closed at the other end which represents the sum total of high resistance arterioles in which the elastic arteries terminate. Such a model allows for wave travel along the tube (and back again) after wave reflection at the distal end. In this model, one can see and explain the known properties of the arterial system – delay of the pulse between proximal and distal arteries, difference in shape and amplitude of the pulse in proximal aorta and distal arteries, and wave reflection (Fig. 1.2).

So what is wave reflection? This is best understood by considering the difference between pressure and flow waves in the ascending aorta. The flow wave from the heart shows a single spurt, whereafter flow falls to zero at the incisura, and stays at zero throughout diastole. In contrast, the pressure wave shows two localised peaks, the first corresponding to the peak of flow and the second to the summation of reflection from multiple sites, principally in the trunk and lower body. In children and young adults, the second peak is in diastole, after the incisura caused by aortic valve closure. In older adults, the aorta is stiffened and pulse wave velocity increased, so that the reflected wave returns early from peripheral arterioles, and augments pressure in mid-late systole (Fig. 1.2).

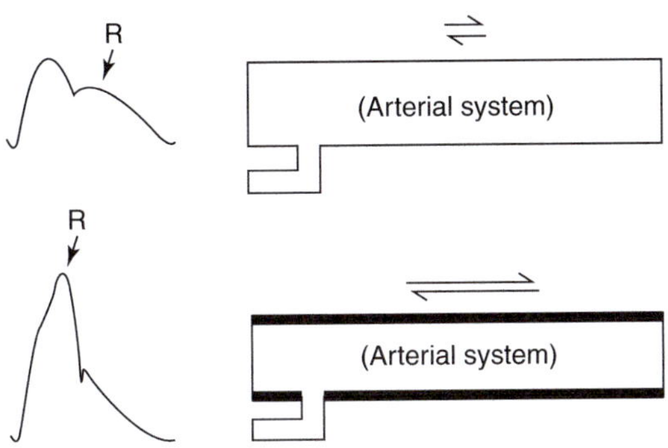

Fig. 1.1 Tubular models of the arterial system with the heart (*left*) and conduit arteries (*right*). Pressure waves in the ascending aorta are shown at *left side*. The normal young arterial tree is represented at *top*, while the old stiffened arterial tree is represented at *bottom*. *Arrows* represent speed of pulse wave travel to the peripheral resistance and back to the heart

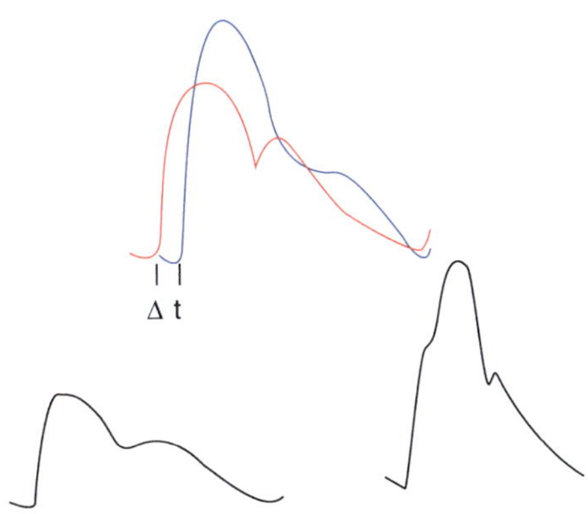

Fig. 1.2 *Top*: The time delay (**Δ**t) due the pressure wave travelling from the ascending aorta (*red*) to the femoral artery (*blue*). The time delay (**Δ**t) is used in the determination of "ascending aortic" pulse wave velocity, where the distance between carotid and femoral arteries is divided by time required for the pressure wave to travel. *Bottom*: Ascending aortic pressure wave in a young individual (*left*) and old subject with stiffened arteries (*right*)

Pulse Wave Velocity: The Best Currently Available Non-invasive Measure of Arterial Stiffness

Pulse wave velocity (PWV) is the speed of the pulse wave generated by the heart, along the arterial tree. It is considerably higher (5–15 M/s) than the blood flow velocity (peak ~1 M/s) and is determined by properties of the arterial wall and of blood within. It is determined by the stiffness of the segments of arterial tree traversed by the pulse according to the Moens-Korteweg equation [1, 2]:

$$PWV = \sqrt{\frac{E/h}{\rho.D}},$$

where "E" is stiffness of the arterial wall as Young's modulus [1], "h" is wall thickness (assuming homogeneity), "ρ" is kinematic viscosity of blood = blood viscosity ÷ density, and "D" is diameter. Typical values of ascending aortic PWV of a child are 3–5 M/s. This can be compared to peak flow velocity in the ascending aorta (~1 M/s) and the height of the human body in a 12 year-old child 1–1.5 M, and distance from heart to resultant peripheral reflecting site of ~0.5 M [1, 2]. A reflected pressure wave would be expected to appear some 300 ms after the foot of the pressure wave and to be most prominent after the aortic valve shuts. In an older adult, with aortic PWV 10 M/s and height 1.5–2 M, the reflected wave would be expected in late systole. Both waves in Fig. 1.2 are typically what one sees in young and old human respectively.

PWV in the aorta can be estimated from measurement of distance from aortic origin to femoral artery, then measuring the delay in the foot of the wave between ascending aorta (or carotid with correction of delay from aorta to carotid site) to femoral artery [13]. Typical values for a young adult are distance 0.6 M, delay 100 ms, and "aortic" PWV of 6 M/s.

Efficiency of the arterial tree, as referred to above, was one of the key interests of pioneers of this field such as Donald McDonald and Michael Taylor, some 50 years ago [2, 3]. It had been alluded to by Hales [12] in 1769 as the cardiovascular "oeconomy". Taylor noted that aortic PWV was always slightly higher than peak flow velocity from the left ventricle (in a child 3 M/s compared to 1 M/s respectively) so there would be no concern about development of shock waves in the aorta, and that there was such correspondence between PWV, body length and heart rate that wave reflection would normally return to the heart after ventricular ejection had ceased, and so would not increase left ventricular load of that beat. On the other hand, the reflected boost to pressure during diastole would maintain coronary perfusion pressure during diastole – the only period when the left ventricular muscle was relaxed and capable of being perfused. Taylor commented on these desirable features of arterial function, showed that they were retained in mammals of different size and responsible for the inverse relationship between body size and heart rate [3]. Milnor [14] and O'Rourke [15] later highlighted these issues, with the latter pointing out how the optimal timing of wave reflection was lost with aging as aortic PWV increased and wave reflection arrived early to augment pressure or suppress flow [1, 2, 6] from the heart in late systole.

Fifty years back [2], the marked increase of aortic PWV with age in humans was not appreciated, nor were the ill-effects this had on the heart. Maximal efficiency of the arterial tree appears to decrease progressively from around age 30. This corresponds to the average life span in earlier times; hence arterial degeneration after age 30 [2, 6] did not pose an evolutionary threat to the human species.

Principles of Measurement, Analysis

Invasive studies of arterial pressure and flow waves were undertaken up till around 1950 by physiologists exclusively, initially by pioneers such as Starling, Frank and Wiggers, then after devastation of Europe by two World Wars and their sequelae, later by luminaries of American Physiology such as Hamilton, Dow and

Remington. Concepts of this time are prominently displayed in the Handbooks of the American Physiological Society [16]. However, physicians of the late nineteenth century (i.e. 60 years before) had sought clinical information through analysing radial and carotid pulse waves as introduced by Marey and Mahomed, using mechanical sensors and smoked drums, but these lapsed with introduction of the cuff sphygmomanometer, and the numbers they provided for brachial cuff systolic and diastolic pressures [17]. Electronic sensors were introduced by Wiggers and Hamilton for measurement of pressure waves, then electromagnetic flow cuffs for direct application to an artery were introduced just prior to World War 2. Physiologists using these devices were generally aware of the shortcomings of the devices they used for measuring pressure and flow, and the potential artefacts that accompanied their use, as well as concerns on frequency response of recording systems. Around this time, and even later, medical device industries were primitive or non-existent, and physiologists needed to make and calibrate their own [18]. As late as 1964, Taylor's laboratory in Sydney made its own cuff electromagnetic flowmeter probes, and callipers for measuring pulsatile diameter change, and calibrated these for steady and pulsatile response. In the process, physiologists became very aware of instrumental and analytic shortcomings [19], but were guided by the traditions of their profession, inherited from European masters including Carl Ludwig that "Die Methode ist Alles" [19].

Shortly after conclusion of World War 2, the field of arterial hemodynamics was taken up again, particularly in the USA with the field of coronary hemodynamics investigated thoroughly by Donald Gregg [20] and colleagues at the Walter Reid Hospital in Washington using cuff electromagnetic flowmeters, then by Braunwald and colleagues [21] at the National Institute of Health for study of animal and human heart function. Enthusiastic development of cardiac surgery and cardiac catheterisation widened the field, introducing more and better instruments, but eventually a degree of laxity on fundamentals – a straying from the dicta of Ludwig. This was later associated with break-up of the American Physiological Society so that Neurophysiology joined Neuroscience, and Cardiovascular Physiology became largely a clinical discipline. Similar changes in allegiance have occurred elsewhere, but for Physiology, incorporation with anatomy or clinical science can be seen as a backward step in medical pre and postgraduate education.

Up until the late 1960s, the strong departments of academic cardiovascular physiology were directed by those who sought to examine cardiovascular physiology in the time domain, as it had been prior to the Second World War [16]. Alternative approaches, developed largely in emerging departments of Biomedical Engineering, were spurred on by physiologists/mathematicians McDonald, Womersley and Taylor in Britain who espoused analysis of pressure and flow in the frequency domain, with pressure wave transmission described in terms of transfer functions of modulus and phase plotted against frequency, and pressure/flow relationships described as modulus and phase of impedance [2, 22, 23]. These analytic principles are now regarded as complementary, but they are often not familiar to the modern conventionally-trained physicians and clinical scientists who now dominate the field of arterial hemodynamics, and are strongly represented in this book.

Modern advances in arterial hemodynamics, as used in clinical departments, were first developed in experimental animals where it was possible to control variables in a way that is not possible in clinical practice. Clinicians work in an environment when advance needs be made in the process of treating patients to the highest possible standards. Corners need be cut and approximations made. Such need is a fact of life, and not necessarily undesirable. Indeed McDonald's new approach was based on the assumption (quantified by Womersley [23]), that non-linearities in pressure/flow relations were sufficiently small to be neglected to a first approximation. However, many problems have arisen in clinical practice with respect to the issues previously discussed in this chapter, and warrant consideration when reading what follows in later chapters.

Wave Reflection

Readers will find considerable confusion on this subject in recent publications [24], and even in this book. The view presented in this chapter is conventional and mainstream – that promoted by Wiggers and other classic physiologists at the time of the peak influence of the American Physiological Society and the (British) Physiological Society [2, 16], and by Taylor and colleagues on the basis of conventional physiology and from analysis of pressure and flow waves in both the time and frequency domain. This view notes studies extending back to Galen and Harvey, implemented by master surgeon John Hunter in 1775 [25] for treatment of popliteal aneurysms. These are interpreted now to show that wave reflection has greatest effect on the low frequency components of flow and pressure waves (i.e. those of greatest magnitude) and least effect on higher harmonics which are highly damped [26]. A different point of view is promoted by groups in Calgary [27] and London [28] who see greatest effect of wave reflection on higher harmonics. The views are based on studies from a single human catheterisation laboratory in London, and are debated sometimes scathingly [29] as reactionary "Cross Talk" in 2013 editions of the Journal of Physiology (London) [27], and in other journal correspondence [29]. Early wave reflection in the ascending aorta, as manifest from pressure wave augmentation, ratio of backward to forward wave or as pressure wave amplification has been shown to predict cardiovascular events in the majority (14/19) of reported studies (Table 1.2). In the five negative studies, amplification was not measured with validated methods.

Another viewpoint on wave reflection is voiced in a series of articles from distinguished authors in the main clinical journal of the American Heart Association where magnitude of wave reflection is gauged from magnitude of aortic augmentation index, without consideration of effects of wave reflection on flow from the heart. Wave reflection can subtract from flow as well as add to pressure [2, 30, 31]. To properly interpret pressure waves in the arterial system one needs to consider not only shape of the pressure wave but the flow wave that generates the pressure wave [2, 9]. This is why the best description of LV hydraulic load is as vascular impedance, and this requires measurement of flow as well as pressure, then describing the relationship in the frequency domain as pioneered by Taylor and Milnor 50 years ago [32, 33].

Another problem in interpretation of impedance and flow waveforms in human studies has been the use of Doppler flowmetry in the left ventricular outflow tract from the envelope of the flow wave and the assumption of laminar flow in the ascending aorta. The envelope of flow represents highest velocities in a turbulent jet and does not represent average flow across the aorta at any point in time. The turbulence can be seen in Magnetic Resonance (MR) studies as forward and backward flow occurring at the same time and as previously mentioned. The MR analysis enables backward and forward flow to be separated, with instantaneous mean flow estimated across the aortic lumen [34, 35]. MR ascending aortic flow shows the predicted pattern, as previously shown in experimental animals and humans with cuff type electromagnetic flowmeters. MR ascending aortic flow (peak and mean) is less than Doppler flow, and decreases with age in line with increase in aortic cross-sectional area. Such differences in flow are not seen in Doppler studies, nor in multiple impedance values reported therefrom [36–38].

Amplification of the Pressure Wave

Amplification of the pressure wave (Fig. 1.3) in the upper limb is expressed as amplitude of radial pulse pressure divided by central aortic pulse pressure. It is independent of brachial cuff pressure since it is a ratio of pressures, and ranges between 0 (in older subjects) and 2 (in younger subjects), and is inversely related to augmentation index, and is caused by wave reflection as this influences the timing of the reflected wave in aorta and radial artery. Wave reflection is known to be high (0.80 estimated by O'Rourke and Taylor in a vascular bed [32, 39, 40] and up to 100 % by Hamilton and others [16]) but cannot

Table 1.2 Wave reflections and risk predictions

Author	Population	n	Method	Endpoint	Independent of	Significant parameter
London	ESRD	180	Carotid PWA	Mortality	DBP	AIx
Takenaka	ESRD	104	Radial PWA	CV events	n/a	AIx
Covic	ESRD	92	Aortic (GTF) PWA	Mortality	bSBP, bPP	–
Verbeke	RTX	512	Aortic (GTF) PWA	CV events	bSBP, MBP, PWV	AP, (AIx)
Weber	CKD 3,4	111	Aortic (GTF) PWA	Cardiorenal events	MBP	AIx, AP
Ueda	Coronary intervent	103	Aortic PWA	Restenosis	n/a	AIx
Weber	Coronary intervent	262	Aortic (GTF) PWA	CV events	bSBP, bPP	AIx
Weber	CAD	520 m	Aortic (GTF) PWA	CV events	MBP, bPP	AIx
Chirinos	CAD	297 m	Aortic PWA	CV events	MBP, bPP	AIx, AP
Weber	CAD	725	Aortic (GTF) PWA, WSA	CV events	MBP, bSBP, DBP	AIx, AP, Pb
Sung	Heart failure hosp	120	Carotid PWA, WSA	CV events	MBP	AP, Pb
Sung	Heart failure hosp	80	Carotid PWA	CV events	n/a	AP
Wang	Community	1,272	Carotid PWA, WSA	CV mortality	MBP, bSBP, bPP, PWV	Pb, (AP)
Mitchell	Community	2,232	Carotid PWA	CV events	bSBP	–
Chirinos	Community	5,960	Radial PWA, WSA	CV events/HF	bSBP, DBP	AIx, RM
Benetos	Very elderly	1,126	Carotid PWA	Mortality	n/a	–
Williams	Hypertensives	2,199	Aortic (GTF) PWA	CV + renal events	n/a	(AP)
Dart	Hypertensives	484 f	Carotid PWA (?)	CV events	n/a	–
Manisty	Hypertensives	259	Carotid PWA	CV events	DBP	–

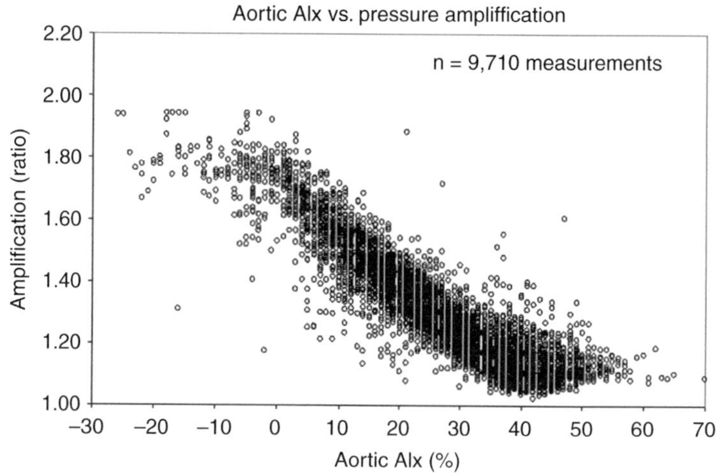

Fig. 1.3 Pulse pressure amplification (brachial pulse pressure/aortic pulse pressure) plotted against aortic augmentation index (AIx) calculated as augmented pressure divided by pulse pressure. There was significant difference in pressure amplification between subjects with aortic AIx more than 0 % and aortic AIx greater than or equal to 50 % ($p<0.0005$). This range contained over 98 % of all data (Reproduced with permission from O'Rourke and Adji [52])

be above unity (or below zero). The greatest value approximating 100 % is seen for positively reflected waves from "closed end" sites where low resistance arteries terminate in high resistance arterioles summate at the periphery (e.g. radial site) [41]. The lowest value approximating zero (Fig. 1.3) is seen when the reflected wave is of similar height in peripheral and central arteries because of high aortic impedance at low frequencies in persons with stiffened arteries [32].

Amplification of the pressure wave in the upper limb as measured invasively or as generated by the SphygmoCor (AtCor) method non-invasively is similar to that measured by the Omron HEM9000 (Omron) non-invasive device, but both are different to amplification described by van Bortel [42] and by Mitchell [43] who base their calibrations on brachial artery tonometry and who find no amplification between brachial and carotid arteries but extreme amplification between the brachial and radial arteries. This anomaly (referred to as the Popeye phenomenon, on the basis of a cartoon character with huge forearms) is not seen in directly recorded pressure waveforms, and is attributable to an inability to applanate (flatten) the anterior surface of the brachial artery when not supported by bone behind, and covered superficially by the rigid brachial aponeurosis [44]. This issue has confused and continues to confuse many clinician scientists, but is explained on the basis of theory and practice of applanation tonometry, and on estimation of amplification from brachial mean and diastolic pressure. The brachial artery wave, measured by tonometry, is blunted at its peak, and shows a Form Factor ((mean pressure – diastolic pressure) ÷ pulse pressure) identical to carotid and aortic pressure. Since amplification is determined by the ratio of Form Factors between the sites, calculated carotid and central pulse pressures appear identical [44].

While wave reflection from the lower body has substantial effect on the ascending aortic pressure wave (as a consequence of more reflecting sites in the lower than upper body), wave reflection in the upper limb has little or no effect on the ascending aortic pressure wave in humans [45]. Amplification in the upper limb is however, of substantial clinical significance since arterial pressure is conventionally measured by cuff sphygmomanometer at the brachial site (providing just peak and nadir of the wave) or when more accuracy or detail is desired, in the radial artery by a catheter or cannula. The principles enunciated above can best be applied to the cardiovascular system by generating the aortic pressure wave from the radial pressure pulse. This can be done by using the transfer function, applied to the radial artery pulse, measured non-invasively by applanation tonometry and calibrated to brachial cuff peak and trough pressures, or from the radial artery pulse recorded directly by invasive cannulation [2]. It is appropriate to use the transfer function technique because the transfer function for pressure wave transmission in the upper limb is applicable in all fully grown humans, irrespective of age, gender, or degree of cardiovascular disease elsewhere, or of drug therapy [2]. Transfer functions used in recent major studies [7, 46] are similar to those in the original SphygmoCor device, which was approved by the US FDA # K002742 and K012487.

While the transfer function remains constant in the upper limb arteries, amplification of the compound pulse (i.e. radial pulse pressure ÷ aortic pulse pressure) is related to augmentation index of the aortic pulse, and to cardiovascular disease elsewhere. Value of pressure amplification in the upper limb depends on the harmonic components of the aortic pulse, and hence on ascending aortic impedance, which is the best possible measure of left ventricular afterload [33]. This can now be determined accurately and non-invasively by relating the ascending aortic pressure wave to the ascending aortic flow wave recorded by MRI [35].

Bodily "Oeconomy"

Stephen Hales, the English clergyman who first measured arterial blood pressure [12], lived in the era of prominent botanists Solander and Banks (who accompanied James Cook on his historic voyage of discovery to the South Pacific in 1770), and was as interested in movement of sap in the bark of trees as in the movement of blood in arteries of animals. His book Statical Essays: containing Haemastatics [12] described "a Matter well worth enquiring into, to find the Force and Velocity with which these Fluids are impelled; as a likely means to give a considerable Insight into Animal Oeconomy". Hales stressed optimal function (oeconomy) as the change of highly pulsatile flow at the aorta's origin from the left ventricle into steady non-pulsatile flow in the smallest arteriolar and capillary vessels. He invoked for the first time the Windkessel (aortic elastic chamber) concept and the concept of peripheral resistance in small vessels of vascular beds as the relationship of steady, non-pulsatile flow to steady, non-pulsatile pressure.

Hales' views on arterial "oeconomy" are taken a step forward by the concepts presented here. The arterial tree was seen by Hales as very efficient as a conduit, with high mean pressure maintained right down to the most peripheral arterial vessels through arterial conduits of low resistance, and with abrupt change into high resistance arterioles whose resistance could be lowered when high flow is required. Taylor [3] pointed to problems of "oeconomy" with a Windkessel. The tubular model utilised by Taylor has wave reflection occurring at multiple junctions of low resistance arterial conduits with high resistance arterioles, and having the effect of confining pulsations to the proximal low resistance conduit arteries. "Oeconomy" also extends to the origin of the tubular model where the heart beat of the animal is such that it is "tuned" to the timely return of reflected waves such that reflected pressure surge in the aorta is least during systole and most during the period of diastole when the coronary patency and perfusion is restored (after compression with closure during systole) and when the relaxed left ventricular myocardium can be perfused [2, 3]. This issue was addressed by McDonald, Taylor, Milnor and O'Rourke, and seen to explain the inverse relationship between heart rate and body length [2, 3, 14, 15]. It was taken further to explain how further tuning can be attained during long distance running, by entraining step rate to heart rate, and utilising vertical body movement that necessarily accompanies horizontal movement to assist left ventricular ejection and coronary flow [2, 47]. Folkow [2, 48, 49] has commented on how such bodily movement, entrained with heart rate, can optimally increase flow to rhythmically contracting large hip and leg muscles during long distance running and with the heart perfused during upward movement, and the leg muscles when the body falls before the next upward step.

Impaired "Oeconomy" with Aging in Man

Bjorn Folkow, recently deceased, was the most recent of a long line of brilliant Scandinavian physiologists, with his name attached to the highest annual prize of the European Society of Hypertension. Folkow wrote extensively on arterial and cardiovascular aging in humans [50].

He described how the oeconomy of arterial function is distorted by aging, with progressive aortic stiffening causing increased aortic impedance and increased pulsatile pressure in the arterial tree. His interest followed the work of Taylor, Glagov, and others [6] as this applied to the non-living components of the arteries – with fracture and disorganisation of elastic fibres and remodelling with collagen.

Stephen Hales' other interest was with botany, and the normal flow of sap with nutrients from the ground to the leaves, flowers, and eventually to the seeds that ensure viability of the species. We see a continuity of interest in an aging human and in an aging or "stressed" tree, in that the aged human has cells which can live on, and can procreate normally (even from a male in his 90s) but whose cells are subject to the carriage of blood in adequate amounts, like the tree's leaves and blooms are subject to carriage of sap. Cells are threatened in the one case by progressive inability of the left ventricle to pump against a progressively increasing impedance [6, 8], and through damage of cerebral arteries of supply by increasing pulsatile tensile and shear stresses ([2, 6, 10, 12], Chap. 24), and in the other case by fatigue and eventual fracture of bark, branches and trunk, with inadequate delivery of sap from the roots to the leaves above. In both cases, degeneration with age is attributable to fatigue and fracture of non-living material (elastin and wood respectively) laid down by cells, and lasting long enough to be damaged by repetitive stretch or bending. This phenomena of aging is not seen in animals who die of other causes before attaining three billion heartbeats; it is seen in some birds who do [2, 51].

References

1. O'Rourke MF. Chapter 1: Principles and definitions of arterial stiffness, wave reflections and pulse pressure amplification. In: Safar ME, O'Rourke MF, editors. Arterial stiffness in hypertension, Handbook of hypertension, vol. 23. Amsterdam: Elsevier; 2006.
2. Nichols WW, O'Rourke MF, Vlachopoulos C. McDonald's blood flow in arteries. 6th ed. London: Arnold Hodder; 2011.
3. Taylor MG. The elastic properties of arteries in relation to the physiological functions of the arterial system. Gastroenterology. 1967;52:358–63.
4. O'Rourke MF, Nichols WW. Aortic diameter, aortic stiffness, and wave reflection increase with age and isolated systolic hypertension. Hypertension. 2005;45:652–8.
5. Laurent S, Cockcroft J, Van Bortel L, et al. On behalf of the European Network for Non-invasive Investigation of Large Arteries. Eur Heart J. 2006;27:2588–605.
6. O'Rourke MF, Hashimoto J. Mechanical factors in arterial aging. J Am Coll Cardiol. 2007;50:1–13.
7. Chirinos JA, Kips JG, Jacobs Jr DR, et al. Arterial wave reflections and incident cardiovascular events and heart failure: MESA (Multi-Ethnic Study of Atherosclerosis). J Am Coll Cardiol. 2012;60:2170–7.
8. Weber T, Wassertheurer S, O'Rourke MF, et al. Pulsatile hemodynamics in patients with exertional dyspnea: potentially of value in the diagnostic evaluation of suspected heart failure with preserved ejection fraction. J Am Coll Cardiol. 2013;61:1874–83.
9. O'Rourke MF, Safar ME. Relationship between aortic stiffening and microvascular disease in brain and kidney: cause and logic of therapy. Hypertension. 2005;46:200–4.
10. Stone J. What initiates the formation of senile plaques? The origin of Alzheimer-like dementias in capillary haemorrhages. Med Hypotheses. 2008;71:347–59.
11. Gorelick PB, Scuteri A, Black SE, Decarli C, American Heart Association Stroke Council, Council on Epidemiology and Prevention, Council on Cardiovascular Nursing, Council on Cardiovascular Radiology and Intervention, and Council on Cardiovascular Surgery and Anesthesia, et al. Vascular contributions to cognitive impairment and dementia: a statement for healthcare professionals from the American Heart Association/American Stroke Association. Stroke. 2011;42:2672–713.
12. Hales S. 1733: Statical essays: containing haemastaticks, History of Medicine Series, Library of New York Academy of Medicine, vol. 22. New York: Hafner Publishing; 1964.
13. Weber T, Ammer M, Rammer M, et al. Noninvasive determination of carotid-femoral pulse wave velocity depends critically on assessment of travel distance: a comparison with invasive measurement. J Hypertens. 2009;27:1624–30.
14. Milnor WR. Aortic wavelength as a determinant of the relation between heart rate and body size in mammals. Am J Physiol. 1979;237:R3–6.
15. O'Rourke MF. Commentary on: Aortic wavelength as a determinant of the relationship between heart rate and body size in mammals. Am J Physiol. 1981;240:R393–5.
16. American Physiological Society. Handbook of physiology. Washington, DC: American Physiology Society; 1963.
17. Postel-Vinay NA. A century of arterial hypertension 1896–1996. Chichester: Wiley; 1996.

18. O'Rourke MF. Dynamic accuracy of the electromagnetic flowmeter. J Appl Physiol. 1965;20:142–7.
19. Ludwig C. Contributions to the knowledge of the influence of the respiratory movements upon the blood flow in the arterial system. In: Ruskin A, Charles CT, editors. Classics in arterial hypertension. Springfield: Charles C. Thomas; 1847.
20. Gregg DE, Fisher LC. Blood supply to the heart. In: Handbook of physiology. Section 2: Circulation, vol. II. Washington, DC: American Physiological Society; 1963.
21. Braunwald E. The determinants of myocardial oxygen consumption. Physiologist. 1969;12:65–93.
22. McDonald DA, Taylor MG. The hydrodynamics of the arterial circulation. Prog Biophys. 1959;9:107–73.
23. Womersley JR. The mathematical analysis of the arterial circulation in a state of oscillatory motion. Technical Report Wade-TR. 56-614. Dayton: Wright Air Development Center; 1957.
24. O'Rourke MF, Nichols WW, Vlachopoulos C. CrossTalk: Wave reflection and the Physiological Society. J Physiol. 2013;591. Comments on the CrossTalk proposal and opposing view: Forward and backward pressure waves in the arterial system.
25. Moore W. The Knife Man: the coach driver's knee. New York: Broadway Books; 2005. p. 1–44.
26. Westerhof N, Sipkema P, van der Bos GC, et al. Forward and backward waves in the arterial system. Cardiovasc Res. 1972;6:648–56.
27. Tyberg JV, Bouwmeester JC, Shrive NG, Wang JJ. CrossTalk opposing view: Forward and backward pressure waves in the arterial system do not represent reality. J Physiol. 2013;591:1171–3; discussion 1175.
28. Sen S, Asrress KN, Nijjer S, Petraco R, et al. Diagnostic classification of the instantaneous wave-free ratio is equivalent to fractional flow reserve and is not improved with adenosine administration. Results of CLARIFY (Classification Accuracy of Pressure-Only Ratios Against Indices Using Flow Study). J Am Coll Cardiol. 2013;61:1409–20.
29. Johnson NP, Kirkeeide RL, Gould KL. Reply: Instantaneous wave-free ratio numerically different, but diagnostically superior to FFR? Is lower always better? J Am Coll Cardiol. 2013;62:566–7.
30. Westerhof N, O'Rourke MF. Haemodynamic basis for the development of left ventricular failure in systolic hypertension and for its logical therapy. J Hypertens. 1995;13:943–52.
31. Miyashita H, Ikeda U, Tsuruya Y, et al. Noninvasive evaluation of the influence of aortic wave reflection on left ventricular ejection during auxotonic contraction. Heart Vessels. 1994;9:30–9.
32. O'Rourke MF, Taylor MG. Vascular impedance of the femoral bed. Circ Res. 1966;18:126–39.
33. Milnor WR. Arterial impedance as ventricular afterload. Circ Res. 1975;36:565–70.
34. Bensalah MZ, Bollache E, Kachenoura N, Giron A, De Cesare A, Macron L, Lefort M, Redheuill A, Mousseaux E. Geometry is a major determinant of flow reversal in proximal aorta. Am J Physiol Heart Circ Physiol 2014;306:H1408–16.
35. O'Rourke M, Adji A, Kachenoura N, Bollache E, Mousseaux E, Avolio A. Effects of aging on ascending aortic flow waveform. Pulse. 2013;1:44–5.
36. Segers P, Rietzschel ER, De Buyzere ML, et al. Noninvasive (input) impedance, pulse wave velocity, and wave reflection in healthy middle-aged men and women. Hypertension. 2007;49:1248–55.
37. Mitchell GF, Parise H, Benjamin EJ, et al. Changes in arterial stiffness and wave reflection with advancing age in healthy men and women. The Framingham Heart Study. Hypertension. 2004;43:1239–45.
38. Mitchell GF. Clinical achievements of impedance analysis. Med Biol Eng Comput. 2009;47:153–63.
39. O'Rourke MF, Taylor MG. Input impedance of the systemic circulation. Circ Res. 1967;20:365–80.
40. Taylor MG. Wave transmission through an assembly of randomly branching elastic tubes. Biophys J. 1966;6:697–716.
41. Karamanoglu M, O'Rourke MF, Avolio AP, et al. An analysis of the relationship between central aortic and peripheral upper limb pressure waves in man. Eur Heart J. 1993;14:160–7.
42. Van Bortel LM, Balkestein EJ, Van Der Heijden-Spek JJ, et al. Non-invasive assessment of local arterial pulse pressure, comparison of applanation tonometry and echo-tracking. J Hypertens. 2001;19:1037–44.
43. Mitchell GF, Hwang SJ, Vasan RS, et al. Arterial stiffness and cardiovascular events: the Framingham Heart Study. Circulation. 2010;121:505–11.
44. Adji A, O'Rourke MF. Brachial artery tonometry and the Popeye phenomenon: explanation of anomalies in generating central from upper limb pressure waveform. J Hypertens. 2012;30:1540–51.
45. Karamanoglu M, Gallagher DE, Avolio AP, et al. Pressure wave propagation in a multibranched model of the human upper limb. Am J Physiol. 1995;269: H1363–9.
46. Cheng HM, Chuang SY, Sung SH, et al. Derivation and validation of diagnostic thresholds for central blood pressure measurements based on long-term cardiovascular risks. J Am Coll Cardiol. 2013;62:1780–7.
47. O'Rourke MF, Avolio AP. Improved cardiovascular performance with optimal entrainment between heart rate and step rate during running in man. Coron Artery Dis. 1992;3:963–9.
48. Folkow B, Gaskell P, Waaler B. Blood flow through limb muscles during heavy rhythmic exercise. Acta Physiol Scand. 1970;80:61–72.
49. Folkow B, Haglund Y, Jodal M, et al. Blood flow in the calf muscle of man during heavy rhythmic exercise. Acta Physiol Scand. 1971;81:157–63.
50. Folkow B, Svanborg A. Physiology of cardiovascular aging. Physiol Rev. 1993;73:725–64.
51. Wheat Jr MW. Acute dissecting aneurysms of the aorta: diagnosis and treatment – 1979. Am Heart J. 1980;99:373–87.
52. O'Rourke MF, Adji A. Basis for use of central blood pressure measurement in office clinical practice. J Am Soc Hypertens. 2008;1:28–38.

2 Large Arteries, Microcirculation, and Mechanisms of Hypertension

Harry A.J. Struijker-Boudier

Abstract

Although the macro- and microcirculation have different embryological origins a constant match in their mechanical behavior is essential for an optimal function of the cardiovascular system. Extrinsic neurohormonal control systems contribute to this match. In addition, blood pressure transfers energy, mechanical signals, and metabolic factors independently of these neurohormonal control mechanisms. The plasticity of vascular structure provides a long-term control mechanism of blood pressure throughout the vascular tree. Hypertension is characterized by vascular structural changes that cause increased arterial stiffness and resistance to flow. This chapter discusses the major structural changes in the vascular tree in hypertension.

Keywords

Hypertension • Microcirculation • Arterial stiffness • Blood pressure • Vascular resistance • Arterial remodeling • Large arteries • Pulse pressure

The hemodynamic characteristics of most forms of hypertension consist of an elevated blood pressure, an increased arterial stiffness, and an elevated peripheral vascular resistance. The description of mechanical forces within the cardiovascular system requires distinction between those that are mainly of a pulsatile nature (pulse pressure, PP) and those that are steady and continuous (mean arterial pressure, MAP). PP is predominantly influenced by the elastic properties of the large conduit arteries, whereas MAP is determined by the resistance to flow in smaller arteries and arterioles [1]. The large conduit arteries are composed of an endothelial cell layer, vascular smooth muscle cells, and a relatively large amount of extracellular elastic tissue. This structure renders them a temporal buffer for blood during the ejection phase of the heart (Windkessel function) and effectively tends to reduce its afterload [1] The small arteries and arterioles are a continuous distal segment of the vascular system consisting of an endothelial cell layer, a relatively large vascular smooth muscle cell layer, and smaller amounts of extracellular

H.A.J. Struijker-Boudier, PhD
Department of Pharmacology,
CARIM, Maastricht University,
616, Maastricht, 6200 MD, The Netherlands
e-mail: h.struijkerboudier@maastrichtuniversity.nl

M.E. Safar et al. (eds.), *Blood Pressure and Arterial Wall Mechanics in Cardiovascular Diseases*,
DOI 10.1007/978-1-4471-5198-2_2, © Springer-Verlag London 2014

elastic tissue. In this segment pulsations gradually disappear and pressure drops. The exact location of the pressure drop may differ per tissue. In the kidney, for example, a relatively high pressure – and associated pulsatility – is maintained to the level of afferent arterioles. In contrast, in the mesentery the pressure drop is located more proximally [2]. For a single vessel, resistance can be calculated as mean pressure divided by flow. However, in the microcirculation vessels are part of a larger network. In such a network resistance is determined by the vascular architecture, the number of vessels, and their interconnections, such as parallel-coupled vessels or arcades.

Mechanical forces at the different levels of the vascular system are determined by various short-term and long-term control mechanisms [3]. Acute mechanisms include the myogenic response, endothelium-dependent paracrine factors, and nervous mechanisms. These mechanisms are predominantly active in the more distal segments of the vascular tree. Long-term control of mechanical forces depends on endocrine systems such as the renin-angiotensin-aldosterone system (RAAS), the renal control of body fluid volumes, and structural regulatory mechanisms. In the classical Guytonian theory of long-term control of blood pressure, renal body fluid control was the predominant mechanism [3]. Cumulating evidence over the last decades shows that structural mechanisms play an equally important role.

Structure of the Vascular System: Developmental Aspects

In the classical control theory of the cardiovascular system, vascular structure was generally regarded as a static phenomenon [3]. We now know that this is not the case: vascular structure is dynamic, although with a relatively slow time constant. The ability to alter its structure (vascular plasticity) is largest during embryological and perinatal growth. In the embryo the large arteries develop from the aortic arches. After entering the embryonic mammalian heart, the blood is pumped into a series of aortic arches that encircle the pharynx to bring the blood dorsally [4]. In mammals only one of these arches survives to reach the aorta. Other arches become the root of the subclavian, the carotid, or the pulmonary arteries, while other arches degenerate. The aorta and pulmonary artery have a common opening to the heart for much of their development. Eventually, partitions form within the truncus arteriosus to create two different vessels. Only when the first breath of the newborn mammal indicates that the lungs are ready to handle the oxygenation of the blood does the heart become modified to pump blood separately to the pulmonary artery [4]. Upon cessation of the placenta blood flow, perfusion of many arteries is approximately halved. This diminution probably reflects the decreased demands for perfusion because arterial pO_2 doubles after lung ventilation starts [1]. The most significant change seen in a major systemic vessel is a more than 90 % decrease in blood flow in the subrenal abdominal aorta [5]. In sheep, this dramatically decreased blood flow is accompanied by a marked reduction in the abdominal aortic diameter and a near arrest due to wall-tissue accumulation that lasts 3 weeks [5]. Around birth a rapid accumulation of elastin in the aorta is necessary to modulate the Windkessel function. Martyn and Greenwald [6] proposed that reduced elastin deposition in low-birth-weight babies might lead to increased stiffness in the major arteries and thus might predict subsequent elevated PP and hypertension. The amount of elastin in large arteries is largely determined during early life with little turnover later in life [6].

The development of microvasculature is the result of a highly complex and plastic process of vasculogenesis and angiogenesis. Vasculogenesis is the de novo formation of blood vessels from the mesoderm. In most tissues capillaries do not arise as smaller and smaller extensions of the major vessels growing from the heart, but are formed independently within the tissues themselves [4]. These organ-specific capillary networks eventually become linked to the extensions of the major blood vessels. Vasculogenesis is not the only way to make blood vessels. In organs like the brain and kidney, existing blood vessels sprout and send endothelial cells into the developing organ. This type of blood vessel growth is referred to as angiogenesis.

Research in the past two decades has led to an explosive increase in knowledge concerning the molecular and cellular processes underlying vasculogenesis and angiogenesis. The reader is referred to several recent review articles for an update on this research [7, 8]. Interestingly the basic mechanical laws underlying the embryological growth of blood vessels were postulated more than 100 years ago by Thoma [9]. Thoma proposed that the rate of blood flow is an important determinant of both the diameter of individual vessels and the growth of vessels in a developing vascular network. Murray [10] subsequently proposed that vascular networks adapt their geometry on the basis of the principle of minimalization of work required to maintain adequate blood flow.

Structure of the Vascular System: Control of Blood Pressure

The plasticity of the vascular system is highest during the embryological and perinatal period, as was discussed above. However, also in adults the vascular tree can adapt its structure to physiological requirements. Two important sources of stimuli can trigger long-term adaptations in vascular structure: (a) metabolic and (b) mechanical triggers. Metabolic stimuli act predominantly at the microvascular level. Microvascular structure can be adapted to an altered metabolic demand both acutely and chronically. The acute response during hyperemia is a dilation of small arteries and arterioles as well as capillary recruitment. Tissues thus have an acute flow reserve. This flow reserve is significantly reduced in patients with hypertension, heart failure, or diabetes mellitus [11]. The long-term mechanism to increase the flow reserve is the growth of new microvessels. The primary trigger for this long-term structural adaptation is the tissue oxygen level. In hypertensive patients this long-term angiogenic response seems suppressed due to a structural rarefaction of the microvasculature [11, 12].

The mechanical triggers involved in structural control of the vascular system are predominantly shear stress and circumferential wall stress. On the basis of Murray's principle of minimalization of work, Zamir [13] proposed that shear stress is the primary driving force for control of blood vessel architecture. For single vessels, adaptation to shear stress implies that an acute reduction in flow is countered by a lumen reduction, whereas an increase in flow is countered by a lumen increase. Shear stress is fairly constant throughout the circulation, with values in the arteriolar tree ranging from 1.0 to 2.6 N/m^2. Experimental studies have shown that long-term increases in tissue flow, during exercise or treatment with vasodilators, many cause a radial outgrowth of arteries, implying a structural lumen increase [12, 14]. Both the flow-induced acute vasodilator response and the long-term structural growth response are mediated by endothelium-derived vasoactive factors. Theoretical (computer modeling) studies suggest that adaptation to shear stress alone is not enough to explain the maintenance of a stable vascular network [12, 15]. Pressure and pressure-related circumferential wall stress are additional important mechanical factors in the control of microvascular network geometry [16]. Wall stress has been known for a long time as an important parameter in the control of wall thickness and the diameter of individual vessels [12]. It is the primary trigger for the remodeling of arteries in hypertension [17]. Apart from these effects on the structure of single vessels, pressure may also have effects on microvascular network architecture. In experimental secondary forms of hypertension, an increase in arteriolar pressure is accompanied by a decrease in the number of perfused arterioles and capillaries [12].

In conclusion, plasticity of the architecture of the vascular tree is a slow, but powerful mechanism of control of blood pressure and its underlying hemodynamic factors, such as blood flow, shear stress, and wall stress. In chronic pathologies of the cardiovascular system, as they occur in hypertension, heart failure, and diabetes, a failure in this plasticity may lie at the root of the altered hemodynamics.

Cross Talk Between the Macro- and Microcirculation

During embryological and perinatal development, a dynamic match between the macro- and microcirculation provides an optimal function of the cardiovascular system. However, even in the full-grown adult organism, a constant match is needed to maintain this function.

Neurohormonal cardiovascular control mechanisms operate constantly to guarantee this match. In addition, blood pressure transfers energy, mechanical signals, and metabolic factors independently of these neurohormonal control mechanisms [1, 18, 19]. The pressure waves travel at fast speed through the arterial system and consist of two components. The first is the high-pressure wave generated by the left ventricle that ejects into the proximal aorta. The second arises from the distal microvascular segment through the creation of wave reflections. This interaction is responsible for a constant cross talk between the macro- and microcirculation. The reader is referred to other chapters in this volume as well as to McDonald's Blood flow in Arteries Handbook [19] for a detailed discussion on the mechanical basis of pulse wave velocity and wave reflections.

Several recent studies have suggested that there is a direct relation between large artery stiffness and peripheral microvascular function. In an analysis of the data from the Framingham Heart Study, Mitchell et al. [20] showed that abnormal aortic stiffness and increased pulse pressure are associated with blunted microvascular reactivity to ischemic stress that is in excess of changes attributable to conventional cardiovascular risk factors alone, including mean arterial pressure. Along the same lines Cheung et al. [21] found that increased aortic stiffness is associated with retinal arteriolar narrowing, independent of measured blood pressure levels and vascular risk factors. Similar results were reported for carotid artery stiffness [22]. Several authors have shown that indices of large artery stiffness are related to wall to lumen ratio of retinal [23] or subcutaneous small arteries [24].

Structural Abnormalities of the Vascular System and Mechanisms of Hypertension

Hypertension is an important cardiovascular risk factor primarily through the long-term damage it exerts on target organs like the kidney, brain, and heart. In this target organ damage structural changes in the arterial and microvascular tree play a dominant role [25]. Age and blood pressure are the two major determinants of increased large artery stiffness in hypertension [26]. The structural basis of large artery stiffness lies in the fibrotic components of the extracellular matrix, mainly elastin, collagen, and fibronectin [26]. As blood vessels become stiffer because of age-related processes, the pulse wave is transmitted more rapidly and returns to the heart during left ventricular contraction, thus causing a greater augmentation of the central aortic systolic pressure [27]. It is now well established that carotid-femoral PWV yields prognostic values beyond and above traditional risk factors [28]. Furthermore, increased aortic augmentation index is associated with coronary artery disease [29].

The structural changes in small arteries in hypertension have been reviewed in detail recently by Rizzoni et al. [27] and Mulvany [17]. In brief, in patients with essential hypertension, small arteries show a greater media thickness and a reduced internal and external diameter with increased media to lumen ratio, without any significant change of the total amount of wall tissue [17, 27]. These changes are usually referred to as eutrophic inward remodeling without net cell growth. In contrast, in some patients with secondary forms of hypertension or animal models of hypertension, hypertrophic forms of remodeling are observed with a more evident contribution of vascular smooth muscle cell hypertrophy [17, 27, 30]. An enhanced activity of the renin-angiotensin system may play an important role in hypertrophic forms of arterial remodeling [31]. Small artery structural changes are a predictor for later cardiovascular events [17, 27]. For a given lumen diameter, a greater cross-sectional area gives increased risk for cardiovascular events.

Mulvany [17] recently suggested that the increased risk may be the consequence of a reduced vascular reserve, in particular in the coronary circulation.

The molecular and cellular basis of the inward remodeling of small arteries in hypertension has been investigated in recent years [17]. A rearrangement of the extracellular matrix seems pivotal. This requires a break and reformation of the protein cross-links which involves the action of integrins [32]. In addition, tissue transglutaminases could be involved in the remodeling process [33, 34].

The third major vascular structural change in hypertension is microvascular rarefaction, in particular of the smallest arterioles and capillaries. We have reviewed the evidence for microvascular rarefaction and its underlying mechanisms elsewhere [1, 11, 35]. Microvascular rarefaction not only is a consequence of long-term hypertension but may even precede it as was shown in borderline hypertensives as well as in offspring from hypertensive parents [36]. In 10–14-year-old children, elevated blood pressure is associated with rarefaction of retinal microvasculature [37]. The molecular and cellular basis of microvascular rarefaction remains enigmatic. Schmid-Schönbein and coworkers [38–40] have implied endothelial cell apoptosis due to oxidative stress mechanisms. Wang et al. [41] recently suggested a role for enhanced matrix metalloproteinases-2 in endothelial cell apoptosis and vascular rarefaction in spontaneously hypertensive rats. An alternative hypothesis is derived from the long-term effects of antiangiogenic drugs on microvascular rarefaction. There is now ample evidence that hypertension is a serious side effect of anti-angiogenic drugs used in cancer therapy [42]. These drugs are inhibitors of vascular growth factors such as VEGF and act via inhibition of tyrosine kinase cellular pathways. This may imply tyrosine kinase as a key molecule in microvascular rarefaction. A recent study by Le Noble and coworkers [43] suggests a role for a specific microRNA, miR-30a, in the rarefaction process. In this elegant study the essential role of miR-30 family members was shown in endothelial tip cell formation and arterioles branching in a zebra fish model. Future studies in mammalian models may reveal the relevance of these microRNAs in the rarefaction process and hypertension. Already there is evidence that selected microRNAs are involved in the balance between angiogenic and apoptotic factors in SHR [44] as well as in hypertension-related target organ damage [45].

Conclusion

Historically, the macro- and microcirculation have been regarded as independent segments of the circulation, even having their own scientific societies and journals. The evidence reviewed above suggests a bidirectional link between the macro- and microcirculation via the communication of pressure and flow between these segments of the vascular tree. A range of mechanical, metabolic, neurohormonal, and structural mechanisms control this communication. The structural mechanisms are the long-term controllers of the hemodynamic stability of the vascular system due to their plasticity. On the other hand, long-term derangements in the hemodynamic stability, such as occurring in hypertension, heart failure, or diabetes, are the consequence of chronic changes in vascular structure, at the level of both macro- and microcirculation.

References

1. Safar ME, Struijker-Boudier HA. Cross-talk between macro-and microcirculation. Acta Physiol (Oxf). 2010;198:417–30.
2. Levy BI, Ambrosio G, Pries AR, Struijker-Boudier HA. Microcirculation in hypertension: a new target for treatment? Circulation. 2001;104:735–40.
3. Guyton AC. Arterial pressure and hypertension. In: Guyton AC, editor. Circulatory physiology III. Saunders: Philadelphia; 1980. p. 30–165.
4. Gilbert SF. Developmental biology. 9th ed. Sunderland: Sinnauer Associates; 2010.
5. Bendeck MP, Langille BL. Changes in blood flow distribution during the perinatal period in fetal sheep and lambs. Can J Physiol Pharmacol. 1992;70:1576–82.
6. Martyn CN, Greenwald S. Impaired synthesis of elastin in walls of aorta and large conduit arteries during early development as an initiating event in pathogenesis of systemic hypertension. Lancet. 1997;350:953–5.

7. Potente M, Gerhardt H, Carmeliet P. Basic and therapeutic aspects of angiogenesis. Cell. 2011;146(6): 873–87.
8. Carmeliet P, Jain RK. Molecular mechanisms and clinical applications of angiogenesis. Nature. 2011; 473:298–307.
9. Thoma R. Untersuchingen über die Histogenesis und Histomechanik das gefassystem. Stuttgart: Enke; 1893.
10. Murray CD. The physiological principle of minimum work. 1 The vascular system and the cost of blood volume. Proc Natl Acad Sci U S A. 1926;12:207–14.
11. Levy BI, Schiffrin EL, Mourad J, Agostini D, Vicaut E, Safar ME, Struijker-Boudier HAJ. Impaired tissue perfusion. Circulation. 2008;118:968–76.
12. Le Noble FAC, Stassen FRM, Hacking WJG, Struijker-Boudier HAJ. Angiogenesis and hypertension. J Hypertens. 1998;16:1563–72.
13. Zamir M. Shear forces and blood vessel radii in the cardiovascular system. J Gen Physiol. 1977;69:449–61.
14. Koller A, Kaley G. Shear stress dependent regulation of vascular resistance in health and disease: role of endothelium. Endothelium. 1996;4:247–72.
15. Hackeng WJG, Van Bavel E, Spaan JAE. Shear stress is not sufficient to control growth of vascular networks: a model study. Am J Physiol. 1996;270:H364–75.
16. Skalak TC, Price RJ. The role of mechanical stresses in microvascular remodeling. Microcirculation. 1996;3:143–65.
17. Mulvany MJ. Small artery remodelling in hypertension. Basic Clin Pharmacol Toxicol. 2011;110:49–55.
18. Safar ME, Levy BI, Struijker-Boudier HA. Current perspectives on arterial stiffness and pulse pressure in hypertension and cardiovascular diseases. Circulation. 2003;107:2864–9.
19. Nichols WW, O'Rourke M, Vlachopoulos C. Mc Donald's blood flow in arteries. 6th ed. Boca Raton: CRC Press; 2011.
20. Mitchell G, Vita JA, Larson MG, Parise H, Keyes MJ, Warner E, Vasa RS, Levy D, Benjamin EJ. Cross-sectional relations of peripheral microvascular function, cardiovascular disease risk factors, and aortic stiffness. Circulation. 2005;112:3722–8.
21. Cheung N, Sharret AR, Klein R, Criqui MH, Islam FMA, Macura KJ, Cotch MF, Klein BEK, Wong TY. Aortic distensibility and retinal arteriolar narrowing. Hypertension. 2007;50:617–22.
22. Liao D, Wong TY, Klein R, Joens D, Hubbard L, Sharret AR. Relationship between carotid artery stiffness and retinal arteriolar narrowing in healthy middle-aged persons. Stroke. 2004;35(4):837–42.
23. Ott C, Raff U, Harazny JM, Michelson G, Schmieder RE. Central pulse pressure is an independent determinant of vascular remodeling in the retinal circulation. Hypertension. 2013;61:1340–5.
24. Muiesan ML, Salvetti M, Rizzoni D, Oaini A, Agabati-Rosei C, Aggiusti C, Bertacchini F, Stassaldi D, Gavazii A, Porteri E, De Ciuceis C, Agabiti-Rosei E. Pulsatile hemodynamics and microcirculation. Hypertension. 2013;61:130–6.
25. Cohuet G, Struijker-Boudier HAJ. Mechanism of target organ damage caused by hypertension: therapeutic potential. Pharmacol Ther. 2006;111:81–98.
26. Boutouyrie P, Laurent S, Briet M. Importance of arterial stiffness as cardiovascular risk factor for future development of new type drugs. Fundam Clin Pharmacol. 2008;22:241–6.
27. Rizzoni D, Muiesan ML, Porteri E, De Ciuceis C, Boari GEM, Salvetti M, Paini A, Rosei EA. Interrelationships between macro and microvascular structure and function. Artery Res. 2010;4: 114–17.
28. Laurent S, Cockcroft J, Van Bortel L, Boutouyrie P, Giannattasio C, Hayoz D, On behalf of the European network for Non-invasive Investigation of Large Arteries, et al. Expert consensus document on arterial stiffness: methodological issues and clinical applications. Eur Heart J. 2006;27:2588–605.
29. Agabiti-Rosei E, Mancia G, O'rourke MF, Roman MJ, Safar ME, Smulyan H, et al. Central blood pressure measurements and antihypertensive therapy: a consensus document. Hypertension. 2007;50:154–60.
30. Schiffrin EL. Remodeling of resistance arteries in essential hypertension and effects of antihypertensive treatment. Am J Hypertens. 2004;17:1192–200.
31. Struijker-Boudier HAJ, van Essen H, Fazzi G, De Mey JG, Qiu HY, Lévy BI. Disproportional arterial hypertrophy in hypertensive mRen-2 transgenic rats. Hypertension. 1996;28:779–84.
32. Heerkens EH, Shaw L, Ryding A, Brooker G, Mullins JJ, Austin C, et al. AlphaV integrins are necessary for eutrophic inward remodeling of small arteries in hypertension. Hypertension. 2006;47:281–7.
33. Bakker EN, Buus CL, Spaan JA, Perree E, Ganga A, Rolf TM, et al. Small artery remodeling depends on tissue-type transglutaminase. Circ Res. 2005;96: 119–26.
34. Bakker EN, Pistea A, Van Bavel E. Transglutaminases in vascular biology: relevance for vascular remodeling and atherosclerosis. J Vasc Res. 2008;45:271–8.
35. Struijker-Boudier HAJ, Heijnen BF, Liu YP, Staessen JA. Phenotyping the microcirculation. Hypertension. 2012;60:523–7.
36. Noon JP, Walker BR, Webb DJ, et al. Impaired microvascular dilation and capillary rarefaction in young adults with a predisposition to high blood pressure. J Clin Invest. 1997;99:1873–9.
37. Kurniawan ED, Cheung N, Cheung CY, Tay WT, Saw SM, Wong TY. Elevated blood pressure is associated with rarefaction of the retinal vasculature in children. Invest Ophthalmol Vis Sci. 2012;53:470–4.
38. Tran ED, Schmid-Schönbein GW. An in-vivo analysis of capillary stasis and endothelial apoptosis in a model of hypertension. Microcirculation. 2007;14: 793–804.
39. Kobayashi N, DeLano FA, Schmid-Schönbein GW. Oxidative stress promotes endothelial cell apoptosis and loss of microvessels in the spontaneously hypertensive rat. Arterioscler Thromb Vasc Biol. 2005;25:2114–21.

40. Vogt CJ, Schmid-Schönbein GW. Microvascular endothelial cell death and rarefaction in the glucocorticoid-induced hypertensive rat. Microcirculation. 2001;8:129–39.
41. Wang B, Li BW, Li HW, Li Al, Yuan XC, Wang Q, Xiu RJ. Enhanced matrix metalloproteinases-2 activates endothelial hyperpermeability, apoptosis and vascular rarefaction in spontaneously hypertensive rat. Clin Hemorheol Microcirc. 2013. doi:10.3233/CH-131713.
42. Mourad JJ, Levy BI. Mechanisms of antiangiogenic-induced arterial hypertension. Curr Hypertens Rep. 2011;13:289–93.
43. Jiang Q, Lagos-Quintana M, Liu D, Shi Y, Helker C, Herzog W, le Noble F. MiR-30a regulates endothelial tip cell formation and arteriolar branching. Hypertension. 2013;62:592–8.
44. Fernandes T, Magalhães, Roque FR, Philips MI, Oliveira EM. Exercise training prevents the microvascular rarefaction in hypertension balancing angiogenic and apoptotic factors role of microRNAs-16, -21, and -126. Hypertension. 2012;59:513–20.
45. Heggermont WA, Heymans S. MicroRNAs are involved in end-organ damage during hypertension. Hypertension. 2012;60:1088–93.

Direct Measurement of Local Arterial Stiffness and Pulse Pressure

3

Luc M. Van Bortel, Tine De Backer, and Patrick Segers

Abstract

Arterial stiffness differs between different sites in the arterial tree. It can, therefore, be of interest to know the stiffness at a particular arterial site. Local arterial stiffness assesses stiffness at a cross section of an artery. At present echo-tracking methods are the gold standard to measure local wall properties of superficial arteries. This technique measures with very high precision the diameter and diameter change of a cross section of an artery. For deep arteries like the aorta, CT and MRI techniques have been developed. Although less than echo tracking, the accuracy of these latter techniques increased over recent years. Assuming the cross section being circular, the change in cross-sectional area can be calculated from diameter and diameter change. From the change in cross-sectional area and change in pressure, the local vessel wall properties distensibility coefficient (DC) and cross-sectional compliance (CC) can be calculated. Distensibility is a measure of wall elasticity and the inverse of stiffness. Compliance reflects the buffering capacity of the artery. Local stiffness assessment is the only method that can assess both wall properties. In addition, if the pressure curve is available, the full pressure–diameter relation can be shown and wall properties at a particular pressure or pressure range (isobaric conditions) can be calculated. Alternative methods have also been developed

L.M. Van Bortel, MD, PhD (✉)
Clinical Pharmacology, Heymans Institute of Pharmacology, Ghent University, De Pintelaan 185, Ghent 9000, Belgium
e-mail: luc.vanbortel@ugent.be

T. De Backer, MD, PhD
Clinical Pharmacology, Heymans Institute of Pharmacology, Ghent University, De Pintelaan 185, Ghent 9000, Belgium

Cardiovascular Diseases, University Hospital Ghent, De Pintelaan 185, Ghent 9000, Belgium
e-mail: tine.debacker@ugent.be

P. Segers, PhD
Institute Biomedical Technology (IBITEch), iMinds Medical IT, Ghent University, Campus Heymans-Blok B, De Pintelaan 185, Ghent 9000, Belgium
e-mail: patrick.segers@ugent.be

M.E. Safar et al. (eds.), *Blood Pressure and Arterial Wall Mechanics in Cardiovascular Diseases*, DOI 10.1007/978-1-4471-5198-2_3, © Springer-Verlag London 2014

and are briefly discussed. The major source of error in calculating local arterial stiffness comes from the assessment of the arterial pressure at the same arterial site. Different methods to calculate this local pressure are discussed.

Keywords
Local arterial stiffness • Distensibility • Compliance • Pulse pressure • Local blood pressure • Methods

Introduction

It has been demonstrated in large cohorts that higher systolic blood pressure is associated with higher cardiovascular risk. For each level of systolic blood pressure, the risk is higher when pulse pressure, i.e., the difference between systolic and diastolic blood pressure, is larger [1–3]. Pulse pressure is directly related to arterial stiffness.

Pulse pressure and arterial stiffness determine, together with the geometrical characteristics of the vessel, the mechanical stress within the arterial wall [4]. Arterial stiffness is involved in 3 out of the 4 major stress factors acting on the arterial wall: peak stress (systolic blood pressure), change in stress (pulse pressure), and velocity of the change in stress and stress frequency (heart rate) [5]. Apart from pressure, the blood flow exerts a low magnitude yet physiologically important mechanical shear stress on the arterial wall. Mechanical stress and the distribution of stress within diseased vessels are hypothesized as major factors determining the susceptibility of plaque to rupture [6–9], which is the underlying cause of a large majority of cardiovascular events and probably also rapidly growing plaques.

The assessment of local arterial stiffness and pulse pressure is the subject of the present chapter.

Local Arterial Stiffness

Different arterial stiffness indices exist and are described in Chap. 1. Three types of arterial stiffness can be considered (Table 3.1): systemic, regional, and local arterial stiffness [10]. This chapter focuses on local arterial stiffness, while systemic and regional arterial stiffness are discussed in other chapters.

Table 3.1 Wall properties measured in different types of arterial stiffness

Wall property →	Distensibility		Compliance	
Type ↓	Operating	Isobaric	Operating	Isobaric
Systemic			X	
Regional	X			
Local	X	X	X	X

Operating at operating pressure, *isobaric* under isobaric condition, this is at a defined pressure (range)

Definitions of Local Wall Properties

Local arterial wall properties are defined as wall properties per unit of length, or cross-sectional area wall properties, and are derived from locally measured pressure and diameter or pressure and area loops. Whereas compliance reflects the buffering capacity of the artery, distensibility reflects the elastic properties of the arterial wall.

In clinical practice, instead of calculating compliance at a specific pressure, compliance is calculated over a pressure range, thereby neglecting the nonlinearity of the pressure–area relation. This approximation of compliance is commonly called the *cross-sectional compliance or compliance coefficient*, $CC(m^2/Pa)$:

$$CC = \Delta A / \Delta P = \pi\left(2D \cdot \Delta D + \Delta D^2\right) / 4\Delta P$$

ΔA is the absolute change in cross-sectional area due to ΔP the local change in pressure. The compliance coefficient can also be calculated from diameter (D) and change in diameter (ΔD) presuming that the cross-sectional area of the artery is circular. In general, the compliance coefficient is calculated at the operating pressure; this is over the full systolic–diastolic pressure interval with ΔP equal to the pulse pressure PP, D the diastolic diameter, and ΔD the diastolic-to-systolic change in diameter. However, when the pressure and diameter curves are available, CC can also be measured over a smaller pressure interval. This may be of particular use when CC has to be compared at isobaric conditions.

Similarly, one can also calculate distensibility using relative changes in dimensions for a pressure change, which then yields the *distensibility coefficient*, *DC (1/Pa)*, defined as

$$\mathrm{DC} = \left(\Delta A / A\right) / \Delta P = \left(2\Delta D \cdot D + \Delta D^2\right) / \left(\Delta P \cdot D^2\right)$$

Methods to Measure Arterial Diameter and Diameter Change

For superficial arteries such as the carotid, femoral, or brachial artery, ultrasound technology is the method of choice to measure the cyclic variation of diameter throughout the cardiac cycle (the diameter distension waveforms). An acoustic ultrasound wave, transmitted by an echo transducer (typically at frequencies of 7–12 MHz for noninvasive vascular ultrasound applications), propagates in the tissue (at a speed of 1,540 m/s) and reflects on interfaces with a discontinuity in acoustic impedance. This reflected ultrasound signal is captured by a receiver and, after processing, translated into an image, for instance, a 2D image of the vessel. In these so-called B-mode images, the magnitude of the echo is displayed as an intensity value; the brighter the image, the stronger the echo. When visualizing the common carotid artery, a strong echo is generated by the vessel adventitia; the intima–media complex is visible as the narrow gray band lining the inner wall of the vessel (Fig. 3.1).

When scanning the vessel with a single ultrasound beam, and displaying the intensity of the echo along the beam as a function of time (i.e., creating an M-mode image, where "M" stands for "motion"), the displacement of the vessel becomes clear. A crude way of obtaining the vessel displacement is to analyze these M-mode images, whereby the accuracy is restricted to the spatial resolution of the M-mode image. To increase accuracy, alternative methods have been elaborated, making use of the received radio frequency (RF) data (see RF line in Fig. 3.1). Hoeks and coworkers were among the first to develop RF data-based algorithms [11] (making use of cross-correlation techniques) that allowed to automatically detect the echo arising from the anterior and posterior vessel wall within the RF signal and to "track" the displacement of these echos in time. Distension waveforms, where vessel diameter is plotted as a function of time, are directly obtained by adding the displacement curves of the anterior and posterior wall. The accuracy of arterial distension obtained from echo tracking is about 20 times higher than the accuracy from M-mode imaging with most of the classical ultrasound devices [11, 12], with an error less than 5 μm and approaching 1 μm with modern ultrasound devices making use of echo tracking based on amplitude and phase information. These algorithms have been embedded in commercially available ultrasound equipment (Wall Track System/ART.LAB (before Pie Medical, Maastricht, the Netherlands), Esaote, Maastricht, the Netherlands, and QAS, MyLab, Esaote, Genova, Italy), and the equipment has gained the status of a reference system for measurement of vessel wall displacement. These Esaote systems measure the changes in arterial diameter simultaneously in 32 equidistant and parallel lines within a rectangular region of interest.

Another commercially available system (Aloka WTS E-track; Prosound Alpha 10, Tokyo, Japan)

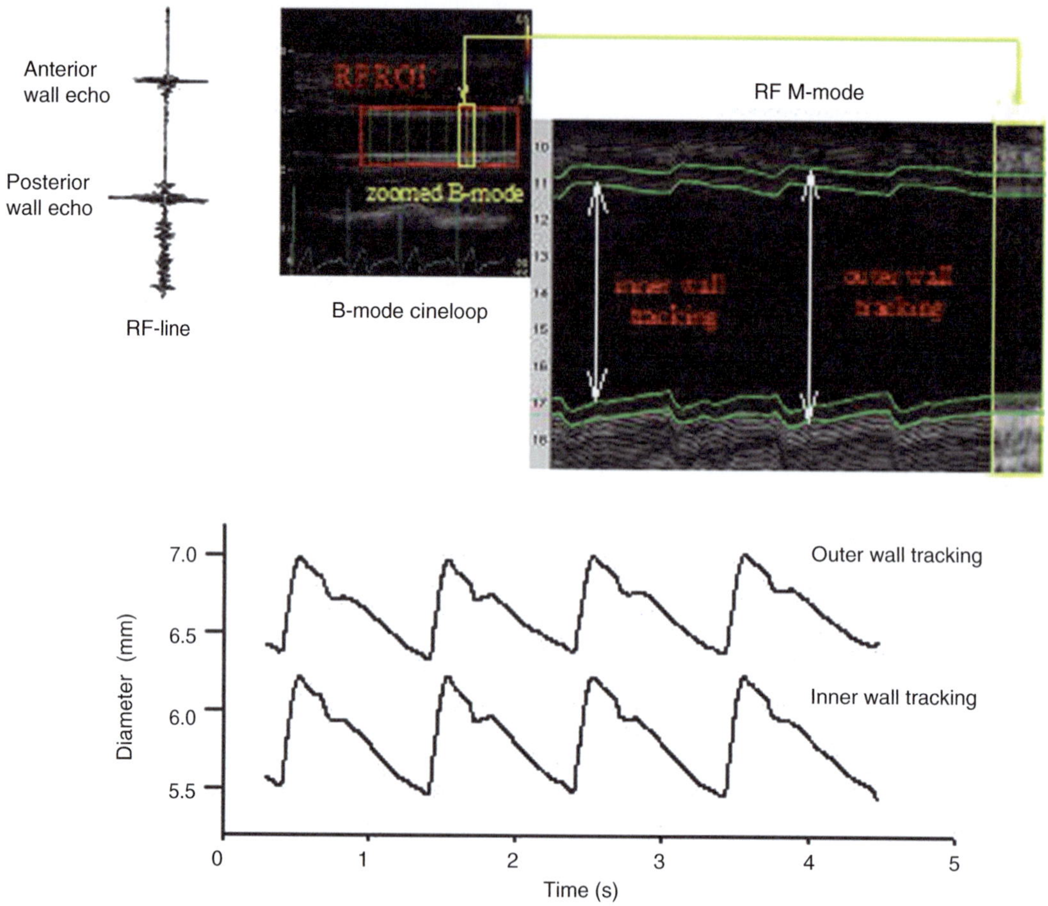

Fig. 3.1 Arterial wall tracking using the Vivid 7 modality. Along with the B-mode image, radio frequency (*RF*; *top left*) data are measured along eight scan lines, evenly spread over a region of interest (*RF ROI*; *top middle*). RF data along a selected scan line are displayed as an M-mode (*RF M-mode*; *top right*). On this image, material points are manually selected (lumen–intima and intima–adventitia transitions) and tracked in time, resulting in cyclic variation of inner and outer diameter (*bottom panels*)

evaluates the diameter changes along a single line. With the Aloka WTS the operator places the calipers at the anterior and posterior walls to enable the wall tracking (cfr Vivid 7 WTS).

Palombo et al. compared the values of carotid distension and stiffness obtained in the same population, both during the same session and during two separate sessions, by the Esaote and by the Aloka WTS, in order to determine whether these two systems may be interchangeable.

Although the correlations between the measures of common carotid artery diameter, distension, and beta-stiffness index provided by the two WTS were high, carotid distension was systematically lower and beta-stiffness index higher with the Esaote system as compared with the Aloka system.

They concluded that the values of carotid distension and stiffness obtained by these two different WTS are not interchangeable and cannot be merged into a common database. However, calibrated distension curves may provide an acceptable estimate of local carotid pressure [13].

With the increasing interest in vascular mechanics, other echo-tracking systems have become available. These systems are based on time integration of the velocity of the vessel wall (obtained

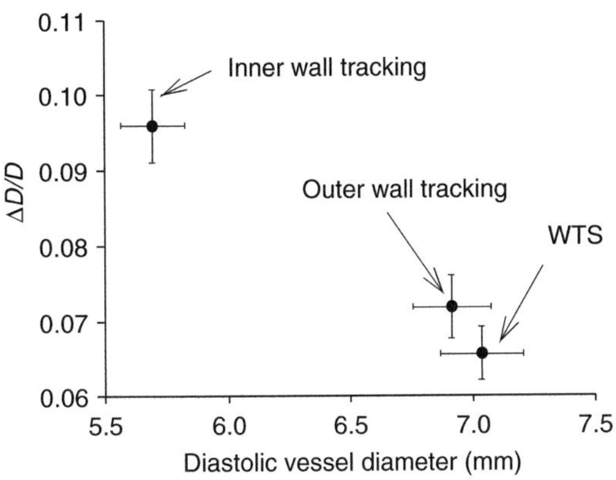

Fig. 3.2 Relative diameter change (**Δ***D*/*D*) in a mixed population when tracking the inner (lumen–intima transition) or outer (media–adventitia transition) wall with the Vivid 7 system and the automated wall tracking modality of the Wall Track System (*WTS*) [17]

with tissue Doppler; e.g., Philips Arterial Wall Motion Analyzer) [14, 15] or make use of alternative RF processing algorithms [16]. An example of a system using alternative RF processing is based on the Vivid 7 platform (GE Medical Ultrasound, Horten, Norway). Whereas the Wall Track System automatically detects the vessel wall, with the Vivid 7 wall track application, the investigator selects the material points within the vessel wall to track. This application allows tracking the lumen–intima interface ("inner wall tracking"), as well as of the media–adventitia interface ("outer wall tracking") as shown in Fig. 3.1. The absolute (ΔD) and relative diameter distension ($\Delta D/D$) are higher on the inner than on the outer wall (Fig. 3.2). In the population studied by Segers et al., ΔD and $\Delta D/D$ were on average 10 and 25 % higher on the inner than on the outer wall, respectively [17]. This heterogeneous deformation is not likely to arise from any structural heterogeneity (e.g., the presence of plaque), but can be explained by simple geometrical considerations. Arterial distension is accompanied by thinning of the arterial wall because of conservation of wall volume, leading to a smaller increase in diameter of the outer compared to the inner wall.

To increase reproducibility of data, the automated wall detection algorithm of the Wall Track System picks the largest echo in the radio frequency signal, generally arising from the adventitia of the near and far wall. As a consequence, the automated wall detection algorithm of the Wall Track System showed larger diameters and smaller distensions than the investigator-guided Vivid 7 wall track application [17]. The place of wall detection is substantially influencing the results. As a consequence of this observation, it appears logical to consider the lumen–intima interface as the most appropriate for wall detection. On the other hand, all studies on cardiovascular risk and local arterial stiffness have been done on the media–adventitia interface. These observations lead to some considerations which require further research: (1) It is not clear whether assessments of arterial stiffness based on lumen–intima interface will have a higher predictive value for cardiovascular risk than the current assessments based on the media–adventitia interface. (2) Theoretically it might be. However, the lumen–intima interface definition is less accurate and reproducible than the media–adventitia interface. (3) In longitudinal studies where vessel wall remodeling may occur, it is not a priori clear which material point should be used to derive the functional parameters reflecting the mechanics of the vessel. It is further expected that for more muscular arteries (brachial, radial, femoral artery) and in vessels subject to wall remodeling, the differences in ΔD and $\Delta D/D$ over the vascular wall will be more pronounced. (4) Particularly in longitudinal trials, reproducible automated investigator-independent wall detection may decrease interpretation bias.

It is clear that in comparing data from different studies or different devices, it is important to know which material point within the vessel wall has been used to calculate diameter and distension parameters. Therefore the tracking point should be clearly mentioned in the methods section.

Finally, other imaging techniques like CT (computer tomography) and MRI (magnetic resonance imaging) are available, with rapidly increasing possibilities for vascular research [18, 19]. These techniques are of particular interest for deep arteries, like the aorta, which cannot yet be measured with appropriate resolution by noninvasive ultrasound. These devices yield, in the first place, morphological information, with MRI allowing full 3-D imaging and reconstructions in all directions are possible. In addition, MRI allows measuring flow throughout the arterial tree. For MRI, 1.5-Tesla machines can measure vessel dimensions with a spatial resolution of 1x1x6 mm and a temporal resolution of 8 milliseconds. With 3-Tesla machines becoming more and more standard, these numbers can only improve. With recent scanning techniques temporal resolution can be increased to 1–6 s at little cost to spatial resolution (1–3 mm^3). These images can be used to represent aortic anatomy as a virtually rendered luminal volume. Source images are used to measure aortic diameters, preferably in a plane perpendicular to the aortic centerline, and at reproducible locations along the aorta (e.g., aortic valve ring; aortic sinus; sinotubular junction; ascending aorta; proximal, mid, and distal aortic arch; descending aorta; and aorta at the level of the diaphragm).

Perpendicular Fast Field Echo (FFE) cine images of the aorta can be used to measure diameters as well, but then only in prospectively determined imaging planes. As these cine images are gathered in a segmented fashion, they represent changes of the aortic wall during the entire cardiac cycle. FFE images are bright blood images, showing excellent contrast between blood and vessel wall. This makes them suitable for perpendicular area measurement in both systole and diastole, from which local distensibility can be calculated. Typically temporal resolution of these images is 20–40 ms, and inplane spatial resolution is 1.2 mm^2.

Recommendations for User Procedures

The accuracy of in vivo measurements is dependent on many different factors, including intrinsic accuracy of the measuring equipment, but also the careful adherence to measuring protocols and patient handling [20]. In this part, some recommendations based on a consensus conference on arterial stiffness measurement in Paris in 2000 are formulated. These play at three different levels [10, 21]: standardization of the participant condition (Table 3.2), standardization of methodological conditions (Table 3.3), and device-specific recommendations. In this chapter, the latter recommendations are limited to local arterial stiffness measurements (Table 3.4).

Table 3.2 Standardization of the subject condition

Subjects will be at rest for at least 10 min in a quiet room at room temperature (*consensus*)
Prolong resting period or cancel measurements in conditions where subjects' basal conditions are substantially altered, like when outside temperature is high or immediately after strenuous exercise (*consensus*)
Subjects have to refrain from smoking, eating, and drinking beverages containing caffeine for at least 3 h before assessments (*consensus*)
Unless measurements are performed early in the morning, advise a light meal 3–4 h before assessments (*large agreement*)
Subjects should refrain from drinking alcohol 10 h prior to measurements (*consensus*)
Subjects may neither speak nor sleep during assessments (*consensus*)
Authors should mention in which position measurements have been done (supine, sitting....) (*consensus*). The supine position is preferred (*large agreement*)
For repeated measures, subject measurements should be performed at the same time of the day and in the same position (*consensus*)
Be aware of possible "white coat" arterial stiffness, and if suspected, perform repeated measurements within 1 visit or in additional visits to detect it (*consensus*)
Be aware of possible disturbance of data due to cardiac arrhythmia (*consensus*)

Level of agreement on the recommendation is mentioned within brackets

Emerging Techniques to Measure Local Stiffness

There is a direct inverse relation between the local distensibility of an elastic tube and the value of local pulse wave velocity (see Chap. 1). As such, another way of assessing local stiffness is measurement of local PWV. At present, different strategies are being explored. One strategy involves the assessment of the local PWV in tubes and arteries from a combination of two of

Table 3.3 Standardization of the methodological conditions

Where possible use validated user-independent automated procedures (*large agreement*)
One observer is preferable, in particular for repeated measures: in each subject measurements should be performed by the same observer (*consensus*)
Perform quality control of data obtained: repeatability within 1 measurement and between two or more consecutive measurements (*consensus*)
When appropriate, correct[a] for differences in blood pressure regardless the device used (*consensus*)
In comparative studies correct for the most important confounding factors: mean arterial pressure, age, and gender, and if necessary also for other confounding factors like body mass index, heart rate, and drug therapy (*large agreement*)
When correcting for confounding factors, always test for (non)linearity of associations, confounding factors, and correct accordingly. When correcting, always give absolute uncorrected values (*consensus*)
In pharmacological intervention studies, time relation to drug intake should be mentioned (*consensus*)

Level of agreement on the recommendation is mentioned within brackets

[a]Correction can be done by statistical methods like covariant analysis. Local wall properties can also be calculated/compared at isobaric conditions

the following measurements: pressure (P), flow (Q), velocity (U), diameter (D), or cross-sectional area (A) waveforms. This led to methods known as the PU-loop [22], QA [23] or $\ln(D)U$ methods [24]. All methods can be applied using noninvasive measuring techniques (applanation tonometry and/or ultrasound), including MRI as demonstrated by Vulliémoz et al. [25]. In the QA method, local PWV is estimated as $\Delta Q/\Delta A$, with ΔQ and ΔA the change in flow and area during early systole, when the relationship between Q and A is linear, as it is not disturbed by wave reflection. The other methods rely on the same principle. These methods have been validated in vitro and using computational methods, but to the best of our knowledge, there is no unequivocal answer as to which of these methods is most accurate. These methods are not interchangeable and lead to different values, hampering their use in clinical practice [26].

With the further development in medical (ultrasound) imaging, techniques have become fast enough to directly measure the propagation of the pressure pulse over the short distance covered by the measuring probe. Hermeling et al. were among the first to demonstrate the feasibility of this technique, but they also referred to the difficulty in tracking the propagation of the foot of the wave, suggesting the dicrotic notch to be the better fiducial point to track [27]. This method of locally measuring the pulse wave propagation is sometimes referred to as "pulse wave imaging" [28]. These novel methods are now only

Table 3.4 Recommendations on user procedures for measuring local arterial stiffness

The investigator has to be well trained[a] (*consensus*)
Do not use simplified formulas[b] (*consensus*)
Do not push or squeeze the artery (*consensus*)
The use of the Langewouters model versus the measurement of isobaric compliance in a small common pressure window has to be discussed[c] (*large agreement*)
Pulse pressure should be measured at the site of distension measurements (*consensus*)
Pulse pressure in the common carotid artery is a valid surrogate for pulse pressure in the ascending aorta. This does not apply to the waveform (*large agreement*)
In the hands of a large number of investigators, pulse pressure data directly obtained from applanation tonometry are not reliable, and if so, they should be avoided (*large agreement*)
Assessment of local pulse pressure using calibrated pressure waves obtained from applanation tonometry appears a valid method. For calibration make use of a validated sphygmomanometer (*consensus*)
If no reliable pressure waves can be obtained using applanation tonometry, the use of distension waves from echo-tracking devices can be a good alternative. Also adding 40 % of the brachial pulse pressure to brachial diastolic pressure is much better than the one-third rule to estimate mean arterial pressure. Whether the use of mean blood pressure and diastolic pressure from oscillometric devices is reliable has to be further investigated (*large agreement*)
Repeated measurements should be done at the same local site: it is advisable that this site is well-defined and reported at the first measurement. For the common carotid and common femoral artery, the distance to the bifurcation can be used as reference

Level of agreement on the recommendation is mentioned within brackets

[a]The investigator should obtain reproducible data comparable with published data [20]

[b]Complete formulas are shown in this chapter, paragraph "Definitions of Local Wall Properties"

[c]Extrapolation of data outside the measured pressure/diameter range should be avoided

emerging. While these methods seem feasible and lead to realistic values of local stiffness, the relation between directly measured local PWV and the distensibility indices still needs to be assessed. Despite the fact that there is a direct theoretical relation, this relation applies to wave propagation in uniform tubes in absence of wave reflections, conditions which are not met neither in normal nor in diseased arteries.

Assessment of Local Pulse Pressure

A large number of studies have shown that pulse pressure at the brachial artery is an important cardiovascular risk factor [2, 3, 29]. There is growing interest in studying local pulse pressure at other arterial sites than the brachial artery for the following reasons: (1) there is increasing evidence in support of the local mechanical stress hypothesis (see section "Introduction") that pulse pressure at other arterial sites (i.e., the ascending aorta) may show stronger associations with cardiovascular events [30, 31]; (2) it has been found that local pulse pressure is a major determinant of large artery remodeling [32]; (3) accurate assessment of local pulse pressure may be needed for the correct calculation of local arterial wall properties.

In contrast to mean arterial pressure (MAP), pulse pressure is not constant throughout the large artery tree [33]. It increases centrifugally [21, 34]. However, this pulse pressure amplification might be attenuated and even lost by early reflected pulse waves due to stiffening of arteries and/or by more proximal reflection sites [21, 34]. As a consequence, use of the pulse pressure obtained at one arterial site as surrogate of the pulse pressure at another arterial site might be erroneous [35].

The most accurate assessment of pressure is obtained invasively using high fidelity pressure transducers, measuring pressure directly at the tip of the catheter. However, this invasive technique is not appropriate for (relative) large populations often needed in clinical studies. In this chapter only noninvasive methods of pressure measurement will be discussed.

Applanation tonometry has been proposed to assess local pulse pressure. It allows noninvasive recording of the arterial pressure waveform and magnitude in both central and peripheral arteries [36, 37]. This technique provides pressure waveforms, being almost identical to those obtained intra-arterially [38]. Although it is theoretically possible to directly measure pulse pressure with tonometry [39, 40], several authors are convinced that the magnitude of the pulse pressure obtained by this internally calibrated applanation tonometry is unreliable [12, 41].

Kelly and Fitchett have proposed an alternative calibration of the tonometer pressure waves [42], a method that has been validated and found accurate [12]. The calibration procedure is based on the observation that the difference between mean and diastolic blood pressure is nearly constant throughout the large artery tree [34, 43]. Pauca et al. [33] showed that (in the absence of stenotic lesions in the arterial pathway) the difference between mean arterial pressure (MAP) and diastolic blood pressure (DBP) was only 0.2 mmHg larger in the radial artery than in the ascending aorta. The radial MAP and DBP are reliable, since in 90 % percent and 92 % percent of the patients, respectively, the pressure differences were within ±3 mmHg of those in the aorta. DBP can easily be obtained at the brachial artery from a validated cuff blood pressure device. For the assessment of mean brachial blood pressure, different approaches can be followed. First, one may rely on an oscillometric blood pressure reader to estimate mean blood pressure. Second, the rule of thumb can be used, estimating MAP from SBP and DBP, e.g., using DBP + PP/3, PP being the brachial systolic–diastolic pressure difference. However, the accuracy of both methods is rather limited. The calculation of MAP from numeric integral of a calibrated accurate pressure wave appears the most reliable method. Bos et al. [44] questioned the general validity of the formula MAP = DBP + PP/3. Using previously recorded resting intrabrachial pressures and Riva-Rocci Korotkoff blood pressure measurements they found that intra-arterially measured real mean pressure was at 39.5 ± 2.5 % of pulse pressure above diastolic pressure in

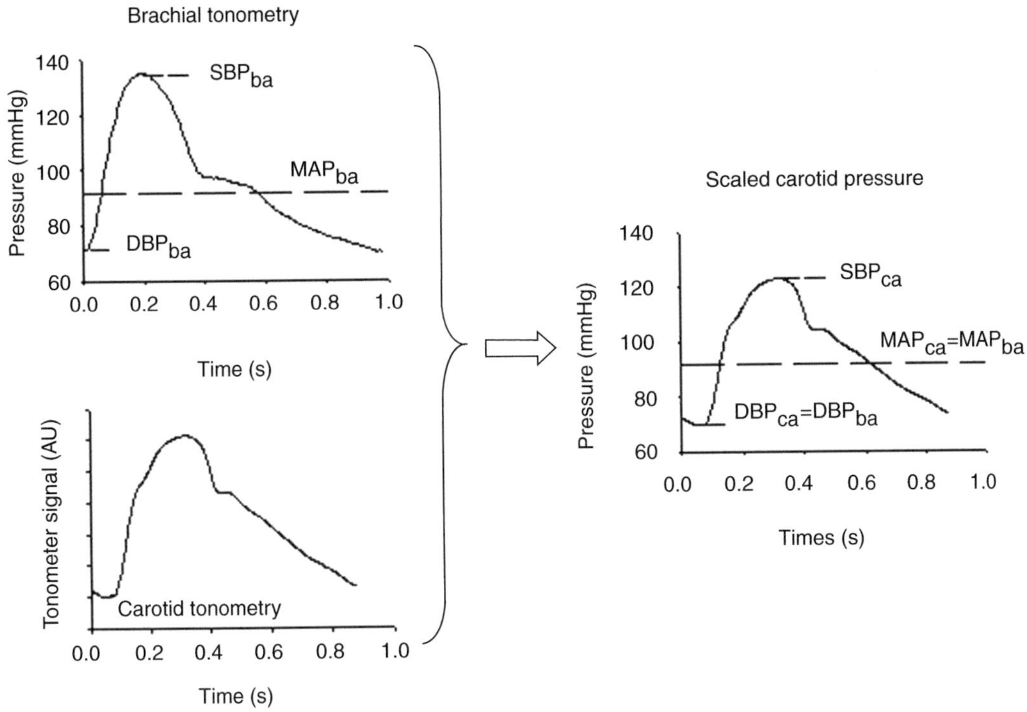

Fig. 3.3 Scaling of carotid pressure wave from brachial artery pressure and wave. See text for description of the calibration scheme. SBP, DBP, and MAP are brachial artery systolic, diastolic, and mean blood pressure, respectively, the subscript "ba" indicating values at the brachial artery and "ca" at the carotid artery. The tonometer signal is in arbitrary units (*AU*)

all individuals. Results were not related to age, blood pressure, pulse pressure, or heart rate levels. Mean pressure calculated with the traditional one-third rule therefore underestimated "real" mean pressure by 5.0 ± 2.3 mmHg ($P<0.01$) when calculated from intra-arterial pressure readings and by 4.9 ± 5.3 mmHg ($P<0.01$) when calculated from Riva-Rocci Korotkoff readings. The conclusion was that mean pressure at the upper arm is underestimated when calculated using the traditional formula of adding one-third of the pulse pressure to the diastolic pressure and that this underestimation can be avoided by adding 40 % of pulse pressure to the diastolic pressure. Langesen et al. confirmed the superiority of the 40 % of pulse pressure rule above the one-third rule. They also concluded that this 40 % of pulse pressure rule was acceptable when studying patient groups but much less reliable on an individual patient level. [45].

As an example of this calibration procedure, the assessment of the carotid pressure is shown (Fig. 3.3): at the reference artery (i.e., brachial artery) peak and nadir of the pressure wave are assigned systolic and diastolic pressures determined by a conventional method (i.e., sphygmomanometry). The mean pressure is calculated from numeric integral of a calibrated accurate pressure wave. With assignment of the same mean and diastolic pressures to the target artery (i.e., carotid artery), the pressure wave at the target artery is calibrated throughout the cardiac cycle. This method has been validated and found accurate [12]. It got grade A according to British Hypertension Society criteria for the evaluation of blood pressure measuring devices [46].

Applanation tonometry cannot be applied to all subjects and at all arterial sites [34]. It requires a stiff or bony structure to flatten the artery wall and a lean skin to avoid cushioning of the pressure pulse [39, 40]. In obese subjects applanation tonometry often is inaccurate at a majority of arterial sites. In contrast to the pressure waves obtained by applanation tonometry, arterial distension waves from echo-tracking devices [11] can be obtained accurately at more arterial sites and also in a majority of obese subjects. Assessment of blood pressure based on calibrated arterial distension waves has been attempted in the past [47, 48] but failed because of lack of accurate arterial distension registration. Echo-tracking devices have shown high accuracy and can measure arterial distension with an error less than 5 μm [11]. Application of the above-described calibration method on distension waves from echo-tracking devices showed an acceptable alternative for sites where use of applanation tonometry is unreliable [12]. This procedure got grade B according to British Hypertension Society criteria for the evaluation of blood pressure measuring devices [46]. The procedure appears valid for pulse pressures up to 70 mmHg. Due to the nonlinear relation between pressure and diameter, it is likely that at high pressures distension waves may not sufficiently reflect pressure waves. Kips et al. [49] examined the use of brachial and carotid diameter distension waveforms as an alternative for tonometric pressure to assess carotid blood pressure. It can be concluded from this study that results are comparable as long as one sticks to one technique on both the brachial and the carotid artery, either tonometry or distension, when assessing carotid blood pressure noninvasively. Combining tonometry on one site and diameter distension on the other leads to larger inter-method differences.

Application of the Fitchett and Kelly procedure assumes that MAP is constant. This is only true in the large artery tree when no hemodynamically relevant stenosis is present. Blood pressure devices making use of smaller arteries such as finger arteries, where increase in resistance due to viscous friction causes mean blood pressure to drop significantly along the artery, are probably not suitable for this procedure.

An alternative method to assess central pulse pressure makes use of peripheral tonometry recordings and a (generalized) transfer function to synthesize central pressure from the peripheral recording [50–52]. This transfer function appears limited to the upper limb and assesses ascending aorta pulse pressure from radial or carotid artery tonometer [34]. The merit of such transfer functions, as is, for instance, built in the SphygmoCor device, is the ease of use, since recordings are obtained at the radial artery, the vascular site which is most appropriate for applanation tonometry. Validation studies by Pauca and O'Rourke [52, 53] demonstrated that pulse pressure is estimated with an accuracy meeting the Association for the Advancement of Medical Instrumentation (AAMI) [54] and British Hypertension Society grade A criteria [46]. The validity of the radial-to-aorta transfer function has, nonetheless, also been debated [55] and found to underestimate central pulse pressure. It is, however, likely that a substantial part of this underestimation is not due to the transfer function itself, but to inaccuracies related to cuff sphygmomanometry [56] and to the use of the brachial artery pressure as surrogate for the radial artery pressure, neglecting a possible brachial-to-radial pulse pressure amplification [35].

The calibration of pressure waveforms from tonometry (or surrogate waveforms from diameter distension measurements) using two discrete blood pressure values (e.g., mean and diastolic blood pressure) directly relates to the shape of the waveform, which can be quantified by the form factor. The form factor (FF) is defined as the ratio of the difference between the mean and minimum value of the wave and its amplitude (maximal–minimal value):

$$FF = \frac{\text{mean} - \text{minimum}}{\text{amplitude}}$$

The lower the FF, the more peaked the waveform. Form factors are thus lowest in peripheral arteries and in younger subjects, while they are highest in central sites and in elderly. Assuming that the difference between mean and diastolic blood pressure remains constant, the ratio of form factors at central over peripheral sites is the amplification. Noninvasive applanation tonometry studies of the brachial and radial artery pressure waves show a substantial amplification between the brachial and radial sites. [57] Adji and O'Rourke consider this amplification to be artificial, explained by an inability to applanate the brachial artery properly resulting in a systematic error in generating brachial waveforms. They termed the apparent amplification the "Popeye" phenomenon [58]. It was reported in Kips et al. [49] that brachial waveforms measured with tonometry are more peaked than the corresponding diameter distension waveforms, but this was expected given the nonlinear relation between pressure and diameter. Anyhow, the relation between the form factor of the tonometer and distension waveforms was not different for the carotid and brachial artery in that study, supporting the feasibility of applanation tonometry as a reliable technique to obtain noninvasive pressure waveforms at the brachial artery.

Estimation of central pressure and particularly the use of radial versus brachial tonometry remain a hot debate where neither party might be right or wrong.

Acknowledgment The authors thank Dan De Vos, MD, for his contribution on MR imaging.

References

1. Haider AW, Larson MG, Franklin SS, Levy D. Systolic blood pressure, diastolic blood pressure, and pulse pressure as predictors of risk for congestive heart failure in the Framingham Heart Study. Ann Intern Med. 2003;138(1):10–6.
2. Benetos A, Zureik M, Morcet J, Thomas F, Bean K, Safar M, et al. A decrease in diastolic blood pressure combined with an increase in systolic blood pressure is associated with a higher cardiovascular mortality in men. J Am Coll Cardiol. 2000;35(3):673–80.
3. Blacher J, Staessen JA, Girerd X, Gasowski J, Thijs L, Liu L, et al. Pulse pressure not mean pressure determines cardiovascular risk in older hypertensive patients. Arch Intern Med. 2000;160(8):1085–9.
4. Van Bortel LM, Hoeks AP, Kool MJ, Struijker-Boudier HA. Introduction to large artery properties as a target for risk reduction by antihypertensive therapy. J Hypertens Suppl. 1992;10(6):S123–6.
5. O'Rourke MF. Basic concepts for the understanding of large arteries in hypertension. J Cardiovasc Pharmacol. 1985;7 Suppl 2:S14–21.
6. Gutstein DE, Fuster V. Pathophysiology and clinical significance of atherosclerotic plaque rupture. Cardiovasc Res. 1999;41(2):323–33.
7. Richardson PD. Biomechanics of plaque rupture: progress, problems, and new frontiers. Ann Biomed Eng. 2002;30(4):524–36.
8. Tang D, Yang C, Kobayashi S, Ku DN. Effect of a lipid pool on stress/strain distributions in stenotic arteries: 3-D fluid-structure interactions (FSI) models. J Biomech Eng. 2004;126(3):363–70.
9. Paini A, Boutouyrie P, Calvet D, Zidi M, Agabiti-Rosei E, Laurent S. Multiaxial mechanical characteristics of carotid plaque: analysis by multiarray echotracking system. Stroke. 2007;38(1):117–23.
10. Van Bortel LM, Duprez D, Starmans-Kool MJ, Safar ME, Giannattasio C, Cockcroft J, et al. Clinical applications of arterial stiffness, task force III: recommendations for user procedures. Am J Hypertens. 2002;15(5):445–52.
11. Hoeks AP, Brands PJ, Smeets FA, Reneman RS. Assessment of the distensibility of superficial arteries. Ultrasound Med Biol. 1990;16(2):121–8.
12. Van Bortel LM, Balkestein EJ, van der Heijden-Spek JJ, Vanmolkot FH, Staessen JA, Kragten JA, et al. Non-invasive assessment of local arterial pulse pressure: comparison of applanation tonometry and echo-tracking. J Hypertens. 2001;19(6):1037–44.
13. Palombo C, Kozakova M, Guraschi N, Bini G, Cesana F, Castoldi G, et al. Radiofrequency-based carotid wall tracking: a comparison between two different systems. J Hypertens. 2012;30(8):1614–9.
14. Bonnefous O, Montaudon M, Sananes J, Denis E. Noninvasive echographic techniques for arterial wall characterization. In: Levy M, Schneider SC, McAvoy BR, editors. IEEE Ultrasonics Symposium, Proceedings Vols 1 and 2. Texas, USA: San Antonio 1996, pp.1059–64.
15. Ramnarine KV, Hartshorne T, Sensier Y, Naylor M, Walker J, Naylor AR, et al. Tissue Doppler imaging of carotid plaque wall motion: a pilot study. Cardiovasc Ultrasound. 2003;1:17.
16. Rabben SI, Baerum S, Sorhus V, Torp H. Ultrasound-based vessel wall tracking: an auto-correlation technique with RF center frequency estimation. Ultrasound Med Biol. 2002;28(4):507–17.
17. Segers P, Rabben SI, De BJ, De SJ, Gillebert TC, Van BL, et al. Functional analysis of the common carotid artery: relative distension differences over the vessel wall measured in vivo. J Hypertens. 2004;22(5):973–81.
18. Resnick LM, Militianu D, Cunnings AJ, Pipe JG, Evelhoch JL, Soulen RL. Direct magnetic resonance determination of aortic distensibility in essential hypertension: relation to age, abdominal visceral fat, and in situ intracellular free magnesium. Hypertension. 1997;30(3 Pt 2):654–9.
19. Danias PG, Tritos NA, Stuber M, Botnar RM, Kissinger KV, Manning WJ. Comparison of aortic elasticity determined by cardiovascular magnetic resonance imaging in obese versus lean adults. Am J Cardiol. 2003;91(2):195–9.
20. Kool MJ, Kool MJ, Van Merode T, Reneman RS, Hoeks AP, Struyker Boudier HA, Van Bortel

LM. Evaluation of reproducibility of a vessel wall movement detector system for assessment of large artery properties. Cardiovasc Res. 1994;28(5):610–4.
21. Laurent S, Cockcroft J, Van Bortel L, Boutouyrie P, Giannattasio C, Hayoz D, et al. Expert consensus document on arterial stiffness: methodological issues and clinical applications. Eur Heart J. 2006;27(21): 2588–605.
22. Khir AW, O'Brien A, Gibbs JS, Parker KH. Determination of wave speed and wave separation in the arteries. J Biomech. 2001;34(9):1145–55.
23. Rabben SI, Stergiopulos N, Hellevik LR, Smiseth OA, Slordahl S, Urheim S, et al. An ultrasound-based method for determining pulse wave velocity in superficial arteries. J Biomech. 2004;37(10):1615–22.
24. Feng J, Khir AW. Determination of wave speed and wave separation in the arteries using diameter and velocity. J Biomech. 2010;43(3):455–62.
25. Vulliemoz S, Stergiopulos N, Meuli R. Estimation of local aortic elastic properties with MRI. Magn Reson Med. 2002;47(4):649–54.
26. Swillens A, Taelman L, Degroote J, Vierendeels J, Segers P. Comparison of non-invasive methods for measurement of local pulse wave velocity using FSI-Simulations and in vivo data. Ann Biomed Eng. 2013;41(7):1567–78.
27. Hermeling E, Reesink KD, Kornmann LM, Reneman RS, Hoeks AP. The dicrotic notch as alternative time-reference point to measure local pulse wave velocity in the carotid artery by means of ultrasonography. J Hypertens. 2009;27(10):2028–35.
28. Luo J, Li RX, Konofagou EE. Pulse wave imaging of the human carotid artery: an in vivo feasibility study. IEEE Trans Ultrason Ferroelectr Freq Control. 2012;59(1):174–81.
29. Benetos A, Thomas F, Joly L, Blacher J, Pannier B, Labat C, et al. Pulse pressure amplification a mechanical biomarker of cardiovascular risk. J Am Coll Cardiol. 2010;55(10):1032–7.
30. Vlachopoulos C, Aznaouridis K, O'Rourke MF, Safar ME, Baou K, Stefanadis C. Prediction of cardiovascular events and all-cause mortality with central haemodynamics: a systematic review and meta-analysis. Eur Heart J. 2010;31(15):1865–71.
31. Huang CM, Wang KL, Cheng HM, Chuang SY, Sung SH, Yu WC, Ting CT, Lakatta EG, Yin FC, Chou P, Chen CH. Central versus ambulatory blood pressure in the prediction of all-cause and cardiovascular mortalities. J Hypertens. 2011;29(3):454–9.
32. Laurent S, Tropeano AI, Lillo-Lelouet A, Jondeau G, Laloux B, Boutouyrie P. Local pulse pressure is a major determinant of large artery remodelling. Clin Exp Pharmacol Physiol. 2001;28(12):1011–4.
33. Pauca AL, Wallenhaupt SL, Kon ND, Tucker WY. Does radial artery pressure accurately reflect aortic pressure? Chest. 1992;102(4):1193–8.
34. Nichols W, O'Rourke M, editors. McDonald's blood flow in arteries. Theoretical, experimental and clinical principles. London/Sydney/Auckland: Arnold; 1998.
35. Verbeke F, Segers P, Heireman S, Vanholder R, Verdonck P, Van Bortel LM. Noninvasive assessment of local pulse pressure: importance of brachial-to-radial pressure amplification. Hypertension. 2005;46(1): 244–8.
36. London G, Guerin A, Pannier B, Marchais S, Benetos A, Safar M. Increased systolic pressure in chronic uremia. Role of arterial wave reflections. Hypertension. 1992;20(1):10–9.
37. Benetos A, Laurent S, Hoeks AP, Boutouyrie PH, Safar ME. Arterial alterations with aging and high blood pressure. A noninvasive study of carotid and femoral arteries. Arterioscler Thromb. 1993;13(1): 90–7.
38. Kelly R, Hayward C, Avolio A, O'Rourke M. Noninvasive determination of age-related changes in the human arterial pulse. Circulation. 1989;80:1652–9.
39. Drzewiecki GM, Melbin J, Noordergraaf A. Arterial tonometry: review and analysis. J Biomech. 1983; 16(2):141–52.
40. Matthys K, Verdonck P. Development and modelling of arterial applanation tonometry: a review. Technol Health Care. 2002;10(1):65–76.
41. Chen CH, Ting CT, Nussbacher A, Nevo E, Kass DA, Pak P, et al. Validation of carotid artery tonometry as a means of estimating augmentation index of ascending aortic pressure. Hypertension. 1996;27(2):168–75.
42. Kelly R, Fitchett D. Noninvasive determination of aortic input impedance and external left ventricular power output: a validation and repeatability study of a new technique. J Am Coll Cardiol. 1992;20(4):952–63.
43. Milnor W, editor. Hemodynamics. The normal hemodynamic state. Baltimore: Williams and Wilkins; 1982.
44. Bos WJ, Verrij E, Vincent HH, Westerhof BE, Parati G, van Montfrans GA. How to assess mean blood pressure properly at the brachial artery level. J Hypertens. 2007;25(4):751–5.
45. Laugesen E, Rossen NB, Peters CD, Mæng M, Ebbehøj E, Knudsen ST, Hansen KW, Bøtker HE, Poulsen PL. Assessment of central blood pressure in patients with type 2 diabetes: a comparison between sphygmocor and invasively measured values. Am J Hypertens. 2014;27(2):169–76.
46. O'Brien E, Petrie J, Littler W, de Swiet M, Padfield PL, Altman DG, et al. An outline of the revised British Hypertension Society protocol for the evaluation of blood pressure measuring devices. J Hypertens. 1993;11(6):677–9.
47. Correll RW. Theoretical analysis and preliminary development of an indirect blood pressure recording system. MS thesis. Cambridge: MIT; 1978.
48. Ghista DN, Jayaraman G, Sandler H. Analysis for the non-invasive determination of arterial properties and for the transcutaneous continuous monitoring of arterial blood pressure. Med Biol Eng Comput. 1978; 16(6):715–26.
49. Kips J, Vanmolkot F, Mahieu D, Vermeersch I, Fabry S, de Hoon J, et al. The use of diameter distension

waveforms as an alternative for tonometric pressure to assess carotid blood pressure. Physiol Meas. 2010;31(4):543–53.
50. Karamanoglu M, O'Rourke MF, Avolio AP, Kelly RP. An analysis of the relationship between central aortic and peripheral upper limb pressure waves in man. Eur Heart J. 1993;14(2):160–7.
51. Chen CH, Nevo E, Fetics B, Pak PH, Yin FC, Maughan WL, et al. Estimation of central aortic pressure waveform by mathematical transformation of radial tonometry pressure. Validation of generalized transfer function. Circulation. 1997;95(7):1827–36.
52. Pauca AL, O'Rourke MF, Kon ND. Prospective evaluation of a method for estimating ascending aortic pressure from the radial artery pressure waveform. Hypertension. 2001;38(4):932–7.
53. O'Rourke MF, Pauca AL. Augmentation of the aortic and central arterial pressure waveform. Blood Press Monit. 2004;9(4):179–85.
54. White WB, Berson AS, Robbins C, Jamieson MJ, Prisant M, Roccella E, Sheps SG. National standard for measurement of resting and ambulatory blood pressures with automated sphygmomanometers. Hypertension. 1993;21:504–9.
55. Davies JI, Band MM, Pringle S, Ogston S, Struthers AD. Peripheral blood pressure measurement is as good as applanation tonometry at predicting ascending aortic blood pressure. J Hypertens. 2003;21(3):571–6.
56. O'Rourke M, Avolio A. Assessment of central arterial pressure? J Hypertens. 2003;21(7):1425–6.
57. Segers P, Mahieu D, Kips J, Rietzschel E, De Buyzere M, De Bacquer D, Bekaert S, De Backer G, Gillebert T, Verdonck P, Van Bortel L. Asklepios investigators. Amplification of the pressure pulse in the upper limb in healthy, middle-aged men and women. Hypertension. 2009;54(2):414–20.
58. Adji A, O'Rourke MF. Brachial artery tonometry and the Popeye phenomenon: explanation of anomalies in generating central from upper limb pressure waveforms. J Hypertens. 2012;30(8):1540–51.

Ventricular-Arterial Coupling and Mechanism of Wave Reflections

4

Julio A. Chirinos and Patrick Segers

Abstract

In this chapter, we discuss two approaches to quantitatively assess ventricular-arterial interaction: (i) the "classic" approach based on matching of ventricular and arterial elastance (analysis in pressure-volume plane) and (ii) a novel approach based on assessment of time-varying myocardial stress. The latter analysis, in the time domain, allows to directly link left ventricular myocardial stress with systemic arterial properties and with the magnitude and timing of arterial wave reflections.

Keywords

Hemodynamics • Arterial function • Ventricular function • Wave reflections • Heart failure

Introduction

The interactions between the left ventricle (LV) and the systemic arteries are key determinants of cardiovascular function, dysfunction, and various cardiovascular disease states. This chapter deals with approaches used for the assessment of ventricular-arterial interactions and coupling, with a focus on underlying hemodynamic principles and the interpretation of commonly used physiologic indices. We also review recent studies assessing the association between ventricular-arterial coupling, myocardial function, and heart failure risk in large populations.

J.A. Chirinos, MD, PhD
Philadelphia Veterans Affairs Medical Center, University of Pennsylvania School of Medicine, Philadelphia, PA, USA
e-mail: julio.chirinos@uphs.upenn.edu

P. Segers, PhD (✉)
Institute Biomedical Technology (IBiTech), iMinds Medical IT, Ghent University, Campus Heymans-Blok B, De Pintelaan 185, Ghent 9000, Belgium
e-mail: patrick.segers@ugent.be

Ventricular-Arterial Coupling: Matching Elastances?

Ventricular-arterial coupling is still most often associated with the study of ventricular (E_{es}) and arterial elastance (E_a) and of their ratio, introduced in the early 1980s [1]. E_{es}, end-systolic elastance, is the slope of the end-systolic pressure-volume relation [2], which is usually considered the gold standard measure of ventricular contractility and chamber function. It is

M.E. Safar et al. (eds.), *Blood Pressure and Arterial Wall Mechanics in Cardiovascular Diseases*, DOI 10.1007/978-1-4471-5198-2_4, © Springer-Verlag London 2014

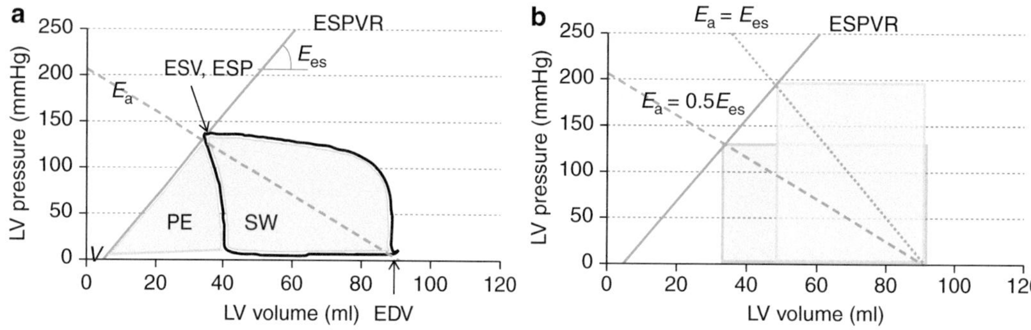

Fig. 4.1 Panel (**a**) Left ventricular pressure-volume (PV) loop with indication of the slope (E_{es}) and intercept (V_0) of the end-systolic pressure-volume relation (*ESPVR*) and the arterial elastance (E_a). The area enclosed by the PV loop represents the stroke work (*SW*), the *gray* area the "potential" energy (*PE*). The sum of SW and PE is the pressure-volume area (PVA). Panel (**b**) Schematic of the PV loop associated with E_a/E_{es} of 1 (maximal SW generation) and E_a/E_{es} of 0.5 (maximal efficiency)

typically measured invasively using a pressure-volume (conductance) catheter, where the preload of the heart is progressively reduced via inflation of a balloon in the inferior vena cava. When considering the pressure-volume (PV) plane and assuming known end-systolic pressure-volume relation and end-diastolic volume (EDV) (and intact cardiac valves), the PV loop – and thus the operating conditions of the cardiovascular system – is fully determined with knowledge of the upper left-hand corner of the PV loop (end-systolic pressure, ESP, and end-systolic volume, ESV). The line connecting this point with the EDV point on the *y*-axis – thus having a slope [ESP/stroke volume] – can be approximated as R/T, with R the systemic vascular resistance and T the cardiac period. The slope, having mmHg/ml as units, has been termed the arterial elastance, E_a [1, 3]. Knowledge of E_a and E_{es} provides an elegant and intuitive (graphical or analytical) way to study the interaction between the heart and the arterial system in the PV plane (Fig. 4.1). The impact of changes in preload, afterload (R), cardiac frequency, and contractility on cardiac function (stroke volume and pressure development) is easily calculated and visualized. In addition, the PV plane provides a straightforward way to link ventricular function to mechanical performance [4]. The area enclosed by the PV loop (Fig. 4.1) is the stroke work (SW), while the area enclosed by the end-diastolic and end-systolic PV relation and descending limb of the PV loop is the "potential energy (PE)," although the terminology "potential" is to be interpreted in a negative sense, as it represents the energy associated with pressurizing the non-ejected volume in the ventricular cavity, and therefore not used for perfusion. Animal studies demonstrated that the sum of the SW and PE (termed the pressure-volume area; PVA) is proportional to the myocardial oxygen consumption when the latter is manipulated by various interventions in single animals [5]. This global PV-based framework now provides a way to study the relation between the energetic output of the ventricle (SW) and the total energy provided to the heart (i.e., the efficiency of conversion of ATP into mechanical work) and this in terms of a "coupling parameter" E_a/E_{es}. This parameter is extensively used in studies considering mechanico-energetic aspects of heart-arterial coupling [4, 6, 7]. E_a/E_{es} varies over the range of 0.5 (optimal efficiency) to 1 (maximal stroke work generation) [4], while in heart failure with reduced ejection fraction, with dilated hearts, E_a/E_{es} becomes larger than one [7, 8]. This approach is highly attractive because of its simplicity, but there are some issues that deserve closer attention:

(i) The concept is based on experimental measurements in open-chest anesthetized animals, which might not be fully representative of normal human physiology. It has been demonstrated that the end-systolic pressure-volume relation is nonlinear rather than linear and sensitive to loading conditions [9].

(ii) The method is difficult to apply in practice. It is, at present, impossible to measure complete left ventricular pressure-volume loops in a noninvasive way. Part of the pressure-volume loop may, however, be obtained from aortic pressure and flow. Ultrasound technology may be used to estimate left ventricular end-systolic and/or end-diastolic dimensions or ejection fraction, though the accuracy is rather limited. In healthy subjects, there is little pressure drop over the aortic valve: aortic and left ventricular pressure can be assumed equal during ejection. Knowing left ventricular end-diastolic volume (EDV) and integrating aortic flow, part of the left ventricular pressure-volume loop can thus be obtained in a noninvasive way. Magnetic resonance imaging may provide a solution for noninvasive measurement of instantaneous ventricular volume. It is, however, difficult to obtain sufficiently large alterations of pre- or afterload without invasive interventions (such as the inflation of a balloon in the inferior vena cava to reduce cardiac filling and preload).

(iii) While the terminology of E_a as arterial elastance suggests that the parameter is related to arterial stiffness, it is not. In addition, E_a is highly determined by heart rate and is therefore not a true arterial parameter [10].

(iv) A major drawback of the analysis in the PV domain is the fact that time is excluded from the analysis. As we will demonstrate further in this chapter, timing of cardiac and vascular events (contraction and relaxation) is important, especially in the context of ventricular-arterial coupling where timing of reflections will be shown to play a major role on their effective impact on myocardial load.

Assessing Arterial Load with Pressure-Flow Analyses

Whereas assessment of ventricular-arterial coupling in the pressure-volume plane is intuitive and intuitively dissects underlying determinants of stroke volume and LV ejection fraction, ventricular-arterial interactions encompass a wide range of phenomena that are not captured by this approach. Assessment of ventricular-arterial interactions in terms of pulsatile pressure-flow relations provides important incremental information about the physiologic status of the ventricular-arterial system.

At the beginning of each cardiac cycle, the heart generates a forward-traveling energy pulse that results in increased pressure and forward flow in the proximal aorta during early systole [11, 12]. The energy wave generated by the LV (incident wave) is transmitted by conduit vessels and partially reflected at sites of impedance mismatch, such as points of branching or change in wall diameter or material properties along the arterial tree (taking place in a continuous manner due to geometric and mechanical tapering). Multiple small reflections are conducted back to the heart and merge into a "net" reflected wave, composed of the contributions of the scattered backward reflections. Wave dynamics are too complex to fully resolve in vivo and are usually simplified, considering only one forward (generated by the heart) and one backward wave (due to reflections in the periphery). Thus, wave reflections are often analyzed as a single discrete wave, originating from an "effective" reflection site, but this wave is actually the result of scattered reflections, originating from distributed reflection sites (see further). In addition to hemodynamic phenomena related to wave transmission and reflections, the arterial system exerts a buffering function, which depends on its compliance, allowing it to accommodate additional blood volume during systole without excessive increases in pressure and to release that excess volume throughout diastole without excessive drops in pressure [13].

Arterial load can be precisely and comprehensively characterized via analyses of pressure-flow relations (Fig. 4.2). The analysis of arterial input impedance obtained in this manner is considered the gold standard method for the assessment of arterial load [14]. Pressure-flow analyses allow the quantification of "steady" or "resistive" load and various components of pulsatile load [14–17]. The steady component of afterload depends

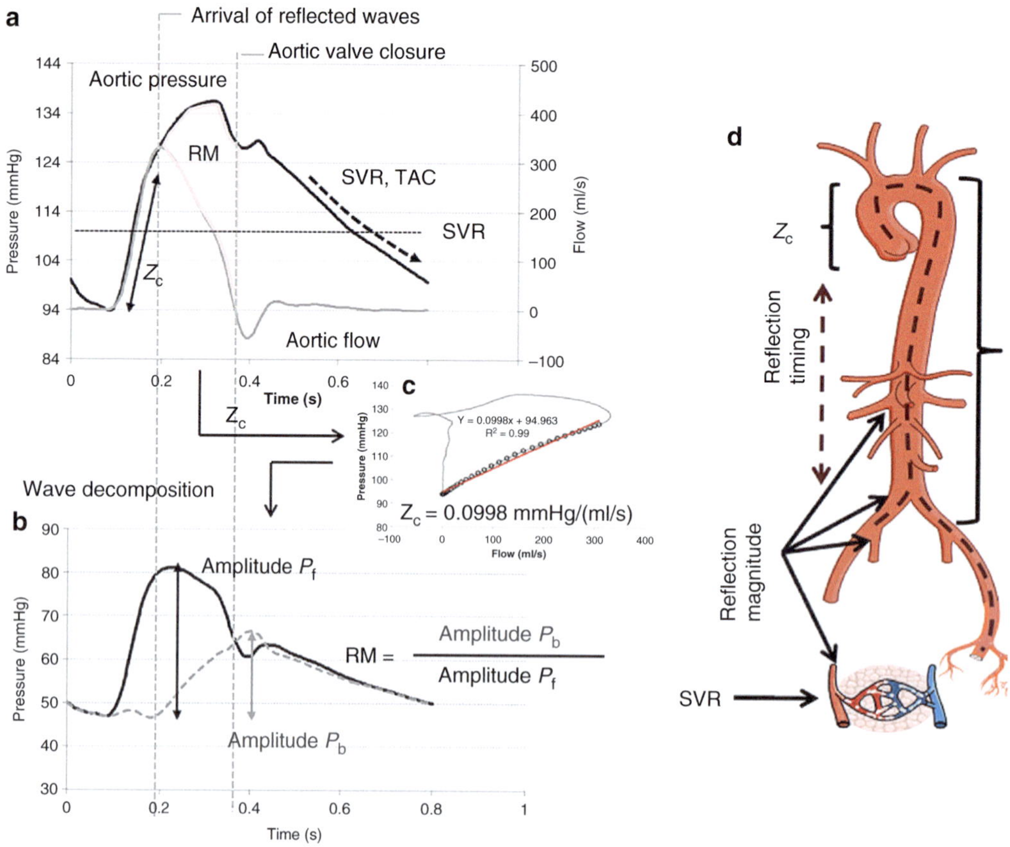

Fig. 4.2 Panel (**a**) Noninvasively acquired carotid pressure and aortic flow waveform, aligned in time. During the early systolic upstroke, in the absence of reflected waves, the pressure and flow waveform are similar in shape, and their ratio determines the characteristic impedance Z_c. When reflected waves kick in, the wave shapes start to deviate, with reflecting generally increasing pressure and decreasing flow. The diastolic pressure decay is determined by the systemic vascular resistance (*SVR*) and total arterial compliance (*TAC*), while SVR also determines the absolute pressure level. Panel (**b**) The result of decomposition of the pressure wave into its forward and backward component. The ratio of their amplitudes is the reflection magnitude (*RM*). Panel (**c**) The computation of RM requires Z_c, which can be estimated from the slope of the linear part of the pressure-flow loop, corresponding to the pressure and flow data prior to the arrival of reflected waves. Panel (**d**) Schematic "anatomical" indication of the components of afterload

largely on the peripheral resistance, which in turn depends on arteriolar caliber, the total number of arterioles that are present "in parallel" and blood viscosity [14, 17]. It can therefore be affected by arteriolar tone, arteriolar remodeling, microvascular rarefaction, and changes in blood viscosity. Pulsatile LV afterload is, in contrast, predominantly influenced by the properties of larger vessels. Although pulsatile LV afterload is fairly complex and cannot be expressed as a single numeric measure, key indices of pulsatile LV afterload can be quantified and summarized using relatively simple principles and mechanical models of the systemic circulation, using time-resolved proximal aortic pressure and flow.

Time-varying aortic pressure and flow can be assessed invasively or noninvasively (Fig. 4.2, panel a). Noninvasive assessments of central pressure can be achieved using high-fidelity applanation arterial tonometry at the carotid or subclavian [18] artery [14]. Aortic flow can also be measured noninvasively, using pulsed wave Doppler echocardiography [19–21] or phase-contrast magnetic resonance imaging [22]. The most convenient method to assess aortic inflow is pulsed wave Doppler interrogation of the LV outflow tract, given that systolic LV volume outflow equals proximal aortic volume inflow [21].

LV afterload can be assessed in the frequency domain from the aortic input impedance spectrum (calculated from the harmonic components of central aortic pressure and flow waves) or estimated in the time domain [14, 23–26]. Input impedance is the "summed" mechanical load imposed by all vessels *downstream a particular point* (and which can be fully assessed by measuring time-varying flow and pressure at that particular point) [14, 15, 21, 24]. Therefore, "aortic input impedance" represents the summed mechanical load impeding LV ejection. It should be noted that aortic input impedance is not exclusively determined by aortic properties, but depends on the properties of the entire arterial system.

Key parameters of pulsatile LV load include the characteristic impedance of the proximal aorta (Z_c), the magnitude and timing of wave reflections, and the total compliance of the arterial tree ("total arterial compliance"). The *characteristic* impedance of an artery can be intuitively measured as the slope of the pulsatile pressure-flow relation (where pressure and flow are measured in the same point within the artery) *in the absence of reflected waves*. Aortic Z_c can thus be computed in the time domain using the slope of the pressure change over flow change in early systole, before the arrival of wave reflections to the proximal aorta (Fig. 4.2, panel c). Z_c is a "local" arterial property (note the difference with *input* impedance); consequently, Z_c measured using proximal aortic pressure and flow represents proximal aortic Z_c. Physically, Z_c reflects the balance between inertial and capacitive effects in the aorta upon cardiac ejection. In a rigid and/or narrowed aorta, blood cannot be stored locally, and blood needs to be accelerated instantaneously throughout the complete aorta, leading to high characteristic impedance. In a wide and/or distensible aorta, blood is stored locally due to the windkessel effect, and acceleration of blood takes place over much shorter lengths and is dampened in time, reducing inertial effects and characteristic impedance.

Wave reflections are usually assessed via *wave separation analysis*, based on the principle that reflected waves, by virtue of adding to pressure and subtracting from forward flow, distort the linear relationship between pulsatile pressure and flow that is seen in early systole (as a result of the forward wave generated by ventricular contraction), when such relationship is governed purely by ascending aortic Z_c (Fig. 4.2, panel b). The ratio of the amplitude of the backward (reflected) and forward wave yields the reflection magnitude (RM).

Making abstraction of wave travel and reflection, one can also consider the arterial tree as a condensed windkessel-like system, of which the "total arterial compliance" (TAC) can be computed using windkessel models of the arterial tree. Frank proposed the original windkessel model as a resistance and compliance (C) pair (2-element windkessel), representing small vessel resistance and large artery compliance. The 3-element windkessel model additionally accounts for aortic characteristic impedance (Z_c) in order to better capture the behavior of the arterial tree for the higher frequency range and to isolate the "slow" effects of compliance in diastole from the "rapid" effects associated with wave dynamics during cardiac ejection [26]. This model, originally proposed by Westerhof et al., can be considered the standard windkessel model for the systemic circulation, although refinements have been proposed by Westerhof [27], as well as several other investigators (see Ref. [13] for review).

Determinants of Pulsatile Arterial Load

The geometric and mechanical properties of the various arterial segments have complex effects on ventricular afterload; through their effects on the early aortic systolic pressure rise, the total compliance of the arterial system and the velocity at which the pulse waves travel forward in the arteries and reflected waves originate and travel backward toward the heart [25, 28]. In early systole, a high proximal aortic characteristic impedance (Z_c) due to a stiff wall, a small aortic diameter, or both increases the amount of pulsatile pressure for any given pulsatile flow [11–14]. The time of arrival of the reflected wave to the proximal aorta depends on the location of reflection sites and on the pulse wave velocity (PWV) of conduit vessels, particularly the aorta, which transmits both the forward and backward traveling waves [12, 14]. Aortic PWV is directly related to the stiffness of the aortic wall (square root of elastic modulus) and inversely proportional to the square root of aortic diameter [12, 14, 29]. Stiffer aortas thus conduct the forward and backward traveling waves at greater velocity and therefore promote an earlier arrival of the reflected wave for any given distance to reflection sites. The distance to the reflection sites is strongly dependent on body height. In the presence of normal LV systolic function, typical effects of the reflected wave on the aortic pressure waveform include a mid-to-late systolic shoulder which determines an increase in peak (systolic) aortic pressure (and pulse pressure) and the area under the pressure curve during systole [14]. When LV systolic function is depressed, however, the reflected wave may induce a reduction on late systolic flow with less prominent effects of pressure augmentation.

The total arterial compliance depends on the summed compliance of the various arterial segments. The compliance of individual vessels is (linearly) proportional to vessel volume (or radius [3]) and, for any given "relative" vessel geometry (wall volume/lumen volume ratio), (linearly and) inversely proportional to wall stiffness (Young's elastic modulus). The interaction between the stiffness and geometry of large and muscular arteries also impacts the magnitude and location of reflection sites. Reflected waves that arrive during LV ejection increase the mid-to-late systolic workload of the LV. Figure 4.2, panel d, illustrates the different components of LV afterload.

A Time-Domain Approach to Ventricular-Arterial Coupling: Time-Varying Myocardial Stress

Pressure-flow analyses thoroughly characterize the interactions between the LV (treated as a hydraulic pump) and the arterial system and provide important indices of arterial load and cardiac function. Various indices of LV afterload are useful because they are meant to be purely reflective of arterial properties [14]. However, arterial load should always be interpreted by considering interactions between arteries and the LV as a pump [14, 30] and also between myocardial elements and instantaneous LV geometry and the time-varying load imposed by the systemic circulation. The generation of pressurized blood flow by the LV can be conceptually represented by a 2-step energy transfer process: first from the contractile elements of the myocardium into the LV chamber and second from the LV chamber to the systemic circulation. However, this process is bidirectional, such that the systemic circulation can also impact the myocardial contractile elements. Wall stress represents the time-varying mechanical load experienced by the contractile elements in the myocardium (myocardial afterload) and is related to the amount of force and work the muscle does during a contraction.

Whereas wall stress has been recognized as a key index of myocardial load, until recently, it was assessed only in end-systole, in analogy to the LV elastance, which reaches a peak in end-systole. However, derivations of Laplace's law indicate that the progressive geometric changes that accompany the ejection of blood from the LV into the arteries will be associated with important changes in wall stress, favoring a reduction of wall stress in late systole. This motivated the development of methods to assess time-resolved myocardial wall stress [31, 32]. There are several methods to estimate wall stress using LV geometric and LV pressure measurements. A particularly useful formula, applicable to axisymmetric ventricles for computation of average LV myocardial fiber stress, was developed by Arts et al. [31] and may be used for calculating time-resolved ejection-phase fiber stress using a central pressure waveform (given that in the absence of aortic stenosis, central arterial pressure is very similar to ventricular pressure) and time-resolved LV geometric information (derived from 2D echocardiography, 3D echocardiography, or magnetic resonance imaging) [25, 31–34]. This method, illustrated in Fig. 4.3, does not neglect radially directed forces or forces generated within the wall that oppose fiber shortening, which vary significantly with cavity and wall

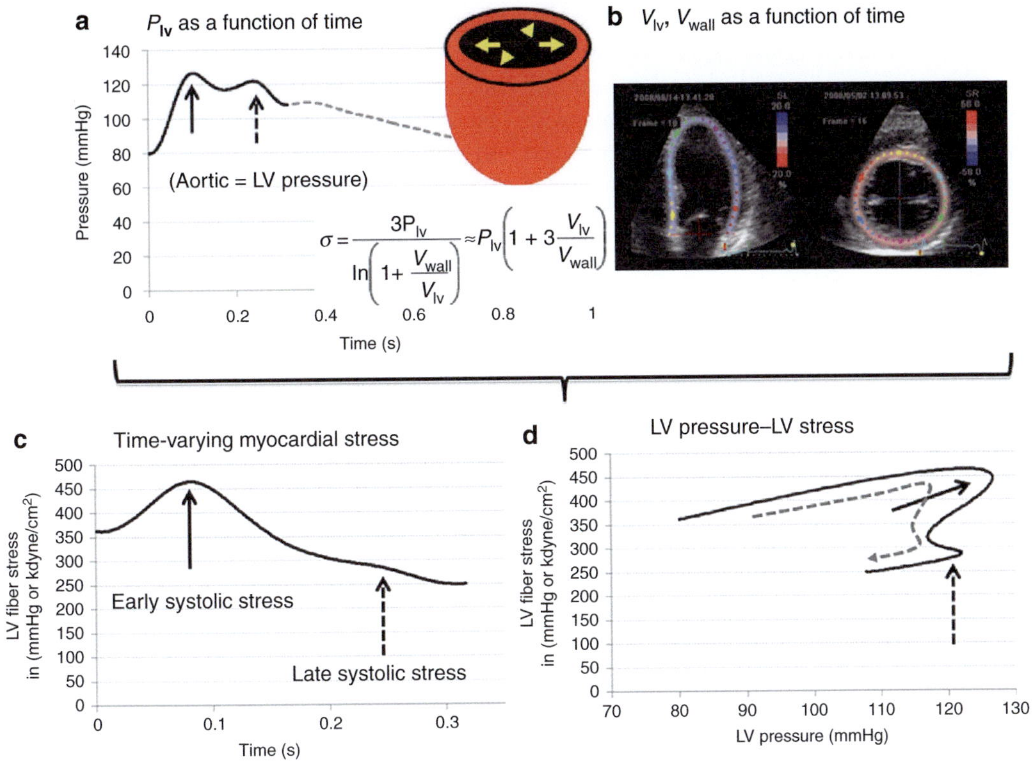

Fig. 4.3 Panel (**a**) Assuming identical aortic and left ventricular pressures during systole, LV pressure can be obtained from a noninvasively measured pressure waveform. Panel (**b**) Combined with time-varying geometric information, which can be measured with ultrasound or MRI, time-varying myocardial stress can be calculated using the formula provided by Arts et al. [31]. Panel (**c**) Time-varying myocardial stress, peaking in early systole. The second pressure peak in late systole does not lead to a high end-systolic stress. Panel (**d**) LV fiber stress plotted as a function of LV pressure, clearly demonstrating the "shift" in stress throughout ejection

thickness and can interfere with direct comparisons of myocardial fiber stress at different times during ejection. The formula is based on LV cavity volume (V_{lv}), LV wall volume (V_{wall}), and pressure:

$$\text{Fiber}\sigma = \frac{P}{\frac{1}{3}\ln\left(1+\frac{V_{\mathrm{wall}}}{V_{\mathrm{lv}}}\right)}$$

It is important to recognize the advantages of assessing time-resolved ejection-phase LV wall stress as opposed to end-systolic wall stress. Throughout systole, myocardial fiber activation results in the development of tension (stress) and shortening of myocardial segments, which results in progressive ejection of blood from the LV cavity and wall thickening. During *early* ejection, active development of fiber crossbridges occurs in the electrically activated myocardium, and peak myocardial wall stress occurs [32], at a time when systolic pressure coexists with quasi-diastolic geometry (relatively thin wall and relatively large cavity) (Fig. 4.3, panel c). Myocardial fiber shortening and ejection of blood determine a progressive change in LV geometry, which causes a drop in myocardial stress (despite rising pressure) during mid-to-late systole. This can be quantified as a clear "shift" in the pressure-stress relation (Fig. 4.3, panel d) and appears to be favorable for the myocardium to handle the additional load imposed by systolic wave reflections, which are "universal" in adults. This shift, however, may be insufficient and/or compromised in the setting of wave reflections of early onset or large magnitude [34–36] and in the presence of a depressed LV ejection fraction [32, 35]. A time-resolved wall stress curve also allows for characterization of the *myocardial* loading sequence, which can be expressed as a ratio of the stress-time integral in late vs. early systole. We note that stress as calculated here encompasses both the active stress generated by active mechanisms in the muscle fibers as well as passively induced stresses in both the cellular and extracellular matrix components of the ventricle.

Determinants of Time-Varying Myocardial Stress: Impact of Wave Reflections

In addition to the well-known role of chronic ventricular geometric changes as determinants of wall stress, as expected from physiologic principles, various arterial properties affect time-varying myocardial wall stress for any given end-diastolic LV geometry [34]. Systemic vascular resistance is a very important determinant of wall stress throughout systole. Z_c selectively affects early systolic and peak systolic wall stress, whereas wave reflections and total arterial compliance impact myocardial stress in mid and late systole and significantly influence the area under the stress curve generated for any given flow output [34]. Interestingly, women seem to demonstrate greater peak and end-systolic wall stress as well as a higher ejection-phase stress-time integral, even after adjustment for arterial properties, which might relate to the differential susceptibility of women to heart failure [34].

Importance of Late Systolic Load: Animal, Epidemiologic, and Clinical Studies of Wave Reflections, Myocardial Function, and Heart Failure Risk

Late Systolic Loading from Wave Reflections Leads to LV Hypertrophy

For any given level of systolic (peak) blood pressure, prominent late systolic loading has been unequivocally demonstrated to exert deleterious effects on LV structure and function in animal models and has been associated with LV hypertrophy in humans [14, 37, 38]. Kobayashi et al. [37] used a Wistar rat model and performed constriction of either the ascending aorta or suprarenal abdominal aorta. Analysis of aortic input impedance demonstrated that constriction of the ascending aorta increased LV load in early systole, whereas constriction of the descending aorta caused prominent late systolic loading from a reflected wave that originated at the distal aortic constriction site, arriving at the heart in late systole [37]. LV pressure profiles induced by proximal aortic constriction demonstrated an early systolic peak, whereas descending aortic constriction induced late systolic peaks. Despite an identical peak LV pressure in rats that underwent ascending vs. descending aortic constriction, rats that underwent descending aortic banding (and were thus exposed to greater late systolic load) demonstrated much greater LV hypertrophy than those undergoing ascending aortic banding (which were exposed to increased early systolic load). Rats that underwent descending aortic banding also demonstrated a greater amount of myocardial fibrosis [37].

These animal causal findings are strongly supported by observational human data. Hashimoto et al. [39] assessed changes in wave reflection magnitude occurring during antihypertensive therapy and observed that the reduction in wave reflections predicted regression of LV mass independently of blood pressure reduction. The association between reflected wave magnitude reduction and LV mass (i.e., hypertrophy) reduction was also independent of age, sex, and use of renin-angiotensin system inhibitors ($\beta=0.41$, $P=0.001$). The correlation was particularly strong in patients with LV hypertrophy at baseline ($R=0.61$; $P<0.001$). Of note, despite the fact that standard antihypertensive therapies reduce wave reflections in some patients, the change is highly unpredictable, with reflection magnitude actually increasing in some subjects in Hashimoto's study, despite blood pressure reduction.

Late Systolic Load Promotes Diastolic Dysfunction

Gillebert et al. [38] used a canine model to study the effect of the *timing* of systolic load on LV relaxation by inflating balloons in the ascending

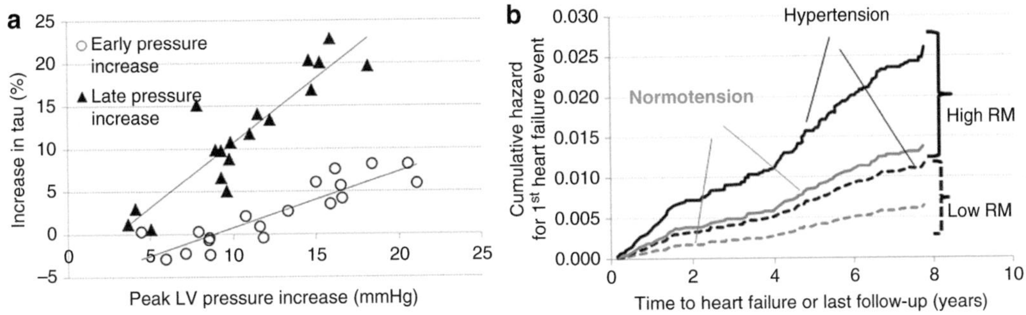

Fig. 4.4 Panel (**a**) Impact of timing of afterload on the time constant of LV relaxation (tau). Late pressure increase has a much more pronounced effect on LV relaxation than an increase in early systole (Modified from Gillebert et al. [38]). Panel (**b**) Impact of reflection magnitude (*RM*) on hazard of heart failure (Modified from Chirinos et al. [47])

aorta during either early vs. late systole. Their study demonstrated that for a given increase in peak (systolic) LV pressure, late systolic inflation (triangles in Fig. 4.4a) prolonged *tau* (i.e., impaired LV relaxation assessed with the gold standard measure) much more than early systolic inflation (circles in Fig. 4.4a), demonstrating a cause-effect relationship between late systolic load and diastolic dysfunction [38].

In support of these causal findings, wave reflections have been independently linked to diastolic dysfunction in human clinical cohorts [40, 41]. Borlaug et al. demonstrated that late systolic load (assessed with the late systolic pressure-time integral) was associated with lower early diastolic mitral annular tissue velocities (a marker of diastolic function) among 48 hypertensive and normotensive subjects [42]. Ikonomidis showed that augmentation index was independently associated with diastolic dysfunction among 143 hypertensive patients [43]. Weber et al. [41] studied 336 patients undergoing coronary angiography and showed that augmentation index and augmented pressure (which are influenced by wave reflections) were associated with lower peak mitral annular systolic velocity, early diastolic velocity, and higher LV filling pressures.

Recently, we used time-resolved stress curves to separate early and late systolic wall stress (i.e., early vs. late myocardial systolic load), which can be quantified as the area under the time-resolved stress curve (stress-time integral, STI) in the first and second halves of ejection, respectively, among [33, 34] middle-aged adults enrolled in the population-based Asklepios study in Belgium [32, 34, 44–46]. We assessed the relationship between the myocardial loading sequence (early vs. late wall stress) and diastolic function [33]. After adjustment for multiple confounders, late systolic load was independently associated with lower mitral annular relaxation velocities, in sharp contrast to early systolic load which was associated with higher mitral annular relaxation velocities, in a multivariate model, implicating the loading sequence as an independent correlate of myocardial relaxation in humans. This model explained 46 % of the variability in mitral annular diastolic (relaxation) velocity.

The Magnitude of Wave Reflections Strongly Predicts New-Onset Heart Failure in the General Population

Based on the data presented above, we hypothesized that wave reflections independently predict the risk of new-onset heart failure (HF) in the general population. To test this hypothesis, we derived aortic pressure waveforms using a transfer function applied to the radial waveform recorded at baseline with arterial tonometry from 5,934 participants in the Multiethnic Study of Atherosclerosis (MESA), who were free of clinically apparent cardiovascular disease. The central pressure waveform was used to assess reflection magnitude [35, 47]. During 7.61 years of follow-up (and after adjustment for systolic and diastolic blood pressure, age, gender, body mass index, diabetes, ethnicity, antihypertensive medication use, total and HDL cholesterol, current smoking, heart rate, and glomerular filtration rate), reflection magnitude strongly predicted HF (hazard ratio per 10 % – increase = 2.69; 95 % CI = 1.79–4.04; $P < 0.0001$) and was a stronger predictor than blood pressure and all other modifiable risk factors listed above.

When we stratified the population based on the presence or absence of hypertension and the presence or absence of high reflection magnitude (Fig. 4.4b), we found that, compared to non-hypertensive subjects with low reflection magnitude (lowest risk category), hazard ratios for hypertensive subjects with low reflection magnitude, non-hypertensive subjects with high reflection magnitude, and hypertensive subjects with high reflection magnitude were 1.81 (95 % CI = 0.85–3.86), 2.16 (95 % CI = 1.04–4.43), and 3.98 (95 % CI = 1.96–8.05), respectively. We also assessed the incremental information provided when various predictors were added to a model containing all other predictors of heart failure, in terms of discrimination (integrated discrimination improvement) and reclassification (net reclassification improvement). Reflection magnitude was associated with the largest Wald statistic of all predictors (including age), the greatest reduction in Akaike's information and Bayesian information criteria (indicating improvement in model fit) and the greatest increases in integrated discrimination improvement (with a 48 % increase in discrimination slope achieved when reflection magnitude was added to a base model containing all other predictors of HF and multiple confounders). With the exception of age, a non-modifiable risk factor, reflection magnitude was associated with the greatest net reclassification improvement for prediction of HF. Therefore, reflection magnitude was a strong predictor of incident HF after adjustment for other known predictors. These findings from a large community-based sample with careful follow-up and event adjudication implicate arterial wave reflections as a novel strong risk factor for HF, thus strongly supporting animal and human mechanistic findings from previous studies and demonstrating the relevance of wave reflections in humans. Based on the strength and biologic plausibility of this association, a high reflection magnitude has been proposed to represent a novel form of stage B HF [35].

The Reflected Wave in Established HF

Early invasive studies demonstrated enhanced wave reflections in patients with systolic HF compared to normal control subjects, with an impaired reduction of wave reflections during exercise [48, 49]. More recently, wave reflections assessed noninvasively have been reported to be increased in patients with established systolic HF and heart failure with preserved ejection fraction (HFpEF). Curtis et al. reported increased wave reflections (assessed via wave intensity analysis) among 67 patients with systolic HF [50]. Recently, Weber et al. demonstrated that a high reflected wave is a good index to identify patients with HFpEF among individuals presenting with dyspnea [51]. Importantly, Sung et al. reported that, among 120 patients hospitalized due to decompensated HF (~56 % with systolic heart failure and 44 % with HFpEF), reflected wave amplitude, but not carotid-femoral pulse wave velocity, was an independent predictor of rehospitalization for HF, all-cause death, nonfatal myocardial infarction and stroke, after adjustment for age, estimated glomerular filtration rate, hemoglobin, and NT-proBNP levels [52].

Where Do Wave Reflections Originate?

Wave reflections arise at any point of impedance mismatch, impedance being here the local characteristic impedance at a given point in the arterial tree. As previously mentioned, it is virtually impossible to unequivocally pinpoint the source(s) of wave reflections. Inspired by the nature of the input impedance and the concept of the "effective length" of the arterial tree [53], researchers attempted to identify "the" dominant reflection site(s) of the arterial tree. The aortoiliac bifurcation [54–57], diaphragm level (and branches toward renal arteries and gastrointestinal organs) [55, 58], and head and upper extremities [57] have been proposed as candidate discrete reflection sites. Nevertheless, the observed reflection patterns do not fully match these of a discrete number of reflection sites [54], suggesting the presence of diffuse reflections, originating all over the arterial tree [59, 60]. These diffuse reflections are due to the branching pattern of the aorta, the effect of geometric and mechanical tapering (leading to a continuous change in local characteristic impedance [61]) but most certainly also due to the resistance vessels, where impedance rapidly increases over very short distances (also leading to an abrupt drop in mean arterial pressure). The presence of reflections close to the heart also seems to obscure reflections arising from further down in the arterial tree, creating sort of a "horizon effect" [62].

It is clear that wave reflections are complex, and this complexity should be considered and taken into account when interpreting hemodynamic data. The paradigm of the arterial tree as a single uniform tube with a discrete reflection occurring at a fixed length is certainly too simple an approach, giving rise to controversies [63–65]. What is also clear is that the sources of wave reflections are not to be sought only distally in the arterial tree, but also closer to the heart. It is well known that wave reflection can be modulated pharmacologically, where the administration of nitroglycerin (NTG) clearly leads to a reduction in wave reflections [66]. NTG is thought to act on peripheral muscular vessels [67]. However, it is possible that NTG also affects vessels closer to the heart. Abdominal organs are relatively close to the heart, and their perfusion is regulated by vasoactive mechanisms. As such, the impact of NTG on wave reflections may be related to vasodilation of splanchnic vessels, as also suggested by Karamanoglu et al. [58]. It is not clear whether there is also an effect on the arterial tone of larger vessels such as the abdominal aorta. We refer to Chap. 40 of this book for an in-depth discussion on the effect of organic nitrates.

Conclusions and Future Directions

Advances in the noninvasive assessment of pressure-flow relations and noninvasive cardiac imaging now allow for a comprehensive noninvasive assessment of ventricular-arterial interactions/coupling and should be more widely applied in clinical research. In particular, whereas analyses of ventricular-arterial coupling in the pressure-volume plane provide a simple, intuitive, and useful framework, it provides limited information, and other comprehensive noninvasive hemodynamic assessments should be more widely applied in human studies. Given the importance of LV afterload and its impact on the heart, afterload should be carefully considered or ruled out as a potential mediator or confounder in a wide variety of observed relationships or therapeutic and adverse effects of interventions related to LV remodeling, LV function, or vasoactive interventions.

Modeling approaches for pressure, flow, and geometric data are likely to continue to evolve, allowing for a more accurate assessment of hemodynamic patterns and their effects on cardiac load and function. This should lead to a better and generally accepted quantification and understanding of wave reflections, their origin, and their role in the pathophysiology of cardiovascular diseases. Carefully designed randomized clinical trials in the next decade may allow these insights to be used in the management of patients at risk for, or those with established, cardiovascular disease.

References

1. Sunagawa K, Maughan WL, Burkhoff D, Sagawa K. Left ventricular interaction with arterial load studied in isolated canine ventricle. Am J Physiol. 1983;245:H773–80.
2. Suga H, Sagawa K. Instantaneous pressure-volume relationships and their ratio in the excised, supported canine left ventricle. Circ Res. 1974;35:117–26.
3. Kelly RP, Ting CT, Yang TM, Liu CP, Maughan WL, Chang MS, Kass DA. Effective arterial elastance as index of arterial vascular load in humans. Circulation. 1992;86:513–21.
4. Burkhoff D, Sagawa K. Ventricular efficiency predicted by an analytical model. Am J Physiol. 1986;250:R1021–7.

5. Suga H, Hayashi T, Shirahata M. Ventricular systolic pressure-volume area as predictor of cardiac oxygen consumption. Am J Physiol. 1981;240:H39–44.
6. Chen CH, Nakayama M, Nevo E, Fetics BJ, Maughan WL, Kass DA. Coupled systolic-ventricular and vascular stiffening with age: implications for pressure regulation and cardiac reserve in the elderly. J Am Coll Cardiol. 1998;32:1221–7.
7. Ishihara H, Yokota M, Sobue T, Saito H. Relation between ventriculoarterial coupling and myocardial energetics in patients with idiopathic dilated cardiomyopathy. J Am Coll Cardiol. 1994;23:406–16.
8. Sasayama S, Asanoi H. Coupling between the heart and arterial system in heart failure. Am J Med. 1991;90:14S–8.
9. van der Velde ET, Burkhoff D, Steendijk P, Karsdon J, Sagawa K, Baan J. Nonlinearity and load sensitivity of end-systolic pressure-volume relation of canine left ventricle in vivo. Circulation. 1991;83:315–27.
10. Segers P, Stergiopulos N, Westerhof N. Relation of effective arterial elastance to arterial system properties. Am J Physiol Heart Circ Physiol. 2002;282:H1041–6.
11. Segers P, Stergiopulos N, Westerhof N. Quantification of the contribution of cardiac and arterial remodeling to hypertension. Hypertension. 2000;36:760–5.
12. Mitchell GF. Arterial stiffness and wave reflection in hypertension: pathophysiologic and therapeutic implications. Curr Hypertens Rep. 2004;6:436–41.
13. Westerhof N, Lankhaar JW, Westerhof BE. The arterial windkessel. Med Biol Eng Comput. 2009;47:131–41.
14. Nichols WW, O'Rourke MF, Vlachopolous C. Mcdonald's blood flow in arteries. Theoretical, experimental and clinical principles. London: Hodder Arnold; 2011.
15. Segers P, Verdonck P. Principles of vascular physiology. In: Lanzer P, Topol E, editors. Panvascular medicine: integrated clinical management. Berlin/Heidelberg: Springer; 2002.
16. O'Rourke MF, Safar ME. Relationship between aortic stiffening and microvascular disease in brain and kidney: cause and logic of therapy. Hypertension. 2005;46:200–4.
17. Ooi H, Chung W, Biolo A. Arterial stiffness and vascular load in heart failure. Congest Heart Fail. 2008;14:31–6.
18. Aakhus S, Soerlie C, Faanes A, Hauger SO, Bjoernstad K, Hatle L, Angelsen BA. Noninvasive computerized assessment of left ventricular performance and systemic hemodynamics by study of aortic root pressure and flow estimates in healthy men, and men with acute and healed myocardial infarction. Am J Cardiol. 1993;72:260–7.
19. Mitchell GF, Lacourciere Y, Arnold JM, Dunlap ME, Conlin PR, Izzo Jr JL. Changes in aortic stiffness and augmentation index after acute converting enzyme or vasopeptidase inhibition. Hypertension. 2005;46:1111–7.
20. Mitchell GF, Lacourciere Y, Ouellet JP, Izzo Jr JL, Neutel J, Kerwin LJ, Block AJ, Pfeffer MA. Determinants of elevated pulse pressure in middle-aged and older subjects with uncomplicated systolic hypertension: the role of proximal aortic diameter and the aortic pressure-flow relationship. Circulation. 2003;108:1592–8.
21. Segers P, Rietzschel ER, De Buyzere ML, Vermeersch SJ, De Bacquer D, Van Bortel LM, De Backer G, Gillebert TC, Verdonck PR. Noninvasive (input) impedance, pulse wave velocity, and wave reflection in healthy middle-aged men and women. Hypertension. 2007;49:1248–55.
22. Gatehouse PD, Keegan J, Crowe LA, Masood S, Mohiaddin RH, Kreitner KF, Firmin DN. Applications of phase-contrast flow and velocity imaging in cardiovascular mri. Eur Radiol. 2005;15:2172–84.
23. Kass DA. Ventricular arterial stiffening: integrating the pathophysiology. Hypertension. 2005;46:185–93.
24. Mitchell GF. Clinical achievements of impedance analysis. Med Biol Eng Comput. 2009;47:153–63.
25. Chirinos JA, Segers P. Noninvasive evaluation of left ventricular afterload: part 2: arterial pressure-flow and pressure-volume relations in humans. Hypertension. 2010;56:563–70.
26. Segers P, Rietzschel ER, De Buyzere ML, Stergiopulos N, Westerhof N, Van Bortel LM, Gillebert T, Verdonck PR. Three- and four-element windkessel models: assessment of their fitting performance in a large cohort of healthy middle-aged individuals. Proc Inst Mech Eng H. 2008;222:417–28.
27. Stergiopulos N, Westerhof BE, Westerhof N. Total arterial inertance as the fourth element of the windkessel model. Am J Physiol. 1999;276:H81–8.
28. Chirinos JA, Segers P. Noninvasive evaluation of left ventricular afterload: part 1: pressure and flow measurements and basic principles of wave conduction and reflection. Hypertension. 2010;56:555–62.
29. Chirinos JA. Arterial stiffness: basic concepts and measurement techniques. J Cardiovasc Transl Res. 2012;5:243–55.
30. Kawaguchi M, Hay I, Fetics B, Kass DA. Combined ventricular systolic and arterial stiffening in patients with heart failure and preserved ejection fraction: implications for systolic and diastolic reserve limitations. Circulation. 2003;107:714–20.
31. Arts T, Bovendeerd PH, Prinzen FW, Reneman RS. Relation between left ventricular cavity pressure and volume and systolic fiber stress and strain in the wall. Biophys J. 1991;59:93–102.
32. Chirinos JA, Segers P, Gupta AK, Swillens A, Rietzschel ER, De Buyzere ML, Kirkpatrick JN, Gillebert TC, Wang Y, Keane MG, Townsend R, Ferrari VA, Wiegers SE, St John Sutton M. Time-varying myocardial stress and systolic pressure-stress relationship: role in myocardial-arterial coupling in hypertension. Circulation. 2009;119:2798–807.
33. Chirinos JA, Segers P, Rietzschel ER, De Buyzere ML, Raja MW, Claessens T, De Bacquer D, St John Sutton M, Gillebert T, Asklepios Investigators. Early and late systolic wall stress differentially relate to myocardial contraction and relaxation in middle-aged adults. The asklepios study. Hypertension. 2013;61:296–303.

34. Chirinos JA, Segers P, Gillebert TC, Gupta AK, De Buyzere ML, De Bacquer D, St John-Sutton M, Rietzschel ER. Arterial properties as determinants of time-varying myocardial stress in humans. Hypertension. 2012;60:64–70.
35. Shah SJ, Wasserstrom JA. Increased arterial wave reflection magnitude: a novel form of stage b heart failure? J Am Coll Cardiol. 2012;60:2178–81.
36. Chowienczyk P, Shah A. Myocardial wall stress: from hypertension to heart tension. Hypertension. 2012;60:10–1.
37. Kobayashi S, Yano M, Kohno M, Obayashi M, Hisamatsu Y, Ryoke T, Ohkusa T, Yamakawa K, Matsuzaki M. Influence of aortic impedance on the development of pressure-overload left ventricular hypertrophy in rats. Circulation. 1996;94:3362–8.
38. Gillebert TC, Lew WY. Influence of systolic pressure profile on rate of left ventricular pressure fall. Am J Physiol. 1991;261:H805–13.
39. Hashimoto J, Westerhof BE, Westerhof N, Imai Y, O'Rourke MF. Different role of wave reflection magnitude and timing on left ventricular mass reduction during antihypertensive treatment. J Hypertens. 2008;26:1017–24.
40. Fukuta H, Ohte N, Wakami K, Asada K, Goto T, Mukai S, Tani T, Kimura G. Impact of arterial load on left ventricular diastolic function in patients undergoing cardiac catheterization for coronary artery disease. Circ J. 2010;74:1900–5.
41. Weber T, O'Rourke MF, Ammer M, Kvas E, Punzengruber C, Eber B. Arterial stiffness and arterial wave reflections are associated with systolic and diastolic function in patients with normal ejection fraction. Am J Hypertens. 2008;21:1194–202.
42. Borlaug BA, Melenovsky V, Redfield MM, Kessler K, Chang HJ, Abraham TP, Kass DA. Impact of arterial load and loading sequence on left ventricular tissue velocities in humans. J Am Coll Cardiol. 2007;50:1570–7.
43. Ikonomidis I, Tzortzis S, Papaioannou T, Protogerou A, Stamatelopoulos K, Papamichael C, Zakopoulos N, Lekakis J. Incremental value of arterial wave reflections in the determination of left ventricular diastolic dysfunction in untreated patients with essential hypertension. J Hum Hypertens. 2008;22:687–98.
44. Chirinos JA, Rietzschel ER, De Buyzere ML, De Bacquer D, Gillebert TC, Gupta AK, Segers P. Arterial load and ventricular-arterial coupling: physiologic relations with body size and effect of obesity. Hypertension. 2009;54:558–66.
45. Chirinos JA, Segers P, De Buyzere ML, Kronmal RA, Raja MW, De Bacquer D, Claessens T, Gillebert TC, St John-Sutton M, Rietzschel ER. Left ventricular mass: allometric scaling, normative values, effect of obesity, and prognostic performance. Hypertension. 2010;56:91–8.
46. Chirinos JA, Segers P, Rietzschel ER, De Buyzere ML, Raja MW, Claessens T, De Bacquer D, St John Sutton M, Gillebert TC. Early and late systolic wall stress differentially relate to myocardial contraction and relaxation in middle-aged adults: the asklepios study. Hypertension. 2013;61:296–303.
47. Chirinos JA, Kips JG, Jacobs Jr DR, Brumback L, Duprez DA, Kronmal R, Bluemke DA, Townsend RR, Vermeersch S, Segers P. Arterial wave reflections and incident cardiovascular events and heart failure: Mesa (multiethnic study of atherosclerosis). J Am Coll Cardiol. 2012;60:2170–7.
48. Laskey WK, Kussmaul WG. Arterial wave reflection in heart failure. Circulation. 1987;75:711–22.
49. Pepine CJ, Nichols WW, Conti CR. Aortic input impedance in heart failure. Circulation. 1978;58:460–5.
50. Curtis SL, Zambanini A, Mayet J, Mc GTSA, Foale R, Parker KH, Hughes AD. Reduced systolic wave generation and increased peripheral wave reflection in chronic heart failure. Am J Physiol Heart Circ Physiol. 2007;293:H557–62.
51. Weber T, Wassertheurer S, O'Rourke MF, Haiden A, Zweiker R, Rammer M, Hametner B, Eber B. Pulsatile hemodynamics in patients with exertional dyspnea: potentially of value in the diagnostic evaluation of suspected heart failure with preserved ejection fraction. J Am Coll Cardiol. 2013;61:1874–83.
52. Sung SH, Yu WC, Cheng HM, Lee CW, Lin MM, Chuang SY, Chen CH. Excessive wave reflections on admission predict post-discharge events in patients hospitalized due to acute heart failure. Eur J Heart Fail. 2012;14:1348–55.
53. Campbell KB, Lee LC, Frasch HF, Noordergraaf A. Pulse reflection sites and effective length of the arterial system. Am J Physiol. 1989;256:H1684–9.
54. Pythoud F, Stergiopulos N, Westerhof N, Meister JJ. Method for determining distribution of reflection sites in the arterial system. Am J Physiol. 1996;271:H1807–13.
55. Latham RD, Westerhof N, Sipkema P, Rubal BJ, Reuderink P, Murgo JP. Regional wave travel and reflections along the human aorta: a study with six simultaneous micromanometric pressures. Circulation. 1985;72:1257–69.
56. Murgo JP, Westerhof N, Giolma JP, Altobelli SA. Aortic input impedance in normal man: relationship to pressure wave forms. Circulation. 1980;62:105–16.
57. O'Rourke MF. Pressure and flow waves in systemic arteries and the anatomical design of the arterial system. J Appl Physiol. 1967;23:139–49.
58. Karamanoglu M, Gallagher DE, Avolio AP, O'Rourke MF. Functional origin of reflected pressure waves in a multibranched model of the human arterial system. Am J Physiol. 1994;267:H1681–8.
59. O'Rourke MF, Taylor MG. Input impedance of the systemic circulation. Circ Res. 1967;20:365–80.
60. Taylor MG. The input impedance of an assembly of randomly branching elastic tubes. Biophys J. 1966;6:29–51.
61. Segers P, Verdonck P. Role of tapering in aortic wave reflection: hydraulic and mathematical model study. J Biomech. 2000;33:299–306.

62. Davies JE, Alastruey J, Francis DP, Hadjiloizou N, Whinnett ZI, Manisty CH, Aguado-Sierra J, Willson K, Foale RA, Malik IS, Hughes AD, Parker KH, Mayet J. Attenuation of wave reflection by wave entrapment creates a "horizon effect" in the human aorta. Hypertension. 2012;60:778–85.
63. Segers P, Mynard J, Taelman L, Vermeersch S, Swillens A. Wave reflection: myth or reality? Artery Res. 2012;6:7–11.
64. Segers P, Kips J, Trachet B, Swillens A, Vermeersch S, Mahieu D, Rietzschel ER, De Buyzere M, Van Bortel L. Limitations and pitfalls of non-invasive measurement of arterial pressure wave reflections and pulse wave velocity. Artery Res. 2009;3:79–88.
65. Westerhof BE, Westerhof N. Magnitude and return time of the reflected wave: the effects of large artery stiffness and aortic geometry. J Hypertens. 2012;30:932–9.
66. Kelly RP, Gibbs HH, O'Rourke MF, Daley JE, Mang K, Morgan JJ, Avolio AP. Nitroglycerin has more favourable effects on left ventricular afterload than apparent from measurement of pressure in a peripheral artery. Eur Heart J. 1990;11:138–44.
67. Pauca AL, Kon ND, O'Rourke MF. Benefit of glyceryl trinitrate on arterial stiffness is directly due to effects on peripheral arteries. Heart. 2005;91:1428–32.

Determination of Systemic and Regional Arterial Structure and Function

5

Pierre Boutouyrie, Laurent Macron, Elie Mousseaux, and Stéphane Laurent

Abstract

Large artery stiffness can be measured through direct and indirect techniques. Measurement of pulse wave propagation is among the most direct techniques, either through pulse wave velocity or through artificial pressure wave propagation. Measurement of strain and stress through echotracking techniques gives also direct, hypothesis-free measurement of arterial stiffness. Other techniques are derived from models of circulation and can approximate arterial stiffness. Details about techniques, parameter definition, are given here to help researchers and practitioners to make the best choice of technique for their applications.

Keywords

Stiffness • Measurement • Distensibility • Compliance • Echotracking • Remodeling • Arteries

Arterial stiffness is a generic word covering the way an elastic artery can accommodate changes in blood pressure. This is a key function in physiology and pathology because elastic artery can relay the cardiac contraction during diastole (Fig. 5.1). There are two main techniques to measure arterial stiffness: direct or indirect from circulation models. Because the physical definition of stiffness (Hooke's law) is the relation between a force applied to a material and the deformation of this material, direct measurement of stiffness is only possible through the measurement of both parameters: force and deformation (Fig. 5.2). Arteries are cylindrical structures exposed to pressure. The force applied to the vessel is called stress, which is three dimensional in nature (longitudinal, radial, and circumferential). For the

P. Boutouyrie, MD, PhD (✉) • S. Laurent, MD, PhD
Department of Pharmacology and Institut National de la Santé et de la Recherche Médicale U970(Eq7)-PARCC, Hôpital Européen Georges Pompidou, Assistance Publique-Hôpitaux de Paris, Université Paris-Descartes, 20 rue Leblanc, Paris 75015, France
e-mail: pierre.boutouyrie@egp.aphp.fr; stephane.laurent@egp.aphp.fr

L. Macron, MD, PhD • E. Mousseaux, MD, PhD
Radiologie, HEGP, APHP, Inserm U970 Eq7, Université Paris Descartes, Paris, France

Radiology, Hopital Europeen Georges Pompidou, 20 rue Leblanc, Paris 75015, France
e-mail: laurent.macron@egp.aphp.fr; elie.moussseaux@egp.aphp.fr

M.E. Safar et al. (eds.), *Blood Pressure and Arterial Wall Mechanics in Cardiovascular Diseases*, DOI 10.1007/978-1-4471-5198-2_5, © Springer-Verlag London 2014

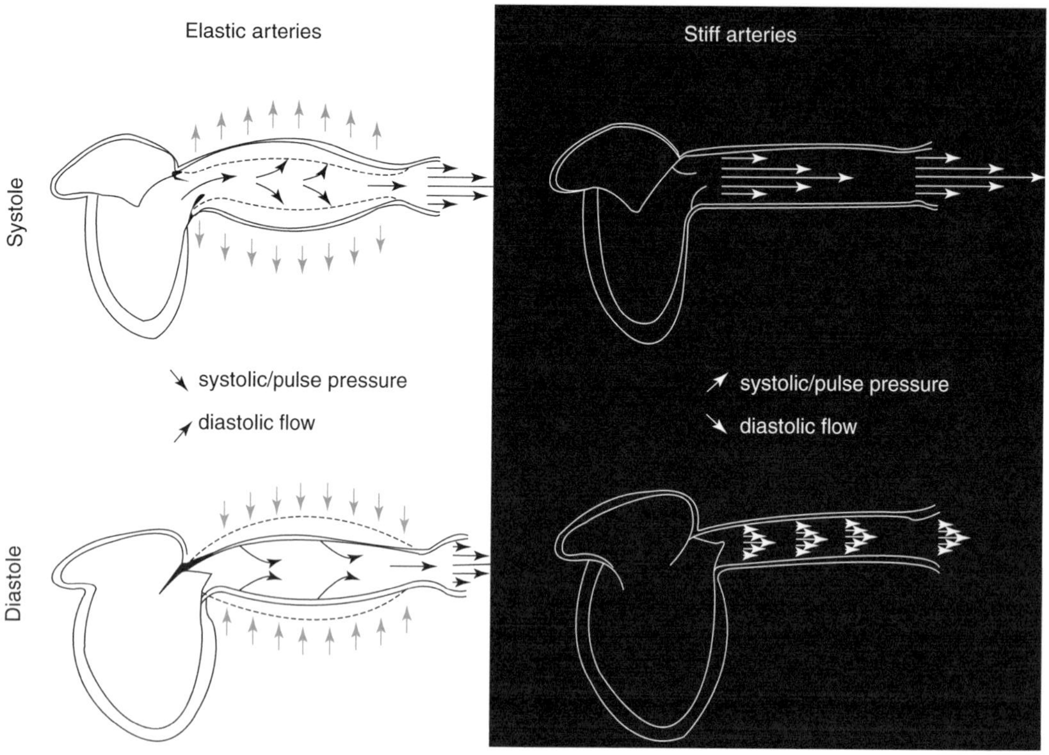

Fig. 5.1 Arterial elasticity and diastolic relay of cardiac contraction

sake of simplicity, circumferential wall stress is usually considered alone and it can only be approximated by the Lamé equation, although arteries are stretched longitudinally by 15–20 % under static conditions [1], and attempts to measure longitudinal stretch variations show significant variations clinically relevant [2]:

$$\sigma_\theta = \frac{P \times R}{h}$$

Because the Lamé equation says that stress is proportional to radius (R) and pressure (P) and inversely proportional to thickness (h), we can understand that it is impossible to interpret stiffness independently of arterial structure. The stress/strain relationship defines the stiffness of the wall material (Einc) (Fig. 5.2). Because the arterial structure is complex, involving smooth muscle cells, elastin, collagen, and many other macromolecules, the mechanical behavior of the arterial wall represents the summation of the individual components behavior, with added complexity due to the distribution of the components and their tridimensional relations [3–5]. Therefore, it is more the 3-D organization of components which can explain the mechanical properties of large arteries [6]. The pressure–diameter or stress–strain relationship is curvilinear; the artery is stiffer at high strain. This is generally associated with the composite nature of the arterial wall and the progressive recruitment of collagen fibers [5]. Whereas technical progress have been outstanding for measuring strain, through ultrasounds or MRI, measurement of stress is still hampered by imprecise noninvasive measurement of blood pressure and the necessity to measure precisely wall thickness. It is also limited by theoretical considerations on which structure in the wall is really carrying the mechanical stress [4]. It remains that the stress–strain relation is considered as the gold standard for assessing arterial stiffness.

Newton's second law of motion implies that the celerity of mechanical waves propagation

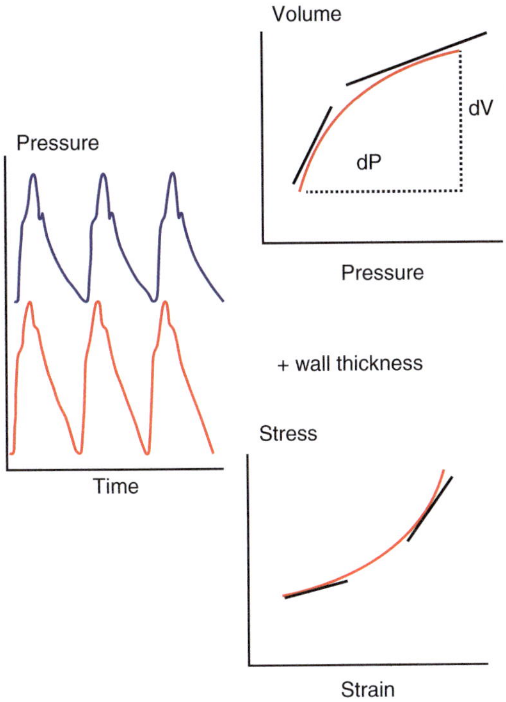

Distension	$Ds{-}Dd$
Stretch/Strain	$\varepsilon=\frac{\partial D}{D_0}\approx\frac{Ds-Dd}{Dd}$
Peterson's modulus	$E_P=\frac{PP\times Dd}{Ds-Dd}$
Compliance	$CC=\frac{\pi}{4}\frac{Ds^2-Dd^2}{PP}$
Distensibility	$DC=\frac{Ds^2-Dd^2}{Dd^2\times PP}$
Beta stiffness index	$\beta=\frac{Ds-Dd}{Dd\times\ln\left(\frac{SBP}{DBP}\right)}$
Circumferential wall stress	$\sigma=\frac{P\times R}{h}$
Young's elastic modulus	$E_{inc}=\frac{\sigma}{\varepsilon}\approx\frac{3}{DC}\left(1+\frac{LCSA}{WCSA}\right)$

Fig. 5.2 Pressure–diameter and stress–strain relationship: definition of main stiffness parameters

is proportional to its elastic modulus (i.e., stiffness). Moens and Korteweg [7, 8] have derived and simplified this relation into the famous equation

$$PWV=\sqrt{\frac{E_{inc}\cdot h}{2r\rho}}.$$

This equation has been further simplified by Bramwell and Hill [9]:

$$PWV=\sqrt{\frac{dP\cdot V}{\rho\cdot dV}}$$

It is noteworthy that PWV is directly related to characteristic impedance in a pure Windkessel model (Fig. 5.3). The relation between the speed of wave propagation and elastic modulus is also used by very modern techniques such as ultrafast imaging [10].

Direct Measurement of Arterial Stiffness

Pulse wave velocity (PWV) is the most widely used technique that Bramwell and Hill introduced to physiology in 1922 [9]. Briefly, a pressure wave's propagation speed in a solid is proportional to its stiffness. If expressed through the elastic modulus (E_{inc}), PWV can be expressed as PWV = $K\times E^{0.5}$, where K reflects tissue density. Thus, when measuring the pressure wave at different sites along an arterial segment or along the arterial tree (dL), the distal wave is recorded later (dt) than the proximal one and PWV = dL/dt. Waveform landmarks, conserved from one site to another, have to be used; the foot of the wave is widely used because it is more clearly identified on all sites. Because early wave reflections can confuse the precise identification of the foot of

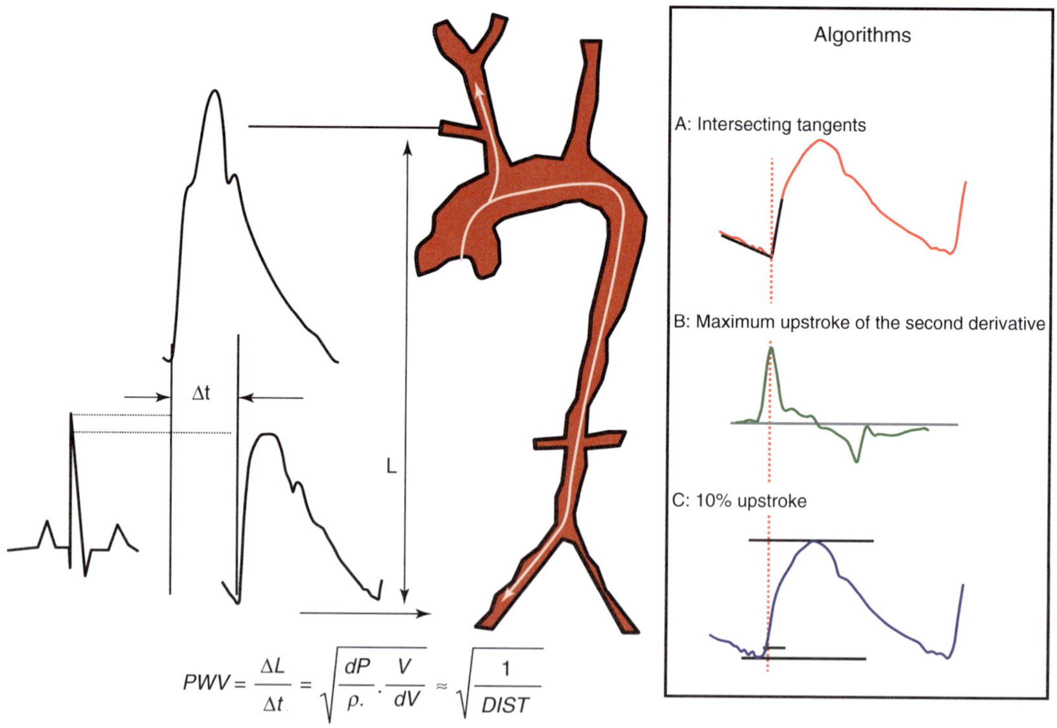

Fig. 5.3 Pulse wave velocity and algorithms for identification of the foot of the wave

the wave, especially if PWV is measured on very short stretches of vessels, it has been proposed to use other landmarks on the pressure wave [11]. The one validated at the site of the carotid is the dichrotic notch, which is not affected by wave reflections [11]. The resulting PWV is nevertheless measured in telesystole and provides higher values than if measured during diastole.

Although PWV can be measured on any artery or between any arterial sites, only carotid-to-femoral [12–15] (or aortic [16], see [17] for meta-analysis) PWV has been shown to have predictive value for morbidity and mortality whereas other arterial pathways have not been associated [18]. Carotid-to-femoral PWV represents stiffness of the aorta and iliofemoral axes. The several commercial devices available differ according to the type of signal (pressure, distension, flow) or whether they simultaneously record both sites or use the ECG for synchronization. When a high-fidelity pressure transducer is used, they may allow pressure-wave analysis and wave-reflection assessment. PWV reference values determined in a very large population are now available, and measurement standardization based on those values was recently proposed [19].

Distance measurement and identification of the foot of the wave are important issues. To have realistic PWV values, the use of intersecting tangents to measure transit time (*dt*) of the foot of the wave and carotid-to-femoral distance (*dL*) is preferred [20]; PWV is then calculated as $PWV = 0.8 \times dL/dt$ [21]. The reason for this correction has to be explained. Because pulse wave reaching the origin of the carotid bifurcates, the time it reaches the carotid site, it has already progressed in the thoracic aorta. Therefore, measurement of distance between the carotid and the femoral site overestimates the distance. The different options to correct for this have been extensively studied [21, 22]. The most logical is the subtraction method, which unfortunately leads to increased error due to duplicate distance measurements but also to underestimation of the pathway length [22, 23]. The optimal method is to use the direct distance correct by a factor 0.8, which is now recommended [19, 21]. Since most, but not all epidemiological studies used the direct distance, some authors question the influence of distance measurements on outcome [24]; however, their analysis is biased by the fact that they used the same fixed threshold of 12 m/s for each of the recalculated pathways which do not have the same metrics.

Because measurement of carotid-to-femoral pulse wave velocity necessitates some training, because the patient has to be reclining, and because exposure of the groin is not acceptable in all culture, manufacturers have developed alternative techniques which allow to approximate CF-PWV on different arterial paths, using either multiple or simple cuffs. Several of the implications of this have been discussed in a recent editorial [25]. Although many devices are now on the market (table from Hypertension 2013), there is up to now no validation of such measurements on hard outcome.

The common view for techniques such as the brachial ankle PWV is that much of the aorta is simply ignored by this parameter because the wave is propagating simultaneously in the arm and the aorta and that this might limit its usefulness and reliability. Despite that, agreement between ankle–brachial PWV is better than expected [26], and ankle–brachial PWV is associated with major CV risk factors and outcome, quite similarly to carotid-to-femoral pulse wave velocity [27]. This indicates that the link between aortic stiffness and brachial–ankle PWV is closer than generally considered. An alternative view of the arterial path is that muscular arteries only contribute for a small part to the compliance of large vessels and that it is rather insensitive to aging and hypertension [28, 29], the major contribution to brachial–ankle pulse wave velocity being provided by the aorta.

Another alternative interesting technique is the Q-KD which measures the time interval between the ECG Q wave and the first Korotkov sound during ambulatory blood-pressure monitoring [30]. This technique provides an estimate of stiffness partly dependent on heart rate because of variable electromechanical coupling time, but it has the major advantages of including mostly the ascending aorta, being ambulatory and minimally invasive. Most importantly, it has been shown to be predictive of events, even on top of LV mass [31]. The method developed by Gosse et al. measures the time delay between the onset of the QRS on the ECG and the detection of the last Korotkoff sound by the microphone placed upon the brachial artery. Thus, the pressure pulse wave travels first along the ascending aorta and the aortic arch, i.e., a short pathway of elastic arteries, and then along the subclavian and brachial arteries, i.e., a much longer pathway of muscular arteries. Since the stiffness of muscular arteries is little influenced by age and hypertension, Gosse et al. attributed the difference in QKD duration to ascending aorta and aortic arch. However, a closer look at the figure shows that the length of the ascending and aortic arch pathway represents a very small part of the total pathway and casts doubt about this statement [25]. Furthermore, in MRI studies, the transit time of flow wave along the aortic arch (average 120 mm length) is often found around 35 ms in young healthy subjects [32], a value which is far from the mean 206 ms QKD duration found in the present study. Thus, part of that QFD duration has to be further explained by both the pre-ejection period and the transit time within muscular arteries.

Local Measurement of Arterial Stiffness

It is also possible to directly measure arterial dimension changes during the cardiac cycle and link them to local pulse pressure changes [33–37] (Figs. 5.2, 5.4, and 5.5). This approach is straightforward and provides the pressure–diameter relationship which is the most closely related to the definition of stiffness, the stress–strain relationship if thickness is also measured, and, thus, yields stiffness indexes at any given blood-pressure level (Fig. 5.2). These techniques are based on high-precision vascular echotracking or magnetic resonance imaging [38–40] coupled with applanation tonometry (Fig. 5.4). The advantage of echotracking technique is its ability

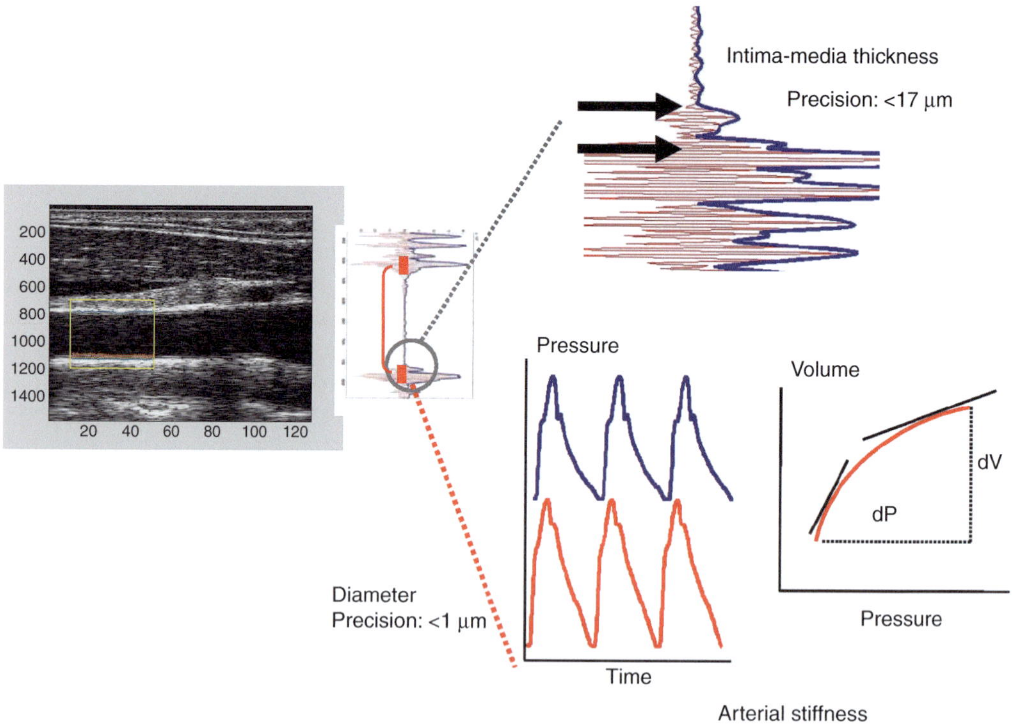

Fig. 5.4 Principle of echotracking

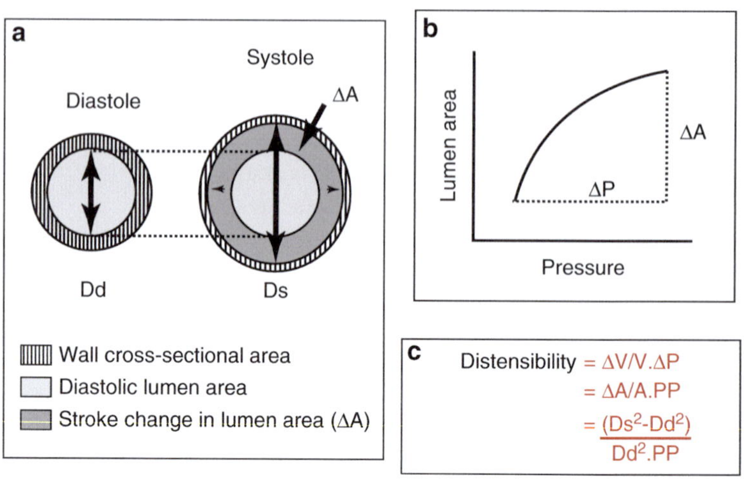

Fig. 5.5 Simplified representation of echotracking of superficial arteries

to track ultrasound radiofrequency signals with a very high time and space resolution. Typically, a 10 MHz probe provides a temporal resolution of 600–1,000 Hz with a spatial resolution of 17 µm for fixed structures and <1 µm for motion [37]. This very high precision is also very useful to quantify arterial structure in terms of diameter, intima media thickness, and related measures. The use of multiframe echotracking makes it possible to assess the heterogeneity of the wall on a segment [37, 41]. We recently applied this approach to the characterization of atherosclerotic plaques, showing that the artery might be more or less distensible at the site of the plaque than beside and that this characteristic was associated with the kind of remodeling (eccentric or concentric) at the site of the plaque [42]. Recent improvement in ultrasound probe quality and in signal processing allows to use dedicated devices based on image analysis since they show a very good agreement with echotracking techniques [43]. Measurement of local arterial stiffness is still limited by the accessibility of the artery to ultrasound (which practically excludes the thoracic aorta) but most importantly limited by the measurement of local pulse pressure. The advantage of MRI is the accessibility of deep arteries, the possibility to investigate the true arterial geometry and blood flow distribution. Its limits are the low temporal and spatial resolution. Both ultrasound and MRI share the same limits for local pressure assessment. Tonometric techniques have been validated against invasive measurements; however, this validation concerns more populations than measurements for individual patients [44]. Calibration of pressure waves is still highly debated, and inaccuracies may lead to errors in interpretation of data [45–47]. It is also likely that the applanation tonometry by itself induces push–pull artifacts due to the motion of the arterial wall and thus might distort the shape of the curve. This explains why it is very difficult to assess arterial wall viscosity in vivo. Experimental data show that in controlled conditions in vivo in animals [48, 49] and in human [50], viscosity is barely measurable and arteries behave as quasi-pure elastic structures. Opposite to that, human data were all obtained with noninvasive pressure and all exhibited large viscoelastic loops [51]. The most likely explanation is the presence of distortions on the pressure recording with tonometry. Analyses have focused on modeling the pressure–diameter relationship which enables to determine arterial stiffness and all parameter for any given blood pressure or wall stress [52–57]. This is of course the most rigorous method but it is not free of caveats. For instance, the reference condition at 0 stress is necessary for any physical model [3, 5] and is considered of crucial importance for characterizing the arterial wall mechanical behavior [58]. The determination of unloaded dimension is quite impossible in vivo, because even if studied at 0 pressure, the artery is still submitted to quantitatively important residual stresses (longitudinal and circumferential). Parameters have then to be "incremental," which means that they are determined within a narrow range of blood pressure (usually diastolic and systolic). It is not warranted that this mechanical behavior can be extrapolated to blood pressure (wall stress) beyond these boundaries, and it usually does not. Experiments have shown that systolic–diastolic variations of diameter and pressure do not follow the whole range, static pressure–diameter relation [59]. Thus usual models are purely phenomenological and do not help to predict behavior outside the experimental conditions. It is possible to partially circumvent these theoretical problems by applying advanced techniques to solve the energy equation of the wall by the reverse problem solving using diameter and pressure data [3]. This has been successfully used in animal and human [4, 60] research. This approach is still highly demanding in terms of calculation power and cannot be applied in routine. The other caveat is that measuring simultaneously pressure and diameter for the carotid artery in human can be done only on right and left or in immediate succession [54]. The last one is that expression of results is very cumbersome and complex, which does not help.

In order to circumvent the limits of applanation tonometry, an interesting approach is to rescale the distension waveform obtained by echotracking since this is a noncontact, high-fidelity technique [61]. By using and extending this method, it is possible to assess arterial stiffness at different time points either in diastole or during systole [62]. The advantage over modeling the whole pressure/diameter curve is that we deal with discrete number of values instead of a continuum. It has also been shown that systolic stiffness might be more associated with target organ damage than diastolic stiffness [62]. Another application of echotracking is local measurement of local pulse wave velocity. For this we take advantage of the measurement of 14 distension waveforms on 2 cm along the vessel. Using adequate landmarks (the dicrotic notch), PWV can be measured and contrasted with the

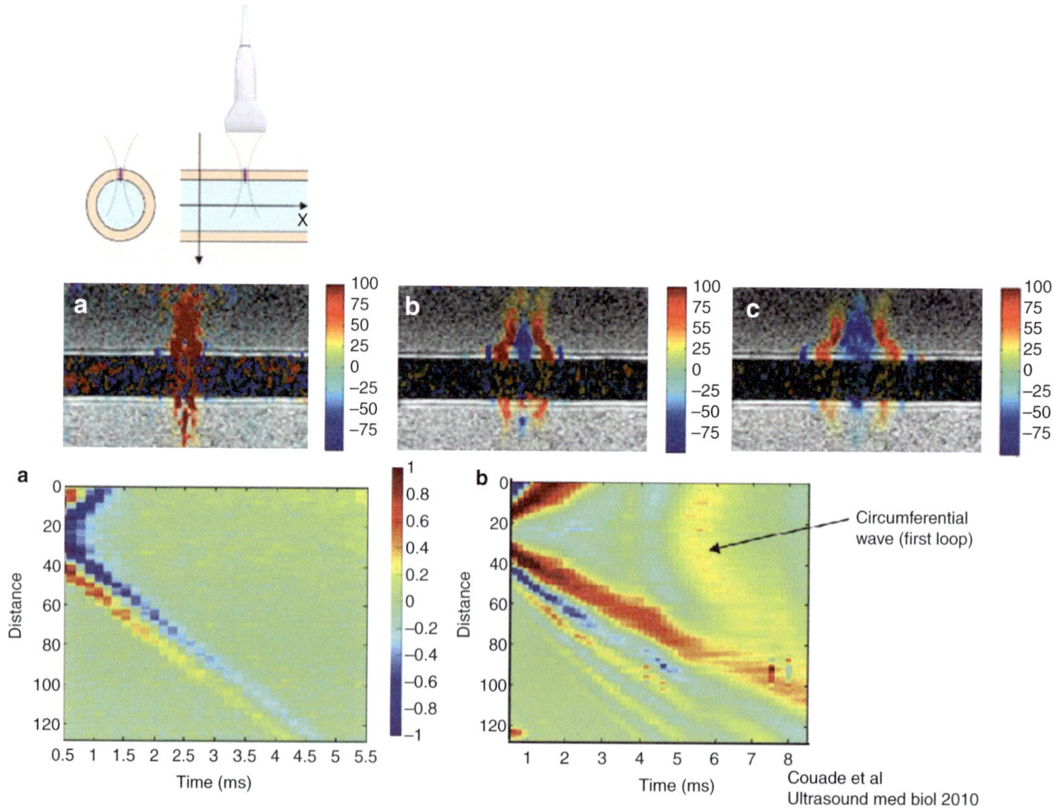

Fig. 5.6 Principles of ultrafast ultrasound scans. Scans are performed on artificial tissues. *Middle panels*: shear wave propagating from the center of the image. *Bottom panels* wave propagation. The slope of each waveform gives the wave speed, i.e., the stiffness of the wall material in a homogenous material (**a**) or in an heterogeneous one (**b**) (Reproduced with permission of Couade et al. [10], Elsevier)

locally measured distensibility from local pressure and distension [11]. To what extent this technique performs better or is complementary to more classical one remains to be determined.

The ultrafast imaging technique is an innovative ultrasound imaging technique. It takes advantage of the very high pulse rate frequency for acquiring plane emission waves [63]. Frequencies up to 20 kHz can be used. At that frequency, it is possible to measure accurately the speed of propagation of spontaneous waves such as the pressure wave. Moreover, it is possible to locally apply short ultrasound impulsion at a very precise place in a tissue and to measure the propagation speed of this pressure wave (Fig. 5.6). By using the Moens–Korteweg equation, propagation speed can be converted into elastic modulus. This method has been applied to the detection of cancer in solid organs and more recently to the heart and the arteries [10]. Because of the complex pattern of pressure wave propagation within laminar structure, there are still some theoretical issues to solve for extracting pressure independent values of elastic modulus. The quality of images obtained from plane wave emission is low, and coupling with echotracking might be necessary for obtaining full potential for this method.

Indirect Estimation of Arterial Stiffness

These techniques rely on simplified circulation models and are being used when a single site for measuring the pressure waveform is required. The most widely used is the Windkessel model [64].

In a "pure" Windkessel, the diastolic blood-pressure decay is exponential, and the constant of this exponential modeling is proportional to stiffness. This model can be made more complex by using two exponential functions: one for large arteries (C1) and the other for small arteries (C2) [65, 66]. To date, only one published study epidemiologically validated this technique in terms of hard clinical endpoints [66], only for small-artery compliance. Sophisticated Windkessel models have been applied to derive PWV from single-point cuff measurements. Although the method takes more than a simple Windkessel [67], the prediction of PWV from a simple brachial cuff waveform seems to provide accurate estimates [68]. Some methods are based on the time flight of the reflected wave. The arteriograph takes advantage of the sharpening of the late systolic peak observed after overinflation of the brachial cuff, which makes it sharper and easier to detect [69–71]. After some assumptions on the pulse wave travel path and distance estimation [72], it is possible to deduce a value for PWV. This method appears to correlate reasonably well with reference techniques [73]. These methods have still to demonstrate their predictive value for hard clinical outcome.

Another indirect technique, aortic characteristic impedance, requires flow and pressure measurement at the aortic root [64, 74, 75]. Characteristic impedance is the minimal impedance for higher frequencies of pressure and flow harmonics. It is proportional to PWV, again if a pure Windkessel model is retained. This technique is rarely used alone, as it is hampered by the difficulty of obtaining reliable noninvasive data for aortic flow and pressure.

Ambulatory Arterial Stiffness Index

On the list are also rigidity estimates derived from blood-pressure measurement, e.g., ambulatory blood-pressure-monitoring-derived ambulatory arterial stiffness index (1/slope of the systolic blood pressure and diastolic blood pressure relationship) or crude brachial pulse pressure [76]. Although these values partially reflect arterial stiffness, they also depend on many other parameters [77], so it is very reductive to interpret them as arterial stiffness. The simple metric of this parameter makes it also difficult to interpret, because it might be confounded by short term variability of blood pressure [78, 79].

Conclusion

There are many techniques to measure arterial stiffness available now. The most validated in terms of association with cardiovascular risk factors, early organ damage, and hard clinical endpoints is carotid-to-femoral pulse wave velocity, measured from tonometry or Doppler. Because they came later than the carotid-to-femoral PWV, for which a tremendous amount of data is available in terms of association with target organ damage and hard clinical endpoints, the alternative techniques will have undergo similar validations and further will have to be scaled against reference techniques, so that thresholds and reference values might be shared. Techniques measuring directly arterial stiffness through the pressure–diameter relationship, although being the most direct, do not have extensive validation in terms of epidemiology; they are limited by measurement of local blood pressure. Learned societies will have to provide clear indications as to which level of agreement is necessary to substitute one technique by another one and finally which alternative technique can be accepted.

References

1. Learoyd BM, Taylor MG. Alterations with age in the viscoelastic properties of human arterial walls. Circ Res. 1966;18(3):278–92.
2. Svedlund S, Eklund C, Robertsson P, Lomsky M, Gan LM. Carotid artery longitudinal displacement predicts 1-year cardiovascular outcome in patients with suspected coronary artery disease. Arterioscler Thromb Vasc Biol. 2011;31(7):1668–74.
3. Humphrey JD, Yin FC. A new constitutive formulation for characterizing the mechanical behavior of soft tissues. Biophys J. 1987;52(4):563–70.
4. Masson I, Beaussier H, Boutouyrie P, Laurent S, Humphrey JD, Zidi M. Carotid artery mechanical properties and stresses quantified using in vivo data

from normotensive and hypertensive humans. Biomech Model Mechanobiol. 2011;10(6):867–82.
5. Zulliger MA, Fridez P, Hayashi K, Stergiopulos N. A strain energy function for arteries accounting for wall composition and structure. J Biomech. 2004;37(7): 989–1000.
6. Laurent S, Boutouyrie P, Lacolley P. Structural and genetic bases of arterial stiffness. Hypertension. 2005; 45(6):1050–5.
7. Moens AI. Over de voortplantingssnelheid van den pols. S.C. Van Doesburgh, Leiden; 1877.
8. Korteveg DJ. Uber die Fortpflanzungsgeschwindigkeit des Schalles in Elastischen Rohren. Annu Phys Chem. 1878;5:52–537.
9. Bramwell LC, Hill AV. Velocity of transmission of the pulse wave. Lancet. 1922;1:891–2.
10. Couade M, Pernot M, Prada C, et al. Quantitative assessment of arterial wall biomechanical properties using shear wave imaging. Ultrasound Med Biol. 2010;36(10):1662–76.
11. Hermeling E, Reesink KD, Reneman RS, Hoeks AP. Confluence of incident and reflected waves interferes with systolic foot detection of the carotid artery distension waveform. J Hypertens. 2008;26(12): 2374–80.
12. Blacher J, Guerin AP, Pannier B, Marchais SJ, Safar ME, London GM. Impact of aortic stiffness on survival in end-stage renal disease. Circulation. 1999; 99(18):2434–9.
13. Shoji T, Emoto M, Shinohara K, et al. Diabetes mellitus, aortic stiffness, and cardiovascular mortality in end-stage renal disease. J Am Soc Nephrol. 2001; 12(10):2117–24.
14. Laurent S, Boutouyrie P, Asmar R, et al. Aortic stiffness is an independent predictor of all-cause and cardiovascular mortality in hypertensive patients. Hypertension. 2001;37(5):1236–41.
15. Guerin AP, Blacher J, Pannier B, Marchais SJ, Safar ME, London GM. Impact of aortic stiffness attenuation on survival of patients in end-stage renal failure. Circulation. 2001;103(7):987–92.
16. Cruickshank K, Riste L, Anderson SG, Wright JS, Dunn G, Gosling RG. Aortic pulse-wave velocity and its relationship to mortality in diabetes and glucose intolerance: an integrated index of vascular function? Circulation. 2002;106(16):2085–90.
17. ben Shlomo Y, Spears M, Boustred C, et al. Aortic pulse wave velocity improves cardiovascular event prediction: an individual participant meta-analysis of prospective observational data from 17,635 subjects. J Am Coll Cardiol. 2014;63:636–46.
18. Pannier B, Guerin AP, Marchais SJ, Safar ME, London GM. Stiffness of capacitive and conduit arteries: prognostic significance for end-stage renal disease patients. Hypertension. 2005;45(4):592–6.
19. Reference values for arterial stiffness' collaboration. Determinants of pulse wave velocity in healthy people and in the presence of cardiovascular risk factors: 'establishing normal and reference values'. Eur Heart J. 2010;31(19):2338–50.
20. Wilkinson I, McEniery CM, Schillaci G, et al. ARTERY society guidelines for validation of non(invasive haemodynamic measurement devices: Part 1, Arterial pulse wave velocity. Artery Res. 2010; 6:1–6.
21. Van Bortel LM, Laurent S, Boutouyrie P, et al. Expert consensus document on the measurement of aortic stiffness in daily practice using carotid-femoral pulse wave velocity. J Hypertens. 2012;30(3):445–8.
22. Sugawara J, Hayashi K, Yokoi T, Tanaka H. Carotid-femoral pulse wave velocity: impact of different arterial path length measurements. Artery Res. 2010;4(1):27–31.
23. Weber T, Ammer M, Rammer M, et al. Noninvasive determination of carotid-femoral pulse wave velocity depends critically on assessment of travel distance: a comparison with invasive measurement. J Hypertens. 2009;27(8):1624–30.
24. Girerd N, Legedz L, Paget V, et al. Outcome associations of carotid-femoral pulse wave velocity vary with different measurement methods. Am J Hypertens. 2012;25(12):1264–70.
25. Laurent S, Mousseaux E, Boutouyrie P. Arterial stiffness as an imaging biomarker: are all pathways equal? Hypertension. 2013;62(1):10–2.
26. Sugawara J, Hayashi K, Yokoi T, et al. Brachial-ankle pulse wave velocity: an index of central arterial stiffness? J Hum Hypertens. 2005;19(5):401–6.
27. Matsuoka O, Otsuka K, Murakami S, et al. Arterial stiffness independently predicts cardiovascular events in an elderly community – Longitudinal Investigation for the Longevity and Aging in Hokkaido County (LILAC) study. Biomed Pharmacother. 2005;59 Suppl 1:S40–4.
28. Boutouyrie P, Laurent S, Benetos A, Girerd XJ, Hoeks AP, Safar ME. Opposing effects of ageing on distal and proximal large arteries in hypertensives. J Hypertens Suppl. 1992;10(6):S87–91.
29. Laurent S, Girerd X, Mourad JJ, et al. Elastic modulus of the radial artery wall material is not increased in patients with essential hypertension. Arterioscler Thromb. 1994;14(7):1223–31.
30. Gosse P, Guillo P, Ascher G, Clementy J. Assessment of arterial distensibility by monitoring the timing of Korotkoff sounds. Am J Hypertens. 1994;7(3):228–33.
31. Gosse P, Cremer A, Papaioannou G, Yeim S. Arterial stiffness from monitoring of timing of Korotkoff sounds predicts the occurrence of cardiovascular events independently of left ventricular mass in hypertensive patients. Hypertension. 2013;62(1):161–7.
32. Dogui A, Redheuil A, Lefort M, et al. Measurement of aortic arch pulse wave velocity in cardiovascular MR: comparison of transit time estimators and description of a new approach. J Magn Reson Imaging. 2011;33(6):1321–9.
33. Hoeks AP, Brands PJ, Smeets FA, Reneman RS. Assessment of the distensibility of superficial arteries. Ultrasound Med Biol. 1990;16(2):121–8.
34. Kawasaki T, Sasayama S, Yagi S, Asakawa T, Hirai T. Non-invasive assessment of the age related changes in stiffness of major branches of the human arteries. Cardiovasc Res. 1987;21(9):678–87.

35. Hirai T, Sasayama S, Kawasaki T, Yagi S. Stiffness of systemic arteries in patients with myocardial infarction. A noninvasive method to predict severity of coronary atherosclerosis. Circulation. 1989;80(1):78–86.
36. Benetos A, Laurent S, Hoeks AP, Boutouyrie PH, Safar ME. Arterial alterations with aging and high blood pressure. A noninvasive study of carotid and femoral arteries. Arterioscler Thromb. 1993;13(1):90–7.
37. Meinders JM, Brands PJ, Willigers JM, Kornet L, Hoeks AP. Assessment of the spatial homogeneity of artery dimension parameters with high frame rate 2-D B-mode. Ultrasound Med Biol. 2001;27(6):785–94.
38. Redheuil A, Yu WC, Wu CO, et al. Reduced ascending aortic strain and distensibility: earliest manifestations of vascular aging in humans. Hypertension. 2010;55(2):319–26.
39. Giannattasio C, Cesana F, Maestroni S, et al. Comparison of echotracking and magnetic resonance assessment of abdominal aorta distensibility and relationships with pulse wave velocity. Ultrasound Med Biol. 2011;37(12):1970–6.
40. Redheuil A, Yu WC, Mousseaux E, et al. Age-related changes in aortic arch geometry: relationship with proximal aortic function and left ventricular mass and remodeling. J Am Coll Cardiol. 2011;58(12):1262–70.
41. Harada A, Okada T, Niki K, Chang D, Sugawara M. On-line noninvasive one-point measurements of pulse wave velocity. Heart Vessels. 2002;17(2):61–8.
42. Beaussier H, Naggara O, Calvet D, et al. Mechanical and structural characteristics of carotid plaques by combined analysis with echotracking system and MR imaging. JACC Cardiovasc Imaging. 2011;4(5):468–77.
43. Bianchini E, Bozec E, Gemignani V, et al. Assessment of carotid stiffness and intima-media thickness from ultrasound data: comparison between two methods. J Ultrasound Med. 2010;29(8):1169–75.
44. Karamanoglu M, O'Rourke MF, Avolio AP, Kelly RP. An analysis of the relationship between central aortic and peripheral upper limb pressure waves in man. Eur Heart J. 1993;14(2):160–7.
45. Verbeke F, Segers P, Heireman S, Vanholder R, Verdonck P, Van Bortel LM. Noninvasive assessment of local pulse pressure: importance of brachial-to-radial pressure amplification. Hypertension. 2005;46(1):244–8.
46. Segers P, Mahieu D, Kips J, et al. Amplification of the pressure pulse in the upper limb in healthy, middle-aged men and women. Hypertension. 2009;54(2):414–20.
47. Soender TK, Van Bortel LM, Moller JE, Lambrechtsen J, Hangaard J, Egstrup K. Impact of calibration on estimates of central blood pressures. J Hum Hypertens. 2012;26(12):706–10.
48. Boutouyrie P, Bezie Y, Lacolley P, et al. In vivo/in vitro comparison of rat abdominal aorta wall viscosity. Influence of endothelial function. Arterioscler Thromb Vasc Biol. 1997;17(7):1346–55.
49. Lacolley P, Challande P, Boumaza S, et al. Mechanical properties and structure of carotid arteries in mice lacking desmin. Cardiovasc Res. 2001;51(1):178–87.
50. Rosset E, Brunet C, Rieu R, et al. Viscoelastic properties of human arteries. Methodology and preliminary results. Surg Radiol Anat. 1996;18(2):89–96.
51. Giannattasio C, Salvi P, Valbusa F, et al. Simultaneous measurement of beat-to-beat carotid diameter and pressure changes to assess arterial mechanical properties. Hypertension. 2008;52(5):896–902.
52. Langewouters GJ, Wesseling KH, Goedhard WJ. The static elastic properties of 45 human thoracic and 20 abdominal aortas in vitro and the parameters of a new model. J Biomech. 1984;17(6):425–35.
53. Tardy Y, Meister JJ, Perret F, Brunner HR, Arditi M. Non-invasive estimate of the mechanical properties of peripheral arteries from ultrasonic and photoplethysmographic measurements. Clin Phys Physiol Meas. 1991;12(1):39–54.
54. Bussy C, Boutouyrie P, Lacolley P, Challande P, Laurent S. Intrinsic stiffness of the carotid arterial wall material in essential hypertensives. Hypertension. 2000;35(5):1049–54.
55. Lacolley P, Glaser E, Challande P, et al. Structural changes and in situ aortic pressure-diameter relationship in long-term chemical-sympathectomized rats. Am J Physiol. 1995;269(2 Pt 2):H407–16.
56. Bezie Y, Lacolley P, Laurent S, Gabella G. Connection of smooth muscle cells to elastic lamellae in aorta of spontaneously hypertensive rats. Hypertension. 1998;32(1):166–9.
57. Galmiche G, Labat C, Mericskay M, et al. Inactivation of serum response factor contributes to decrease vascular muscular tone and arterial stiffness in mice. Circ Res. 2013;112(7):1035–45.
58. Fung YC. What are the residual stresses doing in our blood vessels? Ann Biomed Eng. 1991;19(3):237–49.
59. Glaser E, Lacolley P, Boutouyrie P, et al. Dynamic versus static compliance of the carotid artery in living Wistar-Kyoto rats. J Vasc Res. 1995;32(4):254–65.
60. Wilson JS, Baek S, Humphrey JD. Importance of initial aortic properties on the evolving regional anisotropy, stiffness and wall thickness of human abdominal aortic aneurysms. J R Soc Interface. 2012;9(74):2047–58.
61. Van Bortel LM, Balkestein EJ, van der Heijden-Spek JJ, et al. Non-invasive assessment of local arterial pulse pressure: comparison of applanation tonometry and echo-tracking. J Hypertens. 2001;19(6):1037–44.
62. Hermeling E, Vermeersch SJ, Rietzschel ER, et al. The change in arterial stiffness over the cardiac cycle rather than diastolic stiffness is independently associated with left ventricular mass index in healthy middle-aged individuals. J Hypertens. 2012;30(2):396–402.
63. Sandrin L, Catheline S, Tanter M, Hennequin X, Fink M. Time-resolved pulsed elastography with ultrafast ultrasonic imaging. Ultrason Imaging. 1999;21(4):259–72.
64. Nichols WW, O'Rourke MF. McDonald's blood flow in arteries: theoretical, experimental and clinical principles. 5th ed. London: Hodder Arnold; 2005.

65. London GM, Cohn JN. Prognostic application of arterial stiffness: task forces. Am J Hypertens. 2002;15(8):754–8.
66. Duprez DA, Jacobs Jr DR, Lutsey PL, et al. Association of small artery elasticity with incident cardiovascular disease in older adults: the multi-ethnic study of atherosclerosis. Am J Epidemiol. 2011;174(5):528–36.
67. Wassertheurer S, Mayer C, Breitenecker F. Modeling arterial and left ventricular coupling for non-invasive measurements. Simul Model Pract Theory. 2008; 16(8):988–97.
68. Hametner B, Wassertheurer S, Kropf J, Mayer C, Eber B, Weber T. Oscillometric estimation of aortic pulse wave velocity: comparison with intra-aortic catheter measurements. Blood Press Monit. 2013;18(3):173–6.
69. Baulmann J, Schillings U, Rickert S, et al. A new oscillometric method for assessment of arterial stiffness: comparison with tonometric and piezo-electronic methods. J Hypertens. 2008;26(3):523–8.
70. Jatoi NA, Mahmud A, Bennett K, Feely J. Assessment of arterial stiffness in hypertension: comparison of oscillometric (Arteriograph), piezoelectronic (Complior) and tonometric (SphygmoCor) techniques. J Hypertens. 2009;27:2186–91.
71. Nemcsik J, Egresits J, El Hadj OT, et al. Validation of arteriograph – a new oscillometric device to measure arterial stiffness in patients on maintenance hemodialysis. Kidney Blood Press Res. 2009;32(3):223–9.
72. Rezai MR, Cowan BR, Sherratt N, Finn JD, Wu FC, Cruickshank JK. A magnetic resonance perspective of the pulse wave transit time by the Arteriograph device and potential for improving aortic length estimation for central pulse wave velocity. Blood Press Monit. 2013;18(2):111–18.
73. Horvath IG, Nemeth A, Lenkey Z, et al. Invasive validation of a new oscillometric device (Arteriograph) for measuring augmentation index, central blood pressure and aortic pulse wave velocity. J Hypertens. 2010;28(10):2068–75.
74. Nichols WW, O'Rourke MF. McDonald's blood flow in arteries. 3rd ed. London: Edward Arnold; 1990.
75. Mitchell GF. Effects of central arterial aging on the structure and function of the peripheral vasculature: implications for end-organ damage. J Appl Physiol. 2008;105(5):1652–60.
76. Adiyaman A, Dechering DG, Boggia J, et al. Determinants of the ambulatory arterial stiffness index in 7604 subjects from 6 populations. Hypertension. 2008;52(6):1038–44.
77. Segers P, Kips JG, Vermeersch SJ, Boutouyrie P, Laurent S, Van Bortel LM. A model expression for the ambulatory arterial stiffness index. J Hypertens. 2013; 31(1):211–12.
78. Schillaci G, Parati G, Pirro M, et al. Ambulatory arterial stiffness index is not a specific marker of reduced arterial compliance. Hypertension. 2007;49(5):986–91.
79. Schillaci G, Bilo G, Pucci G, et al. Relationship between short-term blood pressure variability and large-artery stiffness in human hypertension: findings from 2 large databases. Hypertension. 2012;60(2):369–77.

Animal Models for Studies of Arterial Stiffness

6

Patrick Lacolley, Simon N. Thornton, and Yvonnick Bezie

Abstract

Arterial stiffness is a perfect example of translational research spanning the understanding of the molecular determinants of the arterial wall constituents and their organization to the physiology of normal and early vascular ageing.

The most widely used parameter to investigate arterial stiffness in rodents is pulse wave velocity (PWV). The relation between strain and stress is also established to characterize the intrinsic behaviour of the arterial wall independent of geometric factors.

The first attempts to explain arterial stiffness by the properties of the structural components of the arterial wall addressed the role of the principal constituents, elastin and collagen fibres and smooth muscle cells. To complete this approach, the roles of the adhesion molecules, inflammation, blood pressure variability, NO, integrins and metalloproteinases in arterial stiffness were also investigated by attempting to try and interfere directly with these different factors.

Hypertensive rodents were the first experimental models used and employed to test remodelling and vascular function in an environment mimicking human physiology. Then, investigations were completed with other cardiovascular animal models (mainly kidney disease, obesity, blood pressure variability or ageing) to discover more specific therapeutic targets related to other mechanisms that trigger arterial stiffness. Nowadays, the advances in mouse genetics have provided numerous genotypes and phenotypes to study changes in arterial mechanics with disease progression and treatment. The aim of modifying a single gene to understand the

P. Lacolley (✉) • S.N. Thornton, PhD
Faculté de Médecine,
Unité INSERM UL U1116,
9 avenue de la Foret de Haye CS 50184,
Vandoeuvre Les Nancy 54505, France
e-mail: patrick.lacolley@inserm.fr

Y. Bezie, PharmD, PhD
Pharmacy Department, Groupe Hospitalier Paris
Saint – Joseph, 185 re Raymond Losserand,
Paris 75014, France

M.E. Safar et al. (eds.), *Blood Pressure and Arterial Wall Mechanics in Cardiovascular Diseases*,
DOI 10.1007/978-1-4471-5198-2_6, © Springer-Verlag London 2014

mechanism of this polygenic disease has led to complete animal models using in vitro cellular approaches.

The response to these questions will ultimately come from more complete knowledge of the mechanisms involved, using pharmacological and other tools in existing and/or newly emerging animal models.

Keywords
Rodent model • Arterial stiffness • Pulse wave velocity • Hypertension • Elastin • Collagen • Fibronectin • Integrin

Arterial stiffness is a cardiovascular risk factor that is independent of arterial pressure [1]. The possibilities of conducting human research about mechanisms and clinical impact of arterial stiffness are limited. First, arterial stiffness develops often along with confounding factors or pathologies that increase per se cardiovascular risk such as ageing, hypertension, diabetes, obesity, chronic kidney disease, blood pressure variability and atherosclerosis. Second, increased arterial stiffness often needs many years to develop before it can be diagnosed clinically. Third, it is difficult to perform invasive experimental procedures in patients. These drawbacks may be overcome by using animal models where a large variety of vascular processes and therapeutic targets can be studied.

Rodent models have been found very useful for studying arterial mechanics in development and disease. Rats and mice have relatively short lifespan (mature adults by 3 months and aged adults by 2 years), and so studies can be carried out over a limited time course. Animal models were first based on general cardiovascular models initially developed for studying end-organ damage and that have been characterized by a decrease in large artery distensibility. They were initially represented by hypertensive and ageing rodent models and employed to test remodelling and vascular function in an environment mimicking human physiology [2, 3]. Nevertheless, to better elucidate the complex mechanisms leading to arterial stiffness, gene-targeting approaches in mice are now performed. Indeed, the advances in mouse genetics have provided numerous genotypes and phenotypes to study changes in arterial mechanics with disease progression and disease treatment [4]. Mice can also be manipulated experimentally to study the effects of changes in hemodynamic parameters of the arterial remodelling process [5]. One drawback of the mouse model, especially when examining young ages, is the size of the arteries. Nevertheless, the aim of modifying a single gene to understand the mechanism of this polygenic disease has led to complete animal models by in vitro cellular approaches [6]. Testing cell topographic features, and cell and cytoskeletal mechanical properties, is beyond the scope of the present review which will focus on the rodent animal models that have been used to evaluate arterial stiffness principally in large arteries.

Classical Models of Arterial Stiffness

Basic Concepts

Arterial stiffness is an intuitive notion that can be quantified by the measurement of parameters that are different in humans and in animals. Experimentally, the most widely used parameter in rodents is pulse wave velocity (PWV) which is an estimation of the speed of the propagation of the elastic waves between two points of the arterial tree [7, 8]. Diameter/pressure curves are the other major way to evaluate arterial stiffness in small animals [9–13]. This method measures systolo-diastolic changes in carotid or abdominal aorta diameter in response to systolo-diastolic blood pressure excursions. Another animal model used is the domestic fowl where arterial stiffness increases with ageing [14].

The values obtained by these measurements permit calculation of the distensibility. This parameter characterizes the global mechanical behaviour of the arterial wall and is especially dependent on its geometry. To characterize the intrinsic behaviour of the arterial wall independently of geometric factors, it is necessary to establish the relation between strain and stress [15]. This may be done by considering the relation between incremental elastic modulus and circumferential wall stress [15].

Arterial stiffness is a perfect example of translational research spanning from the understanding of its molecular determinants of the constituents of the arterial wall and their organization to the physiology of normal and early vascular ageing. We do not yet know the specific genes involved in arterial stiffness as it is a very multifactorial phenotype. But of course this needs new experimental models that are more specific and represent common sicknesses or specific gene anomalies. This research started with looking at elastin/collagen content (a key element in arterial wall stiffness) with respect to vascular smooth muscle cell (VSMC) tone to being able to measure shear stress and tensile pulsatile circumferential stress as key determinants in arterial wall remodelling. After observing abnormal microcirculation and large/small artery crosstalk as key determinants of target organ damage, now is the time for research into the molecular mechanisms and genes involved.

Rodent Models of Hypertension and Stiffness

It is well established that hypertension is associated with an increase of arterial stiffness. These models helped mainly to describe the structure-function relation of large arteries and to assess the interest of pharmacological interventions on arterial stiffness.

Spontaneously hypertensive rats (SHR) have been extensively used in experimental studies, as a genetic model of hypertension because of their clinical relevance to human hypertension. SHR is characterized by a decreased distensibility at its operational pressure compared to its normotensive control [15]. Nevertheless evaluation of the arterial wall stiffness, assessed by the elastic modulus measurement, shows that for a given level of stress, SHR and Wistar rats have similar mechanical properties. Also, the decrease of distensibility observed in SHR is related rather to the hypertension than to the increased stiffness of the arterial wall.

Other Cardiovascular Models and Stiffness

As in humans, it is now clear that arterial stiffness is included in a cluster of cardiovascular disorders such as kidney disease, obesity and the metabolic syndrome or ageing. Therefore, this research field requires other animal models for the analysis of mechanisms that trigger arterial stiffness and for the discovery of more specific therapeutic targets.

The second generation of models now aims to describe the complex relations between arterial mechanics and the other established cardiovascular risk factors. Indeed, these models have been used mostly to illustrate the impact and the time of occurrence of increased arterial stiffness with respect to other pathologies. These models are designed to determine if the rigidity of a blood vessel is a cause or a consequence of other risk factors such as diabetes, metabolic syndrome, ageing or blood pressure variability. Avian models, such as the pigeon and the turkey, have been used also to study the development of atherosclerosis, as they develop this problem spontaneously despite being grain eaters [16, 17].

Kidney Disease

Arterial stiffness has emerged as an important marker of cardiovascular risk in patients with chronic kidney diseases where it contributes to increased cardiovascular morbidity and mortality. The Lewis polycystic kidney (LPK) rat is a

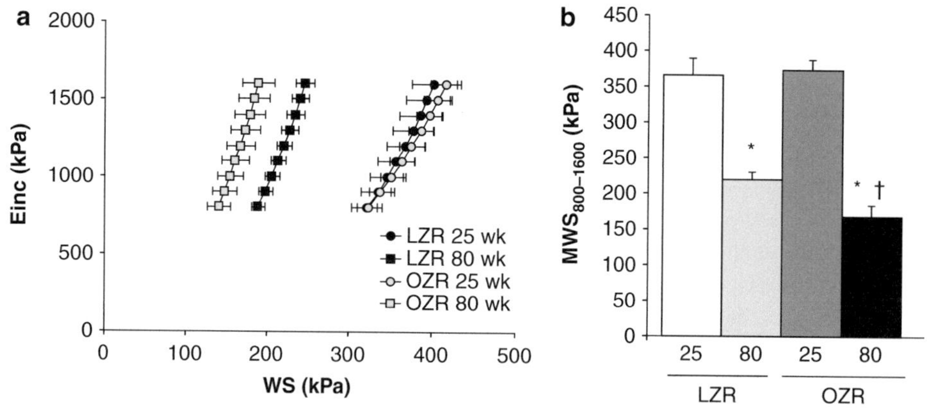

Fig. 6.1 Mechanical properties in carotid arteries in 25- and 80-week-old lean Zucker rat (*LZR*) and obese Zucker rat (*OZR*). Incremental elastic modulus (*Einc*)-wall stress (*WS*) curve (**a**) from 25- to 80-week-old lean and obese rats. (**b**) Carotid artery mean wall stress within the 800- to 1,600-kPa range of Einc (MWS 800–1,600) in the same rats (analysis of variance, age, $p<10\text{–}6$; strain, $p<.05$; interaction, $p=.3$). Values are mean ± standard error of the mean. "*" indicates $p<.05$, 80- vs. 25-week-old in the same strain; "†" indicates $p<.05$, obese vs. lean at the same age ($n=14\text{–}21$ in each group) (Reprinted with permission from Sloboda et al. [19])

model developed from a spontaneous mutation that progresses to end-stage renal disease by 18–24 weeks of age [18]. In this model, hypertension and increased isobaric arterial stiffness associated with increased arterial calcification and media thickness appear as soon as after 12 weeks of age, thus preceding the appearance of kidney disease.

Obesity, Diabetes and Ageing

The obese Zucker rat displays many aspects of metabolic dysfunction, such as insulin resistance, hypertension and increased plasma lipid levels. It represents an ideal model for investigating the mechanisms that contribute to large artery dysfunction which occur with advanced age in obese individuals. The increase in arterial stiffness and the alteration of aortic structure are accentuated by the metabolic disorders present in the obese Zucker rat [19]. In the Zucker fa/fa rat model of type 2 diabetes, mechanical, structural and molecular evidence of increased aortic stiffness before the onset of hyperglycaemia has also been reported [20]. Furthermore, aged obese Zucker rats develop also problems with distensibility with age through a left shift in the carotid elastic modulus-wall stress curves probably due to the changes in aortic composition with an increase in collagen, a decrease in elastin (thus a decrease in the elastin/collagen ratio) and an increase in dry weight due to an increase in protein content [19] (Fig. 6.1).

In another obese model that develops heart failure, the SHHF rat, reduced carotid distensibility and impaired renal function were observed, and with age these obese rats developed eccentric left ventricular hypertrophy from progressive dilation of the left ventricular dimensions (Anne Pizard, personal communication).

Old SHR develop naturally all the pathophysiological and clinical alterations also noted in patients with essential hypertension. Interestingly, chronic administration of the NO synthase inhibitor L-Name at low doses to adult SHR decreases endogenous NO production and promotes aortic stiffening to a similar level as that observed naturally during ageing in hypertensive rats. Aortic stiffening in the SHR L-Name is in part BP independent and due to vascular remodelling and to endothelial dysfunction [21]. Normotensive inbred Wistar or aged Brown Norway (BN) rats (arterial elastin deficient) of 25–30 months old were also used as aged rats [22]. The walls of the large-diameter elastic arteries became progressively stiffer with age [23]. The increased arterial stiffness and dilatation with age were attributable to a progressive increase in collagen and vascular hypertrophy, resulting in a relative decrease in elastin content [24]. Calcification and advanced glycation end-product (AGE) accumulation in arteries accelerated age-induced arterial stiffening. Glycation of collagens induces covalent bridges between fibrils and elastic fibres which undergo also age-related modifications, leading to more stiffness. Receptor-mediated effects of AGEs in VSMCs result in increased proliferation and accumulation of fibronectin [25]. BN rats have a lower aortic elastin to collagen ratio than control rats which at a young age produced an increase in stiffness. However, this stiffness decreased with age probably due to the increase in internal elastic lamina ruptures [24].

Furthermore, treating cultured smooth muscle cells from BN rats with potassium channel blockers, minoxidil, diazide and pinacidil, increased mRNAs that encoded enzymes and proteins involved in elastic fibre formation. Treatment of intact BN rat with minoxidil increased elastic fibre content but induced the undesirable side effect of cardiac hypertrophy [26].

Blood Pressure Variability (BVP)

The association of arterial stiffness with BPV is strengthened by a number of studies showing that increased variability predicts cardiovascular outcome, especially stroke. Pulse pressure and older age, which are both directly associated with arterial stiffness, have also been shown to be independently associated with higher visit to visit variability in SBP. In experimental models such as the SHR, we have previously shown a strong association between increased BPV and increased arterial stiffness [27]. Sinoaortic denervated (SAD) and chemically sympathectomized (SNX) rats, used as experimental models of short-term systolic blood pressure variability, are characterized by an increase of arterial stiffness and a decrease of carotid distensibility without hypertension compared to their respective controls [11, 28, 29]. Another recent study has further demonstrated a relation between BP variability and elastic stiffness-determining components, i.e. a positive correlation with collagen/elastin ratio in SHR [30].

Genetically Modified Models of Arterial Stiffness

Genetically modified animal models provide a unique opportunity to alter the content and organization of key components of the vascular wall. Transgenic mice now allow us to better understand structural modifications related to arterial mechanical alterations to establish new therapeutic targets. These models, more often coupled to in vitro experimental studies, open an important new field of research around intracellular signalling and its consequences on the intrinsic rigidity of vascular smooth muscle.

Influence of Scleroprotein Contents on Arterial Stiffness

The first attempts to explain arterial stiffness by the properties of structural components of the arterial wall addressed the role of the principal constituents, elastic and collagen fibres and smooth muscle cells [31, 32]. The simplest mechanical scheme consists of considering the elastic fibre network, the most distensible component of the arterial wall, in parallel with the collagen fibre network which, in contrast, lacks distensibility but provides rigidity [8, 33].

The quantity of elastic and collagen fibres is appreciated by measuring their relative density and their ratio within the media either by morphometric analysis using elective staining or by biochemical methods.

Studies of elastin-insufficient mice show that there is more flexibility in the building plan than thought previously. Mice with one functional elastin allele (Eln+/−), and thus half as much elastin, live a normal life span and thrive well into adulthood. They have a mean arterial pressure 30–40 mmHg higher than wild-type animals. They have also an increased number of lamellar units in their arteries and a vessel wall with an increased incremental elastic modulus at high pressure [34]. At their higher physiological pressure, arteries in Eln+/− mice are working close to their maximum strain, suggesting that these animals may be more prone to develop hypertensive cardiovascular pathologies when stressed. At maximal strain, there is a lower potential for distension if the blood pressure increases. In contrast, mice with a null mutation in the elastin gene (Eln−/−) die within a few days of birth due to SMC over-proliferation that occludes the vessel lumen. At birth, Eln−/− mice have stiff vessels that show little diameter change between systole and diastole [35].

Fibulin-5 is essential for elastic fibre formation and is expressed in developing arteries as well as in balloon-injured and in atherosclerotic arteries. Mice lacking both alleles of fibulin-5 experience increased arterial stiffness with adequate tropoelastin present in large arteries but not organized into functional elastic lamina in these vessels [36]. It appears clear that, although modifications of the elastic fibre network may contribute to mechanical properties of the arterial wall, these fibres are integrated in a much more complex network, with multiple interactions existing between all of the various components of the arterial wall [37]. Thus the connections between these different components should be considered.

The modifications of stiffness observed in these different models with quantitative or qualitative alterations of elastic fibres appear to be predictable only in the case of HVD, a model of elastocalcinosis induced by chronicle administration of vitamin D (IM injection) and nicotine (per os) and Lox- models (a model of inhibition of lysyl oxidase by administration of beta-aminopropionitrile). In contrast, for IEL rupture, the mechanical consequences are not what would be expected, but it is possible that the decreased elastin content and the presence of IEL ruptures have opposite effects on arterial stiffness and cancel each other out. Indeed, the former should tend to increase stiffness, whereas the latter should decrease it. One explanation for the behaviour in the Fib model, a mouse model of Marfan syndrome by mutation of the fibrillin-1 gene, is the following: fragmentation of the elastic fibre network without change in arterial pressure would lead to distension of the arterial wall and the premature recruitment of collagen fibres. A similar sequence of events may occur in Lox-rats, but as these rats have also decreased collagen cross-linking, the collagen is less rigid and so the effect would be masked. In models where collagen cross-linking is increased, a similar phenomenon is observed: here the collagen fibre network is solicited abnormally in conditions of normal distension, leading to an increase in rigidity.

Vascular Smooth Muscle Cells and Arterial Stiffening

Smooth muscle cells are attached to the elastic fibres and as such are integrated into musculo-elastic units [38–40]. The degree of activation of these cells (muscle tone) can modify the mechanical behaviour of the arterial wall, i.e. by increasing rigidity with increased tone. The elastic properties of the arterial wall may also arise from changes in the structural properties of the vascular smooth muscle (SM) cells. Qiu et al. observed that vascular SM cell stiffness measured both by atomic force microscopy and in a reconstituted tissue model was significantly increased in the aorta from old vs. young monkeys, in association with increased expression of SM α-actin (SMA) and β1 integrin [22]. Serum response factor (SRF) is a major transcription factor regulating SM genes involved in the maintenance of the contractile state of vascular SM cells. A specific knockout mouse of serum response factor (SRF^{SMKO}) has been developed to investigate whether SRF and its target genes regulate intrinsic SM tone and thereby arterial stiffness. The carotid distensibility-pressure curve and elastic modulus-wall stress curves showed a greater arterial elasticity in SRF^{SMKO} mice without modification in the collagen/elastin ratio. These data suggest strongly that the regulatory role of SRF on the differentiation of smooth muscle cells is crucial in the function and structure of elastic arteries and their remodelling during ageing [41, 42] (Fig. 6.2).

Similarly, mice without desmin (DES−/−), the main component of the intermediate filaments in cardiac, skeletal and smooth muscles, showed a lower distensibility and an increase in arterial wall viscosity and a lowered vascular

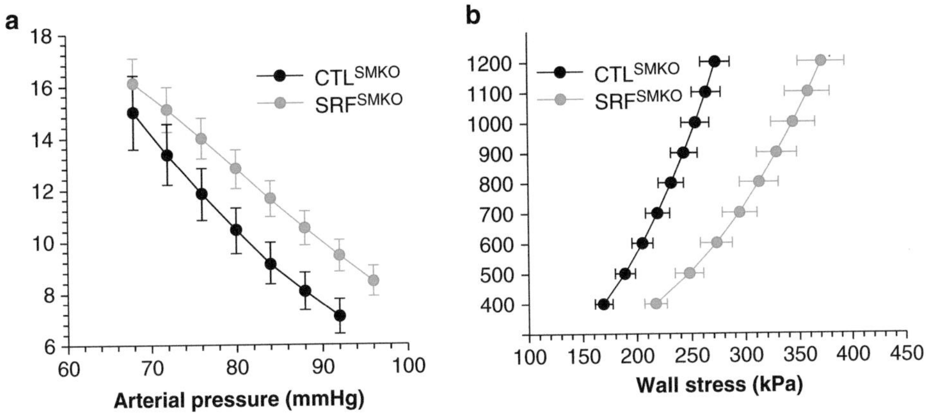

Fig. 6.2 Mechanical properties of carotid arteries from control, smooth muscle-specific knockout of serum response factor (*SRF*^{SMKO}) and smooth muscle-specific overexpression of serum response factor (SRF^{SMTG} mice). Distensibility-arterial pressure (AP) curves (**a**) and incremental elastic modulus (Einc)-wall stress (WS) curves (**b**) in CTL^{SMKO} (control, $n = 19$), SRF^{SMKO} ($n = 22$) (Reprinted with permission from Galmiche et al. [41])

wall mechanical strength compared to wild-type mice [43].

Global arterial stiffness is the sum of passive stiffness, corresponding to the contribution of the inert structural components, and active stiffness provided by the smooth muscle tone [9, 44]. Nevertheless, it has been shown that under basal conditions, the global mechanical behaviour is very close to that of the purely passive elements, indicating that the SMCs are close to their maximal state of relaxation [45]. However, under high distending pressures there is no longer any dependence of the mechanical behaviour on muscle tone, suggesting the preponderance of passive structural elements, probably collagen fibres.

Pseudoxanthoma Elasticum

In this particular inherited multisystem metabolic disorder, there is progressive fragmentation of elastic fibres in the skin, the Bruch membrane of the retina and in the media of the arterial wall. The principal gene affected is the ABCC6, and the knockout mouse model of this disease has a slight increase in arterial stiffness and a significant increase in myogenic tone compared to the wild-type mouse (Kauffenstein, personal communication).

Role of Adhesion Structures

The connections between the components of the media are organized in the form of dense plaques (DP) which represent the principal structures of attachment between the SMCs and the extracellular matrix [46]. By electron microscopy, two types of DP can be distinguished: (1) those in contact with elastic fibres and elastic lamellae (DP-EL) and (2) those in contact with the basal lamina and immediately beyond, with microfibrils and collagen fibrils (DP-M).

From a mechanical point of view, an increase in the number of attachment sites should limit the deformability of the arterial wall. This hypothesis, i.e. that an increase in one or other type of DP is associated with an increase in stiffness, appears to hold true in vivo only in normotensive strains. The relation is not as clear in models of hypertension [15]. However, it is probable that not all attachments should be taken into account, but only those which are mechanically solicited. This number may vary due to both the distension of the arterial wall by the pulsatile arterial pressure and to the increased tension of structures caused by the contraction of the SMCs. This phenomenon of recruitment of cell attachments during deformation of the arterial wall requires further investigation, both at a structural and mechanical level.

The quantification of DPs can only provide a partial explanation of the mechanisms of rigidity. It should be completed by the analysis of the plaque constituents. Among the integrins present in these dense plaques, a large number are capable of forming complexes with fibronectin, a glycoprotein which plays an important role in the organization and assembly of the extracellular matrix [47, 48].

Table 6.1 shows that taking into account variations in fibronectin and/or in collagen allows prediction of the evolution of arterial rigidity in all models except one (SNX). However, the demonstration of the relation between fibronectin content and rigidity does not provide any explanation of the mechanisms intervening at the level of the dense plaques. The integrin composition is important in this respect. In models where the specific receptor for fibronectin, α5β1 integrin, has been studied, this component was shown to follow the same evolution as fibronectin [13]. As for the other integrins present in the arterial wall (α1β1, α3β1, α8β1, αvβ1 αvβ3), which bind to various proteins of the ECM (collagens, fibronectin, laminins, vitronectin, thrombospondin, tenascin, osteopontin, etc.), their role in arterial mechanical properties has been little studied [15, 38, 50]. It has nevertheless been proposed that the increase in αvβ3 observed in the mesenteric artery in the SHR may in part determine rigidity via cell proliferation and ECM remodelling [60, 61].

On the other hand, mice lacking the integrin α1 exhibit reduced mechanical strength at baseline and do not show SMC hypertrophy in response to angiotensin II [62]. The role of the integrins in arterial stiffness is also supported by in vitro manipulations of smooth muscle cells showing that cyclic mechanical stress plays a role in the expression of integrins [63].

Dense plaques form also part of a larger network via their connections with the cytoskeletal proteins. Little is known about this aspect. Some studies have been carried out on one of these proteins, desmin, which is an essential constituent of the intermediate filaments associated with dense plaques. Use of the desmin KO mouse model has shown that the absence of desmin leads to an important reorganization of the ECM with thickening and densification of the spaces between elastic lamellae, cells and basal lamina leading to an increase in arterial stiffness [43].

Table 6.1 Arterial stiffness and fibronectin content

Model (references)	HTA	Arterial stiffness	Arterial FN density	Arterial collagen density
SHR [15, 49]	+	=	↑	↓
SHR-SP [50]	+	↓	↑	↓
SAD [28]	–	↑	↑	↑
SNX [28]	–	↑	=	=
2K1C [51]	+	↑		
L-NAME [52, 53]	+	↑	↑	?
SHR L-NAME [21]	+	↑	↑	↑
SHR-HSD [54, 55]	+	↑	↑	=
Aldo-salt [56]	–	↑	↑	=
DOCA-salt [57–59]	+	↑	↑	?

See the text for other models abbreviations
HTA hypertension, *FN* fibronectin, *2K1C* 2 kidneys-1clip, *HSD* high-salt diet

One final class of constituents which have been implicated in arterial stiffness are the proteoglycans [64, 65]. These molecules represent quantitatively an important part of the ECM. It has been shown that a decrease in glycosaminoglycans is associated with increased wall stiffness, and the hypothesis that proteoglycans take part in cell-matrix attachments has been proposed.

Other Markers

Mice where one of the β-galactoside-binding lectins, Galectin-3, had been knocked out were resistant to aldosterone-induced vascular smooth muscle cell inflammation and the increase in collagen type 1 that would have led to increased fibrosis [66].

Knock out of one of the interleukin-6 family members, cardiotrophin 1, decreases age-dependent arterial stiffness (right shift of the stress-incremental elastic modulus curve) and increases longevity in mice [67] (Fig. 6.3).

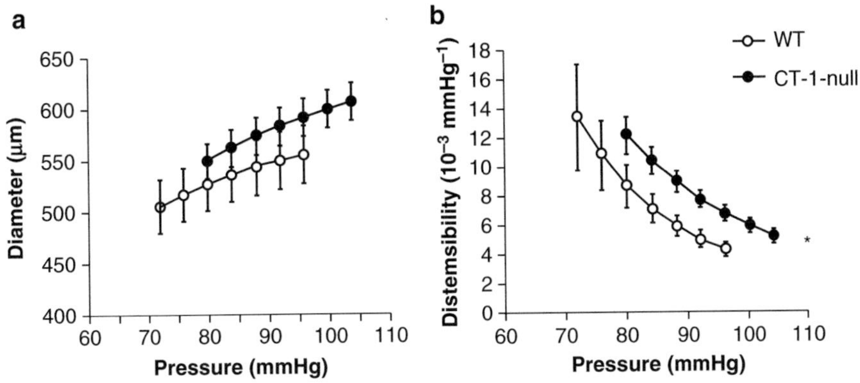

Fig. 6.3 In vivo carotid mechanical properties and vascular morphology and composition in wild-type (*WT*) and cardiotrophin 1 (*CT-1*)-null mice. (**a**) The diameter-arterial pressure curve of the CT-1-null mice group ($n=12$) was shifted upward vs. WT ($n=12$). (**b**) For a given level of arterial pressure, there was a significant upward shift of the distensibility-pressure curve in CT-1-null mice (Reprinted with permission from Lopez-Andres et al. [67])

Aldosterone has been implicated also in stiffness, and two recent papers show the two sides of the effect of aldosterone. In the first, conditional overexpression in mice of aldosterone receptors in endothelial cells showed moderate hypertension independent of renal tubular sodium transport or activation of the smooth muscle receptor [68]. In contrast, in the second, conditional inactivation of the aldosterone receptor leads to a decrease in blood pressure with larger vessel diameter than wild type that did not give increased arterial stiffness in response to an aldosterone/sodium challenge [69].

Conclusion and Perspectives

At present, the therapeutic applications of the studies presented here remain limited. A certain number of currently used antihypertensive drugs have been shown to have beneficial effects on arterial stiffness. However, with the exception of their action on muscular peripheral arteries and arterioles, these agents seem to have little direct influence on central arterial mechanical properties. However, they may act on central arteries through the mechanism of wave reflections (see chapters 1 and 2). Several examples are discussed in this book. Molecules acting on the renin-angiotensin system appear to have a greater effect (independently of the lowering of blood pressure) than the other classes of drug. This is coherent with the fact that these compounds can modulate fibronectin expression.

As mentioned above, it is probable that the adhesion molecules play a major role in arterial stiffness. It is thus tempting to try and interfere directly with these attachments at the level of either collagen or elastin fibres, with the aim of reducing rigidity. Nevertheless, trials for the modulation of these adhesion molecules should be carried out with caution. Indeed, these attachments play also an essential role in determining the mechanical resistance of the arterial wall. It would be counterproductive to decrease parietal mechanical resistance in an attempt to reduce wall stiffness. The difficulty lies at present in the fact that we do not know which molecules within the adhesion structures to target. The integrins, their ligands and their activation pathways represent potential candidates, but the question of their specificity remains open. The response to these questions will ultimately come from more complete knowledge of the mechanisms involved, using pharmacological and other tools in existing or newly emerging animal models.

Although there is an explosion of interest in arterial stiffness with the use of the various animal models mentioned above for the moment, we do not have the exact genes involved in stiffness nor the molecular mechanisms implicated. Several candidate genes are given in another chapter of this book from human studies using modern techniques and very large cohorts. They have confirmed the implication of the renin-angiotensin-aldosterone system and brought to the surface other possible avenues of research, but these future genetic studies must be confirmed by new postgenomic experimental animal models using clear physiological hypotheses concerned with the role of these genes in arterial stiffness.

References

1. Safar ME, Levy BI, Struijker-Boudier H. Current perspectives on arterial stiffness and pulse pressure in hypertension and cardiovascular diseases. Circulation. 2003;107(22):2864–9.
2. Pinto YM, Paul M, Ganten D. Lessons from rat models of hypertension: from Goldblatt to genetic engineering. Cardiovasc Res. 1998;39(1):77–88.
3. Monassier L, Combe R, El Fertak L. Mouse models of hypertension. Drug Discov Today. 2006;3(3): 273–81.
4. Cvetkovic B, Sigmund CD. Understanding hypertension through genetic manipulation in mice. Kidney Int. 2000;57(3):863–74.
5. Amin M, Le VP, Wagenseil JE. Mechanical testing of mouse carotid arteries: from newborn to adult. J Vis Exp. 2012;60:e3733.
6. Sehgel N, Zhu Y, Sun Z, et al. Increased vascular smooth muscle cell stiffness: a novel mechanism for aortic stiffness in hypertension. Am J Physiol Heart Circ Physiol. 2013;305(9):H1281–7.
7. Meaume S, Benetos A, Henry OF, et al. Aortic pulse wave velocity predicts cardiovascular mortality in subjects >70 years of age. Arterioscler Thromb Vasc Biol. 2001;21(12):2046–50.
8. Milnor W. Properties of the vascular wall. In: Collins N, editor. Hemodynamics. Baltimore: Williams and Wilkins; 1989. p. 58–101.
9. Glaser E, Lacolley P, Boutouyrie P, et al. Dynamic versus static compliance of the carotid artery in living Wistar-Kyoto rats. J Vasc Res. 1995;32(4):254–65.
10. Hayoz D, Rutschmann B, Perret F, et al. Conduit artery compliance and distensibility are not necessarily reduced in hypertension. Hypertension. 1992; 20(1):1–6.
11. Lacolley P, Bezie Y, Girerd X, et al. Aortic distensibility and structural changes in sinoaortic-denervated rats. Hypertension. 1995;26(2):337–40.
12. Levy B. Mechanics of the large artery wall. In: Lévy BI, Tedgui A, editors. Biology of the arterial wall. Dordrecht: Kluwer; 1999. p. 13–24.
13. van Gorp AW, van Ingen Schenau DS, Hoeks AP, et al. Aortic wall properties in normotensive and hypertensive rats of various ages in vivo. Hypertension. 1995;26(2):363–8.
14. Ruiz-Feria CA, Yang Y, Thomason DB, et al. Pulse wave velocity and age- and gender-dependent aortic wall hardening in fowl. Comp Biochem Physiol A Mol Integr Physiol. 2009;154(4):429–36.
15. Bezie Y, Lamaziere JM, Laurent S, et al. Fibronectin expression and aortic wall elastic modulus in spontaneously hypertensive rats. Arterioscler Thromb Vasc Biol. 1998;18(7):1027–34.
16. Pauletto P, Scannapieco G, Vescovo G, et al. Catecholamine-induced cardiovascular disease in the spontaneously hypertensive and atherosclerotic turkey. Methods Find Exp Clin Pharmacol. 1988;10(6): 357–62.
17. Hadjiisky P, Bourdillon MC, Grosgogeat Y. Experimental models of atherosclerosis. Contribution, limits and trends. Arch Mal Coeur Vaiss. 1991;84(11): 1593–603.
18. Ng K, Hildreth CM, Phillips JK, et al. Aortic stiffness is associated with vascular calcification and remodeling in a chronic kidney disease rat model. Am J Physiol Renal Physiol. 2011;300(6):F1431–6.
19. Sloboda N, Feve B, Thornton SN, et al. Fatty acids impair endothelium-dependent vasorelaxation: a link between obesity and arterial stiffness in very old Zucker rats. J Gerontol A Biol Sci Med Sci. 2012;67(9):927–38.
20. Sista AK, O'Connell MK, Hinohara T, et al. Increased aortic stiffness in the insulin-resistant Zucker fa/fa rat. Am J Physiol Heart Circ Physiol. 2005;289(2): H845–51.
21. Isabelle M, Simonet S, Ragonnet C, et al. Chronic reduction of nitric oxide level in adult spontaneously hypertensive rats induces aortic stiffness similar to old spontaneously hypertensive rats. J Vasc Res. 2012; 49(4):309–18.
22. Qiu H, Zhu Y, Sun Z, Trzeciakowski JP, et al. Short communication: vascular smooth muscle cell stiffness as a mechanism for increased aortic stiffness with aging. Circ Res. 2010;107(5):615–9.
23. Cantini C, Kieffer P, Corman B, et al. Aminoguanidine and aortic wall mechanics, structure, and composition in aged rats. Hypertension. 2001;38(4):943–8.
24. Osborne-Pellegrin M, Labat C, Mercier N, et al. Changes in aortic stiffness related to elastic fiber network anomalies in the Brown Norway rat during maturation and aging. Am J Physiol Heart Circ Physiol. 2010;299(1):H144–52.
25. Basta G, Schmidt AM, De Caterina R. Advanced glycation end products and vascular inflammation: implications for accelerated atherosclerosis in diabetes. Cardiovasc Res. 2004;63(4):582–92.
26. Slove S, Lannoy M, Behmoaras J, et al. Potassium channel openers increase aortic elastic fiber formation and reverse the genetically determined elastin deficit in the BN rat. Hypertension. 2013;62(4): 794–801.

27. Dabire H, Lacolley P, Chaouche-Teyara K, et al. Relationship between arterial distensibility and low-frequency power spectrum of blood pressure in spontaneously hypertensive rats. J Cardiovasc Pharmacol. 2002;39(1):98–106.
28. Bouissou C, Lacolley P, Dabire H, et al. Increased stiffness and cell-matrix interactions of abdominal aorta in two experimental non-hypertensive models: long-term chemical sympathectomized and sinoaortic-denervated rats. J Hypertens. 2014;32:652–8.
29. Lacolley P, Glaser E, Challande P, et al. Structural changes and in situ aortic pressure-diameter relationship in long-term chemical-sympathectomized rats. Am J Physiol. 1995;269(2 Pt 2):H407–16.
30. Li ZY, Xu TY, Zhang SL, et al. Telemetric ambulatory arterial stiffness index, a predictor of cardio-cerebro-vascular mortality, is associated with aortic stiffness-determining factors. CNS Neurosci Ther. 2013;19(9): 667–74.
31. Cox RH. Basis for the altered arterial wall mechanics in the spontaneously hypertensive rat. Hypertension. 1981;3(4):485–95.
32. Ito H. Vascular connective tissue change in hypertension. In: Lee RE, editor. Blood vessel changes in hypertension: structure and function. Boca Raton: CRC Press; 1989. p. 99–122.
33. Cox RH. Mechanical properties of arteries in hypertension. In: Lee RMKW, editor. Blood vessel changes in hypertension: structure and function. Boca Raton: CRC Press; 1989.
34. Wagenseil JE, Mecham RP. Vascular extracellular matrix and arterial mechanics. Physiol Rev. 2009;89(3):957–89.
35. Wagenseil JE, Ciliberto CH, Knutsen RH, et al. Reduced vessel elasticity alters cardiovascular structure and function in newborn mice. Circ Res. 2009;104(10):1217–24.
36. Wan W, Yanagisawa H, Gleason Jr RL. Biomechanical and microstructural properties of common carotid arteries from fibulin-5 null mice. Ann Biomed Eng. 2010;38(12):3605–17.
37. Small J, North A. Architecture of the smooth muscle cell. In: Schwartz SM, Mecham RP, editors. The vascular smooth muscle cell. New York: Academic; 1995. p. 169–88.
38. Bezie Y, Lacolley P, Laurent S, et al. Connection of smooth muscle cells to elastic lamellae in aorta of spontaneously hypertensive rats. Hypertension. 1998; 32(1):166–9.
39. Clark JM, Glagov S. Structural integration of the arterial wall. I. Relationships and attachments of medial smooth muscle cells in normally distended and hyperdistended aortas. Lab Invest. 1979;40(5):587–602.
40. Osborne-Pellegrin MJ. Some ultrastructural characteristics of the renal artery and abdominal aorta in the rat. J Anat. 1978;125(Pt 3):641–52.
41. Galmiche G, Labat C, Mericskay M, et al. Inactivation of serum response factor contributes to decrease vascular muscular tone and arterial stiffness in mice. Circ Res. 2013;112(7):1035–45.
42. Retailleau K, Toutain B, Galmiche G, et al. Selective involvement of serum response factor in pressure-induced myogenic tone in resistance arteries. Arterioscler Thromb Vasc Biol. 2013;33(2):339–46.
43. Lacolley P, Challande P, Boumaza S, et al. Mechanical properties and structure of carotid arteries in mice lacking desmin. Cardiovasc Res. 2001;51(1): 178–87.
44. Benetos A, Pannier B, Brahimi M, et al. Dose-related changes in the mechanical properties of the carotid artery in WKY rats and SHR following relaxation of arterial smooth muscle. J Vasc Res. 1993; 30(1):23–9.
45. Fridez P, Zulliger M, Bobard F, et al. Geometrical, functional, and histomorphometric adaptation of rat carotid artery in induced hypertension. J Biomech. 2003;36(5):671–80.
46. Gabella G. Structural apparatus for force transmission in smooth muscles. Physiol Rev. 1984;64(2):455–77.
47. Ingber D. Integrins as mechanical transducers. Curr Opin Cell Biol. 1991;3(5):841–8.
48. Wilson E, Sudhir K, Ives HE. Mechanical strain of rat vascular smooth muscle cells is sensed by specific extracellular matrix/integrin interactions. J Clin Invest. 1995;96(5):2364–72.
49. Saouaf R, Takasaki I, Eastman E, et al. Fibronectin biosynthesis in the rat aorta in vitro. Changes due to experimental hypertension. J Clin Invest. 1991;88: 1182–9.
50. Boumaza S, Arribas SM, Osborne-Pellegrin M, et al. Fenestrations of the carotid internal elastic lamina and structural adaptation in stroke-prone spontaneously hypertensive rats. Hypertension. 2001;37(4):1101–7.
51. Zanchi A, Wiesel P, Aubert JF, et al. Time course changes of the mechanical properties of the carotid artery in renal hypertensive rats. Hypertension. 1997;29(5):1199–203.
52. Fitch RM, Vergona R, Sullivan ME, et al. Nitric oxide synthase inhibition increases aortic stiffness measured by pulse wave velocity in rats. Cardiovasc Res. 2001;51:351–8.
53. Kato H, Hou J, Chobanian AV, et al. Effects of angiotensin II infusion and inhibition of nitric oxide synthase on the rat aorta. Hypertension. 1996;28:153–8.
54. Labat C, Lacolley P, Lajemi M, et al. Effects of valsartan on mechanical properties of the carotid artery in spontaneously hypertensive rats under high-salt diet. Hypertension. 2001;38(3):439–43.
55. Mercier N, Labat C, Louis H, et al. Sodium, arterial stiffness, and cardiovascular mortality in hypertensive rats. Am J Hypertens. 2007;20(3):319–25.
56. Lacolley P, Labat C, Pujol A, et al. Increased carotid wall elastic modulus and fibronectin in aldosterone-salt-treated rats: effects of eplerenone. Circulation. 2002;106(22):2848–53.
57. Ammarguellat FZ, Gannon PO, Amiri F, et al. Fibrosis, matrix metalloproteinases, and inflammation in the heart of DOCA-salt hypertensive rats: role of ET(A) receptors. Hypertension. 2002;39(2 Pt 2): 679–84.

58. Cox RH. Effects of deoxycorticosterone on arterial wall properties in two-kidney rats. J Hypertens. 1986;4(5):557–65.
59. Takasaki I, Chobanian AV, Sarzani R, et al. Effect of hypertension on fibronectin expression in the rat aorta. J Biol Chem. 1990;265(35):21935–9.
60. Intengan HD, Schiffrin EL. Structure and mechanical properties of resistance arteries in hypertension: role of adhesion molecules and extracellular matrix determinants. Hypertension. 2000;36(3): 312–8.
61. Intengan HD, Schiffrin EL. Vascular remodeling in hypertension: roles of apoptosis, inflammation, and fibrosis. Hypertension. 2001;38(3 Pt 2):581–7.
62. Louis H, Kakou A, Regnault V, et al. Role of alpha1beta1-integrin in arterial stiffness and angiotensin-induced arterial wall hypertrophy in mice. Am J Physiol Heart Circ Physiol. 2007;293(4): H2597–604.
63. Mao X, Said R, Louis H, et al. Cyclic stretch-induced thrombin generation by rat vascular smooth muscle cells is mediated by the integrin αvβ3 pathway. Cardiovasc Res. 2012;96(3):513–23.
64. Et-Taouil K, Schiavi P, Lévy BI, et al. Sodium intake, large artery stiffness, and proteoglycans in the spontaneously hypertensive rat. Hypertension. 2001;38(5): 1172–6.
65. Gandley RE, McLaughlin MK, Koob TJ, et al. Contribution of chondroitin-dermatan sulfate-containing proteoglycans to the function of rat mesenteric arteries. Am J Physiol. 1997;273(2 Pt 2):H952–60.
66. Calvier L, Miana M, Rebou LP, et al. Galectin-3 mediates aldosterone-induced vascular fibrosis. Arterioscler Thromb Vasc Biol. 2013;33(1):67–75.
67. López-Andrés N, Calvier L, Labat C, et al. Absence of cardiotrophin 1 is associated with decreased age-dependent arterial stiffness and increased longevity in mice. Hypertension. 2013;61(1):120–9.
68. Nguyen Dinh Cat A, Griol-Charhbili V, Loufrani L, et al. The endothelial mineralocorticoid receptor regulates vasoconstrictor tone and blood pressure. FASEB J. 2010;24(7):2454–63.
69. Galmiche G, Pizard A, Gueret A, et al. Smooth muscle cell mineralocorticoid receptors are mandatory for aldosterone-salt to induce vascular stiffness. Hypertension. 2014;63:520–6.

Elastin, Calcium and Age-Related Stiffening of the Arterial Wall

7

Jeffrey Atkinson

Abstract

Mammals, and other vertebrates, adapted to aerobic life on land by developing a closed circulatory system, with separate low (for pulmonary function) and high (for renal and other functions) pressure components. The latter required a change from a low-pressure peristaltic to a high-pressure pulsatile, cardiac function. In this high-pressure system arteries near the heart damp the pulse pressure wave. Damping, which depends upon the visco-elastic properties of the arterial wall elastic fibres, ensures efficient coupling between the heart and the vascular system, reducing shear stress and thus promoting regular downstream flow.

The above system works efficiently in younger mammals. But, as in order to guarantee survival of the species, evolutionary pressure ensures systems' efficiency up to reproductive age – but not beyond, thus as mammals grow older, degenerative processes occur in key functional elements such as the scleroprotein elastin, an essential component of elastic fibres. This deterioration is the basis of many important pathological conditions in man such as stiffening of the arterial wall.

In this article we will examine how ageing can modify elastin and the role of calcification in this process, starting with a description of the organisation and function of elastin.

Keywords

Artery • Age • Mechanics • Stiffening • Calcium • Isolated • Systolic hypertension

Introduction

Mammals, and other vertebrates, adapted to aerobic life on land by developing a closed circulatory system, with separate low (for pulmonary function) and high (for renal and other functions) pressure components. The latter required

J. Atkinson, BA, MA, PhD
Cardiovascular Pharmacology Laboratory, Pharmacy Faculty, Nancy University, Lorraine University, 5 rue Albert Lebrun, Nancy 54000, France
e-mail: jeffrey.atkinson@univ-lorraine.fr

M.E. Safar et al. (eds.), *Blood Pressure and Arterial Wall Mechanics in Cardiovascular Diseases*, DOI 10.1007/978-1-4471-5198-2_7, © Springer-Verlag London 2014

a change from a low-pressure peristaltic to a high-pressure pulsatile, cardiac function. In this high-pressure system arteries near the heart damp the pulse pressure wave. Damping, which depends upon the visco-elastic properties of the arterial wall elastic fibres, ensures efficient coupling between the heart and the vascular system, reducing shear stress and thus promoting regular downstream flow [1].

The above system works efficiently in younger mammals. But, as in order to guarantee survival of the species, evolutionary pressure ensures systems' efficiency up to reproductive age – but not beyond, thus as mammals grow older, degenerative processes occur in key functional elements such as the scleroprotein elastin, an essential component of elastic fibres. This deterioration is the basis of many important pathological conditions in man such as stiffening of the arterial wall.

In this article we will examine how ageing can modify elastin and the role of calcification in this process, starting with a description of the organisation and function of elastin.

Organisation of Elastin and Elastic Fibres

Elastin is organised into an extracellular network of branched fibres. This filamentous aggregation is formed from the soluble precursor tropoelastin (rich in lysine) together with glycoprotein micro-fibrils such as fibrillin [2]. Lysyl oxidase converts lysine into a semi-aldehyde through condensation of aldehyde groups with other peptidyl aldehyde and amino groups giving rise to inter- and intra-molecular covalent cross-linkages essential for the formation of functional insoluble fibres [3]. Studies on the degree of lysyl oxidase-induced cross-linking, using chemical enzyme inhibition of lysyl oxidase or genetic modification, show that a certain degree of cross-linking is required in order to ensure correct mechanical functionality of elastin. The cross-linking amino acids of elastin formed by lysyl oxidase are desmosine, iso-desmosine and lysine-norleucine [4].

The parallel arrangement of a biological material with a relatively low elastic modulus, elastin (10^6 fold less than that of apatite [5]), together with a stiffer material, collagen, produces a curvilinear relationship between intraluminal pressure and diameter. The first part of the diameter/pressure curve is linear; at higher trans-mural pressure levels (>110–125 mmHg) the relationship becomes curvilinear as collagen fibres are recruited [6].

The properties of elastic fibres are not equivalent to those of elastin. Elastin is deposited on a scaffold of micro-fibrils (fibrillin and others) to form elastic fibres that are arranged in elastic lamellae separated by smooth muscle cells [7]. Lamellae are embedded in a viscous mucopolysaccharide ground substance which endows the wall with its visco-elastic behaviour.

Elastin mechanics depend on several factors. Upon stretching, the contact between hydrophobic amino acids and surrounding water increases such that the return to the original form is accompanied by an increase in entropy. The stretching and recoil is thus dependent on the hydration of elastin – dried elastin is brittle and will not stretch. The source of elastin's elasticity – as with other soft tissues – is a decrease in entropy with increasing strain [8]. Factors, such as changes in cross-linking or calcification that modify the decrease in entrophy with increasing strain, will change the mechanical behaviour of elastin.

Arterial wall elasticity is dependent on two factors, the first being the ratio of wall thickness to outer radius (h/Ro [9]). With ageing, arterial dilatation unaccompanied by the compensatory increase in wall thickness [10] transfers strain from elastin onto collagen and increases wall stiffness in the absence of any increase in trans-mural mean pressure. This, however, does not necessarily lead to a fall in arterial compliance as long as a fall in incremental volume occurs.

The second factor – that is independent of h/Ro and of pressure – relates to the proportions of elastin and collagen. The wall of the aortic arch is 70 % water, 1–2 % fat and 30–50 % scleroprotein; elastin represents 60 % of elastin + collagen. This percentage falls to 20–30 % in more distal arteries, and as the percentage of collagen increases so does wall stiffness.

These differences in the ratio of elastin to collagen adapt the arterial wall to local hemodynamic conditions, the distensible proximal aorta having a "*Windkessel*" function and the stiffer, more distal parts a "conduction" function.

Age-Related Quantitative Changes in Elastin and Stiffening of the Arterial Wall

Precise measurement of the wall content of insoluble extracellular matrix proteins is difficult. Thus, indisputable evidence of a net change in a wall component (elastin or any other), responsible for a change in wall mechanics, is difficult to obtain [11]. Arterial wall scleroprotein content can be determined by several methods such as histomorphometry following pressurized perfusion fixation and (more or less) selective staining [12], chemical digestion with isolation, and chemical determination of desmosine and isodesmosine following separation by capillary zone electrophoresis [13]. As these amino acids are essentially for the physiology of elastin, this method provides a measure of "functional" elastin.

Age-Related Changes in Elastin Cross-Linking and Stiffening of the Arterial Wall

As elastin is long-lived with a half-life of several years, age-related changes are generally qualitative [14] rather than quantitative. Qualitative changes involve changes in cross-linking.

Although an optimal degree of peri-natal cross-linking is essential for the physiological function of scleroproteins, age-related cross-linking (glycation, nitration) and calcification have a negative effect of scleroprotein mechanics. Bjorkstein and Champion, after noting that the tanning of a protein gel attenuated the amplitude of its rhythmical stretching, drew an analogy with arterial ageing and put forward the cross-linking hypothesis of ageing: that the formation of supernumerary cross-links leads to physio-pathological changes in scleroprotein function [15].

Many studies have reported an increase in elastin fibre fluorescence with age and related this to glycation and nitration. Bruel et al. [16] reported that the age-related increase in aortic stiffness in rats was associated with an accumulation of fluorescent material in elastin and suggested that this was due to the formation of advanced glycation end-products (AGEs, advanced Maillard products of the terminal phase of non-enzymatic browning). Caution should be used in the interpretation of the results of fluorescence studies. Many factors including dityrosine, products of lipid peroxidation and reactive carbonyl compounds and quinones modify elastin fluorescence. Elastin fluorescence can also be caused by the extraction procedure used. Albeit others have confirmed that elastin can incorporate glucose and ribose and form AGEs [17]. Furthermore "AGE breakers" such as aminoguanidine prevent arterial stiffening in ageing normotensive rats [18], although whether this and similar agents actually break pre-existing AGE cross-links is less certain [19].

Cross-linking can also be affected by nitrite. The nitrite ion reacts with tyrosine in elastin and this non-enzymatic nitration produces marked structural disruption [20]. The effect of this on vascular wall stiffness is not known in detail. However, nitrite effects on the arterial wall are complex. Short-term treatment (3 weeks) of old mice (26–28 months) with sodium nitrite ameliorated oxidative stress, decreased the AGE content of the aortic wall and lowered aortic pulse wave velocity [21].

Age-Related Calcification of Elastic Fibres

Calcification of arteries is a common phenomenon in the elderly. Aortic wall calcium content increases with age [22]. Age-linked medial calcification (elasto-calcinosis) collocates with elastic fibres [23].

Cross-linking may be involved in the calcification of elastin (elasto-calcinosis). Arterial calcification is common in diabetes involving processes such as glycation [24]. In the streptozotocin-induced diabetes rat model, glycation of elastin accelerates calcification [25]. This mechanism may be important in man as the AGE pentosidine collocates with both elastic fibres and calcium deposits in the aortic media of patients with end-stage renal disease [26] again suggesting that modification of elastin by the Maillard reaction is involved in calcification.

Hypertension, which is more prevalent in the elderly, increases intraluminal pressure so promoting elasto-calcinosis [27] suggesting that global degeneration of the arterial wall – of which elasto-calcinosis may be one facet – is due to the fatiguing effects of cyclic stress on medial elastic fibres followed by fracture [28]. As pulse pressure increases in hypertension (especially so in isolated systolic hypertension), cyclic wall stress is increased and so elasto-calcinosis and fracture of elastic fibres would be expected to occur earlier than in normotensive individuals. Other observations strengthen such a link between wall calcification and increased wall stiffness. Asymptomatic hypertensive patients with high aortic pulse wave velocity values show abdominal aortic calcifications [29]. It has been suggested that hypertension and vascular calcification form a vicious cycle with: (1) hypertension activating cellular and matrix remodelling, (2) leading to calcium deposition and elastic fibre fragmentation, (3) producing an increase in arterial wall stiffness, (4) promoting hypertension [30].

Elasto-calcinosis is part of a diffuse medial arteriosclerotic process that is distinct from a localised intimal atherosclerotic process. Diffuse medial elasto-calcinosis is probably a more significant determinant of increased arterial stiffness in ageing then atheroma as shown by the fact that aortic pulse wave velocity evolves in a similar fashion with age in populations with differing prevalence of atheroma [31].

Elasto-calcinosis is complex and involves both polar and apolar processes. The polar nature is suggested by the fact that most molecules regulating biological mineral formation are anionic and that this property facilitates the interaction between minerals and matrix elements [32]. As the calcium content of elastin increases so does that of the acidic groups (glutamic and aspartic acids [33]) and this increase in the base-binding capacity could explain the increase in calcium binding. Albeit, such a change in the primary structure of elastin is difficult to conceive as biochemical ageing of long-lived scleroproteins involves secondary post-synthetic modification. The paradoxical change in the primary structure of elastin may be explained by the accumulation with age of pseudo-elastin with a higher proportion of polar amino acids [34, 35].

Calcification may occur in an apolar environment [36] involving hydrophobic molecules such as cholesterol following lipid infiltration [37]. Cholesterol feeding in animals produces fatty streaks which accumulate calcium [38].

Elasto-calcinosis may be an active process as matrix vesicles similar to those seen in calcification of cartilage, bone and dentin, produced by arterial smooth muscle cells have been observed in wall calcification [39]. Elasto-calcinosis may depend on factors involved in bone formation [40] and other calcium-binding proteins [41] such as S-100 [42]. Circulating calcifying cells have been suggested as regulating the bone-vascular axis [43].

Marked vascular calcification occurs in chronic kidney disease and in this case vascular calcification can be considered as a systemic disease in which both bone and kidney contribute to calcium deposition with fibroblast growth factor 23 (that controls renal phosphate excretion) playing an active role [44]. The link between vascular calcification with elastin fibre degradation and increased aortic wall stiffness has been shown in animal models of chronic kidney disease such as the Lewis polycystic kidney rat model [45]. In this model the angiotensin I converting enzyme inhibitor, perindopril, diminished elasto-calcinosis, elastin degradation and wall stiffness [46].

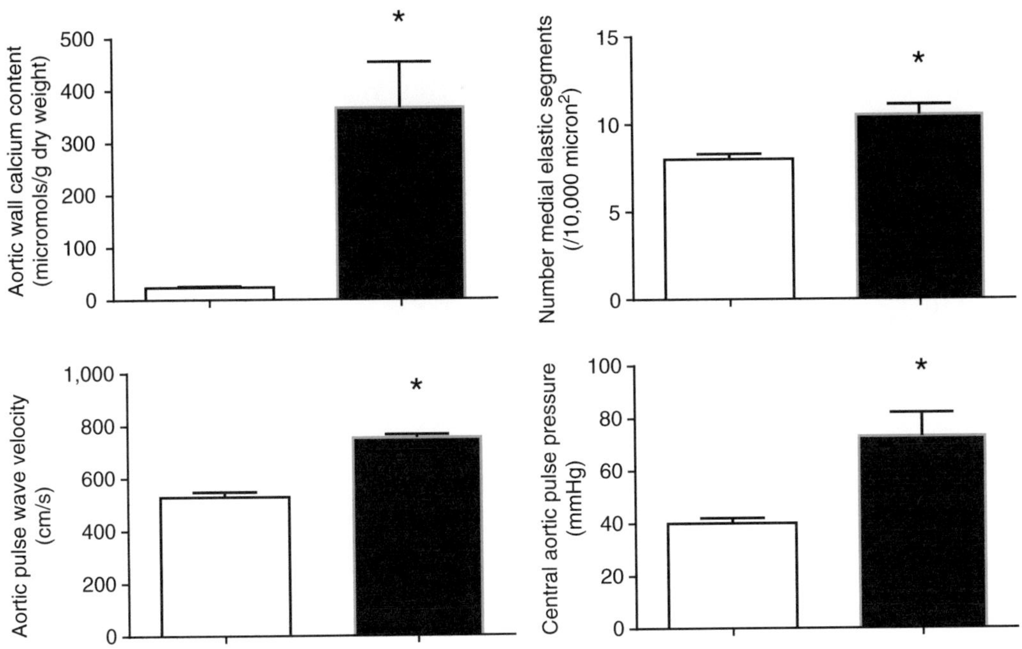

Fig. 7.1 Elasto-calcinosis and its consequences in the VDN rat model (for explanation see text)

An Animal Model of Elasto-Calcinosis

In man age-related elasto-calcinosis promotes a decrease in arterial elasticity. The time course of the increase in aortic wall stiffness [47] closely parallels the rise in medial calcification with age. More direct evidence for proof of the concept that elasto-calcinosis is an important aetiological factor in the development of fibre fragmentation followed by increased arterial wall stiffness has been obtained in animal models.

In "normal" ageing in the rat arterial calcification is not very marked and evolves slowly. Arteries contain up to five times more calcium than other soft tissues and calcify with age (2- to 3-fold) whereas the other soft tissues do not [48]. Calcium bound to elastin increases with age such that elasto-calcinosis and wall stiffness increase in parallel with age [49].

Marked elasto-calcinosis can be produced by hyper-vitaminosis D, alone or in combination with nicotine or cholesterol. Hyper-vitaminosis D plus nicotine (VDN) of the rat produces wall elasto-calcinosis of the same magnitude as that seen in elderly patients. VDN does not modify wall thickness, wall thickness to lumen ratio or wall stress but increases fragmentation of elastic fibres [50]; mean blood pressure remains at a normotensive level, animals suffer from isolated systolic hypertension with increased pulse pressure [51, 52]. VDN increases wall rigidity as shown by increased pulse wave velocity with no change in stroke volume, increased aortic impedance, decreased systemic arterial compliance, decreased *in situ* and *in vitro* carotid artery compliance, increased elastic modulus, increased isobaric elasticity, and decreased pulse amplification [53, 54]. Using confocal microscopy we showed that VDN produces fragmentation of the medial elastic network [55]. These results strongly suggest that elasto-calcinosis-induced damage of the aortic wall produces increased wall stiffness and elevated pulse pressure with isolated systolic hypertension (see Fig. 7.1). However, whilst the model is relevant in terms of phenomenology it is less so in terms of mechanism of production of calcification. In chronic kidney disease, for instance, vascular calcification is associated with vitamin D deficiency [56].

Perspectives

Given the resemblance between vascular calcification and processes occurring in bone, drugs used for the treatment of osteoporosis such as bisphosphonates may prove useful [57]. Certain vascular drugs such as angiotensin I converting enzyme inhibitors may also have their use. Modulation of enzymatic processes such as the activity of matrix metallo-proteinases may be another lead [58]. Such actions and drugs may be able to diminish evolving calcification; whether they can de-calcify calcified elastin is less certain.

References

1. Robert L, Birembaut P. La matrice extra-cellulaire de la paroi artérielle. In: Camillieri JP, Berry CL, Fiessinger JN, et al., editors. Les maladies de la paroi artérielle. Paris: Flammarion; 1987. p. p31–43.
2. Faury G, Pezet M, Knutsen R, et al. Development adaptation of the mouse cardiovascular system to elastin haplo-insufficiency. J Clin Investig. 2003; 112(9):1419–28.
3. Kagan JM, Reddy VB, Narasimhan NK, et al. Catalytic properties and structural component of lysyl oxidase. In: The molecular biology and pathology of elastic tissues. Chichester: Wiley; 1995. p. 100–21.
4. Robert L. Introduction. In: The molecular biology and pathology of elastic tissues. Chichester: Wiley; 1995. p. 1–3.
5. Withers PC. Circulation. In: Comparative animal physiology. Orlando: Saunders; 1992. p. 665–726.
6. Nichols WW, O'Rourke MF. Properties of the arterial wall: practice. In: Nichols WW, O'Rourke MF, editors. McDonald's blood flow in arteries. London: Arnold; 1998. p. 73–97.
7. Wolinsky H. Response of the rat aortic wall to hypertension: importance of comparing absolute amounts of wall components. Atherosclerosis. 1970;11:251–5.
8. Fung YC. Bioviscoelastic solids. In: Fung YC, editor. Biomechanics. Mechanical properties of living tissues. New York: Springer; 1993. p. 242–51.
9. Milnor WR. Properties of the vascular wall. In: Milnor WR, editor. Hemodynamics. Baltimore: Williams & Wilkins; 1989. p. 58–101.
10. Cantini C, Kieffer P, Corman B, et al. Aminoguanidine and aortic wall mechanics, structure and composition in aged rats. Hypertension. 2001;38:943–8.
11. Wolinsky H, Glagov S. Structural basis for the static mechanical properties of the aortic media. Circ Res. 1964;14:400–13.
12. Godeau G, Robert AM. Use of pycnogenols in the histological staining of elastic fibers and their quantification in several tissues by automated image analysis. In: Robert L, Hornebeck W, editors. Elastin and elastases, vol. 1. Boca Raton: CRC Press; 1991. p. 7–20.
13. Giummelly P, Botton B, Friot R, et al. Measurement of desmosine and isodesmosine by capillary zone electrophoresis. J Chromatogr A. 1995;710: 357–60.
14. Sell DR, Monnier VM. Aging of long-lived proteins: extracellular matrix (collagens, elastin and proteoglycans) and lens crystallin. In: Masoro EJ, editor. American physiological society handbook of physiology section 11 aging. New York: Oxford University Press; 1995. p. 235–305.
15. Bjorksten J, Champion WJ. Mechanical influence on tanning. J Am Chem Soc. 1942;64:868–9.
16. Bruel A, Oxlund H. Changes in biomechanical properties, composition of collagen and elastin and advanced glycation end products of the rat aorta in relation to age. Atherosclerosis. 1996;127:155–65.
17. Winlove CP, Parker KH, Avery NC, et al. Interactions of elastin and aorta with sugars in vitro and their effects on biochemical and physical properties. Diabetologia. 1996;39:1131–9.
18. Corman B, Duriez M, Poitevin P, et al. Aminoguandine prevents age-related arterial stiffening and cardiac hypertrophy. Proc Natl Acad Sci U S A. 1998;95: 1301–6.
19. Sell DR, Monnier VM. Molecular basis of arterial stiffening: role of glycation – a mini review. Gerontology. 2012;58:227–37.
20. Paik DC, Ramey WG, Dillon J, et al. The nitrite/elastin reaction: implications for in vivo degenerative effects. Connect Tissue Res. 1997;36(3):241–51.
21. Fleenor BS, Sindler AL, Eng JS, et al. Sodium nitrite de-stiffening of large elastic arteries with aging: role of normalization of advanced glycation end-products. Exp Gerontol. 2012;47:588–94.
22. Zinnser H, Butt EM, Leonard G. Metal content and correlation in aging aorta. J Am Geriatr Soc. 1957;5:20–6.
23. Blumenthal HT, Lansing AI, Wheeler PA. Calcification of the media of the human aorta and its relation to intimal arteriosclerosis, ageing and disease. Am J Pathol. 1944;20:665–79.
24. Fadini GP, Pauletto P, Avogaro A, et al. The good and the bad in the link between insulin resistance and vascular calcification. Atherosclerosis. 2007;193:241–4.
25. Tomizawa H, Yamazaki M, Kunika K, et al. Association of elastin glycation and calcium deposit in diabetic rat aorta. Diabetes Res Clin Pract. 1993;19:1–8.
26. Sakata N, Norma A, Yamamoto Y, et al. Modification of elastin by pentosidine is associated with calcification of aortic media in patients with end-stage renal disease. Nephrol Dial Transplant. 2003;18:1601–9.

27. Megnien JL, Simon A, Lemariey M, et al. Hypertension promotes coronary calcium deposit in asymptomatic men. Hypertension. 1996;27:949–54.
28. O'Rourke MF, Kelly R, Avolio A, et al. Implications of arterial pulsations. In: The arterial pulse. Philadelphia: Lea & Febiger; 1992. p. 228–32.
29. Simon A, Levenson J. Early detection of subclinical atherosclerosis in asymptomatic subjects at high risk for cardiovascular disease. Clin Exp Hypertens. 1993;15:1069–76.
30. Rattazzi M, Bertacco E, Puato M, et al. Hypertension and vascular calcification: a vicious cycle? J Hypertens. 2012;30:1885–983.
31. Avolio AP, Chen SC, Wang RP, et al. Effects of aging on changing arterial compliance and left ventricular load in a northern Chinese urban community. Circulation. 1983;68:50–8.
32. Boskey AL. Matrix protein and mineralization: an overview. Connect Tissue Res. 1996;35:357–63.
33. Lansing AI, Ales M, Rosenthal TB. Calcium and elastin in human arteriosclerosis. J Gerontol. 1949;5:12–9.
34. Hall DA. The ageing of connective tissue. Symp Soc Exp Biol. 1967;21:101–25.
35. Keeley FW, Partridge SM. Amino acid composition and calcification of human aortic elastin. Atherosclerosis. 1974;19:287–96.
36. Urry DW. Molecular perspectives of vascular wall structure and disease: the elastic component. Perspect Biol Med. 1978;21:265–95.
37. Hornbeck W, Partridge SM. Conformational changes in fibrous elastin due to calcium ions. Eur J Biochem. 1975;51:73–8.
38. Kramsch DM, Aspen AJ, Aspen CS. Suppression of experimental atherosclerosis by the Ca antagonist lanthanum. J Clin Invest. 1980;65:967–81.
39. Tanimura A, McGregor DH, Anderson HC. Matrix vesicles in atherosclerotic calcification. Proc Soc Exp Biol Med. 1983;172:173–7.
40. Doherty TM, Detrano RC. Coronary elastocalcinosis as an active process: a new perspective on an old problem. Calcif Tissues Int. 1994;54:224–30.
41. Elliot RJ, McGrath LT. Calcification of the human thoracic aorta during aging. Calcif Tissues Int. 1994;54:268–73.
42. Bobryshev YV, Lord RSA. Detection of vascular dendritic cells and extracellular calcium-binding protein S-100 in foci of calcification in human arteries. Acta Histochem Cytochem. 1995;28:371–80.
43. Fadini GP, Rattazzi M, Matsumoto T, et al. Emerging role of circulating calcifying cells in the bone-vascular axis. Circulation. 2012;125:2722–81.
44. Zoppellaro G, Faggin E, Puato M, et al. Fibroblast growth factor 23 and the bone-vascular axis: lessons learned from animal studies. Am J Kidney Dis. 2012;59:135–44.
45. Ng K, Hildreth CM, Phillips K, et al. Aortic stiffness is associated with vascular calcification and remodelling in a chronic kidney disease rat model. Am J Physiol. 2011;300:F1431–6.
46. Ng K, Hildreth CM, Avolio AP, et al. Angiotensin-converting enzyme inhibitor limits pulse-wave velocity and aortic calcification in a rat model of cystic renal disease. Am J Physiol. 2011;301: F959–66.
47. Wilens SL. The post-mortem elasticity of the adult aorta. Its relation to age and to distribution of intimal atheromas. Am J Pathol. 1937;13:811–34.
48. Kieffer P, Robert A, Capdeville-Atkinson C, et al. Age-related arterial calcification in rats. Life Sci. 2000;66(24):2371–81.
49. Michel JB, Heudes D, Michel O, et al. Effect of chronic ANG I-converting enzyme inhibition on aging processes. II. Large arteries. Am J Physiol. 1994;267:R124–35.
50. Gaillard V, Casellas D, Seguin-Devaux C, et al. Pioglitazone improves aortic wall elasticity in a rat model of elastocalcinotic arteriosclerosis. Hypertension. 2005;46:372–9.
51. Niederhoffer N, Lartaud-Idjouadiene I, Giummelly P, et al. Calcification of medial elastic fibres and aortic elasticity. Hypertension. 1997;29:999–1006.
52. Niederhoffer N, Bobryshev YV, Lartaud-Idjouadiene I, et al. Aortic calcification produced by vitamin D plus nicotine. J Vasc Res. 1997;34:386–98.
53. Atkinson J, Poitevin P, Chillon JM, et al. Vascular Ca overload produced by vitamin D3 plus nicotine diminishes arterial distensibility in rats. Am J Physiol. 1994;266:H540–7.
54. Tatchum-Talom R, Niederhoffer N, Amin F, et al. Aortic stiffness and left ventricular mass in a rat model of isolated systolic hypertension. Hypertension. 1995;26:963–70.
55. Giummelly P, Colas T, Atkinson J, et al. Fluorescence of the medial aortic elastic lamella in elastocalcinotic rats. Naynyn Schemiedebergs Arch Pharmacol. 1998;358:R218.
56. Lee SY, Kim HY, Gu SW, et al. 25-hydroxyvitamin D levels and vascular calcification in predialysis and dialysis patients with chronic kidney disease. Kidney Blood Press Res. 2012;35:349–54.
57. Karwowski W, Naumnik B, Szczepanski M, et al. The mechanism of vascular calcification – a systematic review. Med Sci Monit. 2012;18:R1–11.
58. Bennett BJ, Scatena M, Kirk EA, et al. Osteoprotegerin inactivation accelerates advanced atherosclerotic lesion progression and calcification in older ApoE$^{-/-}$ mice. Arterioscler Thromb Vasc Biol. 2006;26:2117–24.

Genetic and Cellular Aspects of Arterial Stiffness

8

Athanase Benetos, Abraham Aviv, Patrick Lacolley, Michel E. Safar, and Véronique Regnault

Abstract

Increases in arterial stiffness and pulse pressure are typical features of the arterial stiffness during aging and are associated with increased risk of cardiovascular complications. Cellular and molecular determinants of arterial stiffness have not been completely elucidated. Clinically, the carotid-femoral pulse wave velocity (PWV) is the gold standard parameter of arterial stiffness. A recent genome-wide scan of the Framingham Heart Study population has shown that arterial stiffness and mean and pulsatile components of blood pressure are heritable and map to separate the genetic loci in humans, suggesting that distinct genes may modulate these two phenotypes. This chapter details the recent knowledge on the influence of genetic determinants and telomere length on the development of age-related phenotypes. Recent genetic studies have revealed specific genes contributing to arterial stiffening. Available data on genome-wide association (GWA) have been initiated on PWV and have identified common genetic variation in specific loci or single-nucleotide polymorphisms (SNP) significantly associated with PWV. Telomere length at birth is strongly determined genetically and is the main determinant of

A. Benetos, MD, PhD (✉)
Department of Geriatrics, University Hospital of Nancy, Université De Lorraine,
1, allée du Morvan, Vandoeuvre Les Nancy 54500, France

INSERM, U1116, Université de Lorraine, Nancy, France
e-mail: a.benetos@chu-nancy.fr

A. Aviv, MD, PhD
Center of Human Development and Aging Rutgers, The State University of New Jersey, New Jersey Medical School, 185 South Orange Avenue, Newark, NJ 07103, USA
e-mail: avivab@njms.rutgers.edu

P. Lacolley, MD, PhD • V. Regnault, PhD
Unité INSERM U1116, Université de Lorraine, Faculté de Médecine, 9 avenue de la foret de Haye, 54500 Vandoeuvre Les Nancy, France
e-mail: patrick.lacolley@inserm.fr; veronique.regnault@inserm.fr

M.E. Safar, MD
Department of Medicine, Paris Descartes University, Assistance Publique des Hôpitaux de Paris, Hôtel-Dieu Hospital, Diagnosis and Therapeutic Center,
1, place du Parvis Notre-Dame, Paris 75004, France
e-mail: michel.safar@htd.apjp.fr

M.E. Safar et al. (eds.), *Blood Pressure and Arterial Wall Mechanics in Cardiovascular Diseases*,
DOI 10.1007/978-1-4471-5198-2_8,

leukocytes' telomere length (LTL) later in life. Short LTL is associated with increased risk of stiffness and atherosclerosis of the carotid artery, atherosclerotic heart disease, and diminished survival in the elderly.

Keywords
Genetics • Telomere • pulse wave velocity • Arteries • Elasticity, arterial aging

Abbreviations

GWA	Genome-wide association
HPC	Hematopoietic progenitor cell
HSC	Hematopoietic stem cells
LTL	Leukocyte telomere length
PP	Pulse pressure
PWV	Pulse wave velocity
SNPs	Single-nucleotide polymorphisms

Introduction

During the past 10–15 years, modern-era genetics and related molecular biology have progressed rapidly in the field of arterial stiffness. This chapter will focus primarily on telomere length as a real determinant of arterial aging and panels of single-nucleotide polymorphisms (SNPs) covering the whole genome and their incorporation into high-density genotyping microarrays to perform genome-wide association (GWA) studies to investigate the genetic component of quantitative traits of arterial stiffness.

Stiffening of the large arteries leads to an increase in pulse wave velocity (PWV) and pulse pressure (PP). Both of these features of arterial stiffness have independent predictive value for total and cardiovascular (CV) mortality, coronary morbidity and mortality, and fatal stroke in various groups of patients [1–3].

The growing prevalence and associated risk of arterial stiffness provide a substrate to better understand the underlying genetic causes and the resultant physiological impact of this condition. Initially, genetic studies focused on the association between arterial stiffness parameters and common polymorphisms in single candidate genes. Then, genome-wide linkage studies permitted the identification of chromosomal regions associated with arterial stiffness, without relying on any prior biological hypothesis. GWA studies have been recently applied to arterial stiffness parameters. These studies were also conducted using PP as the quantitative trait, which represents an approximation of large-artery stiffness. These approaches provide a rich resource for the future discovery of new causes and mechanisms of disease and open new attractive targets for pharmacological approaches. Among the genetic and molecular factors, telomere dynamics may be a significant determinant of the paces of arterial aging [4, 5]. Telomeres are noncoding double-stranded repetitive structures at the ends of mammalian chromosomes that form protective caps at the ends of eukaryotic chromosomes. They safeguard the ends of chromosomes, maintain genomic integrity, and play a crucial role in replicative senescence. Short LTL is associated with increased risk of stiffness and atherosclerosis of the carotid artery, atherosclerotic heart disease, and diminished survival in the elderly. Telomere length at birth, which is strongly determined genetically, seems to be the main determinant of LTL later in life. Therefore telomere length is a parameter determined early in life with a possible impact on the development of stiffness during aging.

The Possible Role of Telomeres in the Age-Related Arterial Lesions

Telomere Length and Arterial Aging

Telomeres are essential in protecting the terminal ends of chromosomes [4–6]. These noncoding repetitive DNA sequences (TTAGGG) located, as their name indicates, at the ends of chromosomes play a crucial role in cellular replicative capacity and in chromosome stability. Telomere length is genetically determined at birth, decreasing thereafter with age. The reduction in telomere size is due to the fact that during cellular replication, the DNA located at the extreme ends of chromosomes is not replicated, leading to telomere attrition. A reverse transcriptase, telomerase, is capable of adding TTAGGG sequences at the ends of chromosomes and thus offset telomere attrition. Telomerase is active in both embryonic and germ cells, whereas in adult somatic cells in culture, telomerase activity is low or even nonexistent. Short telomeres have consequences on chromosome integrity, chromatin stability, and cellular replicative capacities, the final result being the cessation of cellular replication and cell death [4]. Consequently, telomere length is both an indicator of "the life" of the cell and its future. In humans, telomere length is considered as an indicator of biological age, and although this biological age is largely associated with chronological age, other factors can accelerate the reduction in telomere length [4, 5].

The most powerful factor in the loss of DNA bases by replication is the level of oxidative stress. Indeed, one of the predominant assumptions in the field of aging is that it may be the result of the lifelong accumulation of lesions and that these lesions are essentially due to the actions of chronic inflammation and reactive oxygen species – ROS – at the cellular and tissular level. Chronic inflammation and oxidative stress are evidently major factors of aging-related vascular injury, leading to atherosclerosis and arterial stiffness.

Clinical studies have shown that individuals with shorter telomeres exhibited more frequent manifestations of arterial aging along with increased CV risk [4, 6–10]. LTL is inversely correlated with PP and carotid-femoral PWV [8], both indexes of aortic stiffness. Also, telomere length was shorter in patients with atherosclerotic coronary heart disease [4, 9] and in hypertensives with carotid artery plaques than in their age-matched peers [10]. Type 2 diabetes with microalbuminuria was found to be associated with increased oxidative stress, shorter telomere length, and accrued arterial stiffness [11].

Nevertheless, there is currently an open debate as to whether shorter telomeres increase the risk of developing atherothrombosis or to whether short telomeres are the consequence of increased oxidative stress and the inflammatory condition that are part of the atherothrombotic process. It is therefore important to understand whether LTL at a given age depends mainly on the LTL at birth or to the telomeric attrition during life.

Respective Roles of LTL at Birth and Telomere Attrition During Adulthood in the Determination of LTL (Fig. 8.1)

At a given age, telomere length essentially depends on their initial size at birth and the chronic effects of oxidative stress. In vitro studies show that increased oxidative stress is likely responsible for a higher rate of telomere attrition. However, the role of oxidative stress on telomere regulation in vivo remains poorly understood.

At Birth, TL Shows Characteristics

- *Large interindividual variation in HSC-TL is present at birth.* LTL, and by inference HSC-TL, is highly heritable [12] and shows a wide range of variation among newborns (5 kbp). This variation largely holds in adults, and it might stem in large measure from genetic factors. In fact, recent GWA studies have identified several genes explaining inter-individual variation in LTL in the general population [13].
- *Low inter-tissues variations in the same individual.* In the human fetus and newborn, TL is largely equivalent in all somatic tissues [14]. The inter-tissue equivalence at birth is due in part to the activity of telomerase, which counteracts TL shortening resulting from cell replication during early intrauterine growth.

Telomere Attrition in Extrauterine Life: The Role of Body Growth

Telomerase activity is largely repressed in somatic tissues during extrauterine life, although it is not totally abolished in somatic stem and progenitor cells. However, such activity is not sufficient to prevent TL shortening during replication. Hence, TL varies across somatic tissues in

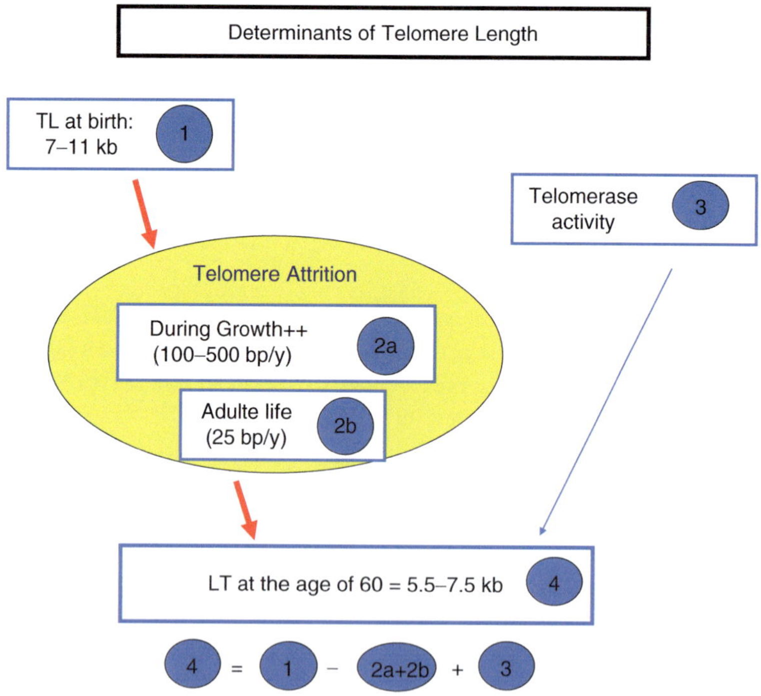

Fig. 8.1 Determinants of leukocyte telomere length (LTL) at the adult life (*4*). At a given age, LTL depends on LTL at birth (*1*) minus the attrition during extrauterine life (*2*). Attrition is much higher during the first years of life (2a > 100 bases/year), dropping during adult life (2b = 20–30 bases/year). Telomerase activity (*3*) contributes very little in most somatic cells

proportion to replicative activity. Notably, LTL, and by inference HSC-TL, is shorter than TLs of minimally proliferative somatic tissues. Yet, the available data from human studies point to strong correlations in TL across somatic tissues, that is, individuals with long (or short) TL in one tissue also have long (or short) TL in other tissues. This "synchrony" in TL across somatic tissues has been observed not only in humans [13, 14] but also in other mammals [15]. Epidemiological reports on age-dependent attrition in TL are based primarily on studies of leukocytes. These studies suggest that the rate of age-dependent LTL shortening is rapid early in life but slows down during adulthood [16], findings that also apply to nonhuman primates. In humans, HSC-TL shortens by approximately 3,000 bp during the first 20 years of life. This massive TL attrition is largely attributed to the expansion of the HSC, and hematopoietic progenitor cell (HPC) pools in tandem with body growth. Thus by the end of the second decade, the difference between LTL and TL in the skeletal muscle, a minimally proliferative tissue, is ~1.5 kbp. Such a difference is largely related to the higher pace of replication of HSCs to expand the HSC and HPC pools [17] in order to accommodate the tremendous turnover rate of blood cells during growth and development and also later in life.

Telomere Attrition During Adult Life

LTL attrition in the course of adult life is estimated at around 25–30 bp/year, which means a total average of 2,000 bp LTL shortening during adult life for an individual reaching the age of 80 years. Several factors have been shown to affect LTL attrition during aging. Smoking, high body mass index [18], and nutritional factors (high-fat, low-fiber diets) have been shown in some studies to be associated with a shorter LTL. The common denominator for these factors associated with a shorter LTL is that they promote inflammation and/or increase oxidative stress, both of which accelerate telomere attrition during cell replications [19]. As we mentioned earlier in this paper, short telomeres have been associated with chronic inflammation probably because inflammation and oxidative stress heighten the rate of telomere attrition. However, the relative contribution of these factors to the overall LTL is relatively small compared to LTL at birth and attrition during the first two decades of life. Further support for this idea comes from our recent longitudinal study, showing that the individual's LTL ranking in relation to his/her peers during adult life is essentially fixed, meaning that having a short or a long LTL is determined prior to adulthood [20]. Moreover, we have shown in a recent study [21] that the difference in TL between leukocytes, representing the highly proliferative hematopoietic system, and the skeletal muscle is established during the two decades of life, suggesting that the bulk of LTL shortening occurs during this time period.

Telomere Length, a Determinant of Repair Capacity of the Endothelial Cells

There is recent evidence that short TL not only is a marker of chronic inflammation and oxidative stress but may also play an active role in the genesis of age-related CV disease because of impaired vascular repair [22]. Compromised ability to repair the vasculature might contribute to diminished survival in the elderly because CV disease, principally atherosclerosis, is the main cause of death in the elderly in modern societies. We propose that TL imposes a limit on HSC-mediated vascular repair. Thus, a shorter leukocyte TL (LTL) denotes diminished HSC-mediated vascular repair capacity.

Genetics of Arterial Stiffness: The Genotype/Phenotype Approach

Since the first study showing the influence of the 1166 A/C polymorphism of the angiotensin II type 1 receptor gene (*AGTR1*) on the regulation of aortic stiffness in hypertensive subjects [23], several studies support a genetic contribution to arterial stiffness with heritability estimates varying from 0.21 to 0.66. Existing genome-wide studies have pointed to distinct chromosomal regions of significant linkage for PP, and genetic association studies have identified a significant number of candidate genes and gene polymorphisms which could modulate arterial stiffness (Table 8.1). We do not focus on candidate gene polymorphisms since these first genetic approaches were previously reviewed. They have led to the exploration of numerous genes affecting the renin-angiotensin-aldosterone system, elastic fiber structural components, metalloproteinases, and the NO pathway. This strategy has provided many interesting results but, to date, only *CYP11B2* and *NOS3* have been confirmed by genome-wide linkage studies as being associated with arterial stiffness. Because arterial stiffness and PP are common complex traits influenced by genomic and environmental factors, GWA studies represent now the most relevant genetic approaches.

In 2001, Atwood et al. [24] found for the first time in a population-based sample four distinct chromosomal regions showing suggestive linkage (logarithm of the odds [LOD] scores >1.9) for PP. The analyses of Camp et al. [25], DeStefano et al. [26], Bielinski et al. [27], and Franceschini et al. [28] confirmed and extended these results. Using multivariate linkage analysis, Turner et al. [29] have identified more statistically significant genetic loci for PP associated with coronary artery calcifications. The demonstration of linkage regions for carotid-femoral PWV was given by the Framingham Heart Study. Potential candidate genes in these regions included the insulin-like growth factor-1 receptor (*IGF1R*), myocyte-specific enhancer factor 2A (*MEF2A*), chondroitin synthase (*CHSY1*), pro-protein convertases (*PACE4* and *FURIN*), β-adducin (*ADD2*), neurokinin-1 receptor (*TACR1*), α-2B adrenergic receptor (*ADRA2B*), and interleukin-6 (*IL6*). *IGF1R*, *MEF2A*, *CHSY1*, and *PACE4* genes had been previously reported as candidate genes for PP in the larger study by DeStefano et al. [26]. The aldosterone synthase (*CYP11B2*) gene was not associated with arterial stiffness and PP in these latter studies although it was identified as a candidate gene in the initial study of Atwood et al. [24].

Contemporary studies are now focusing on analysis of GWA, using dense panels of common

Table 8.1 Genome-wide association for pulse pressure and pulse wave velocity

Population	Number of individuals	Age (years)	Parameter measured	Marker or locus	Candidate gene	Type of association	Reference
San Antonio Family Heart Study (SAFHS)	441	40–60	PP	D7S1799, LOD = 2.04	No information	Suggestive	Atwood et al. [24]
				D8S1100, LOD = 1.98	Aldosterone synthase gene (*CYP11B2*)		
				D18S844, LOD = 1.95	No information		
				D21S1440, LOD = 2.78	No information		
Utah pedigrees	1,454	27.8 ± 18.2	PP	D8S1048, LOD = 2.89	No information	Suggestive	Camp et al. [25]
				PAH, LOD = 2.59	No information		
Framingham Heart Study	1,584	47.5 ± 8.8	PP	Chr 5 at 53 cM, LOD = 2.03	Growth hormone receptor gene (*GHR*)	Suggestive	DeStefano et al. [26]
				Chr 7 at 71 cM, LOD = 2.42, and at 152 cM, LOD = 1.54	Insulinlike growth factor binding protein 1 and 3 genes (*IGFBP1* and *IGFBP3*)		
				Chr 8 at 140 cM, LOD = 1.56	Aldosterone synthase gene (*CYP11B2*) and 11 β-hydroxylase gene (*CYP11B1*)		
				Chr 10 at 81 cM, LOD = 1.83	No information		
				Chr 15 at 122 cM, LOD = 2.94	Insulinlike growth factor-1 receptor		
				Chr 22 at 36 cM, LOD = 1.75	*IGF1R*; myocyte-specific enhancer Factor 2A (*MEF2A*); chondroitin Synthase (*CHSY1*); secretory proprotein convertase (*PACE4*)		
Family blood pressure program (FBPP)	10,798	13–93	PP	D2S1384, LOD = 2.2	No information	Suggestive	Bielinski et al. [27]
				D18S851, LOD = 3.2	No information	Significant	
				D21S2052, LOD = 2.1	No information	Suggestive	

Framingham Offspring Study	590	58 ± 10	CFPWV	Chr 2 at 94 cM, LOD = 2.46	β-adducin (*ADD2*); neurokinin-1 receptor (*TACR1*); α-2B adrenergic receptor (*ADRA2B*)	Suggestive	Mitchell et al. [40]
			Central PP	Chr 7 at 29 cM, LOD = 2.50	Interleukin-6 (*IL6*)		
				Chr 13 at 108 cM, LOD = 2.10	No information		
				Chr 15 at 108 cM, LOD = 2.48	Insulinlike growth factor-1 receptor gene (*IGF1R*); myocyte-specific enhancer factor 2A (*MEF2A*); chondroitin synthase (*CHSY1*); related		
				Chr 15 at 122 cM, LOD = 2.92	Proprotein convertases (*PACE4* and *FURIN*)		
				Chr 7 at 172 cM, LOD = 2.85	No information		
				Chr 9 at 160 cM, LOD = 2.72	No information		
Genetic Epidemiology Network of Arteriopathy (GENOA) of the FBPP	488	64.7 ± 7.5	PP	Chr 7 at 79 cM, LOD = 1.70	No information	Suggestive	Turner et al. [41]
				Chr 11 at 17 cM, LOD = 3.02	Insulin (*INS*); calcitonin gene-related peptide (*CALC*); adrenomedullin (*ADM*)	Significant	
GENOA of the FBPP	948	59.6 ± 9.9	PP	Chr 7 at 85 cM, LOD = 3.03	Insulinlike growth factor binding protein 1 and 3 (*IGFBP1* and *IGFBP3*)	Significant	Turner et al. [29]
Strong Heart Family Study	1,892	14–93	PP	D7S493, LOD = 3.3	Interleukin-6 (*IL6*) and neuropeptide Y (*NPY*)	Significant	Franceschini et al. [28]
				D19S888, LOD = 1.8	Kallikrein 1 (*KLK1*)	Suggestive	

(continued)

Table 8.1 (continued)

Population	Number of individuals	Age (years)	Parameter measured	Marker or locus	Candidate gene	Type of association	Reference
Framingham Offspring Study	644	28–62	CFPWV	rs770189	Myocyte-specific enhancer factor 2C (*MEF2C*)	Suggestive	Levy et al. [30]
				rs10514688	No information		
				rs7042864	No information		
				rs10506440	Ubiquitin-specific peptidase 15 (*USP15*)		
				rs1349721	Rho GTPase-activating protein 24 (*ARHGAP24*)		
				rs3001450	WNK lysine-deficient protein kinase 2 (*WNK2*)		
				rs1389608	No information		
				rs1367248	Contactin-associated protein-like 5 (*CNTNAP5*)		
				sr10521232	Heparan sulfate (glucosamine) 3-O-sulfotransferase 3A1 (*HS3ST3A1*)		
				rs2717594	Aldosterone synthase gene (*CYP11B2*)		
				rs3910046	Nuclear receptor subfamily 3, group C, member 2 (*NR3C2*)		
Samoan Islands	71	44 ± 17	PP	D22S423, LOD = 2.2	No information	Suggestive	Aberg et al. [42]
SardiNIA Study	4,221	14–102	PWV	rs3742207	Collagen type IV alpha 1 (*COL4A1*)		Tarasov et al. [33]
				rs1495448	Membrane-associated guanylate kinase, WW and PDZ domain containing 1 (*MAGI1*)		
San Antonio Family Heart Study	357	19–85	PP	Chr 1 at 200 cM, LOD = 3.82	Selectin genes (*SELP*, *SELL*, *SELF*)	Significant	Kochunov et al. [43]
					Coagulation factor V (*F5*)		
Hypertensive Genetic Epidemiology (HyperGEN) of the FBPP	2,505	50 ± 15	PP	rs898164	No information	Significant	Simino et al. [44]
				rs2876587	No information		
				rs6935795	No information		

Qingdao Twin Registry	630	37 ± 9	PP	rs11603765	No information	Significant	Zhang et al. [45]
				rs2085866	No information		
				rs2576052	No information		

PP indicates pulse pressure, *CFPWV* carotid-femoral pulse wave velocity, *Chr* chromosome

SNPs. They were performed for carotid-femoral PWV or other individual arterial stiffness tonometry phenotypes (carotid-brachial PWV, forward and reflected pressure waves, and mean arterial pressure).

The first study by Levy et al. [30] has identified some interesting candidate genes: myocyte enhancer factor 2C (*MEF2C*), spectrin repeat containing, nuclear envelope 1 (*SYNE1*), tumor necrosis factor ligand superfamily, member 11 (*TNFSF11*), collagen type VIII α1 (*COL8A1*), and transforming growth factor β receptor II (*TGFBR2*). In addition, lysyl oxidase-like 2 (*LOXL2*) involved in extracellular matrix protein cross-linking was also an attractive candidate gene considering the five tonometry phenotypes. On a functional point of view, this latter gene may be linked to those expressed differently by gene expression profiling (integrins, cytoskeleton proteins) between stiff and distensible aortas from patients with coronary heart disease [31, 32]. Further studies have been performed since 2009 using GWAS, and results are summarized in Table 8.1. Some genes appear to be involved in the pathophysiology of arterial stiffness, in particular collagen type IV α1 (*COL4A1*) [33], PR domain containing 6 (*PRDM6*), and selectin genes (*SELP*, *SELL*, and *SELE*) for smooth muscle cell phenotypic regulation and endothelial function. Other PP-associated variants came out from the meta-analysis of Wain et al. [34] for fidgetin (*FIGN*), cysteine-rich hydrophobic domain 2 (*CHIC2*), phosphatidylinositol-4,5-bisphosphate 3-kinase, catalytic subunit gamma (*PIK3CG*), nephroblastoma overexpressed (*NOV*), and ADAM metallopeptidase with thrombospondin type 1 motif, 8 (*ADAMTS8*) involved in platelet aggregation, inflammation, angiogenesis, or cell growth. Interesting meta-analyses resolve the existing evidence on regions linked to PP [34–38]. Finally, Mitchell et al. [39] from the AortaGen Consortium show common genetic variation in a locus in the B-cell CLL/lymphoma 11B (*BCL11B*) gene desert associated with carotid-femoral PWV and expressed in human aorta to regulate the development of the heart and large vessels.

The Perspectives of the Genotype/Phenotype Approach

In recent years, the explosion of genetic studies has revealed several significant associations but has failed to identify any new specific molecular mechanisms of arterial stiffness, probably mainly because of its multifactorial etiology. It appears now that pertinent studies should have only been realized in very large populations with standardized methods for arterial stiffness determination. Similar procedures have been set up for establishment of reference values of PWV and arterial wall thickness from a European consortium.

The biggest challenge for the future will be to follow genetic analysis by a post-genomic approach, which has never been performed in terms of pathophysiology of arterial stiffness.

References

1. Benetos A, Safar M, Rudnichi A, Smulyan H, Richard J-L, Ducimetiere P, Guize L. Pulse pressure: a predictor of long term cardiovascular mortality in a French male population. Hypertension. 1997;30:1410–5.
2. Laurent S, Boutouyrie P, Lacolley P. Structural and genetic bases of arterial stiffness. Hypertension. 2005;45(6):1050–5.
3. Zieman SJ, Melenovsky V, Kass DA. Mechanisms, pathophysiology, and therapy of arterial stiffness. Arterioscler Thromb Vasc Biol. 2005;25(5):932–43.
4. Aviv A. Genetics of leukocyte telomere length and its role in atherosclerosis. Mutat Res. 2012;730(1–2): 68–74.
5. Chang E, Harley CB. Telomere length and replicative aging in human vascular tissues. Proc Natl Acad Sci U S A. 1995;92:11190–4.
6. Aviv A, Levy D, Mangel M. Growth, telomere dynamics and successful and unsuccessful human aging. Mech Ageing Dev. 2003;124:829–37.
7. Cawthon RM, Smith KR, O'Brien E, Sivatchenko A, Kerber RA. Association between telomere length in blood and mortality in people aged 60 years or older. Lancet. 2003;361:393–5.
8. Benetos A, Okuda K, Lajemi M, et al. Telomere length as an indicator of biological aging: the gender effect and relation with pulse pressure and pulse wave velocity. Hypertension. 2001;37:381–5.
9. Brouilette S, Singh RK, Thompson JR, Goodall AH, Samani NJ. White cell telomere length and risk of premature myocardial infarction. Arterioscler Thromb Vasc Biol. 2003;23:842–6.

10. Benetos A, Gardner JP, Zureik M, et al. Short telomeres are associated with increased carotid atherosclerosis in hypertensive subjects. Hypertension. 2004;43:182–5.
11. Tentolouris N, Nzietchueng R, Cattan V, et al. White blood cells telomere length is shorter in males with type 2 diabetes and microalbuminuria. Diabetes Care. 2007;30:2909–15.
12. Youngren K, Jeanclos E, Aviv H, Kimura M, Stock J, Hanna M, et al. Synchrony in telomere length of the human fetus. Hum Genet. 1998;102(6):640–3.
13. Codd V, Nelson CP, Albrecht E, Mangino M, Deelen J, Buxton JL, et al. Identification of seven loci affecting mean telomere length and their association with disease. Nat Genet. 2013;45(4):422–7.
14. Blackburn EH. Telomeres and telomerase: their mechanisms of action and the effects of altering their functions. FEBS Lett. 2005;579(4):859–62.
15. Benetos A, Kimura M, Labat C, Buchoff GM, Huber S, Labat L, et al. A model of canine leukocyte telomere dynamics. Aging Cell. 2011;10(6):991–5.
16. Aubert G, Baerlocher GM, Vulto I, Poon SS, Lansdorp PM. Collapse of telomere homeostasis in hematopoietic cells caused by heterozygous mutations in telomerase genes. PLoS Genet. 2012;8(5):e1002696.
17. Morrison SJ, Kimble J. Asymmetric and symmetric stem-cell divisions in development and cancer. Nature. 2006;441(7097):1068–74.
18. Valdes AM, Andrew T, Gardner JP, Kimura M, Oelsner E, Cherkas LF, et al. Obesity, cigarette smoking, and telomere length in women. Lancet. 2005;366(9486):662–4.
19. von Zglinicki T. Role of oxidative stress in telomere length regulation and replicative senescence. Ann N Y Acad Sci. 2000;908:99–110.
20. Benetos A, Kark J, Susser E, Kimura M, Sinnreich R, Chen W, et al. Tracking and fixed ranking of leukocyte telomere length across the adult life course. Aging Cell. 2013;12:615–21.
21. Daniali L, Benetos A, Susser E, Kark JD, Labat C, Kimura M, et al. Telomeres shorten at equivalent rates in somatic tissues of adults. Nat Commun. 2013;4:1597.
22. Calado RT, Young NS. Telomere diseases. N Engl J Med. 2009;361:2353–65.
23. Benetos A, Gautier S, Ricard S, Topouchian J, Asmar R, Poirier O, et al. Influence of angiotensin-converting enzyme and angiotensin II type 1 receptor gene polymorphisms on aortic stiffness in normotensive and hypertensive patients. Circulation. 1996;94(4):698–703.
24. Atwood LD, Samollow PB, Hixson JE, Stern MP, MacCluer JW. Genome-wide linkage analysis of pulse pressure in Mexican Americans. Hypertension. 2001;37(2 Part 2):425–8.
25. Camp NJ, Hopkins PN, Hasstedt SJ, Coon H, Malhotra A, Cawthon RM, et al. Genome-wide multipoint parametric linkage analysis of pulse pressure in large, extended Utah pedigrees. Hypertension. 2003;42(3):322–8.
26. DeStefano AL, Larson MG, Mitchell GF, Benjamin EJ, Vasan RS, Li J, et al. Genome-wide scan for pulse pressure in the National Heart, Lung and Blood Institute's Framingham Heart Study. Hypertension. 2004;44(2):152–5.
27. Bielinski SJ, Lynch AI, Miller MB, Weder A, Cooper R, Oberman A, et al. Genome-wide linkage analysis for loci affecting pulse pressure: the Family Blood Pressure Program. Hypertension. 2005;46(6):1286–93.
28. Franceschini N, MacCluer JW, Rose KM, Rutherford S, Cole SA, Laston S, et al. Genome-wide linkage analysis of pulse pressure in American Indians: the Strong Heart Study. Am J Hypertens. 2008;21(2):194–9.
29. Turner ST, Peyser PA, Kardia SL, Bielak LF, Sheedy 3rd PF, Boerwinkle E, et al. Genomic loci with pleiotropic effects on coronary artery calcification. Atherosclerosis. 2006;185(2):340–6.
30. Levy D, Larson MG, Benjamin EJ, Newton-Cheh C, Wang TJ, Hwang SJ, et al. Framingham Heart Study 100K Project: genome-wide associations for blood pressure and arterial stiffness. BMC Med Genet. 2007;8 Suppl 1:S3.
31. Durier S, Fassot C, Laurent S, Boutouyrie P, Couetil JP, Fine E, et al. Physiological genomics of human arteries: quantitative relationship between gene expression and arterial stiffness. Circulation. 2003;108(15):1845–51.
32. Fassot C, Briet M, Rostagno P, Barbry P, Perret C, Laude D, et al. Accelerated arterial stiffening and gene expression profile of the aorta in patients with coronary artery disease. J Hypertens. 2008;26(4):747–57.
33. Tarasov KV, Sanna S, Scuteri A, Strait JB, Orru M, Parsa A, et al. COL4A1 is associated with arterial stiffness by genome-wide association scan. Circ Cardiovasc Genet. 2009;2(2):151–8.
34. Wain LV, Verwoert GC, O'Reilly PF, Shi G, Johnson T, Johnson AD, et al. Genome-wide association study identifies six new loci influencing pulse pressure and mean arterial pressure. Nat Genet. 2011;43(10):1005–11.
35. Ganesh SK, Tragante V, Guo W, Guo Y, Lanktree MB, Smith EN, et al. Loci influencing blood pressure identified using a cardiovascular gene-centric array. Hum Mol Genet. 2013;22(8):1663–78.
36. Hong KW, Oh B. Recapitulation of genome-wide association studies on body mass index in the Korean population. Int J Obes (Lond). 2012;36(8):1127–30.
37. Kelly TN, Takeuchi F, Tabara Y, Edwards TL, Kim YJ, Chen P, et al. Genome-wide association study meta-analysis reveals transethnic replication of mean arterial and pulse pressure Loci. Hypertension. 2013;62(5):853–9.
38. Zintzaras E, Kitsios G, Kent D, Camp NJ, Atwood L, Hopkins PN, et al. Genome-wide scans meta-analysis for pulse pressure. Hypertension. 2007;50(3):557–64.

39. Mitchell GF, Verwoert GC, Tarasov KV, Isaacs A, Smith AV, et al. Common genetic variation in the 3′-BCL11B gene desert is associated with carotid-femoral pulse wave velocity and excess cardiovascular disease risk: the AortaGen Consortium. Circ Cardiovasc Genet. 2012;5(1):81–90.
40. Mitchell GF, DeStefano AL, Larson MG, Benjamin EJ, Chen MH, Vasan RS, et al. Heritability and a genome-wide linkage scan for arterial stiffness, wave reflection, and mean arterial pressure: the Framingham Heart Study. Circulation. 2005;112(2):194–9.
41. Turner ST, Fornage M, Jack CR Jr., Mosley TH, Kardia SL, Boerwinkle E, et al. Genomic susceptibility loci for brain atrophy in hypertensive sibships from the GENOA study. Hypertension. 2005;45(4):793–8.
42. Aberg K, Dai F, Viali S, Tuitele J, Sun G, Indugula SR, et al. Suggestive linkage detected for blood pressure related traits on 2q and 22q in the population on the Samoan islands. BMC Med Genet. 2009;10:107.
43. Kochunov P, Glahn D, Lancaster J, Winkler A, Kent JW, Jr., Olvera RL, et al. Whole brain and regional hyperintense white matter volume and blood pressure: overlap of genetic loci produced by bivariate, whole-genome linkage analyses. Stroke. 2010;41(10):2137–42.
44. Simino J, Shi G, Arnett D, Broeckel U, Hunt SC, Rao DC. Variants on chromosome 6p22.3 associated with blood pressure in the HyperGEN study: follow-up of FBPP quantitative trait loci. Am J Hypertens. 2011;24(11):1227–33.
45. Zhang D, Pang Z, Li S, Jiang W, Wang S, Thomassen M, et al. Genome-wide linkage and association scans for pulse pressure in Chinese twins. Hypertens Res. 2012;35(11):1051–7.

Part II

Blood Pressure and Sodium Balance: Pathophysiological Mechanisms and Cardiovascular Risk

Mechanical Stress and the Arterial Wall

9

Ernesto L. Schiffrin, Alain Tedgui, and Stephanie Lehoux

Abstract

Mechanical stress on the vascular wall comprises shear stress and circumferential strain. The former, due to blood flow, acts principally on the endothelium and influences vessel diameter. The latter encompasses blood pressure and the cyclic strain generated by the contraction of the heart; it creates radial and tangential forces that are sensed by all cells in the vessel wall. Changes in blood pressure or pulsatility will typically influence wall thickness, which counterbalances intraluminal pressure. In hypertensive patients and animals models of high blood pressure, the resulting thicker, stiffer vessels are better adjusted to handle the added strain, but this remodeling may itself contribute to disease progression. Also significant to vascular pathology is pulse pressure, the difference between systolic and diastolic blood pressures. Both large and small arteries are exposed to changes in the mechanical environment and are remodeled in response to it.

Keywords

Hypertension • Collagen • Elastin • Extracellular matrix • Matrix metalloproteinases • Circumferential strain

E.L. Schiffrin, MD, PhD • S. Lehoux, PhD (✉)
Department of Medicine, McGill University,
Lady Davis Institute for Medical Research,
Sir Mortimer B. Davis Jewish General Hospital,
3755 Chemin de la Côte-Ste-Catherine, Montréal,
QC H3T 1E2, Canada
e-mail: ernesto.schiffrin@mcgill.ca;
stephanie.lehoux@mcgill.ca

A. Tedgui, PhD
Institut National de la Santé et de la Recherche
Médicale (Inserm), Unité 970, Paris Cardiovascular
Research Center, Université Paris-Descartes,
56 rue Leblanc, Paris 750737, France
e-mail: alain.tedgui@inserm.fr

M.E. Safar et al. (eds.), *Blood Pressure and Arterial Wall Mechanics in Cardiovascular Diseases*,
DOI 10.1007/978-1-4471-5198-2_9, © Springer-Verlag London 2014

Abbreviations

AT1	Angiotensin II type 1
ECM	Extracellular matrix
MMP	Matrix metalloproteinase
SHR	Spontaneously hypertensive rat
TIMP	Tissue inhibitor of metalloproteinase
VSMC	Vascular smooth muscle cell
WKY	Wistar Kyoto rat

Tensile Stress in the Arterial Wall

Blood pressure produces strain on the vessel wall in a direction perpendicular to the endoluminal surface. This is offset by the intraparietal tangential forces in both longitudinal and circumferential direction exerted by different elements of the vessel wall, opposing the distending effects of blood pressure. Each element across the whole thickness of the arterial wall bears part of this circumferential tension. The parietal tension (T, the force per unit length of the vessel) is related to the blood pressure (P) and the vessel radius (r) by Laplace's law: T=P • r. The tension per unit of thickness (h) represents the stress exerted on the wall in the circumferential direction. It is expressed as: T=P • r//h. Hence, when stress increases due to an increase in blood pressure, smooth muscle cell hypertrophy and increases in collagen and fibronectin content follow. Inversely, when the circumferential stress falls, the wall undergoes atrophy. Such changes in the arterial wall compensate for changes in blood pressure and maintain a normal level of circumferential stress (Fig. 9.1).

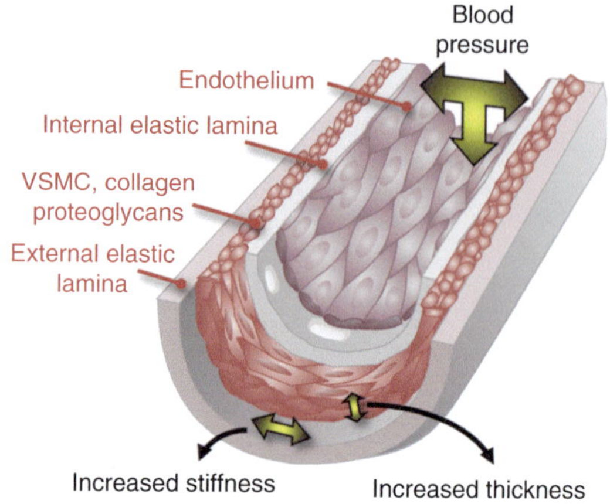

Fig. 9.1 Blood pressure produces strain on the vessel wall in a direction perpendicular to the endoluminal surface. When blood pressure is increased, thickening and/or stiffening of the arterial wall increases intraparietal tangential forces in both longitudinal and circumferential direction, thus maintaining a normal level of circumferential stress

The effects of mechanical tensile stress on the arterial wall have been extensively described and have been applied to the understanding of hypertension. Tensile stress is a strong determinant of the vascular structure among other factors including sympathetic activity and autocrine and paracrine mediators. In the early phase of essential hypertension, it is generally recognized that the vessel wall is subjected to increased pressure because of elevated peripheral resistance related to genetic, humoral, hormonal, nervous, and/or structural factors. Over the course of the disease, injury to large arteries is involved in triggering cardiovascular morbidity and mortality that is associated with hypertension. Animal and human studies have shown that sustained hypertension is associated with structural and functional alterations to both large and small arteries and arterioles. There is good evidence that hypertension leads to increased arterial wall thickness, mostly due to vascular smooth muscle cell (VSMC) hypertrophy, accompanied by polyploidism, hyperplasia, and proportional changes in contractile and matrix proteins, all associated with altered arterial function [1, 2] (Fig. 9.2).

Large Vessels

The aorta and major conduit vessels must sustain and also dampen the large variations in blood pressure that occur as a consequence of the cardiac cycle. As a result, large conduit arteries are composed of many layers of smooth muscle that depend on the size of the animal and diameter of the particular vessel, intercalated within an extracellular matrix (ECM) composed for the most part of type 1 collagen, fibronectin, and elastin. Elastin is the essential component that allows

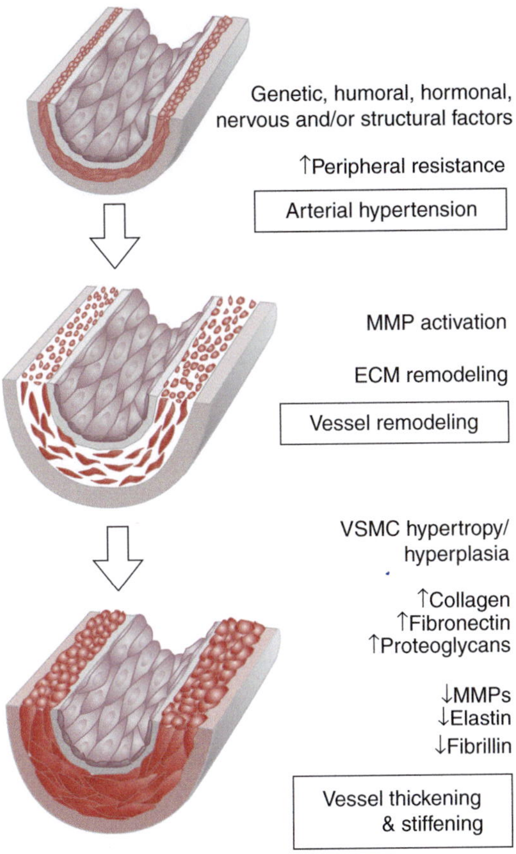

Fig. 9.2 Multiple factors can lead to elevated peripheral resistance, which increases blood pressure. In the early stages of hypertensive remodeling, activation of MMPs and modulation of ECM components may allow the vessel to expand. Over the course of the disease, smooth muscle cell proliferation and growth and remodeling of the ECM in favor of stiffer components yields a stiffer, thicker vessel

conduit vessels to expand and retract as blood pulses between systole and diastole. Pulsatility is accordingly mostly eliminated by the time the blood reaches the smaller arterioles and capillaries. Since it has a very low turnover rate, elastin is susceptible to fatigue and cannot be restored efficiently once it becomes fragmented [3, 4]. It is therefore vulnerable to physical and enzymatic damage that may occur when arteries are exposed to changes in mechanical load, or with ageing. Loss of elasticity in conduit arteries is associated with increased stiffness and pulse pressure, such that greater pulsatility is propagated to downstream arteries [5]. This injures smaller vessels, promoting organ damage. Collagen, on the other hand, is synthesized continually. It provides a strong structural backbone that is little solicited at low pressure but limits maximal arterial expansion during systole. The collagen fiber network must therefore be disrupted when arterial remodeling requires vessel expansion.

Small Vessels

Small arteries are resistance vessels. They have 100–300 μm in lumen diameter, and their wall is composed of three to four layers of smooth muscle cells surrounding the endothelial monolayer. The smooth muscle cells are surrounded by variable amounts of adventitia, and the latter, depending on the tissue being perfused, by variable amounts of perivascular fat. These small arteries are intercalated between larger muscular arteries and arterioles. Both small arteries and arterioles are associated with significant energy dissipation and accordingly, with resistance to blood flow. Small arteries probably provide about 30 % of peripheral resistance, and arterioles another 30–40 %, with the rest originating in larger vessels and a small proportion in pre-capillary vessels. Vasoconstriction and stiffness of vessels are responsible via the effect of a smaller lumen for most of the peripheral resistance to blood flow. A small proportion of the resistance to flow depends on rarefaction, initially due to active constriction of pre-capillary arterioles, and anatomical changes in the long run, with reduction of the capillary bed. The vessel wall of small arteries has small amounts of extracellular matrix composed of collagen and elastin as well as glycoproteins, which contribute to vascular stiffness.

Vascular Stiffness in Hypertension

Increased stiffness of blood vessels has often been considered a characteristic of hypertension (Fig. 9.2). Increased stiffness of the aorta and conductance arteries, discernible by greater pulse wave velocity, is an independent predictor of mortality in patients with hypertension, but also patients with end-stage renal failure, diabetes and in older individuals [6–9]. The stiffness of the wall of arteries is altered in some rat models of hypertension and in essential hypertensive patients, and by influencing lumen diameter, may affect peripheral resistance to blood flow. Distensibility and compliance measure the ability of a vessel to buffer changes in pressure. Both of these measures depend on the stiffness of wall components and the geometry of the vessel and intraluminal pressure to which it is exposed. For this reason it is important to compare vessels under isobaric conditions. Another important consideration is the level of the vasculature, branching order or size of the lumen of vessel. There may be considerable heterogeneity in distensibility with respect to vessel size. Whereas second order cerebral small arteries from stroke-prone spontaneously hypertensive rat (SHR-sp) exhibit decreased distensibility accounting for their apparent reduction in external diameter, third order small arteries of less than 200 μm exhibit remodeling with normal wall mechanics [10]. In genetic and experimental rat models of salt-sensitive hypertension such as Dahl-salt sensitive rats [11] and the deoxycorticosterone acetate-salt rats [12], respectively, mesenteric resistance artery stiffness was normal compared with normotensive controls. In peripheral resistance arteries, namely mesenteric arteries, vessel wall stiffness was increased in SHR [13], associated with increased volume density of collagen and/or collagen/elastin ratio [14, 15]. There may be other examples of this type of heterogeneity. This might also reflect the content of elastin relative to collagen, which diminishes as vessel caliber decreases.

The slope of incremental elastic modulus plotted versus vascular wall stress is a geometry-independent measure of the stiffness of wall components, which includes connective tissue, smooth muscle cells, endothelial cells, and more importantly, collagen and elastin (less and more distensible components, respectively). Thybo et al. found that elastic modulus was not increased in resistance vessels from hypertensive subjects, independently of the presence of arterial wall remodeling, using the wire-myograph technique [16]. This is of particular relevance when one considers that elastin haploinsufficiency alone is sufficient to reduce vessels compliance and raise blood pressure in mice [17]. On the contrary, accumulation of collagen is likely to contribute to arterial stiffness associated with hypertension. In genetic hypertensive rats, conduit artery stiffness is not only influenced by hypertension *per se*, but also by differences in the contents of collagen subtypes [18]. Indeed, the subtypes of collagen present in the vascular wall and other matrix components may also be important determinants of stiffness. Moreover, stiffness may be compounded by changes in the nature and tightness of attachments of cells and extracellular fibrillar components. In the normal artery, fibrillar collagen (types I and III) are the major constituents of the intima, media, and adventitia, whereas types IV and V collagens are situated in the endothelial and smooth muscle cell basement membranes [19], along with collagen types I and III . Increases in collagen type I, III and IV have been quantified in hypertensive patients [14] as well as in animal models of hypertension [13]. Aortae of 6- and 20-week old SHR were stiffer than in age-matched normotensive Wistar Kyoto rats (WKY), in association with a two-fold increase of type V collagen [20] and/or fibronectin [21], consistent with the finding that matrix metalloproteinase 2 (MMP-2), that degrades primarily types IV and V collagen and fibronectin, was lower [22]. Fibronectin gene expression was not increased [21]. Overproduction of collagen upsets the collagen to elastin ratio, contributing to stiffer arteries [3, 23].

Extracellular constituents other than collagen and elastin, such as proteoglycans, may modulate vascular stiffness. These molecules are non-fibrillar matrix components present in increased amounts in resistance artery smooth muscle cells from SHR [24]. Sixty five percent removal of chondroitin-dermatan sulfate-containing glycosaminoglycans from mesenteric resistance arteries increased their stiffness [25]. Similarly, absence of fibrillin-1 in mice leads to abnormal elastin distribution and results in greater arterial stiffness [26]. However, synthesis of proteoglycans was greater in 10 and 28 week-SHR carotid arteries than WKY arteries [27], and was also enhanced in response to angiotensin II in smooth muscle cells from mesenteric resistance arteries of SHR compared with Wistar rats [24]. Finally, abnormal interactions between extracellular matrix proteins, smooth muscle cells, and adhesion receptors may be the most important element by which stiffness is modulated via changes in cell attachment to fibrillar components of the extracellular matrix. Hence, changes in matrix components may contribute not only to stiffening of ECM but also thickening of the vascular wall [28].

Another matter to consider when evaluating arterial remodeling in the setting of hypertension is the stage of the disease. In two-kidney one clip renal hypertensive rats 1 and 5 weeks after renal artery clipping, carotid arteries had normal mechanics under isobaric conditions, whereas after 9 and 24 weeks they had become stiffer [29]. Moreover, we found a paradoxicaal slight decrease in the stiffness of wall components in resistance arteries that had been dissected from subcutaneous tissue biopsies from mild hypertensive patients and studied on a pressurized myograph, despite increased collagen deposition [14]. This was hypothesized to reflect a pressure-dependent fibrillar collagen recruitment or changes in VSMC-matrix anchoring as hypertension progresses [1]. An early increase in proteoglycans in such conditions was also reported [14]. In hypertensive rats, the stiffness of mesenteric small arteries may likewise be reduced initially [30]. A similar observation of decreased wall stiffness in cerebral arterioles from SHR-sp [31] was attributed to increased elastin content [32]. It was concluded that early in the disease, collagen fibers may be recruited at higher distending pressures in small arteries from mild hypertensive patients than in vessels from normotensives, due to closer alignment and changes in the adhesive properties of cellular and fibrillar structures of the remodeled arteries. Later in the evolution of hypertension, vascular compliance of small arteries from hypertensive patients may be reduced in part due to their smaller lumen and greater collagen/elastin ratio [14], and the engagement of collagen fibers and resulting tensing of the collagen jacket that may occur at different portions of the pressure curve.

MMPs and ECM Balance in Hypertension

More recently, a role for matrix degrading enzymes in the early stages of hypertensive vascular remodeling was revealed. MMPs are Zn^{2+}- and Ca^{2+}-dependent proteolytic enzymes that degrade extracellular matrix proteins [33]. In the vasculature, MMPs include collagenases (e.g. interstitial collagenase: MMP-1) that digest structural or fibrillar collagens (types I to III); gelatinases (e.g. gelatinase A {MMP-2} and B {MMP-9}) that digest denatured collagen (gelatin) as well as types IV and V collagen found in the subendothelial basement membrane; and stromelysins (e.g. MMP-3) that digest adhesive molecules like laminin, fibronectin, non-fibrillar collagens and proteoglycans [34]. Matrix metalloproteinases are known to be activated in vascular smooth muscle cells submitted to stationary stretch [35] or cyclic stretch [36], or in arteries exposed to longitudinal tension [37]. In carotid arteries exposed to high intraluminal pressure and in acute models of hypertension, elevated MMP-9 activity was detected, and MMP-9 was found to contribute to increased vessel distensibility [38, 39]. In another study, MMP-2, MMP-9, tissue inhibitor of metalloproteinase (TIMP)-2 and serum elastase activity were measured in patients with isolated systolic hypertension. MMP-9 levels correlated with aortic and brachial pulse wave velocity, and even in healthy subjects serum elastase activity and MMP-9 correlated independently with pulse wave velocity [40]. MMP activation and enhanced distensibility may be hallmarks of early hypertensive remodeling, allowing the vessel to expand to accommodate the new pressure setting (Fig. 9.2). In fact, we demonstrated that blocking MMP production in the setting of an acute hypertensive challenge was associated with an even greater enhancement of blood pressure, suggesting that the initial increase in conducance vessel distensibility may counteract the pro-hypertensive effects of contractile agonists [39].

If high MMP activity characterizes the very early stages of hypertension, the hypertension-related accumulation of extracellular matrix proteins in resistance arteries is most likely facilitated by diminished matrix metalloproteinase activity in the long term. In serum from SHR with extensive myocardial fibrosis [41] and in humans with essential hypertension [42], enhanced synthesis of type I collagen is not balanced by increased type I collagen degradation. In fact, serum concentrations of MMP-1 were diminished in hypertensive patients in who type I collagen was augmented [43]. In aortae and mesenteric arteries of stroke-prone SHR, gene expression of types I, III, and IV collagen is upregulated [44], but as pointed out earlier this is not balanced by an increased MMP-2 activity [22]. In the mesenteric arterial bed, MMP-1 activity was decreased in young SHR before hypertension was established. Hence, lower MMP activity in hypertension may very well be compounded by destabilized production of matrix proteins, upsetting the balance between collagen and elastin content in favor of the former [45]. Interestingly, MMP inhibition with doxycyclin was recently found to reduce established high blood pressure in SHR, further supporting the notion that prolonged low MMP activity is detrimental in hypertension [46]. By modulating extracellular matrix profile and their interactions with adhesive receptors, altered MMP activity may contribute to remodeling of arteries in hypertension. Remodeling of the extracellular matrix would also promote new cell-matrix interactions that facilitate phenotypic modulation and proliferation of smooth muscle cells [47].

Smooth Muscle Cell Hypertrophy/ Hyperplasia

When the circumferential stress increases due an increase in arterial pressure, growth of the media of blood vessels may involve increased smooth muscle cell number and/or size, and even result in lumen encroachment, although these have not been detected consistently [48–50]. Increased stiffness of the VSMCs themselves may also contribute to the overall characteristics of the hypertensive artery [51]. Smooth muscle cell growth may be facilitated by several extracellular matrix proteins; in particular, collagen synthesis was found to correlate with vascular hypertrophy and blood pressure load in hypertensive subjects [52]. Another putative key player in hypertension-related vascular remodeling is tenascin-C, an extracellular matrix glycoprotein that reportedly modulates vascular smooth muscle cell proliferation. Tenascin-C co-localizes with proliferating smooth muscle cells in SHR and human hypertensive pulmonary arteries [53]. Moreover, interactions between $\alpha_v\beta_3$ integrins and tenascin-C promote epidermal growth factor-dependent growth and survival of rat pulmonary artery smooth muscle cells [54, 55]. Thus, tenascin-C and/or other ligands for $\alpha_v\beta_3$ integrins possibly protect smooth muscle cells from apoptosis and promote proliferation. Fibronectin matrix assembly may likewise facilitate VSMC growth. Total fibronectin and $\alpha_5\beta_1$ integrins are increased in arteries of SHR [13, 21]. This suggests that fibronectin matrix assembly, which requires the interaction between the arginine-glycine-aspartate (RGD) site of fibronectin and $\alpha_5\beta_1$ integrins [56] is also elevated in SHR vessels. Moreover, disruption of fibronectin matrix assembly inhibits VSMC growth [57], underlining its potential importance in hypertrophic remodeling. Another RGD-containing protein that may be associated with proliferation is osteopontin, a secreted glycoprotein that is adhesive for vascular smooth muscle cells via $\alpha_v\beta_3$ integrins [58]. *In vitro* studies have demonstrated that osteopontin overexpression is associated with arterial smooth muscle cell proliferation [59] and may be involved in determining the synthetic/proliferative phenotype of these cells previously described in hypertension [60]. Finally, proteoglycans, nonfibrillar matrix components that carry glycosaminoglycans, are synthesized by vascular smooth muscle cells in response to growth factors [61], and may function as modulators of cell proliferation and differentiation.

The intimate relationship between matrix composition and smooth muscle cell response therefore probably depends in the capacity of cells to sense mechanical forces through specific integrin-extracellular matrix interactions, which is itself influenced by matrix composition. The reverse is also true. The synthetic phenotype of vascular smooth muscle cells that predominates in hypertension [62] predisposes these vessels to augmented extracellular matrix deposition – a second component of hypertrophic remodeling. In SHR, the expression of adhesion molecules, specifically integrins, is abnormal. Integrins act as physical joints between extracellular matrix and cytoskeletal components and as signal-transducing receptors. Based on the importance of their actions, we hypothesized that vascular remodeling may involve changes in these anchorage sites. Indeed, with aging from 6 to 20 weeks, mesenteric arteries from SHR exhibited an increase in expression of $\alpha_v\beta_3$ and $\alpha_5\beta_1$ integrins, and in adult SHR arteries, the volume density of collagen was also markedly increased [13]. Bézie et al. [21] also reported an increase in α_5 integrins and their main ligand, fibronectin in SHR aortae. Such changes may represent an increase in cell-matrix attachment sites and their topographical localization that may modulate arterial structure. Indeed, stretching of VSMCs grown on fibronectin or vitronectin induces cellular proliferation, which is prevented by anti-β5 or anti-αvβ3 antibodies [63]. We have proposed that due to changes in extracellular matrix components and corresponding adhesion receptors, interactions between smooth muscle cells and matrix proteins shift, quantitatively and/or topographically, resulting in a rearrangement of smooth muscle cells and a restructured vascular wall.

Mechanisms of Disease

What are the mechanisms that lead to all the changes that we have described above? As already stated, increases in volume density of collagen occur in mesenteric resistance arteries of hypertensive rats [13, 15] and subcutaneous resistance arteries of patients with mild essential hypertension [14]. This may be stimulated by humoral factors whose levels or actions are enhanced in hypertension, for example, by angiotensin II [64]. Angiotensin II activation may implicate a role of generation of superoxide and inflammation [65]. Blocking angiotensin II type 1 (AT1) receptors in humans with hypertension is associated with improved vascular remodeling of resistance arteries [66] and reduced stiffness compared to equieffective BP lowering effects of a beta-blocker [67]. The AT1 receptor is an interesting target since it may be directly activated by mechanical strain in artery cells, independently of agonist [68, 69]. Another mechanically induced pro-fibrotic pathway involves activation of the epidermal growth factor receptor by its ligand transforming growth factor α. Both *in vitro*, in isolated arteries [70] and *in vivo*, in angiotensin II-stimulated mice [71], activation of this pathway by hypertensive conditions and subsequent induction of inflammation is associated with collagen deposition and vessel remodeling. Aldosterone, by triggering inflammation [72] induces fibrosis and increases stiffness of blood vessels and mineralocorticoid receptor blockade reduces stiffness of small arteries in humans with hypertension [73]. In a mouse overexpressing human pre-proendothelin-1 selectively in the endothelium, there was increased stiffness of small arteries. The immune system may contribute through the action of cytokines and inflammation on the production of extracellular matrix components to vascular stiffness. Indeed, in aldosterone-infused osteopetrotic mice, which bear a mutation of the *mcsf* or *csf1* gene and accordingly have functionally deficient monocyte macrophages and therefore a deficient innate immune system, reactive oxygen species generation was impaired but vessels still were stiffer [74]. However, when aldosterone induced increased stiffness of small arteries in wild type mice, adoptive transfer of T regulatory lymphocytes corrected the stiffening of small arteries [75].

Conclusion

In summary, abnormalities of endothelial or smooth muscle cells, adhesion molecules, and extracellular matrix in the vasculature may contribute to structural, mechanical or functional changes that reduce lumen size of small arteries and arterioles, thereby increasing vascular resistance in hypertension. Understanding these vascular alterations and the mechanisms whereby they are generated may offer important insights that may help in the development of therapies contributing to the prevention of vascular-initiated end-organ damage in cardiovascular disease.

Acknowledgments The work of the authors has been supported by grants 13570, 13922, 37917, 82790, 102489, 102606, 130324 from the Medical Research Council of Canada and/or the Canadian Institutes for Health Research (CIHR), Canada Research Chairs (CRC) from the CIHR/Government of Canada CRC Program, and grants from the Canada Fund for Innovation (CFI).

References

1. Intengan HD, Schiffrin EL. Vascular remodeling in hypertension: roles of apoptosis, inflammation, and fibrosis. Hypertension. 2001;38(3 Pt 2):581–7.
2. Lemarie CA, Tharaux PL, Lehoux S. Extracellular matrix alterations in hypertensive vascular remodeling. J Mol Cell Cardiol. 2009;48(3):433–9.
3. Hu JJ, Ambrus A, Fossum TW, Miller MW, Humphrey JD, Wilson E. Time courses of growth and remodeling of porcine aortic media during hypertension: a quantitative immunohistochemical examination. J Histochem Cytochem. 2008;56(4):359–70.
4. O'Rourke MF. Arterial aging: pathophysiological principles. Vasc Med. 2007;12(4):329–41.
5. O'Rourke MF, Hashimoto J. Mechanical factors in arterial aging: a clinical perspective. J Am Coll Cardiol. 2007;50(1):1–13. Epub 2007/07/03.
6. Laurent S, Boutouyrie P, Asmar R, Gautier I, Laloux B, Guize L, et al. Aortic stiffness is an independent predictor of all-cause and cardiovascular mortality in hypertensive patients. Hypertension. 2001;37(5):1236–41.
7. Blacher J, Safar ME, Guerin AP, Pannier B, Marchais SJ, London GM. Aortic pulse wave velocity index and mortality in end-stage renal disease. Kidney Int. 2003;63(5):1852–60.
8. Stork S, van den Beld AW, von Schacky C, Angermann CE, Lamberts SW, Grobbee DE, et al. Carotid artery plaque burden, stiffness, and mortality risk in elderly men: a prospective, population-based cohort study. Circulation. 2004;110(3):344–8.
9. Mattace-Raso FU, van der Cammen TJ, Hofman A, van Popele NM, Bos ML, Schalekamp MA, et al. Arterial stiffness and risk of coronary heart disease and stroke: the Rotterdam Study. Circulation. 2006;113(5):657–63.
10. Hajdu MA, Baumbach GL. Mechanics of large and small cerebral arteries in chronic hypertension. Am J Physiol. 1994;266(3 Pt 2):H1027–33. Epub 1994/03/01.
11. Intengan HD, Schiffrin EL. Mechanical properties of mesenteric resistance arteries from Dahl salt-resistant and salt-sensitive rats: role of endothelin-1. J Hypertens. 1998;16(12 Pt 2):1907–12. Epub 1999/01/14.
12. Intengan HD, He G, Schiffrin EL. Effect of vasopressin antagonism on structure and mechanics of small arteries and vascular expression of endothelin-1 in deoxycorticosterone acetate salt hypertensive rats. Hypertension. 1998;32(4):770–7. Epub 1998/10/17.
13. Intengan HD, Thibault G, Li JS, Schiffrin EL. Resistance artery mechanics, structure, and extracellular components in spontaneously hypertensive rats: effects of angiotensin receptor antagonism and converting enzyme inhibition. Circulation. 1999; 100(22):2267–75.
14. Intengan HD, Deng LY, Li JS, Schiffrin EL. Mechanics and composition of human subcutaneous resistance arteries in essential hypertension. Hypertension. 1999;33(1 Pt 2):569–74.
15. Sharifi AM, Li JS, Endemann D, Schiffrin EL. Effects of enalapril and amlodipine on small-artery structure and composition, and on endothelial dysfunction in spontaneously hypertensive rats. J Hypertens. 1998; 16(4):457–66.
16. Thybo NK, Mulvany MJ, Jastrup B, Nielsen H, Aalkjaer C. Some pharmacological and elastic characteristics of isolated subcutaneous small arteries from patients with essential hypertension. J Hypertens. 1996;14(8):993–8. Epub 1996/08/01.
17. Faury G, Pezet M, Knutsen RH, Boyle WA, Heximer SP, McLean SE, et al. Developmental adaptation of the mouse cardiovascular system to elastin haploinsufficiency. J Clin Invest. 2003;112(9):1419–28.
18. Chamiot Clerc P, Renaud JF, Blacher J, Legrand M, Samuel JL, Levy BI, et al. Collagen I and III and mechanical properties of conduit arteries in rats with genetic hypertension. J Vasc Res. 1999;36(2):139–46. Epub 1999/04/24.
19. Shekhonin BV, Domogatsky SP, Muzykantov VR, Idelson GL, Rukosuev VS. Distribution of type I, III, IV and V collagen in normal and atherosclerotic human arterial wall: immunomorphological characteristics. Coll Relat Res. 1985;5(4):355–68. Epub 1985/09/01.
20. Bashey RI, Cox R, McCann J, Jimenez SA. Changes in collagen biosynthesis, types, and mechanics of aorta in hypertensive rats. J Lab Clin Med. 1989;113(5):604–11. Epub 1989/05/01.
21. Bezie Y, Lamaziere JM, Laurent S, Challande P, Cunha RS, Bonnet J, et al. Fibronectin expression and aortic wall elastic modulus in spontaneously hypertensive rats. Arterioscler Thromb Vasc Biol. 1998; 18(7):1027–34.
22. Yong VW, Krekoski CA, Forsyth PA, Bell R, Edwards DR. Matrix metalloproteinases and diseases of the CNS. Trends Neurosci. 1998;21(2):75–80. Epub 1998/03/14.
23. Xu C, Zarins CK, Pannaraj PS, Bassiouny HS, Glagov S. Hypercholesterolemia superimposed by experimental hypertension induces differential distribution of collagen and elastin. Arterioscler Thromb Vasc Biol. 2000;20(12):2566–72.

24. Castro CM, Cruzado MC, Miatello RM, Risler NR. Proteoglycan production by vascular smooth muscle cells from resistance arteries of hypertensive rats. Hypertension. 1999;34(4 Pt 2):893–6. Epub 1999/10/16.
25. Gandley RE, McLaughlin MK, Koob TJ, Little SA, McGuffee LJ. Contribution of chondroitin-dermatan sulfate-containing proteoglycans to the function of rat mesenteric arteries. Am J Physiol. 1997;273(2 Pt 2):H952–60. Epub 1997/08/01.
26. Marque V, Van Essen H, Struijker-Boudier HA, Atkinson J, Lartaud-Idjouadiene I. Determination of aortic elastic modulus by pulse wave velocity and wall tracking in a rat model of aortic stiffness. J Vasc Res. 2001;38(6):546–50.
27. Walker-Caprioglio HM, Koob TJ, McGuffee LJ. Proteoglycan synthesis in normotensive and spontaneously hypertensive rat arteries in vitro. Matrix. 1992;12(4):308–20. Epub 1992/08/01.
28. Lakatta EG. Arterial and cardiac aging: major shareholders in cardiovascular disease enterprises: Part III: cellular and molecular clues to heart and arterial aging. Circulation. 2003;107(3):490–7.
29. Zanchi A, Wiesel P, Aubert JF, Brunner HR, Hayoz D. Time course changes of the mechanical properties of the carotid artery in renal hypertensive rats. Hypertension. 1997;29(5):1199–203. Epub 1997/05/01.
30. Laurant P, Touyz RM, Schiffrin EL. Effect of pressurization on mechanical properties of mesenteric small arteries from spontaneously hypertensive rats. J Vasc Res. 1997;34(2):117–25. Epub 1997/03/01.
31. Baumbach GL, Dobrin PB, Hart MN, Heistad DD. Mechanics of cerebral arterioles in hypertensive rats. Circ Res. 1988;62(1):56–64. Epub 1988/01/01.
32. Baumbach GL, Hajdu MA. Mechanics and composition of cerebral arterioles in renal and spontaneously hypertensive rats. Hypertension. 1993;21:816–26.
33. Galis ZS, Muszynski M, Sukhova GK, Simonmorrissey E, Unemori EN, Lark MW, et al. Cytokine-stimulated human vascular smooth muscle cells synthesize a complement of enzymes required for extracellular matrix digestion. Circ Res. 1994;75:181–9.
34. Palombo D, Maione M, Cifiello BI, Udini M, Maggio D, Lupo M. Matrix metalloproteinases. Their role in degenerative chronic diseases of abdominal aorta. J Cardiovasc Surg (Torino). 1999;40(2):257–60. Epub 1999/06/01.
35. Asanuma K, Magid R, Johnson C, Nerem RM, Galis ZS. Uniaxial strain upregulates matrix-degrading enzymes produced by human vascular smooth muscle cells. Am J Physiol Heart Circ Physiol. 2003; 284(5):H1778–84.
36. Grote K, Flach I, Luchtefeld M, Akin E, Holland SM, Drexler H, et al. Mechanical stretch enhances mRNA expression and proenzyme release of matrix metalloproteinase-2 (MMP-2) via NAD(P)H oxidase-derived reactive oxygen species. Circ Res. 2003;92(11):e80–6.
37. Jackson ZS, Gotlieb AI, Langille BL. Wall tissue remodeling regulates longitudinal tension in arteries. Circ Res. 2002;90(8):918–25.
38. Lehoux S, Lemarie CA, Esposito B, Lijnen HR, Tedgui A. Pressure-induced matrix metalloproteinase-9 contributes to early hypertensive remodeling. Circulation. 2004;109(8):1041–7.
39. Flamant M, Placier S, Dubroca C, Esposito B, Lopes I, Chatziantoniou C, et al. Role of matrix metalloproteinases in early hypertensive vascular remodeling. Hypertension. 2007;50(1):212–8.
40. Yasmin, Wallace S, McEniery CM, Dakham Z, Pusalkar P, Maki-Petaja K, et al. Matrix metalloproteinase-9 (MMP-9), MMP-2, and serum elastase activity are associated with systolic hypertension and arterial stiffness. Arterioscler Thromb Vasc Biol. 2005;25(2):372.
41. Diez J, Panizo A, Gil MJ, Monreal I, Hernandez M, Pardo Mindan J. Serum markers of collagen type I metabolism in spontaneously hypertensive rats: relation to myocardial fibrosis. Circulation. 1996;93(5):1026–32. Epub 1996/03/01.
42. Diez J, Laviades C, Mayor G, Gil MJ, Monreal I. Increased serum concentrations of procollagen peptides in essential hypertension. Relation to cardiac alterations. Circulation. 1995;91(5):1450–6. Epub 1995/03/01.
43. Laviades C, Varo N, Fernandez J, Mayor G, Gil MJ, Monreal I, et al. Abnormalities of the extracellular degradation of collagen type I in essential hypertension. Circulation. 1998;98(6):535–40.
44. Kim S, Kawamura M, Wanibuchi H, Ohta K, Hamaguchi A, Omura T, et al. Angiotensin II type 1 receptor blockade inhibits the expression of immediate-early genes and fibronectin in rat injured artery. Circulation. 1995;92:88–95.
45. Lee HW, Karam J, Hussain B, Winer N. Vascular compliance in hypertension: therapeutic implications. Curr Diab Rep. 2008;8(3):208–13.
46. Antonio RC, Ceron CS, Rizzi E, Coelho EB, Tanus-Santos JE, Gerlach RF. Antioxidant effect of doxycycline decreases MMP activity and blood pressure in SHR. Mol Cell Biochem. 2014;386:99–105.
47. Thyberg J, Blomgren K, Roy J, Tran PK, Hedin U. Phenotypic modulation of smooth muscle cells after arterial injury is associated with changes in the distribution of laminin and fibronectin. J Histochem Cytochem. 1997;45(6):837–46.
48. Bomberger RA, Zarins CK, Taylor KE, Glagov S. Effect of hypotension on atherogenesis and aortic wall composition. J Surg Res. 1980;28:402–9.
49. Lee RM. Vascular changes at the prehypertensive phase in the mesenteric arteries from spontaneously hypertensive rats. Blood Vessels. 1985;22(3):105–26. Epub 1985/01/01.
50. Mulvany MJ, Baandrup U, Gundersen HJG. Evidence for hyperplasia in mesenteric resistance vessels of spontaneously hypertensive rats using a three-dimensional dissector. Circ Res. 1985;57:794–800.
51. Sehgel NL, Zhu Y, Sun Z, Trzeciakowski JP, Hong Z, Hunter WC, et al. Increased vascular smooth muscle cell stiffness; a novel mechanism for aortic stiffness in hypertension. Am J Physiol Heart Circ Physiol. 2013;305:H1281–7.

52. Olsen MH, Christensen MK, Wachtell K, Tuxen C, Fossum E, Bang LE, et al. Markers of collagen synthesis is related to blood pressure and vascular hypertrophy: a LIFE substudy. J Hum Hypertens. 2005;19(4):301–7.
53. Jones PL, Cowan KN, Rabinovitch M. Tenascin-C, proliferation and subendothelial fibronectin in progressive pulmonary vascular disease. Am J Pathol. 1997;150(4):1349–60. Epub 1997/04/01.
54. Hahn AW, Kern F, Jonas U, John M, Buhler FR, Resink TJ. Functional aspects of vascular tenascin-C expression. J Vasc Res. 1995;32(3):162–74. Epub 1995/05/01.
55. Jones PL, Crack J, Rabinovitch M. Regulation of tenascin-C, a vascular smooth muscle cell survival factor that interacts with the alpha v beta 3 integrin to promote epidermal growth factor receptor phosphorylation and growth. J Cell Biol. 1997;139(1):279–93. Epub 1997/10/06.
56. Fogerty FJ, Akiyama SK, Yamada KM, Mosher DF. Inhibition of binding of fibronectin to matrix assembly sites by anti-integrin (alpha 5 beta 1) antibodies. J Cell Biol. 1990;111(2):699–708. Epub 1990/08/01.
57. Mercurius KO, Morla AO. Inhibition of vascular smooth muscle cell growth by inhibition of fibronectin matrix assembly. Circ Res. 1998;82(5):548–56. Epub 1998/04/07.
58. Liaw L, Almeida M, Hart CE, Schwartz SM, Giachelli CM. Osteopontin promotes vascular cell adhesion and spreading and is chemotactic for smooth muscle cells in vitro. Circ Res. 1994;74(2):214–24. Epub 1994/02/01.
59. Gadeau AP, Campan M, Millet D, Candresse T, Desgranges C. Osteopontin overexpression is associated with arterial smooth muscle cell proliferation in vitro. Arterioscler Thromb. 1993;13(1):120–5. Epub 1993/01/01.
60. Yamamoto M, Aoyagi M, Azuma H, Yamamoto K. Changes in osteopontin mRNA expression during phenotypic transition of rabbit arterial smooth muscle cells. Histochem Cell Biol. 1997;107(4):279–87. Epub 1997/04/01.
61. Emoto N, Onose H, Yamada H, Minami S, Tsushima T, Wakabayashi I. Growth factors increase pericellular proteoglycans independently of their mitogenic effects on A10 rat vascular smooth muscle cells. Int J Biochem Cell Biol. 1998;30(1):47–54. Epub 1998/05/23.
62. Fukuda N, Hu WY, Satoh C, Nakayama M, Kishioka H, Kubo A, et al. Contribution of synthetic phenotype on the enhanced angiotensin II-generating system in vascular smooth muscle cells from spontaneously hypertensive rats. J Hypertens. 1999;17(8):1099–107.
63. Wilson E, Sudhir K, Ives HE. Mechanical strain of rat vascular smooth muscle cells is sensed by specific extracellular matrix/integrin interactions. J Clin Invest. 1995;96:2364–72.
64. Kato H, Suzuki H, Tajima S, Ogata Y, Tominaga T, Sato A, et al. Angiotensin II stimulates collagen synthesis in cultured vascular smooth muscle cells. J Hypertens. 1991;9:17–22.
65. Marchesi C, Paradis P, Schiffrin EL. Role of the renin-angiotensin system in vascular inflammation. Trends Pharmacol Sci. 2008;29(7):367–74. Epub 2008/06/27.
66. Schiffrin EL, Park JB, Intengan HD, Touyz RM. Correction of arterial structure and endothelial dysfunction in human essential hypertension by the angiotensin receptor antagonist losartan. Circulation. 2000;101(14):1653–9. Epub 2000/04/12.
67. Park JB, Intengan HD, Schiffrin EL. Reduction of resistance artery stiffness by treatment with the AT(1)-receptor antagonist losartan in essential hypertension. J Renin Angiotensin Aldosterone Syst. 2000;1(1):40–5. Epub 2002/04/23.
68. Zou Y, Akazawa H, Qin Y, Sano M, Takano H, Minamino T, et al. Mechanical stress activates angiotensin II type 1 receptor without the involvement of angiotensin II. Nat Cell Biol. 2004;6(6):499–506.
69. Ramkhelawon B, Rivas D, Lehoux S. Shear stress activates extracellular signal-regulated kinase 1/2 via the angiotensin II type 1 receptor. FASEB J. 2013;27(8):3008–16. Epub 2013/04/16.
70. Lemarie CA, Esposito B, Tedgui A, Lehoux S. Pressure-induced vascular activation of nuclear factor-kappaB: role in cell survival. Circ Res. 2003;93(3):207–12.
71. Lemarie CA, Tharaux PL, Esposito B, Tedgui A, Lehoux S. Transforming growth factor-alpha mediates nuclear factor kappaB activation in strained arteries. Circ Res. 2006;99(4):434–41.
72. Savoia C, Schiffrin EL. Vascular inflammation in hypertension and diabetes: molecular mechanisms and therapeutic interventions. Clin Sci (Lond). 2007;112(7):375–84. Epub 2007/02/28.
73. Savoia C, Touyz RM, Amiri F, Schiffrin EL. Selective mineralocorticoid receptor blocker eplerenone reduces resistance artery stiffness in hypertensive patients. Hypertension. 2008;51(2):432–9. Epub 2008/01/16.
74. Leibovitz E, Ebrahimian T, Paradis P, Schiffrin EL. Aldosterone induces arterial stiffness in absence of oxidative stress and endothelial dysfunction. J Hypertens. 2009;27(11):2192–200. Epub 2009/08/06.
75. Kasal DA, Barhoumi T, Li MW, Yamamoto N, Zdanovich E, Rehman A, et al. T regulatory lymphocytes prevent aldosterone-induced vascular injury. Hypertension. 2012;59(2):324–30. Epub 2011/12/08.

10 Pulsatile Stress, Arterial Stiffness, and Endothelial Function

Robinson Joannidès, Jérémy Bellien, and Christian Thuillez

Abstract

Vascular endothelium contributes in humans to the regulation of conduit artery mechanical properties at baseline and during the increase in flow. This effect results from the shear stress-dependent release of vasoactive factors, as nitric oxide (NO) and endothelium-derived hyperpolarizing factors as epoxyeicosatrienoic acids (EETs) to modify arterial tone, geometry, and trophicity and to optimize vascular functions and cardiovascular coupling. Endothelial dysfunction appears as a major determinant of arterial stiffening, increased pulse pressure, and systolic hypertension, and in turn strategies protecting the endothelium prevent these abnormalities. In addition, endothelium also integrates pulsatile stimuli (pulse pressure and flow) to increase NO and EET release under physiological conditions, and the reduced pulse pressure-dependent strain in stiff conduits may suppress this adaptive response, thus amplifying the stiffening process. This article details fundamental experiments and clinical studies supporting these mechanisms.

Keywords

Artery • Endothelium • Stiffness • NO • EETs • Pulse pressure • Shear stress

Introduction

Vascular endothelium is continuously exposed to pulsatile stretch and shear stress during the cardiac cycle. These mechanical forces are sensed and converted into chemical signals that regulate the release of vasoactive factors as nitric oxide (NO) and prostacyclin, but also endothelium-derived hyperpolarizing factors (EDHFs) as epoxyeicosatrienoic acids (EETs), reactive oxygen species (ROS), and growth factors. These factors, in turn, participate to the regulation of the mechanical properties throughout the changes in

R. Joannidès, MD, PhD (✉)
Department of Pharmacology, INSERM U1096
Institute for Research and Innovation in Biomedicine, CHU de Rouen, Rouen 76031, France
e-mail: robinson.joannides@chu-rouen.fr

J. Bellien, PharmD, PhD • C. Thuillez, MD, PhD
Department of Pharmacology, INSERM U1096
Institute for Research and Innovation in Biomedicine, CHU de Rouen, Rouen 76031, France
e-mail: jeremy.bellien@chu-rouen.fr; christian.thuillez@univ-rouen.fr

M.E. Safar et al. (eds.), *Blood Pressure and Arterial Wall Mechanics in Cardiovascular Diseases*, DOI 10.1007/978-1-4471-5198-2_10, © Springer-Verlag London 2014

arterial tone, geometry and trophicity, to limit pulsatile stress thus, contributing to optimize vascular functions and cardiovascular coupling. Indeed, endothelial dysfunction will result in the release of profibrotic factors, inflammatory cytokines and in the expression of various adhesion molecules in response to normal or excessive pulsatile stretch, and to the associated shear stress. Hence, in addition to direct smooth muscle cell–stretch activation and extracellular damage, as elastin fatigue and fragmentation, endothelial dysfunction increases arterial stiffness through extracellular matrix fibrosis and calcification. As a result of the increase in arterial stiffness, from the increase in forward pulse pressure, pulse wave velocity (PWV), and/or the magnitude of reflected wave, pulse pressure and pulsatile stress increase along the arterial tree, facilitating early arteriosclerosis and plaque formation. Moreover, at central site, this phenomenon increases left ventricular afterload and oxygen consumption and decreases coronary perfusion pressure. To prevent endothelial dysfunction and the related increase in pulsatile stress may be thus, converted into clinical benefit by reducing the arterial stiffening-associated cardiovascular events. This chapter details fundamental experiments and clinical studies supporting these mechanisms.

Pulsatile Stress and Endothelial Factor Release

Mechanotransduction

Mechanical forces generated by pressure and flow during the cardiac cycle are applied to the various arterial wall components, extracellular matrix, and cells, leading to internal stresses and stretch. These signals are sensed and converted into biochemical response (mechanotransduction) to accommodate new hemodynamic conditions, acutely or chronically, and restore the basal tensile and shear stress through adaptive changes in arterial geometry, smooth muscle tone, or passive wall components [1–4]. Endothelium is particularly exposed to pulsatile fluid shear stress but also to stretch, whose magnitude, in turn, depends on the arterial wall mechanical properties and particularly of arterial wall stiffness [5, 6]. The release of endothelium-derived relaxing and growth factors is thus upregulated by the mean levels of shear stress [3] but also increases with the augmentation in pulsatile stresses and stretch, particularly that of NO and EETs [3, 7–9]. In addition, the expression of vasoconstrictors as endothelin-1 (ET-1) is decreased by steady flow and is increased by oscillatory shear stress in cultured bovine aortic endothelial cells (BAEC) [3], while pulsatile flow decreases the circulating ET-1 levels during cardiopulmonary bypass in humans [10]. Endothelial mechanosensors are of various nature, i.e., ion channels, tyrosine kinase receptors, G-protein-coupled receptors and G-protein itself, caveolae, adhesion proteins as integrins located at the site of cell–cell and cell–matrix attachment, cytoskeleton, glycocalyx, and primary cilia as shown more recently [3]. The signal is transmitted through downstream transduction pathways such as the mitogen-activated protein kinase cascade, via sequential phosphorylations, the activation of target effectors as endothelial NO-synthase (eNOS), or transcription factors with subsequent gene expression [2–4]. In addition, membrane-bounded nicotinamide adenine dinucleotide phosphate-oxidase (NADPH oxidase) can directly release ROS in response to pressure and flow [11]. Superoxide anions released in these conditions can interact with NO to regulate flow-mediated dilatation in response to the acute increase in shear stress but also can interfere with the regulation of matrix metalloproteinases after peroxynitrite formation, to promote adaptive wall remodeling during the chronic increase in flow [12]. Furthermore, oscillatory shear stress favoring atherosclerosis development [4, 13–15] has been reported to markedly increase ROS production by this way, whereas laminar flow enhances the expression of antioxidant enzymes as superoxide dismutase (SOD) and peroxiredoxin [16]. More recently, the role of ciliary proteins polycystin-1 and polycystin-2 in the mechanotransduction of both shear stress and pressure changes in arteries has been put forward. Polycystin-1 is transmembranary protein with a prominent extracellular domain and a short intracellular domain that interacts with polycystin-2, a member of the transient receptor potential (TRP) channels, in the renal epithelium, sensing urinary flow variation and promoting calcium entry to control renal tubular cell maturation and function [17]. Mutations in the genes *PKD1* and *PKD2* encoding these proteins are responsible for autosomal dominant polycystic kidney disease, a common hereditary disorder characterized by the development of multiple cysts in the kidneys, causing a progressive impairment of renal function [17]. However, experimental evidence suggests that these proteins are also present in vascular endothelial and smooth muscle cells [4, 18]. In endothelial cells, the polycystin complex contributes to activate, in a transient calcium-dependent manner, eNOS in response to the increase in shear stress [4]. In vascular smooth muscle, it is rather the ratio between polycystin-1 and polycystin-2 that regulates pressure sensing and thereby myogenic tone notably by affecting stretch-activated channel activity [18].

Endothelial NO Release

Humoral factors control eNOS activity mainly based on the increase in intracellular calcium and calcium–calmodulin interaction. In contrast the fluid shear stress, a main physiological stimulus, regulates the basal and stimulated release of NO by phosphorylation-dependent mechanisms that only necessitate a low basal level of calcium. Sustained increase in shear stress thus enhances eNOS activity after only a transient increase in calcium followed by an apparently "calcium-independent" phase after calcium has returned to basal level [3, 4, 19]. In this context, integrins can be directly activated by shear stress and, through focal adhesion kinase (FAK) activation, promote the serine/threonine kinase Akt (PKB) phosphorylation, which phosphorylates human eNOS at the stimulatory site ser1177 and increases NO release [20, 21]. However, eNOS ser1177 phosphorylation is also mainly induced by Akt/PKB [19, 20] and protein kinase A (PKA) [22] once activated by phosphoinositide-3 kinase (PI3K). In this case, tyrosine kinase receptor as vascular endothelial growth factor receptor 2 (VEGFR2) [23] and, to a lesser extent, G-protein-coupled receptor [3] is involved in the ligand-independent shear stress-mediated transduction and activation of PI3K. In addition, a major mechanosensor involved in the PI3K/Akt activation in response to shear stress is the platelet endothelial cell adhesion molecule-1 (PECAM-1). In fact, PECAM-1 activates integrins in response to shear stress, after forming a complex with VEGFR2 and vascular endothelial cadherin of adherens junctions, the latter being an adaptor protein between PECAM-1 and the PI3K activator VEGFR2 [24]. Regarding the transient release of NO mediated by the ciliary polycystin complex, acting as a shear stress mechanosensor, a calcium/calmodulin-dependent, PI3K-independent Akt activation by protein kinase C (PKC) appears to be involved [3, 17, 18].

As mentioned earlier, the pulsatile flow enhances in an acute manner the release of NO. This effect was first demonstrated in animal models where coronary [7] or systemic flow [8] was manipulated by local servo pump device or during extracorporeal left heart bypass, through the increase in pulse pressure. Thus, the increase in flow pulsatility in coronary arteries enhances coronary flow at stable mean blood pressure, and this effect is abolished by the nonselective NOS inhibitor N^G-nitro-L-arginine methyl ester (L-NAME) [7]. Moreover, the increase in systemic pulse pressure decreases systemic vascular resistance and increases the plasma value of the NO metabolite nitrite [8]. In parallel, the increase in pulsatile strain associated with pulsatile pressure was demonstrated to enhance Akt phosphorylation in bovine aortic vascular smooth muscle cells (VSMC) in culture [25] and more recently in BAEC cultured in compliant tubes, together with eNOS phosphorylation at the bovine stimulatory site ser1179 [6].

In vivo evidences for the presence of a basal release of NO resulting in a permanent NO-dependent vasodilatory influence have been largely demonstrated at the arteriolar level [26]. At the level of the conduit arteries, the basal release of NO is generally accepted although less apparent. In proximal elastic arteries, NOS inhibition is thus generally associated with an increase in isometric tone without change in diameter at stable pressure, the diameter being more pressure dependent than in peripheral muscular conduit arteries. Furthermore, at the distal site of epicardial coronary arteries of subjects with normal angiogram, local administration of the nonselective NOS inhibitor, N^G-monomethyl-L-arginine (L-NMMA), was associated in most of the studies with a decrease in artery diameter [27, 28]. However, this effect was associated with a local decrease in flow, thus confounding the proper effect of NOS inhibition on conduit and resistance arteries. In this context, Puybasset et al. analyzed the effect of systemic infusion of L-NMMA in conscious dogs at the level of the left circumflex coronary artery diameter and flow [29]. The acute NOS inhibition was associated with an increase in blood pressure and a decrease in heart rate suggesting a reduction in sympathetic activity from baroreflex deactivation. Simultaneously, the coronary artery diameter decreased without change in flow as a consequence of the increase in aorta blood pressure, thus demonstrating in vivo the basal release NO at this level [29]. Less constant results were obtained in humans at the level of the proximal coronary artery site, despite the presence of a significant decrease in flow after local NOS inhibition [27, 28], and no decrease in diameter was reported at the level of segmental pulmonary arteries [26]. These divergent results suggest some heterogeneity regarding the role of NO in muscular conduit arteries. Nevertheless, they could be also explained by the presence of local compensating mechanisms that could be more or less effective through the arterial tree. If present, it might rather consist in a compensating switch between NO and other endothelium-derived relaxing factor, emerging after eNOS inhibition, as suggested in atherosclerotic coronary arteries [28, 29]. Concerning the peripheral muscular arteries, most of the experiments performed using noninvasive high-resolution echographic methods reported no significant decrease in diameter after local administration of high doses of L-NMMA. This was observed despite a concomitant decrease in forearm flow and no significant change in blood pressure [26]. Conversely, by using intravascular ultrasound imaging and invasive arterial pressure measurement, it was reported that local NO-synthase inhibition decreases the diastolic brachial artery lumen cross-sectional area, measured at different levels of transmural pressure (these ones obtained by inflating step by step a brachial cuff until the diastolic blood pressure) [30]. This suggests that invasive methods used to evaluate arterial stiffness could provide higher sensitivity but they also may modify the vascular reactivity and potentiate the vascular effect of NOS inhibition, by majoring the local decrease in flow or by interfering with compensating mechanisms maintaining resting arterial diameter [31]. In fact, according to the magnitude and/or the ability to develop these compensatory mechanisms after eNOS inhibition, the effect of L-NMMA on diameter could vary depending on the investigated population and/or measurement sites explaining the apparent divergences observed. More recently, the selective inhibitor of neuronal NOS (nNOS), S-methyl-L-thiocitrulline, was shown to cause a reduction in basal blood flow in the forearm of healthy humans and coronary circulation of subjects without coronary atheroma [32]. These results were obtained without affecting the stimulated eNOS-mediated vasodilatation elicited by acetylcholine, substance P, or increase in shear stress. Inhibition of nNOS reduced proximal epicardial coronary diameter concomitantly to the local flow decrease [32]. Although the exact localization of nNOS isoform remains unknown in healthy subjects, nNOS may be predominantly located in VSMC, as reported from ex vivo studies of mammary arteries obtained from coronary artery disease patients. In situ nNOS may be located also at the level of perivascular nerves; however, nNOS inhibition did not appear to modify the forearm blood flow in healthy volunteers during sympathetic activation testing [33]. These experiments suggest that different sources of NO may juxtapose through the arterial wall and could have different roles and mechanisms of regulation. In fact, NO release from nNOS may mostly contribute to the basal release of NO, while

NO from eNOS activity may mostly contribute to the stimulated response, particularly shear stress. Indeed, NO was shown to mediate flow-dependent dilatation of resistance and conduit arteries in response to postischemic hyperemia and hand skin heating [34, 35].

EDH(F)

In addition to NO and prostacyclin, a third endothelium-dependent pathway mediates the rapid adaptation of vasomotor tone in arteries in response to changes in shear stress and/or pressure. This pathway includes in fact a multitude of complex and juxtaposed processes that have a final common response, i.e., the hyperpolarization and subsequent relaxation of smooth muscle cells [36]. In brief, the "classical" mechanism referred as EDH (endothelium-dependent hyperpolarization) involves first the hyperpolarization of endothelial cells, due to the opening of small- and intermediate calcium-activated potassium (K_{Ca}) channels and efflux of potassium ions, and secondly this hyperpolarization is transmitted electrically to the smooth muscle cell layer through the gap junction, without the obligatory action of a chemical messenger [36]. This mechanism is notably prominent in resistance arteries where it contributes equally with NO to the control of the vasomotor tone [36]. One alternative mechanism is the release by the endothelium of one or more diffusive factor(s), called EDHFs, which induce the opening of smooth muscle large-conductance K_{Ca} channels, promoting potassium efflux and hyperpolarization of smooth muscle cells. Several factors have been identified as EDHFs, but the EETs, synthesized by endothelial cytochrome P450 (CYP450) epoxygenases from arachidonic acid, appear to be important mediators in human conduit arteries [34–36]. The EDH(F) phenomenon was only first described as a compensatory mechanism maintaining endothelium-dependent responses notably during reduced NO availability in pathology or because only studied in the presence of NO and prostacyclin synthesis inhibitors, but accumulating evidence shows that it also plays a major role under physiological conditions.

In human forearm resistance arteries, EETs and, to a larger extent, EDH appear to contribute to the control of the resting tone, as shown by the reduction in basal blood flow with the local infusion of the CYP450 inhibitor fluconazole and the further reduction obtained with the nonspecific K_{Ca} channel blocker tetraethylammonium (TEA) [37]. Similarly, both mechanisms appear to regulate endothelium-dependent dilatations in response to endothelial agonists at this level and these basal and stimulated contributions increase under conditions of impaired NO availability [36, 37].

In conduit arteries, the activation of muscular K_{Ca} channels by pulse pressure was mainly dependent of the basal release of a diffusive EDHF in porcine coronary arteries, and increasing the magnitude of the pulse pressure imposed to the artery leads to a parallel increase in the magnitude of the resulting EDHF-mediated hyperpolarization [9]. More recently [38], it was shown that acute application of cyclic strain to coronary endothelial cell and human umbilical vascular endothelial cells (HUVEC) elicited the release of the 8,9-, 11,12-, and 14,15-EET isoforms and that prolonged stimulation of these cells, but also of epicardial porcine coronary arteries perfused under pulsatile conditions, was associated with an increased mRNA expression and activity of CYP450 2C. All together, these results support the major role of EETs as the diffusible EDHFs released in response to an increase in pulsatile strain in porcine coronary arteries to regulate arterial compliance. At the same time, it was reported that the pulse pressure-dependent increase in the dog coronary artery flow was reduced by half by L-NMMA to inhibit NOS or by the endothelial K_{Ca} channels inhibitors charybdotoxin/apamin and fully abolished by their combination [39]. In contrast, the inhibitor of SMC large-conductance K_{Ca} channels iberiotoxin was without effect, rather supporting the role of the classical EDH than that of a diffusible factor at this level.

In humans in vivo, L-NMMA and fluconazole decreased the basal radial artery diameter of young healthy volunteers when infused in combination but not when used alone, supporting the hypothesis that EETs as NO are continuously

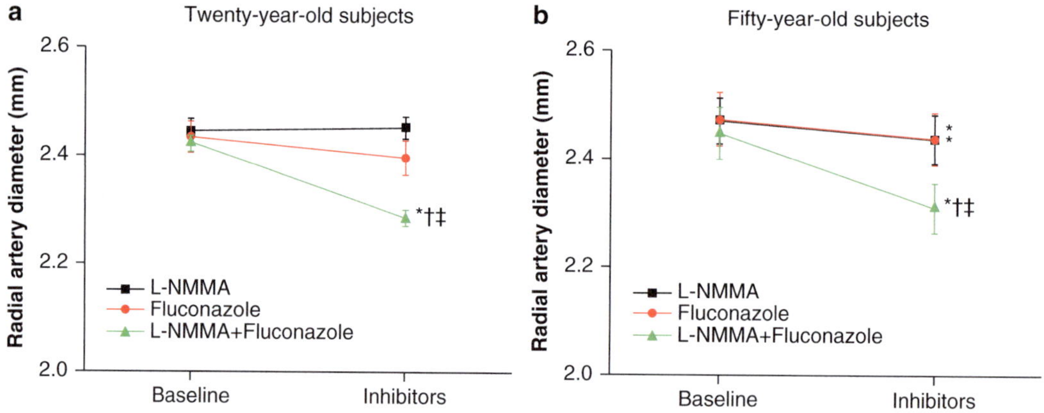

Fig. 10.1 Basal radial artery diameter was not significantly affected by the local infusion of the NO-synthase inhibitor L-NMMA nor by fluconazole alone but was reduced by their combination in 20-year-old healthy subjects (**a**; $n = 8$). In contrast, L-NMMA and fluconazole alone, and, to a larger extent, their combination reduced radial artery diameter in 50-year-old healthy subjects (**b**; $n = 14$). These results suggest that the interaction between NO and EETs to maintain conduit artery diameter at rest decreases with aging. *$P < 0.05$ vs. baseline, †$P < 0.05$ vs. L-NMMA, ‡$P < 0.05$ vs. fluconazole

released in response to pulsatile forces acting on the endothelium and that both pathways can compensate for each other to maintain arterial diameter (Fig. 10.1) [40]. Interestingly, the compensation of NO deficiency by EETs appears to decrease during aging (Fig. 10.1) and is completely lost in essential hypertensive patients [41]. Finally, using combined biological and functional approaches based on local infusion of pharmacological inhibitors and local blood sampling during hand skin heating, EETs were effectively identified as the EDHF release during the increase in shear stress, mediating with NO the sustained flow-mediated dilatation of peripheral conduit arteries in healthy subjects (Fig. 10.2) [35]. Remarkably, this mechanism is also absent in essential hypertensive patients, and, therefore, the restoration of EET pathway emerges as a promising pharmacological target to prevent endothelial dysfunction in these patients [35, 41].

Thus, based on these results, it appears that endothelium-derived relaxing factors, notably NO and EDHF, are continuously released by the vascular endothelium in response to pulsatile strain and that the increase in the forces applied to the endothelium enhances their release and thus may represent a major mechanism involved in the control of arterial mechanics.

Impact of Endothelial Factors on Arterial Stiffness

Analyzing the impact of endothelium-derived factors on arterial mechanics is complex. Indeed, smooth muscle cell relaxation, as expected from NO and/or EDH(F), decreases the arterial wall elastic modulus (which represents wall stiffness) through a reduction in isometric tone. In parallel, the associated increase in diameter and decrease in wall thickness increases wall stiffness at stable levels of arterial pressure, by increasing the mid-wall stress (i.e., close to the pressure radius/wall thickness product in sectional plan) applied to the arterial wall, and thereby by recruiting the stiffer peripheral elements of the vascular wall to support this stress (i.e., the recruitment function) [42]. Thus, the final change in arterial wall stiffness will result from these two opposites influences. At last, the change in arterial compliance, which represents the arterial chamber elasticity, will result from the increase in diameter and the decrease in wall elastic modulus. Furthermore, the chronic suppression of the anti-hypertrophic and antiproliferative influences of the normal endothelium could be associated, independently from changes in arterial tone and geometry, with structural modifications within the arterial wall,

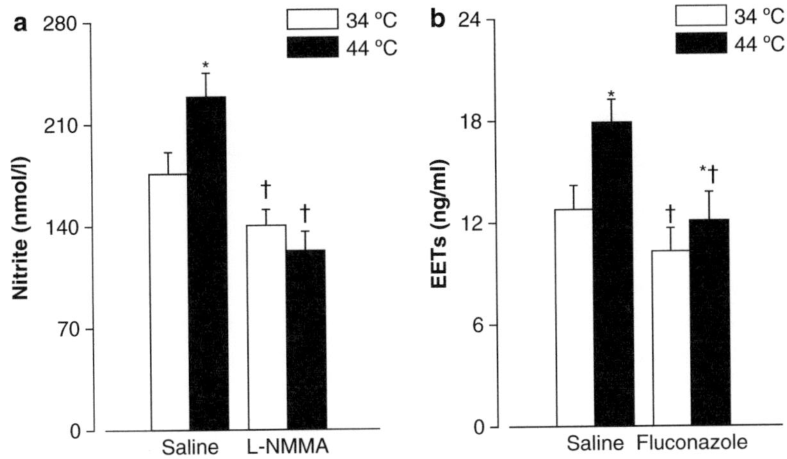

Fig. 10.2 Local plasma levels of the NO metabolite nitrite (**a**) and epoxyeicosatrienoic acids (*EETs*) (**b**) during the endothelium-dependent flow-mediated dilatation of the radial artery induced by the hand skin heating method (from 34 to 44 °C) during the brachial infusion of saline and pharmacological inhibitors of their production. Hand skin heating induced an increase in the local plasma levels of nitrite that was abolished by the NO-synthase inhibitor L-NMMA. In the same way, hand skin heating increased the local plasma EETs that was reduced by the CYP450 epoxygenases inhibitor fluconazole. $*P<0.05$ vs. 34 °C, $†P<0.05$ vs. saline

notably an enhanced contain of stiffer elements, i.e., collagen, leading to an increase in intrinsic arterial stiffness [43]. This mechanism could explain the inappropriate arterial stiffening observed in aging, systolic hypertension, end-stage renal disease, or diabetes despite arterial wall hypertrophy, developed to normalize the arterial wall stress [44].

Evidence for a Role of the Endothelium in the Control Arterial Mechanics

First of all, deendothelialization experiments in animals provide some evidence for a role of the endothelium in the regulation of arterial mechanics. However, because this method may differentially affect the balance between vasoconstrictor and vasodilator influences, according to species and vascular territories, variable associated increase in arterial diameter were reported. Thus, endothelial removal was shown to decrease the distensibility index (compliance/diastolic diameter ratio as a wall stiffness estimate) in coronary arteries [9, 45]. However, as the result of the change in diameter and the decrease in distensibility, arterial compliance decreases [9], remains unchanged [46], or increases depending of experimental models. Importantly, endothelial denudation also increases the aortic wall viscosity [46], a main regulator of the efficiency of heart–vessel coupling in terms of energetics balance [46–48]. In fact, arteries are not purely elastic but exhibit a markedly viscous behavior and thus have a greater diameter at any given pressure during unloading than during the loading phase. This behavior determines a hysteresis loop on the pressure–volume relationship that has a dimension of energy. Thus, while part of the energy stored by the arterial wall during elastic distension is fully restored, the remaining part of the energy corresponding to the viscous deformation (area of the hysteresis loop) is dissipated within the arterial wall [46]. In these respects, arterial wall viscosity is an energy-dissipating mechanism that reduces the efficiency of heart–vessel coupling, when present in excess [46], but that also may prevent the deleterious effect of increased pulsatile stress on the arterial wall in particular during essential hypertension [46, 47].

In vivo in humans, cross-sectional and more recently prospective studies revealed a close correlation between biological and functional markers of endothelial dysfunction and the decrease in arterial compliance or increase in PWV in cardiovascular diseases [49–51]. More direct evidence comes from the demonstration for an endothelium-dependent flow-mediated regulation of arterial mechanic. Thus, a progressive downward shift of the radial artery modulus–midwall stress relationship toward low values of modulus when shear stress increased was demonstrated by using the distal skin heating procedure. [52]. Interestingly, when assessed at operational pressure, mean elastic modulus appears not modified because of the opposite effects of the decrease in tone and increase in arterial wall stress resulting from vasodilatation [52]. Using the same methodology, it was shown that chronic angiotensin-converting-enzyme inhibition restores not only endothelium-dependent dilatation but also the altered flow-dependent increase in distensibility of peripheral conduit arteries in patients with heart failure [53]. Furthermore, one interventional study demonstrated that independently from the drugs used, the normalization of blood pressure in hypertensive postmenopausal women is associated with a higher decrease in cardiovascular events when endothelial function is also restored, as compared to women with persistent endothelial dysfunction [54]. More recently, we observed in a preliminary prospective study that immunosuppressive therapy allowing the prevention of endothelial dysfunction reduces brachial artery systolic and pulse pressure in renal recipients [55]. Additionally, a decrease in aortic PWV and in the magnitude of the forward and backward pressure waves associated with a decrease in plasma ET-1 was obtained using a close to similar immunosuppressive strategy, and this result was further confirmed after a 4-year follow-up period [55]. Altogether these results support the hypothesis that endothelial dysfunction is an important contributor of arterial stiffening in humans and that its correction may be converted into clinical benefit. At present, the NO and EDH(F) pathways that have been shown to be altered in human with cardiovascular diseases appear to be the main endothelium-derived regulators of arterial mechanical properties.

Impact of NO Availability on Arterial Mechanics

In animals, acute and chronic administration of NOS inhibitors are associated with carotid and aortic stiffening that is at least partly independent of the associated increase in blood pressure [56–58]. In this context, eNOS knockout mice and only old spontaneously hypertensive rats (SHR) with a depressed basal NO release have a striking increase in central pulse pressure, providing evidence for a link between altered NO bioavailability, arterial stiffening, and systolic hypertension [43, 59]. In humans, acute systemic administration of the NOS inhibitor L-NMMA is effectively associated with an increase in carotid–femoral PWV, but this appears rather due to the associated increase in blood pressure due to suppression of basal NO release in resistance arteries than to the suppression of a basal vasorelaxing effect of NO in proximal conduit arteries [60, 61]. Indeed, this increase in PWV with L-NMMA is mimicked when using equi-hypertensive doses of norepinephrine and dopamine [60]. These data, however, do not exclude a role for NO in the regulation of the aortic mechanical properties but strongly suggest that under these experimental conditions carotid-to-femoral PWV could be rather influenced by changes in arterial pressure than arterial wall smooth muscle tone. Moreover, as previously stressed [61], this small impact of arterial wall smooth muscle tone on aortic PWV could result from the predominantly elastic nature of this vessel that could minimize in the short term the effects of acute change in pressure and tone and maintain the PWV close to a more appropriate physiological value. Thus, the impact of NOS inhibition may be more important in distal conduit arteries. In this respect, it was shown, using a non-propagative derived Windkessel model to analyze the arterial pulse pressure waveform, that systemic administration of gradual doses of L-NMMA does not decrease the proximal component of systemic compliance despite significantly increasing mean arterial pressure and decreasing peripheral compliance [62]. In this respect, some associations between eNOS gene polymorphisms, decreasing NO availability, and increases in peripheral femoral-to-tibial PWV but not in central carotid-to-femoral PWV [63], as well as with the increase with age of pulse pressure in hypertensive subjects, have been found [64].

More evidence for a role of NO in the control of basal arterial mechanical properties comes from local NOS inhibition experiments at low doses devoid of confounding systemic effects. However, it should be keep in mind that even under these conditions, there was a concomitant decrease in flow resulting from the distal arteriolar NOS inhibition and thus, because shear stress stimulates the release of endothelial factors, the effects on the studied conduit artery could be partly flow dependent. As previously stressed (see section "Endothelial NO Release"), the effects of local NOS inhibition on proximal coronary artery diameter is controversial probably due to the emergence of compensating mechanisms, and these experiments have not assessed the impact on arterial mechanics [27]. Nonetheless, a decrease in epicardial coronary artery distensibility index following NOS inhibition has been reported in anesthetized dogs [45]. In addition, a leftward shift of the stress-strain relationship and an upward shift of the modulus–transmural pressure relationship were observed after local NOS inhibition in the brachial artery, demonstrating an increase in artery wall stiffness [30]. However, by using the distal flow clamp method, a similar upward shift in the modulus–midwall stress curve was reported as a result of the decrease in flow without change in blood pressure [52]. In fact, the role of NO in vivo in the control of arterial mechanics, as for baseline diameter [29], was first demonstrated in animal experiments. Indeed, local L-NMMA infusion increases the common iliac artery PWV, carefully measured by intra-arterial catheter, in anesthetized lamb without change in systemic blood pressure. Importantly, this result was controlled for the effect of the expected concomitant decrease in flow by repeating the infusion of L-NMMA distal to the site of iliac artery measurements, and the absence of change in PWV under these conditions confirmed that NO regulates arterial stiffness in peripheral conduit arteries at baseline. This result was then demonstrated in human iliac artery under local anesthesia with a similar methodology [65].

In more distal muscular conduit arteries such as the radial artery, local infusion of L-NMMA surprisingly decreased arterial stiffness and this, despite the concomitant decrease in flow observed. However, it was further demonstrated that this paradoxical effect is in fact due to the emerging of compensatory mechanisms, in particular of EDH(F) pathway, and that blocking these mechanisms unmasks the role of NO in the control of arterial mechanics [31]. At this level, it can also be demonstrated using the hand skin heating method that the adaptation of arterial mechanics, in particular the decrease in arterial stiffness in response to the increase in shear stress, is notably mediated by NO [34]. Indeed, infusion of L-NMMA at increasing doses, to compensate for the diluting effect of flow increase during the procedure, reduced the downward shift of the modulus–midwall stress relationship and the upward shift of the compliance–midwall stress relationship in response to the increase in shear stress (Fig. 10.3) [34].

Finally, the conclusions obtained from these experiments based on NO suppression were also confirmed by interventional studies evaluating the impact of intervention majoring NO pathway on arterial mechanics. Indeed, the inhibition of arginase, supplementation with the eNOS cofactor tetrahydrobiopterin, or more directly administration of NO donors or phosphodiesterase 5 inhibitor improves the mechanical properties of conduit arteries in animals and humans [30, 31, 66, 67].

Physiological and Compensatory Role of EDH(F)

In contrast to NO, the role of EDH(F) in the regulation of arterial mechanics has been poorly investigated mainly due to the lack of specific inhibitors in particular in humans. Nonetheless, as previously described, the basal release of a diffusive EDHF in porcine coronary arteries participates

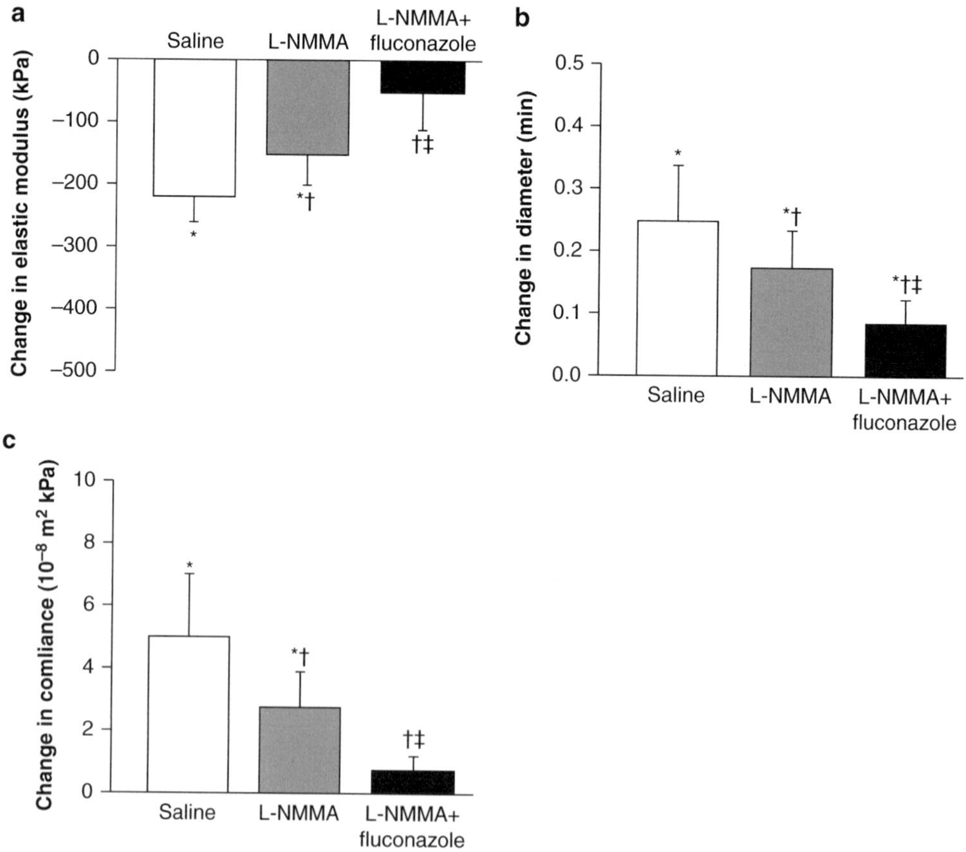

Fig. 10.3 The mean decrease in radial artery elastic modulus, calculated during hand skin heating (from 34 to 44 °C) at each level of midwall stress illustrating the decrease in arterial stiffness during blood flow increase, was reduced by the local infusion of the NO-synthase inhibitor L-NMMA and abolished by the combination of L-NMMA with the CYP450 epoxygenases inhibitor fluconazole (**a**). In addition, L-NMMA and, to a larger extent, L-NMMA + fluconazole reduced the increase in radial artery diameter, i.e., the flow-mediated dilatation, in response to hand skin heating (**b**). As a result, the mean upward shift of the arterial compliance–midwall stress relationship was reduced by L-NMMA and suppressed by L-NMMA + fluconazole (**c**). $*P<0.05$ vs. baseline, $\dagger P<0.05$ vs. saline, $\ddagger P<0.05$ vs. L-NMMA

to the regulation of arterial compliance [9]. Indeed, in the presence of cyclooxygenase and NOS inhibitors, iberiotoxin and deendothelialization resulted in a decrease in the diameter distension of isolated porcine coronary artery in response to an imposed pulse pressure. Similar results were reported concerning the endothelial release of NO in response to the increase in pulsatile pressure [7, 8]. More recently, it was shown by using transgenic mice that the constitutive protein of endothelial gap junction, connexin40, attenuates the myogenic tone in response to intraluminal increase in blood pressure in mesenteric resistance arteries by mediating endothelium-derived hyperpolarization [68]. In addition, an increase in the stiffness of these arteries was observed in the single point mutant animals, demonstrating that connexin40 mediates the EDH phenomenon not only to regulate endothelium-dependent dilatation in resistance arteries but also the stiffness of these arteries [68].

In humans, the effect of the acute blockade of vascular K_{Ca} channels by local tetraethylammonium (TEA) infusion on arterial mechanics was also investigated at the level of the radial artery, before and after inhibition of NOS with L-NMMA [31]. In addition, to reduce radial diameter, TEA increased the modulus and decreased the compliance at all levels of stress, thus supporting a role for EDH(F) in the regulation of the mechanical properties of peripheral conduit arteries at this level in vivo. In addition, while L-NMMA alone paradoxically improved the arterial mechanical properties, the combination of L-NMMA and TEA synergistically enhanced the increase in modulus and decrease in compliance. This demonstrates that EDH(F) is the compensatory mechanism maintaining arterial mechanics during the loss of NO synthesis [31]. Using the local infusion of L-NMMA alone and combined with TEA and the inhibitor of cytochrome P450 epoxygenases fluconazole during hand skin heating, it can be demonstrated that EETs act as EDHF, not only to regulate with NO endothelium-dependent flow-mediated dilatation, but also the adaptation of arterial mechanics to the increase in flow [34]. Indeed, the combination of L-NMMA with TEA or with fluconazole similarly abolished the downward shift of the modulus–midwall stress relationship and the upward shift of the compliance midwall stress relationship (Fig. 10.3) [34].

Taken together, these results indicate that endothelium-derived NO and EDH(F), notably EETs during flow increase, regulate the stiffness of conduit arteries and that, in turn, endothelial dysfunction is probably a main contributor of arterial stiffening during aging and in cardiovascular diseases. However, it should be emphasize that the alteration in the mechanical properties of conduit arteries reinforces the alteration in endothelial function by modifying pulsatile strain thereby creating a vicious circle.

Impact of Arterial Stiffness on Endothelial Function

One mechanism by which endothelium-derived factors release may be reduced is the increase in arterial wall stiffness itself. First, the increase in arterial wall stiffness during aging and pathological conditions is associated with an outward remodeling to maintain arterial compliance in most of the human studies [69, 70]. At the level of the carotid but also in the brachial artery, this increased diameter results in a decrease in the local mean, systolic, and diastolic flow velocities and in the corresponding wall shear stresses, thus probably affecting the endothelium-dependent shear stress-mediated release of vasorelaxant factors [71–73]. This phenomenon juxtaposes with the abnormal blood pressure pulsatility along the arterial tree from the aorta to the capillary. According with the pressure–flow relationship, the conduit artery stiffening along the vascular tree, resulting from the increase in forward pulse pressure, PWV, and/or the magnitude of reflected wave, elevates pulse pressure and flow in the main branches of the aorta, and this elevation is transmitted to the microcirculation. This will be particularly deleterious in the vascular beds characterized by low vascular resistance as the brain and kidney, thus contributing to the high occurrence of cardiovascular events associated with arterial stiffening [74, 75].

Furthermore, a second mechanism has been originally suggested in BAEC, i.e., the direct modulation of pulse pressure/flow mechanosignaling by the reduction in stretch related to the increase in arterial stiffness. Thanks to a servo-pump system, BAEC were cultured within no flow or stable mean flow and pressure but under nonpulsatile or pulsatile conditions. Thus, while in compliant tubes, the increase in pulse pressure enhances pulse flow and elicits pulsatile strain, in stiff tubes, this increase in pulse pressure (PP: 90 mmHg) was associated with an increase in pulse flow and a very reduced strain (from 7 to 1 % radial stretch [6]). As compared with no-flow conditions, steady flow increased Akt phosphorylation in a similar manner in stiff and compliant conduits. In contrast, pulsatile conditions increased the Akt/eNOS-phosphorylation in a PI3K-dependent manner only in compliant tubes. Similarly, it was reported in BAEC a decreased Akt phosphorylation in stiff conduits under less pulsatile conditions (PP: 70 mmHg) as compared with compliant conduits [5]. This effect was accompanied by a Akt-dependent decrease in protection against hydrogen peroxide-stimulated apoptosis in stiff tubes and restored after BAEC transfection with a constitutive active form of Akt. Moreover, additional information were provided concerning the mechanotransduction pathways involved upstream from Akt activation in response to pulsatile stresses in compliant and stiff conduits. Indeed, it was demonstrated that AKt activation by pulse pressure and flow in compliant conduits was VEGFR2/caveolin-independent, whereas the steady shear stress activation in all conduits and the residual activation of AKt in stiff conduits were VEGFR2/caveolin dependent. Although this requires to be confirmed, a major stretch-sensitive mechanism of endothelial protection mediated by Akt may be suppressed in noncompliant arteries, and this could contribute to the high cardiovascular risk provided by arterial stiffening.

Conclusions

Vascular endothelium is continuously exposed to mechanical stimuli that are sensed and integrated to regulate the release of endothelium-derived factors, thus leading to adaptive responses, i.e., changes in arterial tone, geometry, or structural wall content. By modifying these parameters, the endothelium participates to the regulation of the underlying resistance and conduit artery mechanical properties and, moreover, contributes to the adaptation of the whole vascular tree to changes in systemic hemodynamics and cardiovascular coupling. In this respect convincing data are now available in humans to support the presence of an endothelium-dependent flow-mediated regulation of conduit artery mechanics, particularly related to the release of NO and more recently EDHFs such as EETs. Furthermore, the endothelium differentially integrates steady or pulsatile stresses according to their magnitude. Thus, whereas low oscillatory shear stress promotes an unbalance between vasorelaxant and vasoconstrictor influences, the latter becoming predominant, the increase in pulse pressure and flow is associated to the opposite effects in compliant vessels. Thus, by increasing the release of relaxant factors in response to the increase in pulsatile stresses, the endothelium helps to maintain arterial stiffness and reflectivity and to prevent the increase in central pulse pressure. Subsequently, these adaptive responses are suppressed in the presence of endothelial dysfunction, favoring inflammation and wall stiffening through notably a decrease in NO and increase in the release of profibrotic factors. The development of endothelial dysfunction, although limited at an early stage by compensating mechanisms such as EDH(F), is thus a major contributor to systolic hypertension and to the enhanced pulsatility along the vascular tree, ultimately damaging the more distal microvascular territories. Finally, the decrease in pulse strain resulting from the conduit artery stiffening appears to suppress these endothelial protective mechanisms, further amplifying the alteration in arterial mechanical properties.

References

1. Busse R, Fleming I. Pulsatile stretch and shear stress: physical stimuli determining the production of endothelium-derived relaxing factors. J Vasc Res. 1998; 35:73–84.
2. Lehoux S, Tedgui A. Signal transduction of mechanical stresses in the vascular wall. Hypertension. 1998; 32:338–45.
3. Ando J, Yamamoto K. Vascular mechanobiology: endothelial cell responses to fluid shear stress. Circ J. 2009;73:1983–92.
4. Lu D, Kassab GS. Role of shear stress and stretch in vascular mechanobiology. J R Soc Interface. 2011;8:1379–85.
5. Li M, Chiou KR, Bugayenko A, Irani K, Kass DA. Reduced wall compliance suppresses Akt-dependent apoptosis protection stimulated by pulse perfusion. Circ Res. 2005;97:587–95.
6. Peng X, Haldar S, Deshpande S, Irani K, Kass DA. Wall stiffness suppresses Akt/eNOS and cytoprotection in pulse-perfused endothelium. Hypertension. 2003;41:378–81.
7. Recchia FA, Senzaki H, Saeki A, Byrne BJ, Kass DA. Pulse pressure-related changes in coronary flow in vivo are modulated by nitric oxide and adenosine. Circ Res. 1996;79:849–56.
8. Nakano T, Tominaga R, Morita S, Masuda M, Nagano I, Imasaka K, Yasui H. Impacts of pulsatile systemic circulation on endothelium-derived nitric oxide release in anesthetized dogs. Ann Thorac Surg. 2001;72:156–62.
9. Popp R, Fleming I, Busse R. Pulsatile stretch in coronary arteries elicits release of endothelium-derived hyperpolarizing factor: a modulator of arterial compliance. Circ Res. 1998;82:696–703.
10. Zhao J, Yang J, Liu J, Li S, Yan J, Meng Y, Wang X, Long C. Effects of pulsatile and nonpulsatile perfusion on cerebral regional oxygen saturation and endothelin-1 in tetralogy of fallot infants. Artif Organs. 2011;35:E54–8.

11. Godbole AS, Lu X, Guo X, Kassab GS. NADPH oxidase has a directional response to shear stress. Am J Physiol Heart Circ Physiol. 2009;296:H152–8.
12. Castier Y, Brandes RP, Leseche G, Tedgui A, Lehoux S. p47phox-dependent NADPH oxidase regulates flow-induced vascular remodeling. Circ Res. 2005;97:533–40.
13. Li M, Stenmark KR, Shandas R, Tan W. Effects of pathological flow on pulmonary artery endothelial production of vasoactive mediators and growth factors. J Vasc Res. 2009;46:561–71.
14. Koskinas KC, Feldman CL, Chatzizisis YS, Coskun AU, Jonas M, Maynard C, Baker AB, Papafaklis MI, Edelman ER, Stone PH. Natural history of experimental coronary atherosclerosis and vascular remodeling in relation to endothelial shear stress: a serial, in vivo intravascular ultrasound study. Circulation. 2010;121:2092–101.
15. Vion AC, Ramkhelawon B, Loyer X, Chironi G, Devue C, Loirand G, Tedgui A, Lehoux S, Boulanger CM. Shear stress regulates endothelial microparticle release. Circ Res. 2013;112:1323–33.
16. De Keulenaer GW, Chappell DC, Ishizaka N, Nerem RM, Alexander RW, Griendling KK. Oscillatory and steady laminar shear stress differentially affect human endothelial redox state: role of a superoxide-producing NADH oxidase. Circ Res. 1998;82:1094–101.
17. Patel A, Honoré E. Polycystins and renovascular mechanosensory transduction. Nat Rev Nephrol. 2010; 6:530–8.
18. Sharif-Naeini R, Folgering JH, Bichet D, Duprat F, Lauritzen I, Arhatte M, Jodar M, Dedman A, Chatelain FC, Schulte U, Retailleau K, Loufrani L, Patel A, Sachs F, Delmas P, Peters DJ, Honoré E. Polycystin-1 and –2 dosage regulates pressure sensing. Cell. 2009;139:587–96.
19. Fisslthaler B, Dimmeler S, Hermann C, Busse R, Fleming I. Phosphorylation and activation of the endothelial nitric oxide synthase by fluid shear stress. Acta Physiol Scand. 2000;168:81–8.
20. Muller JM, Chilian WM, Davis MJ. Integrin signaling transduces shear stress–dependent vasodilation of coronary arterioles. Circ Res. 1997;80:320–6.
21. Koshida R, Rocic P, Saito S, Kiyooka T, Zhang C, Chilian WM. Role of focal adhesion kinase in flow-induced dilation of coronary arterioles. Arterioscler Thromb Vasc Biol. 2005;25:2548–53.
22. Boo YC, Sorescu G, Boyd N, Shiojima I, Walsh K, Du J, Jo H. Shear stress stimulates phosphorylation of endothelial nitric-oxide synthase at Ser1179 by Akt-independent mechanisms: role of protein kinase A. J Biol Chem. 2002;277:3388–96.
23. Jin ZG, Ueba H, Tanimoto T, Lungu AO, Frame MD, Berk BC. Ligand-independent activation of vascular endothelial growth factor receptor 2 by fluid shear stress regulates activation of endothelial nitric oxide synthase. Circ Res. 2003;93:354–63.
24. Tzima E, Irani-Tehrani M, Kiosses WB, Dejana E, Schultz DA, Engelhardt B, Cao G, DeLisser H, Schwartz MA. A mechanosensory complex that mediates the endothelial cell response to fluid shear stress. Nature. 2005;437:426–31.
25. Chen AH, Gortler DS, Kilaru S, Araim O, Frangos SG, Sumpio BE. Cyclic strain activates the pro-survival Akt protein kinase in bovine aortic smooth muscle cells. Surgery. 2001;130:378–81.
26. Joannides R, Richard V, Haefeli WE, Linder L, Lüscher TF, Thuillez C. Role of basal and stimulated release of nitric oxide in the regulation of radial artery caliber in humans. Hypertension. 1995;26:327–31.
27. Lefroy DC, Crake T, Uren NG, Davies GJ, Maseri A. Effect of inhibition of nitric oxide synthesis on epicardial coronary artery diameter and coronary blood flow in humans. Circulation. 1993;88:43–54.
28. Duffy SJ, Castle SF, Harper RW, Meredith IT. Contribution of vasodilator prostanoids and nitric oxide to resting flow, metabolic vasodilation, and flow-mediated dilation in human coronary circulation. Circulation. 1999;100:1951–7.
29. Puybasset L, Bea ML, Ghaleh B, Giudicelli JF, Berdeaux A. Coronary and systemic hemodynamic effects of sustained inhibition of nitric oxide synthesis in conscious dogs. Evidence for cross talk between nitric oxide and cyclooxygenase in coronary vessels. Circ Res. 1996;79:343–57.
30. Kinlay S, Creager MA, Fukumoto M, Hikita H, Fang JC, Selwyn AP, Ganz P. Endothelium-derived nitric oxide regulates arterial elasticity in human arteries in vivo. Hypertension. 2001;38:1049–53.
31. Bellien J, Joannides R, Iacob M, Arnaud P, Thuillez C. Calcium-activated potassium channels and nitric oxide regulate human peripheral conduit artery mechanics. Hypertension. 2005;46:210–6.
32. Seddon M, Melikian N, Dworakowski R, Shabeeh H, Jiang B, Byrne J, Casadei B, Chowienczyk P, Shah AM. Effects of neuronal nitric oxide synthase on human coronary artery diameter and blood flow in vivo. Circulation. 2009;119:2656–62.
33. Shabeeh H, Seddon M, Brett S, Melikian N, Casadei B, Shah AM, Chowienczyk P. Sympathetic activation increases NO release from eNOS but neither eNOS nor nNOS play an essential role in exercise hyperemia in the human forearm. Am J Physiol Heart Circ Physiol. 2013;304:H1225–30.
34. Bellien J, Favre J, Iacob M, Gao J, Thuillez C, Richard V, Joannidès R. Arterial stiffness is regulated by nitric oxide and endothelium-derived hyperpolarizing factor during changes in blood flow in humans. Hypertension. 2010;55:674–80.
35. Bellien J, Iacob M, Remy-Jouet I, Lucas D, Monteil C, Gutierrez L, Vendeville C, Dreano Y, Mercier A, Thuillez C, Joannides R. Epoxyeicosatrienoic acids contribute with altered nitric oxide and endothelin-1 pathways to conduit artery endothelial dysfunction in essential hypertension. Circulation. 2012;125: 1266–75.
36. Bellien J, Joannides R, Richard V, Thuillez C. Modulation of cytochrome-derived epoxyeicosatrienoic acids pathway: a promising pharmacological approach to prevent endothelial dysfunction in cardiovascular diseases? Pharmacol Ther. 2011;131: 1–17.

37. Ozkor MA, Murrow JR, Rahman AM, Kavtaradze N, Lin J, Manatunga A, Quyyumi AA. Endothelium-derived hyperpolarizing factor determines resting and stimulated forearm vasodilator tone in health and in disease. Circulation. 2011;123:2244–53.
38. Fisslthaler B, Popp R, Michaelis UR, Kiss L, Fleming I, Busse R. Cyclic stretch enhances the expression and activity of coronary endothelium-derived hyperpolarizing factor synthase. Hypertension. 2001;38:1427–32.
39. Paolocci N, Pagliaro P, Isoda T, Saavedra FW, Kass DA. Role of calcium-sensitive K(+) channels and nitric oxide in vivo coronary vasodilation from enhanced perfusion pulsatility. Circulation. 2001;103:119–24.
40. Bellien J, Joannides R, Iacob M, Arnaud P, Thuillez C. Evidence for a basal release of a cytochrome-related endothelium-derived hyperpolarizing factor in the radial artery in humans. Am J Physiol Heart Circ Physiol. 2006;290:H1347–52.
41. Bellien J, Remy-Jouet I, Iacob M, Blot E, Mercier A, Lucas D, Dreano Y, Gutierrez L, Donnadieu N, Thuillez C, Joannides R. Impaired role of epoxyeicosatrienoic acids in the regulation of basal conduit artery diameter during essential hypertension. Hypertension. 2012;60:1415–21.
42. Joannides R, Richard V, Moore N, Godin M, Thuillez C. Influence of sympathetic tone on mechanical properties of muscular arteries in humans. Am J Physiol. 1995;268:H794–801.
43. Chamiot-Clerc P, Renaud JF, Safar ME. Pulse pressure, aortic reactivity, and endothelium dysfunction in old hypertensive rats. Hypertension. 2001;37:313–21.
44. London GM. Role of arterial wall properties in the pathogenesis of systolic hypertension. Am J Hypertens. 2005;18(1 Pt 2):19S–22.
45. Sudhir K, Mullen WL, Hausmann D, Fitzgerald PJ, Chou TM, Yock PG, Chatterjee K. Contribution of endothelium-derived nitric oxide to coronary arterial distensibility: an in vivo two-dimensional intravascular ultrasound study. Am Heart J. 1995;129:726–32.
46. Boutouyrie P, Bezie Y, Lacolley P, Challande P, Chamiot-Clerc P, Benetos A, de la Faverie JF, Safar M, Laurent S. In vivo/in vitro comparison of rat abdominal aorta wall viscosity. Influence of endothelial function. Arterioscler Thromb Vasc Biol. 1997;17: 1346–55.
47. Armentano RL, Barra JG, Santana DB, Pessana FM, Graf S, Craiem D, Brandani LM, Baglivo HP, Sanchez RA. Smart damping modulation of carotid wall energetics in human hypertension: effects of angiotensin-converting enzyme inhibition. Hypertension. 2006;47: 384–90.
48. Hodis S, Zamir M. Mechanical events within the arterial wall: the dynamic context for elastin fatigue. J Biomech. 2009;42:1010–6.
49. Kobayashi K, Akishita M, Yu W, Hashimoto M, Ohni M, Toba K. Interrelationship between non-invasive measurements of atherosclerosis: flow-mediated dilation of brachial artery, carotid intima-media thickness and pulse wave velocity. Atherosclerosis. 2004;173: 13–8.
50. Palombo C, Kozakova M, Morizzo C, Gnesi L, Barsotti MC, Spontoni P, Massart F, Salvi P, Balbarini A, Saggese G, Di Stefano R, Federico G. Circulating endothelial progenitor cells and large artery structure and function in young subjects with uncomplicated type 1 diabetes. Cardiovasc Diabetol. 2011;10:88.
51. van Bussel BC, Schouten F, Henry RM, Schalkwijk CG, de Boer MR, Ferreira I, Smulders YM, Twisk JW, Stehouwer CD. Endothelial dysfunction and low-grade inflammation are associated with greater arterial stiffness over a 6-year period. Hypertension. 2011;58:588–95.
52. Joannides R, Costentin A, Iacob M, Bakkali e-H, Richard MO, Thuillez C. Role of arterial smooth muscle tone and geometry in the regulation of peripheral conduit artery mechanics by shear stress. Clin Exp Pharmacol Physiol. 2001;28:1025–31.
53. Joannides R, Bizet-Nafeh C, Costentin A, Iacob M, Derumeaux G, Cribier A, Thuillez C. Chronic ACE inhibition enhances the endothelial control of arterial mechanics and flow-dependent vasodilatation in heart failure. Hypertension. 2001;38:1446–50.
54. Modena MG, Bonetti L, Coppi F, Bursi F, Rossi R. Prognostic role of reversible endothelial dysfunction in hypertensive postmenopausal women. J Am Coll Cardiol. 2002;40:505–10.
55. Joannidès R, Monteil C, de Ligny BH, Westeel PF, Iacob M, Thervet E, Barbier S, Bellien J, Lebranchu Y, Seguin SG, Thuillez C, Godin M, Etienne I. Immunosuppressant regimen based on sirolimus decreases aortic stiffness in renal transplant recipients in comparison to cyclosporine. Am J Transplant. 2011;11:2414–22.
56. Delacretaz E, Hayoz D, Osterheld MC, Genton CY, Brunner HR, Waeber B. Long-term nitric oxide synthase inhibition and distensibility of carotid artery in intact rats. Hypertension. 1994;23:967–70.
57. Soucy KG, Ryoo S, Benjo A, Lim HK, Gupta G, Sohi JS, Elser J, Aon MA, Nyhan D, Shoukas AA, Berkowitz DE. Impaired shear stress-induced nitric oxide production through decreased NOS phosphorylation contributes to age-related vascular stiffness. J Appl Physiol. 2006;101:1751–9.
58. Isabelle M, Simonet S, Ragonnet C, Sansilvestri-Morel P, Clavreul N, Vayssettes-Courchay C, Verbeuren TJ. Chronic reduction of nitric oxide level in adult spontaneously hypertensive rats induces aortic stiffness similar to old spontaneously hypertensive rats. J Vasc Res. 2012;49:309–18.
59. Safar ME, Laurent P. Pulse pressure and arterial stiffness in rats: comparison with humans. Am J Physiol Heart Circ Physiol. 2003;285:H1363–9.
60. Stewart AD, Millasseau SC, Kearney MT, Ritter JM, Chowienczyk PJ. Effects of inhibition of basal nitric oxide synthesis on carotid-femoral pulse wave velocity and augmentation index in humans. Hypertension. 2003;42:915–8.
61. Kelly RP, Millasseau SC, Ritter JM, Chowienczyk PJ. Vasoactive drugs influence aortic augmentation index independently of pulse-wave velocity in healthy men. Hypertension. 2001;37:1429–33.

62. McVeigh GE, Allen PB, Morgan DR, Hanratty CG, Silke B. Nitric oxide modulation of blood vessel tone identified by arterial waveform analysis. Clin Sci (Lond). 2001;100:387–93.
63. Mayer Jr O, Filipovský J, Pesta M, Cífková R, Dolejsová M, Simon J. Synergistic effect of angiotensin II type 1 receptor and endothelial nitric oxide synthase gene polymorphisms on arterial stiffness. J Hum Hypertens. 2008;22:111–8.
64. Mourad JJ, Ducailar G, Rudnicki A, Lajemi M, Mimran A, Safar ME. Age-related increase of pulse pressure and gene polymorphisms in essential hypertension: a preliminary study. J Renin Angiotensin Aldosterone Syst. 2002;3:109–15.
65. Schmitt M, Avolio A, Qasem A, McEniery CM, Butlin M, Wilkinson IB, Cockcroft JR. Basal NO locally modulates human iliac artery function in vivo. Hypertension. 2005;46:227–31.
66. Kim JH, Bugaj LJ, Oh YJ, Bivalacqua TJ, Ryoo S, Soucy KG, Santhanam L, Webb A, Camara A, Sikka G, Nyhan D, Shoukas AA, Ilies M, Christianson DW, Champion HC, Berkowitz DE. Arginase inhibition restores NOS coupling and reverses endothelial dysfunction and vascular stiffness in old rats. J Appl Physiol. 2009;107:1249–57.
67. Attinà TM, Drummond ID, Malatino LS, Maxwell SR, Webb DJ. Phosphodiesterase type 5 inhibition improves arterial stiffness after exercise but not exercise capacity in hypertensive men. Am J Hypertens. 2013;26:342–50.
68. Chaston DJ, Baillie BK, Grayson TH, Courjaret RJ, Heisler JM, Lau KA, Machaca K, Nicholson BJ, Ashton A, Matthaei KI, Hill CE. Polymorphism in endothelial connexin40 enhances sensitivity to intraluminal pressure and increases arterial stiffness. Arterioscler Thromb Vasc Biol. 2013;33:962–70.
69. Boutouyrie P, Laurent S, Benetos A, Girerd XJ, Hoeks AP, Safar ME. Opposing effects of ageing on distal and proximal large arteries in hypertensives. J Hypertens Suppl. 1992;10:S87–91.
70. van der Heijden-Spek JJ, Staessen JA, Fagard RH, Hoeks AP, Boudier HA, van Bortel LM. Effect of age on brachial artery wall properties differs from the aorta and is gender dependent: a population study. Hypertension. 2000;35:637–42.
71. Simon AC, Levenson J. Abnormal wall shear conditions in the brachial artery of hypertensive patients. J Hypertens. 1990;8:109–14.
72. Samijo SK, Willigers JM, Barkhuysen R, Kitslaar PJ, Reneman RS, Brands PJ, Hoeks AP. Wall shear stress in the human common carotid artery as function of age and gender. Cardiovasc Res. 1998;39:515–22.
73. Duivenvoorden R, Vanbavel E, de Groot E, Stroes ES, Disselhorst JA, Hutten BA, Laméris JS, Kastelein JJ, Nederveen AJ. Endothelial shear stress: a critical determinant of arterial remodeling and arterial stiffness in humans–a carotid 3.0-T MRI study. Circ Cardiovasc Imaging. 2010;3:578–85.
74. O'Rourke MF, Safar ME. Relationship between aortic stiffening and microvascular disease in brain and kidney: cause and logic of therapy. Hypertension. 2005; 46:200–4.
75. Hirata K, Yaginuma T, O'Rourke MF, Kawakami M. Age-related changes in carotid artery flow and pressure pulses: possible implications for cerebral microvascular disease. Stroke. 2006;37:2552–6.

Hypoxia, Arterial Blood Pressure, and Microcirculation

11

Jean-Jacques Mourad, Jean-Sébastien Silvestre, and Bernard I. Lévy

Abstract

The larger part of the systemic hemodynamic resistance is located in the microcirculation. The microcirculatory networks, especially its arteriolar and capillary components, are subjected to angiogenesis in relation to the activation of the HIF-VEGF-NO pathways. In the present chapter we report experiments performed in young and adult spontaneously hypertensive rats maintained for several weeks under chronic hypoxic conditions. Chronic hypoxia resulted in activation of VEGF-induced angiogenesis, increases in myocardial and skeletal muscle capillary density, and normalization of arterial blood pressure in both young prehypertensive rats and old rats with established hypertension.

In parallel and in contrast, administration of bevacizumab, an antibody directed against the VEGF protein, to patients with metastatic colorectal cancer, induced a significant increase in blood pressure in relation to a significant reduction in capillary density and a complete blunting of the endothelial function.

Taken together, these experimental and clinical results suggest that angiogenesis and antiangiogenesis could have rapid and marked effects on the peripheral resistance. Moreover, the density of the capillary bed seems to play a major role in the control of the arterial pressure.

Keywords

Arterial hypertension • Microcirculation • Angiogenesis • VEGF • Bevacizumab

J.-J. Mourad, MD, PhD
Department of Internal Medicine and Arterial Hypertension, Avicenne University Hospital – APHP, 125 rue de Stalingrad, Bobigny 93000, France
e-mail: jean-jacques.mourad@avc.aphp.fr

J.-S. Silvestre, PhD
Cardiovascular Research Center- Inserm UMRS 970, 56 rue Leblanc, Paris 75015, France
e-mail: jean-sebasiten.silvestre@inserm.fr

B.I. Lévy, MD, PhD (✉)
Cardiovascular Research Center- Inserm UMRS 970, 56 rue Leblanc, Paris 75015, France

Blood and Vessel Institute, 8 rue Guy Patin, Paris 75010, France
e-mail: bernard.levy@inserm.fr

M.E. Safar et al. (eds.), *Blood Pressure and Arterial Wall Mechanics in Cardiovascular Diseases*, DOI 10.1007/978-1-4471-5198-2_11,

In most forms of clinical and experimental hypertension, increased arterial blood pressure is associated with *microvascular rarefaction* and increase in peripheral vascular resistances [1]. The cause-effect relationships of vascular rarefaction and hypertension are still debated. It is speculated that diffuse systemic rarefaction might be a primary defect in essential hypertension [2]. On the other hand, rarefaction can also represent a downstream consequence, as shown by its occurrence in animal models of secondary hypertension [3, 4]. Microvascular density might decrease because of either vessel destruction or insufficient angiogenesis, i.e., growth of new capillaries from preexisting ones. This process proceeds during development and also in adults during physiological and pathological conditions. Abnormally low microvascular density can be seen at a very young age in animals with genetic hypertension [5] and also exists in normotensive humans with a familial predisposition to the disease [6, 7] indicating that alteration in vessel growth could lead to elevation in the peripheral vascular resistance and subsequently trigger the pathogenesis of hypertension.

Hypoxia is usually considered as the major stimulus for angiogenesis. The main mechanism of hypoxia-induced capillary growth involves the rise in hypoxia-inducible factor-1 (HIF-1) protein. HIF-1 binds to specific hypoxia-responsive element in the regulatory regions of several hypoxia-sensitive genes, such as vascular endothelial growth factor (VEGF-A) [8]. VEGF-A is then secreted and binds to its cognate receptor tyrosine kinases, Flt-1 and Flk-1/KDR, located on the surface of the vascular cells. Receptor ligation triggers a cascade of intracellular signaling pathways initiating angiogenesis. Furthermore, VEGF-A has been shown, through Flk-1/KDR, to activate endothelial nitric oxide synthase (eNOS)–related pathways leading to nitric oxide (NO) production [9].

In an attempt to understand the relationship between chronic hypoxia and arterial hypertension, we analyzed the effect of normobaric hypoxia on blood pressure levels in animals with genetic hypertension.

In a second work and in a clinical situation, we applied the results obtained under experimental conditions to explore the mechanisms responsible for hypertension in patients receiving an antiangiogenic treatment.

Effect of Chronic Hypoxia on Arterial Pressure of Spontaneously Hypertensive Rats (SHR)

Experimental Design and Methods

Experiment 1

Prehypertensive young SHRs (5 weeks old) treated with or without VEGF-A–neutralizing antibody (3 mg/kg IP, twice a week) and age-matched normotensive Wistar-Kyoto (WKY) rats were housed for 3 or 7 weeks under normoxic (standard laboratory conditions, i.e., 20.5 % O_2) or hypoxic (12 % O_2) conditions. Hypoxic chamber was maintained at 25 °C and 80 % humidity. CO_2 production by the animals was fixed with soda lime, and PCO_2 remained at the 0 level in the hypoxic chamber.

Experiment 2

Hypertensive adult SHRs (12 weeks old) were housed under normobaric hypoxic conditions for 8 weeks and then under normoxic conditions for 2 h or 3 additional weeks before euthanasia. In an additional set of experiments, hypertensive adult SHRs (12 weeks old) were housed under hypoxic conditions for 1 week and then under normoxic conditions for 1 additional week before euthanasia.

Systolic blood pressure (SBP) was measured weekly in all young and adult conscious rats using a computerized tail-cuff system.

Effect of Hypoxia on Hemodynamic Parameters

We first assessed the effect of hypoxia on the development of hypertension in prehypertensive SHRs. Prehypertensive young SHRs, maintained

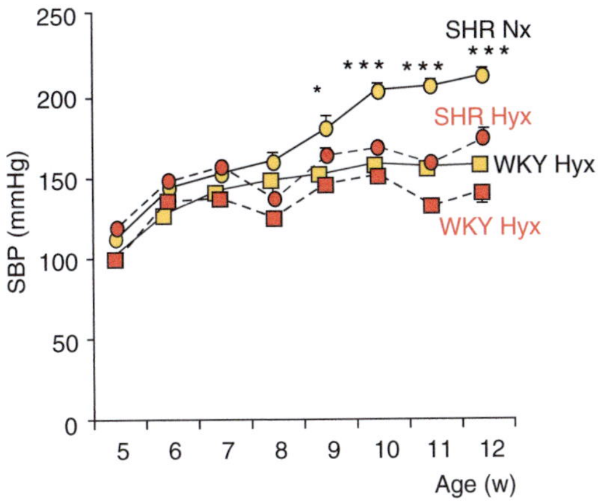

Fig. 11.1 Systolic blood pressure in spontaneously hypertensive rats (*SHR*) and normotensive controls (*WKY*). Five-week-old rats were maintained for 8 weeks under normoxic (*Nx*) or hypoxic (*Hyx*) conditions. Significance of the difference between normoxic and hypoxic values in the SHRs: * $P<0.05$; *** $P<0.001$

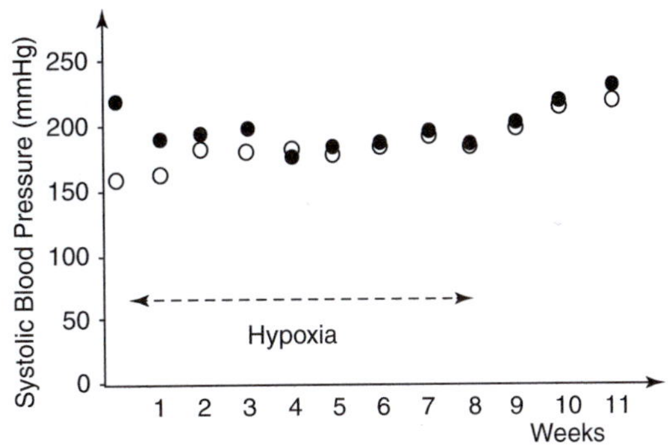

Fig. 11.2 Five- (*open circles*) and 12-week-old (*filled circles*) SHRs were maintained under hypoxia for 8 weeks and then returned to normoxic conditions for 3 additional weeks

under normoxic conditions, showed higher SBP than normoxic WKY rats, throughout the experiment (Fig. 11.1). In WKY rats, hypoxia tended to reduce systolic blood (SBP) pressure when compared to normoxic WKY rats; this difference reached significance after 3 weeks of hypoxia. In SHRs, after 3 weeks of exposure to hypoxia, SBP was lower by 26 % in hypoxic SHRs compared to normoxic SHRs ($P<0.05$). Thereafter, SBP remained lower in hypoxic SHRs compared to normoxic SHRs and was similar to the SBP in normoxic WKY rats during the last 4 weeks of hypoxic period. Cardiac output was not significantly affected by hypoxia in both WKY and SHR strains; total peripheral resistance (TPR) was raised by 30 % in normoxic SHRs compared to normoxic WKY rats ($P<0.001$). In hypoxic SHRs, TPR was reduced by 30 % when compared to normoxic SHRs ($P<0.001$) and returned to WKY levels.

In WKY rats, hypoxia tended to reduce TPR, but this difference did not reach statistical significance. Taken together, these results suggest that hypoxia decreased TPR, preventing the rise in SBP occurring in normoxic SHRs.

We next analyzed the effect of hypoxia in adult SHRs with established hypertension (Fig. 11.2). Interestingly, SBP in adult hypoxic SHRs was also reduced by 16 % ($P<0.001$, versus normoxic SHRs) as early as 1 week of hypoxia, suggesting that hypoxia reversed hypertension in adult SHRs.

In addition, after 8 weeks of hypoxia, return to normoxia was followed by increased SBP in both 5- and 12-week-old SHRs.

These results suggest that:

1. Hypoxia was able to prevent the raise in blood pressure levels in young SHRs and to reverse hypertension in adult SHRs.
2. The hypoxia-related effects were transient and fully abrogated 1–2 weeks after return to normoxia.

Mechanisms of Hypoxia-Induced Reduction in Arterial Pressure in the SHRs

We next attempted to understand the molecular and cellular mechanisms associated with the hypoxia-induced prevention of hypertension development in young SHRs.

We analyzed the effect of hypoxia on blood vessel growth; we first analyzed the density of vascular structure in the hind limb of hypoxic and normoxic animals. Microangiography analysis indicated that arteriole (>200 μm) density was similar in normoxic WKY rats and normoxic SHRs. In addition, hypoxia did not significantly modify arterial angiographic score in

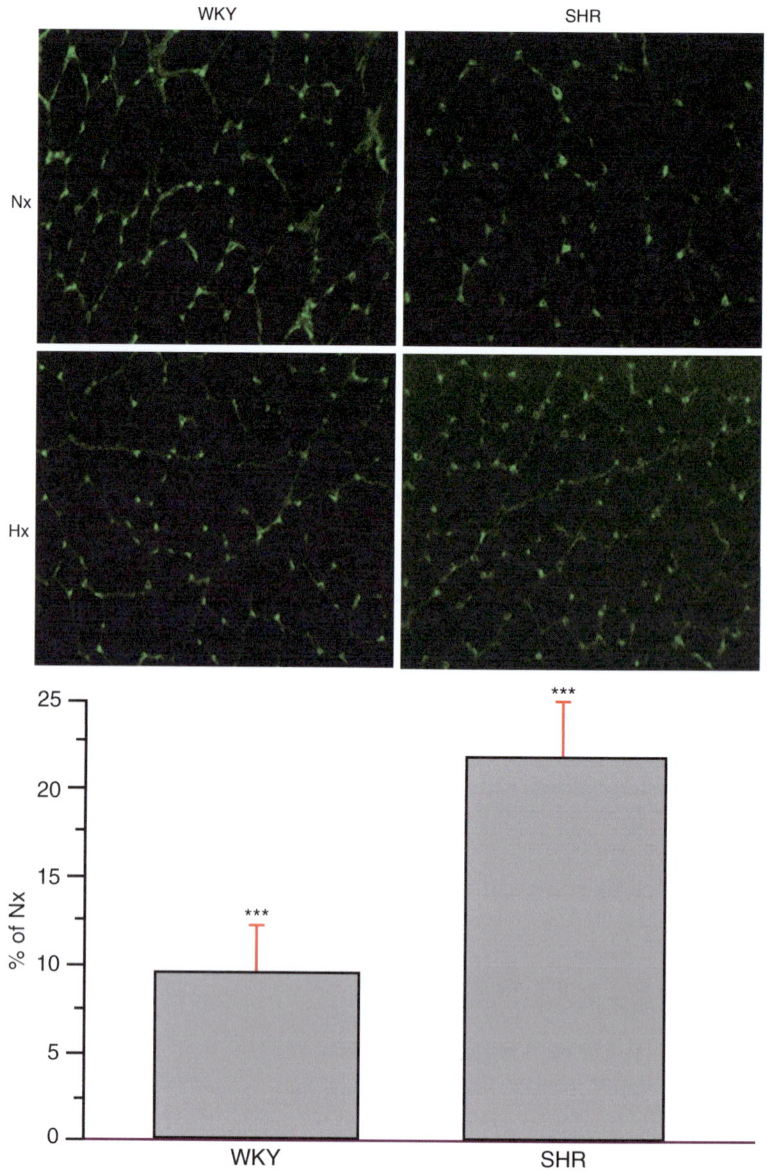

Fig. 11.3 Representative photomicrographs and quantitative evaluation of capillary density in quadriceps muscle (capillaries appears in *green*) in WKY and SHRs under hypoxic (*Hx*) and normoxic (*Nx*) conditions

the hind limb of WKY rats and SHRs. In parallel, arteriole density (measured in skeletal muscle histological sections) was similar in WKY rats and SHRs, regardless of the conditions. In contrast, skeletal muscle capillary density was decreased by 30 % in normoxic SHRs compared to normoxic WKY rats ($P < 0.01$). Interestingly, hypoxia raised capillary density by 30 % in both hypoxic SHRs and WKY rats compared to their normoxic control animals (Fig. 11.3). Capillary density in hypoxic SHRs was then similar to that in normoxic WKY rats.

We analyzed the effect of hypoxia in the left ventricle as well. We did not observe any significant changes in arteriole density in the left ventricle free wall from WKY rats and SHRs, regardless of the experimental conditions. In contrast, capillary density was lower in normoxic SHRs compared to normoxic WKY rats ($P < 0.05$). Capillary density was increased by

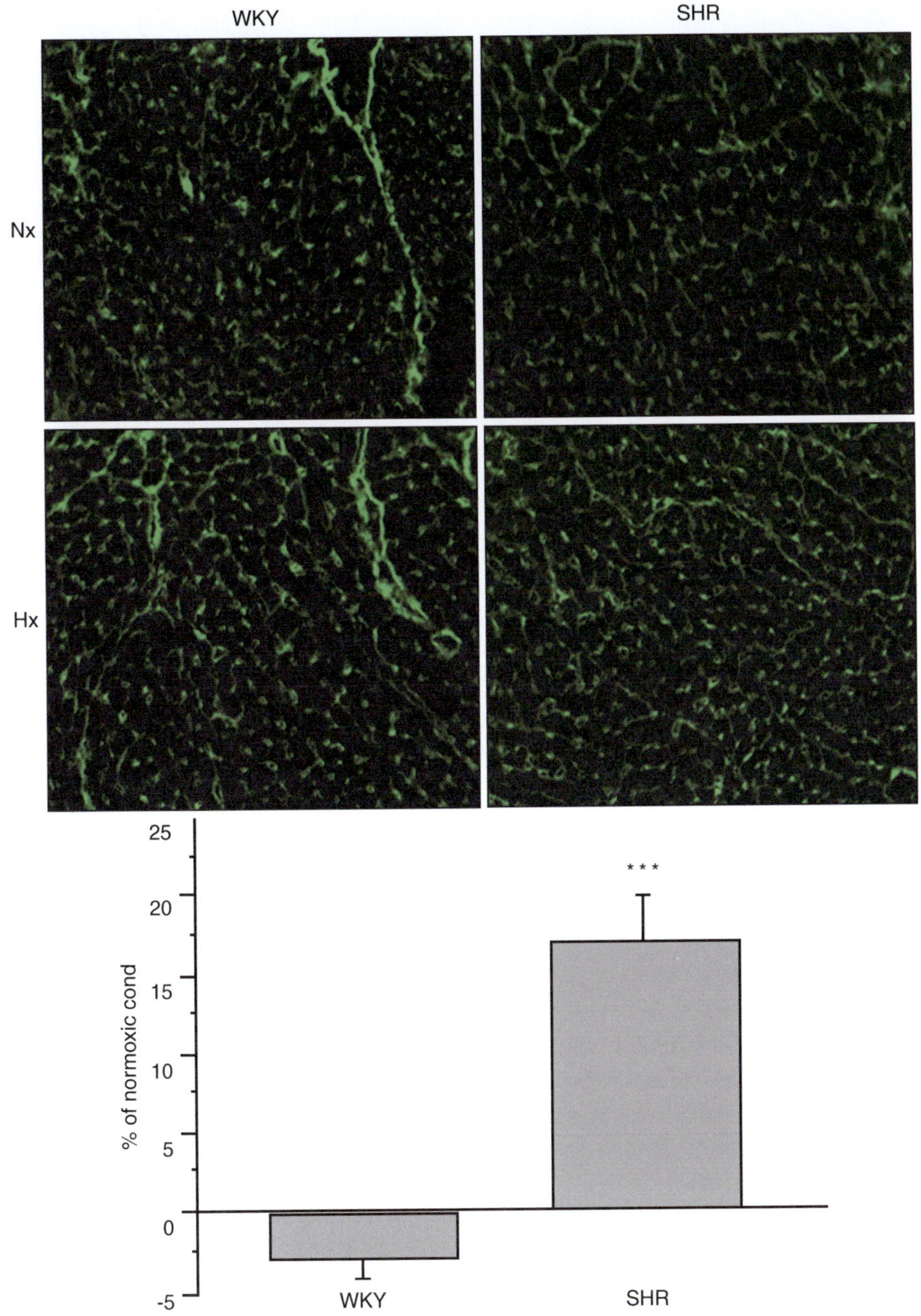

Fig. 11.4 Representative photomicrographs and quantitative evaluation of capillary density in the left ventricular free wall (capillaries appears in *green*) in WKY and SHRs under hypoxic (*Hx*) and normoxic (*Nx*) conditions

20 % in hypoxic SHRs compared to normoxic SHRs ($P<0.001$) and was similar to that of WKY rats (Fig. 11.4).

Finally, return to normoxia for 2 h did not reverse the reduction in blood pressure observed in hypoxic SHRs. This excludes a short-term effect of hypoxia-induced vasoactive substances (especially of VEGF, potent vasodilator peptide) but is, rather, in favor of an effect of the structure of the vascular network on blood pressure.

Nevertheless, changes in blood pressure levels and capillary number were fast. Indeed, we performed additional experiments to analyze the capillary densities in SHRs maintained for 1 week in hypoxia followed or not by 1 additional week under normoxic conditions. We showed that 1 week of hypoxia decreased by 27 % the blood pressure levels and increased capillary number by 1.4-fold in hypoxic SHRs compared to normoxic SHRs. Interestingly, these effects were blunted after return to normoxia for 1 week.

All together, these results suggest that hypoxia triggers angiogenesis within the skeletal muscles and the myocardium, indicating that hypoxia-induced increase in capillary density may reduce TPR and thus SBP in the SHRs.

It is also noteworthy that we did not observe any significant differences in the in vivo and in situ basal and sodium nitroprusside–induced maximal diameters of mesenteric arteries (80–150 μm) in normoxic and hypoxic SHRs, suggesting that chronic hypoxia did not affect the basal diameter of resistance arteries and did not modify their maximal dilation (absence of arteriole remodeling).

We next sought to identify the molecular mechanisms involved in hypoxia-induced angiogenesis. We analyzed the regulations of key genes involved in hypoxia-induced angiogenesis, such as HIF-1α, VEGF-A, its receptor Flk-1/KDR, and eNOS.

We did not observe any significant differences in HIF-1α mRNA levels in our experimental conditions. VEGF-A mRNA expression was reduced by 50 % in the normoxic SHR hind limb compared to normoxic WKY rats.

Interestingly, hypoxia increased VEGF-A mRNA contents in both hind limb and heart of hypoxic SHRs compared to normoxic SHRs. Similarly, Flk-1 mRNA levels were also upregulated in both hind limb and heart of hypoxic SHRs compared to normoxic SHRs (Fig. 11.5a, b).

Changes in mRNA levels were associated with modifications in protein levels. VEGF-A protein levels were decreased by 54 and 43 % in the hind limb and heart, respectively, in normoxic SHRs compared to normoxic WKY rats. Hypoxia increased VEGF-A content by 2.2- and 2.1-fold in the hind limb and heart, respectively, of hypoxic SHRs compared to normoxic SHRs ($P<0.01$). Subsequently, VEGF-A protein levels in hypoxic SHRs returned to normoxic WKY levels.

VEGF-A receptor Flk-1 protein contents were also reduced by 42 % in the hind limb of normoxic SHRs compared to normoxic WKY rats ($P<0.01$). Hypoxia upregulated Flk-1 contents by 2.4-fold in the hind limb of hypoxic SHRs compared to normoxic SHRs ($P<0.01$). Subsequently, Flk-1 protein levels in hypoxic SHRs returned to normoxic WKY levels. In contrast, Flk-1 protein content in heart was similar between normoxic SHRs and normoxic WKY rats and was not modulated by hypoxia in SHRs. Finally, co-treatment with VEGF-A–neutralizing antibody fully abrogated the hypoxia-induced angiogenesis in young prehypertensive SHRs and restored high blood pressure levels in treated hypoxic SHRs (Fig. 11.6).

All together, our results underlined that VEGF-A/Flk-1–related pathway is involved in hypoxia-induced angiogenesis in hypertensive animals.

Discussion

The main result of this study is that hypoxia blunts the development of hypertension in young prehypertensive SHRs and reverses hypertension in adult SHRs with established hypertension. Activation of VEGF-A–dependent angiogenesis plays a major role in these hypoxia-induced modifications of blood pressure levels.

Several authors have previously assessed the effect of hypoxia on hemodynamic parameters in the SHRs. Most were interested by transient pulmonary hypertension [10]. Henley and Tucker reported that chronic hypoxia resulted in decrease systemic blood pressure in young SHRs. Although thyroid status was unchanged, the authors suggested that thyroid hormones might be involved in the hypoxia-related antihypertensive effect [11]. Alternatively, in our present results, the lowering of the arterial pressure could depend on central effects of the hypoxia on the center of the arterial pressure regulation [12]. However, the effects of hypoxia on blood pressure are believed to result in sympathetic activity increase, leading to upregulation of blood pressure and heart rate [13].

The most common clinical form of hypoxia is the *obstructive sleep apnea*. Obstructive sleep apnea, a chronic form of sleep-disordered breathing afflicting millions of patients, has been implicated as a risk factor for an array of cardiovascular diseases including hypertension, stroke, coronary artery disease, and cardiac arrhythmias [14]. Among these comorbidities, evidence is most robust for a direct mechanistic relationship between sleep apnea and hypertension [15]. Extensive ongoing clinical and preclinical research is attempting to decipher the mechanisms of hypertension in patients with sleep apnea. The hallmark of sleep apnea is the recurrent sessions of arterial hypoxia during the brief asphyxiations imposed by airway collapse. Indeed, obstructive sleep apnea is the predominant pathological cause of chronic, intermittent hypoxia affecting the adult population. It is

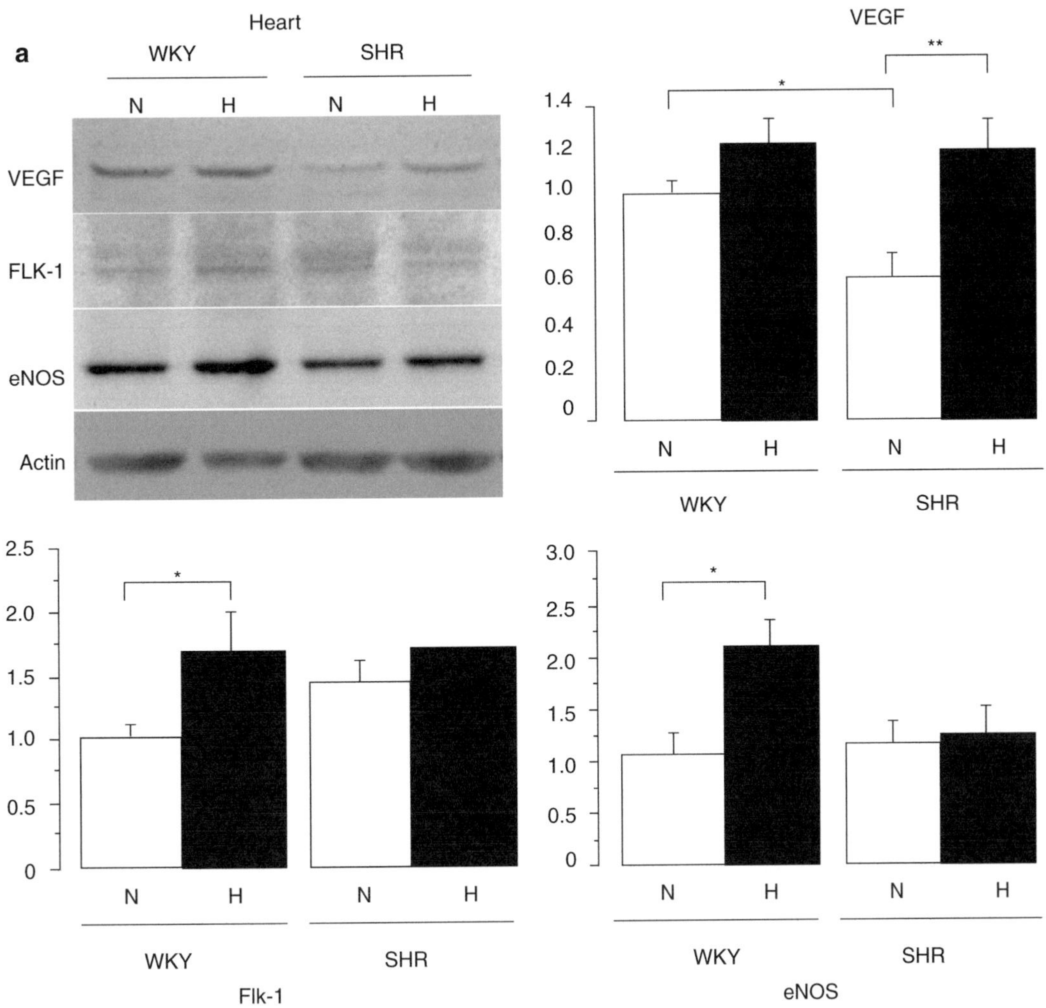

Fig. 11.5 Representative photomicrographs and quantitative evaluation of VEGF-A, Flk-1, and eNOS protein levels in the quadriceps (**a**) and in the left ventricular free wall (**b**) of WKY rats and SHRs under normoxic (*N*) or hypoxic (*H*) conditions

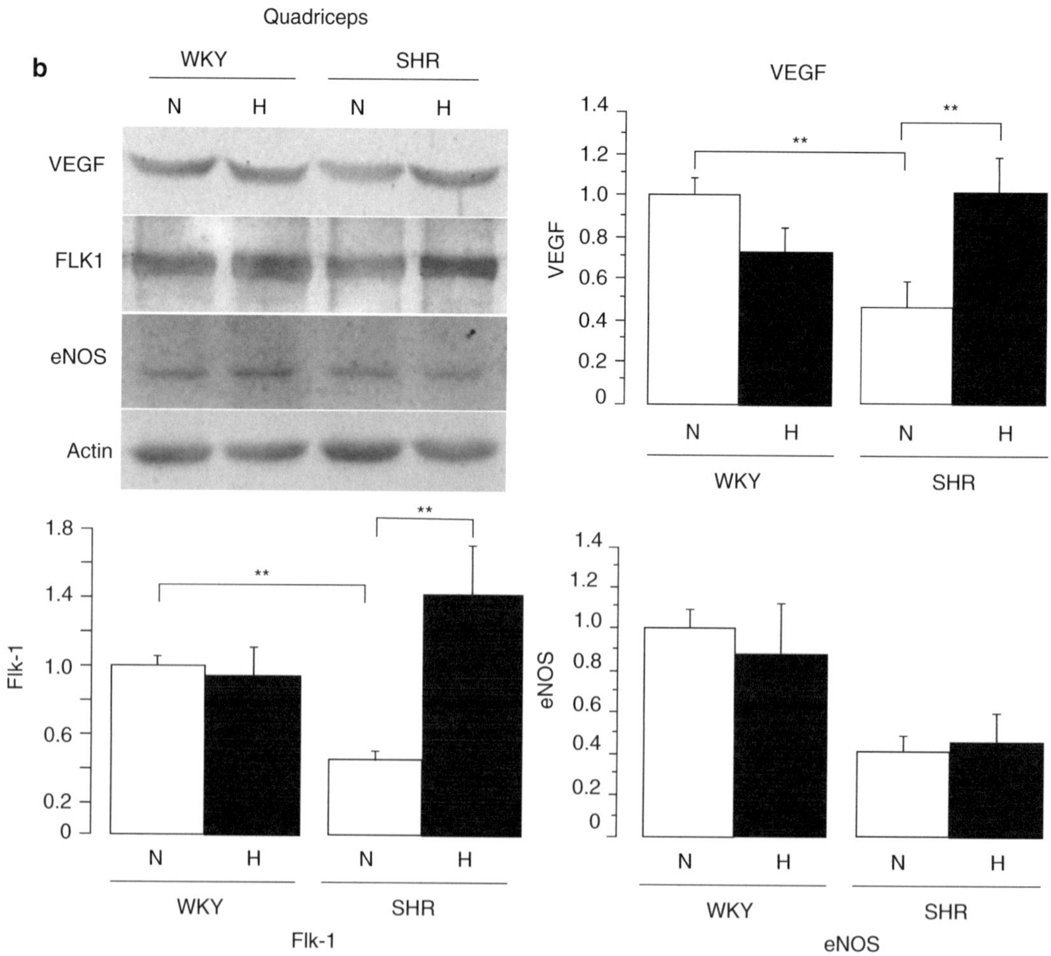

Fig. 11.5 (continued)

noteworthy that pathophysiology of sleep apnea involves intermittent and not chronic hypoxia.

Our results show that hypoxia did not affect cardiac output but decreased TPR and subsequently blood pressure levels. It is widely admitted that microvascular rarefaction contributes to the increase of TPR in hypertension. In support of this view, we suggest that changes in TPR are correlated with modifications of tissue capillary densities. Hence, hypoxia-induced increase in capillary density could reduce TPR and prevent the development of hypertension in SHRs or reduce blood pressure levels in established hypertensive SHRs. Therefore, changes in capillary density might be a key factor involved in the control of blood pressure levels. Previous studies support a primary role for capillary rarefaction in the development of hypertension. In human subjects, skin capillary rarefaction has been reported in normotensive young adults with a genetic propensity to develop high blood pressure [6, 16]. Microvascular rarefaction can be detected in patients with only mild or borderline hypertension [17] and progresses in parallel with the severity of hypertension. In addition, antihypertensive drug treatments increase capillary density in hypertensive subjects [18]. In our present experiments, the effect of hypoxia on blood pressure levels is likely related to activation of VEGF-A–dependent angiogenesis. Hypoxia is a well-known stimulus for angiogenesis through activation of HIF-1 signaling.

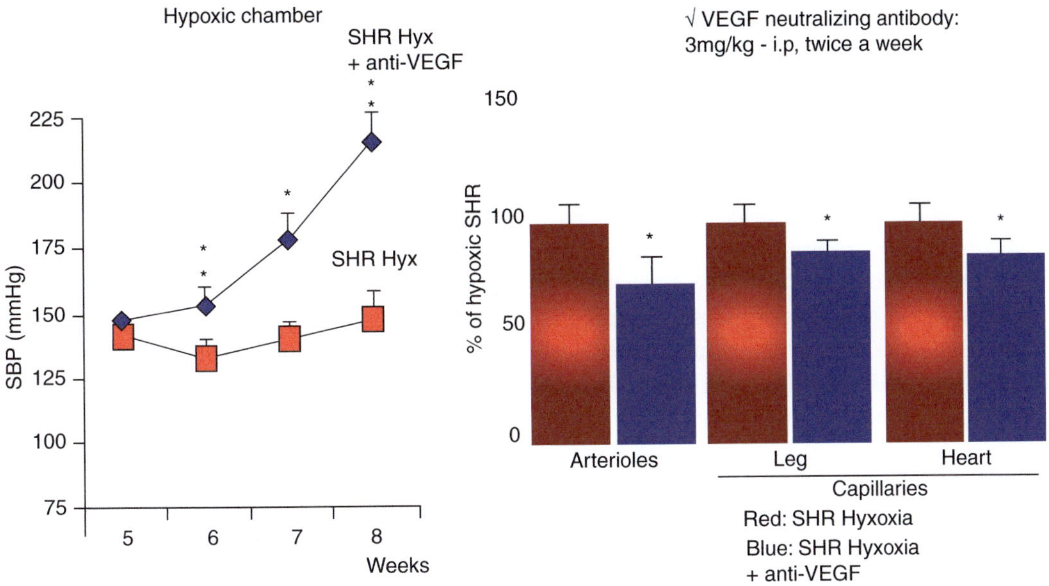

Fig. 11.6 Systolic blood pressure (*SBP*) and quantitative evaluation of arteriolar and capillary densities in 5-week-old SHRs maintained under hypoxic conditions for 3 weeks and treated with or without neutralizing antibody directed against VEGF-A

Although increased levels of HIF-1α mRNA have been reported, most of the studies suggest that HIF-1α is mainly regulated at the translational or posttranslational levels [19]. However, HIF-1α protein contents rapidly undergo proteasomal degradation [20]. Accordingly, we did not find evidence of significant changes in HIF-1α mRNA levels. In contrast, we showed that hypoxia highly stimulates expression of HIF-1–related genes, VEGF-A, and its receptor, Flk-1. Previous reports on the influence of hypoxia on Flk-1 expression are controversial [21–24]. Nevertheless, VEGF-A gene transfer restored Flk-1 mRNA levels in a rat sponge model, suggesting that hypoxia-induced VEGF-A upregulation may enhance Flk-1 contents [25]. Activation of VEGF-A–related pathways has been shown to promote endothelial cells migration, proliferation, survival, and proteolytic activity and may thereby activate angiogenesis. Interestingly, co-treatment with VEGF-A–neutralizing antibody blocked hypoxia-related effects on angiogenesis and blood pressure levels. It is also noteworthy that VEGF-A protein contents are reduced in normoxic SHRs compared to normoxic WKY rats, suggesting that the decrease in VEGF-A levels could be involved in capillary rarefaction in this setting. In addition, antihypertensive agents, such as angiotensin-converting enzyme inhibitor, raise VEGF-A levels and promote angiogenesis [26, 27].

In conclusion, this experimental study shows that hypoxia-induced angiogenesis prevents the microvascular rarefaction, which normally occurs in the course of hypertension and subsequently abrogates the hypertensive status in SHRs.

Therefore, therapeutic strategies designed to affect tissue angiogenesis may change blood pressure levels. In the light of these experimental results, we aimed to explore patients receiving antiangiogenic agents for metastasis colorectal cancer.

Antiangiogenesis and Arterial Hypertension During Cancer Treatment

Arterial hypertension is a commonly reported effect in clinical trials testing inhibitors of angiogenesis and especially inhibitors of VEGF/VEGF receptor-2 (VEGFR-2) signaling, with an incidence ranging from 11 to 43 % in all studies [28]. Whatever their initial level of blood pressure, every patient receiving antiangiogenic treatment evidenced rapid but variable increases in blood pressure. In most cases, the blood pressure values did not reach the levels characterizing clinical hypertension, but cases of malignant hypertension have been reported [29, 30]. The mechanism of elevated blood pressure in patients treated with antiangiogenesis agents is not fully understood, but it is likely to be multifactorial. One of the leading theories is the inhibition or lack of stimulation of the nitric oxide (NO) pathway. VEGF is known to augment the transcription of endothelial NO synthase, leading to the increased production of NO, a potent vasodilator [31, 32]. As anti-VEGF molecules block vascular endothelial NO production, systemic vasoconstriction—and thus hypertension—ensues. NO also plays a more direct role in the kidney, where it participates in sodium homeostasis by controlling the vascular tone of glomerular arterioles, pressure natriuresis, and tubule-glomerular feedback [33]. Thus, decreased NO synthesis results in sodium retention and elevated local and systemic blood pressure. Another postulated mechanism of hypertension induced by antiangiogenesis therapy is reduction in the density of microvascular beds, i.e., microvascular rarefaction. The reduction in microvessel density, which is thought to increase vascular resistance and elevate blood pressure, may be another mechanism by which antiangiogenic drugs promote hypertension.

Preclinical studies of VEGF inhibitors have helped to elucidate the mechanism of some adverse events found in the clinic and considered to be consequences of blocking actions of VEGF in normal physiology. The essential role of VEGF on vessels was thought not to persist into adult life, but rather to be limited to fetal development. Yet actions of VEGF have been identified in normal organs of adults, especially the role of VEGF in the function and survival of normal blood vessels and blood pressure regulation [34, 35]. Studies in mice of the effects of VEGF antibody, analogous to bevacizumab, indicate that VEGF participates in blood vessel survival and plasticity in adult life. In vivo examination of the capillary network of the mouse trachea, treated with an antibody directed against VEGF, revealed rapid regression of normal mucosal capillaries [36, 37]. After only 1 day of treatment, fibrin accumulated and patency was lost in some capillaries. By 2 days, endothelial cells underwent apoptosis and regression. The magnitude of capillary loss after 10 days of treatment depended on the age of the mice, being up to 39 % in young animals and 14 % in adult mice.

After inhibition of VEGF signaling for 1–3 weeks, significant capillary regression occurred in pancreatic islets, thyroid, adrenal cortex, pituitary, villi of the small intestine, choroid plexus, adipose tissue, and trachea; all these tissues evidenced a high rate of capillary genesis and regression under normal physiological conditions. The amount of regression was dose dependent and varied from organ to organ, with a maximum of 68 % in thyroid [38].

Capillary Rarefaction in Experimental and Human Hypertension

We reported the occurrence of capillary rarefaction in the finger skin in patients with metastatic colorectal cancer receiving bevacizumab treatment (Fig. 11.7). The reduction in capillary density at the level of the dorsal finger skin was correlated with the total dose of bevacizumab received by the patients and was closely associated with the rise in blood pressure observed in all patients [39]. Similar results were obtained in the mucosal surface of the inner lip of patients with advanced solid tumors receiving another antiangiogenic agent: telatinib, a small molecule tyrosine kinase inhibitor of VEGF receptors 2 and 3, platelet-derived growth factor (PDGF) receptor, and c-KIT [40].

Both clinical studies suggested a pathophysiological link between the microvascular rarefaction and the appearance and severity of arterial hypertension. It remains unclear whether the key problem is impaired NO synthesis leading to microvascular rarefaction, an imbalance

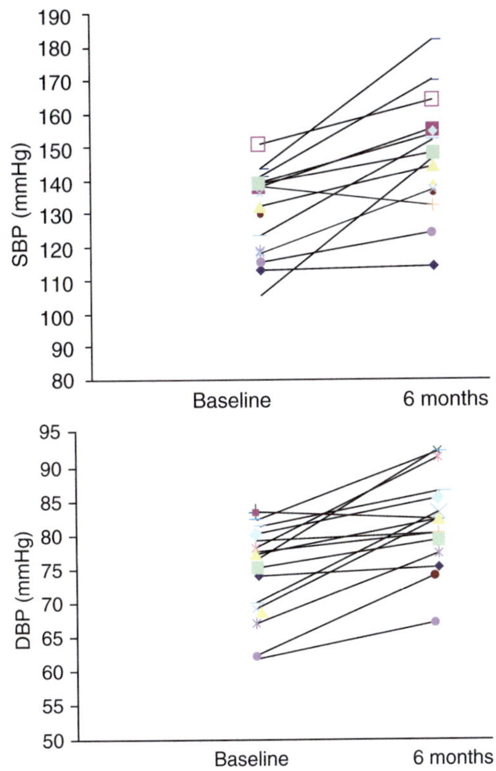

Fig. 11.7 Systolic blood pressure (*SBP*) and structural skin capillary density before and after 6 months of treatment with bevacizumab (Adapted from Mourad et al. [39])

between angiogenesis and endothelial cell apoptosis leading to capillary rarefaction, or a combination of both.

Capillary rarefaction is a constant finding in both experimental and clinical hypertension. Because microvessels (arterioles and capillaries) are a major contributor (>90 %) to total peripheral vascular resistance, functional rarefaction (decreased number of perfused microvessels) or anatomic rarefaction (a reduction in microvascular structures density) may play an important role in the development of hypertension. Under physiological resting conditions, 10–15 % of the microvascular network of most organs remains closed, constituting a flow reserve for adaptation to increased metabolic needs. It was first noted that hypertensive patients had an abnormally low number of small conjunctival vessels [16, 41]. Using venous occlusion capillaroscopy, the nail fold capillary density was also reported to be significantly lower (by 10 %) in nondiabetic patients with never-treated essential hypertension than in healthy, normotensive control subjects matched for age, sex, and lipid profile [42]. Analogous results (20 % difference) were obtained on the dorsal finger skin [43] and on the forearm skin [44] of hypertensive versus normotensive subjects. Finally, in hypertensive patients, whether treated or not, we reported that the Framingham score for cardiovascular risk was negatively correlated with capillary skin density [18]. It is increasingly believed that diffuse systemic microvascular rarefaction may be a primary defect in essential hypertension; however, the cause-effect relationships of rarefaction and hypertension are still debated. Interestingly, microvascular rarefaction exists in normotensive humans with a familial predisposition to the disease, suggesting an imbalance—that is, an inability of vascular growth to keep pace with organ growth [7]. Another powerful reason to link abnormalities in the long-term control of angiogenesis and blood pressure is the crucial role played by NO and the renin-angiotensin system in both processes. NO not only is a vasorelaxant but also is required for appropriate vascular budding in wound healing [45] and stimulates the expression of vascular growth factors, notably vascular VEGF. Impaired angiogenesis has been directly demonstrated in experimental hypertension induced by chronic pharmacologic inhibition of NO synthesis [46]. Several mechanisms should be discussed to explain microvascular rarefaction in patients treated with anti-VEGF molecules. Rarefaction may be structural, associated with decreased angiogenesis and/or increased capillary apoptosis, or functional, associated with local arteriole vasoconstriction and thus with impaired recruitment of non-perfused capillaries. The concept of functional versus structural rarefaction was first developed by Prewitt and colleagues [47]. It was proposed that in hypertension, arterioles first undergo functional rarefaction and then structural rarefaction. Actually, the absence of blood flow and endothelial shear stress in a non-perfused vessel results, in few days, in the activation of the apoptosis pathway. The authors postulated that functional rarefaction is caused by microvascular constriction to the point of non-perfusion of the vessel, whereas structural rarefaction represents a true anatomic absence of the vessels. The facts that blood pressure rises very early (within a few days) after treatment initiation and that capillary rarefaction is reversible after discontinuation of bevacizumab [48] suggest that functional alterations are more likely than structural rarefaction to explain the rise in blood pressure. However, the long-term (>6 months) effect of such treatments on structural capillary density and its putative reversibility have not yet been determined.

The hypertensive and cardiovascular effects of antiangiogenic treatments need thorough surveillance and reporting, and future studies will be needed to identify the mechanisms and appropriate management of treatment-induced hypertension. Preclinical studies of newer anti-VEGF molecules now include parallel evaluation of the simultaneous administration of antihypertensive agents. Franklin et al. demonstrated that hypertension could be both prevented and reversed at therapeutic or even sub-therapeutic doses of antihypertensive agents and that control of hypertension did not attenuate the antitumor efficacy of the multitargeted receptor tyrosine kinase inhibitor, ABT-869 [49]. Finally, interesting features have emerged with post hoc analysis of phase III trials that correlate the occurrence of arterial hypertension with antitumoral efficacy and prognosis [50, 51].

Apparently paradoxically, extensive preclinical and clinical research, conducted primarily in the nations of the former Soviet Union, has shown that intermittent hypoxia can be applied therapeutically to lower blood pressure in hypertensive patients, including those with a genetic predisposition to develop hypertension. An extensive review reports these results often difficult to obtain in the western world [52]. The central question addressed in this review is why the intermittent hypoxia imposed by obstructive sleep apnea versus that administered therapeutically can produce such divergent effects on systemic arterial blood pressure. In summary, obstructive sleep apnea ignites a crescendo of factors activating the sympathetic nervous system and systemic inflammation, culminating in persistent hypertension. In contrast, therapeutic intermittent therapeutic hypoxia minimally activates or even dampens these factors. These distinct differences are likely responsible for the divergent effects of these hypoxia paradigms on systemic arterial pressure and other comorbidities of occlusive sleep apnea. The authors conclude that appropriate application of intermittent hypoxia can produce sustained reductions in systemic arterial pressure in hypertensive subjects.

Our present chapter tries to conciliate both experimental and clinical research and to detail the rare occurrence in a researcher life of basic and clinical research. The words "translational research" are often used but rarely observed. Our results could be summarized:

1. Chronic hypoxia decreased the arterial pressure in the hypertensive rat by activation of VEGF-related angiogenic processes.
2. Pharmaceutical blockade of the VEGF pathway in patients receiving antiangiogenic treatments results in arterial hypertension in relation with microvascular rarefaction.

Our observations are strengthened by epidemiological data published by the Swiss National Cohort Study Group [53]. The 1.64 million German Swiss residents born in Switzerland provided 14.5 million person-years. Mortality from coronary heart disease (−22 % per 1,000 m) and stroke (−12 % per 1,000 m) significantly decreased with increasing altitude. The protective effect of living at higher altitude on coronary heart disease and stroke mortality was consistent and became stronger after adjustment for potential confounders. The effect is unlikely to be due to classic cardiovascular disease risk factors and rather could be explained by factors related to altitude.

References

1. Feihl F, Liaudet L, Waeber B, Levy BI. Hypertension: a disease of the microcirculation? Hypertension. 2006;48:1012–7.
2. Levy BI, Ambrosio G, Pries AR, Struijker-Boudier HA. Microcirculation in hypertension: a new target for treatment? Circulation. 2001;104:735–40.

3. Levy BI, Duriez M, Samuel JL. Coronary microvasculature alteration in hypertensive rats. Effect of treatment with a diuretic and an ACE inhibitor. Am J Hypertens. 2001;14:7–13.
4. Sabri A, Samuel JL, Marotte F, Poitevin P, Rappaport L, Levy BI. Microvasculature in angiotensin II-dependent cardiac hypertrophy in the rat. Hypertension. 1998;32:371–5.
5. Chen II, Prewitt RL, Dowell RF. Microvascular rarefaction in spontaneously hypertensive rat cremaster muscle. Am J Physiol. 1981;241:H306–10.
6. Antonios TF, Rattray FM, Singer DR, Markandu ND, Mortimer PS, MacGregor GA. Rarefaction of skin capillaries in normotensive offspring of individuals with essential hypertension. Heart. 2003;89:175–8.
7. Noon JP, Walker BR, Webb DJ, Shore AC, Holton DW, Edwards HV, Watt GC. Impaired microvascular dilatation and capillary rarefaction in young adults with a predisposition to high blood pressure. J Clin Invest. 1997;99:1873–9.
8. Carmeliet P. Angiogenesis in health and disease. Nat Med. 2003;9:653–60.
9. Blanes MG, Oubaha M, Rautureau Y, Gratton JP. Phosphorylation of tyrosine 801 of the VEGFR-2 is necessary for AKT-dependent eNOS activation and nitric oxide release from endothelial cells. J Biol Chem. 2007;282:10660–9.
10. Janssens SP, Thompson BT, Spence CR, Hales CA. Functional and structural changes with hypoxia in pulmonary circulation of spontaneously hypertensive rats. J Appl Physiol. 1994;77:1101–7.
11. Henley WN, Tucker A. Hypoxic moderation of systemic hypertension in the spontaneously hypertensive rat. Am J Physiol. 1987;252:R554–61.
12. Mifflin S. New insights into the electrophysiology of brainstem circuits controlling blood pressure. Curr Hypertens Rep. 2007;9:236–41.
13. Hainsworth R, Drinkhill MJ, Rivera-Chira M. The autonomic nervous system at high altitude. Clin Auton Res. 2007;17:13–9.
14. Rice TB, Strollo Jr PJ, Morrell MJ. Update in sleep medicine 2011. Am J Respir Crit Care Med. 2012;185:1271–4.
15. Kapa S, Sert Kuniyoshi FH, Somers VK. Sleep apnea and hypertension: interactions and implications for management. Hypertension. 2008;51:605–8.
16. Sullivan JM, Prewitt RL, Josephs JA. Attenuation of the microcirculation in young patients with high-output borderline hypertension. Hypertension. 1983;5:844–51.
17. Gasser P, Buhler FR. Nailfold microcirculation in normotensive and essential hypertensive subjects, as assessed by video-microscopy. J Hypertens. 1992;10:83–6.
18. Debbabi H, Uzan L, Mourad JJ, Safar M, Levy BI, Tibirica E. Increased skin capillary density in treated essential hypertensive patients. Am J Hypertens. 2006;19:477–83.
19. Gleadle JM, Ratcliffe PJ. Hypoxia and the regulation of gene expression. Mol Med Today. 1998;4:122–9.
20. Berra E, Ginouves A, Pouyssegur J. The hypoxia-inducible-factor hydroxylases bring fresh air into hypoxia signalling. EMBO Rep. 2006;7:41–5.
21. Brogi E, Schatteman G, Wu T, Kim EA, Varticovski L, Keyt B, Isner JM. Hypoxia-induced paracrine regulation of vascular endothelial growth factor receptor expression. J Clin Invest. 1996;97:469–76.
22. Marti HH, Risau W. Systemic hypoxia changes the organ-specific distribution of vascular endothelial growth factor and its receptors. Proc Natl Acad Sci U S A. 1998;95:15809–14.
23. Tuder RM, Flook BE, Voelkel NF. Increased gene expression for VEGF and the VEGF receptors KDR/Flk and Flt in lungs exposed to acute or to chronic hypoxia. Modulation of gene expression by nitric oxide. J Clin Invest. 1995;95:1798–807.
24. Waltenberger J, Mayr U, Pentz S, Hombach V. Functional upregulation of the vascular endothelial growth factor receptor KDR by hypoxia. Circulation. 1996;94:1647–54.
25. Wang H, Olszewski B, Rosebury W, Wang D, Robertson A, Keiser JA. Impaired angiogenesis in SHR is associated with decreased KDR and MT1-MMP expression. Biochem Biophys Res Commun. 2004;315:363–8.
26. Silvestre JS, Bergaya S, Tamarat R, Duriez M, Boulanger CM, Levy BI. Proangiogenic effect of angiotensin-converting enzyme inhibition is mediated by the bradykinin B(2) receptor pathway. Circ Res. 2001;89:678–83.
27. Silvestre JS, Kamsu-Kom N, Clergue M, Duriez M, Levy BI. Very low dose combination of the angiotensin-converting enzyme inhibitor perindopril and the diuretic indapamide induces an early and sustained increase in neovascularization in rat ischemic legs. J Pharmacol Exp Ther. 2002;303:1038–43.
28. Sica DA. Angiogenesis inhibitors and hypertension: an emerging issue. J Clin Oncol. 2006;24:1329–31.
29. Ozcan C, Wong SJ, Hari P. Reversible posterior leukoencephalopathy syndrome and bevacizumab. N Engl J Med. 2006;354:980–2.
30. Allen JA, Adlakha A, Bergethon PR. Reversible posterior leukoencephalopathy syndrome after bevacizumab/FOLFIRI regimen for metastatic colon cancer. Arch Neurol. 2006;63:1475–8.
31. Hood JD, Meininger CJ, Ziche M, et al. VEGF upregulates eNOS message, protein, and NO production in human endothelial cells. Am J Physiol. 1998;274:H1054–8.
32. Shen BQ, Lee DY, Zioncheck TF. Vascular endothelial growth factor governs nitric-oxide synthase expression via a KDR/Flk-1 receptor and a protein kinase C signaling pathway. J Biol Chem. 1999;274:33057–63.
33. Zou AP, Cowley AW. Role of nitric oxide in the control of renal function and salt sensitivity. Curr Hypertens Rep. 1999;1:178–86.
34. Horowitz JR, Rivard A, van der Zee R, et al. Vascular endothelial growth factor/vascular permeability factor produces nitric oxide-dependent hypotension. Evidence for a maintenance role in quiescent adult endothelium. Arterioscler Thromb Vasc Biol. 1997;17:2793–800.

35. Kamba T, Tam BY, Hashizume H, et al. VEGF-dependent plasticity of fenestrated capillaries in the normal adult microvasculature. Am J Physiol Heart Circ Physiol. 2006;290:H560–76.
36. Inai T, Mancuso M, Hashizume H, et al. Inhibition of vascular endothelial growth factor (VEGF) signaling in cancer causes loss of endothelial fenestrations, regression of tumor vessels, and appearance of basement membrane ghosts. Am J Pathol. 2004;165:35–52.
37. Baffert F, Le T, Sennino B, et al. Cellular changes in normal blood capillaries undergoing regression after inhibition of VEGF signaling. Am J Physiol Heart Circ Physiol. 2006;290:H547–59.
38. Kamba T, McDonald DM. Mechanisms of adverse effects of anti- VEGF therapy for cancer. Br J Cancer. 2007;96:1788–95.
39. Mourad JJ, des Guetz G, Debbabi H, Levy BI. Blood pressure rise following angiogenesis inhibition by bevacizumab. A crucial role for microcirculation. Ann Oncol. 2008;19:927–34.
40. Steeghs N, Gelderblom H, Roodt JO, et al. Hypertension and rarefaction during treatment with telatinib, a small molecule angiogenesis inhibitor. Clin Cancer Res. 2008;14:3470–6.
41. Ruedemann AD. Conjunctival vessels. JAMA. 1933;101:1477–81.
42. Serne EH, Gans ROB, ter Maaten JC, et al. Impaired skin capillary recruitment in essential hypertension is caused by both functional and structural capillary rarefaction. Hypertension. 2001;38:238–42.
43. Antonios TFT, Singer DRJ, Markandu ND, et al. Structural skin capillary rarefaction in essential hypertension. Hypertension. 1999;33:998–1001.
44. Prasad A, Dunnill GS, Mortimer PS, MacGregor GA. Capillary rarefaction in the forearm skin in essential hypertension. J Hypertens. 1995;13:265–8.
45. Lee PC, Salyapongse AN, Bragdon GA, et al. Impaired wound healing and angiogenesis in eNOS-deficient mice. Am J Physiol. 1999;277:H1600–8.
46. Kiefer FN, Misteli H, Kalak N, et al. Inhibition of NO biosynthesis, but not elevated blood pressure, reduces angiogenesis in rat models of secondary hypertension. Blood Press. 2002;11:116–24.
47. Prewitt RL, Hashimoto H, Stacy DL. Structural and functional rarefaction of microvessels in hypertension. In: Lee R, editor. Blood vessel changes in hypertension: structure and function. Boca Raton: CRC Press; 1990. p. 71–90.
48. Steeghs N, Rabelink TJ, op 't Roodt J, et al. Reversibility of capillary density after discontinuation of bevacizumab treatment. Ann Oncol. 2010;21:1100–5.
49. Franklin PH, Banfor PN, Tapang P, et al. Effect of the multitargeted receptor tyrosine kinase inhibitor, ABT-869, on blood pressure in conscious rats and mice: reversal with antihypertensive agents and effect on tumor growth inhibition. J Pharmacol Exp Ther. 2009;329:928–37.
50. Bono P, Elfving H, Utriainen T, Osterlund P, Saarto T, Alanko T, et al. Hypertension and clinical benefit of bevacizumab in the treatment of advanced renal cell carcinoma. Ann Oncol. 2009;20:393–4.
51. Levy BI. Blood pressure as a potential biomarker of the efficacy angiogenesis inhibitor. Ann Oncol. 2009;20:200–3.
52. Serebrovskaya TV, Manukhina EB, Smith ML, Downey HF, Mallet RT. Intermittent hypoxia: cause of or therapy for systemic hypertension? Exp Biol Med. 2008;233:627–50.
53. Faeh D, Gutzwiller F, Bopp M, Swiss National Cohort Study Group. Lower mortality from coronary heart disease and stroke at higher altitudes in Switzerland. Circulation. 2009;120:495–501.

12 The Reality of Aging Viewed from the Arterial Wall

Majd AlGhatrif and Edward G. Lakatta

Abstract

The main function of central arteries is to transform the pulsatile flow generated by the heart into an almost continuous distal flow. Major changes in the arterial wall ensue with aging, and are characterized by endothelial dysfunction, smooth muscle proliferation, elastin fragmentation, fibrosis, amyloid protein deposition, and calcification. These processes are driven by a proinflammatory microenvironment that features increased production of angiotensin II (Ang II) and its downstream signaling cascade. The aforementioned structural changes result in a loss of the dampening function of central arteries, widening of pulse pressure, and subsequent adverse effects on the heart and end-organ systems, i.e. the brain and kidneys.

Keywords

Arterial aging • Inflammation • Angiotensin • Pulse wave velocity • Pulse pressure

Introduction

Evolutionary biologists proclaim that most of us are wired to be very healthy until around the end of child-bearing age, because the main reason for our reality, they would say, is to perpetually insure the next generation of our species; after that, from an evolutionary perspective, there is no essential reason for us to be alive. However, we do remain alive longer well beyond our evolutionary life expectancy prescription because our environment has protected us by improved hygiene, better nutrition, better health care, etc. But, in outliving our paleolithic gene set, the disorder among the molecules within our body progressively

M. AlGhatrif, MD
Human Cardiovascular Studies Unit, Laboratory of Cardiovascular Science, National Institute on Aging, National Institutes of Health,
251 Bayview Blvd, Baltimore, MD 21114, USA

Department of Medicine, Johns Hopkins School of Medicine, Baltimore, MD, USA
e-mail: majd.alghatrif@nih.gov

E.G. Lakatta, MD (✉)
Laboratory of Cardiovascular Science, Biomedical Research Center, 251 Bayview Boulevard, Suite 100, Room 09B116, Baltimore, MD 21224-6825, USA

Laboratory of Cardiovascular Science, IRP, National Institute on Aging, National Institutes of Health, Baltimore, MD 21224-6825, USA
e-mail: lakattae@grc.nia.nih.gov

M.E. Safar et al. (eds.), *Blood Pressure and Arterial Wall Mechanics in Cardiovascular Diseases*,
DOI 10.1007/978-1-4471-5198-2_12,

increases and functional declines accumulate, and with advancing age we become vulnerable to what are referred to as "degenerative chronic diseases of aging". Arterial aging and its diseases are no exception.

The Evolution of Central Arteries

To understand arterial aging, it is instructive to explore the evolutionary course of this arterial apparatus and the "purpose" of its structure and function. The development of advanced circulatory system that secures a regular irrigation of cells was a necessary step in the evolution of complex organisms. While the heart generates pulsatile flow and pressure, it is the central arteries that receive this pulsation and, via a Windkessel effect, dampen it into an almost continuous distal flow [1]. To achieve this function, central arteries provide resilience "elasticity" over a physiological pressure range of a given organism, in order to achieve dampening of pulsatililty, and tensile strength "stiffness" to contain the stroke volume and avoid rupture at higher pressure.

In early evolutionary steps, invertebrates with low-pressurized systems have arteries composed of fibrin microfibers, along with other extra cellular matrix components, like collagen, which satisfy both functions [2]. However, the appearance of vertebrates with a high-pressurized circulation mandated a more advanced structure, since the microfibrils alone become very stiff in such pressure range [2]. While collagen provides the tensile strength needed at extreme pressures, the evolution of another extra-cellular matrix element that provides elasticity to the microfibril network at physiological higher pressure range was needed; this element is tropoelastin, which forms elastin fibers when combined with the microfibril network and other ECM components [2]. Hence, a balanced structure of elastin and collagen fibers is essential for normal function of the central arteries. Alterations in the function, structure, and balance of these components evolve with aging and lead to dramatic hemodynamic changes.

Characteristics of the Aged Central Arterial Wall

Arterial aging consists of a myriad of progressive structural and functional changes that occur throughout life ranging from changes in molecules to cells to arterial tissue, the blood it transports, and the hormonal and neural factors that modulate molecules, cells, tissues, etc. that comprise our cardiovascular system.

Our textbooks usually describe the characteristics of central arterial changes that accompany advancing age as "Physiologic" arterial aging (Fig. 12.1). Characteristically, there is fragmentation and calcification of elastic fibers, increased deposition of collagen and collagen cross linking, amyloid deposition in the medial layer, and migration/proliferation of vascular smooth muscle cells (VSMC) leading to intimal and medial thickness. These processes are driven by a proinflammatory microenvironment, mediated by mechanical and humoral factors (Fig. 12.1). Oxidative stress and low grade inflammation, by effecting posttranslational modification of molecules that lead to cellular and matrix structural and functional changes, are important factors that accelerate arterial aging. These events act in concert to reduce central arterial distensibility and render the arterial wall stiffer, which results in a more rapid pulse wave velocity and early return of the reflection wave to occur during systolic ejection (Fig. 12.1). As a result, the systolic blood pressure increases, diastolic pressure decreases and the pulse pressure increases with aging. The chronic increase in pulse pressure transmitted to the brain and kidney damage the arterial supply of those organs, leading to vascular encephalopathy and chronic renal failure (Fig. 12.1).

Arterial Aging, a "Set Up" for Vascular Diseases

Chronic arterial diseases, e.g. atherosclerosis, hypertension, diabetes, kidney disease and heart failure (Fig. 12.1), increase exponentially with advancing age and become rampant within our society. Should arterial aging, then,

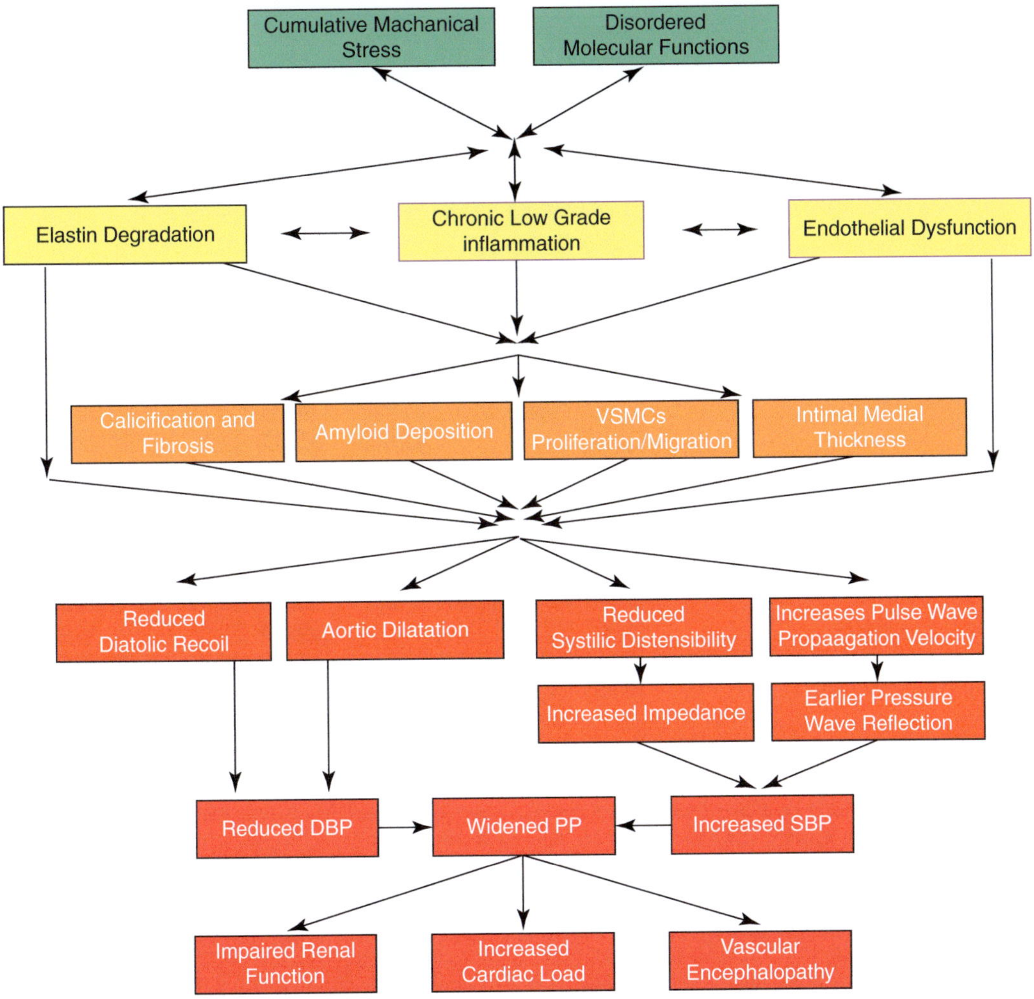

Fig. 12.1 Conceptual model of arterial aging. Age-associated molecular disorders and cumulative mechanical stress lead to a state of chronic inflammation, elastin degradation, and endothelial and VSMC dysfunction. These processes interact and lead to arterial wall calcification, fibrosis, amyloid deposition, VSMCs proliferation, and increased intimal medial thickness. These structural changes lead to functional alterations resulting in widened pulse pressure. The increase in pulsatililty leads to increase left ventricular load, chronic kidney disease, and vascular dementia

be construed as a "disease"? Although clinical medicine focuses mainly on arterial disease diagnoses and treatment of these quintessential cardiovascular diseases, these are only at the tip of an iceberg, with age-associated arterial wall changes comprised the extensive iceberg base. Because the likelihood for predominantly systolic hypertension and atherosclerosis to occur increases in epidemic proportion among older persons [3, 4], it is reasonable to hypothesize that specific mechanisms that underlie alterations in the sub-clinical arterial substrate that accompany "aging" may be intimately linked to the age-associated exponential increase in chronic arterial diseases, predominantly systolic hypertension and atherosclerosis [3]. Thus, in this context, arterial aging may be considered to be latent arterial disease. Indeed, recent studies show that pulse wave velocity, an index of arterial stiffness that increases with age, is an independent predictor of the future increases in SBP and of incident hypertension [5].

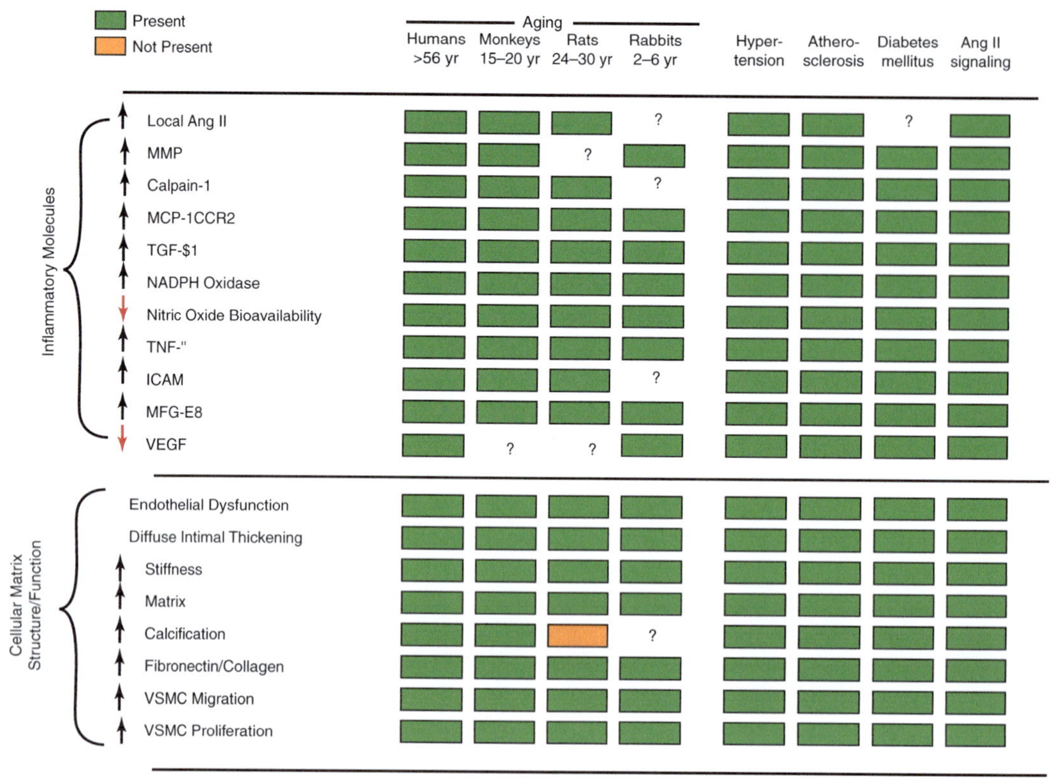

Fig. 12.2 Molecular and cellular remodeling observed with aging in different species, and various vascular diseases. A universal upregulation of Angiotensin (Ang II) pathway, increase in inflammatory molecules, reduction in NO bioavailability, and arterial wall ultrastructure are observed with aging in various species. Interestingly, similar alterations are observed in vascular diseases, e.g. hypertension, atherosclerosis, and diabetes (Reproduced with permission from Wang et al. [6], Elsevier)

A Chronic Arterial Proinflammatory Profile Characterizes the Aging Arterial Wall

In order to determine whether or not to consider arterial aging a disease, we must understand the mechanisms that lead to age-associated changes in the arterial wall. But there is a substantial gap between our knowledge about what's going on in the arterial wall under the microscope with respect to structure or function of the large arteries and what can be measured in vivo.

Under the microscope, the aged artery is characterized by the disruption of the endothelium, increased VSMC migration/proliferation /senescence, extracellular matrix deposition, elastin fracture, and matrix calcification/amyloidization/glycation. Arterial wall aging is quite similar in humans, non-human primates, rabbits and rats (Fig. 12.2) and involves inflammatory processes associated with oxidative stress. The inflammatory patterns are the same for most species that have been studied (Fig. 12.2). Our body's initial response to stress is moderated by increased adrenergic signaling; the downstream receptor signaling cascade results in increased activation of renin-angiotensin-aldosterone, and endothelial dysfunction (Fig. 12.2), ways by which our body responds to chronic stress.

The proinflammatory profile of the aged central arterial wall features increased production of angiotensin II (Ang II) and increased vascular smooth muscle cell expression and secretion of downstream Ang II/AT$_1$, mineralocorticoid and

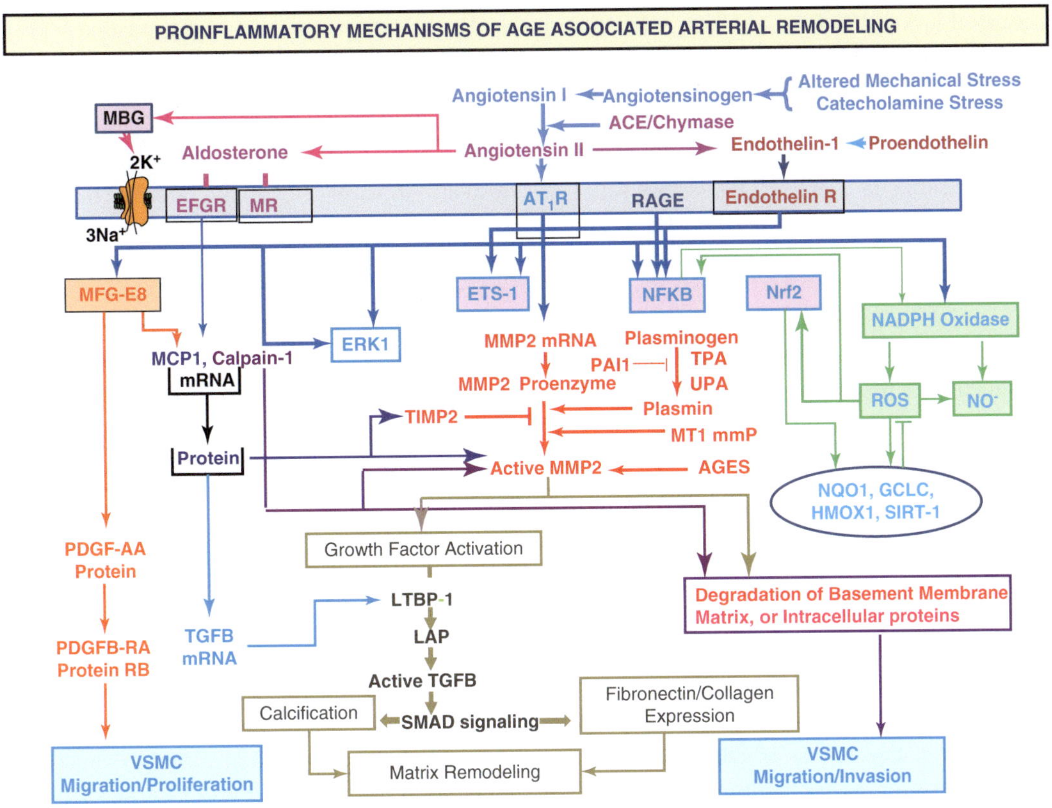

Fig. 12.3 Proinflammatory mechanisms of age-associated arterial remodeling (Reproduced with permission from Lakatta [7], Elsevier)

endothelin receptor signaling molecules (Fig. 12.3), e.g., matrix metalloproteases (MMPs), calpain-1 and monocyte chemoattractant protein (MCP-1), transforming growth factor β1 (TGF-β1) NFκb, TNFα, iNOS, and VCAM. Activation of calpain-1, MMPs, TGF-β, and NADPH oxidase within the arterial wall is increased, and nitric oxide bioavailability is reduced [3, 8–11]. Invasive, proliferative and secretory capacities of early passage vascular smooth muscle cells (VSMC) isolated from the aged arterial wall are increased, and are linked to augmented Ang II signaling. This Age-Associated Arterial proinflammatory Secretory Profile (AAASP) within the grossly appearing arterial wall and related structural/functional remodeling of cells and matrix is reproduced in young rats by chronic infusion of Ang-II [12].

The aortic wall remodeling induced by aging, however, likely results from the concerted effects of numerous signaling proteins that have yet to be identified. The expression of one such recently discovered arterial wall protein, milk fat globule protein epidermal growth factor 8 (MFG-E8), increases 2.3-fold in abundance in aortae of humans, non-human primates and rats (Fig. 12.2). Milk fat globule E-8 (MFG-E8), aka lactadherin, SED1, colocalizes with both angiotensin II and monocyte chemoattractant protein (MCP)-1 within vascular smooth muscle cells (VSMCs) and matrix of the thickened aged aortic wall and is a pivotal relay element within the angiotensin II/MCP-1/VSMC signaling cascade (Fig. 12.2). Exposure of early passage VSMCs from young aorta to angiotensin II markedly increases MFG-E8 and enhances invasive capacity to levels observed in VSMCs from old rats. MFG-E8 not only induces VSMC invasion, but also affects VSMC proliferation, which is a salient feature of arterial inflammation. An MFG-E8 degradation product, medin, is an amyloid protein that accumulates within the aging arterial matrix wall (see below). Thus, the increase in MFG-E8 is a novel pivotal relay element within the angiotensin II/MCP-1/ERK, CDK4 VSMC signaling cascades.

It remains to be debatable whether age-associated changes in arterial structure and/or function initiates a reparative chronic inflammation, or whether chronic inflammation from increasing molecular disorder with advancing age initiates alterations in arterial structure and function with aging. It is likely that both of these views are correct, i.e. that chronic reparatory inflammation, a mechanism to cope with chronic disease, may accelerate arterial aging. In other terms, an overshoot in mechanisms designed to cope with chronic stress, i.e. angiotensin II signaling and that of other related molecules, i.e. endothelin or aldosterone, which effect many signaling pathways across the arterial wall, have a feed-forward effect that enhances the proinflammatory arterial wall phenotype that evolves with advancing age.

A megacept emerges with the realization that in arteries of younger animals, in response to experimental induction of hypertension or early atherosclerosis or diabetes, parts of this proinflammatory profile within the arterial wall are strikingly similar to the profile that occurs with advancing age [3] (Fig. 12.2).

Aging of the Different Components of the Arterial Wall: Origins and Consequences of Arterial Proinflammation

Endothelial Dysfunction with Aging

Arterial endothelium has been long recognized to be more than a barrier separating the vessel wall from blood stream; it plays a major regulatory role in several arterial properties, including vascular reactivity to flow, permeability, angiogenesis, and the response to inflammation [13]. Endothelial-derived vasodilators (e.g., nitric oxide [NO], prostacyclin) and vasoconstrictors (e.g. endothelin-1, angiotensin II (Ang II) and thromboxane A2) control arterial dilatation in response to sheer stress, and modulate the structure of underlying layers. While age-associated changes in endothelial function of the central arteries have not been directly assessed, alterations in endothelial function of the muscular arteries are observed with increasing age in healthy humans. In the brachial artery, endothelial function, as assessed by flow-mediated dilatation (FMD), has been shown to decline with advancing age in the absence of clinical disease [14]. That dilatation in response to glyceryl nitrate is not reduced with aging emphasizes that these age-associated changes are related to a reduced NO bioavailability rather than to impaired intrinsic relaxation of the vascular smooth muscle cells (Fig. 12.2). Cumulative oxidative stress, due, in part, to an increase in Ang II signaling-induced NADPH oxidase (Fig. 12.3) within dysfunctional endothelial cells, is thought to be a major player in decreased endothelial NO bioavailability [15, 16]. In addition, plasma levels of asymmetric dimethyl arginine (ADMA), which reduces NO synthase (NOS) activity, also increases with age in humans, making it another culprit in endothelial dysfunction; in fact increasing L-arginine/ADMA ratio by L-arginine oral supplementation partially improves vasoreactivity [17]. An age-associated decline in number and function of circulating endothelial progenitor cells (EPC) may be implicated in endothelial dysfunction with aging [16, 18]. The blunted vasodilatation and additional structural changes stemming from endothelial dysfunction are thought to contribute to reduced aortic compliance and increased impedance with aging (see below).

Age-Associated Increase in Central Arterial Intimal-Medial Thickness

Common carotid intima-medial thickness, assessed by B-mode ultrasound, which has been used as a surrogate for central arterial intimal thickness [19], increases with age in cross-sectional studies [20]. A post-mortem study indicates that the age-associated increase in aortic wall thickness in humans is mainly attributable to increased intimal thickness [21]. Intimal-medial thickening is associated with increased number of vascular smooth muscle cells (VSMC), likely due to migration from the tunica media, and production of fibronectin, and collagen within the thickened intima [10]. VSMCs within the arterial wall media plays a major role in the arterial wall inflammation via the production and secretion of cytokines and other inflammatory substances that have been referred to as Age-Associated Arterial proinflammatory Secretory Profile (AAASP) [12].

While intimal medial thickness has been considered by some to be equivalent to preclinical atherosclerosis [19], it is important to note that the aforementioned age-associated changes are independent from atherosclerosis, as evidenced by its occurrence with advanced age in rodents and non-human primates that are not prone to atherosclerosis [10, 22]. In fact, intima-medial thickness in humans is only weakly associated with the severity of coronary artery disease [23]. Hence, an increased intima-medial thickness mainly reflects age-associated inflammation [13].

Age-Associated Changes in the Arterial Wall Matrix

Senescence of Elastic Fibers

Elastin, the most abundant protein in central arteries, is mainly synthesized early in life and goes through slow turnover with aging, making it one of the most inert proteins [10]. Elastin is formed of tropoelastin monomers that are organized and cross-linked in a pattern that gives rise to its rubber-like properties [11]. Two primary processes are involved in elastin damage with aging: mechanical injury to elastin fibers with repetitive cycles of stretching [12], and active enzymatic elastolysis by elastases, e.g. MMP II (see below), that could be activated with high oxidative stress and unfavorable medial environment as a result of endothelial and VSMC dysfunction [13]. Elastin fragmentation results in loss of its rubber-like properties [11], and manifests as a reduction in the capacitance of arterial wall in systole and decreased recoil in diastole [14]. In addition, elastin fragments subsequently activate a process of repair "inflammation" that further changes the structure of the arterial wall [15].

Calcification and Fibrosis

Central arterial fibrosis and calcification are features of age-associated arterial extracellular remodeling and also linked to Ang II signaling and AAASP. Angiotensin II induces arterial wall matrix metalloproteinase 2 (MMP2) and calpain-1 expression and activity. Cross-talk of these two proteases leads to secretion of active MMP2, which modulates ECM remodeling via enhancing collagen production and facilitating vascular calcification. Calpain-1 induces MMP2 transcripts, protein levels and activity, in part, by increasing the ratio of membrane-type 1 MMPs to tissue inhibitor of metalloproteinases 2. These effects of calpain-1-induced MMP2 activation are linked to increased collagen I, II and III production and vascular calcification via TGF-β1 (Fig. 12.3). In addition to increased collagen content, advanced glycation end product (AGE) formation that occurs with aging and diabetes leads to the cross-linking of proteins and subsequent changes in the physicochemical properties of tissues [24].

Over-expression of calpain-1 also induces transforming growth factor-beta 1/Smad signaling, elastin degradation, alkaline phosphatase activation and total calcium content, but reduces the expression of calcification inhibitors, osteopontin and osteonectin, in cultured vascular smooth muscle cells in vitro and in carotid artery rings ex vivo. Furthermore, both calpain-1 and collagen II increase with aging within human aortic intima [25]. Similarly, both calpain-1 and collagen II are highly expressed in atherosclerotic plaques than non-plaque areas [25].

Other molecules have been implicated in medial calcification, tissue transglutaminase (TG2), is a multifunctional protein that has been found to play a central role in programming chondro-osseous SMC differentiation, a major process in arterial calcification [26]. TG2 localization and function seems to be regulated by

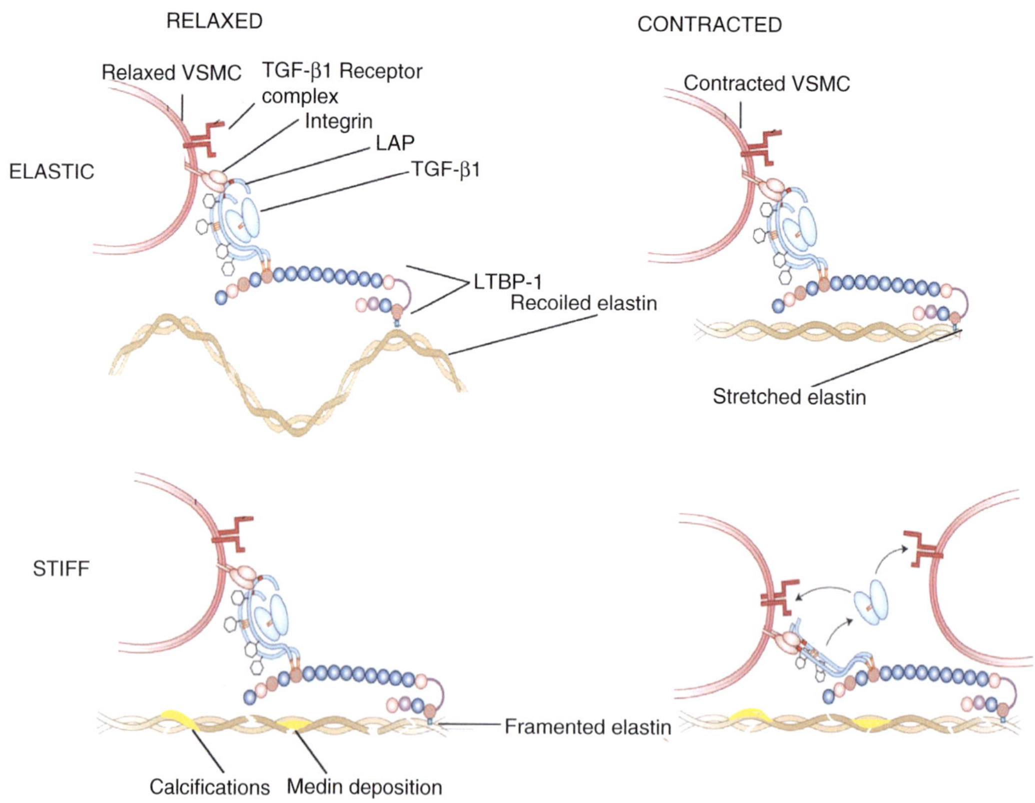

Fig. 12.4 A schematic model illustrating the mechanism of TGF-β1 activation with loss of elasticity. TGF-β1 is secreted in a large latent complex, consisting of TGF-β1 associated with the latency associated peptide (*LAP*) and the latent TGF-β1–binding protein (*LTBP-1*). This structure links VSMCs to elastic fibers. In normal-functioning elastic arteries, VSCMs contraction pulls the whole compound with elastic fiber connected to it. With the loss of elasticity due to calcification, amyloidization, and other factors, the elastic fiber is less mobile and traction forces exerted by the VSMCs is transferred to LAP potentially resulting in a conformation change that liberates active TGF-β1 (Adapted with permission from Hinz [28])

NO; hence the decline in NO bioavailability with aging, and subsequently over activation of TG2 could contribute to the medial calcification with aging [27].

The Transforming Growth Factor Beta 1: A Bridge Between Elastin Senescence and Fibrosis/Calcification?

The stable nature of elastin and its fine organization make it prone to cumulative alterations and fragmentation with aging [14]. Considering that inflammation and fibrosis are in general, reparative processes, it is possible that arterial wall inflammation, fibrosis and calcification are rather reparative mechanisms in origin for the failing elastin under mechanical stress. However, the mechanism by which mechanical stress is translated in biochemical signaling is not fully understood. An interesting structure of the profibrotic transforming growth factor-β1 (TGF- β1), latency associated peptide (LAP), and latent TGF – β1 binding protein (LTBP) connects elastin fibers to VSMC/myofibrolasts and other ECM components (Fig. 12.4); contraction of VSMCs against a stiff ECM leads to stretching of this structure and the release of activated TGF- β1 [16]. Hence, given that TGF- β1 signalizing generates fibronectin and collagen (Fig. 12.3), this system could serve as a mechanical-sensor that translates mechanical stress into biochemical signaling leading to fibrosis.

This model is supported by findings in Marfan syndrome that mimics by far fast-forward arterial aging. Marfan syndrome is an autosomal dominant disorder of connective tissue due to abnormal fibrillin-1 caused by mutations in the *FBN1* gene on chromosome 15 [17]. In addition to that fibrillin-1 forms the scaffold of elastin fibers and connects with LTBP/LAP/TGF-β1 structure [18]. Dysregualtion of TGF- β signaling due to defective fibrilin-1 is a major player in Marfan syndrome, and blocking of TFG-β1 attenuates or prevents the disease in animal models [19]. Considering that TGF- β1 is increased with aging in animals and humans (Fig. 12.2) [20, 21], its plausible that "elastic fatigue, a less intense phenomenon than defective fibrilin-1 in Marfan Syndrome, occurs at a slower rate with aging contributing to more remarkable fibrosis of the arterial wall.

Amyloid Protein Deposition

The incidence of aortic amyloidosis averages 79 % in 224 human autopsy cases. Prior to the fifth decade, the incidence is 51 % and it rises sharply with age and reached over 95 % in the eighth decade. The incidence of aortic amyloidosis is always higher than in the heart, in which amyloidosis also increases with age. The aortic media exhibits the majority of amyloid content, which consists of numerous minute deposits without a relationship to atheromata [29].

Intracellular processing of proteins that leads to their degradation involves a change in their tertiary structure, i.e. folding geometry. Misfolding of extracellular proteins to form amyloid deposits is a dynamic process, occurring in parallel with, or as an alternative to physiologic folding, generates insoluble protein aggregates that are deposited in tissues [30]. Specific amyloid types are defined on the basis of its assembled protein fibril patterns. Initially, localized amyloid deposits, limited to certain organs or tissues, were formerly regarded as innocent bystanders, or by-products of diseases, rather than having involvement in their pathogenesis. This view has changed radically during the last decade [31]. Small amyloid deposits, or oligomeric pre-amyloid aggregates of specific amyloid fibril proteins, are now believed to be critical factors with toxic cellular effects involved in the pathogenesis of common disorders, e.g. the amyloid b-peptide (Ab) in Alzheimer's disease or islet amyloid polypeptide (IAPP) in type II diabetes [31]. Although mechanisms by which protein aggregates lead to cell injury and death are poorly understood, and fibrils are potential cytotoxins [32], β sheet peptides (e.g., amyloid β) are known to form ion channels in lipid bilayers possibly through aggregation, though the channel structure is not clear [33].

MFG E8 is a secreted protein (see above) and the precursor protein of medin amyloid, which becomes deposited in the aortic media in almost 100 % of the Caucasian population over 50 years of age [34]. Medin amyloid (AMed) is not restricted to the aorta but also occurs in other arteries, mainly in the upper part of the body, including temporal intracranial vessels [35]. In vitro aggregated medin induces death of aortic smooth muscle cells, and cells incubated together with medin increased the production of metalloproteinase-2, i.e. a protease that degrades elastin and collagen matrix metalloproteinase-2 [35]. There is some evidence to indicate that non-amyloid pre-fibrillar medin oligomeric aggregates may also be toxic to the surrounding cells.

In human aortae, medin amyloid co-localizes with elastic fibers of arteries [36] and is also associated with other elastic structures [34]. Both medin and MFGE8 bind to tropoelastin (Fig. 12.4) in a concentration-dependent fashion. It has been suggested that the medin domain mediates the MFGE8-tropoelastin interaction is a cell adhesion protein and its medin domain may connect smooth muscle cells to the elastic fibers of arteries (Fig. 12.4) [37]. Given that both medin and MFGE8 interact with elastic fibers, elastin may be an important component in the formation of medin amyloid [34]. It has been hypothesized that medin may be a factor involved in the increased aortic stiffness that accompanies advancing age [34, 36, 38]. Indeed, correlations between serum MFG-E8 and pulse wave velocity and cardiovascular risk factors have been observed in older normal subjects and in elderly patients with type 2 diabetes mellitus [39].

Age-Associated Changes in Aortic Geometry and Function

Strain and Distensibility

The aforementioned age-associated changes in endothelial and VSMC function, arterial matrix and arterial wall remodeling result in reduced aortic distensibility in response to the pulsatile flow generated by the left ventricle [31]. Aortic elastic properties are quantified by a set of parameters including aortic strain, the relative change in AoD in systole to its diastolic diameter, and distensibility, which is strain indexed to pulse pressure, and other parameters [32]. It is quite interesting that, in large, the age-associated decline in aortic strain and distensibility occurs prior to the age of 50, after which a pronounced change in other marker of arterial stiffness, pulse wave velocity, ensues [33]. This suggests that loss of central arterial function occurs much early in life with strain approaching a minimum around the age of 50, giving rise to significant changes in pulse pressure.

Aortic Diameter

Dilatation of proximal aorta with aging has been long recognized in post-mortem and via echocardiography studies in vivo [34–36]. The exhaustion of aortic strain and distensibility reserve that reaches a nadir by the age of 50 is likely to initiate a remodeling process with more pronounced aortic dilatation in response to cumulative effect of pulsatile blood pressure that is not accommodated by distensibility. Aortic root diameter (AoD) increases with age in both men and women, however, men have accelerated dilatation of the aortic root compared to women, adjusting for body habitus and blood pressure [40].

Pulse Wave Velocity and Elevated Blood Pressure

A very important hemodynamic consequence of the stiffening of the arterial wall is a more rapid propagation of the pulse wave generated by the left ventricle known as pulse wave velocity (PWV). Longitudinal data on PWV with extended follow up showed that both men and women experience a non-linear increase in PWV with aging, accompanied by a steep increase in PWV beyond the age of 50 (Fig. 12.5b) [41]. Although there is no gender difference in PWV in early adulthood, men have a much steeper increase in the PWV rates of change with aging, leading to higher PWV in men than women beyond the age of 50. In addition to age, systolic blood pressure (SBP) is a major determinant of the longitudinal increase in arterial stiffness, with less impressive contributions of other factors such as heart rate and BMI. Prior studies have also shown that PWV predicts the longitudinal increase in SBP, and the incidence of hypertension [5, 42]. Hence, the relationship between SBP and PWV is best described as feed forward (i.e. vicious cycle). However, this relationship might be even more complex; concurrent longitudinal tracking of SBP and PWV in the SardiNIA project showed that SBP and PWV diverge in advanced age (Scuteri et al. 2014, unpublished data). Longitudinal increase in PWV beyond the age of 60 in both genders was accompanied by a decrease in SBP in men, and a less pronounced increase than PWV in women. Data from the Baltimore Longitudinal Study on Aging with concurrent tracking of PWV and blood pressure showed the same pattern of separation between PWV and blood pressure: in men longitudinal increase in PWV was not accompanied by longitudinal increase in PP [43] (Fig. 12.5a, b). On the other hand, in women, the accelerated longitudinal increase in PWV was accompanied only by a steady longitudinal increase in PP. These serial studies of concurrent trajectories of PWV, SBP, and PP shed light on the conundrum of relationship of blood pressure and PWV, which given these recent longitudinal data diverge with aging.

Aortic Impedance

Impedance refers to the relationship between pulse pressure and pulsatile flow, hence it is a major determinant of PP and is instrumental to attempts aiming to understand the conundrum of

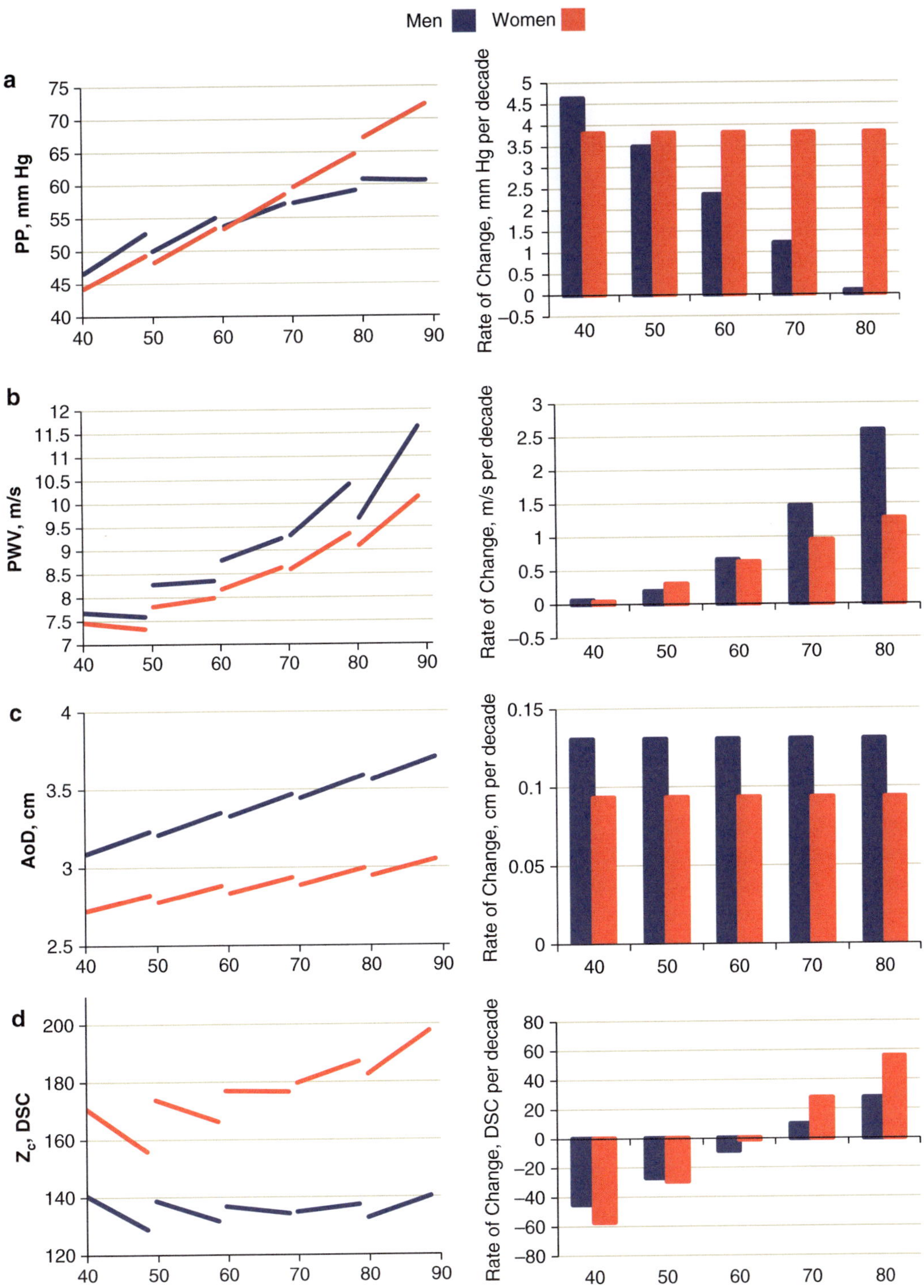

Fig. 12.5 Concurrent longitudinal trajectories (*left*), and rate of change per decade (*right*) of (**a**) pulse pressure, (**b**) pulse wave velocity (m/s), (**c**) aortic root diameter (*AoD*), and (**d**) calculated aortic impedance (Z_c), from the Baltimore Longitudinal Study on Aging. There was dissociation in the trajectories of PP and PWV that is more pronounced in men. This dissociation was accompanied by a more pronounced increase in AoD with aging in men than women. The net effect of the longitudinal changes in PWV and AoD produced a greater increase in Z_c among women with aging, likely contributing to their higher pulse pressure

PWV and PP. Characteristic impedance (Z_c), which represents the initial opposition of the flow in the proximal aorta, but do not account for wave reflection, increases by two fold between the age of 20 and 80. Input impedance, on the other hand, which integrates the effect of wave reflection on the forward flow, increases by four fold [44, 45]. Z_c is determined by PWV and AoD (D) based on the water hammer equation: $Z_c = 4 \times PWV/\rho\pi D^2$ [46]. Hence, it has been proposed that an increase in PWV leads to an increase in Z_c, and subsequently the increased in pulse pressure with aging. Because the increase wave reflection plateaus with aging, the evolution of the conventional wisdom was that the increase in PWV is the main driver for the increase in Z_c and PP and the epidemic of predominant systolic hypertension.

However, in advanced, this conventional wisdom is challenged by the dissociation between the trajectories of PWV and PP; hence, another determinant of Z_c, i.e. AoD, might be a factor separating the trajectories of PWV and PP. In fact, data from the BLSA shows a greater rate of the longitudinal increase in AoD in men than women (Fig. 12.5c) [43]. While Z_c was not directly measured in the BLSA, Z_c was calculated using the water hammer equation to approximate the net effect of the longitudinal changes in PWV and AoD. Women had greater longitudinal increase in calculated Z_c, (Fig. 12.5d), despite men having a greater rate of increase in PWV (AlGhatrif et al. 2014, Unpublished data). These differences in the longitudinal change in PWV and AoD and their relative effect on Z_c may explain in part the age- and gender-related dissociation in PWV and PP trajectories.

Pressure Wave Reflection

As the incident, forward pulse wave propagates down the arterial tree, it becomes reflected at sites of impedance change, producing a "reflected wave" that propagates back to the proximal aorta and left ventricle. In young adults, this pulse wave reaches the left ventricle in diastole, augmenting diastolic pressure, augmenting coronary filling pressure, and theoretically augmenting myocardial perfusion. Increased arterial stiffness and an accelerated PWV with advanced age cause both the amplitude and timing of reflected wave to change, with aging, such that larger reflected waves reach the heart earlier during late systole, augmenting systolic rather than diastolic arterial pressure [1]. Augmentation index (AIx), an integrative measure of wave reflection, is expressed as pressure augmentation, i.e. the pressure increase due to reflected wave, divided by pulse pressure [47]. In contrast to PWV, which increases exponentially with age, data from cross-sectional studies shows that AIx increases steeply in men and women before the age of 50, while it plateaus thereafter in women, and increase modestly in men with aging [47–49].

Wave reflection is thought to have a major role in the increased pulse pressure with aging; prospective studies have shown that augmentation index predicts future pulse pressure and incidence of hypertension [42, 50]. However, that AIx plateaus beyond the age of 50 has created some controversy regarding its relationship to the major hemodynamic changes that ensue beyond this age [51]. It is important to recognize, however, that AIx indicates the ratio of the reflected pressure wave to the forward pressure wave, rather than the absolute value of pressure augmentation. Hence, AIx is analogous to "interest rate" paid on the incident pressure, i.e. the principal of a loan, generating augmented pressure, i.e. interest, and the pulse pressure being analogous to the total payment, i.e. principal plus interest. Following this analogy, even if the interest rate, i.e. AIx, was not increased, an increase in the principal, i.e. the incident pressure, would generate a greater amount of interest paid, i.e. the augmented pressure, and the sum of principal and interest, i.e. pulse pressure, would increase at a greater magnitude compared to the increase in principal itself. Hence, both two sides of the continuous debate about the contribution of reflected wave vs. the forward wave to an increase in PP might be correct.

Interventions to Prevent or Retard Arterial Stiffness to Lower Blood Pressure

Currently, several interventions at the level of endothelial function and peripheral vascular tone result in improvement in central pressures, mainly by improving wave reflection dynamics and improving endothelial function and response to sheer stress. However, interventions directed at the more pronounced structural changes in the arterial wall are lacking. Hereby we will briefly review current interventions and their effect of central arterial properties in addition to investigational intervention ns in progress.

Lifestyle Modification

Similar to other major cardiovascular risk factors, there is some evidence that life style modification could improve some measurements of arterial stiffness. Weight loss, low-salt and low fat diet have been found to improve PWV beyond that of blood pressure control [52–54]. Regular endurance exercise training [55–57], and brisk walking [58, 59] are associated with slower progression of arterial stiffness, as well as improvement of arterial stiffness parameters; this improvement is likely secondary to improved endothelial function and NO bioavailability [60, 61]

Anti-Hypertensive Medications

Anti-hypertensive medications have a differing impact on wave reflection and central pulse pressure. Vasoactive medications such as angiotensin converting enzyme inhibitors (ACE-I) and angiotensin II blockers (ARBs), dihydropyridine calcium-channel blockers, and nitrate favorably change wave reflection, leading to a lower augmentation index and lower central pulse pressure; In contrast, non-vasodilating beta-blockers, appear to paradoxically increase central pulse pressure [50, 62–64]. The effect of beta blockers is thought to be secondary to a prolongation of the cardiac cycle (reduction in heart rate), which causes (1) prolonged relaxation, leading to increased stroke volume, and subsequently larger reflected wave amplitude, and (2) a relatively prolonged ejection period, allowing earlier wave reflection arrival during systole. This explains the differences in central pulse pressures but similar peripheral pulse pressure observed between beta blockers vs. ARBs and calcium channel blockers in the Losartan Intervention For Endpoint Reduction in Hypertension Study (LIFE) and the Conduit Artery Function Evaluation Study (CAFE), respectively, resulting in different outcomes [65, 66]. Whether anti-hypertensive medications further improve arterial wall properties beyond that of blood pressure control and wave reflection is not clear. ACE-I/ARB have the strongest potential to modify arterial wall property, by blocking the angiotensin-renin-aldosterone system, an active pathway in this process [67, 68]; however, a study in patients with isolated systolic hypertension showed no change in PWV with short-term use of ACE-I [62]; similar results were seen with long-term use of ACE-I as well [69]

Statin Therapy

Several studies have shown some improvement in arterial stiffness with long-term statin therapy [70–72]. But, short-term treatment with statin appears to increase PWV in humans and non-human primates, an effect that has been attributed to rapid decline in vascular lipid inclusion which could soften the artery [70, 73]. Hyperlipidemia, per se, does not seem to play a major role in development of arterial stiffness as it does in atherosclerosis [74]. Hence, the long-term effects of statin might be mediated through it is anti-inflammatory effect rather than lipid lowering effect.

Therapeutic Strategies in the Pipeline

ALT-711, advanced-glycation end products (AGE) cross-link breaker has been shown to decrease arterial stiffness beyond decrease in blood pressure in animals and elderly humans [24, 75]. Additional clinical studies to determine the utility of ALT-711 in treating arterial stiffness and with aging are in progress [75]. Resveratrol, a natural compound in grapes and red wine, has antioxidant and anti-inflammatory properties and was associated with improved health and increased lifespan of mice on high-caloric diet [76]; current investigations is ongoing to assess its effect on arterial stiffness parameters. While it is likely that Resveratrol would not develop into a pharmaceutical product, chemically modified Resveratrol-based molecule could play a role in the future [67]

Recent studies also demonstrate that inhibition of MMP activity can decelerate age-associated arterial proinflammation [77]. Chronic administration of a broad-spectrum MMP inhibitor PD, via a daily gavage, to 16-month-old rats for 8 months inhibits the age-associated increases in aortic gelatinase and interstitial collagenase activity in situ; preservation of the elastic fiber network integrity; a reduction of collagen deposition; a reduction of monocyte chemoattractant protein 1 and transforming growth factor-β1 activation; a diminution in the activity of the profibrogenic signaling molecule SMAD-2/3 phosphorylation [10]; inhibition of proendothelin 1 activation [78]; downregulation of expression of ets-1; and marked blunting of the expected age-associated increases in arterial pressure.

Summary

In summary, increasing molecular disorder with advancing age begets chronic arterial inflammation, which drives arterial cell phenotypic shifts, adverse arterial wall remodeling, and alteration of arterial function; the later may lead to exaggerated chronic inflammation. Proinflammatory mechanisms that drive arterial aging are intertwined with hypertension and atherosclerosis at the molecular and cellular levels. Thus, the inflamed arterial wall that accompanies advancing age confers the major risk for hypertension and atherosclerosis. In humans, other well-known risk factors (e.g., excess food intake, altered dietary lipid and metabolism, smoking, and lack of exercise) likely interact with this arterial substrate, and increase the inflammatory process, rendering the aging artery a "fertile soil" that facilitates the initiation and progression of these arterial diseases such as hypertension, atherosclerosis, and diabetes. Interventions to suppress chronic arterial inflammation may beneficially impact on the rampant epidemic of age-associated arterial diseases in our society. The cellular/molecular proinflammatory mechanisms driven by Ang II and other growth factors (Fig. 12.3) that underlie arterial aging are novel putative candidates to be targeted by interventions aimed at attenuating arterial aging, and thus possibly attenuating the major risk factor for hypertension and atherosclerosis.

Some lifestyle and pharmacologic interventions have already proved to be effective in preventing or ameliorating hypertension associated with aging. Much larger future interventional studies are required to delineate whether, and to what extent age-related arterial stiffening, inflammation, and subsequent abnormalities, can be retarded with interventions on the Ang II, aldosterone, endothelin, norepinephrine signaling cascades.

References

1. Lakatta EG. Arterial and cardiac aging: major shareholders in cardiovascular disease enterprises: part I: aging arteries: a "set up" for vascular disease. Circulation. 2003;107(1):139–46.
2. Faury G. Function-structure relationship of elastic arteries in evolution: from microfibrils to elastin and elastic fibres. Pathol Biol (Paris). 2001;49(4):310–25.
3. Lakatta EG, Wang M, Najjar SS. Arterial aging and subclinical arterial disease are fundamentally intertwined at macroscopic and molecular levels. Med Clin North Am. Elsevier Ltd; 2009 ;93(3):583–604.
4. Lloyd-Jones D, Adams RJ, Brown TM, Carnethon M, Dai S, De Simone G, et al. Heart disease and stroke statistics–2010 update: a report from the American Heart Association. Circulation. 2010;121(7):e46–215.
5. Najjar SS, Scuteri A, Shetty V, Wright JG, Muller DC, Fleg JL, et al. Pulse wave velocity is an independent predictor of the longitudinal increase in systolic blood pressure and of incident hypertension in the Baltimore Longitudinal Study of Aging. J Am Coll Cardiol. 2008;51:1377–83.

6. Wang M, et al. Proinflammation: the key to arterial aging. TEM. 2014;25(2):72.
7. Lakatta EG. The reality of aging viewed from the arterial wall. Artery Research. 2013;7(2):73.
8. Najjar SS, Scuteri A, Lakatta EG. Arterial aging: is it an immutable cardiovascular risk factor? Hypertension. 2005;46(3):454–62.
9. Wang M, Lakatta EG. Altered regulation of matrix metalloproteinase-2 in aortic remodeling during aging. Hypertension. 2002;39(4):865–73.
10. Spinetti G, Wang M, Monticone R, Zhang J, Zhao D, Lakatta EG. Rat aortic MCP-1 and its receptor CCR2 increase with age and alter vascular smooth muscle cell function. Arterioscler Thromb Vasc Biol. 2004;24(8):1397–402.
11. Wang M, Zhang J, Jiang L-Q, Spinetti G, Pintus G, Monticone R, et al. Proinflammatory profile within the grossly normal aged human aortic wall. Hypertension. 2007;50(1):219–27.
12. Ong K-T, Delerme S, Pannier B, Safar ME, Benetos A, Laurent S, et al. Aortic stiffness is reduced beyond blood pressure lowering by short-term and long-term antihypertensive treatment: a meta-analysis of individual data in 294 patients. J Hypertens. 2011;29(6):1034–42.
13. Lakatta EG. Central arterial aging and the epidemic of systolic hypertension and atherosclerosis. J Am Soc Hypertens. 2007;1:302–40.
14. Celermajer DS, Sorensen KE, Spiegelhalter DJ, Georgakopoulos D, Robinson J, Deanfield JE. Aging is associated with endothelial dysfunction in healthy men years before the age-related decline in women. J Am Coll Cardiol. 1994;24(2):471–6.
15. Paneni F, Osto E, Costantino S, Mateescu B, Briand S, Coppolino G, et al. Deletion of the AP-1 transcription factor JunD induces oxidative stress and accelerates Age-related endothelial dysfunction. Circulation. 2013;127(11):1229–40.
16. Higashi Y, Kihara Y, Noma K. Endothelial dysfunction and hypertension in aging. Hypertens Res. 2012;35(11):1039–47. The Japanese Society of Hypertension.
17. Bode-Böger SM, Muke J, Surdacki A, Brabant G, Böger RH, Frölich JC. Oral L-arginine improves endothelial function in healthy individuals older than 70 years. Vasc Med. 2003;8(2):77–81.
18. Williamson KA, Hamilton A, Reynolds JA, Sipos P, Crocker I, Stringer SE, et al. Age-related impairment of endothelial progenitor cell migration correlates with structural alterations of heparan sulfate proteoglycans. Aging Cell. 2013;12(1):139–47.
19. Stein JH, Korcarz CE, Hurst RT, Lonn E, Kendall CB, Mohler ER, et al. Use of carotid ultrasound to identify subclinical vascular disease and evaluate cardiovascular disease risk: a consensus statement from the American Society of Echocardiography Carotid Intima-Media Thickness Task Force. Endorsed by the Society for Vascula. J Am Soc Echocardiogr. 2008;21(2):93–111.
20. Nagai Y, Metter EJ, Earley CJ, Kemper MK, Becker LC, Lakatta EG, et al. Increased carotid artery intimal-medial thickness in asymptomatic older subjects with exercise-induced myocardial ischemia. Circulation. 1998;98(15):1504–9.
21. Yan SF, Ramasamy R, Naka Y, Schmidt AM. Glycation, inflammation, and RAGE: a scaffold for the macrovascular complications of diabetes and beyond. Circ Res. 2003;93(12):1159–69.
22. Wang M, Takagi G, Asai K, Resuello RG, Natividad FF, Vatner DE, et al. Aging increases aortic MMP-2 activity and angiotensin II in nonhuman primates. Hypertension. 2003;41(6):1308–16.
23. Adams MR, Nakagomi A, Keech A, Robinson J, McCredie R, Bailey BP, et al. Carotid intima-media thickness is only weakly correlated with the extent and severity of coronary artery disease. Circulation. 1995;92(8):2127–34.
24. Kass DA, Shapiro EP, Kawaguchi M, Capriotti AR, Scuteri A, deGroof RC, et al. Improved arterial compliance by a novel advanced glycation end-product cross-link breaker. Circulation. 2001;104(13):1464–70.
25. Jiang L, Zhang J, Monticone RE, Telljohann R, Wu J, Wang M, et al. Calpain-1 regulation of matrix metalloproteinase 2 activity in vascular smooth muscle cells facilitates age-associated aortic wall calcification and fibrosis. Hypertension. 2012;60(5):1192–9.
26. Johnson KA, Polewski M, Terkeltaub RA. Transglutaminase 2 is central to induction of the arterial calcification program by smooth muscle cells. Circ Res. 2008;102(5):529–37.
27. Jandu SK, Webb AK, Pak A, Sevinc B, Nyhan D, Belkin AM, et al. Nitric oxide regulates tissue transglutaminase localization and function in the vasculature. Amino Acids. 2013;44(1):261–9.
28. Hinz B. Tissue stiffness, latent TGF-beta1 activation, and mechanical signal transduction: implications for the pathogenesis and treatment of fibrosis. Curr Rheumatol Rep. 2009;11(2):120–6.
29. Iwata T, Kamei T, Uchino F, Mimaya H, Yanagaki T, Etoh H. Pathological study on amyloidosis–relationship of amyloid deposits in the aorta to aging. Acta Pathol Jpn. 1978;28(2):193–203.
30. Merlini G, Bellotti V. Molecular mechanisms of amyloidosis. N Engl J Med. 2003;349(6):583–96.
31. Westermark P. Aspects on human amyloid forms and their fibril polypeptides. FEBS J. 2005;272(23):5942–9.
32. Sciarretta KL, Gordon DJ, Meredith SC. Peptide-based inhibitors of amyloid assembly. Methods Enzymol. 2006;413:273–312.
33. Thundimadathil J, Roeske RW, Jiang H-Y, Guo L. Aggregation and porin-like channel activity of a beta sheet peptide. Biochemistry. 2005;44(30):10259–70.
34. Larsson A, Peng S, Persson H, Rosenbloom J, Abrams WR, Wassberg E, et al. Lactadherin binds to elasti-- starting point for medin amyloid formation? Amyloid. Informa UK Ltd UK; 2006;13(2):78–85.

35. Peng S, Glennert J, Westermark P. Medin-amyloid: a recently characterized age-associated arterial amyloid form affects mainly arteries in the upper part of the body. Amyloid. 2005;12(2):96–102.
36. Mucchiano G, Cornwell GG, Westermark P. Senile aortic amyloid. Evidence for two distinct forms of localized deposits. Am J Pathol. 1992;140(4):871–7.
37. Morrell CH, Brant LJ, Ferrucci L. Model choice can obscure results in longitudinal studies. J Gerontol A Biol Sci Med Sci. 2009;64(2):215–22.
38. Häggqvist B, Näslund J, Sletten K, Westermark GT, Mucchiano G, Tjernberg LO, et al. Medin: an integral fragment of aortic smooth muscle cell-produced lactadherin forms the most common human amyloid. Proc Natl Acad Sci U S A. 1999;96(15):8669–74.
39. Cheng M, Li B, Li X, Wang Q, Zhang J, Jing X, et al. Correlation between serum lactadherin and pulse wave velocity and cardiovascular risk factors in elderly patients with type 2 diabetes mellitus. Diabetes Res Clin Pract. 2012;95(1):125–31.
40. Lam CSP, Xanthakis V, Sullivan LM, Lieb W, Aragam J, Redfield MM, et al. Aortic root remodeling over the adult life course: longitudinal data from the Framingham Heart Study. Circulation. 2010;122(9): 884–90.
41. AlGhatrif M, Strait JB, Morrell CH, Canepa M, Wright J, Elango P, et al. Longitudinal trajectories of arterial stiffness and the role of blood pressure: the Baltimore longitudinal study of aging. Hypertension. 2013;62(5):934–51.
42. Kaess BM, Rong J, Larson MG, Hamburg NM, Vita JA, Levy D, et al. Aortic stiffness, blood pressure progression, and incident hypertension. JAMA. 2012;308(9):875–81.
43. AlGhatrif M, Strait JB, Morrell CH, Canepa M, Wright J, Elango P, et al. Attenuated aortic dilatation, not increased wall stiffness best explains the rise in pulse pressure in women with aging: results from the Baltimore longitudinal study of aging. Circulation. 2013;128:A18061.
44. O'Rourke MF, Hashimoto J. Mechanical factors in arterial aging: a clinical perspective. J Am Coll Cardiol. 2007;50(1):1–13.
45. Nichols W, O'Rourke MF, Vlachopoulos C. McDonald's blood flow in arteries: theoretical, experimental and clinical principles. Boca Raton: CRC Press; 2011.
46. Mitchell GF, Lacourciere Y, Ouellet JP, Izzo Jr JL, Neutel J, Kerwin LJ, et al. Determinants of elevated pulse pressure in middle-aged and older subjects with uncomplicated systolic hypertension: the role of proximal aortic diameter and the aortic pressure-flow relationship. Circulation. 2003;108:1592–8.
47. Vaitkevicius PV, Fleg JL, Engel JH, O'Connor FC, Wright JG, Lakatta LE, et al. Effects of age and aerobic capacity on arterial stiffness in healthy-adults. Circulation. 1993;88:1456–62.
48. Redheuil A, Yu W-C, Mousseaux E, Harouni AA, Kachenoura N, Wu CO, et al. Age-related changes in aortic arch geometry: relationship with proximal aortic function and left ventricular mass and remodeling. J Am Coll Cardiol. 2011;58(12):1262–70.
49. Mitchell GF, Parise H, Benjamin EJ, Larson MG, Keyes MJ, Vita JA, et al. Changes in arterial stiffness and wave reflection with advancing age in healthy men and women: the Framingham Heart Study. Hypertension. 2004;43(6):1239–45.
50. Cecelja M, Jiang B, Spector TD, Chowienczyk P. Progression of central pulse pressure over 1 decade of aging and its reversal by nitroglycerin a twin study. J Am Coll Cardiol. 2012;59(5):475–83.
51. Mitchell GF. Impedance progress: aortic diameter rears its head again? Hypertension. 2007;49(6): 1207–9.
52. Van de Laar RJJ, Stehouwer CDA, van Bussel BCT, Prins MH, Twisk JWR, Ferreira I. Adherence to a Mediterranean dietary pattern in early life is associated with lower arterial stiffness in adulthood: the Amsterdam Growth and Health Longitudinal Study. J Intern Med. 2013;273(1):79–93.
53. Cooper JN, Buchanich JM, Youk A, Brooks MM, Barinas-Mitchell E, Conroy MB, et al. Reductions in arterial stiffness with weight loss in overweight and obese young adults: potential mechanisms. Atherosclerosis. 2012;223(2):485–90.
54. Hummel SL, Seymour EM, Brook RD, Kolias TJ, Sheth SS, Rosenblum HR, et al. Low-sodium dietary approaches to stop hypertension diet reduces blood pressure, arterial stiffness, and oxidative stress in hypertensive heart failure with preserved ejection fraction. Hypertension. 2012;60(5):1200–6.
55. DeSouza CA, Shapiro LF, Clevenger CM, Dinenno FA, Monahan KD, Tanaka H, et al. Regular aerobic exercise prevents and restores age-related declines in endothelium-dependent vasodilation in healthy men. Circulation. 2000;102(12):1351–7.
56. Austin BA, Popovic ZB, Kwon DH, Thamilarasan M, Boonyasirinant T, Flamm SD, et al. Aortic stiffness independently predicts exercise capacity in hypertrophic cardiomyopathy: a multimodality imaging study. Heart. 2010;96(16):1303–10.
57. Tanaka H, Dinenno FA, Monahan KD, Clevenger CM, DeSouza CA, Seals DR. Aging, habitual exercise, and dynamic arterial compliance. Circulation. 2000;102(11):1270–5.
58. Seals DR, Desouza CA, Donato AJ, Tanaka H. Habitual exercise and arterial aging. J Appl Physiol Soc. 2008;105(4):1323–32.
59. Kearney TM, Murphy MH, Davison GW, O'Kane MJ, Gallagher AM. Accumulated brisk walking reduces arterial stiffness in overweight adults: evidence from a randomised control trial. J Am Soc Hypertens. 2014;8(2):117–26.
60. Heckman GA, McKelvie RS. Cardiovascular aging and exercise in healthy older adults. Clin J Sport Med. 2008;18(6):479–85.
61. d'Alessio P. Aging and the endothelium. Exp Gerontol. 2004;39(2):165–71.

62. Mackenzie IS, McEniery CM, Dhakam Z, Brown MJ, Cockcroft JR, Wilkinson IB. Comparison of the effects of antihypertensive agents on central blood pressure and arterial stiffness in isolated systolic hypertension. Hypertension. 2009;54(2):409–13.
63. Morgan T, Lauri J, Bertram D, Anderson A. Effect of different antihypertensive drug classes on central aortic pressure. Am J Hypertens. 2004;17(2):118–23.
64. Asmar RG, London GM, O'Rourke ME, Safar ME. Improvement in blood pressure, arterial stiffness and wave reflections with a very-low-dose perindopril/indapamide combination in hypertensive patient: a comparison with atenolol. Hypertension. 2001; 38(4):922–6.
65. Williams B, Lacy PS, Thom SM, Cruickshank K, Stanton A, Collier D, et al. Differential impact of blood pressure-lowering drugs on central aortic pressure and clinical outcomes: principal results of the Conduit Artery Function Evaluation (CAFE) study. Circulation. 2006;113(9):1213–25.
66. Dahlöf B, Devereux RB, Kjeldsen SE, Julius S, Beevers G, de Faire U, et al. Cardiovascular morbidity and mortality in the losartan intervention for endpoint reduction in hypertension study (LIFE): a randomised trial against atenolol. Lancet. 2002;359(9311):995–1003.
67. Benetos A, Vasmant D, Thiéry P, Safar M. Effects of ramipril on arterial hemodynamics. J Cardiovasc Pharmacol. 1991;18 Suppl 2:S153–6.
68. Safar ME, Jankowski P. Antihypertensive therapy and de-stiffening of the arteries. Expert Opin Pharmacother. Informa UK, Ltd. London; 2010; 11(16):2625–34.
69. Mitchell GF, Dunlap ME, Warnica W, Ducharme A, Arnold JMO, Tardif J-C, et al. Long-term trandolapril treatment is associated with reduced aortic stiffness: the prevention of events with angiotensin-converting enzyme inhibition hemodynamic substudy. Hypertension. 2007;49(6):1271–7.
70. Raison J, Rudnichi A, Safar ME. Effects of atorvastatin on aortic pulse wave velocity in patients with hypertension and hypercholesterolaemia: a preliminary study. J Hum Hypertens. 2002;16(10):705–10.
71. Ott C, Schneider MP, Schlaich MP, Schmieder RE. Rosuvastatin improves pulse wave reflection by restoring endothelial function. Microvasc Res. 2012;84(1):60–4.
72. Tousoulis D, Oikonomou E, Siasos G, Chrysohoou C, Zaromitidou M, Kioufis S, et al. Dose-dependent effects of short term atorvastatin treatment on arterial wall properties and on indices of left ventricular remodeling in ischemic heart failure. Atherosclerosis. 2013;227(2):367–72.
73. Farrar DJ, Bond MG, Riley WA, Sawyer JK. Anatomic correlates of aortic pulse wave velocity and carotid artery elasticity during atherosclerosis progression and regression in monkeys. Circulation. 1991;83(5):1754–63.
74. Cecelja M, Chowienczyk P. Dissociation of aortic pulse wave velocity with risk factors for cardiovascular disease other than hypertension: a systematic review. Hypertension. 2009;54(6):1328–36.
75. Bakris GL, Bank AJ, Kass DA, Neutel JM, Preston RA, Oparil S. Advanced glycation end-product cross-link breakers. A novel approach to cardiovascular pathologies related to the aging process. Am J Hypertens. 2004;17(12 Pt 2):23S–30.
76. Baur JA, Pearson KJ, Price NL, Jamieson HA, Lerin C, Kalra A, et al. Resveratrol improves health and survival of mice on a high-calorie diet. Nature. 2006;444(7117):337–42.
77. Wang M, Zhang J, Telljohann R, Jiang L, Wu J, Monticone RE, et al. Chronic matrix metalloproteinase inhibition retards age-associated arterial proinflammation and increase in blood pressure. Hypertension. 2012;60(2):459–66.
78. Wang M, Zhang J, Spinetti G, Jiang L-Q, Monticone R, Zhao D, et al. Angiotensin II activates matrix metalloproteinase type II and mimics age-associated carotid arterial remodeling in young rats. Am J Pathol. 2005;167(5):1429–42.

13 Emerging Aspects of Angiotensin Biology and Their Potential Role in the Vasculature

Richard N. Re and Julia L. Cook

Abstract

Angiotensin II, a major effector protein of the renin-angiotensin, system plays important roles in the regulation of arterial pressure and intravascular volume. In addition, operating at the systemic, tissue, and cellular levels it modifies vascular structure and inflammation, thereby participating in the pathogenesis of hypertension, atherosclerosis, and vascular stiffening. Here recent findings regarding angiotensin II biology and their potential relevance for vascular biology and disease are discussed

Keywords

Angiotensin • Receptors • Vascular Biology • Intracrine • Target Organ Damage

Introduction

The vasculature is a major target of hypertension. Arterial stiffening, vascular remodeling and other pathologic processes are associated with elevated arterial pressure. The mechanisms by which these processes develop are slowly coming to light. Here evidence bearing on the possible participation of angiotensin II in hypertension-related vascular disease will be briefly reviewed [1].

Infusion of angiotensin II, a principle effector peptide of the renin angiotensin system (RAS), has been shown to result in vascular remodeling, vascular hyalinization and fibrinoid necrosis in one or another animal model. That is, angiotensin-induced hypertension can be associated with many of the features of human malignant hypertension. Moreover, therapy with angiotensin converting enzyme inhibitors [1–7] (ACEIs) or angiotensin receptor blockers (ARBs) in human essential hypertension is associated with a reversal of small artery remodeling in gluteal biopsies. This reversal of remodeling was not seen in patients treated with beta blockers making it likely that angiotensin was determinative in inducing the pathological change and that interrupting angiotensin synthesis (with an ACEI) or its action at the AT1 receptor, could lead to reversal [8]. Importantly, angiotensin increases fibrosis in both the heart and the vasculature and therefore potentially plays a role in the development of arterial stiffening [1–7].

R.N. Re, MD (✉) • J.L. Cook, PhD
Research Division,
Ochsner Health System, 1514 Jefferson Highway,
New Orleans, LA 70121, USA
e-mail: rre@ochsner.org; jcook@ochsner.org

M.E. Safar et al. (eds.), *Blood Pressure and Arterial Wall Mechanics in Cardiovascular Diseases*,
DOI 10.1007/978-1-4471-5198-2_13,

Hypertension, like atherosclerosis, is associated with vascular inflammation. Perivascular infiltration of inflammatory cells occurs in the adventitia of arteries in hypertension. Macrophages in the inflammatory cell mass likely produce oxidative stress leading to vascular pathology. Recently it was discovered that T lymphocyte infiltration also occurs. Indeed, animal models show that the absence of T cells results in a blunting of the hypertensive response to angiotensin II, DOCA salt administration, and norepinephrine. It has also been reported that T cells synthesize angiotensin II and display AT1 receptors. In vitro studies suggest that angiotensin II interaction with these cells drives them toward a more pathogenic Th phenotype rather than the inflammation blunting Treg phenotype. Although the picture is not entirely clear, these data suggest a role for angiotensin II in vascular inflammation and secondarily, therefore, in vascular function, and structure as well [9–11].

The RAS also plays a role in atherosclerosis—longer term consequence of hypertension evolving through the phases of fatty streaks, vascular inflammation, plaque formation and in some cases plaque rupture. Studies in primate models of atherosclerosis have shown that blockade of the AT1 angiotensin II receptor leads to marked reduction in large artery fatty streak production. Moreover, monocyte adherence to vascular wall was diminished in these animals and remained reduced for some weeks after AT1 blockade was stopped. This suggested an effect of angiotensin, acting through the AT1 receptor, on monocyte differentiation [12, 13]. Angiotensin II induces oxidative stress in the arterial wall and up-regulates mediators of inflammation [2, 14]. ACE is up-regulated in the shoulders of atherosclerotic plaques where it could lead to inflammatory changes, enhanced generation of metalloproteases, and possibly plaque rupture [15, 16]. In cell culture, angiotensin II can produce vascular smooth muscle proliferation or hypertrophy depending on cell culture conditions. These results potentially are relevant to both vascular remodeling and the formation of athersclerotic plaques [17, 18]. Thus there is substantial evidence linking the RAS and angiotensin II to vascular pathology in both hypertension and atherosclerosis. The mechanisms by which angiotensin II acts to produce these pathologies appear to be multiple and are poorly understood. However, recent studies have suggested an expanded repertoire of angiotensin action and some of these newly defined functions could be at work in the genesis of vascular pathology.

Receptor Biology

Angiotensin II acts through the AT1 receptor to produce vasoconstriction, aldosterone secretion, hypertrophy, hyperplasia, fibrosis, enhanced renal tubular sodium re-absorption, and other responses. There also exists a second G-protein coupled angiotensin II receptor, AT2, which although widely expressed in the fetus decreases in abundance after birth. The effects of angiotensin II binding the AT2 are not as well established as actions at AT1 but it is generally felt that AT2 action tends to offset AT1 action. Binding of angiotensin II to the AT2 receptor up-regulates bradykinin and nitric oxide leading to vasodilatation. AT2 stimulation also enhances sodium excretion and blunts cell proliferation in some circumstances. However, in some cases AT2 stimulation appears to enhance hypertrophy and so the precise role of AT2 in hypertensive remodeling or atherosclerosis is as yet unknown [19–23].

For its part, the AT1 receptor, in addition to its canonical signaling via second messengers, participates in a variety of direct protein interactions at the cell surface with potentially important effects. For example, AT1 can physically contact the bradykinin B2 receptor at the cell surface resulting in enhanced AT1 signaling. It has been proposed that this interaction plays a role in the blood pressure elevation and vascular pathology that occurs in preeclampsia. Direct AT-1 interaction with the AT2 receptor on the cell surface also can occur resulting in reduced AT1 signaling; thus AT2 is an AT1 antagonist [22, 23]. AT1 also engages in crosstalk with the epidermal growth factor (EGF) receptor [21]. Binding of angiotensin II to AT1 causes release of bound EGF from the cell surface and this EGF then can interact with its own receptor to further stimulate cell growth. AT1 action also interfaces with the lectin-like oxidized low density lipoprotein receptor, LOX-1. Low density lipoprotein (LDL) is a risk factor for atherosclerosis and can be oxidized enabling it to bind to LOX-1. Angiotensin II produces oxidative stress in the arterial wall leading to increased oxidized LDL production which in turn is taken up by macrophages leading to increased lipid accumulation; it also can produce endothelial cell apoptosis in a LOX-1 dependent fashion. Moreover, angiotensin II up-regulates LOX-1 and oxidized LDL up-regulates AT1 expression. Thus the potential exists for AT1 and LOX-1 to act in concert to produce vascular pathology [23–25].

Although angiotensin II is widely regarded as the major effector peptide of the RAS, other peptides derived from angiotensinogen have been shown to be biologically active. In particular angiotensin (1–7) is a vasodilating peptide cleaved from angiotensin II by ACE2, an ACE homologue [25–31]. ACE2 does not produce angiotensin II from angiotensin I but rather generates angiotensin (1–7) from angiotensin II. Angiotensin (1–7) acts via the *mas* receptor. Because angiotensin (1–7) has both vasodilating and antiproliferative actions, tissue levels of angiotensin (1–7) and *mas* very likely play an important role in vascular structure. Of note, angiotensin II infusion produces increased fibrosis in heart and aorta in ACE 2 knockout mice compared to wild type animals, likely indicating a beneficial effect of Angiotensin (1–7) on angiotensin II induced fibrosis and remodeling in the heart and arteries [30].

AT1 receptors are dynamic circulating between the cell surface and intracellular locations such as endosomes. Several chaperone proteins regulate this receptor trafficking. Angiotensin Receptor Associated Protein (ATRAP) associates with the receptor on the cell surface and leads to its internalization [32]. This in turn leads to reduced responsiveness to extracellular angiotensin II. For example, transgenic mice over-expressing ATRAP are protected from the RAS dependent hypertension that develops following intrauterine protein deprivation [33]. A second AT1 chaperone is ARAP1. This protein facilitates AT1 trafficking to the cell surface and thereby enhances cellular responsiveness to angiotensin II. It also influences epidermal growth factor trafficking [34, 35].

We recently reported that Gamma Amonobutyric Acid (GABA) Receptor Associated Protein (GABARAP) is an AT1 associated protein and serves as a chaperone that enhances steady state AT1 levels at the cell surface [36–39]. When GABARAP and an AT1 fluorescent fusion protein were co-transfected into PC-12 cells, surface expression of the receptor increased sixfold. Similarly GABARAP expression in CHO-K1 cells already expressing AT1 receptor increased angiotensin II binding more than threefold and also increased AT1 signaling as well as cellular proliferation. Conversely, knockdown of GABARAP by small interfering RNAs resulted in decreased cell surface receptor expression. These studies suggested that GABARAP, and possibly ARAP1 as well, could be an important therapeutic target in that targeted reduction could potentially have important effects on hypertension and cellular proliferation/hypertrophy [36]. To follow up on this possibility we identified the AT1 receptor sequence to which GABARAP binds and developed fusion proteins fusing this sequence with the cell-penetrating peptide penetratin (a modified intracrine factor utilized to introduce peptides into cells; see Intracrine Biology below). Application of active decoy peptides, but not scrambled control peptides, to cells co-transfected with AT1 receptor and GABARAP dramatically reduced accumulation of AT1 at the cell surface, suggesting that these cell-penetrating peptides, or small molecule analogues capable of entering cells and disrupting the AT1/GABARAP interaction could be therapeutically useful [38]. To test this idea we studied normal mice placed on a low sodium diet to induce modest angiotensin dependence of blood pressure. Decoy and control peptides were injected via a jugular catheter and blood pressure was measure by telemetry. As expected, the active decoy peptide, but not control peptide, lowered blood pressure in these animals [39]. Two lessons emerged from these studies. First AT1 receptor trafficking (and likely the trafficking of other receptors) is a viable therapeutic target for lowering blood pressure and likely for mitigating angiotensin II-induced structural changes in the cardiovascular system. Second, intracrine functionality is becoming increasing useful as a research and, likely, as a therapeutic tool.

Studies employing AT1 fluorescent protein fusion protein have shown that these receptors not only cycle between cell surface and endosomes, but like other receptors—including G-protein coupled receptors—they can traffick to nucleus and other intracellular sites after exposure to ligand [40–42]. Interestingly, we observed that in some cases the AT1 receptor is cleaved and its carboxy-terminus trafficks to nucleus in a manner enhanced by ligand binding at the cell surface. Follow on studies showed that this cleavage occurs between Leu(305) and Gly(306) at the junction of the seventh transmembrane domain and the intracellular cytoplasmic carboxy-terminal domain. To evaluate the function of the carboxy fragment distinct from the holoreceptor, cells were transfected with a construct encoding the carboxy fragment as an in-frame yellow fluorescent protein fusion. The fragment accumulated in nuclei and induced apoptosis in CHO-K1 cells, rat aortic smooth muscle cells (RASMCs), MCF-7 human breast adenocarcinoma cells, and H9c2 rat cardiomyoblasts [40]. This observation suggests a previously unsuspected additional mechanism by which angiotensin II can produce cell death and pathology in the cardiovascular system. It potentially plays a role in congestive heart failure and may provide an additional mechanism by which ACEIs improve outcomes in these patients. In addition, it could well play a role in angiotensin II remodeling in the vasculature and potentially in hypertensive arteriolar rarefaction as well.

Intracrine Biology

The renin-angiotensin system is a well established regulator of vascular tone, intravascular volume, and cardiovascular structure. In addition to the well-studied circulating RAS, local systems exist in multiple tissues and can be regulated independent of the circulating system [3, 4]. For example, high salt diet up-regulates angiotensin II production by the heart in normal man while suppressing plasma renin activity [43]. This is potentially important given emerging evidence suggesting that high salt intake *per se* can up-regulate cardiac and vascular RASs and produce fibrosis [44]. These local RASs, their regulation and function, likely play an important role in the development of vascular pathology including arterial stiffening.

Over the last four decade considerable evidence has also been developed to indicate that angiotensin II can act not only at cell surface receptors but also at intracellular locations. We termed this kind of action *intracrine* to imply action of a peptide extracellular signaling moiety in its cell of synthesis or in a target cell after internalization. Thus, angiotensin II is an intracrine because it is a peptide hormone that can be internalized by target cells, bind to nucleus, and based on *in vitro* and *in vivo* experiments, alter gene expression. In fact, a wide variety of peptide signaling molecules including hormones, cytokines, growth factors, enzymes, and others qualify as intracrines [45–48]. Interestingly, homeodomain transcription factors are intracrines: they traffick between nearby cells, are taken up, and affect gene transcription in the target cells. This process is important, for example, in the development of the retina. A sequence within the homeodomain protein antennopedia is responsible for the internalization of the transcription factor and this sequence is currently being utilized as a cell penetrating peptid--penetratin [49, 50].

We have developed an hypothesis regarding the evolution, biological function, and physiology of intracrines and this intracrine biology is reviewed elsewhere. One characteristic of these entities is the creation of intracellular feedforward loops [43–48]. For example, intracellular angiotensin II has been reported to up-regulate renin and angiotensinogen in cardiac fibroblasts thereby potentially creating a positive feedback loop that could well play a role in cardiac fibrosis and in cardiovascular fibrosis in general [51]. This system is up-regulated by glucose a finding that may have clinical significance given the finding of elevated angiotensin II levels in the hearts of patients suffering from diabetic cardiomyopathy [52].

Of note is the fact that intracrines can act in cells in what we have termed canonical or non-canonical fashions [53]. By canonical we mean that the intracrine acts in the cell via one or more of its established cell surface receptors, the receptor often being located in a membrane environment and often acting via traditional second messengers. By non-canonical we mean action other than via a traditional receptor. For example, angiotensin II has been shown to act at nuclear membrane AT1 and AT2 receptors and to generate second messengers such as nitric oxide [54]. Also AT1-like receptors have been shown in association with euchromatin [55, 56]. These finding imply canonical angiotensin II action, although AII action at euchromatin may not involve the traditional signaling system. At the same time some intracellular angiotensin II actions have been reported to be independent of the AT1 receptor and these are not prevented by ACEI administration [57]. These actions likely are non-canonical.

Non-canonical and canonical angiotensin II intracrine action may well turn out to be important determinants of cardiovascular biology. The generation of oxidative stress is a hall mark of angiotensin pathological action in the cardiovascular system. Although much attention has focused on the role of NADPH oxidase in the generation of reactive oxygen species, attention has also recently turned to the mitochondria [58, 59]. Moreover, a connection between the RAS and mitochondria has been demonstrated by both *in vivo* and *in vitro* work demonstrating the trafficking of angiotensin II from the extracellular space to mitochondria [56–60]. Angiotensin II receptors have been reported on mitochondria early as the 1970s [61]. Also, a long line of investigation has demonstrated that chronic treatment of rodents with ACEIs prolongs life span in association with the preservation of mitochondrial number [62]. It is unclear from these reports, however, if angiotensin II affects mitochondrial biology via binding to its cell surface receptor or by way of interaction with mitochondrial receptors. Recently, small numbers of AT1 and AT2 receptors have been shown to be associated with mitochondria [63]. These authors studied a variety of cell types including mouse cardiomyocytes, endothelial cells, and renal tubule cells. They showed AT2 receptor in all these cells using immunogold staining. AT1 receptors were rare in young animals but increased in number with age. AT2 expression decreased with age and this decrease was blunted by chronic treatment with the ARB losartan. Also mitochondrial AT2 was shown to be coupled to mitochondrial nitric oxide production. This report demonstrated a canonical action of angiotensin II at mitochondria and suggests a pathological mechanism by which angiotensin II can produce mitochondrial and cellular damage. This report is also consistent with other studies showing an increase in AT1R/AT2R ratio in sheep proximal tubule cell nuclei with age and this changed was accompanied by enhanced ROS generation by these nuclei following angiotensin II treatment [64]. The observation that high glucose up-regulates intracellular angiotensin II in both cardiomyocytes and vascular smooth muscle cells, at least partially in an AT1R-dependent fashion, suggests the possibility that canonical angiotensin II intracellular action plays a role in the cardiovascular pathologies associated with diabetes [57].

At the same time, our group continued its studies of intracrine angiotensin action through the production of cell lines expressing a non-secreted angiotensinogen which served as the substrate for the production in a hepatoma cell line of intracellular angiotensin II by an endogenous intracellular renin; these cells proliferated in response to the up-regulation of angiotensinogen in the absence of secreted angiotensin. Knockdown of endogenous renin with renin antisense eliminated the proliferation [65]. Also, we showed that a fluorescent fusion protein consisting of Angiotensin II fused downstream and in-frame with cyan fluorescent protein ECFP, when transfected into a variety of cell lines, stimulated cell proliferation, CREB stimulation, and redistribution of the Angiotensin II receptor AT_1 [41, 66]. The angiotensin II encoded by this construct was not secreted and therefore the proliferation was the result of angiotensin II acting within the cell. Thus, these studies collectively defined some of the pathways by which intracellular angiotensin II can alter cellular physiology.

More recently we extended this work by developing a transgenic mouse line expressing an intracellular angiotensin II/cyan fluorescent fusion protein (that is not secreted) driven by a metallothionein promoter [67, 68]. Whereas, in most of the transfected cell lines we had studied the nucleus was the intracellular organelle most heavily labeled by the fusion protein, in these transgenic animals, labeling was most prominent over the mitochondria with lesser labeling of the nuclei. These animals developed hypertension and, in time, thrombotic microangiopathy. Remarkably, they also displayed clear mitochondrial pathology with loss of cristae. Moreover, direct binding of angiotensin II to electron transport chain proteins with effects on ATP synthesis and reactive oxygen species (ROS) generation were observed. Given the importance of oxidative stress in mediating the pathological actions of angiotensin II, these findings suggest that non-canonical angiotensin II action at the mitochondria could be an important determinant of pathology. It is important to note that if this is the case, angiotensin receptor blockers could not produce maximal protection against pathological angiotensin actions. Rather a new class of agents directed at non-canonical binding targets would be required [69].

Conclusion

The biology of the heart and vasculature is now seen to be extremely complex with a wide variety of factors regulating cardiovascular function and structure. As has been shown here, angiotensin II is one such factor---one that regulates cardiovascular function and structure in multiple ways. However, it also must be noted that other components of the RAS also influence the development of pathology. The beneficial effects of ARBs and ACEIs on cardiovascular structure suggest that a better understanding of angiotenin II and other RAS components function could lead to improved therapeutics. There is no shortage of experimental leads in that angiotensin (1–7), the (pro)renin receptor, receptor crosstalk, ACE2, *mas*, and other RAS components all offer therapeutic targets. Moreover, given the fact that renin, angiotensinogen, angiotensin, and ACE are intracrines, the intracellular actions of these RAS components must be considered. It may well be that therapies targeting only cell surface hormone/receptor interactions are inadequate to completely block the deleterious effects of angiotensin II and other intracrines, and only combined cell surface and intracellular blockade will provide complete protection from the deleterious actions of the peptides. But the complexity may go even further. There is compelling support for both canonical and non-canonical RAS action and so traditional RAS blockers such as ARBs may be incapable of blocking all pathologic intracellular mechanisms. This then implies that atypical binding partners for RAS components like angiotensin II will have to be identified before the workings of the RAS will be established sufficiently to optimally convert current knowledge to useful therapies for the prevention of vascular pathologies including arterial stiffening.

References

1. Re RN. New insights into target organ involvement in hypertension. Med Clin North Am. 2009;93:559–67.
2. Re RN. The renin-angiotensin systems. Med Clin North Am. 1987;71:877–95.
3. Re RN. Tissue renin angiotensin systems. Med Clin North Am. 2004;88:19–38.
4. Re RN. The clinical implication of tissue renin angiotensin systems. Curr Opin Cardiol. 2001;16:317–27.
5. Wolf G. Novel aspects of the renin-angiotensin-aldosterone-system. Front Biosci. 2008;13:4993–5005.
6. Burchfiel CM, Tracy RE, Chyou PH, et al. Cardiovascular risk factors and hyalinization of renal arterioles at autopsy. The Honolulu Heart Program. Arterioscler Thromb Vasc Biol. 1997;17:760–8.
7. Johnson RJ, Alpers CE, Yoshimura A, et al. Renal injury from angiotensin II-mediated hypertension. Hypertension. 1992;19:464–74.
8. Schiffrin EL. Vascular remodeling and endothelial function in hypertensive patients: effects of antihypertensive therapy. Scand Cardiovasc J Suppl. 1998;47:15–21.

9. Harrison DG, Marvar PJ, Titze JM. Vascular inflammatory cells in hypertension. Front Physiol. 2012;3:128. Epub 2012 May 7.
10. Harrison DG, Guzik TJ. Studies of the T-cell angiotensin receptor using cre-lox technology: an unan-T-cellpated result. Circ Res. 2012;110:1543–5.
11. Zhang JD, Patel MB, Song YS, Griffiths R, Burchette J, Ruiz P, Sparks MA, Yan M, Howell DN, Gomez JA, Spurney RF, Coffman TM, Crowley SD. A novel role for type 1 angiotensin receptors on T lymphocytes to limit target organ damage in hypertension. Circ Res. 2012;110:1604–17.
12. Strawn WB, Richmond RS, Ann Tallant E, et al. Renin-angiotensin system expression in rat bone marrow haematopoietic and stromal cells. Br J Haematol. 2004;126:120–6.
13. Strawn WB, Ferrario CM. Angiotensin II AT1 receptor blockade normalizes CD11b1 monocyte production in bone marrow of hypercholesterolemic monkeys. Atherosclerosis. 2008;196:624–32. Epub 2007 Aug 9.
14. Re RN. Cellular biology of the renin-angiotensin systems. Arch Intern Med. 1984;144:2037–41.
15. Ribichini F, Pugno F, Ferrero V, et al. Cellular immunostaining of angiotensinconverting enzyme in human coronary atherosclerotic plaques. J Am Coll Cardiol. 2006;47:1143–9. Epub 2006 Feb 23.
16. Diet F, Pratt RE, Berry GJ, et al. Increased accumulation of tissue ACE in human atherosclerotic coronary disease. Circulation. 1996;94:2756–67.
17. Geisterfer AA, Peach MJ, Owens GK. Angiotensin II induces hypertrophy, not hyperplasia, of cultured rat aortic smooth muscle cells. Circ Res. 1988;62:749–56.
18. Campbell-Boswell M, Robertson Jr AL. Effects of angiotensin II and vasopressin on human smooth muscle cells in vitro. Exp Mol Pathol. 1981;35: 265–76.
19. Levy BI. How to explain the differences between renin angiotensin system modulators. Am J Hypertens. 2005;18(9 Pt 2):134S–41.
20. Jones ES, Vinh A, McCarthy CA, et al. AT(2) receptors: functional relevance in cardiovascular disease. Pharmacol Ther. 2008;120:292–316.
21. Tang H, Nishishita T, Fitzgerald T, et al. Inhibition of AT1 receptor internalization by concanavalin A blocks angiotensin II-induced ERK activation in vascular smooth muscle cells. Involvement of epidermal growth factor receptor proteolysis but not AT1 receptor internalization. J Biol Chem. 2000;275:13420–6.
22. AdbAlla S, Abdel-tawab AM, Quitterer U. The angiotensin II AT2 receptor is an AT1 receptor antagonist. J Biol Chem. 2001;276:39721–6.
23. AbdAlla S, Lother H, el Massiery A, et al. Increased AT(1) receptor heterodimers in preeclampsia medicate enhanced angiotensin II responsiveness. Nat Med. 2001;7:1003–9.
24. Singh BM, Mehta JL. Interactions between the renin-angiotensin system and dyslipidemia: relevance in the therapy of hypertension and coronary heart disease. Arch Intern Med. 2003;163:1296–304.
25. Hu C, Dandapat A, Sun L, et al. Modulation of angiotensin II-mediated hypertension and cardiac remodeling by lectin-like oxidized low-density lipoprotein receptor-1 deletion. Hypertension. 2008;52:556–62. Epub 2008 Jul 21.
26. Chappel MC, Ferrario CM. ACE and ACE2: their role to balance the expression of angiotensin II and angiotensin-(1–7). Kidney Int. 2006;70:8–10.
27. Varagic J, Ahmad S, Brosnihan KB, Groban L, Chappell MC, Tallant EA, Gallagher PE, Ferrario CM. Decreased cardiac Ang-(1–7) is associated with salt-induced cardiac remodeling and dysfunction. Ther Adv Cardiovasc Dis. 2010;4:17–25.
28. Trask AJ, Ferrario CM. Angiotensin-(1–7): pharmacology and new perspectives in cardiovascular treatments. Cardiovasc Drug Rev. 2007;25:162–74.
29. Xue H, Zhou L, Yuan P, Wang Z, Ni J, Yao T, Wang J, Huang Y, Yu C, Lu L. Counteraction between angiotensin II and angiotensin-(1–7) via activating angiotensin type I and Mas receptor on rat renal mesangial cells. Regul Pept. 2012;177:12–20.
30. Patel VB, Bodiga S, Fan D, Das SK, Wang Z, Wang W, Basu R, Zhong J, Kassiri Z, Oudit GY. Cardioprotective effects mediated by angiotensin II type 1 receptor blockade and enhancing angiotensin 1–7 in experimental heart failure in angiotensin-converting enzyme 2-null mice. Hypertension. 2012;59:1195–203.
31. Fraga-Silva RA, Ferreira AJ, Dos Santos RA. (1–7)/ mas receptor pathway in hypertension. Curr Hypertens Rep. 2013;15:31–8.
32. Tamura K, Wakui H, Maeda A, Dejima T, Ohsawa M, Azushima K, Kanaoka T, Haku S, Uneda K, Masuda SI, Azuma K, Shigenaga AI, Koide Y, Tsurumi-Ikeya Y, Matsuda M, Toya Y, Tokita Y, Yamashita A, Umemura S. The physiology and pathophysiology of a novel angiotensin receptor-binding protein ATRAP/ Agtrap. Curr Pharm Des. 2013;19:3043–8.
33. Tsukuda K, Mogi M, Iwanami J, Min LJ, Jing F, Ohshima K, Horiuchi M. Influence of angiotensin II type 1 receptor-associated protein on prenatal development and adult hypertension after maternal dietary protein restriction during pregnancy. J Am Soc Hypertens. 2012;6:324–30.
34. Guo DF, Chenier I, Tardif V, Orlov SN, Inagami T. Type 1 angiotensin II receptor-associated protein ARAP1 binds and recycles the receptor to the plasma membrane. Biochem Biophys Res Commun. 2003;310:1254–65.
35. Daniele T, Di Tullio G, Santoro M, Turacchio G, De Matteis MA. ARAP1 regulates EGF receptor trafficking and signalling. Traffic. 2008;9:2221–35.
36. Cook JL, Re RN, de Haro DL, Abadie JM, Peters M, Alam J. The trafficking protein GABARAP binds to and enhances plasma membrane expression and function of the angiotensin II type 1 receptor. Circ Res. 2008;102:1539–47.
37. Alam J, Deharo D, Redding KM, Re RN, Cook JL. C-terminal processing of GABARAP is not required for trafficking of the angiotensin II type 1A receptor. Regul Pept. 2010;159:78–86.

38. Vitko JR, Re RN, Alam J, Cook JL. Cell-penetrating peptides corresponding to the angiotensin II Type 1 receptor reduce receptor accumulation and cell surface expression and signaling. Am J Hypertens. 2012;25:24–8.
39. Re RN, Chen B, Alam J, Cook JL. Reduction of blood pressure by AT1 receptor decoy peptides. Ochsner J. 2013;13:33–6.
40. Cook JL, Mills SJ, Naquin RT, Alam J, Re RN. Cleavage of the angiotensin II type 1 receptor and nuclear accumulation of the cytoplasmic carboxy-terminal fragment. Am J Physiol Cell Physiol. 2007;292:C1313–22. Epub 2006 Nov 22.
41. Cook JL, Mills SJ, Naquin R, Alam J, Re RN. Nuclear accumulation of the AT1 receptor in a rat vascular smooth muscle cell line: effects upon signal transduction and cellular proliferation. J Mol Cell Cardiol. 2006;40:696–707. Epub 2006 Mar 6.
42. Re RN. Lysosomal action of intracrine angiotensin II. Focus on "Intracellular angiotensin II activates rat myometrium". Am J Physiol Cell Physiol. 2011;301:C553–4.
43. Neri Serneri GG, Boddi M, Coppo M, Chechi T, Zarone N, Moira M, Poggesi L, Margheri M, Simonetti I. Evidence for the existence of a functional cardiac renin-angiotensin system in humans. Circulation. 1996;94:1886–93.
44. Frohlich ED, Susic D. Sodium and its multiorgan targets. Circulation. 2011;124:1882–5.
45. Re RN. Toward a theory of intracrine hormone action. Regul Pept. 2002;106:1–6.
46. Re RN. The intracrine hypothesis and intracellular peptide hormone action. Bioessays. 2003;25:401–9.
47. Re RN, Cook JL. The intracrine hypothesis: an update. Regul Pept. 2005;133:1–9.
48. Re RN. The implications of intracrine hormone action for physiology and medicine. Am J Physiol Heart Circ Physiol. 2003;284:H751–7.
49. Spatazza J, Di Lullo E, Joliot A, Dupont E, Moya KL, Prochiantz A. Homeoprotein signaling in development, health, and disease: a shaking of dogmas offers challenges and promises from bench to bed. Pharmacol Rev. 2013;65:90–104.
50. Dupont E, Prochiantz A, Joliot A. Penetratin story: an overview. Methods Mol Biol. 2011;683:21–9.
51. Singh VP, Le B, Bhat VB, et al. High-glucose-induced regulation of intracellular ANG II synthesis and nuclear redistribution in cardiac myocytes. Am J Physiol Heart Circ Physiol. 2007;293:H939–48.
52. Frustaci A, Kajstura J, Chimenti C, Jakoniuk I, Leri A, Maseri A, Nadal-Ginard B, Anversa P. Myocardial cell death in human diabetes. Circ Res. 2000;87:1123–32.
53. Re RN, Cook JL. Noncanonical intracrine action. J Am Soc Hypertens. 2011;5:435–48.
54. Gwathmey TM, Alzayadneh EM, Pendergrass KD, Chappell MC. Novel roles of nuclear angiotensin receptors and signaling mechanisms. Am J Physiol Regul Integr Comp Physiol. 2012;302:R518–30.
55. Re RN, Vizard DL, Brown J, Bryan SE. Angiotensin II receptors in chromatin fragments generated by micrococcal nuclease. Biochem Biophys Res Commun. 1984;119: 220–7.
56. Erdmann B, Fuxe K, Ganten D. Subcellular localization of angiotensin II immunoreactivity in the rat cerebellar cortex. Hypertension. 1996;28:818–24.
57. Singh VP, Le B, Khode R, Baker KM, Kumar R. Intracellular angiotensin II production in diabetic rats is correlated with cardiomyocyte apoptosis, oxidative stress, and cardiac fibrosis. Diabetes. 2008;57:3297–306.
58. Dikalov SI, Dikalova AE, Bikineyeva AT, Schmidt HH, Harrison DG, Griendling KK. Distinct roles of Nox1 and Nox4 in basal and angiotensin II-stimulated superoxide and hydrogen peroxide production. Free Radic Biol Med. 2008;45:1340–51.
59. Takeuchi K, Yamamoto K, Ohishi M, Takeshita H, Hongyo K, Kawai T, Takeda M, Kamide K, Kurtz TW, Rakugi H. Telmisartan modulates mitochondrial function in vascular smooth muscle cells. Hypertens Res. 2013;36:433–9. doi:10.1038/hr.2012.199.
60. Robertson Jr AL, Khairallah PA. Angiotensin II: rapid localization in nuclei of smooth and cardiac muscle. Science. 1971;172:1138–9.
61. Goodfriend TL, Fyhrquist F, Gutmann F, Knych E, Hollemans H, Allmann D, Kent K, Cooper T. Clinical and conceptual uses of angiotensin receptors. In: Genest J, Koiw E, editors. Hypertension '72. Berlin: Springer; 1972. p. 549–63.
62. Husain K, Suarez E, Isidro A, Ferder L. Effects of paricalcitol and enalapril on atherosclerotic injury in mouse aortas. Am J Nephrol. 2010;32:296–304.
63. Abadir PM, Foster DB, Crow M, Cooke CA, Rucker JJ, Jain A, Smith BJ, Burks TN, Cohn RD, Fedarko NS, Carey RM, O'Rourke B, Walston JD. Identification and characterization of a functional mitochondrial angiotensin system. Proc Natl Acad Sci U S A. 2011;108:14849–54.
64. Gwathmey TM, Pendergrass KD, Reid SD, Rose JC, Diz DI, Chappell MC. Angiotensin-(1–7)-angiotensin-converting enzyme 2 attenuates reactive oxygen species formation to angiotensin II within the cell nucleus. Hypertension. 2010;55:166–71.
65. Cook JL, Zhang Z, Re RN. In vitro evidence for an intracellular site of angiotensin action. Circ Res. 2001;89:1138–46.
66. Cook JL, Giardina JF, Zhang Z, Re RN. Intracellular angiotensin II increases the long isoform of PDGF mRNA in rat hepatoma cells. J Mol Cell Cardiol. 2002;34:1525–37.
67. Redding KM, Chen BL, Singh A, Re RN, Navar LG, Seth DM, Sigmund CD, Tang WW, Cook JL. Transgenic mice expressing an intracellular fluorescent fusion of angiotensin II demonstrate renal thrombotic microangiopathy and elevated blood pressure. Am J Physiol Heart Circ Physiol. 2010;298:H1807–18.
68. Cook JL, Re RN. Lessons from in vitro studies and a related intracellular angiotensin II transgenic mouse model. Am J Physiol Regul Integr Comp Physiol. 2012;302:R482–93.
69. Re RN, Cook JL. The mitochondrial component of intracrine action. Am J Physiol Heart Circ Physiol. 2010;299:H577–83.

14 Arterial Stiffness and the Sympathetic Nervous System

Gianfranco Parati and Paolo Salvi

Abstract

This chapter addresses the complex relationship between sympathetic activity and the main factors affecting arterial distensibility. Sympathetic nervous system is considered one of the major elements involved in the regulation of mean arterial pressure, affecting heart rate, left ventricular contractility, and systemic vascular resistance. Actually, in hypertensive patients a permanent increase in mean arterial pressure may cause structural changes in viscoelastic properties of arterial wall, causing a permanent reduction in arterial distensibility. Moreover, heart rate, left ventricular function, and mean arterial pressure can also be considered major functional factors which can cause transient changes in arterial viscoelastic properties. Evidence is available that sympathetic activity plays a major role in modulating the mechanical properties of muscular arteries. This explains the reduction in distensibility of muscular arteries shown under particular conditions of stress, such as exposure to high altitude and, in general, to hypoxia. Changes in sympathetic activity may be influenced by baroreflex regulation of cardiovascular homeostasis. Reflex changes of arterial tone and modifications of cardiac output are the result of this regulation. A carotid and aortic stiffness may be associated with reduced cardiovagal baroreflex sensitivity, with a consequent increase in blood pressure variability, and also with a higher speed of changes in beat-to-beat systolic blood pressure fluctuations typical of hypertension.

Keywords

Arterial stiffness • Blood pressure • Pulse wave velocity • Pulse wave analysis • Sympathetic nervous system • Vascular hemodynamics • Blood pressure variability

G. Parati, MD (✉)
Department of Health Sciences,
University of Milano-Bicocca, Milan, Italy

Department of Cardiology, S. Luca Hospital,
Istituto Auxologico Italiano, Milan, Italy
e-mail: gianfranco.parati@unimib.it

P. Salvi, MD, PhD
Department of Cardiology,
S. Luca Hospital, Istituto
Auxologico Italiano, Milan, Italy
e-mail: psalvi.md@gmail.com

M.E. Safar et al. (eds.), *Blood Pressure and Arterial Wall Mechanics in Cardiovascular Diseases*,
DOI 10.1007/978-1-4471-5198-2_14, © Springer-Verlag London 2014

Sympathetic Nervous System, Pulsatile Blood Pressure, and Arterial Distensibility

Sympathetic nervous system (SNS) is known to be one of the major factors involved in the regulation of blood pressure and cardiovascular hemodynamics, extensively affecting mean arterial pressure. Indeed, SNS activation is responsible for an increase in heart rate, an increase in ventricular contractility, and peripheral vasoconstriction, that can selectively or diffusely increase peripheral vascular resistances, leading to a mean arterial pressure increase.

However, blood pressure cannot be characterized only in terms of mean arterial pressure. Actually two distinct but interdependent components define arterial blood pressure: a steady state component, namely, mean arterial pressure, and a pulsatile component, defined as pulse pressure, which represents the fluctuation in blood pressure around its mean value throughout the cardiac cycle [1] (Fig. 14.1).

While the modulation exerted by SNS on mean arterial pressure is well known, the role of SNS activation in modulating changes in the variables determining pulse pressure, such as arterial distensibility, left ventricle-aorta interaction, and reflection of pulse waves in the aorta, is still less clearly defined. The action of SNS on pulse pressure is complex, and there are numerous and complex interactions between the factors affecting mean arterial pressure and those affecting pulse pressure.

The main parameter determining pulse pressure values is the distensibility of the aorta and large arteries, due to the viscoelastic properties of the arterial wall. Aortic distensibility can be easily evaluated by measuring the carotid-femoral pulse wave transit time. Indeed, carotid to femoral pulse wave velocity (PWV) is the acknowledged gold standard method to assess arterial distensibility.

Large artery distensibility depends on structural characteristics and on transient functional changes in the arterial wall.

Structural characteristics are relatively stable and depend on the elastin/collagen fiber ratio in the arterial wall. The increase of arterial stiffness with age is a well-established phenomenon which

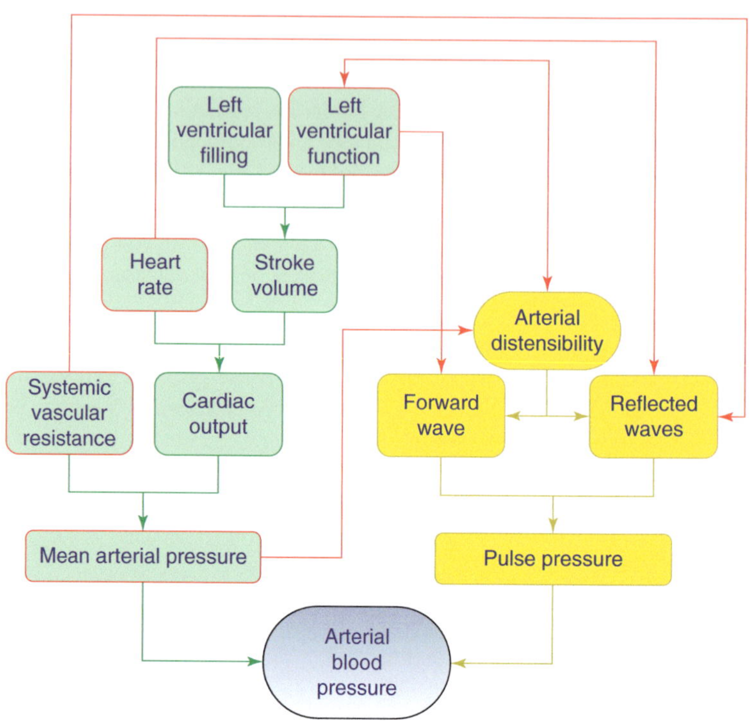

Fig. 14.1 Schematic description of the main factors involved in blood pressure regulation

depends on alterations in such a ratio. The aging process causes histological alterations in the arterial wall, and the degeneration of elastin fibers is accompanied by a boost in collagen fibers. Also a condition characterized by steady increase in blood pressure values causes structural alterations in the arterial wall. The arterial wall tends to increase biosynthesis of collagen fibers in order to face increasing pressures in the vascular lumen, and further changes of the elastin/collagen ratio occur. Structural alterations in the wall of large elastic arteries have been described even in metabolic diseases such as diabetes, kidney failure, liver failure, and alterations in calcium metabolism. Some metabolic disorders can indeed be accompanied by an increase in oxidative stress, by appearance of areas of arterial wall calcifications and by inflammation of the arterial wall. Inflammation may cause both arterial stiffening and endothelial dysfunction.

The role of factors affecting functional and transient changes in arterial distensibility is less clearly defined. We can identify three major functional factors which can cause transient changes in arterial viscoelastic properties: (1) heart rate and left ventricular function, (2) mean arterial pressure level, and (3) tonic activity of smooth muscle cell within the arterial wall. All these parameters can be affected by SNS. Even if the role of functional factors in determining distensibility of large arteries may be weaker as compared to organic, structural alterations, however the relationship between PWV (i.e., arterial distensibility) and functional changes in arterial wall properties could affect the reproducibility and, in the end, the reliability of the PWV values.

Heart Rate and Left Ventricular Function

Left ventricular function affects the forward pulse waveform, originating from the interaction between the left ventricular ejection activity and the mechanical properties of large arteries. Thus SNS activation, increasing ventricular contractility, makes changes in forward waveforms, determining a steeper slope in the protosystolic phase of aortic pulse waveform. In order to better understand the role of ventricular function in affecting blood pressure waveform, it is sufficient to consider the well-known typical changes in arterial pulse waveform occurring in subjects affected by aortic stenosis or insufficiency.

A number of cross-sectional studies showed a significant association between heart rate and PWV (commonly assumed as an index of aortic distensibility), independent of blood pressure levels [2–6]. On the background of the evidence that heart rate is, at least in part, an index of sympathetic activity and, to some extent, also of renin-angiotensin-aldosterone system activity [7], it has been suggested that both sympathetic activation and activation of the renin-angiotensin-aldosterone system could contribute to increase both heart rate and arterial stiffness in parallel. This hypothesis, however, has been challenged by Mircoli et al. [8] and Mangoni et al. [9], who showed that the reduction in arterial distensibility associated with tachycardia occurred even in the absence of a sympathetic activation. Moreover, the results obtained in subjects with permanent cardiac pacing suggest that the association between PWV and heart rate is at least partially related to a direct mechanical effect of heart rate on PWV. Another possible explanation for the relationship between PWV and heart rate comes from the viscous and inertial properties of arterial wall: an increase in heart rate shortens the time available for recoil, which results in arterial stiffening [10, 11]. In spite of these observations, however, the actual mechanisms responsible for the relationship between heart rate and arterial stiffness are still largely unknown [12].

Recently a significant and inverse association between carotid-femoral PWV and left ventricular ejection time was found [13]. The shorter the left ventricular ejection time, the higher the aortic PWV. Left ventricular ejection time is a composite index of left ventricular performance affected by cardiac inotropic function and influenced by preload and afterload [14, 15] and it seems to be more closely and inversely associated with PWV than R-R interval (the inverse of heart rate). This strong inverse link between PWV and left ventricular ejection time can be in part explained by a simple energetic model. At a given heart rate, in case of reduction in systolic ejection time, mechanical work of left ventricle is carried out in a shorter time, thus with a greater power. Power (*P*) represents the work (*W*) of blood pressure on the arterial wall during a given time (*t*) interval ($P = \Delta W / \Delta t$). Given that power is proportional to mean arterial pressure and to velocity of traveling waves, an increase in power corresponds to an increase in PWV. Thus, for a given value of heart rate, a reduction in left ventricular ejection time determines an increase in PWV. Conversely, since left ventricular ejection time depends on the capability of the left ventricle to eject blood, and thus on left ventricular inotropic function and loading conditions [16], an alteration in any of these variables may influence the left ventricular ejection time. Taking into account both these two plausible mechanisms, the relationship between left ventricular ejection time and PWV should not be considered only as a result of a direct modulation of arterial distensibility induced by changes in heart rate, but could rather be the result of a mutual interaction between left ventricular ejection function and aortic and large arteries distensibility [13]. Thus it can be hypothesized that in young people with distensible arteries, PWV shows a prevalent association with mean arterial pressure and left ventricular ejection time, suggesting a stronger dependence of aortic PWV on left ventricular performance than on vascular distensibility. On the contrary, with advancing age, when age progressively becomes the most powerful predictor of PWV, the inverse relation between left ventricular ejection time and PWV may be an epiphenomenon of an age-related increase in large artery stiffness contributing to an increased aortic impedance which ultimately tends to limit ejection duration [13].

The SNS activation, raising heart rate and increasing left ventricular contractility, may therefore cause a decrease in arterial distensibility also through these mechanisms, thus resulting in an increase in pulse pressure. This implies that, under specific conditions characterized by significant changes in heart rate, the changes in heart rate should be taken into serious consideration when analyzing aortic PWV values. For example, exposure to high altitude or sport activity may cause considerable increase in heart rate and may significantly affect PWV values.

Nevertheless, the effects of increasing heart rate on reflected waves cause an opposite result on pulse pressure. Even if heart rate is directly related to PWV, and an increased PWV causes an accelerate return of reflected waves in the ascending aorta, however, there is a predominant action of heart rate which is not due to the early arrival of reflected wave but rather due to the complex relationship between the forward waveform and the timing of the backward wave. An increase in heart rate is accompanied by a relative decrease in diastolic time of the cardiac cycle and a small change in systolic time. The main consequence of the decrease in diastolic time, therefore, will be a decrease in left ventricular diastolic filling time. The result is a change in pulse waveform, characterized by a quick systolic peak followed by a sharp and shorter lasting fall in blood pressure values. When the backward wave travels to the center, it will tend to superimpose onto the forward wave in its "descending phase." Thanks to this process and to the high heart rate, the reflected wave does not participate much in defining aortic systolic blood pressure values. As a consequence, we do not have an increase in pulse pressure, as expected. On the contrary, for low heart rate, the decrease in pulse wave velocity, and therefore the delay in reflected wave, is counterbalanced by the complete superimposition of the backward wave on the systolic peak of the forward wave. As a result, there is an increase in pulse pressure at low heart rates in ascending aorta. This phenomenon which occurs with low heart rate is considered to be the main (but not the only) cause of the lower decrease in central arterial pressure with β-blocker treatment.

Mean Arterial Pressure

As we have highlighted above, SNS is considered one of the major elements in the regulation of mean arterial pressure, affecting heart rate, left ventricular contractility, and systemic vascular resistance.

In hypertensive patients a permanent increase in mean arterial pressure may cause structural changes in viscoelastic properties of arterial wall. An increased biosynthesis of collagen occurs in order to counterbalance the increase in transmural pressure. This process can be associated with

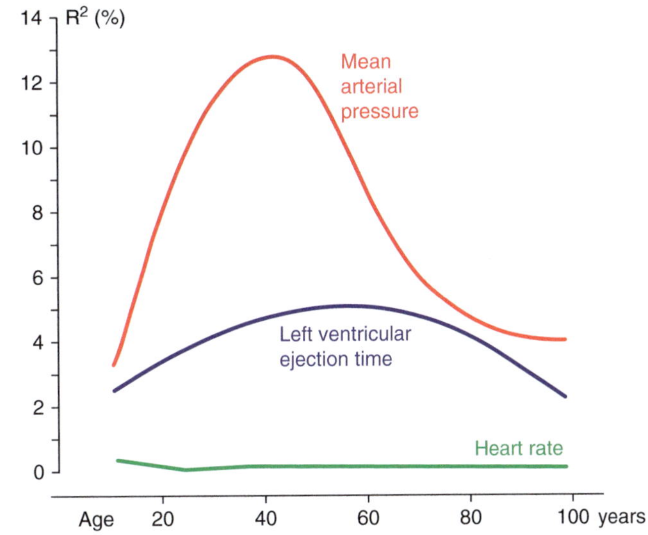

Fig. 14.2 Contribution of mean arterial pressure and other functional parameters in determining pulse wave velocity values at different ages (From Salvi [1], modified by permission)

alterations in the endothelial function and with a remodeling process of the arterial wall, characterized by hypertrophy and hyperplasia of smooth muscle cells. These alterations in mechanical properties of arterial wall cause a permanent reduction in arterial distensibility, and the PWV values are increased independently of the blood pressure values recorded at the moment of the test.

However also blood pressure values during the test may contribute to change arterial distensibility, by means of a functional modulation in vascular properties. The relative weight of mean arterial pressure and other functional parameters in determining pulse wave velocity values at different ages is shown in Fig. 14.2 [1, 13]. Mean arterial pressure explains up to 13 % of the variance in aortic PWV in young adults, and its contribution decreases with age to nearly 4 % in the elderly. Left ventricular ejection time explains between 2 and 5 % of the variance in PWV values. Actually, with the exception of age and hypertension, it is very unusual to detect functional variables that have a stronger effect on variations of aortic PWV.

Sympathetic Nervous System and Arterial Function

We may identify two types of arteries, in relation to the prevalence of elastic fibers or smooth muscle cells, respectively, in their walls: (1) the elastic arteries, including the large vessels emerging from the heart ventricles, such as aorta, pulmonary artery, brachiocephalic trunk, common carotid, and subclavian arteries, and (2) the muscular arteries, including the main branches of the arterial tree, like radial, femoral, and cerebral arteries.

The shift between these types of arterial vessels is gradual, rather than abrupt. The amount of elastic tissue decreases from the center to the periphery of the arterial tree, whether the smooth muscle component assumes gradually more and more prominence in the peripheral arteries. Through the controlled variation in the diameter of the peripheral arteries, these arteries distribute blood flow to different parts of the body according to regional needs. This function is performed by modulation of the smooth muscle cells circumferentially arranged within the vessel walls and is principally under the control of the SNS.

Action on Muscular Arteries

Several studies showed that in humans the SNS exerts a pronounced restraint on distensibility of medium-size and large muscular arteries not only when its activity is phasically increased in a short term by behavioral influences or emotional stimuli [17–19], but also when the vessel is exposed to long-term modulation of the smaller degree of existing sympathetic tone [20, 21].

Procedures or situations that acutely increase sympathetic activity are associated with reduction in distensibility of muscular arteries, such as brachial, radial, or femoral arteries [20, 17]. This explains the presence of high carotid-radial PWV values under particular conditions of stress, such as altitude or hypoxia.

Action on Elastic Arteries

Whether the sympathetic activity plays a major role in modulating the mechanical properties of muscular arteries, the activity of SNS on visco-elastic properties of central arteries remains still widely unknown.

Actually, some studies showed that mechanical properties of the human abdominal aorta remain unaltered during sympathetic stimulation [22, 23]. The pressure-diameter relationship and the distensibility indices, stiffness (beta), and pressure strain elastic modulus of the abdominal aorta were widely studied by Sonesson et al. [22]. Sympathetic stimulation induced by lower body negative pressure did not change aortic wall mechanics. The authors concluded that sympathetic modulation of the aortic smooth muscle contractile activity seems to be unimportant in the blood pressure regulation [22]. Similarly Lydakis et al. did not demonstrate any change in measures of central large artery stiffness and wave reflection caused by SNS activation during lower body negative pressure [23].

However even if the role of SNS on aortic stiffness is weak, we should not conclude that SNS has not any effect on pulse pressure. Actually it is necessary to highlight how high sympathetic activity may also affect pulse pressure by increasing systemic vascular resistance, thus modifying amplitude and distribution of reflected pressure waves [24, 25]. An increase in backward pressure waves can increase central systolic blood pressure and reduce blood pressure amplification in the periphery even without change in aortic distensibility.

Different Meaning of Upper Limb and Aortic Pulse Wave Velocity

Probably functional factors, including SNS activity, play a significant role in affecting arterial stiffness in muscular arteries, whereas structural factors play the major role in modulating the elastic properties of large arteries [1]. This different contribution by functional and structural factors in affecting arterial distensibility in muscular and elastic arteries may help explain the different behavior of arterial distensibility and PWV during life.

Carotid-femoral PWV, marker of the distensibility of the aorta (an elastic artery), increases with age. Actually the aging process causes well-known histological alterations in the elastic large arteries. An increased elastase activity and a reduced elastin synthesis cause thinning and breakage of elastin fibers, and the result is a decrease in the elastin/collagen ratio. However, the relationship between age and PWV is not linear. PWV values change insignificantly in the first decades of life, and then they tend to increase as age advances, by an average of 70 mm/s per year from 45 to 65 years and of 200 mm/s per year after 65 years. On the contrary, the PWV in upper limb muscular arteries (axillo-brachial-radial axis) does not significantly change with age [1] (Fig. 14.3). Young adults have the same mean values of carotid-radial PWV than subjects over 80 years old. Most likely, upper limb PWV reflects the functional condition of the arterial tree, which is closely related to the modulation by the SNS. Thus it is not surprising that carotid-radial PWV values generally increase together with diastolic blood pressure, mean arterial pressure, and heart rate, whereas carotid-femoral PWV values are more closely associated with systolic blood pressure.

As an example of these different modulations, we mention below two situations in which the dissociation in PWV changes between elastic and muscular arteries is particularly evident: namely, the influence of birth weight and postnatal growth on hemodynamic parameters assessed in adult age and the changes in mechanical properties of arteries after acute exposition at high altitude.

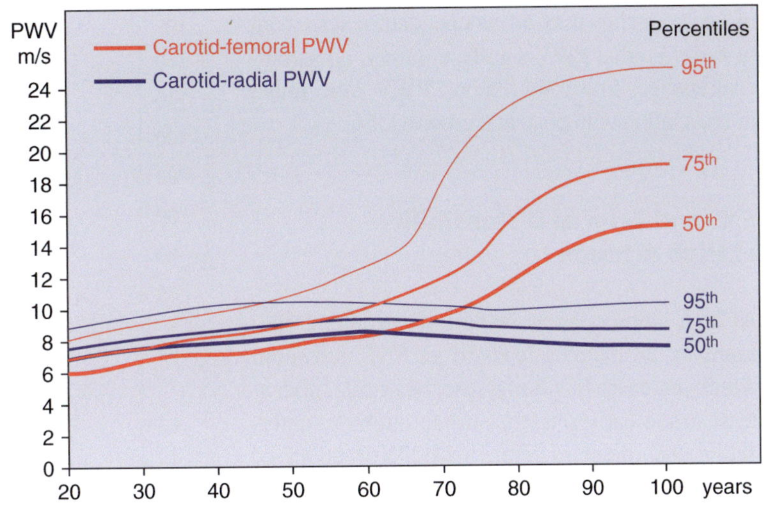

Fig. 14.3 Carotid-femoral and carotid-radial pulse wave velocity at different ages (From Salvi [1], modified by permission)

SNS Activity: Relationship with Birth Weight and Postnatal Growth

Low birth weight and accelerated postnatal growth are known to be associated with impairment of endothelial function [26, 27] and insulin resistance [28]. Moreover, the association between low birth weight related to gestational age and increased sympathetic activity is consistent with several clinical [29] and experimental studies [30, 31]. All these factors can influence arterial tone and distensibility of large muscular arteries [32, 33]. Low birth weight is also associated with high resting heart rate in adult life, in middle-aged individuals [34].

Recently our research group evaluated if birth weight and postnatal growth may affect hemodynamic parameters in adolescents and young adults [35]. Several factors were evaluated, including birth weight, postnatal growth, timing of adiposity rebound, lifestyle, anthropometric characteristics, and hemodynamic parameters. No association between low birth weight or accelerated postnatal growth and carotid-femoral PWV was found. Conversely, carotid-radial PWV, mean arterial pressure, diastolic blood pressure, and heart rate were significantly higher in adolescents characterized by a birth weight ≤2 kg (Fig. 14.4). Moreover, a strong association between accelerated growth from 0 to 12 months and carotid-radial PWV in adolescent age was also found, and the weight gain in the first year

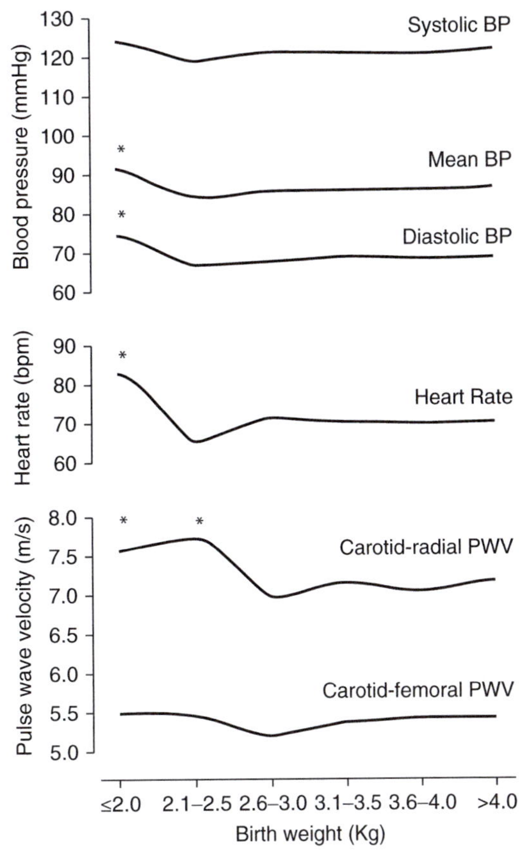

Fig. 14.4 Blood pressure, heart rate, and pulse wave velocity in relation to birth weight in healthy teenagers. $*p<0.05$, probabily level versus birth weight groups characterized by a birth weight between 2.5 and 4.0 Kg

of age was shown as an independent determinant of carotid-radial PWV. On the contrary, no significant changes in carotid-femoral PWV were found in association with postnatal growth [35].

SNS and Arterial Distensibility at High Altitude

At high altitude, an activation of peripheral chemoreflex by hypoxia leads to an SNS activation which increases blood pressure, heart rate, and, at least in the early phases, cardiac output counteracting the direct systemic vasodilator effect of hypoxia [36–40]. An increased sympathetic activity, reflected by changes in blood pressure variability spectral indices, has been shown to characterize also subjects with acute mountain sickness, suggesting a potential role of an exaggerated individual chemoreflex vasoconstrictive response to hypoxia also in the genesis of this condition [41].

The HIGHCARE (HIGH altitude CArdiovascular REsearch) Alps Project studied the effects of acute exposure to hypobaric hypoxia at altitude on the main hemodynamic parameters in a group of normotensive volunteers. The results of this study showed a significant increase in SNS activity during exposure to high- and very-high-altitude hypobaric hypoxia [42]. The SNS activation induced by acute high-altitude exposure was associated not only with a significant increase in mean arterial pressure, diastolic blood pressure, and heart rate, as expected, but also with an increase in carotid-radial PWV. On the contrary, no significant changes in carotid-femoral PWV were found (Fig. 14.5) [42].

Actually, hypoxia might also have a direct effect on renin-angiotensin-aldosterone system (RAAS), and retention of fluid and sodium has been proposed as one of the mechanisms involved in the pathogenesis of high-altitude pulmonary edema [43]. One of the aims of the HIGHCARE Himalaya Project was to evaluate the hemodynamic effects of RAAS at high altitude. This was a randomized, double-blind, parallel group, placebo-controlled study which had among its aims the investigation of the hemodynamic effects at high altitude of RAAS and of its blockade by telmisartan, an angiotensin II receptor AT1 blocker. This study, however, did not show

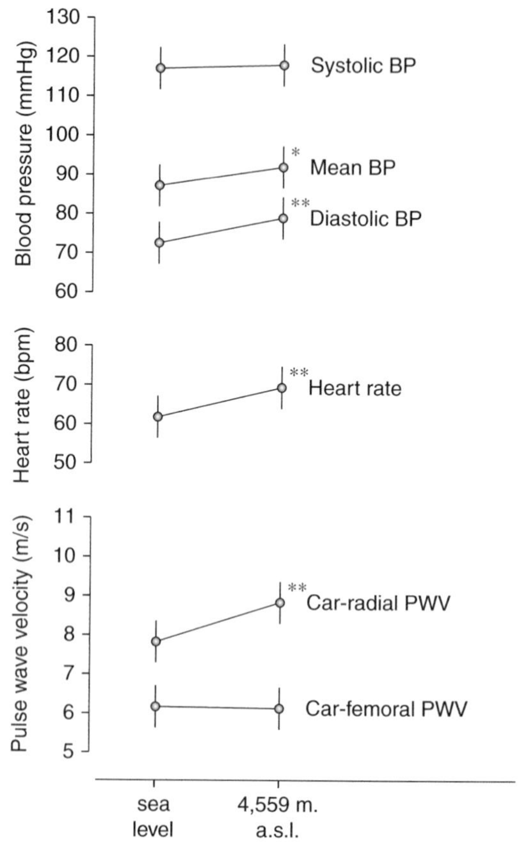

Fig. 14.5 Effects of acute high-altitude exposure on systolic, diastolic, and mean blood pressure (*BP*), heart rate, and carotid-femoral and carotid-radial pulse wave velocity (*PWV*) * $p<0.05$; ** $p<0.001$ (From Parati et al. [42], modified by permission)

any role of RAAS on hemodynamic changes during acute and prolonged exposition at very high altitude, where renin and angiotensin II levels were significantly reduced. In spite of this, after 2 weeks of very-high-altitude exposure, not only carotid-radial but also carotid-femoral PWV and augmentation index were significantly increased.

Taking into account the results of these two studies (HIGHCARE Himalaya and HIGHCARE Alps), we may hypothesize that the changes in distensibility of muscular arteries observed after acute exposure to very high altitude were secondary to a direct SNS activation. Also in this case SNS affects blood pressure and vascular hemodynamics modulating diastolic blood pressure, mean arterial pressure, and heart rate together with muscular arteries distensibility, without any direct action on mechanical properties of elastic arteries, if not under more prolonged exposure to hypobaric hypoxia.

Arterial Stiffness, Baroreflex Sensitivity, and Blood Pressure Variability

Changes in sympathetic activity [44] may be also influenced by baroreflex regulation of cardiovascular homeostasis. Reflex changes of arterial tone and modifications of cardiac output (including vagally mediated changes in heart rate) are the result of this regulation. Baroreflex influences stemming from stretch receptors located mainly in the carotid arteries and in the aortic arch are triggered by changes in transmural pressure of these vessels.

The overall baroreflex modulation of cardiovascular parameters has two distinct components. The first one is the relationship between changes in carotid/aortic transmural pressure and the corresponding changes in carotid/aortic diameter. This component depends on arterial wall stiffness, which represents one of the principal determinants of the degree of baroreceptor stretching/relaxation in response to a given pressure change (mechanical component). The second one is the link between changes in carotid/aortic diameter and the subsequent reflex changes in cardiac and vascular responses, which depend on the features of afferent neural inputs to brain stem centers, on the central integration of these inputs, and on the efferent neural firing to cardiac and vascular targets (neural component).

Recently the development of noninvasive techniques for the study of arterial properties has made it possible to investigate more in depth the relationship between the arterial wall stiffness and baroreflex function [45]. In fact, given that baroreceptors respond to the extent of stretching/relaxation of carotid/aortic arterial walls rather than to blood pressure, per se, one may expect that, in subjects with stiff arteries, which distend less than more elastic vessels in response to blood pressure changes, baroreflex responsiveness will be reduced. This reasonable pathophysiological hypothesis was supported by studies showing that, in humans, increased local carotid stiffness may be associated with reduced cardiovagal baroreflex sensitivity [46, 47].

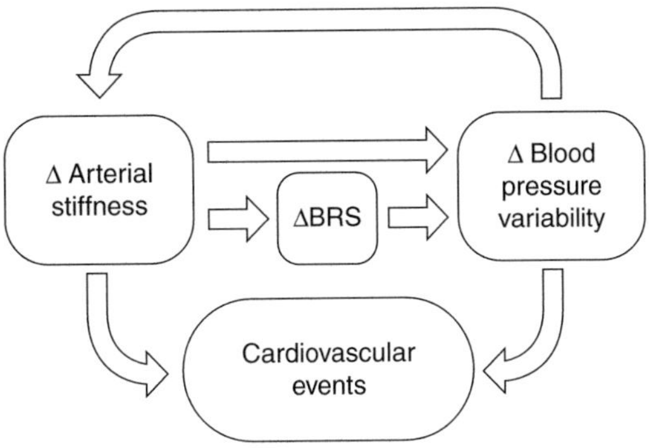

Fig. 14.6 Schematic drawing illustrating the complex links between arterial stiffness, baroreflex sensitivity (BRS), blood pressure variability, and the associated risk of cardiovascular events

Okada et al. [48] clearly demonstrated a significant inverse correlation between the sympathetic baroreflex sensitivity and degree of carotid stiffness and between sympathetic baroreflex sensitivity and carotid-femoral PWV.

A significant relation between large artery stiffness, as assessed by carotid-femoral PWV, and short-term SBP variability over the 24 h was clearly shown, independent of the influence of age, average BP, and other variables [49]. Short-term blood pressure variability reflects sympathetic nerve activation [50], impaired baroreflex sensitivity [44, 51], and other intrinsic and environmental factors [52, 53]. The favoring effect of aortic stiffness in determining an increased short-term blood pressure variability might be mediated by a reduced arterial baroreflex sensitivity, a rigid carotid and aortic wall being responsible for a reduced stimulation of arterial baroreceptors located in these vascular areas by pulsatile blood pressure, with a consequent reduced sensitivity of the baroreflex and its resulting reduced efficacy in buffering blood pressure fluctuations [46, 54] (Fig. 14.6). Such a reduced baroreflex sensitivity, which is a characteristic feature of autonomic cardiac modulation in hypertension, might be one of the factors, together with the accompanying increase in arterial stiffness, responsible not only for the increased blood pressure variability typical of hypertension [55], but also for the higher speed of changes in beat-to-beat systolic blood pressure fluctuations reported to occur in hypertensive patients as compared with normotensive individuals [56].

References

1. Salvi P. Pulse waves. How vascular hemodynamics affects blood pressure. Milan: Springer; 2012.
2. Lantelme P, Khettab F, Custaud MA, Rial MO, Joanny C, Gharib C, et al. Spontaneous baroreflex sensitivity: toward an ideal index of cardiovascular risk in hypertension? J Hypertens. 2002;20(5):935–44.
3. Lantelme P, Mestre C, Lievre M, Gressard A, Milon H. Heart rate: an important confounder of pulse wave velocity assessment. Hypertension. 2002;39(6):1083–7.
4. Albaladejo P, Copie X, Boutouyrie P, Laloux B, Declere AD, Smulyan H, et al. Heart rate, arterial stiffness, and wave reflections in paced patients. Hypertension. 2001;38(4):949–52.
5. Sa Cunha R, Pannier B, Benetos A, Siche JP, London GM, Mallion JM, et al. Association between high heart rate and high arterial rigidity in normotensive and hypertensive subjects. J Hypertens. 1997;15(12 Pt 1): 1423–30.
6. Weissler AM, Harris WS, Schoenfeld CD. Systolic time intervals in heart failure in man. Circulation. 1968;37(2):149–59.
7. Campese VM, Shaohua Y, Huiquin Z. Oxidative stress mediates angiotensin II-dependent stimulation of sympathetic nerve activity. Hypertension. 2005; 46(3):533–9.
8. Mircoli L, Mangoni AA, Giannattasio C, Mancia G, Ferrari AU. Heart rate-dependent stiffening of large arteries in intact and sympathectomized rats. Hypertension. 1999;34(4 Pt 1):598–602.
9. Mangoni AA, Mircoli L, Giannattasio C, Mancia G, Ferrari AU. Effect of sympathectomy on mechanical properties of common carotid and femoral arteries. Hypertension. 1997;30(5):1085–8.
10. Mangoni AA, Mircoli L, Giannattasio C, Ferrari AU, Mancia G. Heart rate-dependence of arterial distensibility in vivo. J Hypertens. 1996;14(7):897–901.
11. Armentano RL, Barra JG, Levenson J, Simon A, Pichel RH. Arterial wall mechanics in conscious dogs. Assessment of viscous, inertial, and elastic moduli to characterize aortic wall behavior. Circ Res. 1995;76(3):468–78.
12. Tan I, Butlin M, Liu YY, Ng K, Avolio AP. Heart rate dependence of aortic pulse wave velocity at different arterial pressures in rats. Hypertension. 2012;60(2): 528–33.
13. Salvi P, Palombo C, Salvi GM, Labat C, Parati G, Benetos A. Left ventricular ejection time, not heart rate, is an independent correlate of aortic pulse wave velocity. J Appl Physiol. 2013;115(11):1610–7.
14. Boudoulas H. Systolic time intervals. Eur Heart J. 1990;11(Suppl I):93–104.
15. Reant P, Dijos M, Donal E, Mignot A, Ritter P, Bordachar P, et al. Systolic time intervals as simple echocardiographic parameters of left ventricular systolic performance: correlation with ejection fraction and longitudinal two-dimensional strain. Eur J Echocardiogr. 2010;11(10):834–44.
16. Boudoulas H, Karayannacos PE, Lewis RP, Leier CV, Vasko JS. Effect of afterload on left ventricular performance in experimental animals. Comparison of the pre-ejection period and other indices of left ventricular contractility. J Med. 1982;13(5–6):373–85.
17. Boutouyrie P, Lacolley P, Girerd X, Beck L, Safar M, Laurent S. Sympathetic activation decreases medium-sized arterial compliance in humans. Am J Physiol. 1994;267(4 Pt 2):H1368–76.
18. Giannattasio C, Mangoni AA, Stella ML, Carugo S, Grassi G, Mancia G. Acute effects of smoking on radial artery compliance in humans. J Hypertens. 1994;12(6):691–6.
19. Perret F, Mooser V, Waeber B, Yanik T, Jean-Jacques M, Mooser E, et al. Effect of cold pressor test on the internal diameter of the radial artery. Am J Hypertens. 1989;2(9):727–8.
20. Failla M, Grappiolo A, Emanuelli G, Vitale G, Fraschini N, Bigoni M, et al. Sympathetic tone restrains arterial distensibility of healthy and atherosclerotic subjects. J Hypertens. 1999;17(8):1117–23.
21. Grassi G, Giannattasio C, Failla M, Pesenti A, Peretti G, Marinoni E, et al. Sympathetic modulation of radial artery compliance in congestive heart failure. Hypertension. 1995;26(2):348–54.
22. Sonesson B, Vernersson E, Hansen F, Lanne T. Influence of sympathetic stimulation on the mechanical properties of the aorta in humans. Acta Physiol Scand. 1997;159(2):139–45.
23. Lydakis C, Momen A, Blaha C, Herr M, Leuenberger UA, Sinoway LI. Changes of elastic properties of central arteries during acute static exercise and lower body negative pressure. Eur J Appl Physiol. 2008;102(6):633–41.
24. Palatini P, Julius S. The role of cardiac autonomic function in hypertension and cardiovascular disease. Curr Hypertens Rep. 2009;11(3):199–205.
25. Tentolouris N, Argyrakopoulou G, Katsilambros N. Perturbed autonomic nervous system function in metabolic syndrome. Neuromolecular Med. 2008;10(3):169–78.
26. Goodfellow J, Bellamy MF, Gorman ST, Brownlee M, Ramsey MW, Lewis MJ, et al. Endothelial function is impaired in fit young adults of low birth weight. Cardiovasc Res. 1998;40(3):600–6.
27. Leeson CP, Kattenhorn M, Morley R, Lucas A, Deanfield JE. Impact of low birth weight and cardiovascular risk factors on endothelial function in early adult life. Circulation. 2001;103(9):1264–8.
28. Phipps K, Barker DJ, Hales CN, Fall CH, Osmond C, Clark PM. Fetal growth and impaired glucose tolerance in men and women. Diabetologia. 1993;36(3):225–8.
29. IJzerman R, Stehouwer CD, de Geus EJ, van Weissenbruch MM, Delemarre-van de Waal HA, Boomsma DI. Low birth weight is associated with increased sympathetic activity: dependence on genetic factors. Circulation. 2003;108(5):566–71.
30. Jansson T, Lambert GW. Effect of intrauterine growth restriction on blood pressure, glucose tolerance and sympathetic nervous system activity in the rat at 3-4 months of age. J Hypertens. 1999;17(9):1239–48.

31. Ruijtenbeek K, le Noble FA, Janssen GM, Kessels CG, Fazzi GE, Blanco CE, et al. Chronic hypoxia stimulates periarterial sympathetic nerve development in chicken embryo. Circulation. 2000;102(23):2892–7.
32. Westerbacka J, Vehkavaara S, Bergholm R, Wilkinson I, Cockcroft J, Yki-Jarvinen H. Marked resistance of the ability of insulin to decrease arterial stiffness characterizes human obesity. Diabetes. 1999;48(4):821–7.
33. Wilkinson IB, Qasem A, McEniery CM, Webb DJ, Avolio AP, Cockcroft JR. Nitric oxide regulates local arterial distensibility in vivo. Circulation. 2002; 105(2):213–7.
34. Phillips DI, Barker DJ. Association between low birthweight and high resting pulse in adult life: is the sympathetic nervous system involved in programming the insulin resistance syndrome? Diabet Med. 1997;14(8):673–7.
35. Salvi P, Revera M, Joly L, Reusz G, Iaia M, Benkhedda S, et al. Role of birth weight and postnatal growth on pulse wave velocity in teenagers. J Adolesc Health. 2012;51(4):373–9.
36. Richalet JP, Larmignat P, Rathat C, Keromes A, Baud P, Lhoste F. Decreased cardiac response to isoproterenol infusion in acute and chronic hypoxia. J Appl Physiol (1985). 1988;65(5)):1957–61.
37. Koller EA, Drechsel S, Hess T, Macherel P, Boutellier U. Effects of atropine and propranolol on the respiratory, circulatory, and ECG responses to high altitude in man. Eur J Appl Physiol Occup Physiol. 1988;57(2):163–72.
38. Marshall JM. Peripheral chemoreceptors and cardiovascular regulation. Physiol Rev. 1994;74(3):543–94.
39. Salvi P, Revera M, Faini A, Giuliano A, Gregorini F, Agostoni P, et al. Changes in subendocardial viability ratio with acute high-altitude exposure and protective role of acetazolamide. Hypertension. 2013;61(4):793–9.
40. Bilo G, Caldara G, Styczkiewicz K, Revera M, Lombardi C, Giglio A, et al. Effects of selective and nonselective beta-blockade on 24-h ambulatory blood pressure under hypobaric hypoxia at altitude. J Hypertens. 2011;29(2):380–7.
41. Lanfranchi PA, Colombo R, Cremona G, Baderna P, Spagnolatti L, Mazzuero G, et al. Autonomic cardiovascular regulation in subjects with acute mountain sickness. Am J Physiol Heart Circ Physiol. 2005;289(6):H2364–72.
42. Parati G, Revera M, Giuliano A, Faini A, Bilo G, Gregorini F, et al. Effects of acetazolamide on central blood pressure, peripheral blood pressure, and arterial distensibility at acute high altitude exposure. Eur Heart J. 2013;34(10):759–66.
43. Bartsch P, Maggiorini M, Schobersberger W, Shaw S, Rascher W, Girard J, et al. Enhanced exercise-induced rise of aldosterone and vasopressin preceding mountain sickness. J Appl Physiol (1985). 1991;71(1):136–43.
44. Mancia G, Mark A. Arterial baroreflexes in humans. In: Shepherd J, Abboud F, editors. Handbook of physiology, section 2. The cardiovascular system IV, vol. 3, Part 2. Bethesda: American Physiologic Society; 1983. p. 755–93.
45. Boutouyrie P. New techniques for assessing arterial stiffness. Diabetes Metab. 2008;34 Suppl 1:S21–6.
46. Mattace-Raso FU, van den Meiracker AH, Bos WJ, van der Cammen TJ, Westerhof BE, Elias-Smale S, et al. Arterial stiffness, cardiovagal baroreflex sensitivity and postural blood pressure changes in older adults: the Rotterdam Study. J Hypertens. 2007;25(7):1421–6.
47. Parati G, Lantelme P. Mechanical and neural components of the cardiac baroreflex: new insights into complex physiology. J Hypertens. 2005;23(4):717–20.
48. Okada Y, Galbreath MM, Shibata S, Jarvis SS, VanGundy TB, Meier RL, et al. Relationship between sympathetic baroreflex sensitivity and arterial stiffness in elderly men and women. Hypertension. 2012;59(1):98–104.
49. Schillaci G, Bilo G, Pucci G, Laurent S, Macquin-Mavier I, Boutouyrie P, et al. Relationship between short-term blood pressure variability and large-artery stiffness in human hypertension: findings from 2 large databases. Hypertension. 2012;60(2):369–77.
50. Narkiewicz K, Winnicki M, Schroeder K, Phillips BG, Kato M, Cwalina E, et al. Relationship between muscle sympathetic nerve activity and diurnal blood pressure profile. Hypertension. 2002;39(1):168–72.
51. Parati G, Saul JP, Di Rienzo M, Mancia G. Spectral analysis of blood pressure and heart rate variability in evaluating cardiovascular regulation. A critical appraisal. Hypertension. 1995;25(6):1276–86.
52. Parati G, Ulian L, Santucciu C, Tortorici E, Villani A, Di Rienzo M, et al. Clinical value of blood pressure variability. Blood Press Suppl. 1997;2:91–6.
53. Parati G, Di Rienzo M, Omboni S, Ulian L, Mancia G. Blood pressure variability over 24 hours: its different components and its relationship to the arterial baroreflex. J Sleep Res. 1995;4(S1):21–9.
54. Monahan KD, Dinenno FA, Seals DR, Clevenger CM, Desouza CA, Tanaka H. Age-associated changes in cardiovagal baroreflex sensitivity are related to central arterial compliance. Am J Physiol Heart Circ Physiol. 2001;281(1):H284–9.
55. Mancia G, Ferrari A, Gregorini L, Parati G, Pomidossi G, Bertinieri G, et al. Blood pressure and heart rate variabilities in normotensive and hypertensive human beings. Circ Res. 1983;53(1):96–104.
56. Mancia G, Parati G, Castiglioni P, Tordi R, Tortorici E, Glavina F, et al. Daily life blood pressure changes are steeper in hypertensive than in normotensive subjects. Hypertension. 2003;42(3):277–82.

Oxidative Stress and Hypertension 15

Jing Wu and David G. Harrison

Keywords
Oxidation • Reduction • Hypertension • Chronic hypertension • Reactive oxygen species

Introduction

In the past 20 years, it has become clear that reactive oxygen species (ROS) contribute to the development of hypertension via myriad effects. While ROS are essential for normal cell function, they mediate pathological changes in the brain, the kidney and blood vessels associated with the genesis of chronic hypertension.

Reactive Oxygen Species

Reactive oxygen species are intermediates in oxidation-reduction reactions in which an electron from one molecule is removed (oxidation) and transferred to a recipient molecule (reduction). ROS are generally recognized as two major groups: free radicals and non-radical derivatives. The former possess an unpaired electron in their outer orbital, which is highly reactive. These include superoxide ($O_2^{\cdot-}$), the hydroxyl radical (HO·), lipid peroxy-radicals (LOO·) and alkoxy- radicals (LO·). Nitric oxide (NO) is also a free radical, and often referred to as a reactive nitrogen species (RNS) (Fig. 15.1). The non-radical derivatives are more stable with a longer half-life but can have strong oxidant properties, these include hydrogen peroxide (H_2O_2), peroxynitrite ($ONOO^-$), hypochlorous acid ($HOCl^-$). These reactions have been reviewed previously [1].

Normal Cell Function

Although originally considered toxic by-products of cellular metabolism, ROS are now recognized to have signaling roles that are critical for normal cell function, including proliferation, differentiation, aging, defense and repair processes [2]. Physiological levels of ROS are required for the maintenance of hematopoietic stem cell function and therefore hematopoiesis. Recent studies show that ROS, including H_2O_2, may drive pro-survival signaling and protect from the aging process. ROS also contribute to the innate

J. Wu • D.G. Harrison, MD (✉)
Division of Clinical Pharmacology, Departments of Medicine and Pharmacology, Vanderbilt University School of Medicine, Nashville, TN 37232-6602, USA
e-mail: david.g.harrison@vanderbilt.edu

M.E. Safar et al. (eds.), *Blood Pressure and Arterial Wall Mechanics in Cardiovascular Diseases*, DOI 10.1007/978-1-4471-5198-2_15, © Springer-Verlag London 2014

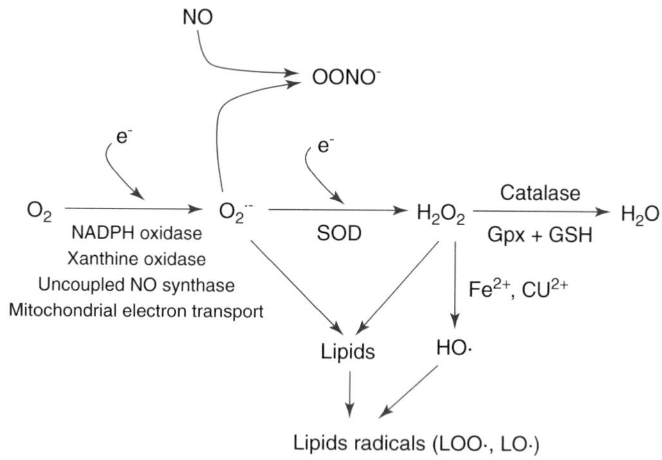

Fig. 15.1 Pathways for production of ROS in mammalian cells. Shown are enzymes thought important in hypertension, which can donate electrons to oxygen to form O_2^-. H_2O_2 can be formed by a two electron donation to oxygen and also be formed by the action of (SOD) on O_2^-. H_2O_2 is further reduced to water by either catalase or glutathione peroxidases (Gpx). O_2^- and H_2O_2 can undergo reactions with transition metals to form OH. ROS can react with lipids to form biologically active lipid radicals. *Gpx* glutathione peroxidases, *H_2O_2* hydrogen peroxide, *OH* hydroxyl radical, *SOD* superoxide dismutase

immune response via respiratory the bursts in phagocytes [3], and also by signaling chemotaxis of inflammatory cells to sites of infection or injury. ROS also participate in tissue repair and remodeling by inducing expression of matrix metalloproteinases (MMPs). These responses, which are vital for normal cell function, become exaggerated in disease states and promote pathological processes.

Oxidative Stress

The term oxidative stress has traditionally referred to an imbalance between the production of reactive oxygen species and antioxidant defenses [4]. This can lead to an increase in ambient levels of ROS that can damage various cellular components including DNA, protein and lipids. It is now clear that this imbalance can be localized to subcellular compartments such the mitochondria, the nucleus or localized at the cellular membrane [5]. This localized ROS generation might not be reflected by total cellular oxidant levels but functionally affect redox signaling specific to these domains. Thus, localized alterations of ROS production in the mitochondria can affect energy homeostasis, while localized ROS production in the nucleus can affect transcriptional events and epigenetic control.

Major ROS Molecules

Superoxide Radical

Superoxide (O_2^-), produced by 1-electron reduction of molecular oxygen, can act both as an oxidant and as a reductant in biological systems, depending on the redox potential of the molecule with which it is reacting [1]. Superoxide is important as it serves as the progenitor for many other biologically relevant ROS, including hydrogen peroxide (H_2O_2), the hydroxyl radical ($HO^·$) and peroxynitrite ($OONO^-$) (Fig. 15.1). Importantly, $OONO^-$ is formed by the diffusion-limited reaction of O_2^- with nitric oxide (NO).

Hydrogen Peroxide

Hydrogen peroxide is formed by dismutation of O_2^-, which can occur either spontaneously or can be catalyzed by the superoxide dismutases. In contrast to O_2^-, H_2O_2 is relatively stable under physiological conditions. Because it is uncharged and lipophilic, H_2O_2 can readily diffuse across membranes and thus can react with targets in organelles and cells apart from where it is formed. In this regard, H_2O_2 has been implicated as a signaling molecule that can, among other actions, promote vasodilatation, activate gene transcription, modify phosphatase activity, and activate other sources of ROS. H_2O_2 is formed by the dismutation of $O_2^{\cdot-}$, which can occur spontaneously but is catalyzed by the superoxide dismutases. The antioxidants enzymes catalase and glutathione peroxidase (Gpx) can further reduce H_2O_2 to H_2O (Fig. 15.1). Myeloperoxidase catalyzes the reaction of H_2O_2 with the chloride ion to generate hypochlorous acid ($HOCl^-$), which is a strong oxidant with high reactivity. The eosinophil peroxidase utilizes bromide in a similar reaction to form $HOBr^-$.

Hydroxyl Radical

The hydroxyl is formed $O_2^{\cdot-}$ donates one electron to H_2O_2 in a reaction classically referred to as the Haber Weiss Reaction (Fig. 15.1). Hydrogen peroxide can also accept one electron from the ferrous cation (Fe^{2+}) in the Fenton reaction to generate $OH^{\cdot}$ and a ferric cation (Fe^{3+}). The hydroxyl radical is a highly reactive oxidant that can attack a variety of biomolecules including lipids, proteins and DNA.

Peroxynitrite

As mentioned above, $OONO^-$ is the product of the spontaneous reaction between $O_2^{\cdot-}$ and NO (Fig. 15.1). This reaction is essentially diffusion limited, and its rate has been estimated to be 9×10^9 mol × s^{-1}, which is faster than that of the reaction of $O_2^{\cdot-}$ with the superoxide dismutases. At physiological pH, $OONO^-$ exists in the protonated form, HOONO or peroxynitrous acid, which is uncharged and can diffuse across cell membranes. Moreover, HONOO undergoes homolysis to yield hydroxyl, and in fact might serve as a more important source of this radical that the Fenton reaction mentioned above. Like hydroxyl, $OONO^-$ is a very strong oxidant and can react with lipids, DNA and proteins. It is also considered a reactive nitrogen species (RNS) that are closely relevant to ROS. Peroxynitrite often reacts and modify proteins and other cellular structures causing oxidative damage to these molecules. In particular, $OONO^-$ modifies protein tyrosine residues to form 3-nitrotyrosine, a biomarker for $OONO^-$ in tissues and blood. These properties of $OONO^-$ have been reviewed in depth [6].

Sources of ROS

NADPH Oxidase

The NADPH oxidases are major sources of ROS in mammalian cells [7]. The catalytic subunits of these enzyme complexes are the NOX proteins. Seven Nox proteins have been identified with differential tissue distribution, diverse function and regulation mechanisms. Nox1 is known to exist in colon, muscle, prostate, uterus and blood vessels and plays important roles in host defense and blood pressure regulation. Nox2 is found in phagocytes, where it is responsible for the oxidative burst. It is also present in endothelial cells and the tubular cells of the kidney. Nox3 is present in fetal tissue and inner ear and is essential for vestibular function. Nox4, expressed in kidneys, vessels and bone, is involved in vasoregulation and erythropointin synthesis. Nox5, not present in rodents, is a Ca^{2+}-dependent homolog that produces $O_2^{\cdot-}$ in response to intracellular Ca^{2+} mobilization in lymph nodes, testes and blood vessels. Nox5 is also expressed in atherosclerotic lesions and seems to be higher in more complex lesions [8]. Duox1/2 are Nox homologues involved in thyroid hormone biosynthesis.

The NADPH oxidases are activated by a variety of physiological and pathophysiological stimuli, including inflammatory cytokines, growth factors, mechanical forces and various G protein coupled receptor agonists. The manner in which the Nox isoforms are activated varies and often involves translocation of the cytoplasmic subunits to the membrane Nox proteins. Of particular importance to cardiovascular disease, angiotensin II activates the NADPH oxidases via the AT1 receptor and stimulation of a signaling pathway involving c-Src, protein kinase C (PKC), phospholipase D (PLD) and phospholipase A_2 (PLA_2). As mentioned, NOX5 is activated by calcium, and thus can be activated by signals that increase this divalent cation [9].

Nitric Oxide Synthase Uncoupling, Tetrahydrobiopterin and Arginine

The nitric oxide synthase (NOS) enzymes are the endogenous sources of NO in mammalian cells. By producing NO, these enzymes have myriad effects on cardiovascular function, including modulation of vascular tone, blood pressure, sympathetic outflow, renal renin release and renal sodium excretion [10]. In the absence of their critical cofactor tetrahydrobiopterin (H_4B), or their substrate L-arginine, the NOS enzymes become uncoupled, such that they produce $O_2^{·-}$ rather than NO. NOS uncoupling has been documented as a source of ROS in diseases such as hypertension, atherosclerosis, diabetes and following ischemia and reperfusion injury. In several of these diseases, oral supplementation of H_4B reverses NOS uncoupling, and improves endothelial function. Importantly, oral H_4B blunts the elevation of blood pressure in angiotensin II- and salt-induced hypertension in animals and has been shown to lower blood pressure in humans with hypertension [11]. Moreover, administration of H_4B also prevents the development of endothelium dysfunction, vascular inflammation and atherosclerosis induced by disturbed flow. Thus, reversing NOS uncoupling is an attractive approach to improve endothelium function and prevent the pathogenesis of vascular diseases.

A major cause of NOS uncoupling is oxidation of tetrahydrobiopterin by oxidants such as peroxynitrite [12]. Interestingly, ROS produced by the NADPH oxidase play a role in this process, and mice lacking the NADPH oxidase are protected against tetrahydrobiopterin oxidation in the setting of hypertension [12].

Xanthine Oxidase

Xanthine oxidoreductase (XOR) is another important source of ROS in mammalian cells [13]. XOR exists in two forms, including xanthine dehydrogenase (XDH), and xanthine oxidase (XO). XDH transfers electrons from hypoxanthine and xanthine to NAD^+ yielding NADH and uric acid, whereas XO transfers electrons to oxygen from these same substrates to generate $O_2^{·-}$ and H_2O_2. The cellular ratio of XO to XDH is therefore critical in modulating ROS production by these enzymes. XDH is converted to XO when a critical cysteine residue is oxidized by peroxynitrite. This conversion is also favored in several pathophysiological settings including inflammation, hypoxia, and radiation exposure, and likely contributes to increased ROS production and in these situations. Interestingly, although XO has been shown to contribute to experimental hypertension in animal models, there is no evidence supporting a role of xanthine oxidase in human hypertension [14].

Mitochondria

The mitochondria are responsible for the majority of ATP production in the cell. These organelles contain 5 enzyme complexes that comprise the electron transport chain. Electrons are transported sequentially from NADH through complexes I to V, the site of ATP generation. During normal mitochondrial function, this electron transfer from one complex to the next is efficient and there is minimal loss or leak from electron transport, however in various disease states, electron leak is increased and can lead to reduction of oxygen and formation of $O_2^{·-}$ and H_2O_2. Electron leak can occur at complexes I to IV, but occurs predominantly at complexes I and III, due to defects in these complexes. A recurring paradigm is that oxidative damage to mitochondrial DNA promotes deficiency in components of the electron transport chain, promoting electron leak. An important phenomenon is reverse electron transport, which occurs particularly in complex I in various pathophysiological states. Mitochondrial dysfunction has arisen as a major source of cellular ROS production in various pathophysiological states. Importantly, ROS from the NADPH oxidase have been shown to enter the mitochondria and promote electron leak and ROS production from the electron transport chain in hypertension [15]. Of note, antioxidants have been engineered that are targeted to the mitochondria and have proven effective in both preventing and reversing experimental hypertension [16]. The reader is referred to an excellent comprehensive review of mitochondrial function and ROS production for in depth details of mitochondrial function [17].

Antioxidant Defense Mechanisms

Because of our oxygen rich atmosphere, all living organisms, including bacteria, plants and animals have adapted and developed enzymatic and non-enzymatic defenses against chronic oxidative stress. In mammalian cells, the major intracellular antioxidant enzymes include superoxide dismutase, catalase and glutathione peroxidase. As mentioned above, SOD catalyzes the dismutation of $O_2^{\cdot-}$ to H_2O_2 and molecular O_2. Catalase and glutathione peroxidase further decompose H_2O_2 into H_2O and O_2. Glutathione peroxidase requires glutathione as a co-substrate, yielding oxidized GSSG upon reaction. In addition to H_2O_2, glutathione peroxidase also reduces lipid hydroperoxides to their respective alcohols and thus protects the cell membrane from lipid peroxidation. Glutathione peroxidase also is protective against $OONO^-$, which it efficiently reduces to nitrite [18]. Unlike $O_2^{\cdot-}$ or H_2O_2, the there are no enzymatic antioxidants that scavenge hydroxyl, but a variety of non-enzymatic antioxidants including vitamin C (ascorbic acid), vitamin E (α-tocopherol) and glutathione react with and eliminate this radical.

Mammalian cells have the capacity to modulate their antioxidant levels by transcriptional modulators such as Nrf2 and DJ-1. The former is a transcription factor that binds to the antioxidant response element of many genes, including the glutathione-S transferases, heme oxygenase 1 and glutamate-cysteine ligase which controls glutathione synthesis. Nrf2 is activated in the setting of oxidative stress, and moves to the nucleus to induce these and other important antioxidant genes. DJ-1 is a recently discovered protein that has antioxidant properties, and translocates to either the nucleus or the mitochondria upon oxidative stress. As discussed below, DJ-1 plays a major role in the response of proximal tubular cells to dopamine, and ultimately regulates blood pressure [19].

Limitations of Antioxidant Therapy

Although basic studies have strongly supported a role of ROS in cell dysfunction and animal models of disease, clinical trials with high dose antioxidants have been disappointing. Several large clinical trials have failed to show beneficial effects of either vitamin C or vitamin E supplementation in cancer, cardiovascular disease and neurodegenerative diseases. A recent meta-analysis of 50 randomized trials including almost 300,000 patients confirmed the futility of treatment with a variety of antioxidants in cardiovascular disease [20]. In hypertensive subjects, a few small trials initially showed benefit, but later large clinical trials, including the SU.VI.MAX study, showed no improvement in blood pressure with antioxidant therapy [21]. Surprisingly, large doses of beta-carotene, vitamin A and vitamin E have paradoxically worsened cardiovascular outcomes in some studies [22]. The failure of antioxidants in humans might reflect the low rate constant of vitamins such as E and C with superoxide and related ROS, the inability to target subcellular sites where ROS are formed, and the fact that some ROS have beneficial effects. Prevention of ROS generation by inhibiting specific enzymatic sources might be more efficient than nonspecific antioxidants such as vitamin C and E. In this regard, a recent study showed that a Nox 1 inhibitor is effective in reducing atherosclerosis in mice with experimental diabetes [23]. It is also possible that these trials were negative because they did not target patients that actually have oxidative stress. As an example, the effect of vitamin E vs. placebo was studied on cardiovascular outcomes in almost 1,500 middle-aged diabetic patients with the haptaglobin 2/2 genotype [24]. The 2/2 genotype is associated with a reduction of haptaglobin's antioxidant properties and therefore these patients were deemed to be at risk for oxidative stress. Vitamin E reduced all cardiovascular events, myocardial infarction and stroke by

50 % in this population. Because of this striking benefit of vitamin E, the study was stopped prematurely. It is also possible that more potent, catalytic agents such as tempol or targeted agents such as mitoTempol, which scavenges radicals specifically in the mitochondria, would have greater efficacy. This topic has been reviewed previously [25].

Role of Reactive Oxygen Species in Hypertension

A large body of literature has shown that excessive production of ROS contributes to hypertension and that scavenging of ROS decreases blood pressure. In an initial study, Nakazono and colleagues showed that bolus administration of a modified form of SOD acutely lowered blood pressure in hypertensive rats. Membrane-targeted forms of SOD and SOD mimetics such as tempol lower blood pressure and decrease renovascular resistance in hypertensive animal models. There is ample evidence suggesting that ROS not only contribute to hypertension but that the NADPH oxidase is their major source. Components of this enzyme system are up-regulated by hypertensive stimuli, and NADPH oxidase enzyme activity is increased by these same stimuli. Moreover, both angiotensin II-induced hypertension and deoxycorticosterone acetate (DOCA)-salt hypertension are blunted in mice lacking this enzyme.

Despite the evidence that oxidative stress contributes to hypertension, the mechanisms involved are not well understood. Hypertension is associated with increased ROS production by multiple organs, including the brain, the vasculature, and the kidney, all of which are likely important. A major problem is that we currently lack a complete understanding of which of these organs or cell types predominate in the genesis of hypertension or if there is important interplay between them that causes this disease. In the next sections, we discuss evidence that hypertension is associated with oxidative stress that occurs in the central nervous system (CNS), the kidney, and the vasculature and attempt to provide evidence for how this contributes to hypertension.

Renal Oxidative Stress and Hypertension

There is ample evidence supporting that ROS generated in the kidney and its blood vessels contribute to the development and maintenance of hypertension. Virtually all cells in the kidney, including vessels, glomeruli, podocytes, interstitial fibroblasts, the medullary thick ascending limb (mTAL), the macula densa, the distal tubule, and the collecting duct express components of the NADPH oxidase, and various stimuli have been shown to activate these. Several of the effects of ROS in the kidney are summarized in Fig. 15.2. For purposes of discussion, we first focus on oxidative events in the renal cortex and then in the medulla.

Several studies have examined the effect of various hypertensive stimuli on the renal cortex and how these are modulated by ROS. The structures that are targets of oxidant stress include the afferent arteriole, the glomerulus, the proximal tubule, and the cortical collecting duct (CCD). As with other vessels, an increase in $O_2^{\cdot-}$ in the afferent arteriole can oxidatively degrade NO, which would enhance afferent arteriolar vasoconstriction and reduce glomerular filtration rate (GFR). Indeed, studies in rabbits have shown that angiotensin II-induced hypertension increases expression of the NADPH oxidase subunit $p22^{phox}$, activates the NADPH oxidase, and causes endothelial dysfunction in afferent arterioles [26]. Studies of isolated afferent arterioles have also shown that $O_2^{\cdot-}$ generated by the NADPH oxidase potentiates intracellular calcium [27]. ROS are also generated in the afferent arterioles of spontaneous hypertensive rats and in the kidney of animals in response to other vasoconstrictors such as endothelin-1 (ET-1) and thromboxane prostanoids [28]. Intrarenal and afferent arteriolar ROS promote vasoconstriction, reduces GFR and contribute to hypertension. These effects are markedly augmented by genetic deletion of SOD-1 and are ameliorated by administration of polyethylene glycol (PEG)-SOD or efforts to block NADPH oxidase [29]. Therefore, the beneficial effects of $O_2^{\cdot-}$ scavenging in hypertensive animals have, at least in part,

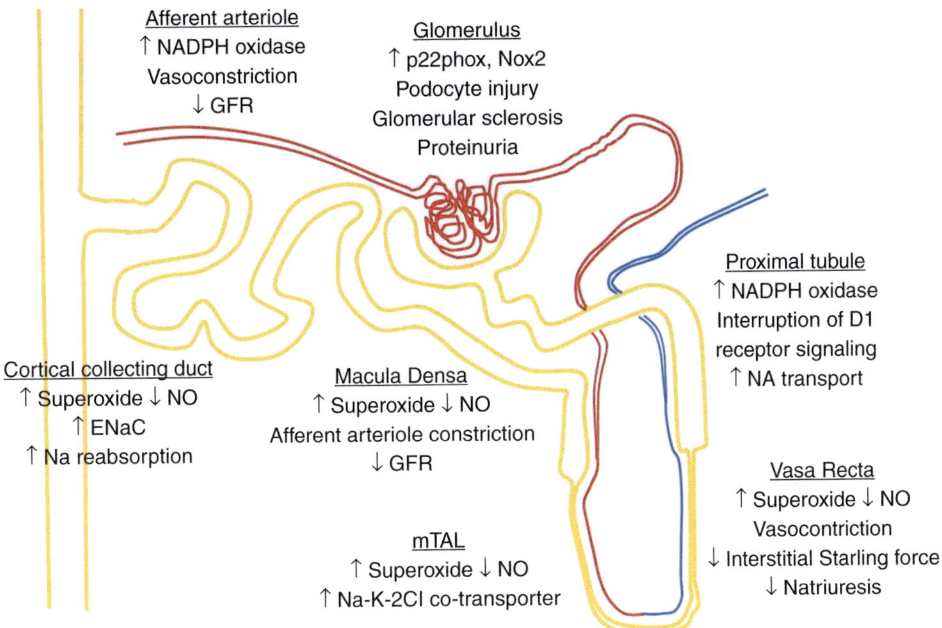

Fig. 15.2 Schematic representation of a juxtamedullary glomerulus showing sites of ROS production and potential roles in sodium transport, reabsorption, and blood pressure regulation. *D1* Dopamine type 1 receptor, *GFR* glomerular filtration rate, *mTAL* medullary thick ascending limb, *Na* sodium, *NO* nitric oxide, *ENaC* epithelial Na channel

been attributed to alleviation of renal vasoconstriction and improved renal perfusion.

Podocyte injury, a precursor to glumerulosclerosis and proteinuria, occurs early after salt loading in Dahl salt-sensitive rats. There is up-regulation of glomerular p22^{phox} and Nox2 in the glomeruli of these animals. The antioxidant tempol reduces glomerular sclerosis and proteinuria in Dahl salt-sensitive rats, further supporting a role for ROS in glomerular injury [30]. In addition, angiotensin II also causes podocyte injury by stimulating mitochondria ROS generation and inducing podocyte autophagy [31]. Increased ROS in podocytes disrupt the crosstalk between nephrin and caveolin-1, which is required for maintenance of the glomerular filtration barrier [32]. ROS also mediate mesangial cell proliferation, migration and extracellular matrix deposition, which are characteristic of glomerulosclerosis induced by angiotensin II or aldosterone [33]. Thus, glomerular oxidative stress is a common occurrence in several forms of experimental hypertension and a likely cause of proteinuria and renal failure in this disease.

Cells of the proximal tubule also contain components of the NADPH oxidase, particularly in lipid rafts, where they are maintained in an inactive state. Dopamine-1 (D_1) receptor agonists inhibit, whereas disruption of lipid rafts and angiotensin II stimulate the proximal tubule NADPH oxidase. An important role of ROS and the NADPH oxidase in the proximal tubule is modulation of sodium transport via altering Na/K ATPase and Na/H exchange-3 (NHE-3) function on the basal and apical membranes of the proximal tubular cells, respectively [34]. Sodium transport is stimulated by angiotensin II and inhibited by dopamine, and oxidant stress enhances the effect of angiotensin II and disrupts dopamine signaling, thus increasing proximal tubular sodium transport. In keeping with these observations, Cuevas et al. recently showed that stimulation of the Dopamine D_2 receptor (D_2R) inhibits ROS production in renal proximal tubular cells and that mice lacking one D_2R allele have increased ROS in the proximal tubule and are hypertensive [19]. These authors also showed that an antioxidant protein, known as DJ-1 associates with D_2R and that if either D_2R or DJ-1 is knocked down, proximal tubule ROS are increased. This is at least in part due to increased expression of Nox4, but DJ-1 is an antioxidant transcriptional regulator that also modulates expression of many antioxidant proteins, including the superoxide dismutases [35].

One of the important mechanisms by which ROS in the cortex modulate sodium handling and ultimately blood pressure is via tubuloglomerular feedback. This is a phenomenon mediated by the interaction of the macula densa of the thick ascending limb as it makes contact with its own glomerulus in the cortex. The macula densa senses sodium concentration in the proximal tubule via its apical Na/K/2Cl co-transporter, which in turn stimulates signaling molecules, one of which is NO produced by the neuronal nitric oxide synthase. This dilates afferent arterioles and increases glomerular filtration [36]. An increase in $O_2^{\cdot-}$ within or in the vicinity of the macula densa likely inactivates NO, leading to afferent arteriolar vasoconstriction and a reduction of GFR [37]. In this regard, an elegant study of isolated, single nephrons by Nouri and colleagues showed that in vivo silencing RNA of the NADPH oxidase subunit $p22^{phox}$ enhances single tubular glomerular filtration in angiotensin II-treated rats but not in control rats. By either including or excluding the distal tubule, these authors showed that this effect was likely mediated by ROS produced in the macula densa [38].

The epithelial Na^+ channel (ENaC) is responsible for the final tubular adjustment of Na^+ reabsorption in the cortical collecting duct (CCD). Angiotensin II activates the NADPH oxidase in the CCD, and this stimulates ENaC activity [39]. This is likely mediated by aldosterone, the principle regulator of ENaC activity. Aldosterone induces superoxide generation in A6 epithelial cells, which in turn reduces the inhibitory effect of NO on the ENaC [40]. In addition, angiotensin II-induced H_2O_2 diminishes the ability of arachidonic acid (AA) to inhibit ENaC in the CCD [39].

There is ample evidence linking oxidative stress in the renal medulla with sodium reabsorption and modulation of blood pressure. As in the blood vessel, there is a balance between $O_2^{\cdot-}$ and NO produced by cells within the medulla, including the epithelial cells of the mTAL and the pericytes of the vasa recta. Interestingly, there is markedly more NO synthase activity in the renal medulla compared with that in the cortex. This likely contributes to independent regulation of medullary and cortical perfusion. Elegant studies by Cowley's group have shown that cells of the mTAL release NO that diffuses to nearby pericytes of the adjacent vasa recta to promote dilation of these vessels. This increases medullary flow, and by increasing interstitial Starling forces, promotes sodium movement to the tubule and thus natriuresis and diuresis. Inhibition of NO synthase in the medulla with L-nitroarginine methyl ester (L-NAME) markedly reduces medullary perfusion and promotes sodium reabsorption without changing cortical flow [41]. As discussed earlier, all of the components of the NADPH oxidase are present in the renal medulla and can be activated by either systemic or locally produced angiotensin II. The consequent increase in medullary $O_2^{\cdot-}$ leads to vasoconstriction of the vasa recta and reduces Starling forces such that sodium movement into the vasa recta is favored, reducing natriuresis and increasing blood pressure. Another important mechanism whereby medullary $O_2^{\cdot-}$ could affect renal sodium relates to changes in medullary sodium transport [42]. Direct exposure of mTAL preparations to $O_2^{\cdot-}$ enhances Na/K/2Cl cotransporter activity via a protein kinase C activation [43]. Infusion of angiotensin II in vivo mimics this effect and is prevented by administration of the $O_2^{\cdot-}$ scavenger tempol. Nitric oxide also regulates NaCl transport in the mTAL. In isolated thick ascending limb, NO generated by NOS3 inhibits the Na/K/2Cl cotransporter and NHE-3 [44]. The inhibitory effect on Na/K/2Cl cotransporter is mediated by phosphodiesterase-mediated degradation of cyclic AMP while NHE-3 is directly inhibited by NO.

These considerations regarding the role of ROS in the control of renal function emphasize an important function of these molecules in that they seem to play a critical role in normal renal physiology and are not simply mediators of

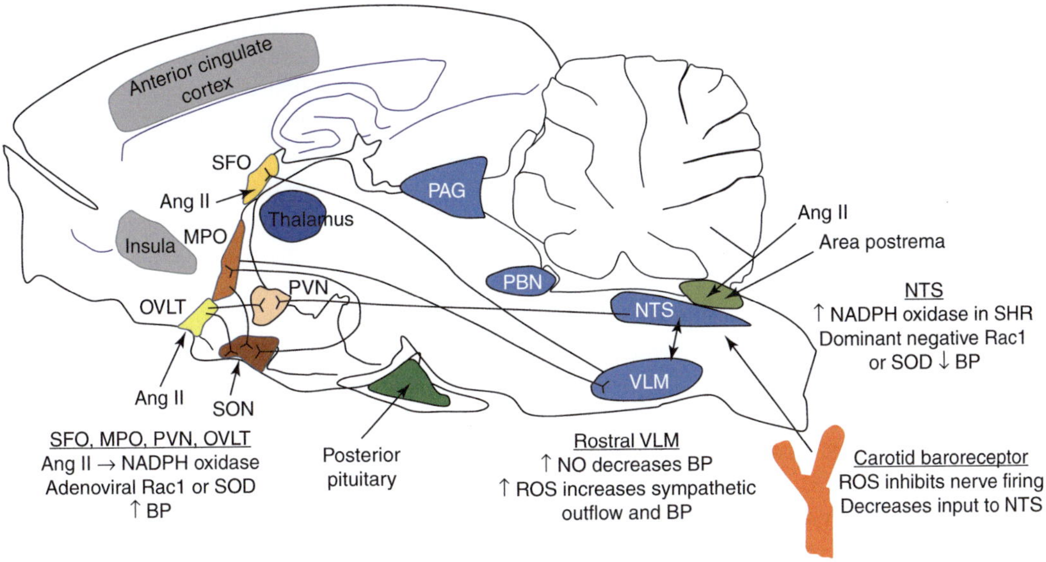

Fig. 15.3 Schematic representation of the brain showing centers affected by ROS that are thought to participate in hypertension. *NTS* nucleus tractis solitarius, *OVLT* organum vasculosum lateral terminalis, *PAG* periaquaductal gray, *PBN* parabrachial nucleus, *PVN* paraventricular nucleus, *SFO* subfornical organ, *VLM* ventral lateral medulla, *MPO* median preoptic eminence

pathophysiological events. The ability of the kidney to retain sodium and water during times of salt restriction is an extremely important function in land-dwelling mammals, without which survival would be impossible. It is likely that $O_2^{\cdot-}$ and other ROS are generated as needed to modulate sodium balance.

Reactive Oxygen Species, the Central Nervous System and Hypertension

It is well established that the CNS is necessary for production and maintenance of most forms of experimental hypertension, principally by sympathetic efferent nerves, and that even hormones like angiotensin II and aldosterone, which have myriad systemic effects, causes hypertension via action on central sites [45]. The most compelling evidence supporting this is that destruction of a region of the forebrain surrounding the anteroventral third cerebral ventricle (AV3V) prevents development of many forms of experimentally induced hypertension in rodents [46]. This region of the forebrain includes the median preoptic eminence, the organum vasculosum of the lateral terminalis, and the preoptic periventricular nucleus (Fig. 15.3). Following disruption of this region of the brain, virtually all of the central actions of angiotensin II, including drinking behavior, vasopressin secretion and increased sympathetic outflow, are abrogated. These portions of the brain are also reciprocally connected to other regions involved in central cardiovascular regulation. Important among these is the subfornical organ (SFO), a circumventricular organ (CVO) lacking a blood-brain barrier, allowing peripheral hormonal signals sent to the AV3V to be translated into increased sympathetic outflow and hypertension [47]. This region also communicates with other important cardiovascular control centers in the mid- and hindbrain, including the parabrachial nucleus, the nucleus tractus solitarius (NTS) and the rostral ventral lateral medulla (VLM) (see Fig. 15.3).

In the past several years, a convincing body of evidence has emerged suggesting that signaling in these brain centers is modulated by local production of ROS and can contribute to hypertension [48]. As an example, intracerebroventricular (ICV) injection of an adenovirus encoding SOD markedly attenuates the hypertension caused by either local injection or systemic infusion of angiotensin II [49]. Zimmerman and colleagues have shown that angiotensin II increases $\cdot O_2^-$ production and intracellular calcium in cultured neurons [50]. An important regulator of the NADPH oxidase is the small G protein Rac-1, and these investigators showed that the increase in neuronal intracellular calcium caused by angiotensin II was blocked by administration of adenoviruses expressing either a dominant negative form of Rac-1 or SOD. Moreover, these investigators have also shown that dominant negative Rac1 gene transfer in the CNS prevents the acute hypertensive response to angiotensin II [51]. Recently, Peterson et al., using selective siRNA-expressing adenoviruses, have shown that Nox2 and Nox4 have different roles in the SFO, such that both are linked to blood pressure regulation, but only Nox2 modulates drinking behavior [52]. A very recent study by Lob et al. has shown that Cre-Lox deletion of p22*phox* in the SFO completely abrogates the long-term hypertensive response to angiotensin II [53].

As mentioned here, projections from the circumventricular organ interact with centers in the hypothalamus. There is evidence that ROS derived from the NADPH oxidase enhances nerve traffic in this region. Erdos and colleagues have shown that ICV injection of angiotensin II increases NADPH oxidase-mediated $O_2^{\cdot-}$ production not only in the SFO but also in anterior hypothalamic nuclei such as the median preoptic eminence and in the paraventricular nucleus of the hypothalamus [54]. These effects were blocked by the NADPH oxidase inhibitor apocynin as were the hemodynamic effects of centrally administered angiotensin II. Thus, angiotensin II and its effects on the NADPH oxidase seem to coordinate activation of several forebrain centers to promote a hypertensive response.

There is also important signaling between the forebrain and pontomedullary cardiovascular control centers in the hindbrain. An important nucleus in the hindbrain that regulates blood pressure is the NTS, which receives input from the CVO and relays inhibitory stimuli from baroreceptors. Angiotensin II inhibits the negative feedback from the baroreceptors to the NTS. In studies of neurons from the NTS, angiotensin II has been shown to augment L-type calcium channel activity via ROS generated by the NADPH oxidase [55]. Nozoe and colleagues showed that the activities of NADPH oxidase and Rac1 are increased in the NTS of stroke-prone, spontaneously hypertensive rats. These investigators further showed that injection of an adenovirus that inhibits Rac-1 or an adenovirus to increase SOD into the NTS reduced blood pressure, heart rate, urinary norepinephrine, and a marker of oxidative stress in these animals [56]. This elegant study provides strong evidence for oxidative stress in the NTS in this model of hypertension.

An important consequence of increased $O_2^{\cdot-}$ production is a loss of NO, which has a critical role in the central regulation of blood pressure. A site that has been studied in this regard is the ventral lateral medulla (VLM). The VLM lies below the NTS and receives and sends signals to the NTS and, as a result, importantly regulates cardiovascular sympathetic tone. NO in this region stimulates release of the inhibitory neurotransmitter γ-amino butylic acid (GABA) while a reduction of NO bioavailability in the VLM causes sympathoexcitation [57]. Experimental interventions that increase NO in the rostral VLM lower blood pressure, whereas increased in oxidative stress in this region raises blood pressure [58].

There is also evidence that ROS modulate baroreflex function, which is routinely abnormal in the setting of chronic hypertension. Normally, an increase in blood pressure activates the carotid baroreflex, resulting in bradycardia and sympathetic withdrawal. This response is blunted in chronic hypertension, a phenomenon referred to as baroreflex resetting. Elegant studies by Li and colleagues have shown that ROS generated in the carotid bulb of atherosclerotic rabbits reduce carotid sinus nerve responses to elevations of pressure and that this could be mimicked by exogenous administration of ROS and prevented by ROS scavenging [59].

The efferent sympathetic renal nerves govern both the vasculature and tubular segments of the kidney. Renal sympathetic stimulation promotes afferent arteriolar vasoconstriction, renin release and increases Na+reabsorption [60]. ROS generated in response to α1 adrenergic receptor activation enhance constriction of the afferent arterioles and reduce renal blood flow (RBF) in angiotensin II-infused rabbits. In contrast, β1 adrenergic receptor activation inhibits ROS generation and promotes vasodilation. In keeping with these important roles of renal sympathetic nerves in controlling renal ROS production, renal denervation blunts blood pressure elevation in multiple experimental hypertensive models, including angiotensin II-induced, DOCA-salt and two kidney one clip hypertension as well as SHR and SHRSP rats [61]. Moreover, renal denervation has recently become widely employed to treat resistant hypertension in humans [62].

A consequence of renal denervation is ablation of the renal afferent nerves. These are mainly located in the renal pelvis and are activated by various physical and chemical stimuli. During kidney injury, increased input from these afferent nerves activates central sympathetic nuclei in a ROS-dependent manner [63]. For instance, renal denervation prevents release of norepinephrine from the posterior hypothalamic nuclei and the elevation of blood pressure following kidney injury induced intrarenal injection of phenol [64]. These changes are mediated by increased NADPH oxidase expression in the central nuclei but are prevented by intracerebroventricular (ICV) injection of the SOD mimetic tempol or PEG-SOD. Interestingly, a vitamin E-fortified diet blunts the increase of sympathetic nerve activity and hypertension in response to interrenal phenol injection [65]. These data indicate that ROS modulate activity of both efferent and afferent renal nerves and therefore promote development of hypertension.

Vascular Oxidative Stress and Hypertension

Elevated vascular ROS promotes the development of hypertension in various animal models, including angiotensin II-induced and DOCA-salt hypertension, Dahl salt-sensitive hypertension and the spontaneous hypertensive rat (SHR). Humans with hypertension have alterations of vascular reactivity [66].

The endothelium regulates vascular tone via releasing of endothelium-derived relaxing factors (EDRFs) and endothelium-derived contractile factors (EDCFs). Oxidative stress causes imbalanced production and bioavailability of these molecules leading to endothelial dysfunction. NO is one of the most important mediators of endothelium-dependent relaxation in blood pressure regulation. The major mechanism for alteration of NO bioavailability when superoxide is increased is that this radical reacts with NO at an extremely rapid rate, as discussed above (see Fig. 15.4).

As mentioned above, uncoupling of endothelial nitric oxide synthase (eNOS), due to deprivation

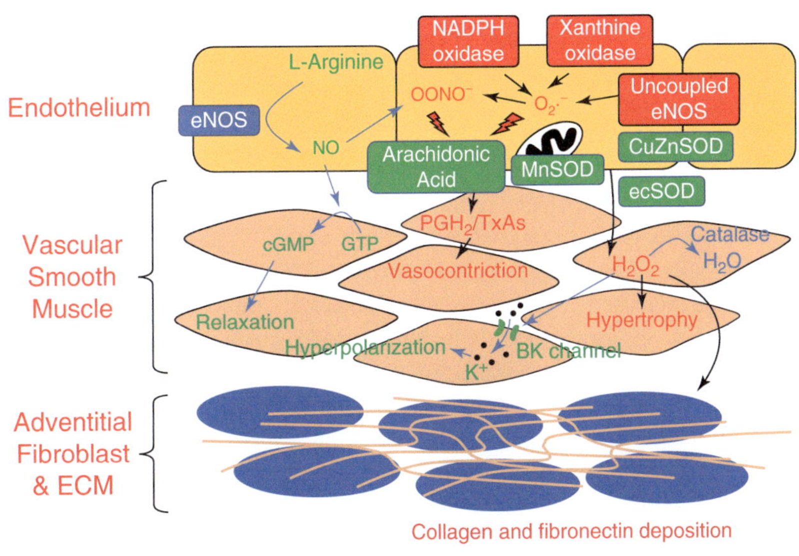

Fig. 15.4 Vascular effects of ROS contributing to hypertension

of cofactor tetrahydrobiopterin, results in reduced NO release, increased superoxide production, impaired endothelium-dependent relaxation and elevated arterial pressure. Similarly, lack of eNOS substrate L-arginine also reduces NO bioavailability and impairs NO-induced dilation. L-arginine is the substrate for both eNOS and arginase, and increased arginase activity reduces the local bioavailability of L-arginine. Interestingly, peroxinitrite and hydrogen peroxide have recently been shown to increase the expression and activity of arginase in endothelial cells, potentially contributing to endothelial dysfunction [67].

Oxidation of membrane fatty acids and in particular arachidonic acid can lead to formation of F2-isoprostanes, which are present in the blood of patients with oxidative stress (e.g. those with hypercholesterolemia, diabetics, and cigarette smokers). Importantly, plasma F2-isoprostanes are increased in animals with experimental hypertension and in humans with renovascular hypertension [68]. These oxidatively modified fatty acids act on prostaglandin H/thromboxane receptors to enhance vasoconstriction.

Superoxide and other ROS can also affect the structure and function of the vascular media. An important consequence of ROS formation is vascular smooth muscle hypertrophy. In particular, H_2O_2 has been implicated in the hypertrophic effect of angiotensin II in cultured cells and vascular smooth muscle hypertrophy is strikingly increased in mice overexpressing the NADPH oxidase in the vascular smooth muscle [69]. The hypertrophic response of vascular smooth muscle is a critical component of vascular remodeling in hypertension. Vascular ROS also stimulate the production of collagen and fibronectin both in vitro and in vivo [70], and removal of vascular ROS prevents these fibrotic changes. Structural changes such as these in resistance vessels could add to the increased systemic vascular resistance that occurs in established hypertension and, therefore, worsen the disease.

Endothelium-dependent hyperpolarization is an NO-independent mechanism of vasodilatation in resistance vessels, involving opening of vascular smooth muscle potassium channels and a reduction of intracellular calcium concentrations. The nature of the endothelium-derived hyperpolarizing factor (EDHF) remains a topic of study, but H_2O_2 produced by the mitochondria is likely one EDHF that acts by activating the Ca^{2+}-dependent potassium (BK) channel. This seems to be an important mechanism of flow mediated vasodilatation in human coronary arterioles. The production of H_2O_2 seems to be mediated by calcium entry into endothelial cells through the TRP vanilloid type 4 (TRPV4) channel in several vascular beds [71]. Another EDHF is likely a cytochrome p450 epoxide metabolite of arachidonic acid, which also opens the TRPV4 channel [72].

H_2O_2 also affects the NO-cGMP pathway. H_2O_2 acutely stimulates NO production and over the long term induces expression of the endothelial nitric oxide synthase (eNOS) [73]. H_2O_2 also activates protein kinase G (PKG) by inducing cross-linking two alpha subunits of this enzyme via disulfide bond formation, and therefore promotes vasodilation independent of NO.

Reactive Oxygen Species, Inflammation and Hypertension

Diverse stimuli common to the hypertensive milieu, including angiotensin II, aldosterone, catecholamines, increased vascular stretch, and endothelin promote ROS production, which then increases expression of proinflammatory molecules that cause rolling, adhesion, and transcytosis of inflammatory cells. As a result, there is a striking accumulation of inflammatory cells in the vessel and kidney. In keeping with this, there is an increase in plasma markers of inflammation in hypertensive humans [74].

Although macrophages are commonly considered important in the genesis of cardiovascular disease, increasing evidence has accumulated suggesting that the adaptive immune response and, in particular, T lymphocytes are important in hypertension. Mice and rats lacking the RAG-1 gene are partly protected against the blood pressure elevation and renal damage caused by angiotensin II or salt [75–77]. Effector T cells enter the

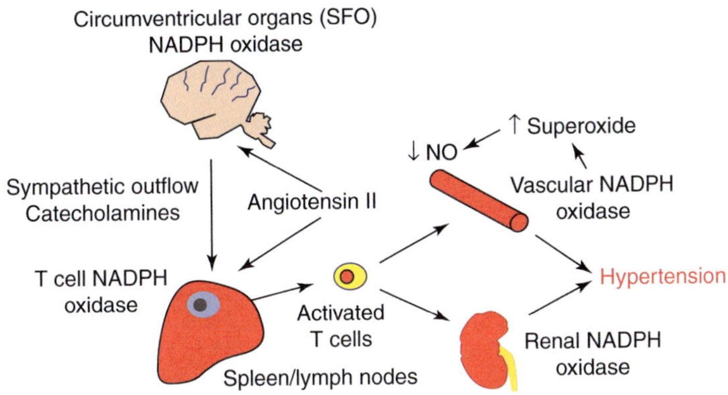

Fig. 15.5 Proposed role of T cells in the genesis of hypertension and the role of the NADPH oxidase in multiple cells/organs in modulating this effect. In this scenario, angiotensin II stimulates an NADPH oxidase in the CVOs of the brain, increasing sympathetic outflow. Sympathetic nerve terminals in lymph nodes activate T cells, and angiotensin II also directly activates T cells. These stimuli also activate expression of homing signals in the vessel and likely the kidney, which attract T cells to these organs. T cells release cytokines that stimulate the vessel and kidney NADPH oxidases, promoting vasoconstriction and sodium retention. *SFO* subfornical organ

kidney and the perivascular fat, where they release cytokines that promote salt retention and vasoconstriction, ultimately promoting hypertension. An important cytokine seems to be interleukin 17a. Mice lacking this are protected against angiotensin II-induced hypertension, and infusion of the IL17 soluble receptor C lowers blood pressure and prevents oxidative stress in rats with experimental pre-eclampsia [78, 79]. Moreover, IL17 induces endothelial dysfunction and ROS production in isolated vessels and raises blood pressure when infused in mice [80].

The observation that a circulating cell, such as the T cell, is important in the genesis of hypertension might help provide a unifying link between oxidative events in the CNS, the vasculature, and the kidney. These interactions, illustrated in Fig. 15.5, are dependent on activation of the NADPH oxidase in all of these sites. Centrally, in the SFO, and other CVOs, NADPH oxidase activation increases neuronal firing increases sympathetic nerve stimulation of peripheral lymphoid tissues, leading to T cell activation. The NADPH oxidase is essential for T cell activation in hypertension, as T cells lacking this enzyme mediate this response in an incomplete fashion [81]. The NADPH oxidase in the kidney and vessels initiates signals that cause T cell homing and infiltration [82]. Finally, cytokines released by T cells diffuse to renal and vascular cells, promoting further NADPH oxidase activation, sodium retention, and vasoconstriction, leading to overt hypertension.

Summary

This review has summarized some of the data supporting a role of ROS and oxidant stress in the genesis of hypertension. There is evidence that hypertensive stimuli, such as high salt and angiotensin II, promote production of ROS in the brain, the kidney, and the vasculature and that each of these sites contributes either to hypertension or to the untoward sequelae of this disease. Although the NADPH oxidase in these various organs is a predominant source, other enzymes likely contribute to ROS production and signaling in these tissues. A major clinical challenge is that the routinely used antioxidants are ineffective in preventing or treating cardiovascular disease and hypertension. This is likely because these drugs are either ineffective or act in a non-targeted fashion, such that they remove not only injurious ROS but also those involved in normal cell signaling. A potentially important and relatively new direction is the concept that inflammatory cells such as T cells contribute to hypertension. Future studies are needed to understand the interaction of T cells with the CNS, the kidney, and the vasculature and how this might be interrupted to provide therapeutic benefit.

References

1. Afanas Ev IB. Superoxide ion chemistry and biological implications. Boca Raton: CRC Press; 1989.
2. Ray PD, Huang BW, Tsuji Y. Reactive oxygen species (ROS) homeostasis and redox regulation in cellular signaling. Cell Signal. 2012;24:981–90.
3. Nauseef WM. How human neutrophils kill and degrade microbes: an integrated view. Immunol Rev. 2007;219:88–102.
4. Sies H. Oxidative stress: from basic research to clinical application. Am J Med. 1991;91:31S–8.
5. Go YM, Jones DP. Redox compartmentalization in eukaryotic cells. Biochim Biophys Acta. 2008;1780: 1273–90.
6. Halliwell B, Zhao K, Whiteman M. Nitric oxide and peroxynitrite. The ugly, the uglier and the not so good: a personal view of recent controversies. Free Radic Res. 1999;31:651–69.
7. Lassegue B, Griendling KK. NADPH oxidases: functions and pathologies in the vasculature. Arterioscler Thromb Vasc Biol. 2010;30:653–61.
8. Guzik TJ, Chen W, Gongora MC, Guzik B, Lob HE, Mangalat D, Hoch N, Dikalov S, Rudzinski P, Kapelak B, Sadowski J, Harrison DG. Calcium-dependent NOX5 nicotinamide adenine dinucleotide phosphate oxidase contributes to vascular oxidative stress in human coronary artery disease. J Am Coll Cardiol. 2008;52:1803–9.
9. Banfi B, Tirone F, Durussel I, Knisz J, Moskwa P, Molnar GZ, Krause KH, Cox JA. Mechanism of Ca2+ activation of the NADPH oxidase 5 (NOX5). J Biol Chem. 2004;279:18583–91.
10. Forstermann U, Sessa WC. Nitric oxide synthases: regulation and function. Eur Heart J. 2012;33: 829–37, 837a–d.
11. Porkert M, Sher S, Reddy U, Cheema F, Niessner C, Kolm P, Jones DP, Hooper C, Taylor WR, Harrison D, Quyyumi AA. Tetrahydrobiopterin: a novel antihypertensive therapy. J Hum Hypertens. 2008;22:401–7.
12. Landmesser U, Dikalov S, Price SR, McCann L, Fukai T, Holland SM, Mitch WE, Harrison DG. Oxidation of tetrahydrobiopterin leads to uncoupling of endothelial cell nitric oxide synthase in hypertension. J Clin Invest. 2003;111:1201–9.
13. Cantu-Medellin N, Kelley EE. Xanthine oxidoreductase-catalyzed reactive species generation: a process in critical need of reevaluation. Redox Biol. 2013;1:353–8.
14. Butler R, Morris AD, Belch JJ, Hill A, Struthers AD. Allopurinol normalizes endothelial dysfunction in type 2 diabetics with mild hypertension. Hypertension. 2000;35:746–51.
15. Doughan AK, Harrison DG, Dikalov SI. Molecular mechanisms of angiotensin II-mediated mitochondrial dysfunction: linking mitochondrial oxidative damage and vascular endothelial dysfunction. Circ Res. 2008;102:488–96.
16. Dikalova AE, Bikineyeva AT, Budzyn K, Nazarewicz RR, McCann L, Lewis W, Harrison DG, Dikalov SI. Therapeutic targeting of mitochondrial superoxide in hypertension. Circ Res. 2010;107:106–16.
17. Stowe DF, Camara AK. Mitochondrial reactive oxygen species production in excitable cells: modulators of mitochondrial and cell function. Antioxid Redox Signal. 2009;11:1373–414.
18. Arteel GE, Briviba K, Sies H. Protection against peroxynitrite. FEBS Lett. 1999;445:226–30.
19. Cuevas S, Zhang Y, Yang Y, Escano C, Asico L, Jones JE, Armando I, Jose PA. Role of renal DJ-1 in the pathogenesis of hypertension associated with increased reactive oxygen species production. Hypertension. 2012;59:446–52.
20. Myung SK, Ju W, Cho B, Oh SW, Park SM, Koo BK, Park BJ. Efficacy of vitamin and antioxidant supplements in prevention of cardiovascular disease: systematic review and meta-analysis of randomised controlled trials. BMJ. 2013;346:f10.
21. Czernichow S, Bertrais S, Blacher J, Galan P, Briancon S, Favier A, Safar M, Hercberg S. Effect of supplementation with antioxidants upon long-term risk of hypertension in the SU.VI.MAX study: association with plasma antioxidant levels. J Hypertens. 2005;23:2013–8.
22. Bjelakovic G, Nikolova D, Gluud LL, Simonetti RG, Gluud C. Mortality in randomized trials of antioxidant supplements for primary and secondary prevention: systematic review and meta-analysis. JAMA. 2007;297:842–57.
23. Gray SP, Di Marco E, Okabe J, Szyndralewiez C, Heitz F, Montezano AC, de Haan JB, Koulis C, El-Osta A, Andrews KL, Chin-Dusting JP, Touyz RM, Wingler K, Cooper ME, Schmidt HH, Jandeleit-Dahm KA. NADPH oxidase 1 plays a key role in diabetes mellitus-accelerated atherosclerosis. Circulation. 2013;127: 1888–902.
24. Milman U, Blum S, Shapira C, Aronson D, Miller-Lotan R, Anbinder Y, Alshiek J, Bennett L, Kostenko M, Landau M, Keidar S, Levy Y, Khemlin A, Radan A, Levy AP. Vitamin E supplementation reduces cardiovascular events in a subgroup of middle-aged individuals with both type 2 diabetes mellitus and the haptoglobin 2–2 genotype: a prospective double-blinded clinical trial. Arterioscler Thromb Vasc Biol. 2008;28:341–7.
25. Robinson I, de Serna DG, Gutierrez A, Schade DS. Vitamin E in humans: an explanation of clinical trial failure. Endocr Pract. 2006;12:576–82.
26. Wang D, Chen Y, Chabrashvili T, Aslam S, Borrego Conde LJ, Umans JG, Wilcox CS. Role of oxidative stress in endothelial dysfunction and enhanced responses to angiotensin II of afferent arterioles from rabbits infused with angiotensin II. J Am Soc Nephrol. 2003;14:2783–9.

27. Fellner SK, Arendshorst WJ. Angiotensin II, reactive oxygen species, and Ca2+ signaling in afferent arterioles. Am J Physiol Renal Physiol. 2005;289:F1012–9.
28. Araujo M, Wilcox CS. Oxidative stress in hypertension: role of the kidney. Antioxid Redox Signal. 2014;20:74–101.
29. Lai EY, Wellstein A, Welch WJ, Wilcox CS. Superoxide modulates myogenic contractions of mouse afferent arterioles. Hypertension. 2011;58:650–6.
30. Meng S, Cason GW, Gannon AW, Racusen LC, Manning Jr RD. Oxidative stress in Dahl salt-sensitive hypertension. Hypertension. 2003;41:1346–52.
31. Jia J, Ding G, Zhu J, Chen C, Liang W, Franki N, Singhal PC. Angiotensin II infusion induces nephrin expression changes and podocyte apoptosis. Am J Nephrol. 2008;28:500–7.
32. Ren Z, Liang W, Chen C, Yang H, Singhal PC, Ding G. Angiotensin II induces nephrin dephosphorylation and podocyte injury: role of caveolin-1. Cell Signal. 2012;24:443–50.
33. Hua P, Feng W, Rezonzew G, Chumley P, Jaimes EA. The transcription factor ETS-1 regulates angiotensin II-stimulated fibronectin production in mesangial cells. Am J Physiol Renal Physiol. 2012;302:F1418–29.
34. Banday AA, Lokhandwala MF. Loss of biphasic effect on Na/K-ATPase activity by angiotensin II involves defective angiotensin type 1 receptor-nitric oxide signaling. Hypertension. 2008;52:1099–105.
35. Duan X, Kelsen SG, Merali S. Proteomic analysis of oxidative stress-responsive proteins in human pneumocytes: insight into the regulation of DJ-1 expression. J Proteome Res. 2008;7:4955–61.
36. Vallon V, Traynor T, Barajas L, Huang YG, Briggs JP, Schnermann J. Feedback control of glomerular vascular tone in neuronal nitric oxide synthase knockout mice. J Am Soc Nephrol. 2001;12:1599–606.
37. Liu R, Ren Y, Garvin JL, Carretero OA. Superoxide enhances tubuloglomerular feedback by constricting the afferent arteriole. Kidney Int. 2004;66:268–74.
38. Nouri P, Gill P, Li M, Wilcox CS, Welch WJ. p22phox in the macula densa regulates single nephron GFR during angiotensin II infusion in rats. Am J Physiol Heart Circ Physiol. 2007;292:H1685–9.
39. Sun P, Yue P, Wang WH. Angiotensin II stimulates epithelial sodium channels in the cortical collecting duct of the rat kidney. Am J Physiol Renal Physiol. 2012;302:F679–87.
40. Yu L, Bao HF, Self JL, Eaton DC, Helms MN. Aldosterone-induced increases in superoxide production counters nitric oxide inhibition of epithelial Na channel activity in A6 distal nephron cells. Am J Physiol Renal Physiol. 2007;293:F1666–77.
41. Dickhout JG, Mori T, Cowley Jr AW. Tubulovascular nitric oxide crosstalk: buffering of angiotensin II-induced medullary vasoconstriction. Circ Res. 2002;91:487–93.
42. Beltowski J, Marciniak A, Jamroz-Wisniewska A, Borkowska E. Nitric oxide – superoxide cooperation in the regulation of renal Na(+), K(+)-ATPase. Acta Biochim Pol. 2004;51:933–42.
43. Silva GB, Ortiz PA, Hong NJ, Garvin JL. Superoxide stimulates NaCl absorption in the thick ascending limb via activation of protein kinase C. Hypertension. 2006;48:467–72.
44. Garvin JL, Herrera M, Ortiz PA. Regulation of renal NaCl transport by nitric oxide, endothelin, and ATP: clinical implications. Annu Rev Physiol. 2011;73:359–76.
45. Guyenet PG. The sympathetic control of blood pressure. Nat Rev Neurosci. 2006;7:335–46.
46. Brody MJ. Central nervous system and mechanisms of hypertension. Clin Physiol Biochem. 1988;6:230–9.
47. Brody M, Fink G, Buggy J, Haywood J, Gordon F, Knuepfer M, Mow M, Mahoney L, Johnson A. Critical role of the AV3V region in development and maintenance of experimental hypertension. In: Schmitt H, Meyers P, editors. Perspectives in nephrology and hypertension. New York: Wiley and Flammarion; 1978. p. 76–84.
48. Zimmerman MC, Lazartigues E, Lang JA, Sinnayah P, Ahmad IM, Spitz DR, Davisson RL. Superoxide mediates the actions of angiotensin II in the central nervous system. Circ Res. 2002;91:1038–45.
49. Zimmerman MC, Lazartigues E, Sharma RV, Davisson RL. Hypertension caused by angiotensin II infusion involves increased superoxide production in the central nervous system. Circ Res. 2004;95:210–6.
50. Zimmerman MC, Sharma RV, Davisson RL. Superoxide mediates angiotensin II-induced influx of extracellular calcium in neural cells. Hypertension. 2005;45:717–23.
51. Zimmerman MC, Dunlay RP, Lazartigues E, Zhang Y, Sharma RV, Engelhardt JF, Davisson RL. Requirement for Rac1-dependent NADPH oxidase in the cardiovascular and dipsogenic actions of angiotensin II in the brain. Circ Res. 2004;95:532–9.
52. Peterson JR, Burmeister MA, Tian X, Zhou Y, Guruju MR, Stupinski JA, Sharma RV, Davisson RL. Genetic silencing of Nox2 and Nox4 reveals differential roles of these NADPH oxidase homologues in the vasopressor and dipsogenic effects of brain angiotensin II. Hypertension. 2009;54:1106–14.
53. Lob HE, Schultz D, Marvar PJ, Davisson RL, Harrison DG. Role of the NADPH oxidases in the subfornical organ in angiotensin II-induced hypertension. Hypertension. 2013;61:382–7.
54. Erdos B, Broxson CS, King MA, Scarpace PJ, Tumer N. Acute pressor effect of central angiotensin II is mediated by NAD(P)H-oxidase-dependent production of superoxide in the hypothalamic cardiovascular regulatory nuclei. J Hypertens. 2006;24:109–16.
55. Wang G, Anrather J, Huang J, Speth RC, Pickel VM, Iadecola C. NADPH oxidase contributes to angiotensin II signaling in the nucleus tractus solitarius. J Neurosci. 2004;24:5516–24.
56. Nozoe M, Hirooka Y, Koga Y, Sagara Y, Kishi T, Engelhardt JF, Sunagawa K. Inhibition of Rac1-derived reactive oxygen species in nucleus tractus solitarius decreases blood pressure and heart rate in stroke-prone spontaneously hypertensive rats. Hypertension. 2007;50:62–8.

57. Nishihara M, Hirooka Y, Matsukawa R, Kishi T, Sunagawa K. Oxidative stress in the rostral ventrolateral medulla modulates excitatory and inhibitory inputs in spontaneously hypertensive rats. J Hypertens. 2012;30:97–106.
58. Kishi T, Hirooka Y, Kimura Y, Ito K, Shimokawa H, Takeshita A. Increased reactive oxygen species in rostral ventrolateral medulla contribute to neural mechanisms of hypertension in stroke-prone spontaneously hypertensive rats. Circulation. 2004;109:2357–62.
59. Li Z, Mao HZ, Abboud FM, Chapleau MW. Oxygen-derived free radicals contribute to baroreceptor dysfunction in atherosclerotic rabbits. Circ Res. 1996;79: 802–11.
60. Grassi G, Seravalle G, Brambilla G, Mancia G. The sympathetic nervous system and new nonpharmacologic approaches to treating hypertension: a focus on renal denervation. Can J Cardiol. 2012;28:311–7.
61. DiBona GF, Esler M. Translational medicine: the antihypertensive effect of renal denervation. Am J Physiol Regul Integr Comp Physiol. 2010;298:R245–53.
62. Esler MD, Krum H, Sobotka PA, Schlaich MP, Schmieder RE, Bohm M. Renal sympathetic denervation in patients with treatment-resistant hypertension (The Symplicity HTN-2 Trial): a randomised controlled trial. Lancet. 2010;376:1903–9.
63. Chan SH, Tai MH, Li CY, Chan JY. Reduction in molecular synthesis or enzyme activity of superoxide dismutases and catalase contributes to oxidative stress and neurogenic hypertension in spontaneously hypertensive rats. Free Radic Biol Med. 2006;40:2028–39.
64. Ye S, Zhong H, Yanamadala S, Campese VM. Oxidative stress mediates the stimulation of sympathetic nerve activity in the phenol renal injury model of hypertension. Hypertension. 2006;48:309–15.
65. Campese VM, Ye S. A vitamin-E-fortified diet reduces oxidative stress, sympathetic nerve activity, and hypertension in the phenol-renal injury model in rats. J Am Soc Hypertens. 2007;1:242–50.
66. Dharmashankar K, Widlansky ME. Vascular endothelial function and hypertension: insights and directions. Curr Hypertens Rep. 2010;12:448–55.
67. Chandra S, Romero MJ, Shatanawi A, Alkilany AM, Caldwell RB, Caldwell RW. Oxidative species increase arginase activity in endothelial cells through the RhoA/Rho kinase pathway. Br J Pharmacol. 2012; 165:506–19.
68. Minuz P, Patrignani P, Gaino S, Degan M, Menapace L, Tommasoli R, Seta F, Capone ML, Tacconelli S, Palatresi S, Bencini C, Del Vecchio C, Mansueto G, Arosio E, Santonastaso CL, Lechi A, Morganti A, Patrono C. Increased oxidative stress and platelet activation in patients with hypertension and renovascular disease. Circulation. 2002;106:2800–5.
69. Laude K, Cai H, Fink B, Hoch N, Weber DS, McCann L, Kojda G, Fukai T, Schmidt HH, Dikalov S, Ramasamy S, Gamez G, Griendling KK, Harrison DG. Hemodynamic and biochemical adaptations to vascular smooth muscle overexpression of p22phox in mice. Am J Physiol Heart Circ Physiol. 2005;288:H7–12.
70. Patel R, Cardneau JD, Colles SM, Graham LM. Synthetic smooth muscle cell phenotype is associated with increased nicotinamide adenine dinucleotide phosphate oxidase activity: effect on collagen secretion. J Vasc Surg. 2006;43:364–71.
71. Kohler R, Heyken WT, Heinau P, Schubert R, Si H, Kacik M, Busch C, Grgic I, Maier T, Hoyer J. Evidence for a functional role of endothelial transient receptor potential V4 in shear stress-induced vasodilatation. Arterioscler Thromb Vasc Biol. 2006; 26:1495–502.
72. Zheng X, Zinkevich NS, Gebremedhin D, Gauthier KM, Nishijima Y, Fang J, Wilcox DA, Campbell WB, Gutterman DD, Zhang DX. Arachidonic acid-induced dilation in human coronary arterioles: convergence of signaling mechanisms on endothelial TRPV4-mediated Ca2+ entry. J Am Heart Assoc. 2013;2:e000080.
73. Cai H, Li Z, Davis ME, Kanner W, Harrison DG, Dudley Jr SC. Akt-dependent phosphorylation of serine 1179 and mitogen-activated protein kinase kinase/extracellular signal-regulated kinase 1/2 cooperatively mediate activation of the endothelial nitric-oxide synthase by hydrogen peroxide. Mol Pharmacol. 2003;63:325–31.
74. Sesso HD, Buring JE, Rifai N, Blake GJ, Gaziano JM, Ridker PM. C-reactive protein and the risk of developing hypertension. JAMA. 2003;290: 2945–51.
75. Guzik TJ, Hoch NE, Brown KA, McCann LA, Rahman A, Dikalov S, Goronzy J, Weyand C, Harrison DG. Role of the T cell in the genesis of angiotensin II induced hypertension and vascular dysfunction. J Exp Med. 2007;204:2449–60.
76. Crowley SD, Frey CW, Gould SK, Griffiths R, Ruiz P, Burchette JL, Howell DN, Makhanova N, Yan M, Kim HS, Tharaux PL, Coffman TM. Stimulation of lymphocyte responses by angiotensin II promotes kidney injury in hypertension. Am J Physiol Renal Physiol. 2008;295:F515–24.
77. Mattson DL, Lund H, Guo C, Rudemiller N, Geurts AM, Jacob H. Genetic mutation of recombination activating gene 1 in Dahl salt-sensitive rats attenuates hypertension and renal damage. Am J Physiol Regul Integr Comp Physiol. 2013;304:R407–14.
78. Madhur MS, Lob HE, McCann LA, Iwakura Y, Blinder Y, Guzik TJ, Harrison DG. Interleukin 17 promotes angiotensin II-induced hypertension and vascular dysfunction. Hypertension. 2010;55:500–7.
79. Cornelius DC, Hogg JP, Scott J, Wallace K, Herse F, Moseley J, Wallukat G, Dechend R, Lamarca B. Administration of interleukin-17 soluble receptor C suppresses TH17 cells, oxidative stress, and hypertension in response to placental ischemia during pregnancy. Hypertension. 2013;62:1068–73.
80. Nguyen H, Chiasson VL, Chatterjee P, Kopriva SE, Young KJ, Mitchell BM. Interleukin-17 causes Rho-kinase-mediated endothelial dysfunction and hypertension. Cardiovasc Res. 2013;97: 696–704.

81. Hoch NE, Guzik TJ, Chen W, Deans T, Maalouf SA, Gratze P, Weyand C, Harrison DG. Regulation of T-cell function by endogenously produced angiotensin II. Am J Physiol Regul Integr Comp Physiol. 2009;296:R208–16.

82. Liu J, Yang F, Yang XP, Jankowski M, Pagano PJ. NAD(P)H oxidase mediates angiotensin II-induced vascular macrophage infiltration and medial hypertrophy. Arterioscler Thromb Vasc Biol. 2003;23:776–82.

Heart Failure with Preserved Ejection Fraction

16

Scott L. Hummel

Abstract

Of the millions of heart failure heart failure patients worldwide, approximately half present with preserved left ventricular ejection fraction (HFPEF). HFPEF has high rates of morbidity and mortality, yet therapy remains empirical due to incomplete understanding of disease pathophysiology. Systemic hypertension is the most prominent risk factor for HFPEF. Patients often have multiple other comorbid conditions, which may contribute to symptom burden and the HFPEF syndrome itself. The classic paradigm of ventricular diastolic dysfunction has expanded, and vascular dysfunction likely contributes to HFPEF in many patients. Pressure-volume loop analysis identifies three distinct hemodynamic phenotypes for HFPEF, a finding which may have significant implications for clinical trial enrollment and individual patient treatment.

Keywords

Heart Failure • Diastolic • Vascular Stiffness • Hypertension • Elderly • Endothelial dysfunction

Introduction

Over five million Americans currently have heart failure, and of these approximately half have preserved left ventricular ejection fraction (HFPEF) [1]. The clinical signs and symptoms, substantial morbidity burden, and long-term mortality rates in HFPEF patients are similar to those observed in heart failure with reduced ejection fraction (HFREF). Over 50 % of HFPEF patients die within 5 years after diagnosis [1, 2], and over a third of patients hospitalized for decompensated HFPEF die or are readmitted within 90 days of discharge [3]. Mortality rates in HFREF have decreased in recent years with the advent of evidence-based medication and device therapies. In contrast, large clinical trials in HFPEF have not clearly established evidence-based treatments, therapy remains empirical, and outcomes have not improved [1].

Systemic hypertension is a major risk factor for the development of HFPEF, but the specific aspects of hypertension that promote HFPEF are

S.L. Hummel
Division of Cardiovascular Medicine,
Department of Internal Medicine,
University of Michigan, Ann Arbor, MI, USA
e-mail: scothumm@med.umich.edu

M.E. Safar et al. (eds.), *Blood Pressure and Arterial Wall Mechanics in Cardiovascular Diseases*,
DOI 10.1007/978-1-4471-5198-2_16,

still undefined. The epidemiology of HFPEF differs from that of HFREF in several notable ways, including female predominance, older age, and a lower prevalence of known coronary artery disease [3, 4]. Patients with HFPEF commonly have multiple comorbidities such as obesity, sleep apnea, anemia, diabetes, and chronic renal insufficiency. These conditions make diagnosis challenging as they can mimic heart failure signs and symptoms (e.g. fatigue, edema, dyspnea), but also may contribute directly to the pathophysiology of HFPEF [5, 6].

Some question the concept of HFPEF as a distinct clinical disorder, but overall mortality and hospitalization for decompensated heart failure is clearly higher than in age-matched patients with similar comorbidities who do not have heart failure [7]. Clinical trials in HFPEF have typically defined the threshold for 'preserved' left ventricular ejection fraction as 40–45 %, primarily due to the exclusion of such patients from HFREF trials. Due to the bimodal distribution of ejection fraction in large heart failure registries [3], current diagnostic guidelines for HFPEF mandate left ventricular ejection fraction ≥50 %. Early HFPEF guidelines required invasive confirmation of left ventricular diastolic dysfunction. The 2007 European Society of Cardiology criteria also allow for echocardiographic determination of diastolic dysfunction, as well as the diagnosis of HFPEF with indeterminate diastolic function but other supportive structural (e.g. left ventricular hypertrophy, left atrial enlargement) or neurohormonal evidence [8]. The classic paradigm of 'diastolic' heart failure [9] has recently been expanded to incorporate additional mechanisms. The importance of vascular structural and functional abnormalities in HFPEF is increasingly recognized, and the HFPEF syndrome provides an opportunity to integrate several topics described elsewhere in this book.

Pressure-Volume Loop Analysis in HFPEF

The hemodynamic contributors to HFPEF may be explored through considering the cardiac pressure-volume loop (Fig. 16.1), which provides important information on ventricular performance and ventricular-arterial interactions. The arterial elastance (Ea; green line in Fig. 16.1), is a lumped arterial afterload parameter that combines the net effects of steady and pulsatile components. The Ea is defined as the central end-systolic pressure divided by the ventricular stroke volume (SV) and is dependent on arterial resistance, proximal aortic stiffness, and heart rate. The ventricular end-systolic elastance (Ees; red line in Fig. 16.1) is defined as the central end-systolic pressure divided by the end-systolic volume (ESV) minus the 'unstressed' ventricular volume (V_O, generally considered negligible under physiologic loading conditions). The Ees is classically assessed by constructing multiple pressure-volume loops with a conductance catheter while varying ventricular preload, but single-beat echocardiographic methods have been devised and invasively validated [10]. The Ees intersects with Ea at the central end-systolic pressure, defines the end-systolic pressure-volume relationship (ESPVR), and governs the systolic contours of the cardiac pressure-volume loop along with the end-diastolic volume (EDV)

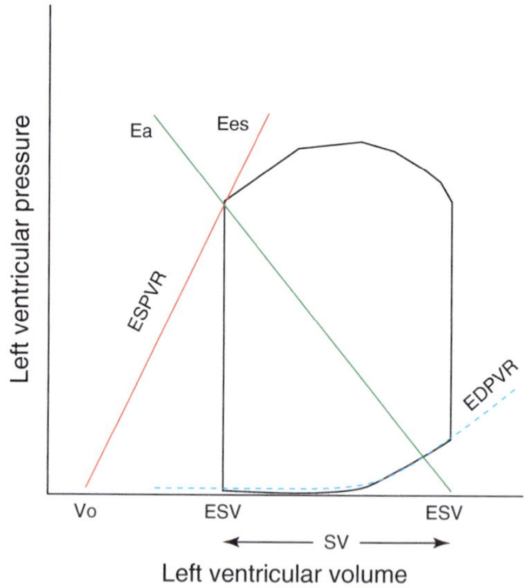

Fig. 16.1 Cardiac pressure-volume loop. Abbreviations: *Ea* arterial elastance, *Ees* ventricular end-systolic elastance, *EDV* end-diastolic volume, *EDPVR* end-diastolic pressure-volume relationship, *ESV* end-systolic volume, *ESPVR* end-systolic pressure-volume relationship, *SV* stroke volume, *Vo* unstressed ventricular volume

and ESV. The ratio Ea/Ees describes ventricular-arterial 'coupling,' a measure of how efficiently ventricular work transfers blood volume to the arterial system during systole. The non-linear end-diastolic pressure-volume relationship (EDPVR; blue dotted line in Fig. 16.1) is defined by the pressure required to fill the ventricle to a given volume.

The traditional paradigm of diastolic heart failure is characterized by a leftward and upward shift of the EDPVR and increased left ventricular end-diastolic pressure in the setting of concentric left ventricular hypertrophy, 'trouble filling the heart,' and resultant small EDV and SV [9]. The presence of diastolic dysfunction increases concomitantly with age and hypertension, and over one-quarter of American adults over the age of 45 have echocardiographic evidence of left ventricular diastolic dysfunction [11]. In longitudinally followed community cohorts, the presence of even mild diastolic dysfunction independently increases long-term mortality [11]. Diastolic dysfunction predicts incident heart failure across diverse U.S. populations, including the primarily Caucasian Olmstead County, Minnesota community cohort [12], the African American Study of Kidney Disease and Hypertension cohort [13], and the Cardiovascular Health Study of community-living older adults [14].

However, it is crucial to note that diastolic dysfunction overlaps significantly between HFPEF patients and asymptomatic hypertensives with left ventricular hypertrophy [15]. The presence of ventricular diastolic dysfunction does not necessarily signify HFPEF, which remains a clinical diagnosis requiring the specific signs and/or symptoms of heart failure. Interestingly, in the archetypal model of diastolic heart failure, described above and shown in Fig. 16.2a, the constraints of the pressure-volume loop dictate normal or reduced systolic blood pressure. The observation that most HFPEF patients have systemic hypertension [1, 4], rather than low blood pressure, suggests that additional mechanisms beyond ventricular diastolic dysfunction contribute to HFPEF.

Maurer and colleagues used the pressure-volume loop concept to propose two additional possible hemodynamic phenotypes for HFPEF, assuming ventricular SV ≥50 % of EDV and normal or increased ESPVR slope (i.e., left ventricular ejection fraction ≥50 % and normal ventricular contractile function). One model includes tandem increases in Ea and Ees, leading to elevated end-systolic pressure, and concentric left ventricular remodeling with diastolic dysfunction and upward/leftward shift of the EDPVR (Fig. 16.2b). Another proposed phenotype involves ventricular 'overfilling,' with elevated systemic and left ventricular end-diastolic pressures despite normal Ea, Ees, and EDPVR in the setting of elevated EDV (Fig. 16.2c). Using sophisticated three-dimensional echocardiographic analysis, their group noninvasively confirmed these three phenotypes in a small group of HFPEF patients [16].

Mechanistic Studies in Human HFPEF

While diastolic dysfunction may not be the sole mechanism in all patients with HFPEF, several contemporary studies do validate its importance. Lam and colleagues, evaluating the Olmstead County echocardiographic cohort, noted that HFPEF patients had delayed ventricular relaxation and increased ventricular stiffness when compared with hypertensives without heart failure [17]. Westermann et al. studied 70 HFPEF patients using conductance catheters to construct pressure-volume loops. In comparison to controls, HFPEF patients had increased left ventricular stiffness and an upward and leftward shifted EDPVR at rest and during rapid atrial pacing [18]. Borlaug's group studied HFPEF patients during cycle ergometry, a more physiologic exercise stimulus. They also linked increased filling pressures and an upward shift of the EDPVR to intrinsic ventricular stiffness and reduced diastolic filling time at higher heart rates [19].

The effects of hypertension and arterial afterload on ventricular diastolic function are often underappreciated. Ventricular relaxation is an energy-dependent process that requires calcium re-sequestration and uncoupling of myosin-actin

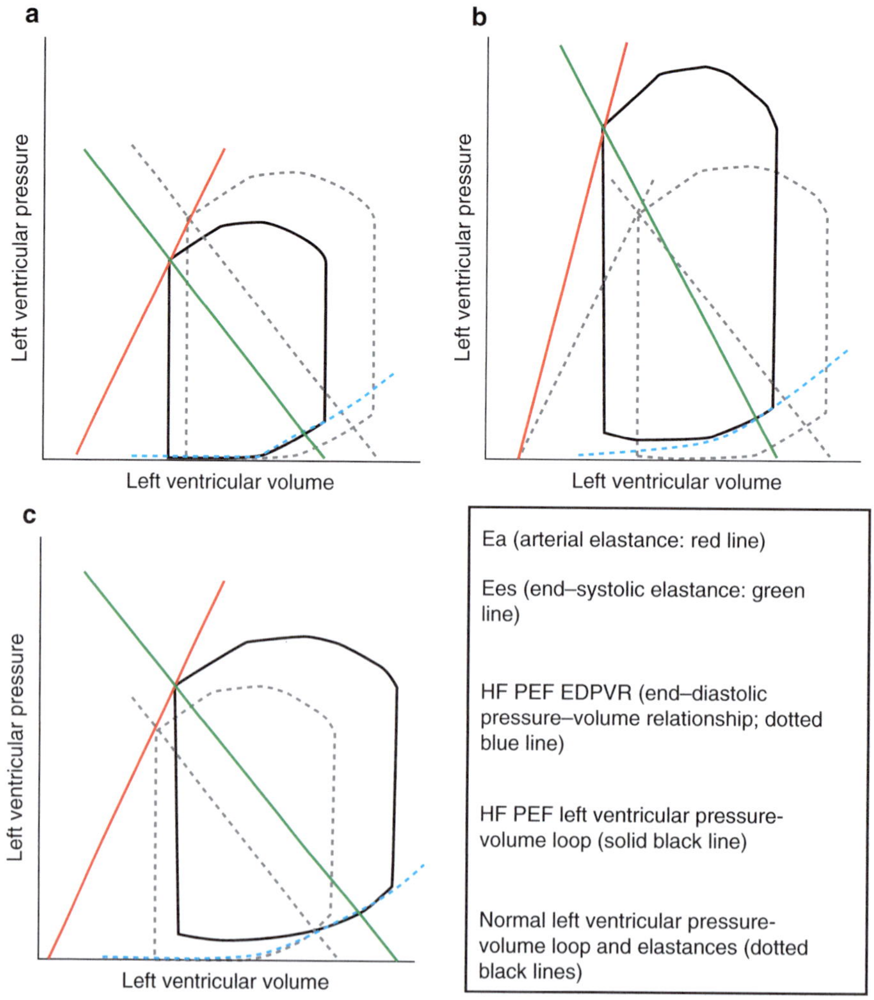

Fig. 16.2 Possible hemodynamic phenotypes of HFPEF. (**a**) Isolated diastolic dysfunction, (**b**) Combined ventricular-vascular stiffening, (**c**) Increased plasma volume (Adapted from Maurer et al. [16])

cross-bridges. Not only are more cross-bridges engaged during systole to generate pressure in patients with uncontrolled hypertension, such patients may have prolonged cross-bridge attachment time due to altered phosphorylation of troponin [20]. Gandhi et al. studied 38 patients with hypertensive pulmonary edema (presenting systolic blood pressure >160 mmHg), finding that 18 had normal left ventricular ejection fraction and mitral valve function during and after the episode. The authors of this report hypothesized that in these patients, acute increases in blood pressure exacerbated diastolic dysfunction [21]. This concept is supported by the work of Leite-Moreira and colleagues, who altered ventricular preload (via caval occlusion or dextran infusion) and afterload (by graded aortic occlusion) in rabbits. They found that acute increases in afterload delayed ventricular relaxation and shifted the EDPVR upward, i.e. induced ventricular diastolic dysfunction. These effects were particularly evident under conditions of high ventricular preload, as would be expected in volume-expanded HFPEF patients [22]. Westermann and colleagues invasively studied HFPEF patients during handgrip exercise, and confirmed that this acute afterload stimulus increased left ventricular end-diastolic pressure [18].

Systemic hypertension and aging are commonly associated with increased proximal arterial stiffness, but HFPEF patients have markedly reduced aortic distensibility [23] even after adjustment for these factors. Redfield and colleagues observed that Ea and Ees both increased with age in the Olmstead County cohort, particularly in women. They hypothesized that age-and gender-related arterial stiffening contributed to incident HFPEF and might explain its female predominance [24]. However, subsequent analysis of the same cohort revealed that the magnitude of increase in Ea and Ees was similar among HFPEF patients and hypertensives without heart failure even after adjustment for age, gender, and body size. Noting impaired ventricular relaxation and increased ventricular stiffness, the authors concluded that diastolic dysfunction, rather than arterial stiffness, was the key determinant of progression from compensated hypertensive heart disease to HFPEF [17].

Combined increases in Ees and proximal arterial stiffness amplify the effects of small changes in ventricular preload, as shown in Fig. 16.2b, and markedly increase the energy cost for cardiac output [25]. While Ees is often described as a measure of ventricular contractile function, it is important to remember that this parameter also incorporates intrinsic ventricular stiffness (e.g. due to fibrosis and myocyte hypertrophy) [26]. A 'normal' Ees may not actually reflect normal ventricular contractile reserve. Indeed several studies demonstrate that echocardiographic indices of whole-chamber and mid-myocardial contractility are decreased in HFPEF [26, 27]. Moderate-intensity and peak cycle ergometry exercise clearly illustrate the disproportionate impact of proximal arterial stiffness on ventricular afterload and cardiac output in patients with HFPEF [28, 29]. Part of the mechanism for exertional limitations, particularly in hypertensive HFPEF, may be an inability to augment left ventricular contractile function to match arterial load during exercise [25, 28–30].

With normal aging, conduit artery endothelial function declines in tandem with exercise capacity. Reduced vasodilator reserve contributes to exercise intolerance in HFREF, but the additive role of endothelial dysfunction in HFPEF is currently controversial. Haykowsky and colleagues studied 48 older HFPEF patients during upright cycle ergometry, and noted that the arteriovenous oxygen difference from rest to peak exercise was the strongest predictor of peak oxygen consumption. They suggested that peripheral, non-cardiac factors partially govern exercise intolerance in HFPEF [31]. However, the same group later found that brachial and femoral flow-mediated dilation did not differ between HFPEF patients and age-matched controls [32, 33], leading them to conclude that conduit artery endothelial dysfunction did not relate to reduced exercise capacity.

Several lines of evidence suggest that microvascular endothelial dysfunction contributes significantly to HFPEF. Aging, hypertension, and left ventricular hypertrophy are associated with decreased coronary flow reserve in the absence of epicardial coronary artery disease [34]. Endomyocardial biopsy specimens in human HFPEF show robust expression of endothelial adhesion molecules in the coronary microvasculature [35]. Using laser Doppler imaging, Balmain and colleagues found that HFPEF patients had cutaneous microvascular endothelial dysfunction equivalent to HFREF subjects and beyond that seen in controls with coronary artery disease [36]. Borlaug et al. studied HFPEF patients and age-matched hypertensives, and noted that both groups had similarly impaired reactive hyperemic blood flow following arm occlusion when compared with controls. However, HFPEF patients alone had a blunted increase in digital pulse amplitude (i.e. impaired vasodilation) during cycle exercise [30]. Finally, in a large prospective Japanese HFPEF cohort, the reactive hyperemia index strongly predicted cardiovascular events, independent of other traditional risk factors [37].

At least some patients with clinical HFPEF have normal EDPVR curves and elevated ventricular end-diastolic pressure due to increased EDV (Fig. 16.2c) [5, 16]. Large cohort studies confirm that a proportion of HFPEF patients has eccentric, rather than concentric, left ventricular hypertrophy and increased, rather than decreased,

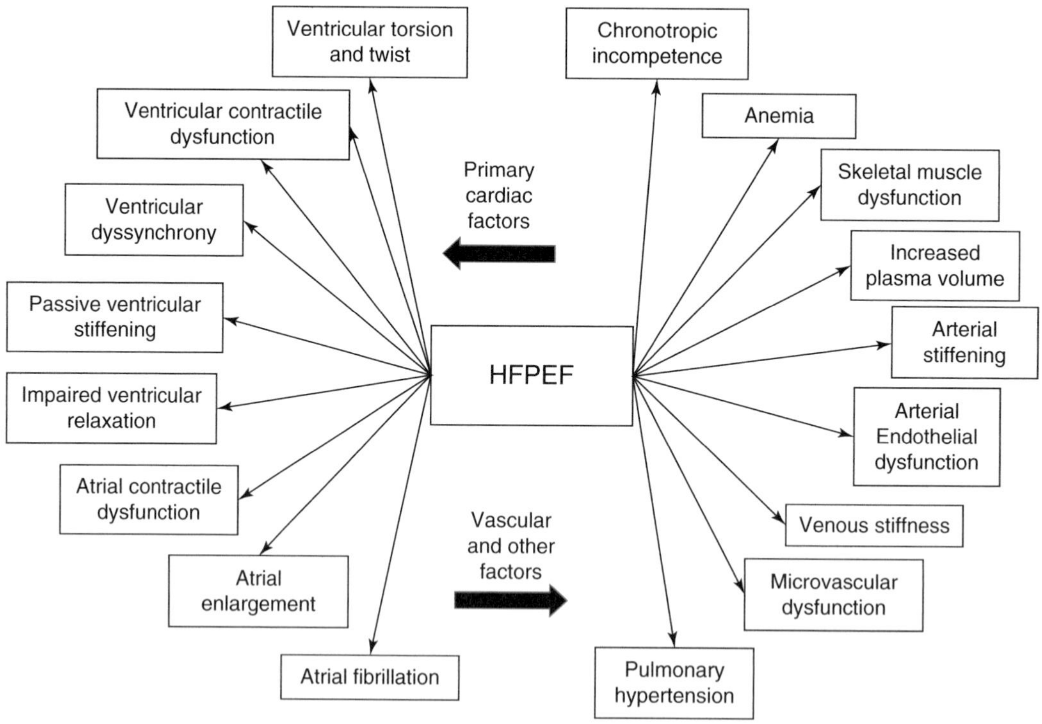

Fig. 16.3 Cardiac, vascular, and other contributors to HFPEF

EDV [38]. This ventricular 'overfilling' often occurs in the setting of comorbidities that increase plasma volume (e.g., anemia, chronic kidney disease, obesity) [5, 6]. Moreover, patients with HFPEF have reduced peripheral venous capacitance even when compared with HFREF subjects [36]. In humans with HFREF [39] and dogs with normal ejection fraction undergoing volume loading [40], venous stretch is associated with oxidative stress, pro-inflammatory gene expression, and endothelial dysfunction. Since the peripheral venous reservoir contains over 70 % of the systemic blood volume, even a small redistribution of blood to the central circulation could have amplified effects on cardiac filling pressure and systemic blood pressure lability (e.g., Fig. 16.2b), greatly increasing the risk for heart failure decompensation [41].

In addition to the mechanisms described above, many other potential contributors to the HFPEF syndrome have recently been explored (Fig. 16.3); a partial list includes pulmonary hypertension with or without right heart failure [42], chronotropic incompetence [30, 43] as well as inappropriate tachycardia during exercise [44], left atrial contractile dysfunction [45], impaired natriuretic peptide function [46], anemia [47], and skeletal muscle metabolic dysfunction [48, 49].

Implications for HFPEF Management

Given the phenotypic heterogeneity outlined above, it is perhaps unsurprising that HFPEF remains without universal, evidence-based treatment. Clinical treatment trials in HFPEF have been reviewed elsewhere [50, 51], and extensive discussion is beyond the scope of this chapter. However, several general principles can be outlined based on this experience.

First, systemic hypertension is clearly a strong risk factor for adverse cardiovascular remodeling and subsequent HFPEF. Treatment of systolic hypertension, even in very elderly subjects, markedly reduces incident heart failure [52]. Blood pressure reduction, regardless of agent or mechanism, improves ventricular diastolic function [53–55]. Pharmacological blood pressure treatment also reduces Ea and Ees, improves ventricular-arterial coupling, and increases ventricular systolic performance [55]. Current guidelines recommend aggressive control of systolic blood pressure to prevent and manage HFPEF [56, 57], although this must be balanced against the likelihood of orthostatic hypotension, reduced coronary perfusion, and other concerns in the setting of advanced age and combined ventricular-vascular stiffening with attendant blood pressure lability (e.g. Fig. 16.2b).

The rationale for blockade of the renin-angiotensin-aldosterone system (RAAS) in HFPEF is strong based on data from numerous HFPEF animal models and studies demonstrating benefits in human HFREF. Unfortunately, large clinical trials of angiotensin-converting enzyme inhibition (ACEI) and angiotensin-receptor blockade (ARB) failed to improve mortality or cardiovascular morbidity, although these studies were plagued by a lower-than-expected event rate and a high rate of crossover to open-label agents [58–60]. Aldosterone blockade reduces collagen production and diastolic dysfunction in animal models and humans, but did not affect exertional capacity or quality of life in the 450-patient ALDO-DHF study [54]. Moreover, the multinational Treatment Of Preserved Cardiac function heart failure with an Aldosterone anTagonist (TOPCAT) study recently demonstrated a neutral effect of spironolactone on combined death and heart failure hospitalization in 3,445 HFPEF patients [61].

Of note, HFPEF patients with eccentric ventricular hypertrophy have reduced contractility and increased ventricular compliance when compared to those patients having concentric hypertrophy [62]. These characteristics (e.g., Fig. 16.2c vs. Fig. 16.2b) are more similar to those seen in HFREF, and suggest a potential subgroup that could benefit from RAAS inhibition. In support of this concept, a recent propensity-adjusted analysis of the Swedish Heart Failure Registry suggested that ACEI/ARB modestly reduce mortality in HFPEF, particularly in patients with ejection fraction 40–49 % [63]. However, this favorable signal was not seen in a propensity-matched analysis of hospitalized HFPEF patients from the Organized Program to Initiate Lifesaving Treatment in Hospitalized Patients with Heart Failure (OPTIMIZE-HF) study, in which aldosterone antagonists had no effect on all-cause mortality or hospitalization [64]. Further subgroup analysis of TOPCAT may reveal specific phenotypes of HFPEF that are more likely to benefit from RAAS blockade.

Other small, mechanism-oriented studies further highlight the importance of physiological phenotyping in HFPEF. For example, phosphodiesterase-5 inhibition with sildenafil had neutral effects on quality of life and functional capacity in 216 HFPEF patients [65]. In contrast, Guazzi et al. found that in 44 HFPEF patients with pulmonary hypertension and hemodynamics consistent with right heart dysfunction, sildenafil markedly improved left ventricular diastolic function, right heart pressures, and quality of life over 12 months of therapy [42]. Studying 17 previously hospitalized HFPEF patients, Borlaug and colleagues observed that chronotropic incompetence was a major factor limiting cardiac output and maximal exertional capacity [43]. However, Kosmala et al. recently treated 61 less ill HFPEF patients with exercise-induced diastolic dysfunction to 7 days of placebo or ivabradine, which reduces heart rate without impairing contractile function, and found that peak treadmill oxygen consumption increased by more than 20 % in the ivabradine group [44]. Data from HFREF patients suggest that at least part of this effect may have been due to reductions in Ea and improved ventricular-arterial coupling [66].

The disappointment of large pharmacological trials to date in HFPEF has nonetheless enabled a rethinking of treatment strategies and underlying mechanisms. Intriguing early data suggest that skeletal muscle metabolic abnormalities are present in HFPEF [49], and medically-supervised exercise training increases peak exercise oxygen uptake, 6-min walk distance, and physical quality-of-life scores in HFPEF patients [67, 68].

Chronic oxidative stress and vascular dysfunction are key driving mechanisms for HFPEF in 'salt-sensitive' animal models [69–71]. In a recent pilot study in 13 hypertensive HFPEF patients, Hummel and colleagues found that the sodium-restricted DASH diet reduced blood pressure and oxidative stress while improving ventricular diastolic function and ventricular-arterial coupling [72, 73]. Systemic inflammatory markers strongly predict HFPEF in cohort studies of older adults [74, 75], and some propose coronary microvascular inflammation, driven by multiple pro-oxidant comorbidities, as the central defect in HFPEF [71]. This paradigm could lead to innovative anti-inflammatory or anti-oxidant therapeutic strategies.

Conclusions

A growing body of evidence portrays HFPEF as a heterogeneous and multifactorial syndrome which may have similar clinical manifestations but quite different underlying causes depending on the patient (Fig. 16.3). Recent studies indicate that HFPEF patients often have failure of cardiovascular reserve in multiple domains beyond diastolic function [26, 29, 30], and non-cardiac factors are likely important in some patients [47–49]. Physiological phenotyping may help choose the proper treatment regimen for a given HFPEF patient as well as guide the selection of appropriate participants for future HFPEF clinical trials.

References

1. Owan TE, Hodge DO, Herges RM, Jacobsen SJ, Roger VL, Redfield MM. Trends in prevalence and outcome of heart failure with preserved ejection fraction. N Engl J Med. 2006;355:251–9.
2. Tribouilloy C, Rusinaru D, Mahjoub H, Souliere V, Levy F, Peltier M, Slama M, Massy Z. Prognosis of heart failure with preserved ejection fraction: a 5 year prospective population-based study. Eur Heart J. 2008;29:339–47.
3. Fonarow GC, Stough WG, Abraham WT, Albert NM, Gheorghiade M, Greenberg BH, O'Connor CM, Sun JL, Yancy CW, Young JB. Characteristics, treatments, and outcomes of patients with preserved systolic function hospitalized for heart failure: a report from the OPTIMIZE-HF registry. J Am Coll Cardiol. 2007;50:768–77.
4. Yancy CW, Lopatin M, Stevenson LW, De Marco T, Fonarow GC, ADHERE Scientific Advisory Committee and Investigators. Clinical presentation, management, and in-hospital outcomes of patients admitted with acute decompensated heart failure with preserved systolic function: a report from the Acute Decompensated HEart failure national REgistry (ADHERE) database. J Am Coll Cardiol. 2006;47:76–84.
5. Abramov D, He K-L, Wang J, Burkhoff D, Maurer MS. The impact of extra cardiac comorbidities on pressure volume relations in heart failure and preserved ejection fraction. J Card Fail. 2011;17:547–55.
6. Mohammed SF, Borlaug BA, Roger VL, Mirzoyev SA, Rodeheffer RJ, Chirinos JA, Redfield MM. Comorbidity and ventricular and vascular structure and function in heart failure with preserved ejection fraction: a community-based study. Circ Heart Fail. 2012;5:710–9.
7. Campbell RT, Jhund PS, Castagno D, Hawkins NM, Petrie MC, McMurray JJV. What have we learned about patients with heart failure and preserved ejection fraction from DIG-PEF, CHARM-preserved, and I-PRESERVE? J Am Coll Cardiol. 2012;60:2349–56.
8. Paulus WJ, Tschope C, Sanderson JE, Rusconi C, Flachskampf FA, Rademakers FE, Marino P, Smiseth OA, De Keulenaer G, Leite-Moreira AF, Borbely A, Edes I, Handoko ML, Heymans S, Pezzali N, Pieske B, Dickstein K, Fraser AG, Brutsaert DL. How to diagnose diastolic heart failure: a consensus statement on the diagnosis of heart failure with normal left ventricular ejection fraction by the Heart Failure and Echocardiography Associations of the European Society of Cardiology. Eur Heart J. 2007;28:2539–50.
9. Zile MR, Baicu CF, Gaasch WH. Diastolic heart failure – abnormalities in active relaxation and passive stiffness of the left ventricle. N Engl J Med. 2004;350:1953–9.
10. Chen CH, Fetics B, Nevo E, Rochitte CE, Chiou KR, Ding PA, Kawaguchi M, Kass DA. Noninvasive single-beat determination of left ventricular end-systolic elastance in humans. J Am Coll Cardiol. 2001;38:2028–34.
11. Redfield MM, Jacobsen SJ Jr CBJ, Mahoney DW, Bailey KR, Rodeheffer RJ. Burden of systolic and diastolic ventricular dysfunction in the community: appreciating the scope of the heart failure epidemic. JAMA. 2003;289:194–202 [see comment].
12. Lam CSP, Lyass A, Kraigher-Krainer E, Massaro JM, Lee DS, Ho JE, Levy D, Redfield MM, Pieske BM, Benjamin EJ, Vasan RS. Cardiac dysfunction and noncardiac dysfunction as precursors of heart failure with reduced and preserved ejection fraction in the community/clinical perspective. Circulation. 2011;124:24–30.
13. Peterson GE, de Backer T, Contreras G, Wang X, Kendrick C, Greene T, Appel LJ, Randall OS, Lea J, Smogorzewski M, Vagaonescu T, Phillips RA. Relationship of left ventricular hypertrophy and

diastolic function with cardiovascular and renal outcomes in African-Americans with hypertensive chronic kidney disease. Hypertension. 2013;62:518–25.
14. Aurigemma GP, Gottdiener JS, Shemanski L, Gardin J, Kitzman D. Predictive value of systolic and diastolic function for incident congestive heart failure in the elderly: The Cardiovascular Health Study. J Am Coll Cardiol. 2001;37:1042–8.
15. Melenovsky V, Borlaug BA, Rosen B, Hay I, Ferruci L, Morell CH, Lakatta EG, Najjar SS, Kass DA. Cardiovascular features of heart failure with preserved ejection fraction versus nonfailing hypertensive left ventricular hypertrophy in the urban Baltimore community: the role of atrial remodeling/dysfunction. J Am Coll Cardiol. 2007;49:198–207.
16. Maurer MS, King DL, El-Khoury Rumbarger L, Packer M, Burkhoff D. Left heart failure with a normal ejection fraction: identification of different pathophysiologic mechanisms. J Card Fail. 2005;11:177–87.
17. Lam CSP, Roger VL, Rodeheffer RJ, Bursi F, Borlaug BA, Ommen SR, Kass DA, Redfield MM. Cardiac structure and ventricular-vascular function in persons with heart failure and preserved ejection fraction from Olmsted County, Minnesota. Circulation. 2007;115:1982–90.
18. Westermann D, Kasner M, Steendijk P, Spillmann F, Riad A, Weitmann K, Hoffmann W, Poller W, Pauschinger M, Schultheiss H-P, Tschope C. Role of left ventricular stiffness in heart failure with normal ejection fraction. Circulation. 2008;117:2051–60.
19. Borlaug BA, Jaber WA, Ommen SR, Lam CSP, Redfield MM, Nishimura RA. Diastolic relaxation and compliance reserve during dynamic exercise in heart failure with preserved ejection fraction. Heart. 2011;97:964–9.
20. Donaldson C, Palmer BM, Zile M, Maughan DW, Ikonomidis JS, Granzier H, Meyer M, VanBuren P, LeWinter MM. Myosin cross-bridge dynamics in patients with hypertension and concentric left ventricular remodeling. Circ Heart Fail. 2012;5:803–11.
21. Gandhi SK, Powers JC, Nomeir A-M, Fowle K, Kitzman DW, Rankin KM, Little WC. The pathogenesis of acute pulmonary edema associated with hypertension. N Engl J Med. 2001;344:17–22.
22. Noumi B, Teruya S, Salomon S, Helmke S, Maurer MS. Blood volume measurements in patients with heart failure and a preserved ejection fraction: implications for diagnosing anemia. Congest Heart Fail. 2011;17:14–8.
23. Hundley WG, Kitzman DW, Morgan TM, Hamilton CA, Darty SN, Stewart KP, Herrington DM, Link KM, Little WC. Cardiac cycle-dependent changes in aortic area and distensibility are reduced in older patients with isolated diastolic heart failure and correlate with exercise intolerance. J Am Coll Cardiol. 2001;38:796–802.
24. Redfield MM, Jacobsen SJ, Borlaug BA, Rodeheffer RJ, Kass DA. Age- and gender-related ventricular-vascular stiffening: a community-based study. Circulation. 2005;112:2254–62.
25. Kawaguchi M, Hay I, Fetics B, Kass DA. Combined ventricular systolic and arterial stiffening in patients with heart failure and preserved ejection fraction: implications for systolic and diastolic reserve limitations. Circulation. 2003;107:714–20.
26. Borlaug BA, Lam CSP, Roger VL, Rodeheffer RJ, Redfield MM. Contractility and ventricular systolic stiffening in hypertensive heart disease: insights into the pathogenesis of heart failure with preserved ejection fraction. J Am Coll Cardiol. 2009;54:410–8.
27. Zhong L. Attenuation of stress-based ventricular contractility in patients with heart failure and normal ejection fraction. Ann Acad Med Singapore. 2011;40:179–85.
28. Kitzman DW, Herrington DM, Brubaker PH, Moore JB, Eggebeen J, Haykowsky MJ. Carotid arterial stiffness and its relationship to exercise intolerance in older patients with heart failure and preserved ejection fraction. Hypertension. 2013;61:112–9.
29. Tartière-Kesri L, Tartière J-M, Logeart D, Beauvais F, Cohen SA. Increased proximal arterial stiffness and cardiac response with moderate exercise in patients with heart failure and preserved ejection fraction. J Am Coll Cardiol. 2012;59:455–61.
30. Borlaug BA, Olson TP, Lam CSP, Flood KS, Lerman A, Johnson BD, Redfield MM. Global cardiovascular reserve dysfunction in heart failure with preserved ejection fraction. J Am Coll Cardiol. 2010;56:845–54.
31. Haykowsky MJ, Brubaker PH, John JM, Stewart KP, Morgan TM, Kitzman DW. Determinants of exercise intolerance in elderly heart failure patients with preserved ejection fraction. J Am Coll Cardiol. 2011;58:265–74.
32. Hundley WG, Bayram E, Hamilton CA, Hamilton EA, Morgan TM, Darty SN, Stewart KP, Link KM, Herrington DM, Kitzman DW. Leg flow-mediated arterial dilation in elderly patients with heart failure and normal left ventricular ejection fraction. Am J Physiol Heart Circ Physiol. 2007;292:H1427–34.
33. Haykowsky MJ, Herrington DM, Brubaker PH, Morgan TM, Hundley WG, Kitzman DW. Relationship of flow-mediated arterial dilation and exercise capacity in older patients with heart failure and preserved ejection fraction. J Gerontol A Biol Sci Med Sci. 2013;68:161–7.
34. Houghton JL, Frank MJ, Carr AA, von Dohlen TW, Prisant LM. Relations among impaired coronary flow reserve, left ventricular hypertrophy and thallium perfusion defects in hypertensive patients without obstructive coronary artery disease. J Am Coll Cardiol. 1990;15:43–51.
35. Westermann D, Lindner D, Kasner M, Zietsch C, Savvatis K, Escher F, von Schlippenbach J, Skurk C, Steendijk P, Riad A, Poller W, Schultheiss H-P, Tschöpe C. Cardiac inflammation contributes to changes in the extracellular matrix in patients with

heart failure and normal ejection fraction/clinical perspective. Circ Heart Fail. 2011;4:44–52.
36. McMurray JJV, Morton J, Ferrell W, Padmanabhan N, Balmain S. Differences in arterial compliance, microvascular function and venous capacitance between patients with heart failure and either preserved or reduced left ventricular systolic function. Eur J Heart Fail. 2007;9:865–71.
37. Akiyama E, Sugiyama S, Matsuzawa Y, Konishi M, Suzuki H, Nozaki T, Ohba K, Matsubara J, Maeda H, Horibata Y, Sakamoto K, Sugamura K, Yamamuro M, Sumida H, Kaikita K, Iwashita S, Matsui K, Kimura K, Umemura S, Ogawa H. Incremental prognostic significance of peripheral endothelial dysfunction in patients with heart failure with normal left ventricular ejection fraction. J Am Coll Cardiol. 2012;60:1778–86.
38. Maurer MS, Burkhoff D, Fried LP, Gottdiener J, King DL, Kitzman DW. Ventricular structure and function in hypertensive participants with heart failure and a normal ejection fraction: the Cardiovascular Health Study. J Am Coll Cardiol. 2007;49:972–81.
39. Colombo PC, Banchs JE, Celaj S, Talreja A, Lachmann J, Malla S, DuBois NB, Ashton AW, Latif F, Jorde UP, Ware JA, LeJemtel TH. Endothelial cell activation in patients with decompensated heart failure. Circulation. 2005;111:58–62.
40. Colombo P, Rastogi S, Onat D, Zac V, Gupta R, Jorde U, Sabbah H. Activation of endothelial cells in conduit veins of dogs with heart failure and veins of normal dogs after vascular stretch by acute volume loading. J Card Fail. 2009;15:457–63.
41. Colombo PC, Onat D, Sabbah HN. Acute heart failure as "acute endothelitis" – interaction of fluid overload and endothelial dysfunction. Eur J Heart Fail. 2008;10:170–5.
42. Guazzi M, Vicenzi M, Arena R, Guazzi MD. Pulmonary hypertension in heart failure with preserved ejection fraction: a target of phosphodiesterase-5 inhibition in a 1-year study. Circulation. 2011;124:164–74.
43. Borlaug BA, Melenovsky V, Russell SD, Kessler K, Pacak K, Becker LC, Kass DA. Impaired chronotropic and vasodilator reserves limit exercise capacity in patients with heart failure and a preserved ejection fraction. Circulation. 2006;114:2138–47.
44. Kosmala W, Holland DJ, Rojek A, Wright L, Przewlocka-Kosmala M, Marwick TH. Effect of If-channel inhibition on hemodynamics and exercise tolerance in heart failure with preserved ejection fraction: a randomized trial. J Am Coll Cardiol. 2013;62:1330–8.
45. Obokata M, Negishi K, Kurosawa K, Arima H, Tateno R, Ui G, Tange S, Arai M, Kurabayashi M. Incremental diagnostic value of LA strain with leg lifts in heart failure with preserved ejection fraction. JACC Cardiovasc Imaging. 2013;6:749–58.
46. McKie PM, Schirger JA, Costello-Boerrigter LC, Benike SL, Harstad LK, Bailey KR, Hodge DO, Redfield MM, Simari RD, Burnett Jr JC, Chen HH. Impaired natriuretic and renal endocrine response to acute volume expansion in pre-clinical systolic and diastolic dysfunction. J Am Coll Cardiol. 2011;58:2095–103.
47. Maurer MS, Teruya S, Chakraborty B, Helmke S, Mancini D. Treating anemia in older adults with heart failure with a preserved ejection fraction with epoetin alfa: single-blind randomized clinical trial of safety and efficacy. Circ Heart Fail. 2013;6:254–63.
48. Haykowsky MJ, Brubaker PH, Morgan TM, Kritchevsky S, Eggebeen J, Kitzman DW. Impaired aerobic capacity and physical functional performance in older heart failure patients with preserved ejection fraction: role of lean body mass. J Gerontol Series A Biol Sci Med Sci. 2013;68:968–75.
49. Bhella PS, Prasad A, Heinicke K, Hastings JL, Arbab-Zadeh A, Adams-Huet B, Pacini EL, Shibata S, Palmer MD, Newcomer BR, Levine BD. Abnormal haemodynamic response to exercise in heart failure with preserved ejection fraction. Eur J Heart Fail. 2011;13:1296–304.
50. Hummel SL, Kitzman DW. Update on heart failure with preserved ejection fraction. Curr Cardiovasc Risk Rep. 2013;7:495–502.
51. Borlaug BA, Paulus WJ. Heart failure with preserved ejection fraction: pathophysiology, diagnosis, and treatment. Eur Heart J. 2011;32:670–9.
52. Beckett NS, Peters R, Fletcher AE, Staessen JA, Liu L, Dumitrascu D, Stoyanovsky V, Antikainen RL, Nikitin Y, Anderson C, Belhani A, Forette F, Rajkumar C, Thijs L, Banya W, Bulpitt CJ. Treatment of hypertension in patients 80 years of age or older. N Engl J Med. 2008;358:1887–98.
53. Solomon SD, Janardhanan R, Verma A, Bourgoun M, Daley WL, Purkayastha D, Lacourcière Y, Hippler SE, Fields H, Naqvi TZ, Mulvagh SL, Arnold JMO, Thomas JD, Zile MR, Aurigemma GP. Effect of angiotensin receptor blockade and antihypertensive drugs on diastolic function in patients with hypertension and diastolic dysfunction: a randomised trial. Lancet. 2007;369:2079–87.
54. Edelmann F, et al. Effect of spironolactone on diastolic function and exercise capacity in patients with heart failure with preserved ejection fraction: the ALDO-DHF randomized controlled trial. JAMA. 2013;309:781–91.
55. Lam CSP, Shah AM, Borlaug BA, Cheng S, Verma A, Izzo J, Oparil S, Aurigemma GP, Thomas JD, Pitt B, Zile MR, Solomon SD. Effect of antihypertensive therapy on ventricular–arterial mechanics, coupling, and efficiency. Eur Heart J. 2013;34:676–83.
56. Yancy CW, Jessup M, Bozkurt B, Masoudi FA, Butler J, McBride PE, Casey DE, McMurray JJV, Drazner MH, Mitchell JE, Fonarow GC, Peterson PN, Geraci SA, Horwich T, Januzzi JL, Johnson MR, Kasper EK, Levy WC, Riegel B, Sam F, Stevenson LW, Tang WHW, Tsai EJ, Wilkoff BL. ACCF/AHA guideline for the management of heart failure: a report of the American College of Cardiology Foundation/American Heart Association task force on practice guidelines. J Am Coll Cardiol. 2013;2013.

57. Lindenfeld J, Albert N, Boehmer J, Collins S, Ezekowitz J, Givertz M, Katz S, Klapholz M, Moser D, Rogers J, Starling R, Stevenson W, Tang WHW, Teerlink J, Walsh M. HFSA 2010 comprehensive heart failure practice guideline. J Card Fail. 2010;16:e1–194.
58. Yusuf S, Pfeffer MA, Swedberg K, Granger CB, Held P, McMurray JJ, Michelson EL, Olofsson B, Ostergren J, CHARM Investigators and Committees. Effects of candesartan in patients with chronic heart failure and preserved left-ventricular ejection fraction: the CHARM-Preserved trial. Lancet. 2003;362:777–81.
59. Cleland JG, Tendera M, Adamus J, Freemantle N, Polonski L, Taylor J, PEP-CHF Investigators. The perindopril in elderly people with chronic heart failure (PEP-CHF) study. Eur Heart J. 2006;27: 2338–45.
60. Massie BM, Carson PE, McMurray JJ, Komajda M, McKelvie R, Zile MR, Anderson S, Donovan M, Iverson E, Staiger C, Ptaszynska A. Irbesartan in patients with heart failure and preserved ejection fraction. N Engl J Med. 2008;359:2456–67.
61. Pitt B, Pfeffer MA, Assmann SF, Boineau R, Anand IS, Claggett B, Clausell N, Desai AS, Diaz R, Fleg JL, Gordeev I, Harty B, Heitner JF, Kenwood CT, Lewis EF, O'Meara E, Probstfield JL, Shaburishvili T, Shah SJ, Solomon SD, Sweitzer NK, Yang S, McKinlay SM; TOPCAT Investigators. Spironolactone for heart failure with preserved ejection fraction. N Engl J Med. 2014;370:1383–92.
62. Katz DH, Beussink L, Sauer AJ, Freed BH, Burke MA, Shah SJ. Prevalence, clinical characteristics, and outcomes associated with eccentric versus concentric left ventricular hypertrophy in heart failure with preserved ejection fraction. Am J Cardiol. 2013;112:1158–64.
63. Lund LH, Benson L, Dahlström U, Edner M. Association between use of renin-angiotensin system antagonists and mortality in patients with heart failure and preserved ejection fraction. JAMA. 2012;308:2108–17.
64. Patel K, Fonarow GC, Kitzman DW, Aban IB, Love TE, Allman RM, Gheorghiade M, Ahmed A. Aldosterone antagonists and outcomes in real-world older patients with heart failure and preserved ejection fraction. JACC Heart Fail. 2013;1:40–7.
65. Redfield MM, Chen HH. Effect of phosphodiesterase-5 inhibition on exercise capacity and clinical status in heart failure with preserved ejection fraction: a randomized clinical trial. JAMA. 2013;309:1268–77.
66. Reil J-C, Tardif J-C, Ford I, Lloyd SM, O'Meara E, Komajda M, Borer JS, Tavazzi L, Swedberg K, Bohm M. Selective heart rate reduction with ivabradine unloads the left ventricle in heart failure patients. J Am Coll Cardiol. 2013;62(21):1977–85.
67. Edelmann F, Gelbrich G, Düngen H-D, Fröhling S, Wachter R, Stahrenberg R, Binder L, Töpper A, Lashki DJ, Schwarz S, Herrmann-Lingen C, Löffler M, Hasenfuss G, Halle M, Pieske B. Exercise training improves exercise capacity and diastolic function in patients with heart failure with preserved ejection fraction: results of the EX-DHF (exercise training in diastolic heart failure) pilot study. J Am Coll Cardiol. 2011;58:1780–91.
68. Kitzman D, Brubaker P, Morgan T, Stewart K, Little W. Exercise training in older patients with heart failure and preserved ejection fraction: a randomized, controlled, single-blind trial. Circ Heart Fail. 2010; 3:659–67.
69. Klotz S, Hay I, Zhang G, Maurer M, Wang J, Burkhoff D. Development of heart failure in chronic hypertensive Dahl rats: focus on heart failure with preserved ejection fraction. Hypertension. 2006;47:901–11.
70. Ahn J, Varagic J, Slama M, Susic D, Frohlich ED. Cardiac structural and functional responses to salt loading in SHR. Am J Physiol Heart Circ Physiol. 2004;287:H767–72.
71. Paulus WJ, Tschöpe C. A novel paradigm for heart failure with preserved ejection fraction: comorbidities drive myocardial dysfunction and remodeling through coronary microvascular endothelial inflammation. J Am Coll Cardiol. 2013;62:263–71.
72. Hummel SL, Seymour EM, Brook RD, Sheth SS, Ghosh E, Zhu S, Weder AB, Kovacs SJ, Kolias TJ. Low-sodium DASH diet improves diastolic function and ventricular-arterial coupling in hypertensive heart failure with preserved ejection fraction. Circ Heart Fail. 2013;6:1165–71.
73. Hummel SL, Seymour EM, Brook RD, Kolias TJ, Sheth SS, Rosenblum HR, Wells JM, Weder AB. Low-sodium dietary approaches to stop hypertension diet reduces blood pressure, arterial stiffness, and oxidative stress in hypertensive heart failure with preserved ejection fraction/novelty and significance. Hypertension. 2012;60:1200–6.
74. Kalogeropoulos A, Georgiopoulou V, Psaty BM, Rodondi N, Smith AL, Harrison DG, Liu Y, Hoffmann U, Bauer DC, Newman AB, Kritchevsky SB, Harris TB, Butler J. Inflammatory markers and incident heart failure risk in older adults: the Health ABC (Health, Aging, and Body Composition) study. J Am Coll Cardiol. 2010;55:2129–37.
75. Suzuki T, Katz R, Jenny NS, Zakai NA, LeWinter MM, Barzilay JI, Cushman M. Metabolic syndrome, inflammation, and incident heart failure in the elderly: the Cardiovascular Health Study. Circ Heart Fail. 2008;1:242–8.

Structural Alterations in Arterial Stiffness: Role of Arterial Fibrosis

17

Javier Díez

Abstract

The structural changes involved in arterial stiffness include cellular changes (namely, smooth muscle cell differentiation) and noncellular changes affecting the extracellular matrix (namely, increased collagen deposition leading to fibrosis of the arterial wall or arteriosclerosis). By altering the geometry and the biomechanical properties of the arterial wall, these changes will contribute to arterial stiffness. A number of pathophysiologic processes develop within the arterial wall that is responsible for its altered structure and stiffening. For instance, increased activity of fibrogenic neurohormones and proinflammatory cytokines and oxidative stress have been shown to play a role in arterial stiffening through mechanisms that affect the metabolism and function of vascular collagen. The possibility is emerging to target the vascular collagen matrix for future pharmacological interventions on arterial stiffness.

Keywords

Arterial remodeling • Collagen • Cytokines • Extracellular matrix • Fibrosis • Oxidative stress • Vascular smooth muscle cells

Introduction

Increased arterial stiffness is a hallmark of the aging process and the consequence of many disease states such as hypertension, diabetes, atherosclerosis, and chronic renal failure. Accordingly, there is a marked increase in the incidence and prevalence of clinical surrogate markers of arterial stiffness, such as pulse pressure and isolated systolic hypertension, with age and these associated conditions [1–5]. Arterial stiffness is also a marker for increased cardiovascular risk, including myocardial infarction, heart failure, and total mortality, as well as stroke, dementia, and renal disease [6–14]. Arterial stiffness is a multifactorial phenotype and as such is the final result of changes in functional and structural properties of the arterial wall that are

J. Díez, MD, PhD
Program of Cardiovascular Diseases, Centre of Applied Medical Research, Pamplona, Spain

Department of Cardiology and Cardiac Surgery, School of Medicine, University Clinic, University of Navarra, Av. Pío XII 55, Pamplona 31008, Spain
e-mail: jadimar@unav.es

M.E. Safar et al. (eds.), *Blood Pressure and Arterial Wall Mechanics in Cardiovascular Diseases*,
DOI 10.1007/978-1-4471-5198-2_17, © Springer-Verlag London 2014

influenced by multiple factors, including hemodynamic forces [15], as well as by genetic determinants [16], humoral factors such as vasoactive substances, hormones, salt, lipids and glucose [17], and the process of aging [18]. Beyond changes in vascular smooth muscle tone [19] and endothelial function [20], it is classically recognized that structural alterations within the arterial wall are major determinants of arterial stiffness [16]. This chapter is focused on the role of one of these alterations, the fibrosis of the arterial wall (i.e., arteriosclerosis), in arterial stiffness.

Histological Features of Arterial Stiffness

Histological examination of the stiffened vessel wall reveals a number of morphological alterations (Fig. 17.1): abnormal and disarrayed endothelial cells; infiltration of the subintimal space by macrophages, mononuclear cells, and vascular smooth muscle cells (VSMCs); frayed, broken, and frequently calcified elastin fibers of the elastic lamina; increased number of VSMCs within the media; enhanced deposition of collagen type I fibers in the intima and of collagen type III fibers in the media and the adventitia; increased deposition of fibronectin in the media and the adventitia; and diminution of the vasa vasorum network [21]. Collectively, these changes will result in remodeling of arterial geometry (i.e., enlargement of the wall mostly due to intima-media thickening).

More in detail, the above alterations are the result of the phenotypic differentiation of VSMCs (a process characterized by increased proliferation, migration, and ECM synthesis) and of alterations in the regulation of the ECM (resulting in increased deposition of highly cross-linked fibrillar collagens type I and type III leading to fibrosis of the arterial wall, reduction in the elastin/collagen ratio, and altered spatial organization of collagen fibers within the vascular wall) [22, 23].

These alterations are nonuniformly disseminated throughout the vascular tree but are often patchy [24–26] occurring in central and conduit arteries while sparing more peripheral arteries [27, 28].

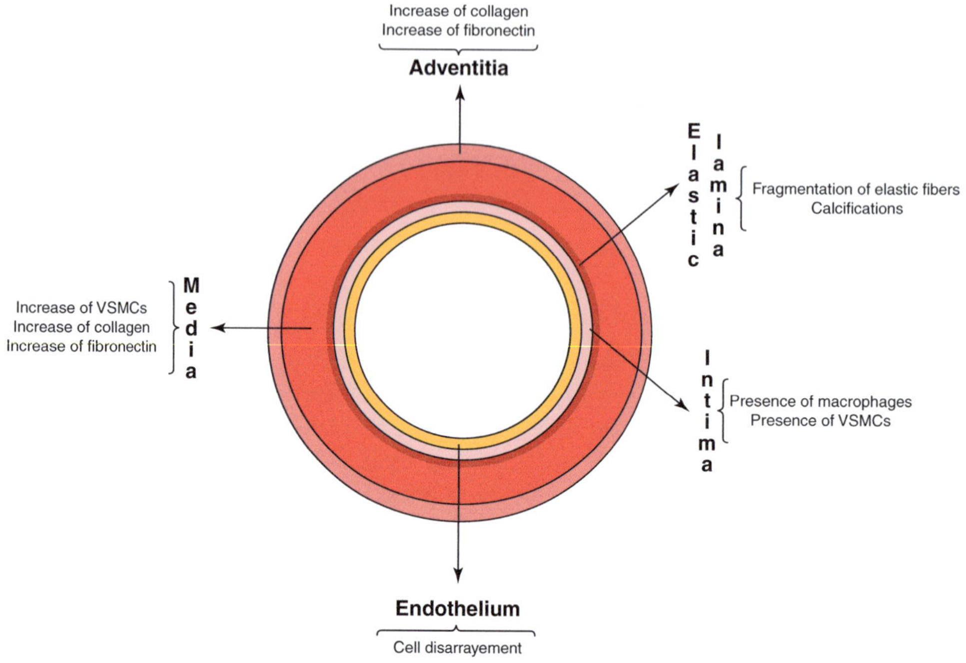

Fig. 17.1 Histological alterations associated with arterial stiffness. *VSMCs* means vascular smooth muscle cells

On the other hand, since ECM volume in large arteries is roughly 40–50 %, whereas in resistance arteries more than 70 % of the tissue volume is occupied by VSMCs, cellular changes are likely to have more impact on stiffness of resistance arteries [15]. In contrast, stiffness of large arteries is more likely influenced by ECM, namely, fibrosis [15].

Arterial Fibrosis and Stiffness

Arterial fibrosis is the result of the excessive accumulation of collagen type I and type III fibers within the arterial wall due to the predominance of their synthesis over their degradation. Beyond this quantitative definition of fibrosis, it is now accepted that the fibrotic tissue is also functionally abnormal due to qualitative alterations of its composition and physicochemical properties. Thus, arterial fibrosis must be approached in terms of the metabolic and functional alterations of its major constituent (i.e., the fibrillar collagen).

Metabolism of Vascular Collagen

Fibrillar collagens type I and type III are the major collagens detectable in vessels, representing more than 60 and 30 % of vascular collagens, respectively [29, 30]. The regulation of fibrillar collagen deposition and turnover in tissue is complex. Firstly, the amount of procollagen precursors secreted by the fibrogenic cells is controlled at the level of transcription [31] and by regulating intracellular degradation [32]. While most of the collagens in the vascular intima and media are synthesized by VSMCs, fibroblasts are responsible for collagen synthesis in the adventitia. VSMCs are, however, phenotypically plastic and can differentiate from a contractile phenotype to a synthetic phenotype. These cells resemble the more immature fetal or neonatal cells and are commonly found in secondary culture and in the arterial intima; they migrate, divide, and produce ECM, namely, fibrillar collagen. Thus, a number of chemical and physical factors influence collagen production by VSMCs through their phenotypic differentiation [33].

After secretion of procollagen molecules in the extracellular compartment, the carboxy- and amino-terminal non-collagenous domains are removed by specific proteinases. The resulting collagen triple helices aggregate in quarter-staggered fibrils. Newly formed collagen fibrils are soluble in salt solutions and dilute acid and have no tensile strength. During the formation of intermolecular cross-linking, collagen fibers become increasingly insoluble and stiff. The cross-linking process is initiated by the enzyme lysyl oxidase (LOX), through the oxidation of specific lysine or hydroxylysine residues in the telopeptide regions. The resulting aldehydes undergo a series of reactions with adjacent reactive residues to give both intermolecular and intramolecular cross-links [34].

The metabolic turnover of mature collagen in adult animals is relatively slow. In fact, only small amounts of these proteins are degraded normally by collagenolytic enzymes. Collagenolytic enzymes are mainly matrix metalloproteinases (MMPs) [35, 36]. The substrate specificity differs for the various MMPs present in the vascular wall with MMP-1 (or collagenase) degrading collagens type I and type III [37]. The proteolytic activity of each MMP is tightly regulated at three levels: first, gene expression and protein secretion levels; second, activation of the inactive proenzyme; and, third, inhibition by the tissue inhibitors of MMPs (TIMPs) or other inhibitors (α_2-macroglobulin). The activation of MMPs and their inhibition by TIMPs are the main regulatory mechanisms of MMP activities in the vascular wall [35, 36].

Functional Properties of Vascular Collagen

The biomechanical properties of the large arteries are mostly dependent not only on the quantity of collagen fibers but also on the quality of the different types of fibrillar collagen (e.g., type I versus type III and highly cross-linked versus non-highly cross-linked), their spatial distribution within the arterial wall, and their relation to the quantity and quality of elastin and other components of the ECM [23, 38] (Table 17.1).

Table 17.1 Factors facilitating the functional impact of arterial fibrosis on arterial stiffness

Increased cross-linking among collagen molecules integrated into collagen fibers
Relative excess of collagen type I fibers over collagen type III fibers
Altered spatial orientation of collagen fibers within the arterial wall
Increased ratio collagen fibers/elastin fibers
Excess of other extracellular matrix components (e.g., fibronectin, proteoglycans, glycosaminoglycans)
Altered expression of integrins (e.g., increased expression of α_{2b} and α_6, reduced expression of β_3 and β_5)

The larger diameter of collagen type I fibers is believed to confer high tensile strength while the thinner collagen type III fibers are associated with increased tissue flexibility [39]. With the increase in cross-links between collagen fibrils, the resulting collagen fiber is characterized by an increased tensile strength, an increased resistance against enzymatic degradation, a higher shrinkage temperature, a lower swelling rate, and an increased diameter [40].

The organization of the vessel wall is characterized by circumferentially oriented collagen fibers/cells and lamellar elastin. Collagen fibers run longitudinally in the intima and adventitia and run spirally between muscle layers in the media [41]. The functional properties of the wall, including stiffness, depend critically on the maintenance of this structural organization [42]. The collagen orientation and location are tightly regulated by other components of the ECM, namely, proteoglycans [43]. In fact, the sulfated saccharide domains of proteoglycan molecules provide numerous docking sites for a multitude of protein ligands, including structural collagens and other ECM molecules [43].

Elastin is an insoluble protein due to the cross-links existing between its lysine residues [34]. This cross-linking confers to elastin its function, i.e., elasticity, essential in large arteries which distend during systole and recoil during diastole. Elastic fibers are degraded and fragmented with age and disease, leading to increased stiffness of the arterial wall [18, 44]. Therefore, the predominance of fibrillar collagen over elastin facilitates arterial stiffening [45]. On the other hand, ample evidence (i.e., animal data and studies of diabetes and chronic kidney disease) has demonstrated that medial calcification of elastic fibers contributes to increased arterial stiffness [46].

In order to explain the respective role of collagen and elastin on the stiffness of the vessel wall, Burton [21] assessed Young's modulus (wall tension per centimeter wall thickness for 100 % diameter increase) of isolated elastic and collagen tissues and showed that the latter made the major contribution to the stiffness of the vessel wall. These data were expanded in the experiments of Dobrin et al. [47] in which human isolated arterial vessels were studied in the presence of elastase and collagenase. With elastase, the pressure-volume relationship of the arterial vessel was shifted towards higher values of arterial diameter and volume, indicating that the loss of elastin greatly influenced the geometry of the vessel without changing its mechanical properties (i.e., the slope of the curve). On the other hand, with collagenase the slope of the curve increased greatly, indicating a decreased stiffness of the vessel wall, without substantial change in its geometry.

Mechanisms of Arterial Fibrosis

As mentioned before the relative content of fibrillar collagen in the vascular wall is normally held stable by a slow, but dynamic, process of synthesis and degradation. Dysregulation of this balance due to the predominance of collagen synthesis over its degradation results in overabundance of collagen type I and type III fibers and thus fibrosis [23] (Fig. 17.2). A number of mechanical and humoral factors may facilitate collagen synthesis in the vascular wall, namely, through the stimulation of the differentiation of VSMC to the synthetic phenotype. For instance, increased luminal and transmural pressure stimulate collagen synthesis and deposition in the vascular wall [48]. In addition, several neurohormonal factors, particularly those related to the renin-angiotensin-aldosterone system [49], and fibrogenic cytokines such as transforming growth factor-β (TGF-β) [50] may also induce collagen

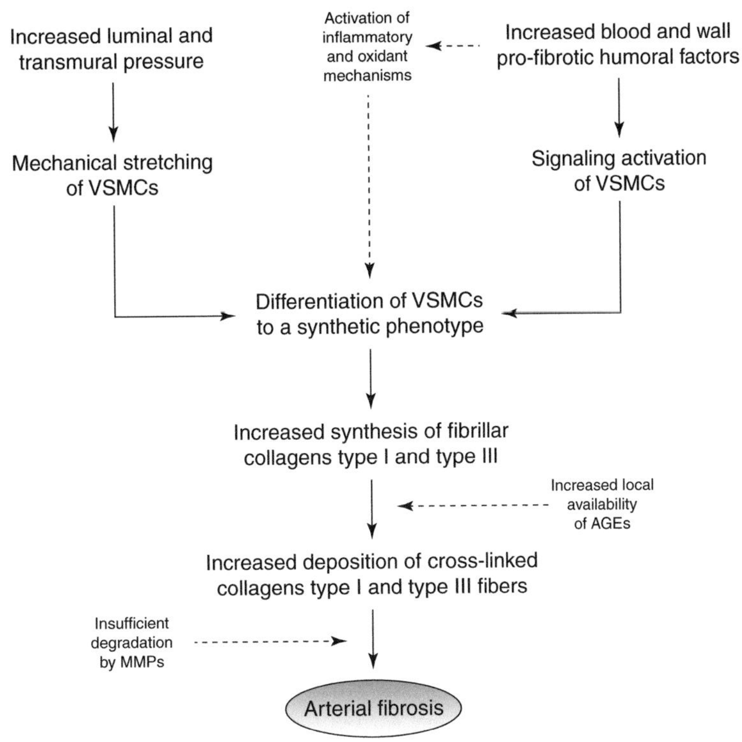

Fig. 17.2 Schematic view of the mechanisms of arterial fibrosis. *VSMCs* means vascular smooth muscle cells, *AGEs* advanced glycation end products, *MMPs* matrix metalloproteinases

accumulation within the vessel wall. In fact, arterial stiffness is associated with the increased signaling activity of angiotensin II leading to activation of MMPs which degrade TGF-β precursors to produce active TGF-β, which then results in increased arterial fibrosis [51]. Angiotensin II signaling also activates cytokines, including monocyte chemoattractant protein-1, TNF-α, interleukin-1, interleukin-17, and interleukin-6, thus facilitating a proinflammatory milieu that, in turn, will enhance fibrosis [51, 52]. Finally, increased angiotensin II results in increased vascular NADPH oxidase activity and increased production of reactive oxygen species (ROS) that also facilitate fibrogenesis [51, 53]. More recently, cardiotrophin-1 (CT-1), a member of the inteleukin-6 family of cytokines, has emerged as a potential mediator of arterial fibrosis and stiffness. In fact, chronic exposure of rats to an excess of exogenous CT-1 was associated with intima-media thickening and fibrosis of large arteries that was accompanied by increased arterial stiffness in the absence of changes in blood pressure [54]. Furthermore, it has been reported that the absence of CT-1 translated into a marked reduction in arterial stiffness associated with aging [55]. CT-1 null mice developed less arterial fibrosis with aging than did wild-type mice. In addition, compared to wild-type mice, CT-1 null mice exhibited decreased arterial stiffness and prolongation of the life span [55].

The expression and activity of the LOX enzyme, responsible for the enzymatic cross-linking of collagen molecules, have been reported to be decreased in the arterial wall of animals and humans with arterial stiffness [56, 57]. Thus, nonenzymatic processes may be determinant of the formation of highly cross-linked collagen in arterial stiffness (Fig. 17.2). The advanced glycation end products (AGEs) formed during the Maillard nonenzymatic reaction of reducing sugars with lysine residues of proteins which occurs slowly in vivo with normal aging and at an accelerated rate in diabetes, hypertension, and chronic kidney disease are able to cause cross-linking of collagen molecules to each other [58]. Interestingly, it has been shown that the age-related increase of AGEs in aorta correlated directly with its stiffness in both control subjects and diabetic patients [59].

Since elastin molecules are stabilized by cross-linking to form desmosine and isodesmosine, disruption of these cross-links by mechanisms triggered by humoral factors (e.g., angiotensin II) and mediated by cytokine- and ROS-mediated pathways contributes to weakening of the elastin array with predisposition to mineralization by calcium and phosphorus, together increasing arterial stiffness [60–62]. In addition, activation of various elastases (i.e., serine proteases and MMPs) produced by VSMCs generates broken and frayed elastin molecules [63]. In this regard, it has been reported recently that aortic stiffness is related to serum MMP-9 levels and serum elastase activity in patients with isolated systolic hypertension and apparently healthy individuals [64]. Furthermore, it has been reported that aortic stiffness is greater in aged subjects homozygous for the 5A promoter polymorphism of MMP-3 than aged subjects homozygous for the 6A promoter polymorphism [65]. Interestingly, both MMP-3 gene and protein expression were higher in 6A subjects than in 5A subjects [65].

Finally, it is important to consider that arterial stiffness creates per se a pathological hemodynamic profile in large arteries that, in turn, exacerbates the mechanisms of fibrosis and other structural alterations involved in stiffening of the vascular wall, thus resulting in a vicious circle. In fact, arterial stiffening will result in increased pulse wave velocity; the forward traveling wave and reflected wave are summated leading to a high pulsatile flow in aorta and branching arteries [66]. High blood pressure pulsatility leads to increased mechanical vascular wall stress that, in turn, leads to increased stretching of VSMCs and elastin fibers in the arterial wall. Whereas stretching induces phenotypic differentiation of VSMCs, thus facilitating further collagen synthesis and deposition, it also contributes to fatigue and accelerated degradation of elastin fibers [67, 68].

Perspectives

Arterial stiffness is an important, independent predictor of cardiovascular risk. Therefore, reduction in arterial stiffness with drugs is an important end point in clinical trials. In this conceptual framework, the effect of available cardiovascular pharmacologic agents on arterial stiffness has been reviewed recently [69]. Although it has been suggested that most antihypertensive drugs exert beneficial effects on arterial stiffness, recent data in patients with isolated hypertension challenge this notion [70] (Table 17.2), highlighting the urgent need for novel strategies to reduce arterial stiffness in hypertension. For instance, experimental and clinical findings suggest that antihypertensive drugs with proven antifibrotic properties beyond their hemodynamic effects (e.g., the angiotensin type 1 receptor blocker losartan) look promising to reduce arterial stiffness [71, 72]. On the other hand, drugs targeting glycemic control have also

Table 17.2 Effects induced by 10-week treatment with several antihypertensive agents on hemodynamic measurements in patients with isolated systolic hypertension

Parameter	Bendrofluazide	Atenolol	Lercanidipine	Perindopril
Peripheral SBP	Significant reduction	Significant reduction	Significant reduction	Significant reduction
Peripheral DBP	Significant reduction	Significant reduction	Significant reduction	Significant reduction
Peripheral PP	Significant reduction	Significant reduction	Significant reduction	Significant reduction
Central SBP	Significant reduction	Significant reduction	Significant reduction	Significant reduction
Central PP	Significant reduction	Nonsignificant reduction	Significant reduction	Significant reduction
Aortic PWV	Nonsignificant increase	Nonsignificant reduction	Nonsignificant increase	Nonsignificant increase

Modified from Ref. [70]

PWV was assessed as the gold standard measurement of arterial stiffness

SBP means systolic blood pressure, *DBP* diastolic BP, *PP* pulse pressure, *PWV* pulse wave velocity shown to improve aortic stiffness. In particular, glitazones decrease aortic stiffness together with intima-media thickness, thus meaning a potential antifibrotic effect in the arterial wall [73]. Finally, although the effects of statins on arterial stiffness are not clinically relevant, it must be mentioned that simvastatin has been shown to reduce inflammation-induced aortic stiffening through a lipid reduction mechanism [74].

Drugs reversing deposits of AGE are good candidates as de-stiffening drugs. α-Aminoguanidine, a first-line compound for reducing AGE deposits, has been shown to reduce arterial stiffness in experimental diabetes [75]. In addition, a thiazolium derivative (ALT-711), which breaks AGE-mediated cross-links between collagen proteins, has been reported to reduce arterial stiffness in hypertensive patients with diabetes [76, 77]. Whether de-stiffening drugs are beneficial in the long term remains to be proven. Indeed, threats are also expected. Collagen-derived stiffness is an important determinant for maintaining wall resistance to distension, and inappropriate arterial distensibility may lead to propensity for dilatation and rupture [78].

Besides the advances in the noninvasive assessment of arterial stiffness obtained in the last 2 decades, the future of this condition must be covered by advances in its therapeutic handling. In this regard, it is probable that structural alterations of the arterial wall, such as fibrosis, involved in its stiffening constitute new targets for novel therapeutic strategies aimed to reduce the cardiovascular risk associated with arterial stiffness. For instance, it has been reported recently that the selective angiotensin type 2 receptor agonist C21 may reduce aortic oxidative stress, inflammatory cell infiltration, collagen content, and stiffness in stroke-prone spontaneously hypertensive rats in the absence of any effect on blood pressure [71].

References

1. Chobanian AV, Bakris GL, Black HR, Cushman WC, Green LA, Izzo Jr JL, et al. The seventh report of the Joint National Committee on Prevention, Detection, Evaluation, and Treatment of High Blood Pressure: the JNC 7 report. JAMA. 2003;289:2560–72.
2. Scuteri A, Najjar SS, Muller DC, Andres R, Hougaku H, Metter EJ, et al. Metabolic syndrome amplifies the age-associated increases in vascular thickness and stiffness. J Am Coll Cardiol. 2004;43:1388–95.
3. Dart A, Kingwell B. Pulse pressure – a review of mechanisms and clinical relevance. J Am Coll Cardiol. 2001;37:975–84.
4. Lakatta EG, Levy D. Arterial and cardiac aging: major shareholders in cardiovascular disease enterprises. I. Aging arteries: a 'set up' for vascular disease. Circulation. 2003;107:139–46.
5. Collins AJ, Li S, Gilbertson DT, Liu J, Chen SC, Herzog CA. Chronic kidney disease and cardiovascular disease in the Medicare population. Kidney Int. 2003;64 suppl 87:S24–31.
6. Chae CU, Pfeffer MA, Glynn RJ, Mitchell GF, Taylor JO, Hennekens CH. Increased pulse pressure and risk of heart failure in the elderly. JAMA. 1999;281: 634–9.
7. Franklin SS, Larson MG, Khan SA, Wong ND, Leip FP, Kannel WB, et al. Does the relation of blood pressure to coronary heart disease risk change with aging? The Framingham Heart Study. Circulation. 2001;103: 1245–9.
8. Mitchell GF, Pfeffer MA, Braunwald E, Rouleau JL, Bernstein V, Geltman EM, et al. Sphygmomanometrically determined pulse pressure is a powerful independent predictor of recurrent events after myocardial infarction in patients with impaired left ventricular function. Circulation. 1997;96:4254–60.
9. Vaccarino V, Berger A, Abramson J, Black H, Setaro J, Davey J, et al. Pulse pressure and risk of cardiovascular events in the systolic hypertension in the elderly program. Am J Cardiol. 2001;88:980–6.
10. Kostis J, Lawrence-Nelson J, Ranjan R, Wilson A, Kostis W, Lacy C. Association of increased pulse pressure with the development of heart failure in SHEP. Systolic Hypertension in the Elderly (SHEP) Cooperative Research Group. Am J Hypertens. 2001;14:798–803.
11. Blacher J, Guerin AP, Pannier B, Marchais SJ, Safar ME, London GM. Impact of aortic stiffness on survival in end-stage renal disease. Circulation. 1999; 99:2434–9.
12. Forette F, Seux ML, Staessen JA, Thijs L, Birkenhager WH, Babarskiene MR, et al. Prevention of dementia in randomised double-blind placebo-controlled Systolic Hypertension in Europe (Syst-Eur) trial. Lancet. 1998;352:1347–51.
13. Benetos A, Safar M, Rudnichi A, Smulyan H, Richard JL, Ducimetière P, et al. Pulse pressure: a predictor of long-term cardiovascular mortality in a French male population. Hypertension. 1997;30:1410–5.
14. Cohn JN, Quyyumi AA, Hollenberg NK, Jamerson KA. Surrogate markers for cardiovascular disease. Functional markers. Circulation. 2004;109(suppl IV): IV-31–46.
15. Et-Taouil K, Safar M, Plante GE. Mechanisms and consequences of large artery rigidity. Can J Physiol Pharmacol. 2003;81:205–11.

16. Laurent A, Boutouyrie P, Lacolley P. Structural and genetic bases of arterial stiffness. Hypertension. 2005; 45:1050–5.
17. Zieman SJ, Melenovsky V, Kass DA. Mechanisms, pathophysiology, and therapy of arterial stiffness. Arterioscler Thromb Vasc Biol. 2005;25:932–43.
18. Lee HY, Oh BH. Aging and arterial stiffness. Circ J. 2010;74:2257–62.
19. Gow BS. The influence of vascular smooth muscle on the viscoelastic properties of blood vessels. In: Bergel DH, editor. Cardiovascular fluid dynamics. London: Academic; 1972. p. 66–97.
20. Wilkinson IB, McEniery CM. Arterial stiffness, endothelial function and novel pharmacological approaches. Clin Exp Pharmacol Physiol. 2004;31:795–9.
21. Burton AC. Relation of structure to function of tissues of the wall of blood vessels. Physiol Rev. 1954;34: 619–24.
22. Mack CP. Signaling mechanisms that regulate smooth muscle cell differentiation. Arterioscler Thromb Vasc Biol. 2011;31:1495–505.
23. Díez J. Arterial stiffness and extracellular matrix. Adv Cardiol. 2007;44:76–95.
24. Galis ZS, Khatri JJ. Matrix metalloproteinases in vascular remodeling and atherogenesis: the good, the bad, and the ugly. Circ Res. 2002;90:251–62.
25. Beattie D, Xu C, Vito R, Glagov S, Whang MC. Mechanical analysis of heterogeneous, atherosclerotic human aorta. J Biomech Eng. 1998;120:602–7.
26. Bassiouny HS, Zarins CK, Kadowaki MH, Glagov S. Hemodynamic stress and experimental aortoiliac atherosclerosis. J Vasc Surg. 1994;19:426–34.
27. Benetos A, Laurent S, Hoeks AP, Boutouyrie PH, Safar ME. Arterial alterations with aging and high blood pressure. A noninvasive study of carotid and femoral arteries. Arterioscler Thromb. 1993;13:90–7.
28. Gillessen T, Gillessen F, Sieberth H, Hanrath P, Heintz B. Age-related changes in the elastic properties of the aortic tree in normotensive patients: investigation by intravascular ultrasound. Eur J Med Res. 1995;1:144–8.
29. Mayne R. Collagenous proteins of blood vessels. Arteriosclerosis. 1986;6:585–93.
30. Seyer JM, Kang AH. Connective tissues of the subendothelium. In: Loscalzo J, Creager MA, Dzau VJ, editors. Vascular medicine. Boston: Little, Brown & Company; 1992. p. 47–78.
31. Slack JL, Liska DJ, Bornstein P. Regulation of expression of type I collagen genes. Am J Med Genet. 1993;45:140–51.
32. Laurent J. Dynamic state of collagen: pathways of collagen degradation in vivo and their possible role in regulation of collagen mass. Am J Physiol. 1987;252:C1–9.
33. Fitzsimmons CM, Shanahan CM. Vascular extracellular matrix. In: Lanzer P, Topol EJ, editors. Panvascular medicine. Berlin: Springer; 2002. p. 217–31.
34. Reiser K, McCormick RJ, Bucker RB. Enzymatic and nonenzymatic cross-linking of collagen and elastin. FASEB J. 1992;6:2439–49.
35. Bode W, Maskos K. Structural basis of matrix metalloproteinases and their physiological inhibitors, the tissue inhibitors of metalloproteinases. Biol Chem. 2003;384:863–72.
36. Visse R, Nagase H. Matrix metalloproteinases and tissue inhibitors of metalloproteinases. Structure, function, and biochemistry. Circ Res. 2003;92:827–39.
37. Palombo D, Maione M, Cifiello BI, Udini M, Maggio D, Lupo M. Matrix metalloproteinases. Their role in degenerative chronic diseases of abdominal aorta. J Cardiovasc Surg. 1999;40:257–60.
38. Robins SP, Farquharson C. Connective tissue components of the blood vessel wall in health and disease. In: Stehbens WE, Lie JT, editors. Vascular pathology. London: Chapman & Hall Medical; 1995. p. 89–127.
39. Barnes MJ, Farndale RW. Collagens in atherosclerosis. Exp Gerontol. 1999;34:513–25.
40. Robins SP. Biochemistry and functional significance of collagen cross-linking. Biochem Soc Trans. 2007;35(Pt 5):849–52.
41. Clarke JM, Glagov S. Transmural organisation of the arterial media. Atherosclerosis. 1985;5:19–34.
42. Wolinsky H, Glagov S. Structural basis for the static mechanical properties of the aortic media. Circ Res. 1967;20:99–111.
43. Lindahl U, Li JP. Interactions between heparan sulfate and proteins – design and functional implications. Int Rev Cell Mol Bio. 2009;276:105–9.
44. Wagenseil JE, Mecham RP. Elastin in large artery stiffness and hypertension. J Cardiovasc Transl Res. 2012;5:264–73.
45. Armentano RL, Levenson J, Barra JG, Fischer EI, Breitbart GJ, Pichel RH, et al. Assessment of elastin and collagen contribution to aortic elasticity in conscious dogs. Am J Physiol. 1991;260(6 Pt 2):H1870–7.
46. Mackey RH, Venkitachalam L, Sutton-Tyrrell K. Calcifications, arterial stiffness and atherosclerosis. Adv Cardiol. 2007;44:234–44.
47. Dobrin PB, Baker WH, Gley WC. Elastolytic and collagenolytic studies of arteries: implications for the mechanical properties of aneurysms. Arch Surg. 1984;119:406–9.
48. Hoefer IE, den Adel B, Daemen MJAP. Biomechanical factors as triggers of vascular growth. Cardiovasc Res. 2013;99:276–83.
49. Mahmud A, Feely J. Arterial stiffness and the renin-angiotensin-aldosterone system. J Renin Angiotensin Aldosterone Syst. 2004;5:102–8.
50. Ruiz-Ortega M, Rodríguez-Vita J, Sanchez-Lopez E, Carvajal G, Egido J. TGF-beta signaling in vascular fibrosis. Cardiovasc Res. 2007;74:196–206.
51. Wang M, Zhang J, Jiang LQ, Spinetti G, Pintus G, Monticone R, et al. Proinflammatory profile within the grossly normal aged human aortic wall. Hypertension. 2007;50:219–27.
52. Park S, Lakatta EG. Role of inflammation in the pathogenesis of arterial stiffness. Yonsei Med J. 2012; 53:258–61.
53. Bachschmid MM, Schildknecht S, Matsui R, Zee R, Haeussler D, Cohen RA, et al. Vascular aging: chronic oxidative stress and impairment of redox signaling-consequences for vascular homeostasis and disease. Ann Med. 2013;45:17–36.

54. López-Andrés N, Rousseau A, Akhtar R, Calvier L, Iñigo C, Labat C, et al. Cardiotrophin 1 is involved in cardiac, vascular, and renal fibrosis and dysfunction. Hypertension. 2012;60:563–73.
55. López-Andrés N, Calvier L, Labat C, Fay R, Díez J, Benetos A, et al. Absence of cardiotrophin 1 is associated with decreased age-dependent arterial stiffness and increased longevity in mice. Hypertension. 2013; 61:120–9.
56. Fornieri C, Quaglino Jr D, Mori G. Role of the extracellular matrix in age-related modifications of the rat aorta. Ultrastructural, morphometric, and enzymatic evaluations. Arterioscler Thromb. 1992;12:1008–16.
57. Chen JY, Tsai PJ, Tai HC, Tsai RL, Chang YT, Wang MC, et al. Increased aortic stiffness and attenuated lysyl oxidase activity in obesity. Arterioscler Thromb Vasc Biol. 2013;33:839–46.
58. Sell DR, Monnier VM. Molecular basis of arterial stiffening: role of glycation – a mini-review. Gerontology. 2012;58:227–37.
59. Sim STJ, Rasmussen LM, Oxlund H, Bailey AJ. The role of glycation cross-links in diabetic vascular stiffening. Diabetologia. 1996;39:946–51.
60. Watanabe M, Sawai T, Nagura H, Suyama K. Age-related alteration of cross-linking amino acids of elastin in human aorta. Tohoku J Exp Med. 1996;180: 115–30.
61. Spina M, Garbin G. Age-related chemical changes in human elastins from non-atherosclerotic areas of thoracic aorta. Atherosclerosis. 1976;24:267–9.
62. Cattell MA, Anderson JC, Hasleton PS. Age-related changes in amounts and concentrations of collagen and elastin in normotensive human thoracic aorta. Clin Chim Acta. 1996;245:73–84.
63. Avolio A, Jones D, Tafazzoli-Shadpour M. Quantification of alterations in structure and function of elastin in the arterial media. Hypertension. 1998;32:170–5.
64. Yasmin, Wallace S, McEniery CM, Dakham Z, Pusalkar P, Maki-Petaja K, et al. Matrix metalloproteinase-9 (MMP-9), MMP-2, and serum elastase activity are associated with systolic hypertension and arterial stiffness. Arterioscler Thromb Vasc Biol. 2005;25:372–8.
65. Medley TL, Kingwell BA, Gatzka CD, Pillay P, Cole TJ. Matrix metalloproteinase-3 genotype contributes to age-related aortic stiffening through modulation of gene and protein expression. Circ Res. 2003;92: 1254–61.
66. Safar ME, Blacher J, Jankowski P. Arterial stiffness, pulse pressure, and cardiovascular disease-is it possible to break the vicious circle? Atherosclerosis. 2011; 218:263–71.
67. Gupta V, Grande-Allen KJ. Effects of static and cyclic loading in regulating extracellular matrix synthesis by cardiovascular cells. Cardiovasc Res. 2006;72: 375–83.
68. Hodis S, Zamir M. Mechanical events within the arterial wall: the dynamic context for elastin fatigue. J Biomech. 2009;42:1010–6.
69. Boutouyrie P, Lacolley P, Briet M, Regnault V, Stanton A, Laurent S, et al. Pharmacological modulation of arterial stiffness. Drugs. 2011;71:1689–701.
70. Mackenzie IS, McEniery CM, Dhakam Z, Brown MJ, Cockcroft JR, Wilkinson IB. Comparison of the effects of antihypertensive agents on central blood pressure and arterial stiffness in isolated systolic hypertension. Hypertension. 2009;54:409–13.
71. Rehman A, Leibowitz A, Yamamoto N, Rautureau Y, Paradis P, Schiffrin EL. Angiotensin type 2 receptor agonist compound 21 reduces vascular injury and myocardial fibrosis in stroke-prone spontaneously hypertensive rats. Hypertension. 2012;59:291–9.
72. Mahmud A, Feely J. Effect of angiotensin II receptor blockade on arterial stiffness: beyond blood pressure reduction. Am J Hypertens. 2002;15:1092–5.
73. Yu J, Jin N, Wang G, Zhang F, Mao J, Wang X. Peroxisome proliferator-activated receptor gamma agonist improves arterial stiffness in patients with type 2 diabetes mellitus and coronary artery disease. Metabolism. 2007;56:1396–401.
74. Wallace SM, Maki-Petaja KM, Cheriyan J, Davidson EH, Cherry L, McEniery CM, et al. Simvastatin prevents inflammation-induced aortic stiffening and endothelial dysfunction. Br J Clin Pharmacol. 2010; 70:799–806.
75. Wolffenbutel BH, Boulanger CM, Crijns FR, Huijberts MS, Poitevin P, Swennen GN, et al. Breakers of advanced glycation end products restore large artery properties in experimental diabetes. Proc Natl Acad Sci U S A. 1998;95:4630–4.
76. Kass DA, Shapiro EP, Kawaguchi M, Capriotti AR, Scuteri A, deGroof RC. Impaired arterial compliance by a novel advanced glycation end-product cross-link breaker. Circulation. 2001;104:1464–70.
77. Zieman SJ, Melenovsky V, Clattenburg L, Corretti MC, Capriotti A, Gerstenblith G, et al. Advanced glycation endproduct crosslink breaker (alagebrium) improves endothelial function in patients with isolated systolic hypertension. J Hypertens. 2007;25: 577–83.
78. Ong KT, Perdu J, De Backer J, Bozec E, Collignon P, Emmerich J, et al. Effect of celiprolol on prevention of cardiovascular events in vascular Ehlers-Danlos syndrome: a prospective randomised, open, blinded endpoints trial. Lancet. 2010;376:1476–84.

Salt and Multiorgan Damage in Hypertension: Vascular Stiffening and Cardiorenal Structural Dysfunction Responses

18

Edward D. Frohlich

Abstract

This chapter focuses on some of the new factors adversely affecting the target organs of hypertensive disease resulting from long-term dietary salt excess including the local renin-angiotensin systems in the arteries, heart, and kidneys. The data presented suggests that the stimulation of these cardiovascular and renal sites is responsible for their damage that alters the structure and function of these organs through other biological systems. These actions may be mediated by the expression of lysyl oxidase formation, oxidative stress, and inflammation that may account for the development of organ fibrosis including collagen and its cross-linking which reduces vascular elasticity and cardiovascular and/or renal stiffening. These latter concepts permit reference to mosaic of multifactorial factors of disease, the concept of which was introduced by Irvine Page. The reader can appreciate how the generation of simple questions in earlier investigative processes leads to more complex problems which, in turn, can provide important clinical answers that continue to stimulate an active investigative scientific medical career.

Keywords

Salt • Heart • Large arteries • Kidneys • Heart failure • Renal failure • Local renin-angiotensin systems • Reactive oxygen species • Inflammation • Fibrosis

Since Ambard and Beaujard first introduced the concept about the role of dietary salt excess in producing hypertension in 1904, most succeeding scientific (and the lay) literature continued to relate this increasingly important clinical problem primarily to hypertension [1]. Since then, a voluminous literature has amassed including an excellent historical monograph written for broad readership dealing with the role of sodium not only to hypertension but also to economics, social behavior, epidemiology, selected scientific contributions, and, of course, the controversy surrounding this long-standing interest [2]. Investigative efforts have since continued to focus almost

E.D. Frohlich, MD, MACP, FACC
Department of Cardiology,
Ochsner Clinic Foundation, 1514 Jefferson Highway,
New Orleans, LA 70121, USA
e-mail: efrohlich@ochsner.org

M.E. Safar et al. (eds.), *Blood Pressure and Arterial Wall Mechanics in Cardiovascular Diseases*,
DOI 10.1007/978-1-4471-5198-2_18,

unabatedly and, perhaps without distraction, on a singular role that salt has played in the pathogenesis of hypertension and, more recently, on cardiovascular and renal functions. In our earlier review on these relationships over 30 years ago, my early attention was focused all too briefly on dietary sodium restriction and its therapeutic interrelationship with diuretics. Perhaps this may not be surprising since much other interest was focused at the time to the number of newer classes of pharmacological agents that were being studied and introduced for antihypertensive therapy. Be that as it may, the main purpose therein was the biological significance of the sodium ion. Furthermore, not surprisingly, less information was available on the broader implications of the renin-angiotensin system (RAS) and, even less, on the local RASs on the structure and function of the major target organs of hypertensive disease [3].

Over subsequent years, much of the story on the role of dietary salt excess and disease became related to its pathophysiological relationships with volume overload, cardiac failure, and end-stage renal disease. During these years, less thought was dedicated to the coexistent development of specific organ involvements that may be promoted by a lifetime of dietary salt excess on its associated pathophysiological changes that are manifested by subclinical promotion of structural and functional disease of the arteries, heart, and kidneys [4, 5]. Much interest in this regard must be credited to current information concerning biological mechanisms, techniques for evaluating functional changes, and biological models employed in evaluating these newer concepts.

Furthermore, less thought has been directed toward the interaction of aging, per se, on the biological processes that may also interact with environmental factors, disease, and therapeutic interventions [6, 7]. It seems that there is very real possibility that the aging process itself could be exacerbated or even directly associated with the progression of hypertensive disease [6]. We are already keenly aware of the increasing prevalence of hypertension in the elderly and the effects of sodium that are related to biological mechanisms and pathophysiological alterations which affect on the target organs of aging and disease. For example, in recent years, a variety of fundamental laboratory and clinical investigative studies have demonstrated progressive cardiovascular and/or renal fibrotic changes that may occur and participate (if not produce) in large arterial stiffening; in ventricular diastolic dysfunction and, later, on systolic cardiac failure; and on similar renal structural and functional alterations that promote eventual renal failure [4, 7]. Of course, it is also reasonable to believe that some of these same endpoints of hypertension and aging may occur independently. Thus, each of the structural and functional changes promoted by sodium, aging, and disease(s) may be independent or even coincident with each other. Indeed, both may be responsible for the coexistence of hypertensive cardiovascular and renal diseases as well as with their concurrence in normotensive individuals. Thus, there seems to be a more complicated and intriguing course of events that can be produced during a lifetime of dietary salt excess that relates to the aging process which may also explain, at least in part, why arterial, cardiac, and/or renal functional and structural impairment in hypertensive patients may also occur in with normotensive individuals [4–7].

For example, the initial renal vascular and parenchymal changes have generally been associated with diminishing renal function or proteinuria in elderly individuals which, in time, may further result in end-stage renal disease resulting from aging and/or associated hypertension. The causative mechanisms have generally been attributed to the development of nephrosclerosis manifested by renal arteriolar, interstitial hyaline deposition or to glomerular arteriolar thickening and fibrosis that may ultimately result in of end-stage renal disease [8, 9]. However, when disease coding is required, these clinical consequences have usually been ascribed to hypertension in the elderly associated diabetes or to the "aging process" itself [8–10].

Background and the "New" Problem

The Problem

As stated above, an etiological relationship between dietary salt excess and hypertension has been well demonstrated alone or in combination in the course of events of cardiovascular and renal diseases and the aging process itself [4, 5, 7]. These changes occur primarily in the large arteries manifested by stiffening, development of impaired distensibility, and pulse wave propagation that participate in developing systolic hypertension (particularly in the elderly) [9–12]. In addition, they also promote fibrosis, left ventricular hypertrophy, and, consequently, more complex arterial, cardiac, and renal structural and functional impairment [4, 5, 11, 12]. These earlier and independent and/or coexistent events seem to have been largely disregarded, and the associated long-term pathophysiological effects of prolonged dietary salt overload have not been fully appreciated until relatively recently. Moreover, the functional effects of chronic salt excess have been primarily related to volume overload rather than to long-term and progressive arterial stiffening and cardiovascular and/or renal dysfunction and failure that occur primarily in patients with essential hypertension and, perhaps, the "very elderly" normotensive individuals [4, 9–13]. On the other hand, salt excess may also result in early ventricular stiffening and diastolic ventricular dysfunction associated with fibrosis and, later, with eventual impaired myocardial contractility and, eventually, systolic failure [13]. These common events have been well recognized epidemiologically and clinically [9–16]. They have also been associated with a progressively increasing number of hospitalizations and end-stage outcomes (i.e., cardiac and/or renal failure) in patients with hypertension or even individuals with a normal blood pressure that occurs with great cost to human life and disability as well as healthcare cost. Indeed, they represent the most common causes of hospitalization and death in the United States and other industrialized societies [7, 9, 10, 13].

We suggest in this discussion that the prolonged dietary salt overload which occurs in our societies has not remained at the forefront of our thinking. Even in the reports of the Joint National Committee and in similar national and world reports, endpoints have focused primarily on improving death rates associated with stroke and coronary heart disease related to effective antihypertensive treatment [7, 9, 10]. In striking contrast, there have been coincident astounding and progressive increases in the annual occurrences of hospitalizations and deaths associated with cardiovascular and renal failure [9, 13]. The purpose of establishing these relationships at the outset of this discussion is to underscore these previously unappreciated relationships. In doing so, our purpose is to promote more vigorous national and international efforts directed to reduce sodium/salt diets. Hopefully, these efforts will result in a further reduction in associated cardiovascular-renal morbidity and mortality. Recent reductions of these end-stage effects of salt-related diseases have already been demonstrated in Great Britain which has been attributed to legislated demonstrations of sodium restrictions in baked, processed, and frozen foods [14].

Evidence

Although much has been written about convincing evidence associating dietary sodium excess with hypertensive disease, much has also been written maintaining controversy. In response, several well-reference reports have responded supporting the relationship of salt and disease [15, 16]. The evidence cited includes a large body of well-designed and conducted epidemiological studies that involve valid statistical design and interpretation of the data [15, 16]. Additionally, in recent years, there has been increasing emphasis demonstrating convincing experimental laboratory and clinical investigative data supporting the existence of the strong relationship between prolonged dietary salt overload and its multiorgan life-threatening structural and functional consequences [7]. The following discussion provides some of that laboratory and clinical experience.

Laboratory Studies

Much of the laboratory and clinical studies have been based on the initial establishment of valid experimental methodology, established meaningful acceptable animal models, and supportive clinical findings. The experimental studies have involved various animal models involving varied species produced surgically or by administration of specific chemical interventions administered acutely or chronically. In more recent years well-disciplined and carefully designed experimental efforts were developed involving confirmed meticulous brother-to-sister inbreeding techniques [17, 18]. Later, more sophisticated methodological methods were developed whereby specific genes were added or deleted selectively involving this approach [19, 20]. Our personal studies have involved the spontaneously hypertensive rat (SHR) and have been reported in peer-reviewed journals over the past five decades involving controlled studies of the SHR compared with their normotensive control rats, the Wistar-Kyoto (WKY) rat. Their findings are discussed below.

Genetically Hypertensive Rat Strains

In the earlier years, prior to initiation of specific genetic studies, investigators employed time-consuming selective brother-to-sister rat inbreeding. These studies were developed in order to provide predictably developed hypertensive or normotensive offspring in 100 % of their respective progenies after many generations; they remain available to this date. One early rat strain was developed by Professor Louis K. Dahl at the Brookhaven National Laboratory, Long Island, New York, and was termed the Dahl "salt-sensitive" or "salt-resistant" rat strains. They have been studied meticulously for over 50 years [21, 22]. These strains correctly use their acronyms by virtue of their strict inbreeding over these many decades. The other broadly used rat strain is that of the spontaneously hypertensive rat (SHR) and its related stroke-prone SHR [18, 23–25]. Two of a variety of other inbred strains have been studied less extensively [17, 26]. The SHR was also bred meticulously, but neither this strain nor its normotensive control strain (the WKY) was bred for "salt-sensitive" purity. However, as its acronym clearly indicates, the SHR was bred for its purity in naturally developed hypertension [18, 23]. And, strikingly, it is to the benefit of the SHR that it is very similar in its characteristics with essential hypertension in man without descriptive nomenclature suggesting "salt sensitivity," but to its pure characteristic of hypertension. These two genetically inbred strains (Dahl and SHR) still remain under frequent study throughout the world.

Spontaneously Hypertensive Rat

The two Kyoto strains that include the SHR and the WKY have many characteristics similar to the most common form of hypertension that occurs in the patient having essential hypertension [18, 23–25]. Their genes are responsible for ensuring their respective characteristics in the SHR or in most patients (i.e., >85 %) having essential hypertension. As suggested above, the control group for the SHR and its normotensive control strain (the WKY) are unlike the Dahl hypertensive and normotensive rats. Thus, the Dahl "salt-sensitive" and "salt-resistant" hypertensive rats were each developed simultaneously and, unlike the SHR, were bred specifically for their responses to salt loading. In contrast, the SHR was bred for its naturally elevated arterial pressure. Several other strains with hypertension have not been as broadly studied as these two pairs of rat strains (Dahl and SHR) that were developed using similar techniques of strict brother-to-sister inbreeding. They have been studied less frequently and are referenced in the peer-reviewed literature.

The SHR strain was developed by Professors Kozo Okamoto and Kyuzo Aoki [18, 23–25] who generously made the male and female representatives of their SHR and WKY strains available to the National Heart Institute (NHI) of the National Institutes of Health (NIH) in Bethesda, Maryland, in latter 1968. Soon thereafter, Professor Aoki (my friend and colleague with whom I related while on the staff of the Research Division, Cleveland Clinic) informed me that he had recently presented male and female SHR and WKY representatives of their strain to the NHI from Kyoto University. He informed me that his

Kyoto colleague at Professor Okamoto's laboratory, Professor Yukio Yamori, was spending his sabbatical leave at the NHI at that time. Dr. Yamori, who had continued his SHR studies in Kyoto, suggested that I contact him at the NHI so that I could obtain several male and female counterparts of the original SHR strains from NHI. I promptly did just that and, shortly thereafter, came to the NHI where I received my gift of SHR and WKY rats. This opened a new chapter of my research activities at the University of Oklahoma Health Sciences Center where I initiated a long history of investigative studies in collaboration with my friends and colleagues in Japan as well as my forthcoming experimental research with my two dear colleagues and doctoral students and lifelong friends, Doctors Marc A. Pfeffer and Janice M. Pfeffer, who, in subsequent years, were on the faculty at Brigham and Women's Hospital, Boston, Massachusetts [27].

In our extended research studies concerning salt loading in the SHR (spanning over 45 years), we consistently found that the SHR strain was uniformly predisposed to develop severely elevated arterial pressure, left ventricular enlargement, and hemodynamics that were exacerbated by salt loading [28–42]. Thus, the meticulous inbreeding of the SHR (and WKY) was similar to that of the "salt-sensitive" Dahl rat. It was thus possible for us to develop and to exacerbate consistently their increased arterial pressure, hemodynamics, and cardiac mass. However, as the Dahl "salt-sensitive" nomenclature implies, a clear-cut nomenclature of "salt sensitivity" is not possible for the inbred SHR. To date, we have continuously studied the Okamoto-Aoki SHR and WKY rat (and the American normotensive Wistar model) and found that they consistently demonstrated significantly elevated arterial pressure from the first time that we were able to measure it directly (i.e., intra-arterially) within days after their birth [18]. Thus, we have favored and continued to use the SHR model. Moreover, when given a dietary salt load chronically (the details are specifically spelled out in each of our reports) for time periods ranging from 3 to 12 and as long as 73 or more weeks. They all demonstrated severely elevated arterial pressure and associated pathophysiological characteristics [18, 31–42] that are very similar to those reported for essential hypertensive patients.

(Parenthetically, and in a very practical and pragmatic sense, the only way to define whether the essential hypertensive patient is or is not truly "salt sensitive" is to have that specific patient discontinue the salt from the diet (and any antihypertensive therapy) to demonstrate that his/her pressure returns to hypertensive levels [4]. It then is possible to know whether the blood pressure of that patient demonstrated pretreatment "salt-sensitive" hypertension. The clinical study to arrive at this necessary conclusion has not yet been reported and, most likely, will not be performed for ethical reasons. Hence, we remain convinced that the SHR is "hypertension" specific, although we have not yet experienced failure for its arterial pressure to increase and, then, to increase further following a prolonged dietary salt load.)

Experimental SHR Studies

At this time, many compelling experimental laboratory studies have accumulated and continue to provide clear-cut evidence that prolonged salt loading has produced structural and functional increasingly more severe hemodynamics, and clear-cut evidence of target organ involvement from hypertension. As indicated above, this chapter focuses on our long-standing and current laboratory studies using strict SHR and WKY brother-to-sister inbreeding of SHR and WKY rats of the same age and gender in each of our specific studies [31–42]. We have previously shown (and have consistently confirmed) studies from the Kyoto group of Professor Okamoto that contrary to some reports, the SHR arterial pressures are always increased significantly with respect to their appropriate normotensive WKY controls. The major condition for our assertion is that the SHR and their WKY controls must be matched for identical age, gender, and laboratory conditions in each study. Several reports from other laboratories have expressed otherwise suggesting that the expected increase of the SHR arterial pressure increases at later ages. Their increased pressures were defined as an arterial pressure level increase to a level usually greater than 150 mmHg (or otherwise specified) systolic rather than comparing with pressure of control WKY rats of the same age and gender.

Thus, over these many years, our studies have continued to provide strong pathophysiological evidence demonstrating that the resulting hemodynamics are common to cardiac, vascular, and renal structural and functional damage that was identical to those findings observed in patients with essential hypertension [43]. (However, unfortunately, none were focused on brain involvement.) Additionally, the specific age, gender, and experimental conditions for each population of rats studied were specifically stated and involved administration of excess dietary salt loading (usually by mouth) to SHR and WKY rats of identical ages and sex specifically indicated in their respective publications. Further, for each of these studies that included normotensive WKY control rats, the methods used in each publication provide detailed evidence related to arterial pressure, gender, and cardiovascular or renal findings. Furthermore, each salt-loading study from our laboratory demonstrated severe perivascular and extravascular parenchymal changes in the target organs that mimic those changes that have been so stated in those patients having essential hypertension with biopsy and postmortem study [33–42]. These changes had been demonstrated in an earlier study in 1998 by Yu et al. clearly demonstrating fibrosis in the coronary and renal circulations [44].

Cardiovascular Involvement

In the above-cited studies, we have consistently demonstrated that prolonged dietary loading of salt was maintained for at least 3 weeks (or up to 12 and to 73 weeks). The directly measured arterial pressures were consistently elevated (systolic, diastolic, and mean arterial pressure) and were directly related to respective increased total peripheral and organ vascular resistances and increased left ventricular masses [35–42]. In addition, we have also found abnormal hemodynamic and cardiac changes demonstrating that left ventricular and cardiac masses increased further with salt loading. Moreover, they developed abnormal coronary vascular hemodynamics (including the left and right ventricular baseline, coronary blood flow and resistance, and respective minimal coronary blood flow and resistance) after dipyridamole administration. These abnormal coronary (and renal) hemodynamic changes were complicated further by fibrosis that occurred surrounding the arterioles of the cardiac and renal parenchyma within the extracellular tissue of both ventricles, large vessels, and kidneys that significantly impaired their respective structure and function [34–36]. These changes were also revealed on myocardial biopsies of patients with essential hypertension which was not complicated by occlusive atherosclerotic coronary artery disease [43]. Moreover, the affected cardiac alterations were associated with significant ischemia of both the hypertrophied left ventricle and the non-hypertrophied right ventricle [35]. Furthermore, the ventricular functional changes were initially manifested by impaired diastolic dysfunction (with preserved systolic function) in all older adult SHR rats although younger adult rats also developed impaired systolic ventricular function that was complicated by overt cardiac failure and death in approximately one-fourth of these younger rats [32, 35, 37]. A number of specific diastolic and systolic functional determinations have been defined in advance of these studies and were specifically identified and related to these ventricular function studies for the SHR [34]. Of importance, the findings obtained were strikingly similar to the most common cause of heart failure and hospitalization encountered in Medicare-aged patients with hypertension (and normotensive patients) in the United States and in most other industrialized nations. Additionally, there was evidence of significant structural and functional changes in the aorta and large arteries that included diminished distensibility and pulse wave propagation, fibrosis, and decreased elasticity which have also been reported in elderly patients with systolic hypertension [11, 12, 32, 34, 44–48].

Clinical Cardiovascular Studies

In recent years, a number of salt-loading investigative studies have been reported involving essential hypertensive individuals who developed increased left ventricular mass [15, 16, 43–51]. Importantly, impaired left ventricular diastolic function with preserved normal systolic ventricular contraction was demonstrated in those with left ventricular hypertrophy [52–55]. Recently these abnormal functions were reversed in a carefully studied group of hypertensive patients with impaired diastolic ventricular function who were treated with a monitored DASH diet [54]. Other studies demonstrated that a salt surfeit diet increased systolic pressure and was associated with diminished large artery distensibility and decreased forward generation of the large arterial pulse wave [11, 12, 46–48].

Experimental and Clinical Renal Involvement

Much experimental evidence has accumulated over the years demonstrating evidence that prolonged salt loading promotes renal control of fluid balance that leads to fluid retention. However, more recently laboratory investigators also have provided compelling results demonstrating specific adverse effects of salt loading on renal structure and function that leads progressively to end-stage renal failure even before these experimental models did not demonstrate reduced blood flow or functional impairment before salt loading [56–59]. These findings have been shown to be consistent with pathophysiological findings in man [8, 60–63].

In our laboratory, we have demonstrated that, in as short time period as 3 weeks of dietary salt excess, end-stage renal failure was produced that was associated with massive proteinuria and significantly impaired function (hypercreatinemia, hyperuricemia, and reduced glomerular filtration rate) [36, 38–42]. These profound renal and intrarenal changes were manifested pathologically by interstitial and perivascular fibrosis of the larger renal and intrarenal arteries and arterioles. In addition, major structural and functional alterations also were demonstrated using direct renal micropuncture [36]. The end-stage renal pathophysiological changes were characterized by significantly increased glomerular hydrostatic and stop-flow pressures, afferent and efferent arteriolar constriction, and reduced total renal and single nephron glomerular filtration rate [36]. Histological studies demonstrated marked arteriolar thickening and damage and severe hyalinization of the tubules and glomeruli [36]. Further, in another study there was dramatic evidence of increased intrarenal production of angiotensinogen by the distal tubules and/or collecting ducts which strongly suggested active stimulation at the distal nephron level (and/or collection duct) by a local renal renin-angiotensin system (RAS) [40]. This local renal RAS is in addition to the classical intrarenal juxtaglomerular (JG) apparatus which may be stimulated or inhibited by specific systemic or local mechanisms responsible for modulation of the initiation or inhibition of the local RAS [40, 64]. These changes appeared to be strikingly similar to those occurring during development of end-stage renal disease in patients with essential hypertension having structural and functional impairment [8]. Finally, those pathophysiological and biological changes have been shown not only experimentally in long-term SHR studies but in normotensive, pre-hypertensive, and established essential hypertensive and diabetic patients who were exposed to a lifetime of a potentially salt surfeit diet [65–67].

Cardiovascular and Renal Pharmacological Studies

The above-cited reports demonstrated that prolonged dietary salt loading impaired cardiovascular-renal structural and functional alterations (Fig. 18.1). In addition, pharmacological intervention studies have recently shown that angiotensin II (type 1) receptor inhibitory agents (ARBs) prevented (or inhibited) those cardiovascular and/or renal structural and functional changes without necessarily changing arterial

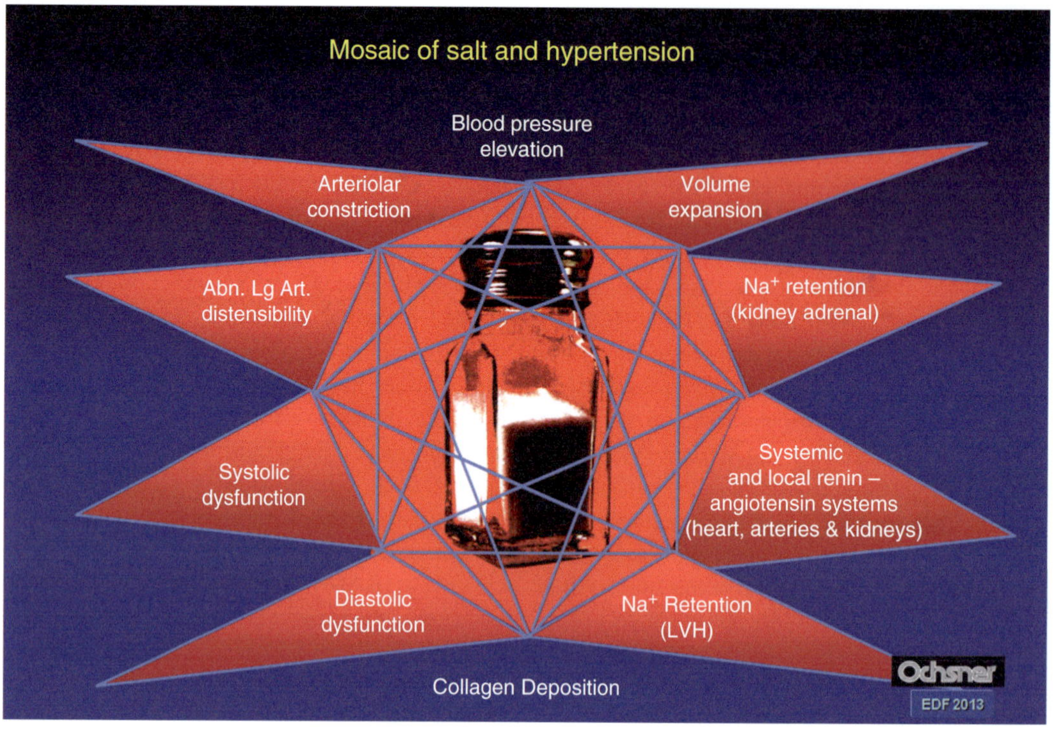

Fig. 18.1 An adaptation of the "Pagean Mosaic" which presents the multiplicity of pathophysiological factors (and others to be identified) that interrelate with each other in a mosaic factor to account for the expression of salt-overload disease

pressure [4, 36–42, 67]. Thus, with respect to cardiac or ventricular function, these agents prevented (or inhibited) the increased ventricular mass as well as hydroxyproline content and fibrosis. These changes were demonstrated by any one of several ARBs, thereby strongly suggesting that their chemical effects were mediated, at least in part, through their local actions expressed through angiotensin type 1 receptors. They were also produced by different beta-adrenergic receptor blocking agents [41, 68] and by one ARB that may act through possibly different mechanisms without affecting arterial pressure [42]. Those findings provide strong evidence that each of these agents operated locally by intervening in the expression of angiotensin II directly or indirectly. Thus, for example, eplerenone (an aldosterone receptor blocking agent) may also operate on the ventricle through local ventricular production of aldosterone and secondarily on the local cardiac RAS system [39]. Furthermore, similar actions in the kidney also suggest inhibition of a local renal angiotensin and/or aldosterone participation in the RAS (RAAS). These local cardiovascular-renal actions suggest a far more complicated action than heretofore conceived; and that they may operate on subsequent more specific biological actions [43, 69]. Further investigation into these possibilities only promotes new and more complicated actions by the RAAS, thereby expanding current considerations of drug actions that may be premature at present.

Epidemiological Trials

A number of prospective epidemiological and clinical trials involving single and multiple centers demonstrated that high-salt diets resulted in elevated arterial pressure and various additional manifestations of cardiovascular and renal functional impairment. Several reports presented pro or con arguments that supported or denied the salt (or sodium) excess responsible for end-stage events in patients with cardiovascular diseases including cardiac failure [15, 16]. Certainly, complicating this controversy have been several reports of therapeutic interventions in patients with cardiac failure who were treated with diuretics, potassium supplements or retaining agents, ACE inhibitors, and other agents that demonstrated impaired or improved cardiac function morbidity.

Therapeutic Inhibition (Prevention or Remodeling) of Target Organ Stiffening

An increasing number of clinical trials have detailed pharmacological cardiovascular reversal of target organ mass, collagen deposition with fibrosis; and this is not a new clinical finding. The value of ACE inhibition in promoting ventricular remodeling and prevention of heart failure or myocardial infarction (in patients with a prior myocardial infarction) was initially demonstrated by Pfeffer and Braunwald [70, 71]. Subsequent multiple confirmations of this innovation were demonstrated using other ACE inhibitors or angiotensin II (type 1) receptor blocking drugs (ARBs) that inhibited systemic and/or local RASs [72]. The precise biological mechanisms whereby these effects were achieved are presently unresolved although a number are presently under intense study. Included among other pharmacological agents that prevent these actions are certain beta-adrenergic receptor blocking agents although their inhibition of the RAS has been employed for many years. Understanding of the actions whereby pharmacological agents of those drug classes that inhibit or prevent cardiovascular and renal stiffening (or remodeling) while not necessarily reducing arterial pressure remain under intense study. Follow-up of these recent observations, investigations should provide further insight into this important question of target organ cardiovascular stiffening or remodeling.

Recent Clinical Experience and the Future

As with any new clinical investigative concept, investigators of an experimental or clinical problem are stimulated by questions generated by ongoing experimental data for further continued research. To this end, well-designed clinical trials have been conducted that raise new questions. Among those that stand out most in my mind relate to the biological mechanisms whereby angiotensin II, produced by salt excess, may stimulate local RASs in the target organs of hypertension to promote adverse clinical endpoints.

In one recent multicenter clinical trial involving volunteer pre-hypertensive subjects in the large multicenter NIH-sponsored, TOPH study [73], one-half of these volunteer subjects agreed to remain on their usual (high-salt) diet. The other half received a prescribed low-salt diet administered by the investigators. After a prolonged and careful follow-up period, the investigators broke the trial's double-blinded protocol. The resulting data demonstrated a highly significant reduction in the number of patients receiving the sodium-restricted diet that resulted in a remarkable and significant number of cardiovascular deaths and endpoints [73]. This was the first prospectively conducted controlled trial that involved individuals with a long-term salt-restricted diet resulting in a significantly decreased number of cardiovascular endpoints of all participants. Results from other similarly designed prospective and controlled clinical trials (as cited by the TOPH investigators) raised certain possible valid reasons that may have negated clear-cut conclusions. Hence, TOPH was the first prospectively conducted clinical trial that demonstrated a reduced cardiovascular morbidity and mortality resulting from a salt-restricted diet.

Hopefully, the long-standing salt controversy will soon abate. However, from my personal view the age-old biblical statement that Lot's wife died from the observation that her heart turned into salt may be corrected. However, it seems clear to me that her heart, vessels, and kidneys may have been severely stiffened by fibrosis and collagen-related biological intermediary effects. There is no doubt in my mind that, following the history of advancing science, this latter conclusion will generate further questions and controversy.

Other Pharmacological and Biological Studies

As stated above, structural and functional pathophysiological alterations involving prolonged salt excess in the SHR and patients on the cardiovascular-renal systems were significantly prevented or improved by several classes of pharmacological agents (e.g., angiotensin-converting enzyme (ACE) inhibitors, ARBs, or beta-adrenergic receptor blocking agents) that inhibit (at the least, in part) systemic or local RASs. These reversals of the pathological, inflammatory, and biological changes strongly suggest a role of local tissue RASs that are apparently promoted by sodium even while, contemporaneously, the renal JG apparatus is suppressed. Indeed, such local biological changes within these organs have been reported to result in stiffness and impaired distensibility of the arteries, ventricular chambers, and kidneys. These findings suggest that the local RASs promote biological events that promote fibrosis within the target organs through local production of collagen or collagen cross-linking fibers through lysyl oxidase and other products within the ventricles, arteries, and kidneys [69]. That these changes were apparently related to specific local RASs is supported by the fact that these changes were locally inhibited (or prevented) pharmacologically within the heart, arteries, or kidneys.

The Mosaic of Salt, Hypertension, and Cardiovascular-Renal Diseases and Stiffness

The Mosaic

As already stated, we have been studying the relationship of dietary salt excess with hypertension, cardiovascular-renal diseases, other complicating clinical problems, and their management for many years. As with many multifactorial and complicated problems, this problem, no doubt, will continue to challenge answers and raise undreamed future questions. It, therefore, was of little surprise to me, upon reflection, that one of my academic role models stimulated my thinking. Thus, I was confronted by Doctor Irvine H. Page about this problem in my reverie, and he promptly responded to my reflection: "Ed, you know just how I would answer. Like any multifactorially complex problem that besets the committed investigator, he/she should return to the laboratory (or patient) and search for answers to those questions that have been raised. Study the answers, and you will find new questions that will continue to challenge you. This is the story of science; and this is the excitement that captured your attention in the first place. I reflected on his response from his mental echo; and, once again, I returned to his Mosaic (Fig. 18.1).

Yes, this is the "stuff" that captures students of medicine, its diseases and problems that constantly beset us. These are the questions that came to mind as I reflected on the problem as to why prolonged dietary salt excess produces increasing morbidity and mortality. How does salt excess account for disease or its exacerbation? What factors, other than hypertension, may account for the production of similar outcomes and hospitalizations even in normotensive individuals? How does a prolonged lifetime of dietary salt excess account for increased vascular stiffness and cardiac and/or renal failure? Why does prolonged dietary salt excess seem to be addictive? And so I charted the salt mosaic and thought – and thought more about this puzzlement over these past four and more decades.

Irvine Page

Irvine Page was stimulated by mathematics and chemistry when he was a young boy. He was a member of the American Chemical Society long before he thought about his future in college and a medical career. Indeed, his father Lafayette Page (a well-known otolaryngologist) insisted that Irvine should first pursue a medical career. He could think later about chemistry and mathematics once he learned a profession that would support him and his family. So young Page went to Cornell University Medical School, graduated, spent 2 years in postgraduate medicine, and then was accepted on the staff of the Kaiser Wilhelm Institute in Germany. He was assigned to a laboratory and program focused on brain chemistry. (Incidentally, he subsequently published on that topic which was the first textbook written on this subject.) However, this young investigator continued to reflect on his primary preoccupation of mathematics and about Josiah Willard Gibbs' (Professor of Chemistry at Yale University) mass system of phases which Gibbs demonstrated to be dependent on the sum total of each of the component masses of that system. It was that very line of thinking that was responsible for Page's Mosaic Theory of Hypertension which, when stated simply, suggested to him that the underlying causation of hypertension was the sum total of underlying mechanisms responsible for the disease [74, 75]. In many discussions with Page, I have thought much about his concept that the causation of any complex (i.e., multifactorial) problem may be explained as a mosaic of interacting factors or mechanisms that are responsible for its causation and maintenance. So, to return to the Mosaic of Salt and the Mosaic Theory of Hypertension.

The Salt Mosaic

We are keenly aware that hypertensive disease is dependent hemodynamically on the product of the height of arterial pressure and on the degree of arterial constriction (i.e., vascular resistance or total peripheral resistance) or the size of the vascular "container" (i.e., its intravascular volume or its "stiffness"). The two factors that are related primarily to its volume are adrenergic input to the cardiovascular system (i.e., the stiff "container") and its intravascular volume (i.e., the "content") which, in turn, is also dependent upon sodium retention or volume expansion, renal function, and their hormonal controls. Cardiac output, in addition, is dependent upon the heart rate and systolic and diastolic ventricular function. Each of the myriad of factors (including sodium or salt) comprise the mosaic result in hypertension (its "Pagean Mosaic").

Page's additional major landmark discoveries include his discovery of angiotensin II and serotonin which he related, in part, determines the state of constriction of the vessels and other systems that account for the increased arterial pressure [75]. Subsequent to Page's death, a number of new humoral factors and hormones were identified that control vascular diameter and volume and, therefore, participate in its mosaic. Among these are the role of oxidative stress and related to reactive oxygen species, inflammation, and other mechanisms under study which may be related to the other underlying mechanisms of hypertension [69]. This, then, brings us to a new multifactorial schema (or mosaic) that permits a revision of our thinking about a Pagean Salt Mosaic.

Conclusion

This discussion has focused on some newer factors underlying salt-induced cardiovascular-renal stiffening including the local renin-angiotensin systems in the arteries, heart, and kidneys. The data presented suggests that stimulation of certain cardiovascular and renal sites may be responsible for the untoward and adverse cardiovascular and renal effects of chronic salt excess. Presented in this discussion are a mosaic of factors that interact with other biological (RAS) systems that may be responsible for the ultimate production of collagen and its cross-linking and fibrosis resulting in reduced cardiovascular elasticity and renal stiffening. These concepts were related to earlier thoughts of Irvine Page's concept of mosaic multifactorial causation of disease. The reader now may understand how the generation of simple questions in earlier investigative processes can lead to more complex problems that maintain an active investigative career. And, so, once again I extend my appreciation to a role model!

References

1. Ambard L, Beaujard E. Causes de l'hypertension arterielle. Arch Gen Med. 1904;1:529.
2. Kurlansky M. SALT: a world history. New York: Penguin Books; 2002. p. 484.

3. Frohlich ED, Messerli FH. Sodium and hypertension. In: Papper S, editor. Sodium, Cations of biologic significance, vol. 2. 2nd ed. Boca Raton: CRC Press; 1982. p. 144–74.
4. Frohlich ED. The salt conundrum: a hypothesis. Hypertension. 2007;50:161–6.
5. Frohlich ED. Are local renin-angiotensin systems the focal points for understanding salt sensitivity in hypertension? In: Frohlich ED, Re RN, editors. The local cardiac renin-angiotensin-aldosterone system. 2nd ed. Federal Republic of Germany: Springer; 2009. p. 1–6.
6. Ferder LE. Renin angiotensin systems and aging. In: De Mello WC, Frohlich ED, editors. Renin angiotensin system and cardiovascular disease. New York: Humana Press; a part of Springer Science & Business Media, LLC; 2009. p. 231–43.
7. Frohlich ED, Susic D. Sodium and its multiorgan targets. Circulation. 2011;124:1882–5.
8. Rule AD, Hatem A, Conell LD, Taler SJ, Cosla FG, Kremers WK, Texter SC, Stegall MD. The association between age and nephrosclerosis on renal biopsy among healthy adults. Ann Intern Med. 2010;152:561–7.
9. Seventh Report of the Joint National Committee on Prevention. Detection, evaluation, and treatment of high blood pressure (JNC-7). JAMA. 2003;289:2560–72.
10. International Society of Hypertension Writing Group. International Society of Hypertension (ISH), statement on blood pressure lowering and stroke prevention. J Hypertens. 2003;21:651–63.
11. Safar ME, Asmar RG, Benetos A, London GM, Levy BL. Sodium, large arteries and diuretic compounds in hypertension. J Hypertens. 1992;10:S133–6.
12. Safar ME, Thuilliez C, Richard V, Benetos A. Pressure independent contribution of sodium to large artery structure and function in hypertension. Cardiovasc Res. 2000;46:269–76.
13. Frohlich ED, Susic D. Pressure overload. Heart Fail Clin. 2012;8:21–32.
14. UK Food Standards Agency. Website. http://www.food.gov.uk. Accessed 18 June 2007.
15. Appel LJ, Frohlich ED, Hall JE, Pearson TA, Sacco RI, Seals DR, Sacks FM, Smith Jr SC, Vafiadis DK, Van Horn LV. The importance of population-wide sodium reduction as a means to prevent cardiovascular disease and stroke: a call to action from the American Heart Association. Circulation. 2011;123:1138–43.
16. Kotchen TA, Cowley Jr AW, Frohlich ED. Salt in health and disease: a delicate balance. N Engl J Med. 2013;368:1229–37.
17. Smirk FH, Hall WH. Inherited hypertension in rats. Nature. 1958;182:717–28.
18. Trippodo NC, Frohlich ED. Controversies in cardiovascular research: similarities of genetic (spontaneous) hypertension. Man and rat. Circ Res. 1981;48:309–19.
19. Graham D, McBride MW, Gaasenbect M, Gilday K, Beattie E, Miller WH, McClure JD, Polke JM, Montezano A, Touyz RM, Dominiczak AF. Candidate genes that determine response to salt in the stroke-prone spontaneously hypertensive rat. Congenic analysis. Hypertension. 2007;50:1134–41.
20. Smithies O. Turning pages (Nobel Lecture). Chembiochem. 2008;9:1342–2359.
21. Dahl LK. Effects of chronic excess salt feeding. Induction of self-sustaining hypertension in rats. J Exp Med. 1961;114:231–6.
22. Dahl LK, Heine M, Tassinari L. Role of genetic factors in susceptibility to experimental hypertension due to chronic excess salt ingestion. Nature. 1962;194:480–2.
23. Okomoto K, Aoki K. Development of a strain of spontaneously hypertensive rats. Jpn Circ J. 1963;27:282–93.
24. Okamoto K, Tabei R, Fukkushima M, Nosaka S, Yamori Y, Ichijima K, Haebara H, Matsumoto M, Maruyama T, Suzuki Y, Tamegai M. Further observations of the development of a strain of spontaneously hypertensive rats. Jpn Circ J. 1966;30:703–16.
25. Aoki K, Yamori Y, Ooshima A, Okamoto K. Effects of high or low sodium intake in spontaneously hypertensive rats. Jpn Circ J. 1972;36:539–45.
26. Bianchi G, Baer PG, Fox U, Duzzi L, Pagetti D, Giovanetti AM. Changes in renin, water balance, and sodium balance during development of high blood pressure in genetically hypertensive rats. Circ Res. 1975;36/37(suppl I):153–61.
27. Pfeffer MA, Frohlich ED. Hemodynamic and myocardial function in young and old normotensive and spontaneously hypertensive rats. Circ Res. 1973;32(I):28–38.
28. Chrysant SG, Walsh GM, Frohlich ED. Hemodynamic changes induced by prolonged NaC1 and DOCA administration in spontaneously hypertensive rats (SHR). Angiology. 1978;29:303–9.
29. Chrysant SG, Walsh GM, Kem DC, Frohlich ED. Hemodynamic and metabolic evidence of salt sensitivity in spontaneously hypertensive rats. Am J Physiol. 1979;236:H403–8.
30. Sesoko S, Pegram BL, Wallis GW, Frohlich ED. DOCA-salt induced malignant hypertension in spontaneously hypertensive rats. J Hypertens. 1984;2:49–54.
31. Frohlich ED, Chien Y, Sesoko S, Pegram BL. Relationships between dietary sodium intake, hemodynamics and cardiac mass in spontaneously hypertensive and normotensive Wistar-Kyoto rats. Am J Physiol. 1993;264:R30–4.
32. Ahn J, Varagic J, Slama M, Susic D, Frohlich ED. Cardiac structural and functional responses to salt loading in SHR. Am J Physiol Heart Circ Physiol. 2004;287:H767–72.
33. Varagic J, Frohlich ED. Hypertension and the multifactorial role of salt. Lab Med. 2005;36:652–5.
34. Slama M, Ahn J, Peltier M, Maizel J, Chemla D, Varagic J, Susic D, Tribouilloy C, Frohlich ED. Validation of echocardiographic and Doppler indices of left ventricular relaxation in adult hypertensive and normotensive rats. Am J Physiol Heart Circ Physiol. 2005;289:H1131–6.
35. Varagic J, Frohlich ED, Diez J, Susic D, Ahn J, Gonzalez A, Lopez B. Myocardial fibrosis, impaired coronary hemodynamics, and biventricular dysfunction in salt-loaded SHR. Am J Physiol Heart Circ Physiol. 2006;290:H1503–9.

36. Matavelli LC, Zhou X, Varagic J, Susic D, Frohlich ED. Salt-loading produces severe renal hemodynamic dysfunction independent of arterial pressure in spontaneously hypertensive rats. Am J Physiol Heart Circ Physiol. 2007;292:H814–9.
37. Varagic J, Frohlich ED, Susic D, Ahn J, Matavelli L, Lopez B, Diez J. AT1 receptor antagonism attenuates target organ effects of salt excess in SHRs without affecting pressure. Am J Physiol Heart Circ Physiol. 2008;294:H853–8.
38. Susic D, Zhou X, Frohlich ED. Angiotensin blockade prevents salt-induced injury of the renal circulation in spontaneously hypertensive rats. Am J Nephrol. 2009; 29:639–45.
39. Susic D, Varagic J, Frohlich ED. Cardiovascular effects of inhibition of renin-angiotensin-aldosterone system components in hypertensive rats given salt excess. Am J Physiol. 2010;298:H1177–81.
40. Susic D, Frohlich ED, Korori H, Shao W, Seth D, Navar LG. Salt-induced renal injury in SHR is mediated by AT1 receptor activation. J Hypertens. 2011;29: 716–23.
41. Susic D, Fares H, Frohlich ED. Nebivolol prevents myocardial fibrosis and diastolic dysfunction in salt-loaded spontaneously hypertensive rats. J Am Soc Hypertens. 2012;6:316–23.
42. Susic D, Fares H, Frohlich ED. Telmisartan prevents salt-excess induced exacerbated (malignant) hypertension in spontaneously hypertensive rats. J Cardiovasc Pharmacol Ther. 2013;18:126–32.
43. Frohlich ED, Diez J. Left ventricular hypertrophy and treatment with renin angiotensin system inhibition. In: DeMello WC, Frohlich ED, editors. Renin angiotensin aldosterone system and cardiovascular disease. New York: Humana Press; 2009. p. 103–19.
44. Yu HCM, Burrel LM, Black J, Wu LL, Dilley RJ, Cooper ME, Johnston CI. Salt induces myocardium and renal fibrosis in normotensive and hypertensive rats. Circulation. 1998;98:2621–8.
45. Frohlich ED. Chapter 63: Evaluation and management of the patient with essential hypertension. In: Chatterjee K, Anderson M, Heistad D, Kerber R, editors. Cardiology – an illustrated text book, vol. 2. New Delhi: Jaypee Brothers Medical Pub. LTD; 2012. p. 1129–44.
46. Partovian C, Benetos A, Pommies JP, Mischler W, Safar ME. Effects of a chronic high-salt diet on large artery structure: role of endogenous bradykinin. Am J Physiol. 1998;274:H1423–8.
47. Labat C, Lacolley P, Lajemi M, deGaspero M, Safar ME, Benetos A. Effects of valsartan on mechanical properties of the carotid artery in spontaneously hypertensive rats under high-salt diet. Hypertension. 2001;38:439–43.
48. Mercier N, Labat C, Louis H, Cattan V, Benetos A, Safar ME, Lacolley P. Sodium, arterial stiffness, and cardiovascular mortality in hypertensive rats. Am J Hypertens. 2007;20:319–25.
49. Stier Jr CT, Chander P, Gutstein WH, Levine S, Itskovitz HD. Therapeutic benefit of captopril in salt-loaded stroke-prone spontaneously hypertensive rats is independent of hypertensive effect. Am J Hypertens. 1991;3:680–7.
50. Kreutz R, Kovacevic L, Schulz A, Rothermund L, Ketteler M, Paul M. Effect of high NaC1 diet on spontaneously hypertension in a genetic rat model with reduced nephron number. J Hypertens. 2000;18:777–82.
51. duCallar G, Ribstein J, Mimran A. Dietary sodium intake and target organ damage in essential hypertension. Am J Hypertens. 2002;15:222–9.
52. Langenfeld MR, Schobel H, Veelken R, Weihprecht H, Schmieder RE. Impact of dietary sodium intake on left ventricular diastolic filling in early essential hypertension. Eur Heart J. 1998;19:951–8.
53. Williams JS, Solomon SD, Crivaro M, Colin PR. Dietary sodium intake modulates myocardial relaxation responsiveness to angiotensin II. Transl Res. 2006;48:49–54.
54. Hummel SL, Seymour M, Brook RD, Kollas TJ, Sheth SS, Rosenblum HR, Wells JM, Weder AB. Low-sodium dietary approaches to stop hypertension diet reduces blood pressure, arterial stiffness, and oxidative stress in hypertensive heart failure with preserved ejection fraction. Hypertension. 2012;60:1200–6.
55. Kalogeropoulous A, Georgiopouloa V, Psaty BM, Rodondi N, Smith AL, Harrison DG, Liu Y, Hoffmann U, Bauer DC, Neuman AB, Kritchevsky SB, Harris TB, Butler J. Inflammatory markers and incident heart failure risk in older adults: the Health ABC (Health, Aging, and Body Composition) study. J Am Coll Cardiol. 2010;55:2129–37.
56. Feld LG, van Leiw JB, Brentjens JR, Boylan JW, Bemben S, Chang H, Manz N. Renal lesions and proteinuria in the spontaneously hypertensive rat model made normotensive by treatment. Kidney Int. 1981; 20:606–14.
57. Hirawa N, Uchara Y, Kawabata Y, Numabe A, Ogawa N, Gomi T, Ikeda T, Goto A, Toyo-oba T, Omata M. High-salt intake potentiates the renal vascular and glomerular damage caused by low doses of angiotensin II in uni-nephrectomized rats. J Hypertens. 1999; 17:923–32.
58. Inada Y, Tazawa S, Murakami M, Akahane M. KRH-594, a new angiotensin AT1 receptor antagonist, prevents end-organ damage in stroke-prone spontaneously hypertensive/Izm rats. Clin Exp Pharmacol Physiol. 2001;28:206–11.
59. Khalil RA. Dietary salt and hypertension: new molecular targets add more spice. Am J Physiol Regul Integr Comp Physiol. 2006;290:R509–13.
60. Price DA, Fisher NDL, Lansang MC, Stevanovic R, Williams GH, Hollenberg NK. Renal perfusion in blacks: alterations caused by insuppressibility of intrarenal renin with salt. Hypertension. 2002;40:186–9.
61. Verhave JC, Hillege HL, Burgerhof JGM, Janssen WMT, Gansevoort RT, Navis GJ, de Zeeuw D, Jong PE. Sodium intake affects urinary albumin excretion especially in overweight subjects. J Intern Med. 2004;256:324–30.
62. Swift PA, Markandu ND, Sagnella GA, He FJ, MacGegor GA. Modest salt reduction reduces blood

pressure and urine protein excretion in black hypertensives: a randomized control trial. Hypertension. 2005;46:308–16.

63. Meneton P, Jeunemaitre X, de Wardener HE, MacGregor GA. Links between dietary salt intake, renal salt handling, blood pressure, and cardiovascular diseases. Physiol Rev. 2005;85:679–715.
64. Schunkert H, Ingelfinger JR, Jacob H, Jackson B, Bouyounes B, Dzau VJ. Reciprocal feedback regulation of kidney angiotensinogen and renin RNA expressions by angiotensin II. Am J Physiol. 1992;263:E863–9.
65. Kobori H, Ohashi N, Katsurada A, Miyata K, Satou R, Saito T, Mamamoto T. Urinary angiotensinogen as a potential biomarker of severity of chronic kidney diseases. J Am Soc Hypertens. 2008;2:349–54.
66. Kobori H, Alper B, Shenava R, Katsurada A, Saito T, Ohashi N, Urushihara M, Miyata K, Satoru R, Hamm L, Navar G. Urinary angiotensinogen as a novel biomarker of the intrarenal renin-angiotensin system in hypertensive patients. Hypertension. 2009;53(part 2): 344–50.
67. Kobori H, Urushhara M, Xu JH, Berenson GS, Navar LG. Urinary angiotensinogen is correlated with blood pressure in men (Bogalusa Heart Study). J Hypertens. 2010;28:1422–8.
68. Arita M, Horinaka S, Frohlich ED. Biochemical components and myocardial performance after reversal of left ventricular hypertrophy in spontaneously hypertensive rats. J Hypertens. 1993;11:951–9.
69. Lopez B, Quenejata R, Gonzalez A, Larman H, Diez J. Collagen cross-linking but not collagen amount associates with elevated filling pressures in hypertensive patients with stage C heart failure. Hypertension. 2013;60:677–83.
70. Pfeffer JM, Pfeffer MA, Braunwald E. Influence of chronic captopril therapy on the infarcted and left ventricle of the rat. Circ Res. 1985;57:84–95.
71. Pfeffer MA, Braunwald E, Moye LA, Basta L, Brown Jr EJ, Cuddy TE, Davis BR, Geltman EM, Goldman S, Flaker GC, Klein M, Lamas GA, Packer M, Rouleau J, Rouleau JL, Rutherford J, Wertheimer JH, Hawkins CM, on behalf of the SAVE Investigators. Effect of captopril on mortality and morbidity in patients with left ventricular dysfunction after myocardial infarction. Results of the Survival and Ventricular Enlargement Trial. N Engl J Med. 1992;327: 669–77.
72. Pfeffer MA, Frohlich ED. Improvements in clinical outcomes with the use of angiotensin converting enzyme inhibitors: cross-fertilization between clinical and basic investigation. Am J Physiol Heart Circ Physiol. 2006;291:H2021–5.
73. Cook NR, Cutler JA, Obarzauck E, Buring JE, Rexrode KM, Kumanyika SK, Appel LJ, Whelton PK. Long term effects of dietary sodium reduction on cardiovascular disease outcomes: observational follow-up of the trials of hypertension prevention (TOHP). Br Med J. 2007;334:885–8.
74. Page IH. Pathogenesis of arterial hypertension. JAMA. 1949;140:451–7.
75. Page IH. Arterial hypertension in retrospect. Circ Res. 1974;34:133–42.

19 Preventive Lessons from Hypertension and Myocardial Infarction: Treating Asymptomatic Individuals to Lower the Risk for Subsequent Cardiovascular Events

Marc A. Pfeffer

Abstract

The establishment of hypertension as a risk factor for premature fatal and nonfatal cardiovascular diseases by epidemiological studies was the first step in developing a management strategy to improve prognosis. The demonstration in randomized, placebo- controlled trials that chronic antihypertensive therapy could reduce this risk provided the impetus for an ongoing educational program to motivate both physicians and patients to use pharmacologic agents to treat this asymptomatic condition in order to prevent future adverse cardiovascular events. The parallelisms between the concepts, surrogate outcomes, and more definitive randomized placebo-controlled trials addressing clinical outcome for the use of angiotensin-converting enzyme (ACE) inhibitors in asymptomatic individuals with left ventricular dysfunction are presented. In both cases, the combination of definitive outcomes and safety data coupled with a supportive educational program are needed for physicians and patients to accept and continue lifelong therapy for asymptomatic conditions.

Keywords

Randomized controlled clinical trial • Framingham Heart Study Hypertension • Risk factors • Left ventricular dysfunction • Antihypertensive agents • Angiotensin-converting enzyme inhibitors • Patient education

Hypertension as a consequence of both its high and increasing prevalence with aging and strong inherent linkage to several adverse pathophysiologic pathways, is undoubtedly the major population attributable risk factor for developing overt cardiovascular morbidities [1]. One third of the adult population of the US has elevated blood pressure or requires antihypertensive agents to control their blood pressure [2]. The adverse impact of chronic hypertension has been demonstrated across the gamut of cardiovascular and renal disorders such as heart failure, stroke, myocardial infarction, aortic aneurysm and/or dissection, peripheral vascular

M.A. Pfeffer, MD, PhD
Division of Cardiology, Department of Medicine, Brigham and Women's Hospital, Harvard Medical School, 75 Francis Street, Boston, MA 02115, USA
e-mail: mpfeffer@rics.bwh.harvard.edu

M.E. Safar et al. (eds.), *Blood Pressure and Arterial Wall Mechanics in Cardiovascular Diseases*, DOI 10.1007/978-1-4471-5198-2_19, © Springer-Verlag London 2014

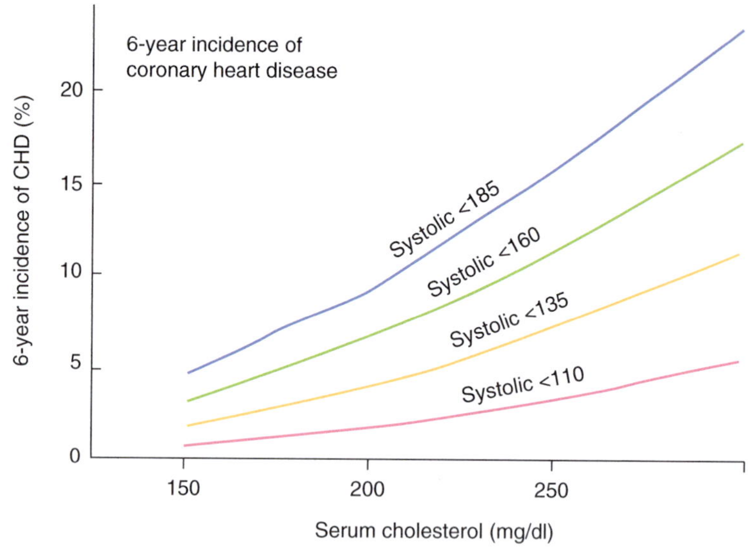

Fig. 19.1 Original figure from Framingham Study providing an early demonstration of the importance of both hypertension and serum cholesterol for subsequent risk of coronary artery disease (Reproduced with permission of Ref. [6])

disease, atrial fibrillation, renal failure and sudden death [3–5]. Although the actuarial data from life-insurance companies had originally shown the negative impact of hypertension on lifespan, the full extent of the morbidity associated with chronically elevated blood pressure from these multiple debilitating and nonfatal as well as fatal events was initially highlighted for the medical community by the Framingham Study [6]. In their now classic paper "Factors of Risk" these pioneering cardiovascular epidemiologists provided data on the incidence of developing coronary heart disease during their initial 6 years of observation, which underscored the importance of elevated blood pressure, serum cholesterol, blood glucose and electrocardiographic left ventricular hypertrophy as independent and additive contributors to manifesting heart disease ([6]; Fig. 19.1).

Confirmation of the Framingham findings has been consistently forthcoming from other even larger emerging major databases, which collectively have solidified the linkage between elevated blood pressure and impaired prognosis. The screening for the Multiple Risk Factor Intervention Trial (MRFIT) created an active registry of approximately 348,000 men between the ages of 35 and 57 years who were then followed for over a decade [7]. This extensive experience generated highly quantitative estimates of the graded adverse impact of blood pressure elevation on the rates of cardiovascular and renal diseases [8]. These risks of both systolic and diastolic blood pressure elevations for experiencing ischemic heart disease deaths were not however, isolated to middle age men. In the Prospective Studies Collaboration, this association between higher blood pressure and greater event rates (all deaths, deaths attributed to stroke or ischemic heart disease) was apparent in women as well as men within each decade of age examined from 40 to 80 years ([9]; Fig. 19.2). The National Health and Nutrition Examination Survey (NHANES) extended this data on hypertension and risks of cardiovascular death across multiple cohorts of race and ethnicity [10].

These and other international epidemiologic studies also produced definitive evidence that hypertension, though an independent hazard, adversely and additively impacts the prognosis of those with other now established classical risk factors such as diabetes, cholesterol and smoking. Indeed, the cumulative adverse outcome from multiple risk factors has reinforced the more holistic approach currently used for a more global overall risk assessment [11–13]. However, estimating an individual's cardiovascular risk would be a clinically shallow activity without the ability to lower their anticipated rates of morbidity and mortality.

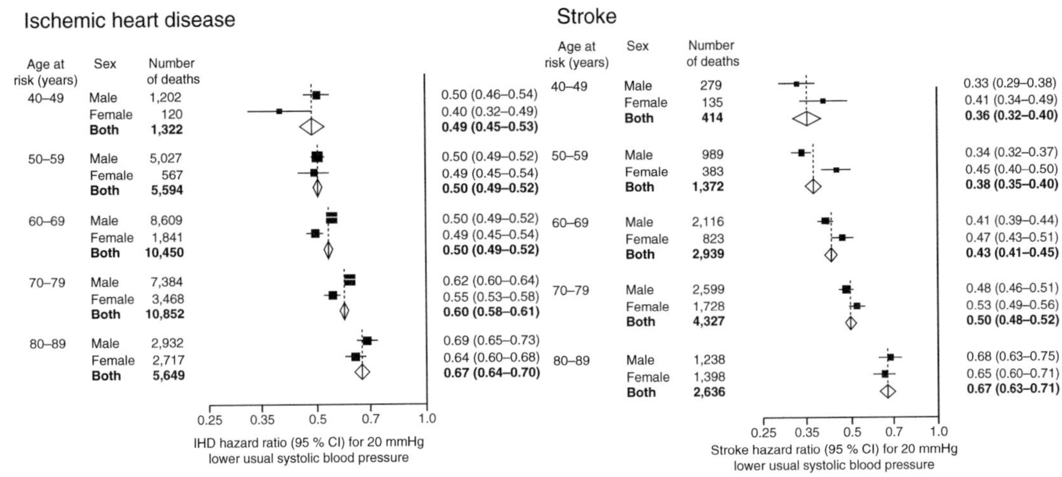

Fig. 19.2 Epidemiologic importance of having lower blood pressure for both risk of ischemic heart disease (*left* panel) and stroke (*right* panel) in both men and women across five decades (Reproduced with permission of Ref. [9])

With the establishment that hypertension augmented rates of adverse cardiovascular events, it remained to be established whether lowering this elevated blood pressure would result in improved prognosis. It is quite fitting that the first major randomized placebo-controlled clinical outcome trials in all of cardiovascular medicine, specifically addressed this issue of determining whether use of antihypertensive therapies could prevent the adverse clinical outcomes observed in the epidemiological studies. Dr. Edward D. Freis accepted this challenge and established and led the Veterans Administration Cooperative Study Group, who then performed the first two major randomized placebo controlled trial testing the effectiveness of antihypertensive agents in altering clinical outcomes not just blood pressure [14, 15]. Utilizing at the time the newly emerging tool of the randomized placebo controlled multicenter trial, the VA Cooperative Study Group on Antihypertensive Agents demonstrated for the first time that lowering blood pressure would result in a reduction in the number of adverse cardiovascular events [14]. By showing that pharmacologic therapy, which reduced blood pressure (combined therapy with hydrochlorothiazide, reserpine and hydralazine) in subjects with marked hypertension (diastolic blood pressure 115–129 mmHg) resulted in lower rates of cardiovascular events and death compared to placebo, the VA investigators provided the first proven rationale to use drugs to treat this risk factor to actually improve prognosis [14]. This blinded trial was stopped prematurely after only 18 months of follow-up at which time 27 of the 70 placebo patients (39 %) had experienced an adverse cardiovascular event or death compared to only 2 of the 73 (3 %) assigned to the active therapy (Table 19.1). In my opinion, the publication of the results of this original VA trial in 1967, represents a watershed moment in cardiovascular medicine. They effectively used the randomized controlled trial to prove that pharmacologic treatment of elevated blood pressure could lower the risk of subsequent major cardiovascular events attributed to hypertension. For the first time, there was evidence that strokes, myocardial infarctions, aortic dissections and heart failure could be prevented! The VA Cooperative Study Group set the stage for the accumulating decades of data justifying the use of antihypertensive therapies in asymptomatic individuals to reduce their risk for subsequent adverse cardiovascular events [14].

On the heels of this ground breaking study, the VA Cooperative Study Group completed a second trial using a similar design but enrolling patients with less severe hypertension (diastolic pressure 90–114 mmHg). With larger numbers of participants and longer follow-up, they again

Table 19.1 VA cooperative study group on antihypertensive agents

	Placebo (n=70)	HCTZ+Reserpine+Hydralazine HCI (n=73)
CV Death	4	0
CVA-Hemorrhage	1	0
CVA-Ischemic	2	1
TIA	1	0
MI	2	0
CCF persisting despite digitalis and mercurial	2	0
CCF responding to digitalis and mercurial	2	0
Worsening renal function	3	0
Hospitalization for Diastolic BP >140 mmHg	3	0
Hypertensive Retinopathy Grade III and IV	10	0
Depression	0	1
Total number of events	30	2
Number of patients with events	27	2

Table constructed from Information from Tables 4, 5 and 6 from *JAMA*. [14]
CV deaths: 2 died of dissecting aortic aneurysm, 1 from ruptured abdominal aortic aneurysm and 1 from sudden cardiac death
Worsening renal function defined as doubling of blood urea nitrogen to levels above 60 mg/100 cc
BP Blood pressure, *CCF* congestive cardiac failure, *CV* cardiovascular

demonstrated that the risk attributed to hypertension could be attenuated by pharmacologic therapy [15]. This additional proof that the ravages of hypertension, so well delineated in prior epidemiologic studies, could be attenuated by pharmacologic antihypertensive therapy became the foundation for our current evidenced-based approach to preventive medicine. By demonstrating an improvement in prognosis with the lowering of blood pressure, Freis and his coworkers provided the first proof that the poor outcomes observed in clinical hypertension, considered inevitable, was amenable to therapy and no longer had to be accepted. This turning point for cardiovascular medicine was achieved with one of the earliest applications of the randomized placebo-controlled trial testing clinical endpoints of morbidity and mortality in cardiovascular medicine [14, 15].

Of interest, Dr. Freis, the leader of these field altering clinical trials also conducted an analogous antihypertensive study in an animal model – the spontaneously hypertensive rat. Employing the same cocktail of pharmacologic agents that the VA study group used in the clinical trials, he and coworkers demonstrated that the lifespan of these genetically hypertensive animals was increased by lowering elevated blood pressure [16]. This study in an animal model of genetic hypertension provided a vivid illustration that it was the elevated blood pressure rather than some other genetic problem producing the negative impact of hypertension since pharmacologic control of elevated blood pressure prolonged life without altering their genetic condition. That pharmacologic blood pressure lowering prolonged survival in this animal model of genetic hypertension reinforced the message that the negative impact of hypertension could be mitigated by control of elevated blood pressure.

With over four decades of additional clinical trial evidence consistently strengthening the importance of treating hypertension to lower cardiovascular event rates, the results of the first two VA studies may now seem intuitive. However, the results of the first two VA antihypertensive trials did not result in a prompt sea change in medical practice. Overcoming inertia and motivating both patients and physicians to initiate and continue early generation antihypertensive agents of the treatment of a generally asymptomatic condition for the elusive promise of reducing future risk, represented a formidable challenge. The importance of acting on the findings from the VA trials to improve public health was however, readily apparent to the then Secretary of Health, Elliot Richardson and Mary Lasker a prominent philanthropist. Together, they led the efforts to launch the National High Blood Pressure Education Program (NHBPEP) with the intent of informing the medical community as well as the general public concerning both the ravages of hypertension and the importance of blood pressure control [17]. This currently existing educational program was established in 1972 by the National Institutes of Health "to reduce death and disability related to high blood pressure through programs a professional, patient and public education [18]." The NHBPEP used the power of emerging multimedia advertising industry to generate, popularize and link terms like "silent killer" to hypertension. The combination of quality data and effective education were needed to initially implement preventive measures. Although progress has been steady, there is still a long road to meet the national and international objectives of reducing premature morbidity from hypertension as the number of untreated and undertreated individuals remain excessive [10–13, 19, 20].

Since the groundbreaking VA Cooperative Studies, there have been over 30 major randomized controlled clinical trials (RCTs) of antihypertensive agents involving over 200,000 participants. The overall results are generally best summarized by the cooperative publications of the Blood Pressure Lowering Treatment Trialist Collaboration (BPLTTC) [21–23]. Collectively, the benefits of treating elevated pressure versus placebo in reducing the incidence of vascular diseases and deaths has been clearly and reproducibly established. As such, many of the more recent RCTs have, for ethical reasons, shifted from use of placebo to comparisons of different active antihypertensive compounds [24–27]. These even larger RCTs are generally designed to attempt to provide evidence of an incremental advantage beyond blood pressure lowering between agents to justify improved market share. The BPLTTC has also conducted several analyses for these comparator trials [22, 28]. The major message for the practitioner is that the extent of sustained blood pressure control is the first and foremost factor in reducing the cardiovascular risks attributed to hypertension [13]. In practical terms, since effective control of arterial pressure commonly requires concurrent use of more than one drug, the potential distinctions on event rates between specific antihypertensive agents is diminished.

Since hypertension is such a widespread condition and affected individuals frequently have other comorbidities, therapeutic decisions regarding choice of antihypertensive agents are also influenced by data on the established effects of the therapy on the other conditions. Some of the perceived benefits of one class of antihypertensive relative to another are derived from data on the favorable actions on morbidity and mortality demonstrated in other cardiorenal disorders commonly coexisting in patients with hypertension. This so called "halo effect" of projecting a benefit shown in another population has influenced key recommendations from authoritative committees [13, 29, 30]. For example, the recommendations for the preferential use of an angiotensin converting enzyme inhibitor (ACE I) or an angiotensin receptor blocker (ARB) as opposed to other classes of antihypertensive agents, are not based predominantly on data from randomized trials in patients with hypertension. In both cases, the direct comparator trials provided conflicting and not convincing information regarding specific clinical outcome advantage versus other classes of drugs to control elevated blood pressure [25, 27, 31, 32]. In the Antihypertensive and Lipid-Lowering Treatment to Prevent Heart Attack Trial (ALLHAT), one of the largest randomized clinical outcome trials, patients assigned to the diuretic chlorthalidone had lower event rates compared to an ACE I as well as a calcium channel blocker [27]. The most recent recommendations stress the importance of the control of elevated blood

Table 19.2 Meta-analysis of the ACE inhibitor placebo-controlled trials in patients with vascular disease without LV dysfunction or heart failure and in the trials of patients with LV dysfunction or heart failure [45]

All-cause mortality	ACE inhibitors events/ patients (%)	Controls events/ patients (%)	OR (95 %CI)	P
Trials without LVSD or heart failure				
HOPE (n=9,297)	482 (10.4)	569 (12.2)	0.83 (0.73–0.95)	0.0047
EUROPA (n=12,218)	375 (6.1)	420 (6.9)	0.89 (0.77–1.02)	0.0979
PEACE (n=8,290)	299 (7.2)	334 (8.1)	0.88 (0.75–1.04)	0.1261
Total	1,156 (7.8)	1,323 (8.9)	0.86 (0.79–0.94)	0.0004
Trials with LVSD or heart failure				
SAVE (n=2,231)	228 (20.4)	275 (24.6)	0.79 (0.64–0.96)	0.0178
AIRE (n=1,986)	170 (16.9)	222 (22.6)	0.70 (0.56–0.87)	0.0015
TRACE (n=1,749)	304 (34.7)	369 (42.3)	0.73 (0.60–0.88)	0.0011
SOLVD-P (n=4,228)	313 (14.8)	334 (15.8)	0.93 (0.79–1.10)	0.3910
SOLVD-T (n=2,569)	452 (35.2)	510 (39.7)	0.82 (0.70–0.97)	0.0173
Total	1,467 (23.0)	1,710 (26.8)	0.80 (0.74–0.87)	<0.0001
Combined total for all-cause mortality	2,623 (12.3)	3,033 (14.3)	0.83 (0.79–0.88)	<0.0001

pressure rather than the specific class of antihypertensive agents to use to lower blood pressure [13, 30]. Despite the lack of direct comparator evidence for superiority in clinical outcomes in patients with hypertension both ACE I and ARBs are often preferentially used in the treatment of patients with hypertension and coexisting diabetes as well as those with hypertension and either left ventricular dysfunction or heart failure [29]. In patients with diabetes and chronic kidney disease, randomized trials of both ACE I and ARBs have shown that these agents can reduce the progression of renal disease [33–36]. Although many of the patients in these RCTs had elevated blood pressure, the studies were not considered as antihypertensive trials. However, the benefit of the inhibitor of the renin angiotensin system on hard clinical end points in these trials enrolling subjects with diabetes and chronic kidney disease appropriately received considerable attention and influenced choices of antihypertensive therapies based on coexisting diseases.

Similarly, the presence of left ventricular dysfunction and or symptomatic heart failure are other coexisting conditions that influence choice of blood pressure lowering medications in selective patients with hypertension [28]. Extrapolations of survival benefits and reductions in hospitalizations in major placebo controlled randomized trials from heart failure [37–39], LV dysfunction [40, 41], post myocardial infarction [41, 42] and vascular disease [43–45] are often considered in this context (Table 19.2). Although each of these now classic trials has a unique and informative background, the parallels between the evidence justifying treating the asymptomatic condition of hypertension (discussed above) and left ventricular dysfunction following myocardial infarction will be elaborated (below).

Use of Renin Angiotensin Inhibitors to Prevent Cardiovascular Events Following Myocardial Infarction

The rationale for the use of inhibitors of the renin-angiotensin system to reduce morbidity and mortality following myocardial infarction are deeply rooted in the comparable use of antihypertensive agents to improve prognosis in the treatment of asymptomatic individuals with hypertension. In longitudinal studies of left ventricular function and geometry in the spontaneously hypertensive rat, a time-dependent transition to ventricular dysfunction and chamber enlargement was observed with aging in untreated animals [46]. The ACE I, captopril, was found to be particularly effective in attenuating these structural changes [47, 48]. In an animal model of myocardial infarction, analogous time-dependent adverse changes in ventricular architecture were shown to occur in relation to the degree of the initial myocardial damage [49]. This process termed "ventricular remodeling" reflects the adverse changes in left ventricular chamber size and shape that began with the initial loss of myocytes and continue well after histologic resolution of replacement fibrosis and wall thinning in the infarcted region [50].

The importance of ventricular enlargement was emerging from other clinical databases. Although left ventricular ejection fraction was the most commonly used assessment of ventricular performance, the few databases which also included quantitative measures of left ventricular cavity size highlighted that a larger ventricular volume as an even more important adverse prognostic factor [51]. In a population of survivors of myocardial infarction, this association was particularly pronounced, since larger end-systolic volume emerged as the most significant prognostic factor for premature death in a multi-variable regression model which included ejection fraction [52]. The observation from the Framingham investigators that although heart failure and pulmonary congestion are frequent complications of acute myocardial infarction, the appearance of chronic heart failure as a consequence of myocardial infarction can commonly take years to become manifest [53] supported the idea that a therapy to mitigate adverse ventricular remodeling may result in the lowering of the risk for a subsequent adverse cardiovascular event (prevention) following myocardial infarction.

As a natural extension of Dr. Janice Pfeffer's thesis work concerning the longitudinal changes in ventricular geometry and function in the spontaneously hypertensive rat and its modification [54], she evaluated the long term alterations in ventricular size and function in an animal model of myocardial infarction via coronary ligation. In a series of studies, she demonstrated that progressive ventricular enlargement occurred following infarction that this process was a modifiable process [55, 56]. Using the same ACE I regimen which was effective in regressing hypertrophy in the spontaneously hypertensive rat, she showed that some of the progressive rightward shift in the ventricular pressure volume relationship to higher volumes at the same filling pressure in the rats with chronic myocardial infarction could also be reduced. In this animal model, captopril therapy resulted in not only a greater preservation of ventricular chamber size, but also improved ventricular pump function and importantly prolonged survival [55–57].

These observations in an animal model provided the impetus for a small surrogate outcome clinical trial to determine the extent of time-dependent ventricular enlargement that occurs in patients following a myocardial infarction and importantly ascertain whether this process could in humans as in animals, be attenuated by ACE I therapy. In a randomized trial of asymptomatic survivors of a recent anterior myocardial infarction resulting in reduced LV ejection fraction (<40 %), ventricular dilatation and changes in geometry were demonstrated during a 1 year follow-up in patients randomized to placebo, while those randomized to the ACE I exhibited more structural stability [58]. Although supportive of the observations from the animals and clearly of clinical interest, the relatively small differences in ventricular volume had to be considered as only a soft end point, not sufficient to guide clinical practice. Just as in hypertension, where the importance of blood pressure lowering had to be demonstrated in a randomized placebo-controlled trial with hard clinical outcomes, so too would the importance of attenuating remodeling require a trial demonstrating translation to improved prognosis.

The Survival And Ventricular Enlargement (SAVE) trial was a direct test of the hypothesis that use of an ACE I compared to placebo in patients with a recent acute myocardial infarction at high risk based on ejection fraction of 40 % or less but without symptomatic heart failure, would reduce the proportion of patients that die of have a major deterioration (nine units) in left ventricular ejection fraction [58]. With 2,231 patients and 3.5 years of observation, the SAVE investigators were able to demonstrate that deaths from all causes and from cardiovascular etiologies were reduced amongst those randomized to the ACE I [58]. Moreover, there were also significant reductions in the proportion of patients that developed symptomatic heart failure or experienced a recurrent myocardial infarction in the captopril assigned group. Mechanistic confirmation was derived from an echocardiographic substudy which showed that the extent of ventricular enlargement was reduced in the ACE I group and, importantly, that adverse cardiovascular events were more likely to be observed in those experiencing ventricular enlargement [59].

In its time, the use of ACE I to treat patients with acute myocardial infarction became one of the most intensely studied areas in cardiovascular medicine. With eight major randomized, placebo-controlled international trials enrolling over 100,000 patients, definitive data was available regarding multiple ACE Is with consistent information that the oral use of these agents was associated with improved long-term survival [42]. Major established international investigative groups such as the Gruppo Italiano por lo Studio della Streptochinasi nell'Infarto Miocardico (GISSI) and the International Study of Infarct Survival (ISIS) had each proven the survival value of the acute use of an ACE I [60, 61]. This new use of an ACE I in acute myocardial infarction then became established therapy with the highest IA recommendation based on multiple randomized placebo controlled trials [62, 63].

Of interest, when the newer ARBs became clinically available, based on the observations of greater tolerability and the hypothetical concept of more complete inhibition by blocking at the receptor rather than at the production level, there was a general presumption that their use would be associated with even greater efficacy. With the clinical benefits of ACE I already demonstrated, use of placebo was no longer considered ethical in patients with acute myocardial infarction. Therefore, as in hypertension, the design of the more recent clinical trials used active comparators rather than placebo. When directly compared to a proven ACE I, use of an ARB in patients with acute myocardial infarction was not found to be superior to an established dose of an ACE I [64, 65]. In a formal test of noninferiority, a dose of the ARB valsartan was, however, found to preserve the clinical benefits associated with captopril [65]. Parenthetically, this study also showed that the combination of an ACE I plus an ARB did not improve clinical outcomes and resulted in more adverse events [65]. As such, this combination which had hypothetical advantages prior to the randomized trials is not recommended for clinical use.

The treatment of an asymptomatic individual with chronic pharmacologic therapy to prevent subsequent adverse cardiovascular events requires a high level of commitment from both the physician and the patient. The justification for this bilateral trust requires definitive evidence beyond extrapolation from surrogate measurements of presumed benefits. In both hypertension and left ventricular dysfunction populations, high-quality randomized placebo-controlled trials demonstrating clear proof of prognosis improving efficacy and simultaneously providing a safety and tolerability profile of the pharmacologic agent in the specific patient cohort, are necessary data to inform clinical decisions. In cardiovascular medicine, the heritage of using randomized controlled trials can be readily traced to hypertension. The lessons that use of chronic pharmacologic therapy for the prevention of subsequent cardiovascular events in asymptomatic conditions requires first and foremost convincing clinical outcome data that must be coupled with patient and physician education is common to both hypertension and the treatment of left ventricular dysfunction following a myocardial infarction. As is often said, prevention is the most effective therapy, however it is also commonly a thankless task, which must be supported by rigorous data.

References

1. Heidenreich PA, Trogdon JG, Khavjou OA, Butler J, Dracup K, Ezekowitz MD, et al. Forecasting the future of cardiovascular disease in the United States: a policy statement from the American Heart Association. Circulation. 2011;123(8):933–44.
2. Go AS, Mozaffarian D, Roger VL, Benjamin EJ, Berry JD, Borden WB, et al. Heart disease and stroke

statistics—2013 update: a report from the American Heart Association. Circulation. 2013;127(1):e6–245.
3. Kannel WB. Blood pressure as a cardiovascular risk factor: prevention and treatment. JAMA. 1996;275(20):1571–6.
4. Criqui MH, Langer RD, Fronek A, Feigelson HS, Klauber MR, McCann TJ, et al. Mortality over a period of 10 years in patients with peripheral arterial disease. N Engl J Med. 1992;326(6):381–6. Epub 1992/02/06.
5. Klag MJ, Whelton PK, Randall BL, Neaton JD, Brancati FL, Ford CE, et al. Blood pressure and end-stage renal disease in men. N Engl J Med. 1996;334(1):13–8. Epub 1996/01/04.
6. Kannel WB, Dawber TR, Kagan A, Revotskie N, Stokes 3rd J. Factors of risk in the development of coronary heart disease–six year follow-up experience. The Framingham Study. Ann Intern Med. 1961;55:33–50. Epub 1961/07/01.
7. Multiple risk factor intervention trial. Risk factor changes and mortality results. Multiple Risk Factor Intervention Trial Research Group. JAMA. 1982;248(12):1465–77. Epub 1982/09/24.
8. Stamler J, Neaton JD, Wentworth DN. Blood pressure (systolic and diastolic) and risk of fatal coronary heart disease. Hypertension. 1989;13(5 Suppl):I2–12. Epub 1989/05/01.
9. Lewington S, Clarke R, Qizilbash N, Peto R, Collins R. Age-specific relevance of usual blood pressure to vascular mortality: a meta-analysis of individual data for one million adults in 61 prospective studies. Lancet. 2002;360(9349):1903–13. Epub 2002/12/21.
10. Gu Q, Burt VL, Dillon CF, Yoon S. Trends in antihypertensive medication use and blood pressure control among United States adults with hypertension: the National Health And Nutrition Examination Survey, 2001 to 2010. Circulation. 2012;126(17):2105–14. Epub 2012/10/24.
11. Smith Jr SC, Jackson R, Pearson TA, Fuster V, Yusuf S, Faergeman O, et al. Principles for national and regional guidelines on cardiovascular disease prevention: a scientific statement from the World Heart and Stroke Forum. Circulation. 2004;109(25):3112–21. Epub 2004/07/01.
12. Mancia G, De Backer G, Dominiczak A, Cifkova R, Fagard R, Germano G, et al. 2007 ESH-ESC Practice Guidelines for the Management of Arterial Hypertension: ESH-ESC Task Force on the Management of Arterial Hypertension. J Hypertens. 2007;25(9):1751–62. Epub 2007/09/01.
13. Mancia G, Fagard R, Narkiewicz K, Redon J, Zanchetti A, Bohm M, et al. 2013 ESH/ESC guidelines for the management of arterial hypertension: the Task Force for the Management of Arterial Hypertension of the European Society of Hypertension (ESH) and of the European Society of Cardiology (ESC). Eur Heart J. 2013;34(28):2159–219. Epub 2013/06/19.
14. Effects of treatment on morbidity in hypertension. Results in patients with diastolic blood pressures averaging 115 through 129 mm Hg. JAMA. 1967;202(11):1028–34. Epub 1967/12/11.
15. Veterans Administration Cooperative Study Group on Antihypertensive Agents. Effects of treatment on morbidity in hypertension: II. Results in patients with diastolic blood pressure averaging 90 through 114 mmHg. JAMA. 1970;213:1143–52.
16. Freis ED, Ragan D. Effect of treatment on longevity in spontaneously hypertensive rats. Proc Soc Exp Biol Med. 1975;150:422–4.
17. The Edward D. Freis papers. The VA Cooperative Study and the beginning of routine hypertension screening, 1964–1980. http://profiles.nlm.nih.gov/ps/retrieve/Narrative/XF/p-nid/172.
18. National High Blood Pressure Education Program (NHBPEP) Working Group Report on Hypertension and Chronic Renal Failure. Washington, DC: US Dept of Health and Human Services, Public Health Service; 1990. NIH publication 90–3032. National High Blood Pressure Education Program. http://www.nhlbi.nih.gov/about/nhbpep/nhbp_pd.htm.
19. O'Donnell MJ, Xavier D, Liu L, Zhang H, Chin SL, Rao-Melacini P, et al. Risk factors for ischaemic and intracerebral haemorrhagic stroke in 22 countries (the INTERSTROKE study): a case–control study. Lancet. 2010;376(9735):112–23. Epub 2010/06/22.
20. Yusuf S, Hawken S, Ounpuu S, Dans T, Avezum A, Lanas F, et al. Effect of potentially modifiable risk factors associated with myocardial infarction in 52 countries (the INTERHEART study): case–control study. Lancet. 2004;364(9438):937–52. Epub 2004/09/15.
21. Neal B, MacMahon S, Chapman N. Effects of ACE inhibitors, calcium antagonists, and other blood-pressure-lowering drugs: results of prospectively designed overviews of randomised trials. Blood Pressure Lowering Treatment Trialists' Collaboration. Lancet. 2000;356(9246):1955–64. Epub 2000/12/29.
22. Turnbull F. Effects of different blood-pressure-lowering regimens on major cardiovascular events: results of prospectively-designed overviews of randomised trials. Lancet. 2003;362(9395):1527–35.
23. Psaty BM, Lumley T, Furberg CD, Schellenbaum G, Pahor M, Alderman MH, et al. Health outcomes associated with various antihypertensive therapies used as first-line agents: a network meta-analysis. JAMA. 2003;289(19):2534–44.
24. Dahlöf B, Devereux RB, Kjeldsen SE, Julius S, Beevers G, Faire U, et al. Cardiovascular morbidity and mortality in the Losartan Intervention For Endpoint reduction in hypertension study (LIFE): a randomised trial against atenolol. Lancet. 2002;359(9311):995–1003.
25. Julius S, Kjeldsen SE, Weber M, Brunner HR, Ekman S, Hansson L, et al. Outcomes in hypertensive patients at high cardiovascular risk treated with regimens based on valsartan or amlodipine: the VALUE randomised trial. Lancet. 2004;363(9426):2022–31. Epub 2004/06/23.
26. Jamerson K, Weber MA, Bakris GL, Dahlöf B, Pitt B, Shi V, et al. Benazepril plus amlodipine or hydrochlorothiazide for hypertension in high-risk patients.

N Engl J Med. 2008;359(23):2417–28. Epub 2008/12/05.
27. ALLHAT Officers and Coordinators for the ALLHAT Collaborative Research Group. The Antihypertensive and Lipid-Lowering Treatment to Prevent Heart Attack Trial. Major outcomes in high-risk hypertensive patients randomized to angiotensin-converting enzyme inhibitor or calcium channel blocker vs diuretic: The Antihypertensive and Lipid-Lowering Treatment to Prevent Heart Attack Trial (ALLHAT). JAMA. 2002;288(23):2981–97.
28. Turnbull F, Neal B, Algert C, Chalmers J, Chapman N, Cutler J, et al. Effects of different blood pressure-lowering regimens on major cardiovascular events in individuals with and without diabetes mellitus: results of prospectively designed overviews of randomized trials. Arch Intern Med. 2005;165(12):1410–9.
29. Chobanian AV, Bakris GL, Black HR, Cushman WC, Green LA, Izzo Jr JL, et al. The Seventh Report of the Joint National Committee on Prevention, Detection, Evaluation, and Treatment of High Blood Pressure: the JNC 7 report. JAMA. 2003;289(19):2560–72. Epub 2003/05/16.
30. James PA, Oparil S, Carter BL, Cushman WC, Dennison-Himmelfarb C, Handler J, et al. 2014 evidence-based guideline for the management of high blood pressure in adults: report from the panel members appointed to the Eighth Joint National Committee (JNC 8). JAMA. 2014;311:507–20.
31. Hansson L, Lindholm LH, Niskanen L, Lanke J, Hedner T, Niklason A, et al. Effect of angiotensin-converting-enzyme inhibition compared with conventional therapy on cardiovascular morbidity and mortality in hypertension: the Captopril Prevention Project (CAPPP) randomised trial. Lancet. 1999;353(9153):611–6.
32. Hansson L, Hedner T, Lund-Johansen P, Kjeldsen SE, Lindholm LH, Syvertsen JO, et al. Randomised trial of effects of calcium antagonists compared with diuretics and beta-blockers on cardiovascular morbidity and mortality in hypertension: the Nordic Diltiazem (NORDIL) study. Lancet. 2000;356(9227):359–65. Epub 2000/09/06.
33. Lewis EJ, Hunsicker LG, Bain RP, Rohde RD. The effect of angiotensin-converting-enzyme inhibition on diabetic nephropathy. The Collaborative Study Group [see comments] [published erratum appears in N Engl J Med 1993 Jan 13; 330(2):152]. N Engl J Med. 1993;329(20):1456–62.
34. Wright Jr JT, Bakris G, Greene T, Agodoa LY, Appel LJ, Charleston J, et al. Effect of blood pressure lowering and antihypertensive drug class on progression of hypertensive kidney disease: results from the AASK trial. JAMA. 2002;288(19):2421–31. Epub 2002/11/21.
35. Lewis EJ, Hunsicker LG, Clarke WR, Berl T, Pohl MA, Lewis JB, et al. Renoprotective effect of the angiotensin-receptor antagonist irbesartan in patients with nephropathy due to type 2 diabetes. N Engl J Med. 2001;345(12):851–60.
36. Brenner BM, Cooper ME, de Zeeuw D, Keane WF, Mitch WE, Parving HH, et al. Effects of losartan on renal and cardiovascular outcomes in patients with type 2 diabetes and nephropathy. N Engl J Med. 2001;345(12):861–9.
37. The SOLVD Investigators. Effect of enalapril on survival in patients with reduced left ventricular ejection fractions and congestive heart failure. N Engl J Med. 1991;325(5):293–302.
38. Cohn JN, Johnson G, Ziesche S, Cobb F, Francis F, Tristani F, et al. A comparison of enalapril with hydralazine – isosorbide dinitrate in the treatment of chronic congestive heart failure. N Engl J Med. 1991; 325:303–10.
39. Granger CB, McMurray JJ, Yusuf S, Held P, Michelson EL, Olofsson B, et al. Effects of candesartan in patients with chronic heart failure and reduced left-ventricular systolic function intolerant to angiotensin-converting-enzyme inhibitors: the CHARM-Alternative trial. Lancet. 2003;362(9386):772–6.
40. The SOLVD Investigators. Effect of enalapril on mortality and the development of heart failure in asymptomatic patients with reduced left ventricular ejection fractions. N Engl J Med. 1992;327:685–91.
41. Pfeffer MA, Braunwald E, Moyé LA, Basta L, Brown Jr EJ, Cuddy TE, et al. Effect of captopril on mortality and morbidity in patients with left ventricular dysfunction after myocardial infarction. Results of the survival and ventricular enlargement trial. The SAVE Investigators. N Engl J Med. 1992;327:669–77.
42. Flather MD, Yusuf S, Køber L, Pfeffer M, Hall A, Murray G, et al. Long-term ACE-inhibitor therapy in patients with heart failure or left-ventricular dysfunction: a systematic overview of data from individual patients. ACE-Inhibitor Myocardial Infarction Collaborative Group. Lancet. 2000;355:1575–81.
43. Yusuf S, Sleight P, Pogue J, Bosch J, Davies R, Dagenais G. Effects of an angiotensin-converting-enzyme inhibitor, ramipril, on cardiovascular events in high-risk patients. The Heart Outcomes Prevention Evaluation Study Investigators. N Engl J Med. 2000;342(3):145–53.
44. Fox KM, Henderson JR, Bertrand ME, Ferrari R, Remme WJ, Simoons ML. The European trial on reduction of cardiac events with perindopril in stable coronary artery disease (EUROPA). Eur Heart J. 1998; 19(Suppl J):J52–5.
45. Dagenais GR, Pogue J, Fox K, Simoons ML, Yusuf S. Angiotensin-converting-enzyme inhibitors in stable vascular disease without left ventricular systolic dysfunction or heart failure: a combined analysis of three trials. Lancet. 2006;368(9535):581–8.
46. Pfeffer JM, Pfeffer MA, Fletcher PJ, Braunwald E. Alterations of cardiac performance in rats with established spontaneous hypertension. Am J Cardiol. 1979;44:994–8.
47. Pfeffer JM, Pfeffer MA, Mirsky I, Braunwald E. Regression of left ventricular hypertrophy and prevention of left ventricular dysfunction by captopril in the spontaneously hypertensive rat. Proc Natl Acad Sci U S A. 1982;79(10):3310–4.
48. Pfeffer JM, Pfeffer MA, Mirsky I, Braunwald E. Prevention of the development of heart failure and the regression of cardiac hypertrophy by captopril in

the spontaneously hypertensive rat. Eur Heart J. 1983; 4(Suppl A):143–8.

49. Pfeffer JM, Pfeffer MA, Fletcher PJ, Braunwald E. Progressive ventricular remodeling in rat with myocardial infarction. Am J Physiol. 1991;260(5 Pt 2):H1406–14.
50. Pfeffer MA, Braunwald E. Ventricular remodeling after myocardial infarction. Experimental observations and clinical implications. Circulation. 1990;81(4): 1161–72.
51. Hammermeister KE, DeRouen TA, Dodge HT. Variables predictive of survival in patients with coronary disease: selection by univariate and multivariate analyses from the clinical, electrocardiographic, exercise, arteriographic, and quantitative angiographic evaluations. Circulation. 1979;59:421–30.
52. White HD, Norris RM, Brown MA, Brandt PWT, Whitlock RML, Wild CJ. Left ventricular end-systolic volume as the major determinant of survival after recovery from myocardial infarction. Circulation. 1987;76:44–51.
53. Cupples LA, D'Agostino RB. Some risk factors related to the annual incidence of cardiovascular disease and death using pooled repeated biennial measurements: Framingham Heart Study, 30-year follow up. In: Kannel WB, Wolf PA, Garrison RI, editors. The Framingham Study: An Epidemiological Investigation of Cardiovascular Disease. Section 34. DHHS publication no. (NIH) 87–2703. Washington DC: U.S. Government Printing Office; 1987. p. 9–20.
54. Pfeffer JM, Pfeffer MA, Fishbein MC, Frohlich ED. Cardiac function and morphology with aging in the spontaneously hypertensive rat. Am J Physiol. 1979;237(4):H461–8.
55. Pfeffer JM, Pfeffer MA, Braunwald E. Influence of chronic captopril therapy on the infarcted left ventricle of the rat. Circ Res. 1985;57(1):84–95.
56. Pfeffer JM, Pfeffer MA, Braunwald E. Hemodynamic benefits and prolonged survival with long-term captopril therapy in rats with myocardial infarction and heart failure. Circulation. 1987;75(1 Pt 2):I149–55.
57. Pfeffer MA, Pfeffer JM, Steinberg C, Finn P. Survival after an experimental myocardial infarction: beneficial effects of long-term therapy with captopril. Circulation. 1985;72(2):406–12.
58. Pfeffer MA, Lamas GA, Vaughan DE, Parisi AF, Braunwald E. Effect of captopril on progressive ventricular dilatation after anterior myocardial infarction. N Engl J Med. 1988;319(2):80–6.
59. St John Sutton M, Pfeffer MA, Plappert T, Rouleau JL, Moye LA, Dagenais GR, et al. Quantitative two-dimensional echocardiographic measurements are major predictors of adverse cardiovascular events after acute myocardial infarction. The protective effects of captopril. Circulation. 1994;89(1):68–75.
60. Effects of lisinopril and transdermal glyceryl trinitrate singly and together on 6-week mortality and ventricular function after acute myocardial infarction. Gruppo Italiano per lo Studio della Sopravvivenza Nell'Infarto Miocardico (GISSI)-3. Lancet. 1994;343:1115–22.
61. Fourth International Study of Infarct Survival (ISIS-4): a randomised factorial trial assessing early oral captopril, oral mononitrate, and intravenous magnesium sulphate in 58,050 patients with suspected acute myocardial infarction. Lancet. 1995;345:669–85.
62. Latini R, Tognoni G, Maggioni AP, Baigent C, Braunwald E, Chen ZM, et al. Clinical effects of early angiotensin-converting enzyme inhibitor treatment for acute myocardial infarction are similar in the presence and absence of aspirin: systematic overview of individual data from 96,712 randomized patients. J Am Coll Cardiol. 2000;35(7):1801–7. Epub 2000/06/07.
63. Antman EM, Anbe DT, Armstrong PW, Bates ER, Green LA, Hand M, et al. ACC/AHA guidelines for the management of patients with ST-elevation myocardial infarction–executive summary: a report of the American College of Cardiology/American Heart Association Task Force on Practice Guidelines (Writing Committee to Revise the 1999 Guidelines for the Management of Patients With Acute Myocardial Infarction). Circulation. 2004;110(5): 588–636.
64. Dickstein K, Kjekshus J. Effects of losartan and captopril on mortality and morbidity in high-risk patients after acute myocardial infarction: the OPTIMAAL randomised trial. Optimal Trial in Myocardial Infarction with Angiotensin II Antagonist Losartan. Lancet. 2002;360(9335):752–60.
65. Pfeffer MA, McMurray JJ, Velazquez EJ, Rouleau JL, Køber L, Maggioni AP, et al. Valsartan, captopril, or both in myocardial infarction complicated by heart failure, left ventricular dysfunction, or both. N Engl J Med. 2003;349(20):1893–906.

Part III

Hypertension: Evaluation of Cardiovascular Risk and Organ Damage

20 Value of Brachial and Central Blood Pressure for Predicting Cardiovascular Events

Stanley S. Franklin, Carmel M. McEniery, John R. Cockcroft, and Ian B. Wilkinson

Abstract

There is overwhelming evidence demonstrating the importance of brachial blood pressure (BP) as a predictor of future cardiovascular disease (CVD) risk. However, BP has a number of components, which show a distinct age-related pattern of change. A number of large observational studies demonstrate that diastolic blood pressure (DBP) is a more powerful predictor of coronary heart disease risk than either systolic blood pressure (SBP) or pulse pressure (PP) in younger individuals (age <50 years). In contrast, considerable evidence demonstrates the superiority of increased PP and decreased DBP to that of elevated SBP in predicting risk in older individuals. Increasing interest in arterial hemodynamics, especially over the past 20–30 years has generated abundant evidence that SBP changes throughout the arterial tree, such that SBP and PP are higher in the brachial artery than in the ascending aorta. Emerging data support the concept that central (aortic) BP may be superior to brachial BP in predicting future risk. However, the inclusion of central BP into routine clinical practice will require more definitive evidence that central BP is superior to brachial BP in risk stratification and prediction of risk.

Keywords

Blood pressure • Hypertension • Epidemiology • Pulse pressure • Mean arterial pressure • Aortic pressure • Brachial pressure • Arterial stiffness • Cardiovascular disease

S.S. Franklin, MD, FACO, FAHA, FASN (✉)
Preventive Cardiology Program, Division of Cardiology, Department of Medicine, C240 Medical Sciences I, University of California, Irvine, CA 92697, USA
e-mail: ssfranklinmd@earthlink.net

C.M. McEniery, PhD
I.B. Wilkinson, FRCP, DM, BM BCh
Clinical Pharmacology Unit, University of Cambridge, Addenbrooke's Hospital, Box 110, Cambridge CB2 OQQ, UK
e-mail: cmm41@cam.ac.uk; ibw20@cam.ac.uk

J.R. Cockcroft, FRCP, FESC
Department of Cardiology, Wales Heart Research Institute, University Hospital, Cardiff University, Heath Park, Cardiff CF14 44X, UK
e-mail: cockcroftjr@cf.ac.uk

M.E. Safar et al. (eds.), *Blood Pressure and Arterial Wall Mechanics in Cardiovascular Diseases*, DOI 10.1007/978-1-4471-5198-2_20,

While hypertension is a well-established risk factor for CVD events, controversy has existed regarding the relative importance of various BP components in predicting risk. Historically, DBP was considered a better predictor than SBP because it was thought to represent the resistance that the heart had to overcome to eject blood [1, 2]. It was not until the 1970s and 1980s that SBP was accepted as a clinically useful predictor of coronary heart disease (CHD), stroke, and heart failure, and in older people it was superior to DBP as a predictor of risk [3–5]. More recently, in the 1990s, PP, a marker of arterial stiffness, was shown to be useful in predicting CVD events in the elderly [6–15]. However, some controversy still persists regarding which BP component is superior as a predictor of CVD events [16–21]. In addition, there is abundant evidence that SBP and PP values are higher in the brachial artery as compared to the ascending aorta and this difference decreases with advancing age. There is also evidence that central artery stiffness is an independent risk factor for CVD [22–24] and that under many conditions central PP may be a superior marker of arterial stiffness than brachial PP in predicting cardiovascular risk. The objective of this chapter is to review the clinical usefulness of various brachial and central BPs as predictors of CVD risk.

Age-Related Changes in Brachial Artery Pressures

Although SBP is the best predictor of future CVD risk for the majority of the hypertensive population, there is much that can be learned from simultaneously assessing diastolic DBP and its relation to levels of SBP. The Framingham Heart Study in untreated subjects showed after 50 years of age that SBP increased disproportionately to DBP, and after 60 years of age DBP falls, resulting in increasing widening of the PP [9]. Furthermore, with the age-related fall in DBP, high SBP, accompanied by a wide PP [isolated SBP (ISH)], becomes the most common form of hypertension from middle-aged onward [9]. The rise in SBP and DBP up to age 50–55 can best be explained by the dominance of peripheral vascular resistance. In contrast, after the sixth decade of life, increasing PP and decreasing DBP are surrogate measurements for central elastic artery stiffness.

The Framingham Heart Study [9] findings also support the concept of an interaction between aging and hypertension in the progressive fall of DBP and rise of SBP. Subjects with mean baseline BPs of 110/70 (Fig. 20.1, group 1) had no rise in PP from age 30–50 years of age. Nevertheless, this

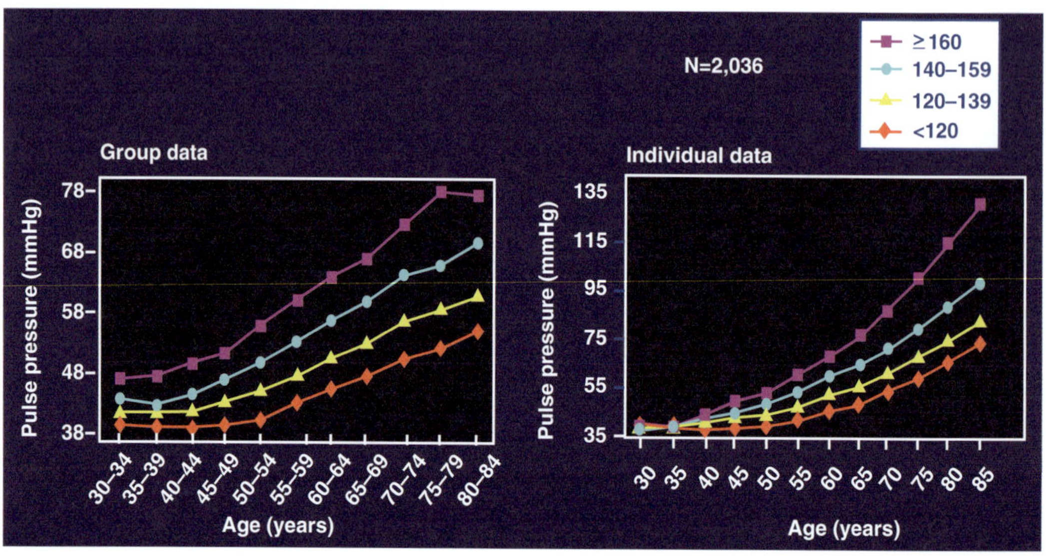

Fig. 20.1 Brachial pulse pressure by age. Group averaged data in *left panel* and averaged individual regression analysis in *right panel* for all subjects and with deaths, MI, and CHF excluded. *Curves* plotted based on blood pressure predicted values at 5-year age intervals by systolic blood pressure groupings (Adapted from Franklin et al. [9])

group of normotensive subjects showed a significant rises in PP and fall in DBP after age 60 years, presumably caused by an increase in large artery stiffness secondary to aging. In contrast, subjects with baseline mean BPs of 130/84 (Fig. 20.1, group 4) showed a steeper rise in PP and a steeper fall in DBP after age 60 than was observed in group 1 subjects. These finding suggest a linkage between the hypertension left untreated and subsequent acceleration of large artery stiffness. Although increased peripheral vascular resistance may initiate essential hypertension, acceleration of large artery stiffness is the driving force leading to the steeper rise of SBP after age 50 in the hypertensive groups 3 and 4 as compared to the normotensive groups 1 and 2.; this, in turn, may set up a vicious cycle of worsening hypertension and further increases in elastic artery stiffness.

The National Health and Nutrition Examination Survey [25] (NHANES III) showed that three out of four adult persons with hypertension are aged ≥50 years. Moreover, 80 % of untreated or inadequately treated persons with hypertension in this age group have isolated systolic hypertension (ISH), which by definition consists of elevated PP [25]. In addition to ISH being the predominant form of geriatric hypertension, there is evidence that widened PP may complement SBP as a predictor of cardiovascular risk.

Brachial BP and CVD Risk

Using almost the same Framingham cohort as in the previous study, 1924 men and women between 50 and 79 years of age at baseline with no clinical evidence of coronary heart disease (CHD) and free from antihypertensive drug therapy, were followed for up to 20 years [11]. In this population, CHD risk was inversely correlated with DBP at any level of SBP >120 mmHg, suggesting that PP was an important component of risk. There was a far greater increase in CHD risk with increments in PP for a given SBP than with increments in SBP with a constant PP. The Framingham study supports the findings of earlier workers [6, 7] that PP may be useful as an adjunct to SBP in predicting risk and that CHD events are more related to the pulsatile stress of elastic artery stiffness during systole (as reflected in a rise in PP) than the steady-state stress of resistance during diastole (as reflected in a parallel rise in SBP and DBP). Furthermore, the value of PP in predicting risk in the elderly has been confirmed by 24 h conventional [26] and intra-arterial [27] ambulatory BP monitoring. Considerable evidence now favors high pulsatile stress caused by sudden rise of pressure from diastolic nadir to systolic peak in early systole and the more gentle change through diastole to the nadir, as seen in stiffened vessels. Indeed, increased PP predicts cardiac complications of left ventricular hypertrophy, atrial fibrillation, systolic/diastolic dysfunction, and heart failure; in addition, increased PP predicts large artery complications of acute myocardial infarction and thrombotic and hemorrhagic stroke in the elderly.

How Does Age Influence the Cuff Pressure Assessment of CHD Risk?

The Framingham Heart Study examined the relationship between BP and CHD risk as a function of age [28]. From the age of 20–79 years there was a continuous, graded shift from DBP to SBP and eventually to PP as predictors of CHD risk. From age 60 onward, when considered with SBP, DBP was negatively related to CHD risk, so that PP emerged as the best predictor [28]. In contrast to the elderly, all three BP indices in the Framingham study were equally predictive of CHD risk in the transition ages of 50–59 year, while in the younger group (<50 years of age) DBP was a more powerful predictor of CHD risk than SBP and PP itself was not predictive [28]. Confirmatory evidence favoring DBP over SBP in predicting CHD risk in young adults was noted in a number of earlier large observational studies [29–31] and in a study utilizing intra-arterial BP measurements [27]. These findings are consistent with the NHANES III BP classification [25], which showed that there were twice as many hypertensive persons <age 50 up-staged by DBP as compared to SBP (moving from a lower to higher BP classification on the basis of incongruence between SBP and DBP values.

The bias towards DBP over SBP by earlier generations of physicians may be, in part, due to the emphasis on hypertension as a young person's condition. However, with the ageing of the population over the past half-century hypertension has become largely a condition affecting older persons, i.e. those with the ISH subtype [25]. Curiously, the underlying hemodynamics that favors DBP as the predominant predictor of CHD risk in young subjects is poorly understood.

Predictors of New-Onset Diastolic Hypertension: Relationship to Obesity

Factors leading to the development of isolated diastolic hypertension (IDH) and systolic-diastolic hypertension (SDH) were studied in the original cohort from the Framingham Heart study [32]. The major findings were that normal and high-normal BP had the highest hazard ratios (HRs) for new-onset of IDH and ISH, whereas IDH had by far the highest HR for new-onset SDH over a 10-year follow up period. The frequent progression from prehypertension to IDH in young adults is consistent with underlying increased peripheral resistance [32]. Brachial DBP and SBP rise with increases in peripheral resistance, but the rise in peripheral SBP, unlike DBP, is partially attenuated by the reduction in peripheral amplification that occurs with the development of hypertension in young adult men and to a lesser extent in young women [33, 34]. There is strong evidence [32] implicating weight gain and obesity as prime factors in the future development of diastolic hypertension. Indeed, both baseline body mass index (BMI) and subsequent weight gain were strong determinants of new-onset IDH and SDH in the Framingham Heart Study [32]. Given the propensity for increased body mass index (BMI) and weight gain in the development of new-onset of IDH, and the high probability of IDH to transition to SDH, it is likely that IDH is not a benign condition [32]. Furthermore, utilizing the US NHANES survey, the IDH population, despite having the lowest mean age of any hypertensive subtype, was associated with the greatest likelihood of having the metabolic syndrome [35]. Indeed, Chirinos et al. [36], again using the NHANES survey population, found obesity to be associated with hypertension in all age groups and both genders. However, the odds for hypertension to be associated with obesity was relatively higher in younger people; conversely, obese hypertensives were younger than lean hypertensives [36]. These findings indicate that IDH and SDH account for most cases of obesity-related HTN in U.S. adult men, a phenomenon that was seen in both representative samples of the U.S. adult population from 1994–1998 to 1999–2004. Therefore, increased mean arterial pressure (MAP, defined as 1/3 SBP + 2/3 DBP) accounts for a large percentage of the public burden of obesity-related hypertension in the U.S. [36].

Predictors of Isolated Systolic Hypertension in Adolescents and Young Adults

Sorof [37] found that ISH was 2.8 times as common as diastolic hypertension in adolescents with increased BMI and echocardiographic left ventricular hypertrophy.

Furthermore, McEniery et al. [38] recruited young adult university students with a mean age of 20 years in the ENIGMA study and confirmed that these persons with ISH had increased BMI, and outnumbered those with diastolic hypertension (elevation in both SBP and DBP, or elevated DBP alone) by a ratio of ~2:1. Whereas university students with diastolic hypertension had elevated peripheral vascular resistance, reduced stroke volume, and isobaric normal PWV, those with ISH showing a 90 % male predominance and had an entirely different hemodynamic profile — increased stroke volume and/or increased pulse wave velocity (PWV) [38]. Furthermore, central SBP was 21–23 mmHg higher in ISH subjects than in normotensives [38]. Although ISH in young adults is probably not a benign condition, long-term follow-up will be necessary to determine ultimate prognosis and ultimate need to begin antihypertensive treatment. This issue remains contentious, as outlined in the latest European Society of Hypertension (ESH) and the European Society of Cardiology (ESC) guidelines [39].

Predictors of Isolated Systolic Hypertension in Middle-Aged and the Elderly

As suggested by their age-dependent divergent patterns of onset, diastolic hypertension and ISH may be two distinct disorders with significant overlap. The conversion from diastolic hypertension to ISH in the older age group has been termed "burned-out" diastolic hypertension. Data from the Framingham Study [32] showed that about 40 % of patients with untreated or poorly treated diastolic hypertension acquired ISH in this manner. In contrast, six out of ten people who developed ISH did so without going through a stage of elevated DBP, but developed ISH *de novo* from normal and high-normal SBP [32]. An incomplete list of *de novo* causes of ISH would include (1) impaired synthesis of elastin as observed in intrauterine fetal growth retardation [40] and successfully repaired coarctation of the aorta [41]; (2) the presence of advanced glycation end products (AGE) that accompanies poorly controlled type 1 diabetes [42] and occasionally type 2 diabetes; and (3) increased aortic calcification as found in chronic kidney disease [43], osteoporosis [44], and premature aging [45].

The Value of Paired BP Components in Predicting CVD Risk

There is still considerable controversy in regard which BP component is the best predictor of CVD risk and whether combined BP components were superior to single ones. For example, the Prospective Studies Collaboration [16] and Asia Pacific Studies Collaboration [17] have concluded that MAP was superior to PP; other studies [18–21] concluded that SBP was superior to PP in predicting CVD risk.

The Framingham Heart Study reexamined this question in a 2009 publication [46] that compared combined versus single BP components. Pooled logistic regression analysis was used within 12 serial 4-year intervals from 1952 to 2000, using a new index examination for determining baseline BP for each 4-year cycle. Continuous and categorical models were compared for prediction of CVD events (CHD, heart failure and stroke) [46].

Categorical models in 6×6 cross-classification bar graphs to test for odds for the likelihood of CVD were constructed for SBP and DBP (Fig. 20.2a) and for PP and MAP (Fig. 20.2b), adjusted for age, sex, total cholesterol, smoking, body mass index, diabetes, and secular trend [46]. Using the combination of BP components in Fig. 20.2a, b, respectively, rather than single BP components separately, improved the fit for predicting CVD risk. Introducing the interaction terms in Fig. 20.2a, b, respectively, further improved the fit over the main effects of the two–component models, indicating that the effect of one BP component on risk varied accordingly to the level of the other. These results confirmed the superiority of combining SBP and DBP as noted in the MRFIT study [47] and extended the findings to older adults and to women.

It was concluded that both two-component models were superior to any single BP component in predicting CVD risk because they assessed both stiffness and resistance (afterload); a single BP component cannot do this. Furthermore, single BP components as predictors of CVD risk in prior studies examined a limited spectrum of the overall hypertensive population by age, sex and other covariates. When PP, a measure of stiffness, was combined with MAP, a measurement of resistance, there is a monotonic relation to risk; one could relate the two major physiologic components of hydraulic load to clinical outcome [46]. Although current 2003 Joint National Committee (JNC-7) guidelines consider both SBP and DBP, which ever is higher, in determining staging of BP, they undervalue the significance of increased arterial stiffness, as manifested by a high SBP and a low DBP [48].

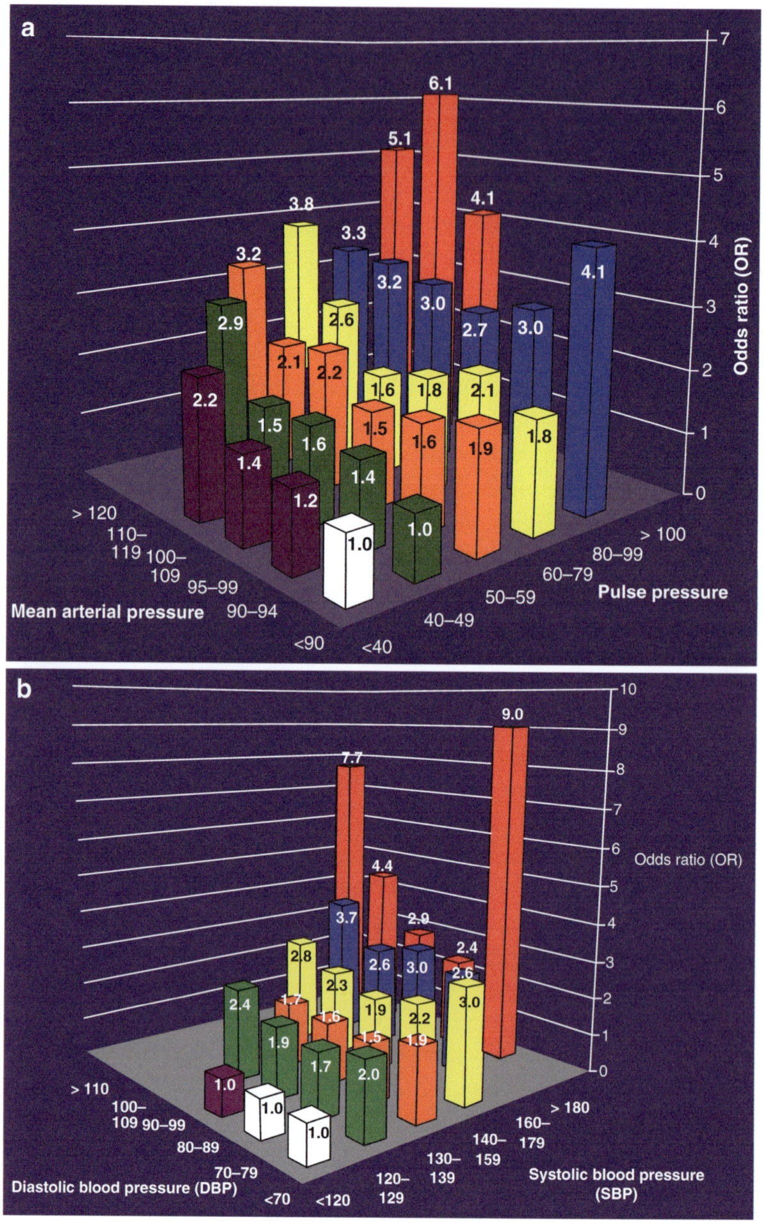

Fig. 20.2 (**a**) Odds for the likelihood of a cardiovascular event with combined brachial PP and MAP (calculated as 1/3 SBP+2/3 DBP) categories in a 6×6 cross-classification bar graph, adjusted for age, sex, total cholesterol, smoking, body mass index, diabetes, and secular trend. An interaction term of PP × MAP improved the model fit ($\Delta X^2 = 43.1$; $p = 0.01$). (**b**) Odds for the likelihood of a cardiovascular event with combined SBP and DBP categories in a 6×6 cross-classification bar graph, adjusted for age, sex, total cholesterol, smoking, body mass index, diabetes, and secular trend. An interaction term of SBP × DBP improved the model fit ($\Delta X^2 = 35.9$; $p = 0.02$) (From Franklin et al. [46], with permission)

The Role of J-Curves in Predicting CVD Risk

Controversy persists regarding the presence and significance of BP "J-curves" of increased CVD risk as they relate to older people with ISH [49]. At present, there are three postulated explanations for the DBP J-curve: (1) This represents the increased CVD risk secondary to increased arterial stiffness; (2) Low DBP may also be an epiphenomenon related to an underlying chronic debilitating illness and/or cardiac dysfunction (this is called reversed causality); lastly (3) This may represent antihypertensive therapy-induced lowering of DBP, which leads to myocardial ischemia and increased risk for an acute coronary event.

The Framingham Heart Study found that CVD risk increased at both the low and high extremes of DBP when combined with increased SBP in the two-component model and these findings were independent of antihypertensive therapy and antecedent CVD events [46]. The J-curve relation to CVD risk presumably reflects increased arterial stiffness as manifested by a low DBP and by definition, a wide PP. In the models based on JNC-6 categories for SBP and DBP groupings, SBP is usually superior to DBP as a predictor of CVD risk; however, a DBP of <70 mmHg versus DBP ≥70–89 mmHg in the absence of antihypertensive therapy could add a risk-equivalent of approximately 20 mmHg rise in SBP—in other words, a potential risk-equivalent shift from prehypertension to stage 1 systolic hypertension or from stage 1 to stage 2 systolic hypertension [46].

Importantly, data from the NHANES [50] confirmed that DBP <70 mmHg with a prevalence of 30 % among untreated persons with ISH was associated with increased CVD risk; advanced age, female sex, and diabetes mellitus, but not treatment status, were associated with this low DBP. Thus, DBP J-curves are common in untreated elderly subjects with ISH, associated with considerable cardiovascular risk, and are most likely representative of increased arterial stiffness.

Secondly, PP may predict CVD risk when SBP is normal or low as a result of ventricular dysfunction or chronic debilitating disease. Indeed, ventricular dysfunction has been described in end-stage-renal disease on hemodialysis [51] and is consistent with "reverse causation", expressed as an increased cardiac mortality in association with a falling SBP. Normally, increased cardiac mortality is associated with elevated BP; in the presence of left ventricular dysfunction, however, there is an inverse relation between BP and cardiac mortality.

Lastly, in the presence of high-grade stenosis of coronary arteries, increased risk of myocardial infarction with antihypertensive therapy-induced decrease in blood pressure may well occur [52], but is by far the least common occurrence of the J-curve phenomenon. Indeed, the risk of plaque disruption that leads to acute coronary syndromes depends more on plaque composition, plaque vulnerability (plaque type), and the degree of pulsatile stress than on the degree of coronary artery stenosis (plaque size) [53]. Not surprisingly, therefore, the majority of myocardial infarctions (>70 %) occur from plaque rupture in coronary arteries that have <50% stenosis [53]. Because of the many factors that result in J-curve risks, only a prospective trial with baseline and pre-event BP determinations can establish the presence and frequency of treatment-induced increase risk. On the other hand, the optimal therapeutic reduction in SBP and DBP in elderly subjects with ISH that maximizes benefit is a separate question from the presence of a therapeutic J-curve of increased cardiovascular risk.

Difference Between Brachial and Central Pressure

Over 50 years ago, Kroeker and Wood [54] observed that although mean and DBPs are relatively constant throughout the arterial tree, there is a gradual increase in SBP (and PP) moving from the aorta to the peripheral arteries. Indeed, the SBP measured at the brachial artery can be ~5–20 mmHg higher than that recorded in the ascending aorta [54–56]. This phenomenon of pressure *amplification* arises principally because of increasing vessel stiffness and changes in vessel geometry, moving away from the central arteries. Importantly, the extent of pressure amplification is not necessarily fixed, either within an individual over time or between individuals. Indeed, data from the Anglo-Cardiff Collaborative Trial, a community based study examining the factors influencing BP and arterial stiffening across the adult age-span in over 10,000 individuals, demonstrated that there was substantial variation in pressure amplification between individuals of a similar age, which remained consistent across the entire adult age spectrum [57]. This variation arises because of the differential impact of wave reflections on the aortic pressure waveform between individuals. Wave reflections are thought to arise from branch points or sites of impedance mismatch throughout the arterial tree, that sum together to produce a single 'effective' reflected wave [58, 59]. As the bulk of these reflections originate from the lower, rather than the upper body, the reflected wave arrives first in the ascending aorta, early in the cardiac cycle, where it tends to *augment,* or increase, SBP in the central arteries, before arriving in the brachial artery after peak SBP. Therefore, any factor increasing wave reflections is likely to influence central pressure independently of brachial pressure.

A number of factors including age [60, 61], gender [60], heart rate [62, 63] and height [64] influence the extent of pressure wave reflections, thus contributing to the differences in pressure amplification observed between individuals. Moreover, CVD risk factors such as hypertension [33], hypercholesterolemia [61, 65], smoking [57, 66] and diabetes [57], together with cardiovascular disease *per se* [57], can also have differential effects on brachial and aortic pressure, largely because of their variable influence on wave reflections. The major implication of these observations is that brachial pressure may not always be a reliable surrogate for central pressure. Indeed, regression models only account for ~70 % of the variability in the difference between brachial and central pressure [57, 67], highlighting the fact that central pressure cannot be predicted with sufficient accuracy from a brachial cuff reading and should be assessed directly, using appropriate methods. This is important since the heart, brain and kidneys are exposed to aortic rather than brachial pressure, and thus cardiovascular risk should relate better to central BP.

The Importance of Central Pressure in Predicting CVD Risk

Evidence published over the last 12 years concerning the relationship between central pressure and both surrogate markers of risk and hard endpoints strongly support the concept that CVD risk may ultimately be more closely related to central, rather than brachial pressure. Observations from cross-sectional studies suggest that central pressure is more closely correlated with widely accepted surrogate measures of CVD risk such as carotid intima-media thickness (CIMT) [68–70] and left ventricular mass (LVM) [70–72], than brachial pressure. Furthermore, longitudinal observations provide greater support for the potential value of central pressure measurement. In the REASON study [73], which compared the effects of atenolol with the fixed-dose combination of the angiotensin converting enzyme (ACE) inhibitor, perindopril and the diuretic, indapamide, regression of LVM was more strongly related to the change in central compared to brachial pressure, after 12 months of active therapy. Moreover, after adjustment for confounding factors, only central pressure remained independently associated with regression of LVM. In addition, in the CELIMENE trial [74] which compared the effects of the partial B1-adrenoceptor antagonist, celiprolol with the ACE inhibitor, enalapril, 9 months of active therapy resulted in a similar reduction in CIMT, which was independently related to the fall in central, but not mean arterial pressure.

Stronger evidence for the importance of central BP comes from outcome studies, which have examined a variety of hard endpoints in different patient cohorts (Table 20.1). Nine out of the eleven published studies report that central pressure was independently related to future cardiovascular events [68, 70, 75–81]. Moreover, four of these studies demonstrate incremental value of central over brachial pressure. Safar et al. [77] found that after adjustment for confounders, only central and not brachial pressure remained predictive of outcome in patients with renal failure. In the larger Strong Heart Study [68], central pressure was more strongly related to future CVD events than brachial pressure, in disease-free individuals. Indeed, after mutual adjustment, brachial pressure ceased to be predictive. Further analyses in this cohort showed that individuals with central PP ≥50 mmHg were at greatest risk of future cardiovascular events [82]. The Dicomano Study in Italy [81] and a community-based Taiwanese study [70] also observed a stronger association between CVD events and central, rather than brachial pressure. In contrast, however, the Australian National Blood Pressure 2 study (ANBP2) [83] and Framingham Heart

Table 20.1 Association between central pressure and outcome

First author	N, population	Duration	Parameter	End-point	Outcome
Nakayama (2000) [75]	53, CAD-PTCA	3-months	Invasive aortic pulsatility	Restenosis	Independent association between aortic pulsatility and restenosis
Lu (2001) [76]	87, CAD-PTCA	6-months	Invasive aortic SBP, PP and pulsatility	Restenosis	Independent association between aortic PP, pulsatility ratio and restenosis
Safar (2002) [77]	180, ESRD	1 year	Carotid PP	All-cause (including CV mortality)	Independent association between carotid PP and all-cause mortality
Chirinos (2005) [78]	324, men with CAD	4 years	Aortic SBP and PP	All-cause mortality and MACE	Independently association between aortic PP and all-cause mortality
Dart (2006) [83]	484, hypertensive women	4.1 years	Carotid SBP and PP	CV events and mortality	No independent association
Williams (2006) [79]	2,199, hypertensives	4 years	Aortic PP	CV events and procedures	Independent association between aortic PP and CV events and procedures
Roman (2009) [82]	2,403, native Americans	4.8 years	Aortic SBP and PP	CV mortality and events	Independent association between aortic SBP, PP and CV mortality and events
Jankowski (2008) [80]	1,109, angiography	4.5 years	Invasive aortic PP and pulsatility	CV mortality and events	Independent association between aortic PP and pulsatility and CV mortality and events
Pini (2008) [81]	173, geriatrics	8 years	Carotid SBP and PP	CV mortality and events	Independent association between carotid SBP, PP and CV events
Wang (2009) [70]	1,272, community	10 years	Carotid SBP and PP	All-cause and CV mortality	Independent association between carotid SBP and CV mortality
Mitchell (2010) [84]	2,232, community	7.8 years	Carotid PP	MACE	No independent association

Study [84] did not show any additional value of carotid BP in the prediction of events. Indeed, the method used in these two studies failed to detect any SBP amplification between the carotid artery and brachial cuff and concluded that there was no advantage in assessing central pressure.

The existing outcome studies of central pressure are small, and thus relatively underpowered to show convincingly that central pressure is meaningfully superior to brachial values in predicting events. This is especially so, given that the correlation between central and brachial pressure is very high (r=0.6–0.9). A recent publication [85] has attempted to address this issue by performing a meta-analysis of the available outcome studies. The meta-analysis confirmed the predictive value of central pressure and suggested that central PP may be a superior predictor, although the analysis did not reach statistical significance (P=0.057). However, the analysis was based on published summary statistics rather than individual patient data and failed to include all of the published data, including some of the larger studies, limiting its practical value. Clearly, a full evidence synthesis with an individual patient meta-analysis of all existing studies is required, together with a definitive outcome study, in order to determine whether central pressure adds meaningfully to brachial pressure-based risk prediction.

Clinical Importance of Central Pressure

Clinically, the assessment of central, rather than brachial pressure has a number of important consequences. In the Anglo-Cardiff Collaborative Trial [57], when healthy, treatment-naive individuals were grouped according to discrete categories of brachial SBP, there were significant overlaps in the corresponding aortic SBP (Fig. 20.3). Over 70 % of males and females with *high-normal* brachial BP and >30 % of males and 10 % of females with *normal* brachial BP had aortic BP in common with individuals with Stage 1 hypertension. These observations suggest that a large proportion of individuals who are classified as being normotensive based on current guidelines, might actually be at increased risk according to their central BP. Conversely, some individuals labeled as being hypertensive or at increased risk of developing hypertension might actually have lower cardiovascular risk, because they have a lower central BP. This has important implications for the way in which hypertension is currently categorized because if central BP is more important in defining an individual's risk and/or the impact of therapy, then categories which are based on central, rather than brachial pressure may be more useful. However, if central BP is ever to replace brachial BP in clinical decision-making, it will be important to determine the precise clinical relevance of the differences in brachial and central BP for the individual patient. Moreover, new guidelines reflecting treatment thresholds for central pressure will be required. Emerging data now support the prognostic value of both 24 h ambulatory [86–88] and home blood pressure monitoring [88] over BP values measured in the clinic setting, because the former minimize the standard deviation of measurements and the well-described white coat effect associated with clinic BP measurement. Similarly, it will be necessary to assess 24 h ambulatory central BP to determine whether this provides even greater prognostic value than corresponding ambulatory brachial BP.

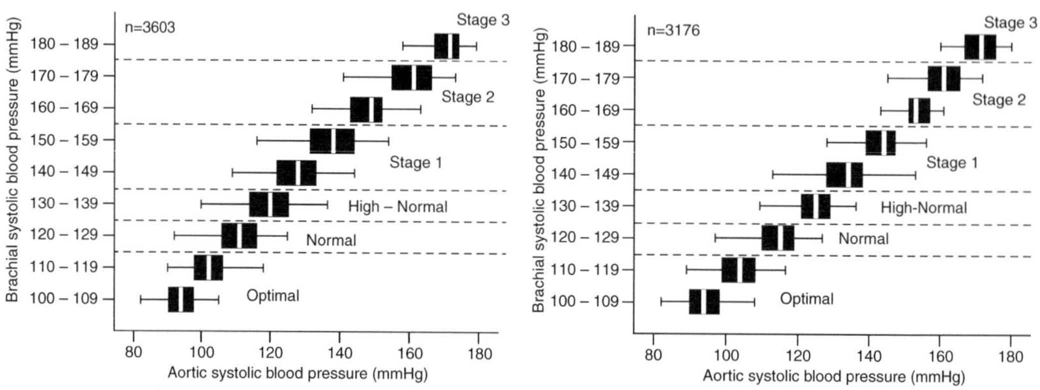

Fig. 20.3 Box plot of aortic systolic pressure per 10 mmHg increments in brachial systolic pressure in healthy males (*left*, n=3,603) and females (*right*, n=3,176). The *vertical line within the box* represents the median, the *box* represents the interquartile range (50 % of the distribution) and the *whiskers* represent the range of values. The *dashed lines* indicate blood pressure classifications (According to the 2007 ESH-ESC guidelines)

References

1. Pachon V. A new approach to sphygmomanometry. Presse Med. 1913;12:229–331.
2. MacWilliams J. Systolic and diastolic blood pressure estimation. Br Med J. 1914;2:693–7.
3. Kannel WB, Gordon T, Schwartz MJ. Systolic versus diastolic blood pressure and risk of coronary heart disease. The Framingham Study. Am J Cardiol. 1971; 27:335–46.
4. Stamler J, Neaton JD, Wentworth DN. Blood pressure (systolic and diastolic) and risk of fatal coronary heart disease. Hypertension. 1989;13:I2–12.
5. Rutan GH, McDonald RH, Kuller LH. A historical perspective of elevated systolic vs diastolic blood pressure from an epidemiological and clinical trial viewpoint. J Clin Epidemiol. 1989;42:663–73.
6. Darne B, Girerd X, Safar M, Cambien F, Guize L. Pulsatile versus steady component of blood pressure: a cross-sectional analysis and a prospective analysis on cardiovascular mortality. Hypertension. 1989;13:392–400.
7. Fang J, Madhavan S, Cohen H, Alderman MH. Measures of blood pressure and myocardial infarction in treated hypertensive patients. J Hypertens. 1995;13:413–9.
8. Franklin SS, Sutton-Tyrrell K, Belle SH, Weber MA, Kuller LH. The importance of pulsatile components of hypertension in predicting carotid stenosis in older adults. J Hypertens. 1997;15:1143–50.
9. Franklin SS, Gustin WT, Wong ND, Larson MG, Weber MA, Kannel WB, Levy D. Hemodynamic patterns of age-related changes in blood pressure. The Framingham Heart study. Circulation. 1997;96: 308–15.
10. Benetos A, Safar M, Rudnichi A, Smulyan H, Richard JL, Ducimetieere P, Guize L. Pulse pressure: a predictor of long-term cardiovascular mortality in a french male population. Hypertension. 1997;30:1410–5.
11. Franklin SS, Khan SA, Wong ND, Larson MG, Levy D. Is pulse pressure useful in predicting risk for coronary heart disease? The Framingham Heart study. Circulation. 1999;100:354–60.
12. Domanski MJ, Mitchell GF, Norman JE, Exner DV, Pitt B, Pfeffer MA. Independent prognostic information provided by sphygmomanometrically determined pulse pressure and mean arterial pressure in patients with left ventricular dysfunction. J Am Coll Cardiol. 1999;33:951–8.
13. Blacher J, Staessen JA, Girerd X, Gasowski J, Thijs L, Liu L, Wang JG, Fagard RH, Safar ME. Pulse pressure not mean pressure determines cardiovascular risk in older hypertensive patients. Arch Intern Med. 2000;160:1085–9.
14. Gasowski J, Fagard RH, Staessen JA, Grodzicki T, Pocock S, Boutitie F, Gueyffier F, Boissel JP. Pulsatile blood pressure component as predictor of mortality in hypertension: a meta-analysis of clinical trial control groups. J Hypertens. 2002;20:145–51.
15. Glynn RJ, L'Italien GJ, Sesso HD, Jackson EA, Buring JE. Development of predictive models for long-term cardiovascular risk associated with systolic and diastolic blood pressure. Hypertension. 2002;39:105–10.
16. Lewington S, Clarke R, Qizilbash N, Peto R, Collins R. Age-specific relevance of usual blood pressure to vascular mortality: a meta-analysis of individual data for one million adults in 61 prospective studies. Lancet. 2002;360:1903–13.
17. Lawes CM, Bennett DA, Parag V, Woodward M, Whitlock G, Lam TH, Suh I, Rodgers A. Blood pressure indices and cardiovascular disease in the Asia pacific region: a pooled analysis. Hypertension. 2003;42:69–75.
18. Antikainen RL, Jousilahti P, Vanhanen H, Tuomilehto J. Excess mortality associated with increased pulse pressure among middle-aged men and women is explained by high systolic blood pressure. J Hypertens. 2000;18:417–23.
19. Psaty BM, Furberg CD, Kuller LH, Cushman M, Savage PJ, Levine D, O'Leary DH, Bryan RN, Anderson M, Lumley T. Association between blood pressure level and the risk of myocardial infarction, stroke, and total mortality: the cardiovascular health study. Arch Intern Med. 2001;161:1183–92.
20. Miura K, Dyer AR, Greenland P, Daviglus ML, Hill M, Liu K, Garside DB, Stamler J. Pulse pressure compared with other blood pressure indexes in the prediction of 25-year cardiovascular and all-cause mortality rates: the Chicago Heart Association Detection Project in Industry study. Hypertension. 2001;38:232–7.
21. Mosley 2nd WJ, Greenland P, Garside DB, Lloyd-Jones DM. Predictive utility of pulse pressure and other blood pressure measures for cardiovascular outcomes. Hypertension. 2007;49:1256–64.
22. Dart AM, Kingwell BA. Pulse pressure – a review of mechanisms and clinical relevance. J Am Coll Cardiol. 2001;37:975–84.
23. Van Bortel LM, Struijker-Boudier HA, Safar ME. Pulse pressure, arterial stiffness, and drug treatment of hypertension. Hypertension. 2001;38:914–21.
24. Safar ME, Levy BI, Struijker-Boudier H. Current perspectives on arterial stiffness and pulse pressure in hypertension and cardiovascular diseases. Circulation. 2003;107:2864–9.
25. Franklin SS, Jacobs MJ, Wong ND, L'Italien GJ, Lapuerta P. Predominance of isolated systolic hypertension among middle-aged and elderly us hypertensives: analysis based on National Health and Nutrition Examination Survey (NHANES) III. Hypertension. 2001;37:869–74.
26. Verdecchia P, Schillaci G, Borgioni C, Ciucci A, Pede S, Porcellati C. Ambulatory pulse pressure: a potent predictor of total cardiovascular risk in hypertension. Hypertension. 1998;32:983–8.
27. Khattar RS, Swales JD, Dore C, Senior R, Lahiri A. Effect of aging on the prognostic significance of ambulatory systolic, diastolic, and pulse pressure in essential hypertension. Circulation. 2001;104:783–9.

28. Franklin SS, Larson MG, Khan SA, Wong ND, Leip EP, Kannel WB, Levy D. Does the relation of blood pressure to coronary heart disease risk change with aging? The Framingham Heart Study. Circulation. 2001;103:1245–9.
29. Lichtenstein MJ, Shipley MJ, Rose G. Systolic and diastolic blood pressures as predictors of coronary heart disease mortality in the Whitehall study. Br Med J (Clin Res Ed). 1985;291:243–5.
30. Tverdal A. Systolic and diastolic blood pressures as predictors of coronary heart disease in middle aged Norwegian men. Br Med J (Clin Res Ed). 1987;294: 671–3.
31. Neaton JD, Kuller LH, Stamler J. Impact of systolic and diastolic blood pressure on cardiovascular mortality. In: Laragh JH, Brenner BM, editors. Hypertension: pathophysiology, diagnosis and management. New York: Raven Press Ltd; 1995. p. 127–44.
32. Franklin SS, Pio JR, Wong ND, Larson MG, Leip EP, Vasan RS, Levy D. Predictors of new-onset diastolic and systolic hypertension: The Framingham Heart Study. Circulation. 2005;111:1121–7.
33. Wilkinson IB, Franklin SS, Hall IR, Tyrrell S, Cockcroft JR. Pressure amplification explains why pulse pressure is unrelated to risk in young subjects. Hypertension. 2001;38:1461–6.
34. Millasseau SC, Ritter JM, Chowienczyk PJ. Relationship between blood pressure and aortic pulse wave velocity in young and old subjects with essential hypertension. J Hypertens. 2003;21 Suppl 4:S253.
35. Franklin SS, Barboza MG, Pio JR, Wong ND. Blood pressure categories, hypertensive subtypes, and the metabolic syndrome. J Hypertens. 2006;24:2009–16.
36. Chirinos JA, Franklin SS, Townsend RR, Raij L. Body mass index and hypertension hemodynamic subtypes in the adult us population. Arch Intern Med. 2009;169:580–6.
37. Sorof JM. Prevalence and consequence of systolic hypertension in children. Am J Hypertens. 2002;15: 57S–60.
38. McEniery CM, Yasmin, Wallace S, Maki-Petaja K, McDonnell B, Sharman JE, Retallick C, Franklin SS, Brown MJ, Lloyd RC, Cockcroft JR, Wilkinson IB. Increased stroke volume and aortic stiffness contribute to isolated systolic hypertension in young adults. Hypertension. 2005;46:221–6.
39. Mancia G, Fagard R, Narkiewiewicz K, Redan J, Zanchetti A, Bohm M, Christiaens T, Cifkova R, De Backer G, Dominiczak A, Galderisi M, Grobbee DE, Jaarsma T, Kirchof P, Kjeldsen SE, Laurent S, Manolis AJ, Nilsson PM, Ruilope LM, Schmieder RE, Sirnes PA, Sleight P, Viigimaa M, Waeber B, Zannad F. Practice guidelines for the management of arterial hypertension of the European Society of Hypertension (ESH) and the European Society of Cardiology (ESC). J Hypertens. 2013;31:1925–38.
40. Martyn CN, Greenwald SE. Impaired synthesis of elastin in walls of aorta and large conduit arteries during early development as an initiating event in pathogenesis of systemic hypertension. Lancet. 1997;350: 953–5.
41. Senzai H, Iwamoto Y, Ishido H, et al. Ventricular-vascular stiffening in patients with repaired coarctation of aorta. Circulation. 2008;118 (Suppl 1):S191–8.
42. Ronnback M, Fagerudd J, Forsblom C, Pettersson-Fernholm K, Reunanen A, Groop PH. Altered age-related blood pressure pattern in type 1 diabetes. Circulation. 2004;110:1076–82.
43. Cheng LT, Gao YL, Gu Y, Zhang L, Bi SH, Tang W, Wang T. Stepwise increase in the prevalence of isolated systolic hypertension with the stages of chronic kidney disease. Nephrol Dialysis Transplant. 2008;23:3895–900.
44. Schulz E, Arfai K, Liu X, Sayre J, Gilsanz V. Aortic calcification and the risk of osteoporosis and fractures. J Clin Endocrinol Metab. 2004;89:4246–53.
45. McEniery CM, McDonnell BJ, So A, Aitken S, Bolton CE, Munnery M, Hickson SS, Yasmin, Maki-Petaja KM, Cockcroft JR, Dixon AK, Wilkinson IB. Aortic calcification is associated with aortic stiffness and isolated systolic hypertension in healthy individuals. Hypertension. 2009;53:524–31.
46. Franklin SS, Lopez VA, Wong ND, Mitchell GF, Larson MG, Vasan RS, Levy D. Single versus combined blood pressure components and risk for cardiovascular disease: The Framingham Heart Study. Circulation. 2009;119:243–50.
47. Domanski M, Mitchell G, Pfeffer M, Neaton JD, Norman J, Svendsen K, Grimm R, Cohen J, Stamler J. Pulse pressure and cardiovascular disease-related mortality: follow-up study of the Multiple Risk Factor Intervention Trial (MRFIT). JAMA. 2002;287:2677–83.
48. Chobanian AV, Bakris GL, Black HR, Cushman WC, Green LA, Izzo Jr JL, Jones DW, Materson BJ, Oparil S, Wright Jr JT, Roccella EJ. The seventh report of the joint national committee on prevention, detection, evaluation, and treatment of high blood pressure: The JNC 7 Report. JAMA. 2003;289:2560–72.
49. Franklin SS. Isolated systolic hypertension and the J-curve of cardiovascular disease risk. Artery Res. 2010;4:1–6.
50. Franklin SS, Chow VH, Mori AD, Wong ND. The significance of low DBP in us adults with isolated systolic hypertension. J Hypertens. 2011;29:1101–8.
51. Klassen PS, Lowrie EG, Reddan DN, DeLong ER, Coladonato JA, Szczech LA, Lazarus JM, Owen Jr WF. Association between pulse pressure and mortality in patients undergoing maintenance hemodialysis. JAMA. 2002;287:1548–55.
52. Messerli FH, Mancia G, Conti CR, Hewkin AC, Kupfer S, Champion A, Kolloch R, Benetos A, Pepine CJ. Dogma disputed: can aggressively lowering blood pressure in hypertensive patients with coronary artery disease be dangerous? Ann Intern Med. 2006;144: 884–93.
53. Falk E, Shah PK, Fuster V. Coronary plaque disruption. Circulation. 1995;92:657–71.
54. Kroeker EJ, Wood EH. Comparison of simultaneously recorded central and peripheral arterial pressure pulses during rest, exercise and tilted position in man. Circ Res. 1955;3:623–32.
55. Pauca AL, O'Rourke MF, Kon ND. Prospective evaluation of a method for estimating ascending aortic

pressure from the radial artery pressure waveform. Hypertension. 2001;38:932–7.
56. Ohte N, Saeki T, Miyabe H, Sakata S, Mukai S, Hayano J, Niki K, Sugawara M, Kimura G. Relationship between blood pressure obtained from the upper arm with a cuff-type sphygmomanometer and central blood pressure measured with a catheter-tipped micromanometer. Heart Vessels. 2007;22:410–5.
57. McEniery CM, Yasmin, McDonnell B, Munnery M, Wallace SM, Rowe CV, Cockcroft JR, Wilkinson IB. Central pressure: variability and impact of cardiovascular risk factors: The Anglo-Cardiff Collaborative Trial II. Hypertension. 2008;51:1476–82.
58. Nichols W, O'Rourke M, Vlachopoulos C, editors. McDonald's blood flow in arteries: theoretical, experimental and clinical principles. 6th ed. London: Hodder Martin; 2011.
59. Westerhof N, Sipkema P, van den Bos GC, Elzinga G. Forward and backward waves in the arterial system. Cardiovasc Res. 1972;6:648–56.
60. McEniery CM, Yasmin, Hall IR, Qasem A, Wilkinson IB, Cockcroft JR. Normal vascular aging: differential effects on wave reflection and aortic pulse wave velocity the Anglo-Cardiff Collaborative Trial (ACCT). J Am Coll Cardiol. 2005;46:1753–60.
61. Sharman JE, McEniery CM, Dhakam ZR, Coombes JS, Wilkinson IB, Cockcroft JR. Pulse pressure amplification during exercise is significantly reduced with age and hypercholesterolemia. J Hypertens. 2007;25:1249–54.
62. Albaladejo P, Copie X, Boutouyrie P, Laloux B, Declere AD, Smulyan H, Benetos A. Heart rate, arterial stiffness, and wave reflections in paced patients. Hypertension. 2001;38:949–52.
63. Wilkinson IB, Mohammad NH, Tyrrell S, Hall IR, Webb DJ, Paul VE, Levy T, Cockcroft JR. Heart rate dependency of pulse pressure amplification and arterial stiffness. Am J Hypertens. 2002;15:24–30.
64. London GM, Guerin AP, Pannier BM, Marchais SJ, Metivier F. Body height as a determinant of carotid pulse contour in humans. J Hypertens Suppl. 1992;10:S93–5.
65. Wilkinson IB, Prasad K, Hall IR, Thomas A, MacCallum H, Webb DJ, Frenneaux MP, Cockcroft JR. Increased central pulse pressure and augmentation index in subjects with hypercholesterolemia. J Am Coll Cardiol. 2002;39:1005–11.
66. Mahmud A, Feely J. Effect of smoking on arterial stiffness and pulse pressure amplification. Hypertension. 2003;41:183–7.
67. Camacho F, Avolio A, Lovell NH. Estimation of pressure pulse amplification between aorta and brachial artery using stepwise multiple regression models. Physiol Meas. 2004;25:879–89.
68. Roman MJ, Devereux RB, Kizer JR, Lee ET, Galloway JM, Ali T, Umans JG, Howard BV. Central pressure more strongly relates to vascular disease and outcome than does brachial pressure: the Strong Heart Study. Hypertension. 2007;50:197–203.
69. Boutouyrie P, Bussy C, Lacolley P, Girerd X, Laloux B, Laurent S. Association between local pulse pressure, mean blood pressure, and large-artery remodeling. Circulation. 1999;100:1387–93.
70. Wang KL, Cheng HM, Chuang SY, Spurgeon HA, Ting CT, Lakatta EG, Yin FC, Chou P, Chen CH. Central or peripheral systolic or pulse pressure: which best relates to target organs and future mortality? J Hypertens. 2009;27:461–7.
71. Roman MJ, Okin PM, Kizer JR, Lee ET, Howard BV, Devereux RB. Relations of central and brachial blood pressure to left ventricular hypertrophy and geometry: the Strong Heart Study. J Hypertens. 2010;28:384–8.
72. Covic A, Goldsmith DJ, Panaghiu L, Covic M, Sedor J. Analysis of the effect of hemodialysis on peripheral and central arterial pressure waveforms. Kidney Int. 2000;57:2634–43.
73. de Luca N, Asmar RG, London GM, O'Rourke MF, Safar ME. Selective reduction of cardiac mass and central blood pressure on low-dose combination perindopril/indapamide in hypertensive subjects. J Hypertens. 2004;22:1623–30.
74. Boutouyrie P, Bussy C, Hayoz D, Hengstler J, Dartois N, Laloux B, Brunner H, Laurent S. Local pulse pressure and regression of arterial wall hypertrophy during long-term antihypertensive treatment. Circulation. 2000;101:2601–6.
75. Nakayama Y, Tsumura K, Yamashita N, Yoshimaru K, Hayashi T. Pulsatility of ascending aortic pressure waveform is a powerful predictor of restenosis after percutaneous transluminal coronary angioplasty. Circulation. 2000;101:470–2.
76. Lu TM, Hsu NW, Chen YH, Lee WS, Wu CC, Ding YA, Chang MS, Lin SJ. Pulsatility of ascending aorta and restenosis after coronary angioplasty in patients >60 years of age with stable angina pectoris. Am J Cardiol. 2001;88:964–8.
77. Safar ME, Blacher J, Pannier B, Guerin AP, Marchais SJ, Guyonvarc'h PM, London GM. Central pulse pressure and mortality in end-stage renal disease. Hypertension. 2002;39:735–8.
78. Chirinos JA, Zambrano JP, Chakko S, Veerani A, Schob A, Willens HJ, Perez G, Mendez AJ. Aortic pressure augmentation predicts adverse cardiovascular events in patients with established coronary artery disease. Hypertension. 2005;45:980–5.
79. Williams B, Lacy PS, Thom SM, Cruickshank K, Stanton A, Collier D, Hughes AD, Thurston H, O'Rourke M. Differential impact of blood pressure-lowering drugs on central aortic pressure and clinical outcomes: principal results of the Conduit Artery Function Evaluation (CAFE) Study. Circulation. 2006;113:1213–25.
80. Jankowski P, Kawecka-Jaszcz K, Czarnecka D, Brzozowska-Kiszka M, Styczkiewicz K, Loster M, Kloch-Badelek M, Wilinski J, Curylo AM, Dudek D. Pulsatile but not steady component of blood pressure predicts cardiovascular events in coronary patients. Hypertension. 2008;51:848–55.
81. Pini R, Cavallini MC, Palmieri V, Marchionni N, Di Bari M, Devereux RB, Masotti G, Roman MJ. Central but not brachial blood pressure predicts cardiovascular

events in an unselected geriatric population: the ICARe Dicomano Study. J Am Coll Cardiol. 2008;51:2432–9.
82. Roman MJ, Devereux RB, Kizer JR, Okin PM, Lee ET, Wang W, Umans JG, Calhoun D, Howard BV. High central pulse pressure is independently associated with adverse cardiovascular outcome the Strong Heart Study. J Am Coll Cardiol. 2009;54:1730–4.
83. Dart AM, Gatzka CD, Kingwell BA, Willson K, Cameron JD, Liang YL, Berry KL, Wing LM, Reid CM, Ryan P, Beilin LJ, Jennings GL, Johnston CI, McNeil JJ, Macdonald GJ, Morgan TO, West MJ. Brachial blood pressure but not carotid arterial waveforms predict cardiovascular events in elderly female hypertensives. Hypertension. 2006;47:785–90.
84. Mitchell GF, Hwang SJ, Vasan RS, Larson MG, Pencina MJ, Hamburg NM, Vita JA, Levy D, Benjamin EJ. Arterial stiffness and cardiovascular events: the Framingham Heart Study. Circulation. 2010;121:505–11.
85. Vlachopoulos C, Aznaouridis K, O'Rourke MF, Safar ME, Baou K, Stefanadis C. Prediction of cardiovascular events and all-cause mortality with central haemodynamics: a systematic review and meta-analysis. Eur Heart J. 2010;31(15):1865–71.
86. Staessen JA, Thijs L, Fagard R, O'Brien ET, Clement D, de Leeuw PW, Mancia G, Nachev C, Palatini P, Parati G, Tuomilehto J, Webster J. Predicting cardiovascular risk using conventional vs ambulatory blood pressure in older patients with systolic hypertension. Systolic hypertension in Europe Trial Investigators. JAMA. 1999;282:539–46.
87. Clement DL, De Buyzere ML, De Bacquer DA, de Leeuw PW, Duprez DA, Fagard RH, Gheeraert PJ, Missault LH, Braun JJ, Six RO, Van Der Niepen P, O'Brien E. Prognostic value of ambulatory blood-pressure recordings in patients with treated hypertension. N Engl J Med. 2003;348:2407–15.
88. Sega R, Facchetti R, Bombelli M, Cesana G, Corrao G, Grassi G, Mancia G. Prognostic value of ambulatory and home blood pressures compared with office blood pressure in the general population: Follow-up results from the Pressioni Arteriose Monitorate e Loro Associazioni (PAMELA) Study. Circulation. 2005;111: 1777–83.

21 Predictive Value of Arterial Stiffness for Cardiovascular Events

Stéphane Laurent, Pierre Boutouyrie, and Francesco Mattace Raso

Abstract

A major reason for measuring arterial stiffness "routinely" in clinical practice comes from the recent demonstration that arterial stiffness has an independent predictive value for cardiovascular events. Several longitudinal epidemiological studies have demonstrated the predictive value of arterial stiffness as intermediate endpoints, i.e. the higher the arterial stiffness, the higher the number of cardiovascular events. The largest amount of evidence has been given for aortic stiffness, measured through carotid-femoral pulse wave velocity which is considered as gold standard. Aortic stiffness has independent predictive value for all-cause and cardiovascular mortality, fatal and nonfatal coronary events and fatal strokes not only in patients with uncomplicated essential hypertension but also in patients with type 2 diabetes or end-stage renal disease, in elderly subjects and in the general population. Currently, as many as 21 studies consistently showed the independent predictive value of aortic stiffness for fatal and nonfatal cardiovascular events in various populations. Aortic stiffness can thus be considered as an intermediate endpoint for cardiovascular events.

Keywords

Arterial stiffness • Cardiovascular events • Epidemiology • Surrogate endpoint

S. Laurent, MD, PhD (✉) • P. Boutouyrie, MD, PhD
Department of Pharmacology and Institut National de la Santé et de la Recherche Médicale U970(Eq7)-PARCC, Hôpital Européen Georges Pompidou, Assistance Publique-Hôpitaux de Paris, Université Paris-Descartes, 20-40- rue Leblanc, Paris 75015, France
e-mail: stephane.laurent@egp.aphp.fr; pierre.boutouyrie@egp.aphp.fr

F.M. Raso, MD, PhD
Department of Internal Medicine, Erasmus MC, University Medical Center, Rotterdam, The Netherlands
e-mail: f.mattaceraso@erasmusmc.nl

M.E. Safar et al. (eds.), *Blood Pressure and Arterial Wall Mechanics in Cardiovascular Diseases*, DOI 10.1007/978-1-4471-5198-2_21,

Introduction

Classical risk scores may underestimate the risk of cardiovascular (CV) events in specific risk groups suitable for primary prevention, such as asymptomatic hypertensive subjects [1]. Particularly, those considered as at intermediate risk may benefit the most from a reassessment of their CV risk using novel biomarkers [2]. In primary prevention, some imaging biomarkers, such as arterial stiffness, enhance risk prediction to a higher extent than circulating biomarkers [3]. Whether novel biomarkers are ready for routine clinical use is a matter of controversy [1–4]. Particularly whether a biomarker can be substituted to clinical events in outcome trials and be considered as surrogate endpoint has rarely been demonstrated [1–4]. The aims of the present chapter are to address the concepts of "imaging biomarker" and "surrogate endpoint", to focus on aortic stiffness as putative surrogate endpoint for future CV events and to suggest additional studies in order to demonstrate its value as surrogate endpoint.

"Circulating" Biomarkers Versus "Tissue" or "Imaging" Biomarkers

Although classical risk scores, such as the Framingham risk score [5] and the European SCORE [6], detect patients at high risk of CV events, they are largely influenced by ageing, leading to undermanagement of CV risk in other risk groups, particularly those considered as at intermediate risk. A very large number of newer biomarkers have been proposed in the literature [2, 4] in order to increase risk prediction beyond classical risk scores. According to the Biomarkers Definition Working Group of the National Institutes of Health (NIH) [7], a biomarker is "a characteristic that is objectively measured and evaluated as an indicator of normal biological processes, pathogenic processes, or pharmacological responses to a therapeutic intervention". Thus, biomarkers could be either "circulating" ones, i.e. requiring blood sampling and specific dosage, or "imaging" ones, i.e. requiring measurements with imaging technology, such as aortic stiffness [2–4].

The use of sophisticated circulating biomarkers has been suggested for increasing the individual prediction of CV risk, beyond the established CV risk factors, such as age, systolic blood pressure, antihypertensive treatment, total cholesterol, high-density lipoprotein cholesterol, lipid-lowering treatment, diabetes, smoking status and body mass index. Results were contrasted. For instance, in the Framingham cohort, using hs-CRP, plasma renin, BNP, homocytein and urinary albumin/creatinine ratio did not improve the prediction of outcome [8]. However, in a community-based cohort of elderly men, a combination of circulating biomarkers reflecting myocardial cell damage, left ventricular dysfunction, renal failure and inflammation (such as troponin I, N-terminal pro-brain natriuretic peptide, cystatin C and C-reactive protein, respectively) improved the risk assessment beyond established CV risk factors and increased the C statistics [9].

As an alternative to using "circulating" biomarkers in hypertensive patients, estimation of CV risk can investigate target organ damage, such as aortic stiffening or left ventricular hypertrophy (LVH) [1]. Thus, target organ damage could play the role of an "imaging" biomarker [2, 10] and may help identify patients at high risk of developing CV disease. This strategy has a strong background since target organ damage, which integrates the long-lasting cumulative effects of all identified and non-identified CV risk factors, can be detected before clinical events occur, at a stage when intervention may reverse damage [11]. By contrast, "circulating" biomarkers may fail to adequately predict the risk of CV events, due to their instantaneous fluctuations, as many "snapshots" of the complex deleterious situation [10]. To underline the structural changes of target organs either directly observed (for instance, left ventricular hypertrophy) or associated with a functional alteration (for instance, aortic stiffening), we added the wording "tissue" for this category of biomarkers. Among "tissue/imaging" biomarkers, aortic stiffness can be considered as a measure of the cumulative influence of CV risk factors with ageing on the arterial tree, having limited acute variability (mainly depending on blood pressure) and enough inertia to reflect the integrated damage of the arterial wall [3, 10]. Recent studies showed that arterial stiffness played an important role in the "large/small artery cross talk" [11] and its damaging effect on the heart, brain, retina and kidney.

"Surrogate endpoints" are a subset of biomarkers. According to the Biomarkers Definition Working Group of the NIH [7], a surrogate endpoint is "a biomarker that is intended to substitute for a clinical endpoint. A surrogate endpoint is expected to predict clinical benefit (or harm or lack of benefit or harm) based on epidemiologic, therapeutic, pathophysiologic, or other scientific evidence" [7]. To avoid confusion with the substitution for a marker, whereas it is really a substitution for a clinical endpoint, the term "surrogate marker" has been discouraged [7]. The next paragraph details how arterial stiffness has demonstrated its usefulness as tissue/imaging biomarker and what should be demonstrated before considering that arterial stiffness is a true surrogate endpoint, i.e. whether the reduction in arterial stiffness translates into a reduction in CV events.

Predictive Value of Aortic Stiffness for CV Event

The predictive value of arterial stiffness for CV events has been initially reported in the late 1990s–early 2000s. The largest amount of evidence has been given for aortic stiffness, measured through carotid-femoral PWV which is considered as gold standard [3]. Aortic stiffness has independent predictive value for several endpoints: all-cause and CV mortality, fatal and nonfatal coronary events, asymptomatic coronary heart disease, fatal strokes, functional outcome after stroke, onset of hypertension and onset of dialysis. Various populations have been studied: general population [12–15], elderly subjects [16, 17], hypertensive patients [18–20], patients with type 2 diabetes [21], patients with chronic kidney disease or end-stage renal disease [22, 23], patients after renal transplant [24] and patients after acute stroke/TIA [25, 26].

Currently, as many as 21 studies consistently showed the independent predictive value of aortic stiffness for fatal and nonfatal CV events in various populations. Seventeen longitudinal studies totalising 15,877 subjects with a mean follow-up of 7.7 years were included in a recent meta-analysis [27] which showed, for one standard deviation (SD) increase in pulse wave velocity, a risk ratio of 1.47 [1.31–1.64] for total mortality, 1.47 [1.29–1.66] for CV mortality and 1.42 [1.29–1.58] for all-cause mortality. Aortic stiffness can thus be considered as an intermediate endpoint for CV events [28].

Although the relationship between aortic stiffness and events is continuous, a threshold of 12 m/s has been suggested as a conservative estimate of significant alterations of aortic function in middle-aged hypertensives and included in the 2007 ESH Guidelines for the management of hypertension [1]. This threshold has been revised in a recent consensus document [29], as 10 m/s, in order to normalise PWV values according to the arterial pathway, as described above. High aortic PWV may thus represent target organ damage, which needs to be detected during estimation of CV risk in hypertensives. Reference values for pulse wave velocity [30] have been established in 1,455 healthy subjects and a larger population of 11,092 subjects with CV risk factors.

Pathophysiology of Cardiovascular Events

A generally accepted mechanistic view is that an increase in arterial stiffness causes a premature return of reflected waves in late systole, increasing central pulse pressure, thus systolic BP. Briefly, since it has been detailed in other chapters of this book, SBP increases the load on the left ventricle, increasing myocardial oxygen demand. In addition, arterial stiffness is associated with left ventricular hypertrophy (LVH) [31], a known risk factor for coronary events, in normotensive and hypertensive patients. The increase in central PP and the decrease in diastolic BP may directly cause subendocardial ischaemia. The measurement of aortic stiffness, which integrates the alterations of the arterial wall, may also reflect parallel lesions present at the site of the coronary arteries [32].

An increased arterial stiffness can increase the risk of stroke through several mechanisms, including an increase in central PP, influencing arterial remodelling at the site of both the extracranial and intracranial arteries, increasing carotid wall thickness and the development of stenosis and plaques [33, 34] and the prevalence and severity of cerebral white matter lesions [35]. Moreover, it has been suggested that the pulsatile mechanical load of PP on the arterial wall, irrespectively of the absolute value of blood pressure, is a major determinant of carotid intraplaque haemorrhage, as recently found in a large population-based study [36]. As seen above, the measurement of aortic stiffness, which integrates the alterations of the arterial wall, may also reflect parallel lesions present at the site of cerebral vasculature. Thus, it is not surprising that aortic stiffness is able to predict the functional outcome after stroke, independently of classical risk factors [25, 26]. Another explanation is given by the differential input impedance in the brain compared with other systemic vascular beds. Finally, coronary heart disease and heart failure, which are favoured by high PP and arterial stiffness, are also risk factors for stroke.

Aortic Stiffness as a Surrogate Endpoint

Several review articles [2, 4, 37] have recently analysed the various methods for estimating the clinical utility of a biomarker. Particularly, a statement from the American Heart Association (AHA) recommended that several steps should be completed for evaluating a novel risk marker and ultimately concluding that the novel risk marker could be used as surrogate endpoint of CV events [37]. Six phases of increasing stringency are described below and in Table 21.1.

Table 21.1 Phases to be completed before aortic stiffness could be considered as a surrogate endpoint of CV events (see Ref. [36]). References (original studies, meta-analyses and reviews) related to each phase are indicated in bracket

Phase	Aortic stiffness
1. Proof of concept	*Yes* [3, 10, 11]
2. Prospective validation	*Yes* [12, 15, 18, 27, 38, 39]
3. Incremental value	*Yes* [12, 15, 18]
4. Clinical utility	*Yes* [12, 15, 38–40]
5. Clinical outcomes	*Weak indirect evidence* [39]
6. Cost-effectiveness	*No*

Phase 1: "Proof of concept: Do novel marker levels differ between subjects with and without outcome?" [37]

This is clearly the case for arterial stiffness, since a large number of pathophysiological conditions are associated with it, as reported in several reviews [3, 41]. In addition to ageing, they included several physiological conditions, the genetic background, classical CV risk factors and established CV disease. Importantly, arterial stiffness is also increased in several disease of non-cardiovascular origin, although complicated by CV events, such as end-stage renal disease (ESRD), moderate chronic kidney disease and disease characterised by chronic low-grade inflammation, such as rheumatoid arthritis, systemic vasculitis, systemic lupus erythematosus, AIDS and inflammatory bowel disease [3].

Phase 2: "Prospective validation. Does the novel marker predict development of future outcomes in a prospective cohort or nested case-cohort study?" [37]

Yes, aortic stiffness has a predictive value for all-cause and CV mortality and total CV events, as detailed above.

Phase 3: "Incremental value: Does the novel marker add predictive information to established, standard risk markers?" [37]

Yes, the predictive value of aortic stiffness for CV events has been demonstrated after adjustment for classical cardiovascular risk factors, including brachial PP. According to this definition, all studies described above showed predictive value of aortic stiffness for CV events independently of classical CV risk factors. The additive value of PWV above and beyond traditional risk factors has been quantified by three separate studies [12, 15, 18]. The first was performed in 1,045 hypertensive patients, with a longitudinal follow-up of 5.9 years for coronary heart disease (CHD) events [18]. The increase in CHD with tertiles of PWV was steeper for patients belonging to the first and second tertiles of the Framingham risk score (FRS). The C statistics (quantifying the area under (AUC) the receiver operating characteristic (ROC) (i.e. sensitivity vs. [1-specificity] curve)) is useful for quantifying discrimination, i.e. the ability of PWV to distinguish patients in whom CV events will occur from those who will remain free of CV complications. In the group of low-to-medium risk patients, the C statistics showed that FRS and PWV had similar predictive value (AUC=0.65±0.07 and 0.63±0.08, respectively), and when combined, the predictive value increased since the AUC significantly rose to 0.76±0.09, indicating that PWV improved the prediction of CV events beyond FRS. This improved ability of aortic stiffness to predict CV mortality was confirmed by Mattace-Raso et al. [12] in the elderly subjects from a general population and by Sehestedt et al. [15] in middle-aged subjects from a general population. The various mechanisms by which an increase in aortic stiffness generates higher risk of cardiac and cerebrovascular events have been described in details in several reviews [3, 11, 41] and above.

Phase 4: "Clinical utility: Does the novel risk marker change predicted risk sufficiently to change recommended therapy?" [37]

In other words, does the addition of PWV result in a substantial proportion of individuals being reclassified across a predefined treatment threshold? The answer is yes, since several studies showed that a substantial amount of patients at intermediate risk could be reclassified into a higher or a lower CV risk, when arterial stiffness was measured [12, 15, 38]. For instance, in the Framingham study, 15.7 % of patients at intermediate risk could be reclassified into a higher (14.3 %) or lower (1.4 %) risk [38]. In a recent unpublished meta-analysis, 19 and 22 % of intermediate risk individuals were reclassified into higher or lower quartiles of risk for coronary heart disease and stroke outcomes, respectively [23, 42].

Phase 5: "Clinical outcomes: Does use of the novel risk marker improve clinical outcomes, especially when tested in a randomised clinical trial?" [37]

An important issue here is whether the reduction in arterial stiffness translates into a reduction in CV events. There is only very little indirect evidence. To our knowledge, only one study reported CV outcomes in patients having repeated measurements of PWV along several years [39]: 150 patients (aged 52±16 years) with end-stage renal disease (ESRD) were monitored for 51±38 months for blood pressure and PWV. Fifty-nine deaths occurred, including 40 cardiovascular and 19 non-cardiovascular events. Cox analyses demonstrated that the lack of PWV decrease in response to BP reduction was a strong independent predictor of all-cause (RR 2.59 [1.51–4.43]) and cardiovascular mortality (RR 2.35 [1.23–4.41]). However, this study suffers several limitations: this was not a randomised clinical trial, rather a post hoc retrospective analysis; baseline PWV was different in the two groups and there is no mention that statistical analysis was adjusted to it; finally this study included patients at very high risk and results cannot be extrapolated to other (milder) clinical situations, as discussed thereafter.

An alternative strategy is to determine whether the change in patient management according to aortic stiffness can improve the outcome. This is the aim of the SPARTE study [28] ("Stratégie de Prévention cardiovasculaire basée sur la rigidité ARTErielle"), which will test the hypothesis that a therapeutic strategy targeting the normalisation of arterial stiffness is more effective in preventing CV events than usual care. The SPARTE study [28] will randomise 3,000 hypertensive patients, aged 55–75 years, who are at medium to very high risk for cardiorenal events, in a parallel group PROBE (prospective randomised open blinded endpoint) study, to receive either a treatment according to international guidelines for the management of blood pressure (control group) or an additional therapeutic strategy aiming at normalising PWV values (active group), during 4 years.

Phase 6: "Cost-effectiveness: Does use of the novel risk marker improve clinical outcomes sufficiently to justify the additional costs?" [37]

Table 21.2 Devices and methods used for determining non-invasively regional arterial stiffness through pulse wave velocity. Arterial pathways and predictive values are indicated

Description of the method: year of first publication	Device	Method	Arterial pathway	Predictive value for CV events (year of first publication)
1984	Complior®	Mechanotransducer	Carotid-femoral	Yes (1999)
1990	SphygmoCor®	Tonometer	Carotid-femoral	Yes (2011)
1994	QKD®	ECG + Korotkoff sounds	Aorta + brachial	Yes (2005)
1997	Cardiov. Eng. Inc®	Tonometer	Carotid-femoral	Yes (2010)
2002	Doppler probes	Doppler probe	Aortic arch + descending aorta	Yes (2002)
2002	VP-1000 Omron®	Brachial and ankle pressure cuffs	Aorta + brachial + lower limbs	Yes (2005)
2004	PulsePen®	Tonometer	Carotid-femoral	No
2006	CAVI-VASERA®	ECG + brachial and ankle pressure cuffs	Aorta + brachial + lower limbs	No
2008	Arteriograph®	Arm pressure cuff	Aorta + brachial	No
2009	MRI-ArtFun®	MRI	Aortic arch	No
2009	Vicorder®	Cuffs	Carotid-femoral	No
2010	Mobil-O-Graph®	Arm pressure cuff	Aorta	No

From Ref. [40] with permission
PWV pulse wave velocity, *MRI* magnetic resonance imaging

The cost-effectiveness issue describes the balance between the additional cost associated with the measurement of aortic stiffness and the subtracted cost due to less CV complications when patients are managed according to aortic stiffness measurement. Cost-effectiveness is a complex public health issue, particularly regarding the quantification of avoided or delayed clinical complication and improved quality of life. This issue is far to be solved, even for well-established tests in other medical specialties (for instance, mammography in breast cancer).

Predictive Values of Arterial Stiffness Measured with Other Devices

Novel devices measuring novel arterial stiffness parameters should show predictive value for CV events [40]. They cannot claim it simply from data showing a significant correlation between the novel stiffness parameter and cfPWV obtained during a cross-sectional validation study. Adequate longitudinal epidemiological studies should be performed. Table 21.2 shows which of the well-established methods and novel ones have demonstrated an independent predictive value of CV events until now. This issue is of major importance at the present time, since several novel apparatus, which were developed for determining arterial stiffness, claim superiority over pioneering methods through either higher simplicity of use, better repeatability or more pertinent arterial pathway.

The question of the functional substratum linking the measured parameter to events is crucial [40]. Carotid-femoral PWV, which is considered as gold standard for determining aortic stiffness [3], is calculated as the ratio of the transit time between the feet of the carotid and femoral pressure waveforms and the carotid-femoral distance, a ratio which is undisputedly recognised as a stiffness parameter. Several studies and a consensus statement [29] have determined the correction factor which should be applied to the carotid-femoral distance, to take into account the fact that, when the pressure wave is recorded at the carotid level, it has already reached the descending thoracic aorta. The pressure wave travels mostly along an aortic segment, including the thoracic descending aorta and the abdominal aorta, and ultimately travels along the iliac and common femoral arteries.

The issue of the arterial pathway is also raised by other methods more recently introduced. The measurement of the brachial-ankle PWV, which includes a much longer trajectory of the pressure wave along the muscular arteries of the upper and lower limbs than along the aortic pathway, has demonstrated a predictive value for CV events [43, 44] including incident hypertension and readmission for heart failure, in several populations: patients with stable angina, acute coronary syndrome or diabetes and elderly subjects [45]. These results extend the findings observed with cfPWV, and it can be concluded that the stiffness of an elastic + muscular arterial segment is predictive of CV events.

The issue of the arterial pathway is even more critical with the QKD [45] method and two novel oscillometric devices. The QKD method [45] measures the time delay between the onset of the QRS on the ECG and the detection of the last Korotkoff sound by the microphone placed upon the brachial artery. Thus, the pressure pulse wave travels first along the ascending aorta and the aortic arch, i.e. a short pathway of elastic arteries, and then along the subclavian and brachial arteries, i.e. a much longer pathway of muscular arteries. Since the stiffness of muscular arteries is little influenced by age and hypertension, Gosse et al. [45] attributed the difference in QKD duration to the ascending aorta and aortic arch. However, the length of the ascending and aortic arch pathway represents a very small part of the total pathway and casts doubt about this statement. These findings suggest that the stiffness of an elastic + muscular arterial segment is predictive of CV events, as discussed also for the brachial-ankle PWV.

The Arteriograph system [46] estimates PWV from a single-site determination of the suprasystolic waveform at the brachial artery site and measures the time elapsed between the first wave ejected from the left ventricle to the aortic root and its reflection from the bifurcation as the second systolic wave, with subtraction of the brachial artery transit time. Arterial stiffness is calculated here from the transit time between two pressure waves, travelling mostly along the thoracic and abdominal aorta, i.e. an elastic arterial segment.

The Mobil-O-Graph system [47] uses an indirect way for determining arterial stiffness. An oscillometric recording of brachial artery pressure waveform allows reconstructing the central pulse wave by applying a transfer function. Central pulse wave is then decomposed into forward and backward waves, and PWV is estimated from their time difference. Although much more indirect than the previous methods, this is again mostly the velocity of the pressure wave along the thoracic and abdominal aorta which is taken into account for measuring arterial stiffness.

These various methods can be ranked as follows, from the most direct method to the most indirect method, all of them claiming the measurement of PWV along the aorta and adjacent muscular arterial segments (either upper or lower limbs): cfPWV > brachial-ankle PWV > QKD method > Arteriograph > Mobil-O-Graph. The first three have already demonstrated a predictive value of PWV measurement for CV events. Epidemiological studies are needed for the novel methods, including both Arteriograph and Mobil-O-Graph, and some listed in Table 21.2.

Conclusion

The measurement of aortic stiffness repeatedly showed predictive value for various CV events in various populations. In addition, aortic stiffness proved to complete a number of criteria for being considered as a true surrogate endpoint for CV events, although not all. This is why its measurement, already recommended by the 2007 [1] and 2013 [48] ESH-ESC Guidelines for the Management of Arterial Hypertension, should be recommended by additional guidelines for the management of CV disease. There is a need for studies comparing aortic stiffness-guided therapeutic strategies with classical guideline-guided strategies for preventing CV events. There is also a need for epidemiological studies showing the predictive value of arterial stiffness, measured with novel devices, for CV events.

Source of Funding INSERM (Institut National de la Santé et de la Recherche Médicale), Assistance-Publique Hôpitaux de Paris, Université Paris Descartes.

Conflict of Interest/Disclosure None

References

1. Mancia G, de Backer G, Cifkova R, Dominiczak A, Fagard R, Germano G, Grassi G, Heagerty AM, Kjeldsen SE, Laurent S, Narkiewicz K, Ruilope L, Rynkiewicz A, Schmieder R, Struijker Boudier HA, Zanchetti A. Guidelines for the management of arterial hypertension. The task force for the management of arterial hypertension of the European Society of Cardiology (ESC) and of the European Society of Hypertension (ESH). J Hypertens. 2007;25: 1105–87.
2. Wang TJ. Assessing the role of circulating, genetic, and imaging biomarkers in cardiovascular risk prediction. Circulation. 2011;123:551–65.
3. Laurent S, Cockcroft J, Van Bortel L, Boutouyrie P, Giannattasio C, Hayoz D, Pannier B, Vlachopoulos C, Wilkinson I, Struijker-Boudier H. Expert consensus document on arterial stiffness: methodological issues and clinical applications. Eur Heart J. 2006;27: 2588–605.
4. Pletcher MJ, Pignone M. Evaluating the clinical utility of a biomarker: a review of methods for estimating health impact. Circulation. 2011;123:1116–24.
5. Wilson PW, D'Agostino RB, Levy D, Belanger AM, Silbershatz H, Kannel WB. Prediction of coronary heart disease using risk factor categories. Circulation. 1998;97:1837–47.
6. Conroy RM, Pyörälä K, Fitzgerald AP, Sans S, Menotti A, De Backer G, De Bacquer D, Ducimetière P, Jousilahti P, Keil U, Njølstad I, Oganov RG, Thomsen T, Tunstall-Pedoe H, Tverdal A, Wedel H, Whincup P, Wilhelmsen L, Graham IM, SCORE project group. Estimation of ten-year risk of fatal cardiovascular disease in Europe: the SCORE project. Eur Heart J. 2003;24:987–1003.
7. Biomarkers Definitions Working Group. Biomarkers and surrogate endpoints: preferred definitions and conceptual framework. Clin Pharmacol Ther. 2001;69:89–95.
8. Wang TJ, Gona P, Larson MG, Tofler GH, Levy D, Newton-Cheh C, Jacques PF, Rifai N, Selhub J, Robins SJ, Benjamin EJ, D'Agostino RB, Vasan RS. Multiple biomarkers for the prediction of first major cardiovascular events and death. N Engl J Med. 2006;355:2631–9.
9. Zethelius B, Berglund L, Sundström J, Ingelsson E, Basu S, Larsson A, Venge P, Arnlöv J. Use of multiple biomarkers to improve the prediction of death from cardiovascular causes. N Engl J Med. 2008;358: 2107–16.
10. Nilsson P, Boutouyrie P, Laurent S. Vascular aging: a tale of EVA and ADAM in cardiovascular risk assessment and prevention. Hypertension. 2009;54:3–10.
11. Laurent S, Briet M, Boutouyrie P. Large/small artery cross talk and recent morbidity mortality trials in hypertension. Hypertension. 2009;54:388–92.
12. Mattace-Raso FU, van der Cammen TJ, Hofman A, van Popele NM, Bos ML, Schalekamp MA, Asmar R, Reneman RS, Hoeks AP, Breteler MM, Witteman JC. Arterial stiffness and risk of coronary heart disease and stroke: the Rotterdam Study. Circulation. 2006;113:657–63.
13. Shokawa T, Imazu M, Yamamoto H, Toyofuku M, Tasaki N, Okimoto T, Yamane K, Kohno N. Pulse wave velocity predicts cardiovascular mortality: findings from the Hawaii-Los Angeles-Hiroshima study. Circ J. 2005;69:259–64.
14. Willum-Hansen T, Staessen JA, Torp-Pedersen C, Rasmussen S, Thijs L, Ibsen H, Jeppesen J. Prognostic value of aortic pulse wave velocity as index of arterial stiffness in the general population. Circulation. 2006;113:664–70.
15. Sehestedt T, Jeppesen J, Hansen TW, Rasmussen S, Wachtell K, Ibsen H, Torp-Pedersen C, Olsen MH. Risk stratification with the risk chart from the European Society of Hypertension compared with SCORE in the general population. J Hypertens. 2009; 27:2351–7.
16. Meaume S, Benetos A, Henry OF, Rudnichi A, Safar ME. Aortic pulse wave velocity predicts cardiovascular mortality in subjects >70 years of age. Arterioscler Thromb Vasc Biol. 2001;21:2046–50.
17. Sutton-Tyrrell K, Najjar SS, Boudreau RM, Venkitachalam L, Kupelian V, Simonsick EM, Havlik R, Lakatta EG, Spurgeon H, Kritchevsky S, Pahor M, Bauer D, Newman A, Health ABC Study. Elevated aortic pulse wave velocity, a marker of arterial stiffness, predicts cardiovascular events in well-functioning older adults. Circulation. 2005;111:3384–90.
18. Boutouyrie P, Tropeano AI, Asmar R, Gautier I, Benetos A, Lacolley P, Laurent S. Aortic stiffness is an independent predictor of primary coronary events in hypertensive patients: a longitudinal study. Hypertension. 2002;39:10–5.
19. Laurent S, Boutouyrie P, Asmar R, Gautier I, Laloux B, Guize L, Ducimetiere P, Benetos A. Aortic stiffness is an independent predictor of all-cause and cardiovascular mortality in hypertensive patients. Hypertension. 2001;37:1236–41.
20. Laurent S, Katsahian S, Fassot C, Tropeano AI, Laloux B, Boutouyrie P. Aortic stiffness is an independent predictor of fatal stroke in essential hypertension. Stroke. 2003;34:1203–6.
21. Cruickshank K, Riste L, Anderson SG, Wright JS, Dunn G, Gosling RG. Aortic pulse-wave velocity and its relationship to mortality in diabetes and glucose intolerance: an integrated index of vascular function? Circulation. 2002;106:2085–90.
22. Blacher J, Guerin AP, Pannier B, Marchais SJ, Safar ME, London GM. Impact of aortic stiffness on

survival in end-stage renal disease. Circulation. 1999; 99:2434–9.

23. Karras A, Haymann JP, Bozec E, Metzger M, Jacquot C, Maruani G, Houillier P, Froissart M, Stengel B, Guardiola P, Laurent S, Boutouyrie P, Briet M, NephroTest study group. Large artery stiffening and remodeling are independently associated with all-cause mortality and cardiovascular events in chronic kidney disease. Hypertension. 2012;60:1451–7.
24. Verbeke F, Maréchal C, Van Laecke S, Van Biesen W, Devuyst O, Van Bortel LM, Jadoul M, Vanholder R. Aortic stiffness and central wave reflections predict outcome in renal transplant recipients. Hypertension. 2011;58:833–8.
25. Gasecki D, Rokek A, Kwarciany M, Kubach M, Boutouyrie P, Nyka V, Laurent S, Narkiewicz K. Pulse wave velocity predicts functional outcome in patients after ischemic stroke. Stroke. 2012;43:543–4.
26. Gasecki D, Rojek A, Kwarciany M, Kowalczyk K, Boutouyrie P, Nyka W, Laurent S, Narkiewicz K. Low pulse wave velocity is associated with early neurological improvement after acute ischemic stroke. Atherosclerosis. 2012;225:348–52.
27. Vlachopoulos C, Aznaouridis K, Stefanadis C. Prediction of cardiovascular events and all-cause mortality with arterial stiffness: a systematic review and meta-analysis. J Am Coll Cardiol. 2010;55:1318–27.
28. Laurent S, Briet M, Boutouyrie P. Arterial stiffness and central pulse pressure as surrogate markers: needed clinical trials. Hypertension. 2012;60(2): 518–22.
29. Van Bortel LM, Laurent S, Boutouyrie P, Chowienczyk P, Cruickshank JK, De Backer T, Filipovsky J, Huybrechts S, Mattace-Raso FU, Protogerou AD, Schillaci G, Segers P, Vermeersch S, Weber T. Expert consensus document on the measurement of aortic stiffness in daily practice using carotid-femoral pulse wave velocity. J Hypertens. 2012;30:445–8.
30. Reference values for carotid-femoral pulse wave velocity in the reference values for arterial stiffness' collaboration database. Eur Heart J. 2010;31:2338–50.
31. Boutouyrie P, Laurent S, Girerd X, Beck L, Abergel E, Safar M. Common carotid artery distensibility and patterns of left ventricular hypertrophy in hypertensive patients. Hypertension. 1995;25(part 1): 651–9.
32. O'Rourke MF, Safar ME, Dzau V. The Cardiovascular Continuum extended: aging effects on the aorta and microvasculature. Vasc Med. 2010;15(6):461–8.
33. Boutouyrie P, Bussy C, Hayoz D, Hengstler J, Dartois N, Laloux B, Brunner H, Laurent S. Local pulse pressure and regression of arterial wall hypertrophy during long term antihypertensive treatment. Circulation. 2000;101:2601–6.
34. Scuteri A, Nilsson P, Tsourio C, Redon J, Laurent S. Microvascular brain damage: pathophysiological consideration and clinical implications. J Hypertens. 2011;29:1469–77.
35. Brisset M, Boutouyrie P, Pico F, Zhu Y, Zureik M, Schilling S, Dufouil C, Mazoyer B, Laurent S, Tzourio C, Debette S. Large-vessel correlates of cerebral small-vessel disease. Neurology. 2013;80:662–9.
36. Selwaness M, van den Bouwhuijsen QJ, Verwoert GC, Dehghan A, Mattace-Raso FU, Vernooij M, Franco OH, Hofman A, van der Lugt A, Wentzel JJ, Witteman JC. Blood pressure parameters and carotid intraplaque hemorrhage as measured by magnetic resonance imaging: The Rotterdam Study. Hypertension. 2013;61:76–81.
37. Hlatky MA, Greenland P, Arnett DK, Ballantyne CM, Criqui MH, Elkind MS, Go AS, Harrell Jr FE, Hong Y, Howard BV, Howard VJ, Hsue PY, Kramer CM, McConnell JP, Normand SL, O'Donnell CJ, Smith Jr SC, Wilson PW, American Heart Association Expert Panel on Subclinical Atherosclerotic Diseases and Emerging Risk Factors and the Stroke Council. Criteria for evaluation of novel markers of cardiovascular risk: a scientific statement from the American Heart Association. Circulation. 2009;119:2408–16.
38. Mitchell GF, Hwang SJ, Vasan RD, Larson MG, Pencina MJ, Hamburg NM, Vita JA, Levy D, Benjamin EJ. Arterial stiffness and cardiovascular events. The Framingham Heart Study. Circulation. 2010;121:505–11.
39. Guerin AP, Blacher J, Pannier B, Marchais SJ, Safar ME, London GM. Impact of aortic stiffness attenuation on survival of patients in end-stage renal failure. Circulation. 2001;20(103):987–92.
40. Laurent S, Mousseaux E, Boutouyrie P. Arterial stiffness as an imaging biomarker: are all pathways equal? Hypertension. 2013;62:10–2.
41. Safar ME. Arterial aging-hemodynamic changes and therapeutic options. Nat Rev Cardiol. 2010;7:442–9.
42. Ben Schlomo Y, Spears M, Boustred C, May M, Anderson S, Boutouyrie P, Cameron J, Chen CH, Cockcroft J, Cruickshank K, Hwang SJ, Lakatta E, Laurent S, Maldonado J, McEniery CM, Mitchell G, Najjar S, Newman A, Ohishi M, Pannier B, Pereira T, Shokawa T, Sutton-Tyrell K, Webb D, Willum-Hansen T, Zoungas S, Wilkinson IB. Aortic pulse wave velocity improves cardiovascular event prediction: an individual participant meta-analysis of prospective observational data from 17,635 subjects. J Am Coll Cardiol. 2014;63(7):636–46.
43. Tomiyama H, Koji Y, Yambe M, Shiina K, Motobe K, Yamada J, Shido N, Tanaka N, Chikamori T, Yamashina A. Brachial – ankle pulse wave velocity is a simple and independent predictor of prognosis in patients with acute coronary syndrome. Circ J. 2005;69:815–22.
44. Vlachopoulos C, Aznaouridis K, Terentes-Printzios D, Ioakeimidis N, Stefanadis C. Prediction of cardiovascular events and all-cause mortality with brachial-ankle elasticity index: a systematic review and meta-analysis. Hypertension. 2012;60:556–62.
45. Gosse P, Cremer A, Papaioannou G, Yeim S. Arterial stiffness from monitoring of timing of Korotkoff sounds predicts the occurrence of cardiovascular events independently of left ventricular mass in hypertensive patients. Hypertension. 2013;62:161–7.
46. Baulmann J, Schillings U, Rickert S, Uen S, Düsing R, Illyes M, Cziraki A, Nickering G, Mengden T.

A new oscillometric method for assessment of arterial stiffness: comparison with tonometric and piezo-electronic methods. J Hypertens. 2008;26:523–8.
47. Weber T, Wassertheurer S, Rammer M, Haiden A, Hametner B, Eber B. Wave reflections, assessed with a novel method for pulse wave separation, are associated with end-organ damage and clinical outcomes. Hypertension. 2012;60:534–41.
48. Mancia G, Fagard R, Narkiewicz K, Redón J, Zanchetti A, Böhm M, Christiaens T, Cifkova R, DeBacker G, Dominiczak A, Galderisi M, Grobbee DE, Jaarsma T, Kirchhof P, Kjeldsen SE, Laurent S, Manolis AJ, Nilsson PM, Ruilope LM, Schmieder RE, Sirnes PA, Sleight P, Viigimaa M, Waeber B, Zannad F. 2013 ESH/ESC Guidelines for the management of arterial hypertension: The Task Force for the management of arterial hypertension of the European Society of Hypertension (ESH) and of the European Society of Cardiology (ESC). Eur Heart J. 2013;34:2159–219.

Heart Rate, Synchrony and Arterial Hemodynamics

22

Alberto P. Avolio, Mark Butlin, and Isabella Tan

Abstract

Heart rate is a conventional index quantifying the pulsatile action of the heart and is a basic parameter used throughout medical history and practice. However, modern science often places relatively little emphasis on heart rate in relation to the oscillatory nature of blood flow in the circulatory system, and the unyielding cyclic stress on the heart and blood vessels. Heart rate is relevant not only as an elemental measure, but also as a statistical entity and a possible confounding factor when considering its interaction with vascular hemodynamics. Pulse pressure amplification from the central aorta to peripheral arteries increases with heart rate. This has significant implications when assessing vascular function based on peripheral (brachial) pressure measurements, as the pressure changes at the central aorta with changes in arterial stiffness (as occurs with age) can be markedly different from changes at the peripheral site at different heart rates. Similarly, heart rate is a significant parameter when assessing cardiac and vascular implications of anti-hypertensive drug treatments. Heart rate, itself an independent parameter of cardiovascular risk, should also be considered in the statistical treatment of cardiovascular risk factors in large epidemiological studies. Disturbance in the regular pulsatile action of the heart due to altered synchrony of the cardiac chambers leads to heart failure, which can be treated with resychronization therapy. Cardiovascular models show that arterial stiffness can significantly affect the modification of parameters associated with cardiac resynchronization therapy. Thus, pulsatile hemodynamic parameters play a significant role when associated with both regular heart rate and with disturbed synchrony of the contracting heart chambers affecting the pump function of the heart.

A.P. Avolio, PhD, BE (✉) • M. Butlin, PhD, BE
I. Tan, BE
The Australian School of Advanced Medicine,
2 Technology Place, Macquarie University,
North Ryde, Sydney, NSW 2109, Australia
e-mail: alberto.avolio@mq.edu.au;
mark.butlin@mq.edu.au; isabella.tan@mq.edu.au

M.E. Safar et al. (eds.), *Blood Pressure and Arterial Wall Mechanics in Cardiovascular Diseases*,
DOI 10.1007/978-1-4471-5198-2_22, © Springer-Verlag London 2014

Keywords
Heart rate • Pulse wave velocity • Pulse pressure • Aorta • Aortic stiffness • Cardiac resynchronization • Hemodynamics • Cardiovascular risk

Introduction

Rhythmic contraction of the heart is the most basic evidence of life. Heart rate is an elementary clinical sign for physicians, having heralded the sphygmomanometer, the sphygmograph, and the stethoscope. Heart rate is a parameter often ignored in modern science, but is a basic parameter in the history of medicine and in medical practice.

This chapter addresses the relevance of heart rate in relation to the pulsatile aspects of hemodynamics in the context of the overall theme of blood pressure and arterial stiffness in cardiovascular prevention. Factors that determine arterial blood pressure and arterial stiffness, as well as their epidemiological relevance to hypertension and cardiovascular risk, are treated in other sections of this volume. Specifically, this chapter examines the association of heart rate with arterial stiffness and its impact on pulse pressure and parameters derived from pulse wave analysis. The importance of pulse pressure amplification between central and peripheral locations related to heart rate is highlighted with respect to proper assessment of arterial hemodynamics by peripheral pressure measurement. In addition, by use of cardiovascular models, the relationship of arterial stiffness and synchrony between the heart chambers is examined in relation to optimizing cardiac output; aspects that have particular relevance to biventricular pacing and cardiac resynchronization therapy.

In general, this chapter highlights the importance of heart rate as a significant parameter that needs to be taken into account when treating physiological, experimental and epidemiological data with regards to quantifying cardiovascular risk, both as a statistical entity and also in terms of measurement of blood pressure when using pulse waveform analysis.

Allometric Nature of Heart Rate

In physiological systems, there are parameters that are related to body weight, for example, heart rate, metabolic rate, heart size, and cardiac output. Other haemodynamic parameters are not related to body weight, for example blood pressure and arterial stiffness. The dependency of a parameter on body weight can be described by an allometric relation as described in Eq. 22.1, where x is the parameter of interest, W is body weight, and A and k are constants.

$$x = A \cdot W^{k} \tag{22.1}$$

The heart rate in mammals is approximately proportional to the cubic root of weight, with small mammals having a high resting rate (e.g. 600 beats/s for mice), and large animals a low resting rate (e.g. 15 beats/min for whales). The reverse relationship of heart rate to length of mammals probably denotes optimization of ventricular-vascular interactions with respect to cardiac diastolic duration and return of wave reflection in the arterial system, as well as to physiological fundamentals of muscular relaxation and contraction.

In an elegant study relating vascular parameters to functional correlates across animal size spanning a range of body weights from the rat (0.2 kg) to the elephant (3,500 kg), Westerhof and Elzinga [1, 2] illustrate the possible mechanism as to why pulse pressure is essentially similar over the whole range of animal body size and weight. Heart period (T) is taken as the characteristic cardiac time and the time constant of the exponential diastolic decay (τ) of the arterial pressure pulse as the characteristic arterial time. It was found that both T and τ increase with body weight with a similar exponent of approximately 0.25 [1]. Hence, the ratio τ/T is essentially independent of animal size.

The arterial system can be modeled in terms of a Windkessel [3, 4], where the exponential diastolic decay of pressure can be expressed in terms of the peripheral resistance (*R*) and the central aortic compliance (*C*, Eq. 22.2). For low values of late systolic augmentation due to wave reflection, compliance is largely related to the ratio of stroke volume (SV) and pulse pressure (PP, Eq. 22.3) [5]. Since mean arterial pressure (MAP) can be expressed as the ratio of stroke volume and resistance to heart period (Eq. 22.4), it follows that the ratio *PP/MAP* is inversely proportional to the ratio τ/T, and is therefore independent of body size. In fact, the ratio τ/T could be considered as a basic coupling parameter between the heart and the arterial system and forms the basis of the interaction between heart rate (*1/T*), pulse pressure and arterial stiffness [1, 2, 5]. Similar matching phenomena across a range of species have been described in terms of impedance spectra normalized for resting heart rate [6, 7]. Milnor's concepts of relating physical body dimensions to wave transmission phenomena in terms of aortic wavelength were further expanded by Iberal [8] and O'Rourke [9] to encompass the earlier work on optimal design proposed by Taylor [10] and McDonald [4].

$$\tau = R \cdot C \tag{22.2}$$

$$C = \frac{SV}{PP} \tag{22.3}$$

$$MAP = \frac{SV \cdot R}{T} \tag{22.4}$$

Heart Rate, Cardiac Function, and Arterial Hemodynamics

The interaction between the ejecting ventricle and the systemic load is described as the coupling between cardiac parameters, such as source impedance [11, 12], myocardial contractility indices [13] and arterial elastance [14]. Since the heart is essentially a self-energizing pump, the output is necessarily intermittent. Power delivery occurs during only a fraction of the periodic cardiac oscillation in which the ventricles are almost emptied of their blood content during systole and are filled during diastole for ejection in the subsequent contraction.

The energy supply to the myocardium is delivered by coronary blood flow occurring predominantly during diastole. Changes in heart rate result in changes in cycle time, which are in turn affected largely by changes in diastolic time with relatively smaller changes in systolic ejection times [15]. The relatively greater effect on the duration of diastole has direct effects on the time available for ventricular filling, hence affecting stroke volume through the Frank-Starling mechanism [13], and also on the time available for diastolic run-off of arterial blood. The rate of run-off is determined by the value of peripheral resistance and the stiffness of the arterial wall. Hence, for a given stroke volume, this mechanism, in addition to the wave reflection phenomenon, will determine the pulse pressure.

The steady state operating point is determined by the properties of the heart in terms of stroke volume, the elastic properties of the large distributing arteries, and the level of peripheral resistance at the microcirculation. Although arterial pressure undergoes instantaneous variation with time, the interaction of the generally periodic nature of the beating heart and the arterial load can be considered to operate at an arterial pressure having a steady component (mean pressure during the cardiac cycle determined by the peripheral resistance) and a superimposed oscillatory component (pulse pressure, determined by the stiffness of the large conduit arteries) [3, 4, 16]. These concepts could explain some of the differences between acute and long-term effects of changes in heart rate on pulse pressure. Acute changes, as seen with pacing studies [17], are essentially passive effects due to changes in diastolic time and so affecting minimum (diastolic) pressure during the cardiac cycle. These short-term changes are different to the long-term changes seen in population studies that may involve sustained effects due to sympathetic or vagal activation. The interaction between heart rate, pulse pressure and arterial stiffness is complex. It involves a closed-loop system with a combination of feedback and feed forward loops, where a change of a parameter in one direction can influence others in the same or opposite direction.

Heart Rate and Arterial Stiffness

Acute Effects

Arterial blood pressure is only a relative measure of arterial function as it is determined by the interaction of cardiac and arterial factors. However, arterial stiffness is entirely determined by vascular characteristics [4]. Of the many indices of arterial stiffness that can be measured non-invasively [18, 19], pulse wave velocity (PWV) has been accepted as an easily measurable parameter and used as a surrogate for arterial stiffness [19]. However, it is important to consider the underlying assumptions. For a uniform arterial segment of a given length, PWV is related to the stiffness of the wall material (Young's Modulus, E), vascular dimensions (radius R, wall thickness, h), and blood density (ρ) by the Moens-Korteweg relation (Eq. 22.5) [3, 4].

$$PWV = \sqrt{\frac{Eh}{2\rho R}} \tag{22.5}$$

It can also be expressed in terms of changes in pressure (ΔP) and volume (ΔV) in closed vessels, as described in the Bramwell-Hill relation (Eq. 22.6) [20].

$$PWV = \sqrt{\frac{\Delta P \cdot V}{\Delta V \cdot \rho}} \tag{22.6}$$

These relations (Eqs. 22.5 and 22.6) essentially express the velocity of the forward going pressure pulse (ΔP) using assumptions of an infinitely long, thin-walled, elastic tube with isotropic elastic properties and containing incompressible fluid. They do not contain terms related to the frequency dependency of the parameters, which would elicit some dependence on heart rate. However, the interaction of the cellular and extracellular matrix components of the arterial wall make it a viscoelastic material [21, 22], thus making the elastic modulus a complex quantity with frequency (ω) dependence (Eq. 22.7) [3, 4, 21, 22] and not a static modulus of elasticity (|E|).

$$E(\omega) = |E| \cdot \exp(j\varphi) \tag{22.7}$$

$$\varphi = arctan(\omega \Delta E) \tag{22.8}$$

This was elegantly demonstrated by Bergel in the early 1960s, using canine arteries cycled at various frequencies, where the stiffness of the vessel (E) was shown to depend on the cycling frequency below 2 Hz [23, 24]. The implication of this is that the frequency dependency of the elastic modulus produces subsequent frequency dependency of PWV (from Eq. 22.5). However, this is not similar in all arteries. From Bergel's classic experiments [23, 24], linear extrapolation from 0 to 2 Hz gives the following average increase in relative dynamic elastic modulus: carotid artery, 30 %/Hz; femoral artery, 16.5 %/Hz; abdominal aorta, 9 %/Hz; thoracic aorta, 3.5 %/Hz. These values indicate that muscular arteries have an increased frequency dependency. Indeed, studies suggest a "smart damping" role of smooth muscle in the artery wall due to viscoelasticity [25]. This is different to the frequency dependency of phase velocity, where the low frequency components have an apparent velocity due to a finite distance of wave propagation in relation to wavelength [4].

Findings from in-vitro experiments are not entirely consistent with some other observations. Accurate pulse transit time measurements in isolated canine carotid arteries showed that over a range of sinusoidal frequency pulses of 1–20 Hz and pressure range of 50–150 mmHg, PWV was independent of frequency and dependent only on pressure [26]. Furthermore, the propagation velocity of the significant harmonic components of the pulsatile pressure waveform did not change for heart rates up to 120 beats/min. Studies of heart rate and arterial stiffness in rats and humans using cardiac pacing found a variety of relations between the parameters [27–31]. The explanation for these findings may be multi-factorial,

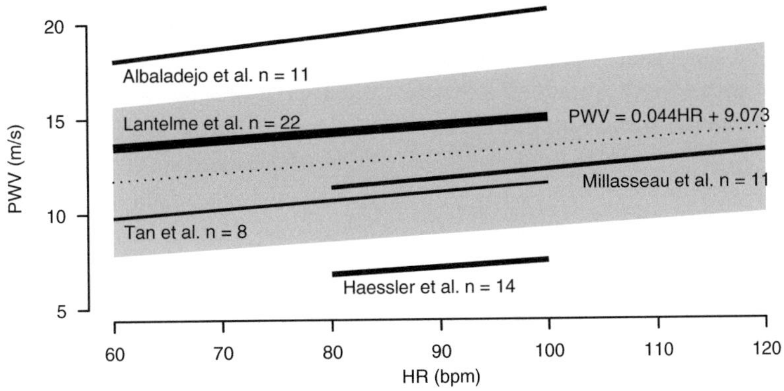

Fig. 22.1 A summary of studies investigating the effect of heart rate on carotid-femoral PWV. The sample size (n) is also indicated by the weight of the lines. The weighted average line (*dashed line*) is plotted, showing a relationship of 0.044 m/s/beat/min. The *shaded area* gives the region ± one standard deviation (Average lines are from Albaladego et al. [17], Haessler et al. [34], Lantelme et al. [27], Millaseau et al. SphygmoCor results [35], and Tan, Butlin, and Avolio [unpublished data]. PWV has not been corrected for any increases in blood pressure with heart rate)

ranging from measurement techniques to determine the fiducial points for transit time measurement to modes of pacing [29, 30]. Spontaneous effects due to sympathetic stimulation of muscular arteries being associated with increased heart rate and arterial stiffness may also play a role [32, 33]. In addition, and this could be an important consideration in clinical measurements in human subjects, measurements over large path lengths may involve different segments with different frequency dependency of the wall elastic modulus.

Figure 22.1 gives relationships between carotid-femoral PWV and heart rate obtained from a number of human studies [17, 27, 34, 35], where heart rate was altered acutely through pacing. The average relationship across the studies gives a change of 0.44 m/s in PWV for every 10 beat/min rise in heart rate. However, in all but the study by Lantelme et al. [27], the paced increase in heart rate was accompanied by a significant rise in arterial pressure, indicating that the mechanism behind the rise in PWV was at least in part, if not entirely, due to changes in distending pressure.

Estimates of expected increases in PWV when transit time measurements are made between the carotid and femoral artery sites may be obtained from values of dynamic modulus change with frequency by Bergel et al. [23, 24]. By applying weights to the slopes according to the respective relative path lengths, the expected increase in PWV is of the order of 5 %/Hz. (that is, a 5 % increase in PWV for heart rate between 60 and 120 beats/min). This is much lower than the average value obtained from the regression equations in Fig. 22.1, ranging from 16 to 35 % increase between heart rate of 60 and 120 beats/min. This indicates that the change in arterial pressure is driving changes in PWV beyond the viscoelastic effect, and again supports the theory that the changes in PWV seen are blood pressure dependent and that the heart rate effect is small.

Chronic Effects

A population regression-based study of carotid-femoral PWV found that age, systolic pressure, weight, and heart rate were predictive of PWV in men, with the relationship between heart rate and PWV being linear. In women, however, only age and systolic pressure were found to be covariates [36]. Another study established a relationship between arterial stiffness and heart rate for both men and women, though heart rate was slightly less predictive in women [37]. Studies to date relating heart rate to PWV within individuals have not been suitably powered to detect differences between males and females [17, 27, 34, 35], though such a study might provide more information on this relationship. An additional chronic effects of heart rate might be related to the cumulative effects of cyclic stress. This has been shown to be associated with the fatiguing effects of cyclic stress on the structural integrity of elastic lamellae in the aortic wall [38].

Heart Rate and Pulse Pressure

Heart rate is measured routinely in conjunction with blood pressure as a conventional procedure. In addition to being a cardiac rhythm parameter, heart rate is related to pulse wave transmission through the frequency characteristics of the arterial propagation system [39, 40]. The transfer function of the brachial arterial system has a monotonic increase in transmission ratio up to around 4 Hz, with a peak ratio of around 3 Hz [39, 40]. Therefore, for an increase in heart rate, or an increase in the frequency of the harmonics of the arterial pulse, the amplification of the pulse pressure increases. Thus, similar values of pulse pressure measured in the arm correspond to different values of pulse pressure at the central aorta. Studies using a brachial transfer function and atrial pacing showed that pulse amplification between the central aorta and radial artery was estimated as 39 % for a heart rate of 65 beats/min and 95 % for 120 beats/min [41]. This amplification ratio is also age dependent, with decreasing amplification with age [42, 43].

Implications of Heart Rate and Pulse Pressure Amplification in Population Studies

There is greater variation of normal resting heart rate in the general population at any age than for blood pressure, yet less notice is taken of heart rate than blood pressure in epidemiological, clinical, and pharmaceutical trials. The arterial vasculature exhibits amplification of the propagating arterial pressure pulse [34] as a function of heart rate. When brachial pulse pressure is used as a surrogate for central, aortic pulse pressure itself, or in determining indices of distensibility for central arteries (carotid artery, proximal aorta), any changes in heart rate can produce profound differences in the results when compared with calculations performed with the central, aortic pulse pressure.

The heart rate effect on pulse pressure amplification can be a potentially important phenomenon in assessing ventricular load (especially peak load due to systolic pressure) for conditions where there are substantial changes in heart rate, such as exercise [44]. It is also important in large-scale studies investigating anti-hypertensive agents that also affect heart rate, as small differences in blood pressure can be statistically significant and may be due to heart rate and not inherent blood pressure changes. The result of the Losartan Intervention For Endpoint reduction in hypertension study (LIFE) in over 9,000 hypertensive subjects followed for 4 years showed that an angiotensin receptor blocking agent (losartan) had reduced brachial blood pressure to an almost identical extent as a beta blocking agent (atenolol) [45]. For a similar reduction in blood pressure, losartan produced additional beneficial and alleged pressure independent effects such as improved regression of left-ventricular hypertrophy [45, 46]. However, atenolol caused a decrease in heart rate of the order of 6 beats/min. This meant that although brachial pulse pressure was identical for both agents, pulse pressure amplification was greater with losartan due to the higher heart rate. Hence, aortic pulse pressure would be lower with losartan. For a given diastolic pressure, and heart rate amplification characteristics [41], the difference in heart rate between the two drug treatments would cause an estimated difference in aortic systolic pressure of 3 mmHg. This, conceivably, would be significant (in a large cohort of over 5,000 subjects) in determining the pressure-related effects on the heart, such as left ventricular hypertrophy. Confirmation of this phenomenon was seen in subsequent studies (e.g. REASON [47], CAFE [48]) showing that the lowering of heart rate with a beta blocker (atenolol) resulted in a sustained higher central aortic pressure despite a similar brachial systolic pressure achieved with other antihypertensive agents.

Neglecting to account for heart rate related changes in pulse pressure amplification also has implications in the calculation of parameters of central arterial stiffness. A recent study [49] conducted in a large cohort (n=6,484) showed that resting heart rate had an independent association

Table 22.1 Distensibility calculated using peripheral and central blood pressure values across different heart rates. Note the low slope and very low r^2 value for carotid distensibility with respect to heart rate calculated using central pressure, and the relatively similar magnitudes of slope, opposite sign and high values of r^2 for aortic distensibility compared to distensibility values calculated using peripheral pressure

			Carotid distensibility (×10^{-3} mmHg)		Aortic distensibility (×10^{-3} mmHg)	
Heart rate quintile	Average heart rate (beats/min)	Pulse amplification	Peripheral pressure	Central pressure	Peripheral pressure	Central pressure
1	50.9	1.18	2.70	3.19	1.90	2.24
2	58.1	1.24	2.62	3.26	1.87	2.33
3	62.9	1.28	2.55	3.27	1.85	2.37
4	68.3	1.33	2.49	3.32	1.85	2.46
5	78.1	1.42	2.22	3.14	1.70	2.41
Slope (10^{-3} mmHg/beat/min)			−0.0174	−0.0012	−0.0067	0.007
Intercept (×10^{-3} mmHg)			3.63	3.31	2.26	1.92
		r^2	0.95	0.03	0.83	0.71

Pulse pressure amplification calculated from the data of Wilkinson et al. [50] using linear regression between heart rate and ratio of peripheral/central pulse pressure. Distensibility using peripheral pressure determined by Whelton et al. [49] using brachial pulse pressure. Distensibility using central pressure uses central pressure estimated with pulse pressure amplification values related to heart rate

with arterial stiffness, even after correction for conventional predictors of arterial stiffness, including brachial systolic, diastolic, and pulse pressure. Arterial stiffness was quantified as distensibility and determined from ultrasound measurements of carotid diameter and MRI measurements of aortic diameter coupled with the pulse pressure in the brachial artery obtained by cuff sphygmomanometry. Central aortic pressures were not used in this study. Distensibility was related to heart rate, which spanned an average range of 50.9–78.1 beats/min between the first and last quintile, respectively (Table 22.1). As so calculated, distensibility showed a marked reduction with heart rate for the carotid artery and less so for the aorta. However, with a change in heart rate, the pulse pressure associated with the measured change in vessel caliber cannot be accurately measured from a peripheral and distal location such as the brachial artery due to the amplification of the pressure pulse between the central and peripheral sites. Furthermore, the difference between central and peripheral pulse pressure increases with heart rate [44, 50].

Using the amplification values reported by Wilkinson et al. [50], which were derived in paced patients, for the range of heart rates in the study by Whelton et al. [49], the average amplification is calculated to increase from 18 % at 50.9 beats/min to 42 % at 78.1 beats/min. Due to pulse amplification, for a given peripheral pulse pressure, the central pulse pressure would decrease with increasing heart rate. Hence, the values of distensibility calculated by Whelton et al. [49] would be increased by the amplification factor for the corresponding heart rate [51]. These values are compared in Table 22.1, showing the calculated carotid and aortic distensibility when corrected for the heart rate dependent pulse amplification. These values are used to determine a linear regression association between heart rate and the carotid and aortic distensibility (Table 22.1). These data demonstrate the significant confounding effect that pulse pressure amplification can produce. When carotid or aortic distensibility is determined from measurements of vessel caliber and peripheral (brachial) pulse pressure, distensibility is inversely related to resting heart rate. However, when distensibility is computed using the central aortic pulse pressure, determined by the specific amplification factors associated with the particular heart rate, the association virtually disappears for the carotid artery and indeed reverses for the aorta.

In the estimation of the corrected values for distensibility shown in Table 22.1, a single value of amplification was used for both carotid artery and aorta. However, this is not unreasonable as both measurement sites are centrally located and close to the heart. In addition, the large cohort in the study of Whelton et al. [49] results in a similar mean age for all heart rate quintiles (mean range 61.8–62.9 years). This is also similar to the mean age of 63 years of the cohort of Wilkinson et al. [50] from which the heart rate dependent pulse wave amplification was determined (Table 22.1). So if peripheral pulse pressure is used as a surrogate for central aortic pressure, the best case is when there is very little or no pulse amplification, a condition that is present for very low heart rates or possibly very old age, in which case the distensibility values using brachial pulse pressure would be valid. In all other cases, even though the vessel caliber measurements using ultrasound or MRI might be accurate, the heart rate effect is overestimated when using brachial pulse pressure and could be significantly different when distensibility is computed using central aortic pulse pressure.

Heart Rate, Arterial Hemodynamics and Cardiovascular Risk

The relationship between heart rate and disease is reciprocal. The physician measures and records heart rate because it may be an indicator of disease – emotional stress, fever, thyroid over or under activity or arrhythmia, for example. In humans, heart rate is generally around 10 % higher in females who are generally 10 % shorter than males. Tall males have a greater life expectancy than shorter males. However, females with faster heart rates outlive males, indicating interaction with other factors. Additionally, change in heart rate can cause disease. Rapid pacing of the heart over a period of days is a method for inducing cardiac failure in experimental models. Tachycardia from any cause can induce dilated cardiomyopathy in humans.

In the animal kingdom, especially among mammals, there is an inverse relationship between heart rate and life expectancy [52]. In human subjects, the epidemiological association between heart rate and cardiovascular mortality was first reported in 1980 in the Chicago People Gas Company Study [53]. The study reported an association between levels of heart rate and coronary heart disease mortality and overall cardiovascular mortality. This was followed by data from a later Framingham longitudinal study showing that an association between heart rate and sudden death existed for both males and females, though it was less marked among females [54].

Other studies such as the Paris Prospective Study [55] and the CORDIS Study [56] from Israel confirmed the relationship between resting heart rate and cardiovascular disease mortality even after adjustment for several other risk factors and other confounding factors. In the CORDIS Study [56], the risk for cardiovascular death was more than doubled in subjects with heart rate greater than 90 beats/min as compared to subjects with heart rate less than 90 beats/min.

A study of over 2,500 subjects (1,407 men and 1,134 women) without major cardiovascular disease at the time of initial examination (65–70 years of age) and followed up at 85 years of age provided evidence that heart rate had a strong predictive value for survival in men [57]. After adjustment for major risk factors (age, systolic blood pressure, smoking, physical activity), men with a heart rate greater than 80 beats/min had a more than 40 % reduction in the probability of reaching 85 years of age compared to men of the same age with a low heart rate (less than 60 beats/min). However, the results of this study [57], along with those from the Framingham Study for subjects over 55 years of age [58], indicated that heart rate was not associated with mortality and longevity in females. A study of 19,386 younger men and women (40–69 years of age) showed that heart rate was a predictor of non-cardiovascular mortality in both men and women, but a predictor of cardiovascular mortality only in men [59]. Interestingly, in men with a brachial pulse pressure greater than 65 mmHg, a high heart rate was not associated with increased cardiovascular mortality. This may be related to the effect of heart rate on aortic pulse pressure relative to brachial aortic pressure, such that for a given brachial pulse pressure, central aortic pulse pressure is lower for higher heart rates [39, 44].

Theoretically, differences between men and women could at least in part be due to the relatively smaller number of cardiovascular disease deaths in the female population, resulting in a lack of statistical power in the studies. However, other risk factors such as blood pressure have similar predictive values for cardiovascular disease and coronary heart disease mortality in both men and women. Similar results were found in a much larger population of more than 96,000 women and 125,000 men [60]. In this cohort, cardiovascular mortality was strongly associated with heart rate and pulse pressure in men. In women, only mean arterial pressure was associated with cardiovascular mortality. Thus, gender differences do not seem to be the exclusive consequence of low death rates in women.

The association of heart rate with cardiovascular disease mortality in men was mainly due to a strong association with coronary heart disease mortality and less with cerebrovascular mortality [59]. The Framingham Study also reported that the relationship between heart rate and cerebrovascular mortality was less significant [58]. The role of heart rate on cardiovascular mortality persisted even after excluding deaths during the first 2 years of the follow-up, thereby eliminating the hypothesis that heart rate was just an indicator of a severe disease [58, 59].

The relationship between heart rate and cardiovascular risk in men has been demonstrated to be linear [59]. After adjustment for age, systolic blood pressure, total cholesterol, smoking, diabetes mellitus, body mass index and physical activity, the increase in risk corresponding to an incremental rise in heart rate of 20 beats/min was 40 % [59]. This is approximately equivalent to the risk of an elevation in systolic blood pressure of 15–20 mmHg.

To date the roles of heart rate and gender-related differences have not been entirely elucidated. Women present a higher heart rate than men, on average between 3 and 7 beats/min greater [61]. Although the mechanisms for this difference are not clearly understood, it is generally believed that they are primarily related to women's average smaller height. Studies in diversified populations [62] have shown a negative relationship between height and heart rate in both genders. Despite these results however, the possibility that other mechanisms regulate heart rate differently in men and in women cannot be excluded.

Cardiac Synchrony and Arterial Hemodynamics

Electromechanical dyssynchrony of the heart chambers, a condition associated with heart failure, results in wasted workload, with internal blood flow ("sloshing") within the ventricle [63]. The dyssynchronous motion of the ventricle walls results in exaggerated sideways movement, and increased work for the same, or reduced, cardiac output. Cardiac dyssynchrony is treated by cardiac resynchronization therapy (CRT) [64, 65], the pacing of two or more heart chambers with a set delay between chamber pacing. The efficacy of CRT is determined by optimizing the appropriate synchrony of the cardiac chambers to maximize cardiac output. Setting of optimum atrio-ventricular (AV) and inter-ventricular (VV) conduction times is often done using echocardiography to maximize atrial inflow [66] and so maximizing cardiac output, or using peripheral pulse measures to maximize arterial pulse pressure [67–69]. However, even with attempts at optimizing timing parameters, not all subjects obtain benefits in terms of increased ejection fraction and improved ventricular function from the different optimal delay strategies [70].

In addition to the optimum time delays for atrial and ventricular filling and contraction to achieve maximal cardiac output, cardiac ejection is also influenced by the arterial load from both the pulmonary and systemic vasculature. The arterial load is determined by the steady component comprising peripheral resistance, and a pulsatile component related to the elastic properties of the large conduit arteries. Hence, with a given set of AV and VV delay times optimized for particular values of load parameters, CRT performance would be altered by changes in either peripheral resistance, arterial compliance, or both.

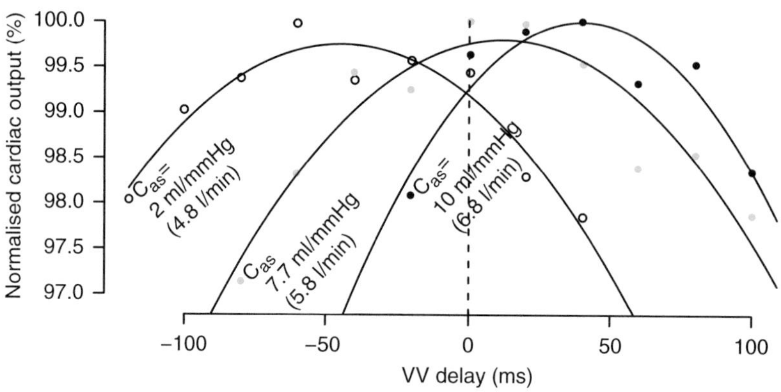

Fig. 22.2 Increase in arterial stiffness (reduction of aortic compliance, C_{as}) casues a left shift in interventricular (VV) delay (shorter delay) of maximal (optimal) cardiac output. Results from a simulation using a lumped parameter cardioavascular model of the cardiac chambers, septum and pulmonary and systemic circulation [71]. For each value of aortic compliance the cardiac output is normalized by the value in *brackets*

To investigate the relationship of changes in arterial load parameters with AV and VV delays to achieve maximal CRT performance, closed-loop computational models of the pulmonary and systemic circulation have been constructed using lumped parameter representation of the arterial load and variable elastance for the cardiac chambers and interventricular septum with incorporation of the Frank-Starling mechanism [70, 71]. Increased arterial stiffness (simulated by reduction in aortic compliance) resulted in a reduction in the VV delay for maximal cardiac output (Fig. 22.2). That is, a decrease in aortic compliance is associated with a relatively earlier activation of the left ventricle compared to right ventricular activation (a negative VV delay indicates that the right ventricle contracts after the left ventricle). This implies that for an arterial system with stiff arteries, the optimum performance of the CRT would not be obtained by the theoretical zero delay between the contraction of the left and right ventricle, but rather with an additional delay of contraction of the right ventricle in relation to the time for contraction of the left ventricle.

The models [70, 71] can be used to assess the sensitivity for maximizing either cardiac output or systolic pressure as functions of large artery stiffness or total peripheral resistance for both VV and AV delays. Simulation results show that vascular effects on AV delay are much less pronounced than that on VV delay for optimal cardiovascular function [71]. Hence, non-invasive measurements of arterial stiffness parameters (aortic pulse wave velocity) can be incorporated in patient specific simulations for synchronisation of chamber contraction by appropriate AV and VV delays so as to maximise pulse pressure or cardiac output.

Conclusions

Although changes in heart rate are inherent in cardiovascular adaptive mechanisms, there is an emerging acceptance of heart rate being associated with cardiovascular risk, high blood pressure, and all-cause morbidity and mortality. The determinants of arterial pressure are related to the interaction of the pulsating ventricle at a given frequency and the elastic and geometric properties of arteries determining arterial stiffness. Hence, a case could be made for heart rate to be considered as an integral parameter when performing the basic measurements of blood pressure and pulse wave velocity. In addition, heart rate is relevant when blood pressure is measured in a peripheral location (as is conventionally measured in the brachial artery) and making conclusion on effects of pressure on the heart since the relation between central aortic and peripheral pulse pressure depends on both the pressure pulse waveform characteristics and heart rate. It follows, therefore, that heart rate should also be taken into account when considering cardiac effects of pharmacological anti-hypertensive agents and in statistical treatment of cardiovascular risk factors in large scale epidemiological studies.

There is also potential for the use of heart rate in other clinical interventional procedures, such as correction of irregular heart rate due to asynchrony of the contracting cardiac chambers through cardiac pacing and CRT. By use of cardiovascular models of the heart and pulmonary and systemic circulation systems, it has been shown that arterial stiffness can have a significant effect in modifying AV and VV delays for optimal CRT performance in maximizing cardiac output.

Acknowledgment The authors acknowledge Professor Athanase Benetos for the contribution of background material on the relevance of heart rate as reported in previous collaborative work [72] and the modeling work conducted by Mr. Xu Ke informing some of the details included in the cardiac synchrony and hemodynamics section [71].

References

1. Westerhof N, Elzinga G. Normalized input impedance and arterial decay time over heart period are independent of animal size. Am J Physiol. 1991;261:R126–33.
2. Westerhof N, Elzinga G. Why smaller animals have higher heart rates. Adv Exp Med Biol. 1993;346:319–23.
3. Milnor WR. Haemodynamics. 2nd ed. Baltimore: Williams and Wilkinson; 1989.
4. Nichols WW, O'Rourke MF, Vlachopoulos C. McDonald's blood flow in arteries. Theoretical, experimental and clinical principles, 6th ed. New York: Oxford University Press; 2011.
5. Chemla D, Hebert JL, Coirault C, et al. Total arterial compliance estimated by stroke volume-to-aortic pulse pressure ratio in humans. Am J Physiol. 1998;274:H500–5.
6. Avolio AP, O'Rourke MF, Mang K, et al. A comparative study of pulsatile arterial hemodynamics in rabbits and guinea pigs. Am J Physiol. 1976;230:868–75.
7. Milnor WR. Aortic wavelength as a determinant of the relation between heart rate and body size in mammals. Am J Physiol. 1979;237:R3–6.
8. Iberal AS. Some comparative scale factors for mammals: comments on Milnor's paper concerning a feature of cardiovascular design. Am J Physiol. 1979;237:R7–9.
9. O'Rourke MF. Aortic wavelength as a determinant of the relationship between heart rate and body size in mammals. Am J Physiol. 1981;240:R393–5.
10. Taylor MG. The elastic properties of arteries in relation to the physiological functions of the arterial system. Gastroenterology. 1967;52:358–63.
11. Elzinga G, Westerhof N. Matching between ventricle and arterial load. An evolutionary process. Circ Res. 1991;68:1495–500.
12. Yin FC. Ventricular/vascular coupling: clinical, physiological and engineering aspects. London: Springer; 1987.
13. Suga H, Sagawa K. Instantaneous pressure-volume relationships and their ratio in the excised, supported canine left ventricle. Circ Res. 1974;35:117–26.
14. Sunagawa K, Sagawa K, Maughan WL. Ventricular interaction with the loading system. Ann Biomed Eng. 1984;12:163–89.
15. Weissler AM, Peeler RG, Roehll Jr WH. Relationships between left ventricular ejection time, stroke volume, and heart rate in normal individuals and patients with cardiovascular disease. Am Heart J. 1961;62:367–78.
16. O'Rourke MF. Arterial function in health and disease. Edinburgh: Churchill Livingstone; 1982.
17. Albaladejo P, Copie X, Boutouyrie P, et al. Heart rate, arterial stiffness, and wave reflections in paced patients. Hypertension. 2001;38:949–52.
18. Gosling RG, Budge MM. Terminology for describing the elastic behavior of arteries. Hypertension. 2003;41:1180–2.
19. O'Rourke MF, Staessen JA, Vlachopoulos C, et al. Clinical applications of arterial stiffness; definitions and reference values. Am J Hypertens. 2002;15:426–44.
20. Bramwell JC, Hill AV. Velocity of transmission of the pulse wave and elasticity of arteries. Lancet. 1922;1:891–2.
21. Armentano RL, Barra JG, Levenson J, et al. Arterial wall mechanics in conscious dogs: assessment of viscous, inertial, and elastic moduli to characterize aortic wall behavior. Circ Res. 1995;76:468–78.
22. Dobrin PB, Rovick AA. Influence of vascular smooth muscle on contractile mechanics and elasticity of arteries. Am J Physiol. 1969;217:1644–51.
23. Bergel DH. Viscoelastic properties of the arterial wall. London: University of London; 1960.
24. Bergel DH. The static elastic properties of the arterial wall. J Physiol. 1961;156:445–69.
25. Armentano RL, Barra JG, Santana DB, et al. Smart damping modulation of carotid wall energetics in human hypertension: effects of angiotensin-converting enzyme inhibition. Hypertension. 2006;47:384–90.
26. Callaghan FJ, Babbs CF, Bourland JD, Geddes LA. The relationship between arterial pulse-wave velocity and pulse frequency at different pressures. J Med Eng Technol. 1984;8:15–8.
27. Lantelme P, Mestre C, Lievre M, et al. Heart rate: an important confounder of pulse wave velocity assessment. Hypertension. 2002;39:1083–7.
28. Mangoni AA, Mircoli L, Giannattasio C, et al. Heart rate-dependence of arterial distensibility in vivo. J Hypertens. 1996;14:897–901.

29. Liang YL, Gatzka CD, Du XJ, et al. Effects of heart rate on arterial compliance in men. Clin Exp Pharmacol Physiol. 1999;26:342–6.
30. Albaladejo P, Challande P, Kakou A, et al. Selective reduction of heart rate by ivabradine: effect on the visco-elastic arterial properties in rats. J Hypertens. 2004;22:1739–45.
31. Tan I, Butlin M, Liu YY, et al. Heart rate dependence of aortic pulse wave velocity at different arterial pressures in rats. Hypertension. 2012;60:528–33.
32. Avolio AP, Butlin M, Liu Y-Y, et al. Regulation of arterial stiffness: cellular, molecular and neurogenic mechanisms. Artery Res. 2011;5:122–7.
33. Mangoni AA, Mircoli L, Giannattasio C, et al. Effect of sympathectomy on mechanical properties of common carotid and femoral arteries. Hypertension. 1997; 30:1085–8.
34. Haesler E, Lyon X, Pruvot E, et al. Confounding effects of heart rate on pulse wave velocity in paced patients with a low degree of atherosclerosis. J Hypertens. 2004;22:1317–22.
35. Millasseau SC, Stewart AD, Patel SJ, et al. Evaluation of carotid-femoral pulse wave velocity: influence of timing algorithm and heart rate. Hypertension. 2005;45: 222–6.
36. Albaladejo P, Laurent P, Pannier B, et al. Influence of sex on the relation between heart rate and aortic stiffness. J Hypertens. 2003;21:555–62.
37. Sa Cunha R, Pannier B, Benetos A, et al. Association between high heart rate and high arterial rigidity in normotensive and hypertensive subjects. J Hypertens. 1997;15:1423–30.
38. Avolio AP, Jones D, Tafazzoli-Shadpour M. Quantification of alterations in structure and function of elastin in the arterial media. Hypertension. 1998;32: 170–5.
39. Karamanoglu M, O'Rourke MF, Avolio AP, Kelly RP. An analysis of the relationship between central aortic and peripheral upper limb pressure waves in man. Eur Heart J. 1993;14:160–7.
40. Chen CH, Nevo E, Fetics B, et al. Estimation of central aortic pressure waveform by mathematical transformation of radial tonometry pressure. Validation of generalized transfer function. Circulation. 1997;95: 1827–36.
41. Wilkinson IB, Mohammad NH, Tyrrell S, et al. Heart rate dependency of pulse pressure amplification and arterial stiffness. Am J Hypertens. 2002;15:24–30.
42. Avolio AP, Van Bortel LM, Boutouyrie P, et al. Role of pulse pressure amplification in arterial hypertension: experts' opinion and review of the data. Hypertension. 2009;54:375–83.
43. O'Rourke MF, Blazek JV, Morreels Jr CL, Krovetz LJ. Pressure wave transmission along the human aorta. Changes with age and in arterial degenerative disease. Circ Res. 1968;23:567–79.
44. Rowell LB, Brengelmann GL, Blackmon JR, et al. Disparities between aortic and peripheral pulse pressures induced by upright exercise and vasomotor changes in man. Circulation. 1968;37:954–64.
45. Dahlof B, Devereux RB, Kjeldsen SE, et al. Cardiovascular morbidity and mortality in the Losartan Intervention For Endpoint reduction in hypertension study (LIFE): a randomised trial against atenolol. Lancet. 2002;359:995–1003.
46. Devereux RB, Palmieri V, Liu JE, et al. Progressive hypertrophy regression with sustained pressure reduction in hypertension: the Losartan Intervention For Endpoint reduction study. J Hypertens. 2002;20:1445–50.
47. De Luca N, Asmar RG, London GM, et al. Selective reduction of cardiac mass and central blood pressure on low-dose combination perindopril/indapamide in hypertensive subjects. J Hypertens. 2004;22:1623–30.
48. Williams B, Lacy PS, Thom SM, et al. Differential impact of blood pressure-lowering drugs on central aortic pressure and clinical outcomes: principal results of the Conduit Artery Function Evaluation (CAFE) study. Circulation. 2006;113:1213–25.
49. Whelton SP, Blankstein R, Al-Mallah MH, et al. Association of resting heart rate with carotid and aortic arterial stiffness: multi-ethnic study of atherosclerosis. Hypertension. 2013;62(3):477–84.
50. Wilkinson IB, MacCallum H, Flint L, et al. The influence of heart rate on augmentation index and central arterial pressure in humans. J Physiol. 2000;525:263–70.
51. Avolio A, Butlin M, Tan I. Importance of pressure pulse amplification in the association of resting heart rate and arterial stiffness. Hypertension. 2013;62:e46.
52. Levine HJ. Rest heart rate and life expectancy. J Am Coll Cardiol. 1997;30:1104–6.
53. Dyer AR, Persky V, Stamler J, et al. Heart rate as a prognostic factor for coronary heart disease and mortality: findings in three Chicago epidemiologic studies. Am J Epidemiol. 1980;112:736–49.
54. Kannel WB, Kannel C, Paffenbarger RS, Cupples LA. Heart rate and cardiovascular mortality: the Framingham Study. Am Heart J. 1987;113:1489–94.
55. Jouven X, Desnos M, Guerot C, Ducimetiere P. Predicting sudden death in the population: the Paris Prospective Study I. Circulation. 1999;99:1978–83.
56. Kristal-Boneh E, Silber H, Harari G, Froom P. The association of resting heart rate with cardiovascular, cancer and all-cause mortality. Eight year follow-up of 3527 male Israeli employees (the CORDIS Study). Eur Heart J. 2000;21:116–24.
57. Benetos A, Thomas F, Bean K, et al. Resting heart rate in older people: a predictor of survival to age 85. J Am Geriatr Soc. 2003;51:284–5.
58. Goldberg RJ, Larson M, Levy D. Factors associated with survival to 75 years of age in middle-aged men and women. The Framingham Study. Arch Intern Med. 1996;156:505–9.
59. Benetos A, Rudnichi A, Thomas F, et al. Influence of heart rate on mortality in a French population: role of age, gender, and blood pressure. Hypertension. 1999;33:44–52.
60. Thomas F, Bean K, Provost JC, et al. Combined effects of heart rate and pulse pressure on cardiovascular mortality according to age. J Hypertens. 2001;19: 863–9.

61. Palatini P, Julius S. Heart rate and the cardiovascular risk. J Hypertens. 1997;15:3–17.
62. Morcet JF, Safar M, Thomas F, et al. Associations between heart rate and other risk factors in a large French population. J Hypertens. 1999;17:1671–6.
63. Fornwalt BK, Gonzales PC, Delfino JG, et al. Quantification of left ventricular internal flow from cardiac magnetic resonance images in patients with dyssynchronous heart failure. J Magn Reson Imaging. 2008;28:375–81.
64. Kirk JA, Kass DA. Electromechanical dyssynchrony and resynchronization of the failing heart. Circ Res. 2013;113:765–76.
65. Abraham WT, Hayes DL. Cardiac resynchronization therapy for heart failure. Circulation. 2003;108: 2596–603.
66. Gorcsan J, Abraham T, Agler DA, et al. Echocardiography for cardiac resynchronization therapy: recommendations for performance and reporting – a report from the American Society of Echocardiography Dyssynchrony Writing Group endorsed by the Heart Rhythm Society. J Am Soc Echocardiogr. 2008;21: 191–213.
67. Whinnett ZI, Davies JER, Willson K, et al. Haemodynamic effects of changes in atrioventricular and interventricular delay in cardiac resynchronisation therapy show a consistent pattern: analysis of shape, magnitude and relative importance of atrioventricular and interventricular delay. Heart. 2006;92:1628–34.
68. Whinnett ZI, Davies JER, Willson K, et al. Determination of optimal atrioventricular delay for cardiac resynchronization therapy using acute non-invasive blood pressure. Europace. 2006;8:358–66.
69. Butter C, Stellbrink C, Belalcazar A, et al. Cardiac resynchronization therapy optimization by finger plethysmography. Heart Rhythm. 2004;1:568–75.
70. Di Molfetta A, Santini L, Forleo GB, et al. Use of a comprehensive numerical model to improve biventricular pacemaker temporization in patients affected by heart failure undergoing to CRT-D therapy. Med Biol Eng Comput. 2010;48:755–64.
71. Xu K, Butlin M, Avolio AP. Assessment of hemodynamic load components affecting optimization of cardiac resynchronization therapy by lumped parameter model. Conf Proc IEEE Eng Med Biol Soc. 2012;2012:6661–4.
72. Avolio AP, Benetos A. Heart rate, pulse pressure and arterial stiffness. In: O'Rourke MF, Safar ME, editors. Handbook of hypertension. Oxford: Elsevier; 2006. p. 279–94.

23 Pulse Pressure Amplification and Arterial Stiffness in Middle Age

Alberto P. Avolio, Mark Butlin, and Athanase D. Protogerou

Abstract

The aging changes in arterial blood pressure that are observed from conventional blood pressure measurement using the brachial cuff sphygmomanometer are not similar to the changes that occur in central aortic pressure, specifically for systolic and pulse pressure. This is due to the phenomenon of pulse pressure amplification that is largely related to aging changes in arterial stiffness. The most pronounced effect of pulse pressure amplification occurs in the middle age range. This chapter assesses the underlying concept and perception of what is considered "middle age" and describes the associated age-related changes in arterial stiffness and pulse pressure and evaluates how the changes observed in middle age (in this context defined between 40 and 60 years) can inform the understanding of cardiovascular risk and treatment and management of hypertension in the aging population.

Keywords

Pulse pressure • Cardiovascular risk • Vascular aging • Pulse velocity

A.P. Avolio, PhD, BE (✉) • M. Butlin, PhD, BE
The Australian School of Advanced Medicine,
2 Technology Place, Macquarie University,
North Ryde 2109, Sydney, NSW, Australia
e-mail: alberto.avolio@mq.edu.au;
mark.butlin@mq.edu.au

A.D. Protogerou, MD, PhD
Cardiovascular Research Laboratory and
Hypertension Center, First Department of
Propedeutic and Internal Medicine,
"Laiko" Hospital, Medical School,
National and Kapodistrian University of Athens,
17 Ag. Thoma str, Athens 117 25, Greece
e-mail: aprotog@med.uoa.gr

Middle age begins when youth fades, hopes, ambitions and delights wane, and the shadows of decay and death are first perceived. Dr John Hunt, President of the Royal College of General Practitioners, *Lancet*, 1967

Introduction

Salient features of age-related changes in arterial pressure are the gradual increase in systolic and diastolic pressure during childhood and adolescence, the relatively smaller rate of increase in systolic pressure during the middle age range

M.E. Safar et al. (eds.), *Blood Pressure and Arterial Wall Mechanics in Cardiovascular Diseases*,
DOI 10.1007/978-1-4471-5198-2_23, © Springer-Verlag London 2014

with relatively stable diastolic pressure, and an accelerated increase in systolic pressure in the elderly, associated with a decrease in diastolic pressure [1, 2]. This is the general age-related profile obtained from brachial cuff sphygmomanometer measurements of arterial blood pressure, suggesting a marked increase in pulse pressure in the young, a slight decrease in pulse pressure during early adulthood due to different rates of systolic and diastolic pressure increase [1], a reduced increase in pulse pressure in the middle age range and a larger increase in the elderly (Fig. 23.1). The importance of pulse pressure in the evolution of cardiovascular disease is highlighted in the extensive analysis of the Framingham data showing that pulse pressure is a more significant predictor of cardiovascular events (e.g. coronary artery disease) after the fifth decade of life, being superior to both systolic and diastolic pressure alone [2].

The determinants of pulse pressure are related to cardiac ejection (stroke volume), stiffness of large conduit arteries, mainly the ascending aorta and the aortic trunk, and peripheral wave reflection. Due to the physiological structure of the arterial vasculature, the central aortic pressure pulse generated in the ascending aorta due to cardiac ejection undergoes change in wave shape such that the pulse pressure becomes amplified as it propagates towards the periphery [4, 5]. The amplification is also age dependent due to the different rate of age-related changes in elastic and geometric properties of central and peripheral conduit arteries [1]. Hence, the age-related changes in pulse pressure as measured by the brachial cuff sphygmomanometer do not represent the changes present in the pulse pressure at the central aorta, the pulse pressure constituting the pulsatile load on the ejecting ventricle. That is, the relatively slow increase in pulse pressure in the middle age range as conventionally measured in the brachial artery is associated with a more pronounced increase in central aortic pulse pressure with age (Fig. 23.1).

This chapter addresses the amplification of the arterial pressure pulse between the central aorta and brachial artery observed in the middle age range, the age range where conventional measurements of blood pressure show the lowest rate of age-related increase in pulse pressure. The amplification will be related to concomitant changes in arterial stiffness in the aortic trunk as assessed by pulse wave velocity (PWV). This chapter will also provide an assessment of whether measurement of pulse pressure amplification and PWV in middle age can offer additional prognostic information in stratifying cardiovascular risk for development of systolic hypertension in the elderly. In addition, the question is posed whether arterial pressure and stiffness related parameters in youth can be useful in assessing the age related changes in middle age.

Aging and the Concept and Perception of Middle Age

The manner in which middle age is perceived in the community varies with both gender and age. Women perceive middle age onset to be older than that perceived by men, and younger people perceive middle age onset to be younger than that perceived by older people [6]. Everyone, on average, perceives the onset of middle age for men to be younger than the onset of middle age for women [6].

Statistically, we enter the middle third of our life in the mid to late 20s, and finish that third of life in the early to mid 50s. This varies between males and females, between regions and with economic status, depending on life expectancy. This variation aside, the statistical middle age or middle third of life is between 25 and 55 years of age. The perceptions of middle age are generally higher than the statistical measurements. In a 1976 study, the average perceived onset of middle age was around 37 years of age, and the onset of old age perceived to be around 62 years of age [6].

This perception of middle age would most likely influence design and analysis of studies concerning middle age. In a survey of publications listed on PubMed under the search terms "middle age" and "blood pressure", or "midlife" and "blood pressure" in the article title, the upper and lower limits of the "middle age" or "midlife"

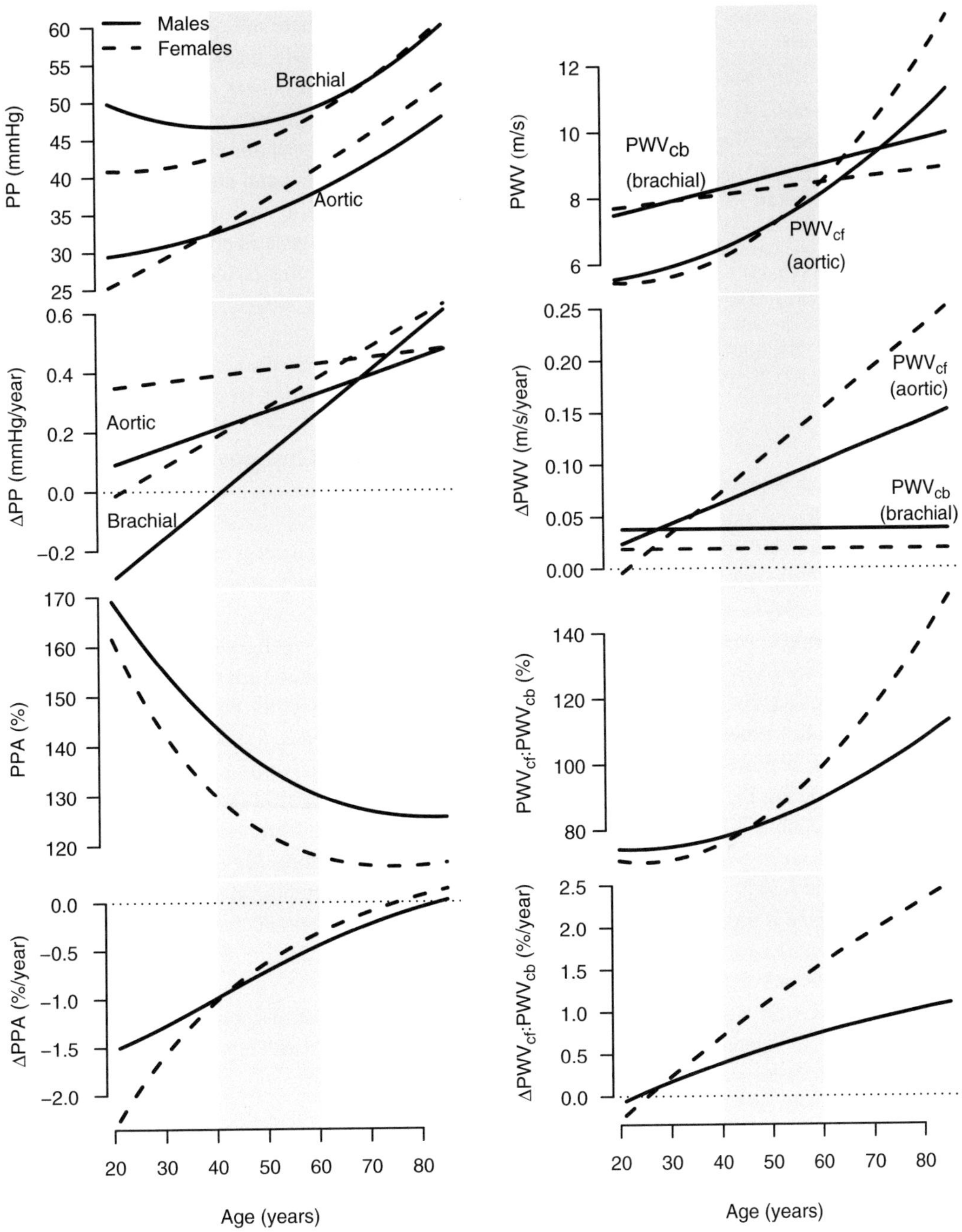

Fig. 23.1 Brachial and aortic pulse pressure, carotid-femoral pulse wave velocity (PWV_{cf}, aortic) and carotid-brachial pulse wave velocity (PWV_{cb}, brachial) changes with age. The ratio of brachial to aortic pulse pressure (pulse pressure amplification, *PPA*) and aortic to brachial PWV (PWV_{cf}:PWV_{cb}) have been calculated. The relationship of pulse pressure and PWV with age is plotted from reported values in the study by McEniery et al. [1] with intercepts for PWV_{cb} calculated using data from Yasmin et al. [3]. The *shaded area* indicates the nominal middle age range (40–60 years)

Table 23.1 Upper and lower limits of "middle age" from blood pressure studies

	Mean	Minimum	Maximum
Lower age limit (years)	41±6	30	47
Upper age limit (years)	57±8	45	68

Studies taken from PubMed under the search terms "middle age" and "blood pressure" or "midlife" and "blood pressure" in the article title (n=33). Studies were omitted if they merged more than one stage of life (e.g. early and midlife), were a sub-section of middle age (e.g. late midlife), were repeated studies from a same population study in another article already included in the analysis, or were comment articles. Data were then included if the paper listed both an upper and lower limit of the recruitment sample (n=12 articles). Publication dates ranged from 1993 to 2012

range was 41±6–7±8 years (Table 23.1). Both the upper and lower limits in studies are markedly higher than that defined by a statistical definition of the middle third of life. The age range also varied greatly between studies, with the lower limit varying between 30 and 47 years, and the upper limit 45–68 years. (It is also plausible that the perception and limits of middle age within a study are influenced by the age of the study's author!). It raises the question: what are the factors that determine the definition of middle age, if it is not upon a strict statistical analysis of life expectancy?

It may be that middle age, as perceived in the general population, is used to describe the stage in life where, generally, life factors have reached a steady state. The second and third decades are often associated with large life changes such as changes in jobs, living circumstances, and having children. The sixth decade onward might be associated with an increasing occurrence of health complications. Indeed, middle age is quite often described in emotive terms as evocatively expressed by Dr John Hunt, president of the Royal College of General Practitioners in 1967: "*Middle age begins when youth fades, hopes, ambitions and delights wane, and the shadows of decay and death are first perceived*" [7]. This 1967 annotation defines middle age as between 40 and 60 years, similar to the range cited in cardiovascular studies of today (Table 23.1), despite increases in life expectancy. In terms of the principle components of the cardiovascular system, the heart and blood vessels, there are ongoing changes during these decades of life, including marked changes in the rate at which indices of arterial stiffness and pulse pressure increase.

The remainder of this chapter reviews changes in arterial stiffness and pulse pressure amplification in middle age, defining middle age as it is perceived in the general population and in cardiovascular studies, that is, the fifth and sixth decade of life (the years between 40 and 60).

Arterial Stiffness in Middle Age

Age Related Changes in Arterial Stiffness

Large arteries generally become stiffer with age, as observed from measures of segmental aortic [8] and carotid-femoral pulse wave velocity [1]. However, these changes are not uniform. The stiffness of peripheral arteries shows a progressive increase with age, but the large arteries show a more rapid increase in stiffness with age [1, 9, 10] (Fig. 23.1). Even within the aorta itself, there are regional differences in the rate of stiffening, with some studies showing more rapid stiffening in the abdominal aorta [8, 11] and others showing predominant stiffening in the proximal aortic arch [12, 13]. The proximal, ascending aorta is exposed to much greater dilation with each heart beat than any other part of the aorta, or any other systemic artery, and is most susceptible to changes in diameter and stiffness with aging [4].

Basic Mechanisms of Arterial Stiffening

Loss of distensibility of conduit arteries is due to changes in mechanical properties of the material of the arterial wall causing alterations in stress/strain characteristics due to modification of properties of load-bearing structural components [14]. The underlying mechanisms responsible for such modifications involve complex interaction between the material properties of connective tissue and cell signaling pathways that alter the intrinsic and combined function of elastin, collagen, proteoglycans and glycoproteins of the extracellular matrix of the artery wall. A number of reviews address these issues [15–18] with the suggestion that the specific mechanisms can interact by way of positive or negative feedback pathways, depending on the extent of the stimulus [19].

Arterial Stiffness and Intra-arterial Distending Pressure

The arterial wall components that bear the wall tension due to the distending pressure interact to produce non-linear wall mechanical properties, such that the wall becomes stiffer with increased distension. That is, the stiffness becomes pressure dependent [20]. This is an important and intrinsic property of arterial design [21, 22] and prevents arterial rupture under high physiological pressures [14]. An increase in distending pressure leads to an increase in stiffness, which then can potentiate a further increase in pulse pressure. This property constitutes a potential positive feedback mechanism in relation to the relevance of arterial stiffness to cardiovascular risk, given the importance of systolic pressure, especially in age-related, isolated systolic hypertension [23, 24].

Thus, arterial stiffness is essentially a blood pressure dependent parameter. As mean arterial pressure increases, so does arterial stiffness. It is therefore expected that as mean pressure increases with age, so will arterial stiffness. Whilst the increase in mean pressure is a factor in the increase seen in large artery stiffness, multiple regression analysis confirms arterial stiffness changes associated with aging are additional to the effect of changes in mean arterial pressure [1, 4, 25].

Mechanical Fatigue and Fracture of Elastin Structures

Fundamental characteristics of elastic materials are found in all structural proteins in biological systems, with some rubber-like proteins (e.g. elastin, resilin) functioning with high resilience, large deformability (strains), and low stiffness, resulting in the ability to store elastic-strain energy [26]. In arteries, this is a characteristic of both elastin and collagen, although elastin is much more extensible at lower strains than collagen. However, just as the efficiency of resilin determines the performance of insect wings during their lifetime [27], the efficiency of elastin is also a significant determinant of the overall stiffness of the arterial wall throughout life. From evolutionary considerations, it is reasonable to assume that the range of properties of elastic proteins will predispose elastic structures that are subjected to repetitive strains to a high resistance to fracture.

Due to the pulsatile nature of circulatory design, arteries are subjected to continuous and repetitive strain throughout life. In human tissue, radiocarbon prevalence data show a range of half-life of 40–174 years (mean of 74 years) [28], making elastin the protein in the human body with the greatest longevity. Having such a stable form with minimal turnover, the question is whether it can be subjected to the mechanical degradation effects of fatigue due to repetitive and unceasing strain throughout life. Such concepts are advanced as a mechanism of arterial stiffening due to elastin degradation, given the 30 million cycles per year to which the arteries are exposed [15] and so passive physical elastin degradation occurs with age, as distinct from active chemical enzymatic processes (due to matrix metalloproteinase activity) [29]. Evidence of increased degree of disorganization and fracture of aortic elastin associated with the total number of cardiac cycles throughout life was found in a cross-sectional study of a range of species with a wide range of body size, heart rate and life span [30]. This is complemented by structural alterations due to embryonic abnormalities affecting the structure of elastin throughout life, with increased predisposition to elevated arterial stiffness and associated cardiovascular risk [31]. These observations have been recently confirmed in the aorta of mice with elastin haploinsufficiency, where increased aortic stiffness precedes elevation of blood pressure during postnatal development [32]. Other evidence of possible effects of fatigue on aortic elastin is obtained from the association of fragmentation and reduction of interlamellar fibers and the formation of aortic aneurysms, and their progression to dissection and/or rupture [33]. Recent investigations in the role of elastin in arterial stiffness of large arteries have suggested means of reversing alterations to elastic fibers as a therapeutic treatment for hypertension [22].

Factors Associated with Arterial Stiffness Changes in Middle Age

There is increasing interest in assessing cardiovascular changes in middle age with longitudinal studies. The Asklepios study is a longitudinal investigation designed to assess the progress of indices of arterial function in middle aged subjects in the age range 35–55 years [34]. In a cohort of 2,026 subjects (974 men), non-invasive measurements were obtained of carotid artery pressure, central aortic blood flow and carotid-femoral PWV from which were derived frequency spectra of aortic input impedance, characteristic impedance, reflection coefficient, reflection magnitude, and augmentation index [35]. Between the extremes of the age range, PWV increased by 15 % (6.1–7.0 m/s) both in men and women. Input impedance spectra suggested differential changes in men and women where, in women, an increase in input impedance in the low frequency range was associated with reduced aortic compliance, changes that were not observed in men. Characteristic impedance did not show any significant increase and was not found to be a major determinant of central aortic pulse pressure in the age range. Carotid augmentation index was higher in women than in men and showed a significant age-related increase. Reflection coefficient and reflection magnitude also increased with age in both genders. Findings of the initial analysis of the Asklepios cohort indicate that in healthy, middle-aged subjects of both genders, age-related increase in arterial stiffness as measured by PWV was not fully explained by changes in aortic impedance. This suggests changes in aortic dimensions, with possible age-related differential increase in wall thickness and cross-sectional area, or that characteristic impedance ought best be expressed in terms of velocity flow, rather than volume flow (i.e. in dynes/s/cm^{-3} rather than dyne/s/cm^{-5}). This is discussed in Chap. 1 of this book and the McDonald text [4].

In a study of middle age men (in this case 30–50 years), the major predictors of carotid-femoral PWV were found to be age, body mass index, and diastolic blood pressure [36]. Whilst the positive association between body mass index and PWV might be expected, other studies have shown a more varied response in investigating body fat percentage. Body fat percentage was shown to have a negative association with thoracic aortic PWV, as measured by magnetic resonance imaging, up until the age of 50 years in men and women [37]. This was reversed for individuals over 50 years, where body fat percentage was positively correlated to thoracic PWV. Mechanistically, this could be due to body fat unloading (compressing) the more distensible, younger aorta, but not the less distensible, older aorta.

Pulse Pressure in Middle Age

Age Related Changes in Pulse Pressure

During middle age, the rate of change of both brachial and aortic pulse pressure increases. In a normotensive early adult population, brachial pulse pressure has been shown to decrease due to greater rates of increase in diastolic pressure than systolic pressure [1]. Following a brief plateau around the third decade of life [2], brachial pulse pressure increases much more rapidly, driven by a continuing increase in systolic pressure, but also a decrease in diastolic pressure [2]. Widening of the brachial pulse pressure is larger in women than it is in men [1]. Aortic pulse pressure shows a similar trend. However, the increase in aortic pulse pressure is greater than the increase in brachial pulse pressure with age, and consistently increases with age including during early adulthood [1]. This pattern of a small but steady increase in aortic pulse pressure in the second and third decade of life, and a more rapid increase in the fourth decade onward, is mimicked in the stiffness of the aorta, as measured by carotid-femoral pulse wave velocity [1] (Fig. 23.1). Comparison of rate of change of pulse pressure associated with the rate of change in central aortic and brachial PWV elucidate the underlying structural mechanisms of the change in pulse amplification during middle age.

Whilst large studies investigate the population average, it is important to consider the environment and lifestyle of the individual on the changes in brachial pulse pressure with age. For example, regular exercise has been shown to decrease resting pulse pressure in individuals over 50 years of age, but has the opposite effect in increasing the resting pulse pressure of individuals under 30 years of age [38]. This again indicates the presence of fundamental changes to the heart and vasculature during middle age that impact on pulse pressure, such as interaction of changes in heart rate and stroke volume.

Determinants of Pulse Pressure

Pulse pressure at the aortic root results from the interaction of ventricular ejection and the vascular load. Under steady state, the vascular load can be expressed as the input impedance and described in the frequency domain. Early in the systolic ejection phase, blood flow and pressure are related by the characteristic impedance (Z_c) determined by the aortic geometry and wall stiffness. Z_c is proportional to the square root of the wall elastic modulus and inversely proportional to cross-sectional area (assuming constant ratio of wall thickness to diameter) [4]. That is, age-related changes in aortic root properties will affect age-related changes in aortic pulse pressure. However, Z_c is not proportional to cross-sectional area if expressed in terms of blood flow velocity (dyne·s·cm^{-3}), which is desirable in terms of scaling [4].

Due to the dispersive nature of wave propagation, the pressure pulse generated at the aortic root is also affected by wave reflection emanating from multiple sites of geometric and elastic mismatch, with the reflection magnitude and time of arrival affecting the amplitude of aortic pulse pressure. Since the ascending aorta constitutes a large part of the storage capacity, that is, the arterial compliance, the aortic pulse pressure is largely determined by the reservoir Windkessel function of the proximal aorta [39, 40]. Indeed, pulse pressure can be modified by a passive elastic wrap around the proximal aorta where the diameter is reduced thereby unloading the stiffened wall, and where the strain is taken up by a more elastic material [41].

Modifications of determinants of aortic pulse pressure in middle age occur in conditions associated with increased cardiovascular risk. Type 1 diabetes has been shown to be associated with an increase in aortic impedance [42]. In the specific middle age cohort of the Asklepios study [43], type 2 diabetes was associated with increased aortic root and carotid-femoral PWV, increased aortic Z_c, reduced total arterial compliance and reduced magnitude of wave reflection.

Pulse Pressure and Cardiac Factors in Middle Age

The increase in pulse pressure in the middle age range (Fig. 23.1) is determined by the age-related changes in cardiac and vascular factors. In general, the changes in cardiac factors (stroke volume, heart rate) predominantly affect the beat-to-beat changes in pulse pressure, whereas the modifications of arterial stiffness properties affect the overall values of pulse pressure in a steady state. However, sustained changes in cardiac parameters will also affect the steady state condition of pulse pressure. The differentiation of age-related contribution of cardiac parameters is important in assessment of cardiovascular function, since high pulse pressure in the young may be predominantly related to a hyperkinetic heart [44] while in the elderly it is largely due to reduced distensibility of the proximal aorta leading to increased incident pressure, augmented by the effects of early return of wave reflection [15].

Stroke Volume

The contribution of stroke volume to aortic pulse pressure is age-dependent. In a study of a cohort of untreated hypertensive males (age 17–76 years) [45], brachial pulse pressure showed lower values in the age range of 30–50 years compared to age <30 and 50–60 years. That is, it exhibited a curvilinear relationship with age with a minimum in the 30–50 year range. The reduced supine pulse pressure was associated with a reduced stroke index (stroke volume normalized for body surface area). There was a relatively larger decrease in stroke index for upright measurements. However, after age 50 years, pulse pressure increased despite a reduction in stroke index. The ratio of stroke volume to pulse pressure was used as an estimate of total arterial compliance, and 24-h pulse pressure was shown to have a positive association with stroke volume and negative association with arterial compliance before age 50. After age 50 there was no association with stroke volume. Although stroke volume was measured non-invasively using bioimpedance techniques, relative changes provide informative comparisons. This study shows that the transition of the fifth to sixth decade, that is, the midpoint of the middle age range as considered in this chapter (40–60 years), marks the transition point where stroke volume does not contribute to the rise in pulse pressure with age. More data are required to confirm the findings from this single study [45].

Heart Rate

Although there is an intrinsic variability in resting heart rate (HR), the average HR generally decreases with age. In a normotensive cohort [1], average resting HR was found to be 73 ± 12 beats/min in men and 76 ± 12 beats/min in women for the second decade. This decreased to 62 ± 10 beats/min and 66 ± 10 beats/min in the eighth decade. In the middle age range of the fifth and sixth decade, it was relatively constant (65 ± 11 beats/min in men; 68 ± 10 beats/min in women) [1]. However, changes during physical activity are highly variable and depend largely on a complex array of parameters that constitute the paradigm of "physical fitness". Hence, studies aimed at assessing the intrinsic effect of aging also assess the age-related differences in HR with exercise [46]. Age is associated with both a decrease in maximal HR during exercise as well as spontaneously recorded HR at night or during the day. Generally, the resting or average HR does not show an apparent age dependency. The average difference between maximum and minimum HR during exercise decreases from 40 to 30 beats/min up to age 40 years. However, after age 40 it remains constant [46]. This implies that the beginning of the middle age range of 40–60 years marks the transition where there is no age effect on the average difference of the extremes of HR at rest and during exercise and may be a reflection of reduced exercise capacity in older persons.

The implications of change in HR are twofold. First, the acute changes in cycle time mainly affect the diastolic portion of the cardiac cycle thus modulating diastolic pressure, and for a given stroke volume would result in increased systolic pressure as well as changes in aortic pulse pressure. Secondly, since pressure pulse amplification between the aorta and periphery is HR dependent [47], this would also result in changes in the measured pulse pressure using the conventional cuff sphygmomanometer.

Pulse Pressure Amplification in Middle Age

Pulse pressure amplification is a measure of the increase in the systolic to diastolic arterial pressure difference (pulse pressure) between two vascular sites. Most commonly, it is the ratio of the arterial pulse pressure at a site distal to the heart to the pulse pressure at a site proximal to the heart (Eq. 23.1).

$$\text{pulse pressure amplification} = \frac{\text{distal pulse pressure}}{\text{proximal pulse pressure}} \quad (23.1)$$

Pulse pressure amplification is also sometimes reported simply as the difference between the pulse pressure at the two sites, or the difference in pulse pressure at the two sites divided by the proximal site pulse pressure. The different methods of calculating pulse pressure amplification yield parameters that shows similar trends, however, whether a normalized (ratio) or absolute (difference) parameter of pulse pressure amplification has stronger clinical significance remains to be established [48]. Throughout this chapter, the more commonly used ratio of distal to proximal pulse pressure will be used.

It must be noted that the notion of "pulse amplification" is not similar to the concept of signal amplification, where the amplified signal contains additional energy (as in amplification of electrical signals by an additional energy source). The pressure wave undergoes a change in wave morphology during propagation towards the periphery, such that the wave undergoes a 'distortion' where the pulse amplitude is higher, and consequently the peaks become narrower with the same energy in the wave. In fact, the peripheral wave contains slightly less energy due to the effects of viscous damping. The 'distortion' is due to the frequency-dependent transfer function characteristics between the two sites [49, 50].

Pulse Pressure Amplification in the Upper Limb

Most commonly, pulse pressure amplification specifically refers to the amplification of the pressure pulse between the aortic arch and the brachial artery. The amplification of the pressure pulse from the aorta to the peripheral large arteries is seen mostly in a higher systolic pressure at the periphery than at the aorta, with diastolic pressure being approximately equal at the two sites [5, 51]. However, because of the frequency dependency of the arterial transfer function, pulse amplification would necessarily depend on the signal spectral content and so on pulse waveform. The important implication of this is that the relationship between central aortic systolic pressure and measured peripheral systolic pressure is variable and depends on the shape of the arterial pulse. Thus, with mathematical quantification and model implementation using non-invasive applanation tomometry or other means of pulse detection, pulse wave analysis techniques have emerged such that the combination of the conventional brachial sphygmomanometer and the peripheral pressure pulse can enhance assessment of cardiovascular function [52]. The quantification of pulse amplification in the upper limb has resulted in value-added information. Non-invasive measurement of central aortic systolic and pulse pressure provide improved assessment of cardiovascular risk [53–55], better understanding of blood pressure guidelines in relation to corresponding values of central aortic systolic pressure for normotensive and hypertensive bands [55] and improved means of guiding anti-hypertensive therapy [56]. Current guidelines, such as those of the European Society of Hypertension and European Society of Cardiology [57] do not yet recommend the adoption of central aortic pressure measurement in clinical practice, except in diagnosis of isolated systolic hypertension in the young, where high brachial systolic pressures may be due to pressure amplification in the presence of normal central, aortic pressures [58].

Although in middle age there is little change in brachial pulse pressure from the end of the fourth to the sixth decade, a much larger change is seen in central aortic pulse pressure [1, 59]. In the Asklepios study [59], a longitudinal investigation specifically designed to assess changes in middle age, pulse pressure amplification varied between 1.08 for women in the oldest category to 1.25 for men in the youngest category of the middle age range. In addition, pulse pressure amplification was generally higher in men (average of 1.20) compared to women (average of 1.13) and decreased with age in both men and women [59].

Pulse Pressure Amplification in the Lower Limb

In the absence of atherosclerotic plaques causing reduction in lumen cross-sectional area, the lower limb also manifests similar pulse wave amplification. Invasive measurements of pressure in the femoral artery and in vessels in the foot show an average pulse amplification of 1.35 for subjects younger than 35 years decreasing to 1.28 in older subjects [60]. Although pulse amplification varied with acute vasoactive interventions and other stimuli (Valsava maneuver), it did not differ in patients with ischemic heart disease [60].

As a diagnostic measurement, lower limb pulse pressure amplification is incorporated in the ankle-brachial index (ABI, ratio of ankle and brachial systolic pressure) for assessment of peripheral arterial disease. While ABI is conventionally obtained using sequential brachial and leg cuff placements with the addition of a Doppler flow measurement, simultaneous brachial and ankle measurement using oscillometric blood pressure sphygmomanometry has been found to give similar results [61]. However, since lower limb pressure amplification is generally confounded by atheromatous lumen encroachment, discussion of hemodynamic and vascular correlates are beyond the scope of this chapter.

Age-Related Changes in Pulse Pressure Amplification and Arterial Stiffness

Amplification of pulse pressure with age between the aorta and brachial artery and change in arterial stiffness as measured by PWV is shown in Fig. 23.1 from a study of a large cohort assessing normal vascular aging in both men and women [1]. The study illustrates the marked gender difference in profiles of changes of brachial and central aorta pulse pressure and brachial and aortic PWV. The specific relevance of middle age is quantified by the association of the pulse pressure amplification (PPA) and the vascular stiffness gradient computed as the ratio of aortic to brachial PWV ($PWV_{carotid\text{-}femoral}$:$PWV_{carotid\text{-}brachial}$). The rate of change of stiffness gradient is greater in women compared to men. This is also associated with a steeper increase in brachial pulse pressure in women compared to men. These associations occur before the onset of middle age in women and during middle age in men (Fig. 23.1). This concept of stiffness gradient has been used in assessment of compensatory mechanisms in dialysis patients [62], however, the potential use of these parameters in age-related predictive models is still not known.

Determinants of Pulse Pressure Amplification

The amplification of the pressure pulse from the aorta to peripheral sites of the arterial tree is due to the progressive vascular impedance mismatch along the arterial path length due to elastic and geometric non-uniformity and to the intensity and timing of wave reflection from peripheral resistance beds [4, 15]. With the assumption of an invariant and stationary system, the relationship of the pulse pressure between a central and peripheral site is described in the frequency domain in terms of a transfer function, where the modulus is the amplification factor of the frequency components and the phase describes the time delay. The transfer function of the upper limb arterial path length (between the aorta and radial artery) exhibits a spectrum where the transmission ratio increases with frequency from unity at zero frequency to a maximum of approximately 3.0 at around 3–4 Hz, after which it decreases towards and below unity with increasing frequency [49, 50].

The implication of the spectral characteristics of arterial transfer functions as observed in the brachial artery is that pulse pressure amplification becomes heart rate dependent. Acute increases in heart rate have been shown in a cardiac pacing study to cause an increase in pulse pressure amplification [47]. Despite no change in brachial pulse blood pressure with increasing heart rate, the study by Wilkinson et al. [47] showed a consistent decrease in aortic pulse pressure with increasing heart rate, resulting in a change in pulse pressure amplification. There was no change in aortic stiffness, and the ratio of the unaugmented aortic pressure to brachial pressure did not change with heart rate. This indicated that pulse pressure amplification changed with heart rate due to changes in the augmentation of the aortic pressure pulse. A cross-sectional study investigating the carotid-brachial pulse pressure amplification showed a heart rate dependent increase in pulse pressure amplification for hypertensive subjects with a heart rate greater than 80 bpm [63], highlighting the interaction between beta-blocker agents and pulse pressure amplification, as was later confirmed in other larger studies [64]. However, these studies did not assess the differential impact of age-related change in pulse amplification, and specifically in the middle age range.

Although the principal determinants of pulse amplification are differential age-related arterial mechanical properties along the arterial tree, there are other associative determinants that have been shown to be independent of age. Pulse pressure amplification is greater in males than in females [1], it is affected by the presence of hypertension [65], diabetes [65], posture [51], body fat [66] and acute exercise [5].

Implications of Pulse Pressure Amplification

Pulse pressure amplification presents a significant confounder in the assessment of central hemodynamics from the conventional brachial cuff sphygmomanometric measurement due to the variable association between brachial and aortic systolic pressure in individual subjects [1, 5, 55]. However, pulse pressure amplification, as a metric in itself, has been proposed as a potential biomarker of cardiovascular risk [54]. This has implications in both the categorization of hypertension in terms of established guidelines as well as in the pharmacological treatment and management of hypertension [55, 65, 67]. Since the advent of techniques for the use of pulse wave analysis and non-invasive measurements of central aortic pressure [52], evidence has emerged of the marked differential effects of antihypertenive agents on peripheral and central aortic systolic pressure [68]. The current general consensus is that there are significant differences between classes of antihypertensive agents on pulse pressure amplification. Generally, angiotensin converting enzyme inhibitors, angiotensin receptor blockers, dihydropyridine calcium blockers, and nitrates, show a greater effect on the difference between central and peripheral systolic pressure than diuretics and beta blockers [64, 68]. These differential effects in combination with the variable gender effects of pulse pressure amplification and arterial stiffness gradient in men and women seen around the middle age range (Fig. 23.1) will present additional challenges for effective treatment and management of hypertension.

Predictive Aspects of Pulse Pressure, Pulse Pressure Amplification, and Arterial Stiffness Changes in Middle Age

Clinical Risk Prediction

To established the validity of central aortic pressure and pulse wave velocity in clinical management, there is an increasing number of meta-analyses aimed at providing quantitative associations with cardiovascular risk [69, 70]. Generally, studies suggest that aortic pulse pressure [53], and pulse pressure amplification [54] are independent predictors of mortality in the general population. However, the data are not consistent. In men aged between 40 and 80 years, pulse pressure amplification is associated with an expected lower carotid to femoral pulse wave velocity, a reduced carotid intima-media thickness, and a lower risk of coronary heart disease by the Framingham risk scale [71]. In elderly patients, greater than 80 years of age, a lower pulse pressure amplification is a predictor of mortality and cardiovascular events, and a stronger metric than brachial blood pressure alone [72]. Although these studies provide substantial information on age-related changes and cardiovascular risk, the capacity of using data in the middle age range for prediction cardiovascular risk in the later years has not yet been established.

Risk Scores and the Concept of "Vascular Age"

Aging is a major determinant of cardiovascular risk. However, the concomitant but variable functional changes that are manifest in age-related changes in arterial pressure are essentially due to changes in the vasculature that are expressed as increase in large artery stiffness and peripheral vascular resistance. There has been increasing interest in the association between the chronological age and the aging of the vasculature to find metrics and parameters that can quantify early vascular aging [73]. There are no data explicitly addressing the relevance of the rate of change in cardiovascular function in the middle age range with respect to early vascular aging. However, there are attempts at identifying accelerated early vascular aging that may be associated with clusters of factors of cardiovascular risk [73]. As in the case where the stiffness gradient between central aorta and peripheral limbs may be a potential biomarker for cardiovascular function [62], a similar metric may be obtained as the age-related relative increase in peripheral resistance and aortic stiffness to be associated with future cardiovascular events. In this context, the changes seen during the middle age range may have a significant role. Indeed, the rate of change during middle age could be an integral part of the complex cardiovascular aging continuum [74].

Conclusions

The changes in large artery stiffness that occur with age were evident from the pulse wave patterns in the early use of the sphygmogram, preceding the use of the sphygmomanometer [4]. Arterial stiffness changes are inherent in the age-related changes in pulse pressure that occur at the onset of middle age (defined in this context between 40 and 60 years). The assessment of arterial pressure using the conventional brachial cuff sphygmomanometer as a major factor of cardiovascular risk and central end organ damage is confounded by the pulse pressure amplification phenomenon, leading to variable differences in peripheral (measured) and central aortic systolic pressure. A significant impact of this is seen in the middle age range where the measured (brachial) change in pulse pressure is relatively small, whereas a much greater change occurs in the same age range for central aortic pulse pressure. There is an increase in available methods and devices for non-invasive measurement of central aortic pressure, both as office and as 24-h measurements, and pulse wave velocity, pulse pressure amplification and arterial stiffness. These parameters in middle age may emerge as significant in improving cardiovascular risk assessment, risk reclassification and risk prediction for the aging population beyond the time in life when ".. *the shadows of decay and death are first perceived*".

References

1. McEniery CM, Hall IR, Yasmin, et al. Normal vascular aging: differential effects on wave reflection and aortic pulse wave velocity: the Anglo-Cardiff Collaborative Trial (ACCT). J Am Coll Cardiol. 2005;46:1753–60.
2. Franklin SS, Gustin W, Wong ND, et al. Hemodynamic patterns of age-related changes in blood pressure. The Framingham Heart Study. Circulation. 1997;96:308–15.
3. Falzone R, Yasmin, Brown MJ. Determinants of arterial stiffness in offspring of families with essential hypertension. Am J Hypertens. 2004;17:292–8.
4. Nichols WW, O'Rourke MF, Vlachopoulos C. McDonald's blood flow in arteries: theoretical, experimental and clinical principles. 6th ed. New York: Oxford University Press; 2011.
5. Rowell LB, Brengelmann GL, Blackmon JR, et al. Disparities between aortic and peripheral pulse pressures induced by upright exercise and vasomotor changes in man. Circulation. 1968;37:954–64.
6. Drevenstedt J. Perceptions of onsets of young adulthood, middle age, and old age. J Gerontol. 1976;31:53–7.
7. Hunt J. Middle age. Lancet. 1967;290:1132.
8. Hickson SS, Butlin M, Graves M, et al. The relationship of age with regional aortic stiffness and diameter. JACC Cardiovasc Imaging. 2010;3:1247–55.
9. Zhang Y, Agnoletti D, Protogerou AD, et al. Characteristics of pulse wave velocity in elastic and muscular arteries: a mismatch beyond age. J Hypertens. 2013;31:554–9.
10. Avolio AP, Chen SG, Wang RP, et al. Effects of aging on changing arterial compliance and left ventricular

load in a northern Chinese urban community. Circulation. 1983;68:50–8.
11. O'Rourke MF, Blazek JV, Morreels Jr CL, et al. Pressure wave transmission along the human aorta. Changes with age and in arterial degenerative disease. Circ Res. 1968;23:567–79.
12. Rogers WJ, Hu YL, Coast D, et al. Age-associated changes in regional aortic pulse wave velocity. J Am Coll Cardiol. 2001;38:1123–9.
13. Nelson AJ, Worthley SG, Cameron JD, et al. Cardiovascular magnetic resonance-derived aortic distensibility: validation and observed regional differences in the elderly. J Hypertens. 2009;27:535–42.
14. Roach MR, Burton AC. The reason for the shape of the distensibility curves of arteries. Can J Biochem Physiol. 1957;35:681–90.
15. O'Rourke MF, Hashimoto J. Mechanical factors in arterial aging: a clinical perspective. J Am Coll Cardiol. 2007;50:1–13.
16. Wang Y-X, Fitch RM. Vascular stiffness: measurements, mechanisms and implications. Curr Vasc Pharmacol. 2004;2:379–84.
17. Zieman SJ, Melenovsky V, Kass DA. Mechanisms, pathophysiology, and therapy of arterial stiffness. Arterioscler Thromb Vasc Biol. 2005;25:932–43.
18. Avolio A. Arterial stiffness. Pulse. 2013;1:14–28.
19. Avolio AP, Butlin M, Liu Y-Y, et al. Regulation of arterial stiffness: cellular, molecular and neurogenic mechanisms. Artery Res. 2011;5:122–7.
20. Cox RH. Pressure dependence of the mechanical properties of arteries in vivo. Am J Physiol. 1975;229:1371–5.
21. Shadwick RE. Mechanical design in arteries. J Exp Biol. 1999;202:3305–13.
22. Wagenseil JE, Mecham RP. Elastin in large artery stiffness and hypertension. J Cardiovasc Transl Res. 2012;5:264–73.
23. Wang JG, Staessen JA. The benefit of treating isolated systolic hypertension. Curr Hypertens Rep. 2001;3:333–9.
24. Staessen J, Fagard R, Amery A. Isolated systolic hypertension in the elderly: implications of Systolic Hypertension in the Elderly Program (SHEP) for clinical practice and for the ongoing trials. J Hum Hypertens. 1991;5:469–74.
25. Mitchell GF, Hwang S-J, Vasan RS, et al. Arterial stiffness and cardiovascular events: the Framingham Heart Study. Circulation. 2010;121:505–11.
26. Gosline J, Lillie M, Carrington E, et al. Elastic proteins: biological roles and mechanical properties. Philos Trans R Soc Lond B Biol Sci. 2002;357:121–32.
27. Elvin CM, Carr AG, Huson MG, et al. Synthesis and properties of crosslinked recombinant pro-resilin. Nature. 2005;437:999–1002.
28. Shapiro SD, Endicott SK, Province MA, et al. Marked longevity of human lung parenchymal elastic fibers deduced from prevalence of D-aspartate and nuclear weapons-related radiocarbon. J Clin Invest. 1991;87:1828–34.
29. Greenwald S. Ageing of the conduit arteries. J Pathol. 2007;211:157.
30. Avolio AP, Jones D, Tafazzoli-Shadpour M. Quantification of alterations in structure and function of elastin in the arterial media. Hypertension. 1998;32:170–5.
31. Martyn CN, Greenwald SE. A hypothesis about a mechanism for the programming of blood pressure and vascular disease in early life. Clin Exp Pharmacol Physiol. 2001;28:948–51.
32. Le VP, Knutsen RH, Mecham RP, Wagenseil JE. Decreased aortic diameter and compliance precedes blood pressure increases in postnatal development of elastin-insufficient mice. Am J Physiol Heart Circ Physiol. 2011;301:H221–9.
33. Nakashima Y, Shiokawa Y, Sueishi K. Alterations of elastic architecture in human aortic dissecting aneurysm. Lab Invest. 1990;62:751–60.
34. Rietzschel E-R, De Buyzere ML, Bekaert S, et al. Rationale, design, methods and baseline characteristics of the Asklepios Study. Eur J Cardiovasc Prev Rehabil. 2007;14:179–91.
35. Segers P, Rietzschel ER, De Buyzere ML, et al. Noninvasive (input) impedance, pulse wave velocity, and wave reflection in healthy middle-aged men and women. Hypertension. 2007;49:1248–55.
36. Lunder M, Janic M, Kejzar N, Sabovic M. Associations among different functional and structural arterial wall properties and their relations to traditional cardiovascular risk factors in healthy subjects: a cross-sectional study. BMC Cardiovasc Disord. 2012;12:29.
37. Corden B, Keenan NG, de Marvao ASM, et al. Body fat is associated with reduced aortic stiffness until middle age. Hypertension. 2013;61:1322–7.
38. McDonnell BJ, Maki-Petaja KM, Munnery M, et al. Habitual exercise and blood pressure: age dependency and underlying mechanisms. Am J Hypertens. 2013;26:334–41.
39. Wang J-J, O'Brien AB, Shrive NG, et al. Time-domain representation of ventricular-arterial coupling as a windkessel and wave system. Am J Physiol Heart Circ Physiol. 2003;284:H1358–68.
40. Westerhof N, Lankhaar J-WW, Westerhof BE. The arterial windkessel. Med Biol Eng Comput. 2009;47:131–41.
41. Giudici F, Qian Y, O'Rourke M, Avolio A. Simulation of reduction of proximal aortic stiffness by an elastic wrap and effects on pulse pressure. Conf Proc IEEE Eng Med Biol Soc. 2012;2012:657–60.
42. Sweitzer NK, Shenoy M, Stein JH, et al. Increases in central aortic impedance precede alterations in arterial stiffness measures in type 1 diabetes. Diabetes Care. 2007;30:2886–91.
43. Chirinos JA, Segers P, Gillebert TC, et al. Central pulse pressure and its hemodynamic determinants in middle-aged adults with impaired fasting glucose and diabetes: the Asklepios study. Diabetes Care. 2013;36:2359–65.

44. McEniery CM, Wallace S, Yasmin, et al. Increased stroke volume and aortic stiffness contribute to isolated systolic hypertension in young adults. Hypertension. 2005;46:221–6.
45. Alfie J, Waisman GD, Galarza CR, Cámera MI. Contribution of stroke volume to the change in pulse pressure pattern with age. Hypertension. 1999; 34:808–12.
46. Kostis JB, Moreyra AE, Amendo MT, et al. The effect of age on heart rate in subjects free of heart disease. Studies by ambulatory electrocardiography and maximal exercise stress test. Circulation. 1982;65:141–5.
47. Wilkinson IB, Mohammad NH, Tyrrell S, et al. Heart rate dependency of pulse pressure amplification and arterial stiffness. Am J Hypertens. 2002;15:24–30.
48. Papaioannou TG, Protogerou AD, Stefanadis C. What to anticipate from pulse pressure amplification. J Am Coll Cardiol. 2010;55:1038–40.
49. Karamanoglu M, O'Rourke MF, Avolio AP, Kelly RP. An analysis of the relationship between central aortic and peripheral upper limb pressure waves in man. Eur Hear J. 1993;14:160–7.
50. Chen CH, Nevo E, Fetics B, et al. Estimation of central aortic pressure waveform by mathematical transformation of radial tonometry pressure. Validation of generalized transfer function. Circulation. 1997;95:1827–36.
51. Kroeker EJ, Wood EH. Comparison of simultaneously recorded central and peripheral arterial pressure pulses during rest, exercise and tilted position in man. Circ Res. 1955;3:623–32.
52. Avolio AP, Butlin M, Walsh A. Arterial blood pressure measurement and pulse wave analysis–their role in enhancing cardiovascular assessment. Physiol Meas. 2010;31:R1–47.
53. Roman MJ, Devereux RB, Kizer JR, et al. High central pulse pressure is independently associated with adverse cardiovascular outcome the strong heart study. J Am Coll Cardiol. 2009;54:1730–4.
54. Benetos A, Thomas F, Joly L, et al. Pulse pressure amplification a mechanical biomarker of cardiovascular risk. J Am Coll Cardiol. 2010;55:1032–7.
55. McEniery CM, McDonnell B, Yasmin, et al. Central pressure: variability and impact of cardiovascular risk factors: the Anglo-Cardiff Collaborative Trial II. Hypertension. 2008;51:1476–82.
56. Sharman JE, Marwick TH, Gilroy D, et al. Randomized trial of guiding hypertension management using central aortic blood pressure compared with best-practice care: principal findings of the BP GUIDE study. Hypertension. 2013;62:1138–45.
57. Mancia G, Fagard R, Narkiewicz K, Redán J, Zanchetti A, Böhm M, Christiaens T, Cifkova R, De Backer G, Dominiczak A, Galderisi M, Grobbee DE, Jaarsma T, Kirchof P, Kjeldsen SE, Laurent S, Man F. 2013 Practice guidelines for the management of arterial hypertension of the European Society of Hypertension (ESH) and the European Society of Cardiology (ESC): ESH/ESC Task Force for the Management of Arterial Hypertension. J Hypertens. 2013;31:1925–38.
58. O'Rourke MF, Adji A. Guidelines on guidelines: focus on isolated systolic hypertension in youth. J Hypertens. 2013;31:649–54.
59. Segers P, Mahieu D, Kips J, et al. Amplification of the pressure pulse in the upper limb in healthy, middle-aged men and women. Hypertension. 2009;54: 414–20.
60. Carter SA. Effect of age, cardiovascular disease, and vasomotor changes on transmission of arterial pressure waves through the lower extremities. Angiology. 1978;29:601–6.
61. Kollias A, Xilomenos A, Protogerou A, et al. Automated determination of the ankle-brachial index using an oscillometric blood pressure monitor: validation vs. Doppler measurement and cardiovascular risk factor profile. Hypertens Res. 2011;34:825–30.
62. Utescu MS, Couture V, Mac-Way F, et al. Determinants of progression of aortic stiffness in hemodialysis patients: a prospective longitudinal study. Hypertension. 2013;62:154–60.
63. Laurent P. Heart rate and pulse pressure amplification in hypertensive subjects. Am J Hypertens. 2003;16: 363–70.
64. Williams B, Lacy PS, Thom SM, et al. Differential impact of blood pressure-lowering drugs on central aortic pressure and clinical outcomes: principal results of the Conduit Artery Function Evaluation (CAFE) study. Circulation. 2006;113:1213–25.
65. Avolio AP, Van Bortel LM, Boutouyrie P, et al. Role of pulse pressure amplification in arterial hypertension: experts' opinion and review of the data. Hypertension. 2009;54:375–83.
66. Wykretowicz A, Rutkowska A, Krauze T, et al. Pulse pressure amplification in relation to body fatness. Br J Clin Pharmacol. 2012;73:546–52.
67. Safar ME, Blacher J, Protogerou A, Achimastos A. Arterial stiffness and central hemodynamics in treated hypertensive subjects according to brachial blood pressure classification. J Hypertens. 2008;26: 130–7.
68. Protogerou AD, Stergiou GS, Vlachopoulos C, et al. The effect of antihypertensive drugs on central blood pressure beyond peripheral blood pressure. Part II: Evidence for specific class-effects of antihypertensive drugs on pressure amplification. Curr Pharm Des. 2009;15:272–89.
69. Vlachopoulos C, Aznaouridis K, O'Rourke MF, et al. Prediction of cardiovascular events and all-cause mortality with central haemodynamics: a systematic review and meta-analysis. Eur Heart J. 2010;31: 1865–71.
70. Ben-Shlomo Y, Spears M, Boustred C, et al. Aortic pulse wave velocity improves cardiovascular event prediction: an individual participant meta-analysis of

prospective observational data from 17,635 subjects. J Am Coll Cardiol. 2014;63(7):636–46.
71. Nijdam M-E, Plantinga Y, Hulsen HT, et al. Pulse pressure amplification and risk of cardiovascular disease. Am J Hypertens. 2008;21:388–92.
72. Benetos A, Gautier S, Labat C, et al. Mortality and cardiovascular events are best predicted by low central/peripheral pulse pressure amplification but not by high blood pressure levels in elderly nursing home subjects: the PARTAGE study. J Am Coll Cardiol. 2012;60:1503–11.
73. Nilsson PM, Khalili P, Franklin SS. Blood pressure and pulse wave velocity as metrics for evaluating pathologic ageing of the cardiovascular system. Blood Press. 2014;23:17–30.
74. O'Rourke MF, Safar ME, Dzau V. The Cardiovascular Continuum extended: aging effects on the aorta and microvasculature. Vasc Med. 2010;15:461–8.

24 Arterial Stiffness, Central Blood Pressure and Cardiac Remodelling: From Cardiac Hypertrophy to Heart Failure

Mary J. Roman and Richard B. Devereux

Abstract

Over the past several decades much has been learned about arterial stiffness and central blood pressure (BP) and their relations to left ventricular (LV) remodelling and hypertrophy. In addition, the impact of central hemodynamics on LV performance and the development of clinical heart failure is under active investigation and is of particular importance from a public health and therapeutic standpoint. The ability to examine these topics has been vastly accelerated by the development of reliable, noninvasive technology to permit evaluation of cardiac and vascular structure and function on an epidemiologic scale. The present review will discuss data regarding the interaction of arterial stiffness and central BP with LV structure and function; the impact of arterial stiffness on the development of heart failure, particularly with preserved ejection fraction, will also be discussed.

Keywords

Arterial stiffness • Central blood pressure • Left ventricular hypertrophy • Heart failure

M.J. Roman, MD (✉) • R.B. Devereux, MD
Greenberg Division of Cardiology,
New York Presbyterian Hospital, Weill Cornell Medical College, 525 East 68th Street, New York, NY 10021, USA
e-mail: mroman@med.cornell.edu;
rbdevere@med.cornell.edu

Abbreviations

AUC	Area under the curve
BP	Blood pressure
HFPEF	Heart failure with preserved ejection fraction
LV	Left ventricular
LVETi	Left ventricular ejection time index
NT-proBNP	N-terminal pro-B-type natriuretic peptides
PP	Pulse pressure
ROC	Receiver operating characteristic

M.E. Safar et al. (eds.), *Blood Pressure and Arterial Wall Mechanics in Cardiovascular Diseases*,
DOI 10.1007/978-1-4471-5198-2_24, © Springer-Verlag London 2014

Over the past several decades much has been learned about arterial stiffness and central blood pressure (BP) and their relations to left ventricular (LV) hypertrophy and geometry. Central arterial BP and measures of arterial stiffness derived therefrom are of particular importance because central BP represents the load placed on the LV and large coronary and cerebral arteries that develop stenosis and occlusion, and because central BP is variably lower than brachial BP due to the invasively-documented phenomenon of pulse-pressure amplification [1–3]. In addition, the impact of central hemodynamics on LV performance and the development of clinical heart failure is under active investigation and is of particular importance from a public health and therapeutic standpoint. The ability to examine these topics has been vastly accelerated by the development of reliable, noninvasive technology to permit evaluation of cardiac and vascular structure and function on an epidemiologic scale. The present review will discuss data regarding the interactions of arterial stiffness and central BP with LV structure and function. The impact of arterial stiffness on the development of heart failure, particularly with preserved ejection fraction, will also be discussed.

Relation of Central BP and Arterial Stiffness to LV Remodelling

Methodologic Considerations

LV remodelling may be characterized an increase in LV mass (hypertrophy) and/or abnormal relative wall thickness (concentric geometry). LV mass and relative wall thickness can be determined by a variety of methods, with almost all data derived from transthoracic echocardiography. LV mass can be accurately calculated from linear measurement of LV wall thicknesses and internal diameter at mid cavity using an autopsy-validated formula [4, 5]. In view of the strong dependence of LV mass on body size in normal individuals, it is optimal to adjust absolute LV mass for differences in body size. Although body surface area is most commonly used, adjustment of LV mass for its allometric relation to height ($ht^{2.7}$) better detects increases in LV mass related to obesity [6].

Relative wall thickness is calculated as posterior wall thickness/chamber radius. It is used to classify LV geometry into one of four patterns (normal, eccentric hypertrophy, concentric hypertrophy, and concentric remodeling [Fig. 24.1]). These patterns reflect differences in underlying hemodynamic abnormalities related to hypertension [7]. Recently, it has been suggested that further subdivision of concentric and eccentric LV hypertrophy into subgroups with or without LV chamber dilatation helps stratify LV function and systemic hemodynamics more precisely [8, 9]. However, whether this classification strengthens relations between arterial stiffness and LV geometry has not yet been evaluated.

Normative values for LV mass vary according to gender. Greater LV mass in men cannot be fully accounted for by larger body size and may relate to differences in fat-free mass [10, 11]. Based on refinements in image quality and cumulative analyses in large international populations, 116 g/m^2 or 48 $g/ht^{2.7}$ in men and 96 g/m^2 or 44 $g/ht^{2.7}$ in women are currently recommended as the upper limits of normal for LV mass index [5]. The upper normal limit for relative wall thickness is 0.42 [5].

Although the importance of blood pressure as a stimulus to LV hypertrophy has long been known, measures of brachial BP account for a relatively modest amount of variability in LV mass. Thus alternate indices of ventricular afterload have been developed, validated, and examined. Central BP, i.e., BP in the ascending aorta, differs from brachial BP to a variable extent based on pulse pressure (PP) amplification. Because central BP more closely reflects loading conditions of the LV myocardium and coronary and cerebral vasculature, it better predicts cardiovascular target organ damage and clinical disease than does brachial BP, as discussed below. Similarly, arterial stiffness and selected measures of pulse wave transmission may better represent changes in physical properties of the conduit arteries. However, the extent to which arterial stiffness promotes LV hypertrophy is strongly influenced by the method by which arterial stiffness is estimated, i.e., the extent to which the stiffness parameter varies with changes in

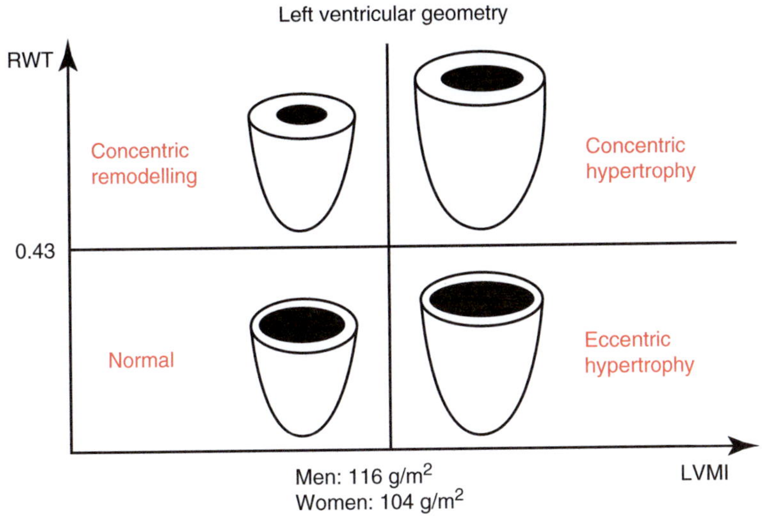

Fig. 24.1 Classification of LV geometric patterns based on LV mass index and relative wall thickness (Adapted from Ref. [7])

distending pressure. This phenomenon will be considered as different measures of arterial stiffness are discussed.

Central BP and LV Remodelling

It has been firmly established that brachial systolic BP (including ambulatory) is more strongly related to LV mass than is brachial PP [12–14]. Similarly, we demonstrated in the Strong Heart Study a stronger relation of central systolic BP than central PP to LV remodelling (both LV mass index and relative wall thickness) [15]. Importantly, central systolic BP bore a significantly stronger relation with LV remodelling than did brachial systolic BP. Central systolic BP was likewise found to correlate better than brachial systolic BP with LV mass in a large Taiwanese population [16], and central PP was found to relate to LV mass independent of brachial PP in a South African population-based study [17].

Arterial Stiffness and LV Remodelling

A variety of techniques are available for noninvasive assessment of arterial stiffness [18]. The extent to which estimates of arterial stiffness promote LV remodelling is largely a function of their dependence on distending pressure. Thus we have found that elastic modulus, a pressure-dependent measure, is significantly related to LV mass index, whereas the arterial stiffness index (β), a pressure-independent measure, is not [19]. However, the arterial stiffness index was directly related to relative wall thickness and thereby to concentric LV geometry. Although younger and older hypertensive subjects had comparable overall LV mass, relative wall thickness was significantly higher in older hypertensive subjects associated with higher arterial stiffness [19]. As a corollary, among 271 untreated hypertensive subjects, we found elastic modulus to track with systolic blood pressure and therefore to be highest in the group with concentric LV hypertrophy [20].

The pattern of LV concentric remodelling (high relative wall thickness and normal LV mass) in hypertensive individuals is also associated with abnormally high effective arterial elastance (Ea), higher peripheral resistance, and lower LV systolic function. In addition, ventriculo-vascular coupling, calculated as Ea/Ees (where Ees is the ratio of end-systolic pressure to LV end-systolic volume), is increased among hypertensive patients with increased effective arterial elastance, indicative of suboptimal mechanical efficiency [21]. Concentric LV remodelling was also directly related to pulse wave velocity – influenced by the level of arterial distending pressure – among middle-aged and older hypertensive patients studied by Schillaci et al. [22].

Among 1,315 normotensive and untreated hypertensive subjects, Chen et al. found echocardiographic LV mass to be directly related to arterial compliance calculated as LV stroke volume/brachial pulse pressure [12], consistent with the known importance of stroke volume as a stimulus to LV hypertrophy [23] but also possible autocorrelation between mass and stroke volume as both were calculated from similar measurements. In addition, LV mass was directly related to elastic modulus and inversely to arterial elastance, similar to our findings [21]. Importantly, in multivariate analyses in this study, the measures of arterial stiffness examined (elastic modulus, carotid augmentation index, and pulse wave velocity) were only independently related to LV mass when blood pressure was excluded from the analyses, underscoring the pressure-dependence of these parameters.

Relations of Arterial Stiffness and Central BP to LV Systolic and Diastolic Function

Invasive measurement of LV pressure and volume and determination of arterial elastance document an age-associated increase in arterial stiffness which is mirrored by an increase in ventricular stiffness, even in the absence of hypertrophy [24]. Although ventriculo-vascular coupling is maintained on average, there is a much greater sensitivity of systolic BP to changes in LV preload. In a rat model of aortic stiffness (induced elastocalcinosis), prolonged exposure to increased aortic stiffness (characteristic impedance) led to LV hypertrophy, fibrosis reflected as increase in collagen content, and a shift in the myosin heavy chain isoform pattern [25]. This latter phenomenon prolongs systolic ejection to maintain contractile performance but shortens diastole in the setting of increased myocardial stiffness. These important experimental observations have been followed by a number of non-invasive investigations of the chronic impact of arterial stiffness on LV function and its clinical implications.

Using non-invasive echocardiographic parameters and estimated end-systolic pressure, Redfield et al. examined ventricular and vascular stiffening in 2,042 participants in a population-based (Olmstead County, Minnesota) study (Rochester Epidemiology Project) [26]. Similar to the earlier invasive study, both ventricular and vascular stiffening–estimated from Doppler echocardiography and brachial BP as vascular (Ea) and ventricular (Ees) elastances–increased with age. Notably, values were higher in women than in men, and ventricular stiffness increased more steeply in women. These findings were independent of symptom status and provided support for the authors' hypothesis that parallel arterial and ventricular stiffening might account for age-related heart failure with preserved ejection fraction (HFPEF), especially in women. Of note, the authors also confirmed age-associated concentric remodelling (increase in relative wall thickness), particularly in women.

As further evidence of a potential link between arterial stiffening and diastolic dysfunction as a potential mechanism for HFPEF, aortic and brachial PPs, but not carotid-femoral pulse wave velocity (influenced by mean arterial pressure), were related to the grade of diastolic dysfunction as well as left atrial volume index, a marker of chronic LV diastolic dysfunction, in older patients at risk for development of atrial fibrillation [27]. In an Austrian study of patients with normal LV systolic function undergoing coronary angiography for suspected coronary artery disease, invasively-determined pulse wave velocity was negatively associated with echocardiographic tissue Doppler measures of diastolic relaxation (septal and lateral E′) and directly related to E/E′, an estimate of LV filling pressure (as well as to measured LV end-diastolic pressure) [28]. Of note, pulse wave velocity was directly related to plasma levels of amino terminal pro-brain natriuretic peptide (NT-proBNP, secreted in response to elevated LV filling pressure) and, along with age and female gender, was an independent predictor of the presence of exertional dyspnea.

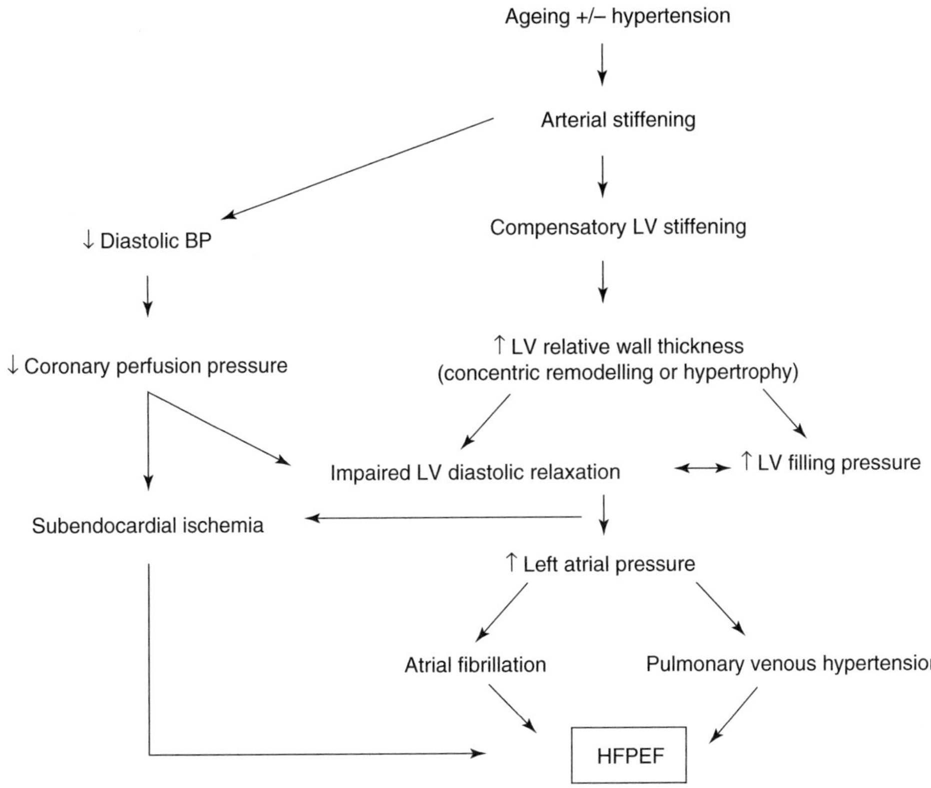

Fig. 24.2 Schematic diagram of potential mechanisms linking arterial stiffness to congestive heart failure (*HFPEF*)

In a subset (n=983) of the population-based Northern Manhattan Study in whom non-invasive pulse wave analysis and echocardiography were performed, "global arterial stiffness" was calculated as: central PP/LV stroke volume index [29]. In confirmation of the Austrian patient-based study, arterial stiffness was negatively related to velocity of myocardial relaxation (E′) and directly related to LV filling pressure (E/E′). In multivariable analyses, arterial stiffness was independently related to the presence of diastolic dysfunction.

Regional LV systolic and diastolic strains were determined using cardiac magnetic resonance imaging in 1,100 asymptomatic participants in the Multi-Ethnic Study of Atherosclerosis (MESA Study) who additionally underwent carotid ultrasound study [30]. Carotid artery compliance (calculated using brachial BP) was directly related to both systolic and diastolic regional performance, even following adjustment for blood pressure, supporting a role for arterial stiffening in the development of ventricular dysfunction.

Relation of Arterial Stiffness and Central BP to Clinical Heart Failure

The interaction between arterial and ventricular stiffening and associated consequences as well as the association between arterial stiffness and abnormal LV function described above has led to the consideration of arterial stiffness as a contributor to heart failure with preserved ejection fraction (HFPEF), particularly when it occurs in the absence of significant epicardial coronary artery disease (Fig. 24.2). Thus, arterial stiffening, in the presence or absence of hypertension, leads to compensatory LV stiffening and remodelling to maintain systolic performance at the expense of diastolic relaxation. Increased pulse wave velocity results in augmentation of late-systolic pressure and reduction of early diastolic aortic pressure. The resultant combination of reduced coronary perfusion pressure during diastole, increased metabolically active myocardial mass, and elevated LV filling pressure may promote subendocardial ischemia. Elevation in left atrial pressure may result in atrial fibrillation, pulmonary hypertension and signs and symptoms of HFPEF may ensue. Understanding the pathophysiology and improving treatment of HFPEF is of major public health importance as recent as HFPEF is now the cause of at least 50 % of congestive heart failure, with outcomes similar to patients with heart failure with reduced ejection fraction [31].

The observation in the Framingham Heart Study [32], the East Boston Senior Health Project [33], the Established Populations for Epidemiologic Study of the Elderly [34], and the Systolic Hypertension in the Elderly Program (SHEP) [35] that brachial PP, a surrogate for arterial stiffness, is independently related to incident clinical heart failure supports the importance of conduit artery stiffness as a marker, if not a cause, of heart failure risk. However assessment of LV function was not systematically included in the evaluation of heart failure in these reports.

In addition, the extent to which pulse pressure is primarily generated by arterial stiffness vs. LV stroke volume may vary based on ejection fraction. Thus in the Studies of Left Ventricular Dysfunction (SOLVD) trials (LV ejection fraction ≤35 % required for study entry), brachial PP was directly related to both ejection fraction and cardiovascular mortality, resulting in the conclusion that arterial stiffness was the mechanism of risk [36]. Similarly, in 135 patients with chronic heart failure over a wide range of ejection fraction, brachial PP was related to ejection fraction in those with reduced and preserved (≥40 %) ejection fraction, whereas carotid-femoral pulse wave velocity, a direct measure of arterial stiffness, was related to ejection fraction in the low ejection fraction group but not in the preserved ejection fraction group [37].

Subsequent invasive and non-invasive studies in patients with HFPEF have supported the contribution of arterial stiffness to overt heart failure, in addition to evidence of abnormal diastolic function. In a small invasive study of 10 patients with HFPEF, Kawaguchi et al. found increased ventricular and vascular stiffness and an upward shift in the diastolic pressure-volume curve in patients compared to control groups [38]. These findings were confirmed in 244 patients with HFPEF studied at the Mayo Clinic [39]. Both asymptomatic hypertensive patients and HFPEF patients had increased ventricular and arterial stiffness (end-systolic ventricular and arterial elastance calculated using estimated end-systolic pressure and Doppler echocardiography) compared to control subjects, whereas diastolic stiffness (curve-fitting constants derived from Doppler echocardiography) was increased in the HFPEF patients compared to the other two groups.

Two studies from Weber and colleagues have provided important data regarding hemodynamic underpinnings of HFPEF as well as diagnostic utility of non-invasive markers [40, 41]. Two hundred and seventy-one patients referred for cardiac catheterization for suspected coronary artery disease were categorized as having definite diastolic dysfunction (LV end-diastolic pressure >16 mmHg with normal end-diastolic volume and NT-proBNP >125 pg/ml; n=44), possible diastolic dysfunction (increased LV end-diastolic pressure or elevated NT-proBNP; n=109), or normal diastolic function [40]. The group with definite diastolic dysfunction had the typical demographic profile of being older and more often female and hypertensive. Patients with diastolic dysfunction had prolonged LV ejection time indexed for heart rate (LVETi) and increased wave reflection (increase in augmentation index and augmented systolic pressure) compared to the other two groups, whereas those with possible diastolic dysfunction had intermediate values (Fig. 24.3). The augmented pressure was directly related to LVETi as well as invasive LV end-diastolic pressure. LVETi was an independent predictor of diastolic dysfunction, as were hypertension, LV mass index, decreased creatinine clearance, and E:E′ ratio from echocardiography. Furthermore, in receiver operating characteristic

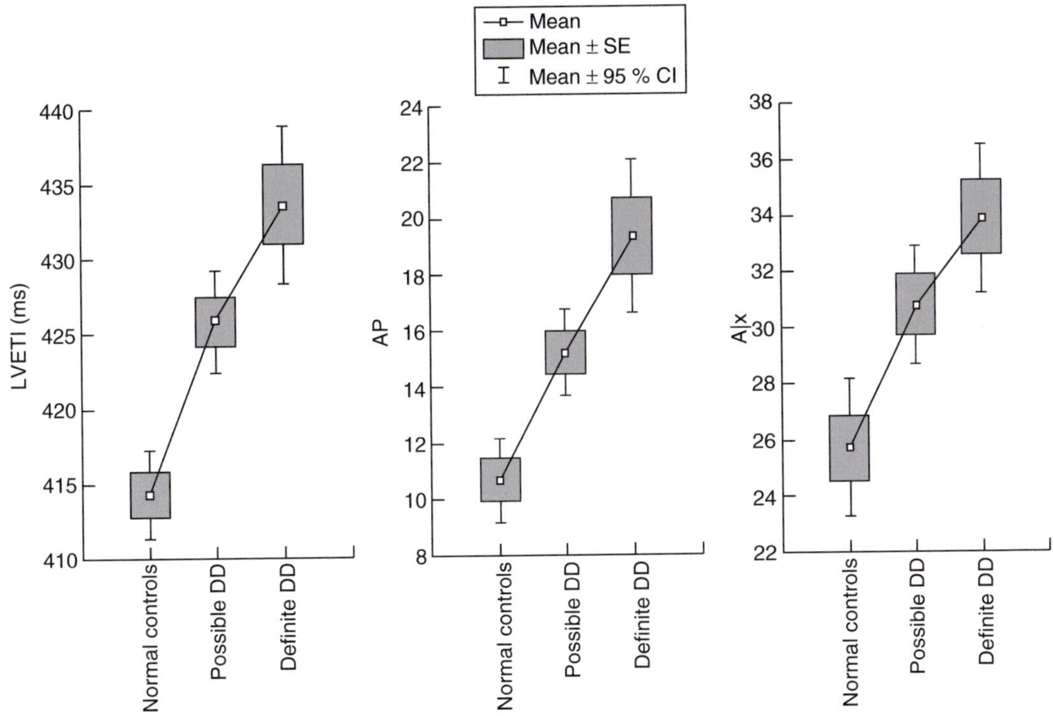

Fig. 24.3 Comparisons of LV ejection time index (*LVETi*), augmentation of central systolic pressure (*AP*), and augmentation index (*Aix*) in normal controls, patients with possible diastolic dysfunction, and patients with definite diastolic dysfunction. See text for definitions (Reproduced with permission from Ref. [40])

(ROC) curve analyses, LVETi and E:E′ ratio were comparable in their ability to detect diastolic dysfunction.

In a subsequent larger study (n = 359), cardiac catheterization, pulse wave analysis and echocardiography were again performed, and HFPEF was defined as LV EF >50 % with end-diastolic pressure >16 mmHg and NT-proBNP >220 pg/ml [41]. In ROC analyses, the areas under the curve (AUC) for brachial PP, E:E′ ratio, central PP from tonometry and invasively-determined aortic pulse wave velocity were 0.816, 0.823, 0.851, and 0.867, respectively (not significantly different). Importantly, in multivariable models, E:E′ correctly classified 77 % as having HFPEF or not, with significant improvement when a measure of arterial function was added to the model. The addition of central PP to E:E′ was significantly superior to the addition of brachial PP (AUC: 0.901 vs. 0.875; Fig. 24.4).

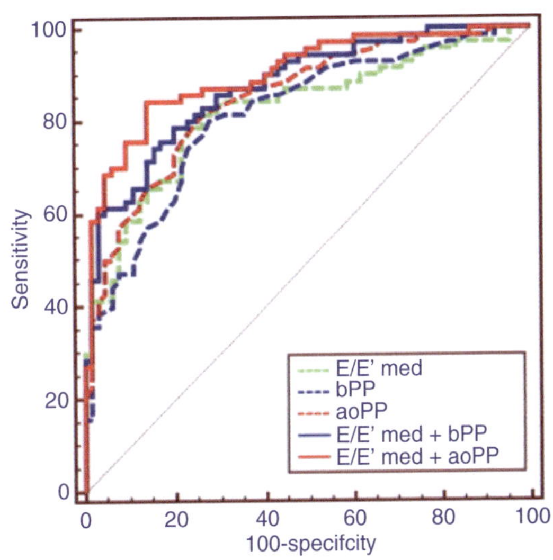

Fig. 24.4 Receiver operating characteristic curves comparing the ability to identify patients with HFPEF. The combination of central PP (*aoPP*) to E:E′ resulted in the highest area under the curve (0.901). *bPP* brachial pulse pressure (Reproduced with permission from Ref. [41])

Vascular stiffness and impaired ventriculo-arterial coupling are exaggerated with exercise in patients with HFPEF. Among 23 patients with HFPEF compared to 15 normal controls, exercise resulted in significant increases in elastic modulus, pulse wave velocity, and arterial elastance (calculated using central pressures derived from carotid applanation tonometry) and a lesser increase in stroke volume measured by echocardiography [42]. Of note, for a given end-diastolic volume, E/E′ ratio, an estimate of LV filling pressure was higher at rest (20 vs. 11, $p<0.001$) and remained elevated with exercise in the HFPEF group.

These results are complemented by a study of 15 patients with HFPEF and 15 matched control subjects who underwent rest and exercise echocardiography and radial applanation tonometry [43]. Exercise in HFPEF patients resulted in an increase in E:E′ which was independently associated with an increase in central pressure augmentation but not with change in brachial systolic or pulse pressure. In contrast, exercise in control subjects resulted in decreases in E:E′, augmentation index and augmented pressure.

In a small study of 10 patients with HFPEF who underwent cardiac magnetic resonance imaging at rest, pulsatile changes in aortic area and distensibility (calculated using brachial blood pressures) were lower than in age-matched controls [44]. Subsequent exercise showed diminished peak exercise oxygen consumption in the patient group that was associated with lower distensibility of the thoracic aorta.

In summary, there is strong support for the importance of increased arterial stiffness and central blood pressure in the development of LV remodelling, abnormal LV function (particularly diastolic relaxation), and clinical manifestations of heart failure, most notably in the presence of apparently preserved systolic function. The inability thus far to identify pharmacologic approaches of clear benefit in patients with HFPEF supports the need to better treat hypertension in the general population, to better identify patients in whom arterial stiffness is a leading pathophysiologic mechanism for diastolic dysfunction and for clinical heart failure, and to identify therapies that are more effective in ameliorating arterial stiffening than current heart failure regimens that have been proven to benefit heart failure patients with systolic dysfunction.

References

1. Karamanoglu M, O'Rourke MF, Avolio AP, Kelly RP. An analysis of the relationship between central aortic and peripheral upper limb pressure waves in man. Eur Heart J. 1993;14:160–7.
2. Westerhof BE, Guelen I, Stok WJ, Lasance HAJ, Ascoop CAPL, Wesseling KH, Westerhof N, Bos WJW, Stergiopulos N, Spaan JAE. Individualization of transfer function in estimation of central aortic pressure from the peripheral pulse is not required in patients at rest. J Appl Physiol. 2008;105:1858–63.
3. Sharman JE, Lim R, Qasem AM, Coombes JS, Burgess MI, Franco J, Garrahy P, Wilkinson IB, Marwick TH. Validation of a generalized transfer function to noninvasively derived central blood pressure during exercise. Hypertension. 2006;47:1203–8.
4. Devereux RB, Reichek N. Echocardiographic determination of left ventricular mass in man. Anatomic validation of the method. Circulation. 1977;55:613–8.
5. Lang RM, Bierig M, Devereux RB, Flachskampf FA, Foster E, Pellikka PA, Picard MH, Roman MJ, Seward J, Shanewise JS, Solomon SD, Spencer KT, St John Sutton M, Stewart WJ. Recommendations for chamber quantification: a report from the American Society of Echocardiography's Guidelines and Standards Committee and the Chamber Quantification Writing Group, developed in conjunction with the European Association of Echocardiography, a branch of the European Society of Cardiology. J Am Soc Echocardiogr. 2005;18:1440–63.
6. de Simone G, Daniels SR, Devereux RB, et al. Left ventricular mass and body size in normotensive children and adults: assessment of allometric relations and of the impact of overweight. J Am Coll Cardiol. 1992;20:1251–60.
7. Ganau A, Devereux RB, Roman MJ, et al. Patterns of left ventricular hypertrophy and geometric remodelling in essential hypertension. J Am Coll Cardiol. 1992;19:1550–8.
8. Khouri MG, Peshock RM, Ayers CR, de Lemos JA, Drazner MH. A 4-tiered classification of left ventricular hypertrophy based on left ventricular geometry: the Dallas Heart Study. Circ Cardiovasc Imaging. 2010;3:164–71.
9. Bang CN, Gerdts E, Aurigemma GP, Boman K, Dahlof B, Roman MJ, Kober L, Wachtell K, Devereux RB. Systolic left ventricular function according to left ventricular concentricity and dilatation in hypertensive patients: the Losartan Intervention For Endpoint reduction in hypertension study. J Hypertens. 2013;31:2060–8.

10. Bella JN, Devereux RB, Roman MJ, et al. Relations of left ventricular mass to fat-free and adipose body mass: the Strong Heart Study. Circulation. 1998;98:2538–44.
11. Kuch B, Hense H-W, Gneiting B, et al. Body composition and prevalence of left ventricular hypertrophy. Circulation. 2000;102:405–10.
12. Chen C-H, Ting C-T, Lin S-J, His T-L, Ho S-J, Chou P, et al. Which arterial and cardiac parameters best predict left ventricular mass? Circulation. 1998;98:422–8.
13. Flack JM, Gardin JM, Yunis C, Liu K, for the CARDIA Research Group. Static and pulsatile blood pressure correlates of left ventricular structure and function in black and white young adults: the CARDIA Study. Am Heart J. 1999;138:856–64.
14. Verdecchia P, Schillaci G, Borgioni C, Gaatobigio R, Ambrosio G, Porcellati C. Prevalent influence of systolic over pulse pressure on left ventricular mass in essential hypertension. Eur Heart J. 2002;23:658–65.
15. Roman MJ, Okin PM, Kizer JR, Lee ET, Howard BV, Devereux RB. Relations of central and brachial blood pressure to left ventricular hypertrophy and geometry: the Strong Heart Study. J Hypertens. 2010;28:384–8.
16. Wang K-L, Cheng H-M, Chuang S-Y, Spurgeon HA, Ting C-T, Lakatta EG, et al. Central or peripheral systolic or pulse pressure: which best relates to target organs and future mortality? J Hypertens. 2009;27:461–7.
17. Norton GR, Majane OHI, Maseko MJ, Libhaber C, Redelinghuys M, Kruger D, Veller M, Sareli P, Woodiwiss AJ. Brachial blood pressure-independent relations between radial late systolic shoulder-derived aortic pressures and target organ changes. Hypertension. 2012;59:885–92.
18. Laurent S, Cockcroft J, Van Bortel L, Boutouyrie P, Giannattasio C, Hayoz D, Pannier B, Vlachopoulos C, Wilkinson I, Struijker-Boudier H, on behalf of the European Network for Non-invasive Investigation of Large Arteries. Expert consensus document on arterial stiffness: methodological issues and clinical applications. Eur Heart J. 2006;27:2588–605.
19. Roman MJ, Ganau A, Saba PS, et al. Impact of arterial stiffening on left ventricular structure. Hypertension. 2000;36:489–94.
20. Roman MJ, Pickering TG, Schwartz JE, et al. Relation of arterial structure and function to left ventricular geometric patterns in hypertensive adults. J Am Coll Cardiol. 1996;28:751–6.
21. Saba PS, Ganau A, Devereux RB, et al. Impact of arterial elastance as a measure of vascular load on left ventricular geometry in hypertension. J Hypertens. 1999;17:1007–15.
22. Schillaci G, Mannarino MR, Pucci G, Pirro M, Helou J, Savarese G, Vaudo G, Mannarino E. Age-specific relationship of aortic pulse wave velocity with left ventricular geometry and function in hypertension. Hypertension. 2007;49:317–21.
23. Ganau A, Devereux RB, Pickering TG, Roman MJ, Schnall PL, Santucci S, Spitzer MC, Laragh JH. Relation of left ventricular hemodynamic load and contractile performance to left ventricular mass in hypertension. Circulation. 1990;81:25–36.
24. Chen C-H, Nakayama M, Nevo E, Fetics BJ, Maughan WL, Kass DA. Coupled systolic-ventricular and vascular stiffening with age: implications for pressure regulation and cardiac reserve in the elderly. J Am Coll Cardiol. 1998;32:1221–7.
25. Lartaud-Idjouadiene I, Lompré A-M, Kieffer P, Colas T, Atkinson J. Cardiac consequences of prolonged exposure to an isolated increase in aortic stiffness. Hypertension. 1999;34:63–9.
26. Redfield MM, Jacobsen SJ, Borlaug BA, Rodeheffer RJ, Kass DA. Age- and gender-related ventricular-vascular stiffening: a community-based study. Circulation. 2005;112:2254–62.
27. Abhayaratna WP, Barnes ME, O'Rourke MF, Gersh BJ, Seward JB, Miyasaka Y, Bailey KR, Tsang TSM. Relation of arterial stiffness to left ventricular diastolic function and cardiovascular risk prediction in patients ≥65 years of age. Am J Cardiol. 2006;98:1387–92.
28. Weber T, O'Rourke MF, Ammer M, Kvas E, Punzengruber C, Eber B. Arterial stiffness and arterial wave reflections are associated with systolic and diastolic function in patients with normal ejection fraction. Am J Hypertens. 2008;21:1194–202.
29. Russo C, Jin Z, Palmieri V, Homma S, Rundek T, Elkind MSV, Sacco RL, Di Tullio MR. Arterial stiffness and wave reflection: sex differences and relationship with left ventricular diastolic function. Hypertension. 2012;60:362–8.
30. Fernandes VRS, Polak JF, Cheng S, Rosen BD, Carvalho B, Nasir K, McClelland R, Hundley G, Pearson G, O'Leary DH, Bluemke DA, Lima JAC. Arterial stiffness is associated with regional ventricular systolic and diastolic dysfunction: The Multi-Ethnic Study of Atherosclerosis. Arterioscler Thromb Vasc Biol. 2008;28:194–201.
31. Borlaug BA, Paulus WJ. Heart failure with preserved ejection fraction: pathophysiology, diagnosis and treatment. Eur Heart J. 2011;32:670–9.
32. Haider AW, Larson MG, Franklin SS, Levy D. Systolic blood pressure, diastolic blood pressure and pulse pressure as predictors of risk for congestive heart failure in the Framingham Heart Study. Ann Intern Med. 2003;138:10–6.
33. Chae CU, Pfeffer MA, Glynn RJ, Mitchell GF, Taylor JO, Hennekens CH. Increased pulse pressure and risk of heart failure in the elderly. JAMA. 1999;281:634–9.
34. Vaccarino V, Holfrod TR, Krumholz HM. Pulse pressure and risk of myocardial infarction and heart failure in the elderly. J Am Coll Cardiol. 2000;36:130–8.
35. Kostis JB, Lawrence-Nelson J, Ranjan R, Wilson AC, Kostis WJ, Lacy CR. Association of increased pulse pressure with the development of heart failure in SHEP. Am J Hypertens. 2001;14:798–803.
36. Domanski MJ, Mitchell GF, Normal JE, Exner DV, Pitt B, Pfeffer MA. Independent prognostic information provided by sphygmomanometrically determined pulse pressure and mean arterial pressure in patients with left ventricular dysfunction. J Am Coll Cardiol. 1999;33:951–8.

37. Tartière J-M, Logaert D, Safar M, Cohen-Solal A. Interaction between pulse wave velocity, augmentation index, pulse pressure and left ventricular function in chronic heart failure. J Hum Hypertens. 2006;20:213–9.
38. Kawaguchi M, Hay I, Fetics B, Kass DA. Combined ventricular systolic and arterial stiffening in patients with heart failure and preserved ejection fraction: implications for systolic and diastolic reserve limitations. Circulation. 2003;107:714–20.
39. Lam CSP, Roger VL, Rodeheffer RJ, Bursi F, Borlaug BA, Ommen SR, Kass DA, Redfield MM. Cardiac structure and ventricular-vascular function in persons with heart failure and preserved ejection fraction from Olmsted County, Minnesota. Circulation. 2007;115: 1982–90.
40. Weber T, Auer J, O'Rourke MF, Punzengruber C, Kvas E, Eber B. Prolonged mechanical systole and increased arterial wave reflections in diastolic dysfunction. Heart. 2006;92:1616–22.
41. Weber T, Wassertheurer S, O'Rourke MF, Haiden A, Zweiker R, Rammer M, Hametner B, Eber B. Pulsatile hemodynamics in patients with exertional dyspnea: potentially of value in the diagnostic evaluation of suspected heart failure with preserved ejection fraction. J Am Coll Cardiol. 2013;61:1874–83.
42. Tartière-Kesri L, Tartière J-M, Logeart D, Beauvais F, Cohen SA. Increased proximal arterial stiffness and cardiac response with moderate exercise in patients with heart failure and preserved ejection fraction. J Am Coll Cardiol. 2012;59:455–61.
43. Holland DJ, Sacre JW, Leano RL, Marwick TH, Sharman JE. Contribution of abnormal central blood pressure to left ventricular filling pressure during exercise in patients with heart failure and preserved ejection fraction. J Hypertens. 2011;29: 1422–30.
44. Hundley WG, Kitzman DW, Morgan TM, Hamilton CA, Darty SN, Stewart KP, Herrington DM, Link KM, Little WC. Cardiac cycle-dependent changes in aortic area and distensibility are reduced in older patients with isolated diastolic heart failure and correlate with exercise intolerance. J Am Coll Cardiol. 2001;38:796–802.

25 The Relationship Between Aortic Stiffness, Microvascular Disease in the Brain and Cognitive Decline: Insights into the Emerging Epidemic of Alzheimer's Disease

Angelo Scuteri, Jonathan Stone, and Michael F. O'Rourke

Abstract

The leading current hypothesis of age-related dementia (Alzheimer's disease) considers this a consequence of the beta-amyloid peptide or of the intracellular skeletal protein tau, causing breakdown of the cerebral capillary bed. External trauma to the head in boxing and football is known to induce similar dementia (*dementia pugilistica*, chronic traumatic encephalopathy), usually showing onset years after the individual's retirement from active sport. At autopsy in *dementia pugilistica*, haemorrhage from cerebral vessels is prominent. This presentation reviews evidence that age-related dementia (ARD) is caused by internal trauma to vascular bed of the brain, by the pulse itself. Between the ages of 50 and 80 years, the heart beats ~10^9 times and, because of the low impedance of the cerebral circulation, each pulse penetrates to the cerebral veins. Further, the stiffness of the walls of the aorta and great arteries increases with age; and the amplitude of the pressure pulse in cerebral vessels (a measure of the cerebral pulse intensity) increases several fold. This pounding of cerebral vessels by the pulse induces (we argue) haemorrhages from cerebral vessels. When the vessel that haemorrhages is large, the patient may display symptoms of stroke and any resulting dementia is designated 'vascular'. When the vessels that haemorrhage are small (capillaries), the patient may experience no acute symptoms; but the cumulative effect of many such haemorrhages becomes evident as loss of memory and of cognition. The pathologies which Alzheimer described in the demented brain (senile

A. Scuteri, MD, PhD
School of Geriatrics – Faculty of Medicine, University of Rome Tor Vergata, Rome, 18-00173, Italy
e-mail: afgeloelefante@interfree.it

J. Stone, BSc (Med), PhD, DSc
Department of Physiology, Bosch Institute, University of Sydney F 13, Sydney, NSW 2006, Australia
e-mail: jonathanstone@sydney.edu.aux

M.F. O'Rourke, MD, DSc (✉)
Department of Cardiovascular and Hypertension, St Vincent's Clinic, University of New South Wales, Victor Chang Cardiac Research Institute, Suite 810 St Vincent Clinic, 438 Victoria Street, Darlinghurst, Sydney, NSW 2010, Australia
e-mail: m.orourke@unsw.edu.au

M.E. Safar et al. (eds.), *Blood Pressure and Arterial Wall Mechanics in Cardiovascular Diseases*, DOI 10.1007/978-1-4471-5198-2_25,

plaques, neurofibrillary tangles and inflammation) occur, we argue, as a result of haemorrhage. The age at which dementia becomes evident is determined by the fragility of cerebral vessels, which may vary between individuals with genetic and lifestyle factors. The hypothesis accounts better than previous proposals for the greatest risk factor for dementia – age.

Keywords
Wave reflection • Dementia • Augmentation index • Pulse wave analysis

Introduction

Just over 100 years ago, Dr. Alois Alzheimer, a German neurologist, described a form of dementia in older persons which was not associated with any macrovascular disease, infarction nor haemorrhage within the cranium, nor with any other cerebral pathology [1, 2]. But it was associated with diffuse arteriosclerosis – generalised dilation and stiffening of the aorta and major elastic arteries elsewhere in the body. William Osler in his contemporary (1906) textbook [3] had referred to this generalised aging arterial disease as "senile arteriosclerosis" and distinguished this from "nodular arteriosclerosis", which we now call "atherosclerosis", emphasising that the former is generalised, associated with dilation and stiffening of major arteries, and with "hardness" of the pulse, while the latter is localised, and causes clinical problems through narrowing or obstruction of smaller predominantly muscular arteries ([4], Table 25.1). Alzheimer did note characteristic histological lesions of plaque and tangles, together with evidence of local inflammation in the white matter of the brain, but he had no reason to consider that these may be the aftermath of any vascular disease. His protégé Kracapetin [5] and others agreed with him [6, 7]. By the 1980s, when incidence of this condition was increasing, attention had switched to the plaques and their beta amyloid content [8, 9] as a primary cause of this condition, and moved further away from vascular disease; the beta amyloid material became a principal research focus as a cause of Alzheimer's disease [8–10]. Senile arteriosclerosis was usually considered to be an innocent bystander, and elevation of systolic pressure, irrelevant. However, hypertension including elevated systolic blood pressure alone (isolated systolic hypertension (ISH)) had increasingly been recognised as a cause of cerebral microvascular disease [11–15] and specific cerebral and renal lesions were described in acute hypertensive crisis [16], as well as in longstanding hypertension [12, 14]. These as well as small asymptomatic lacunar infarcts [11] and micro bleeds [6, 10, 11] were noted in older persons without dementia, while other lesions (white matter hyperintensities) ([6, 11, 17], Fig. 25.1a) were seen more frequently, even in magnetic resonance imaging (MRI) scans of apparently normal older subjects. These were considered to be areas of probable cerebral ischemia and were described initially as "leukoaraiosis" [6, 11]. They were associated with high flow pulsations detected by MRI in adjacent arteries (and venules)

Table 25.1 Contrasts of Atherosclerosis with "Senile" Arteriosclerosis

	Atherosclerosis	Arteriosclerosis
Site	Localised	Generalised
Location in artery	Predominantly intima	Media
Effect on lumen	Narrowed	Distended
Effect on tissue beyond	Ischaemia	Higher pulsations
Effect on tissue upstream	Trivial	Marked ↑ pulse pressure ↑ LV load Cardiac failure Small vessel disease Brain Kidney
Artery type	Predominantly medium sized, muscular arteries	Predominantly large (aorta and elastic) arteries

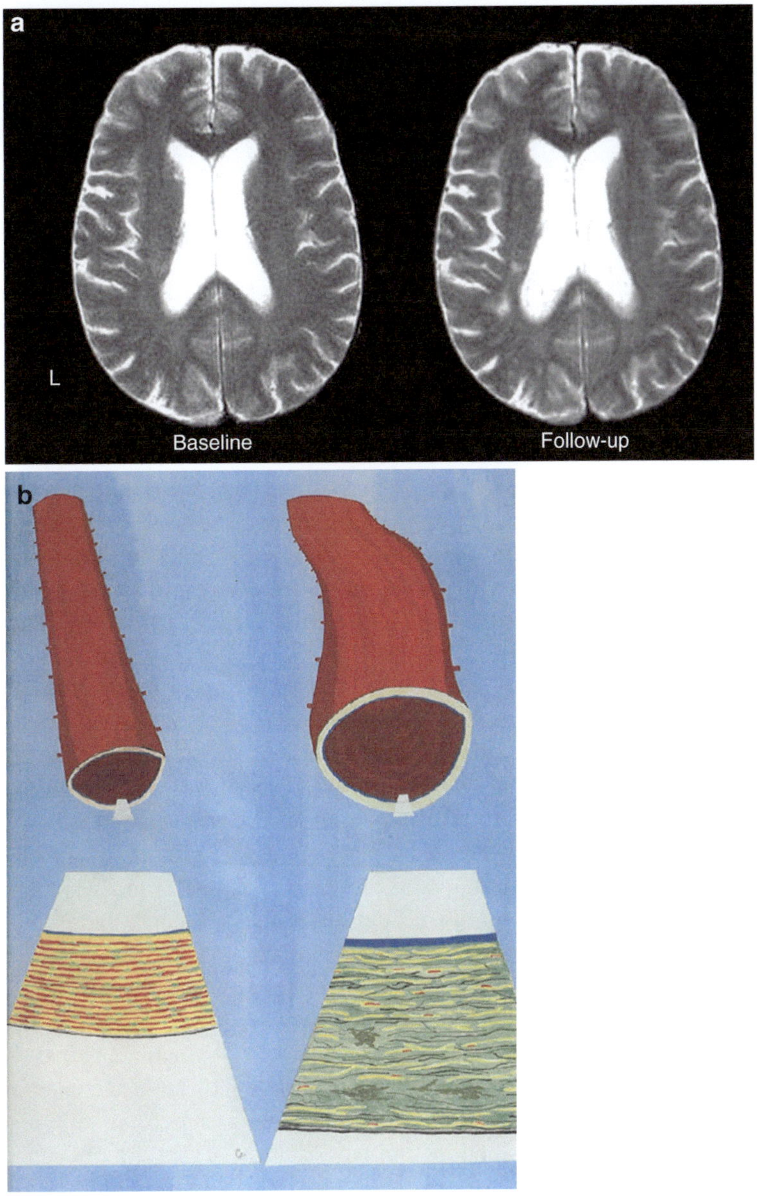

Fig. 25.1 (**a**) Brain MRI showing baseline MRI examination of a patient (*left*). On the *right panel*, the image was recorded at the end of the follow-up on the same patient during PROGRESS study, showing new lesions (white matter hyperintensities) close to the left occipital horn (Reproduced with permission from Ref. [69]). (**b**) Young (*left*) and old (*right*) aorta, with histological structure of the wall of each shown below. In the older aorta, the orderly structure and arrangement of elastic lamellae is disorganised (After Glagov S, personal communications. 1996 From Ref. [42])

[17–21], and the lesions were dubbed as evidence of "pulse wave encephalopathy" by neuroradiologists [19–21]. While white matter hyperintensities were surprisingly common in MRI studies of apparently normal older persons [17], they were more plentiful and extensive in patients with Alzheimer's disease, and were predictive of the development of Alzheimer's disease onset up to 20 or more years later [6, 11]. Over the last 40 years, the line between Alzheimer's disease and vascular dementia has become progressively blurred. Reviewers refer to the "Alzheimerisation" of dementia [6]. The plaques and tangles described by Alzheimer appear to correspond to the "white matter hyperintensities/leucoaurosis/pulse wave encephalopathy" and to be a consequence of microvascular disease, and the cause of dementia through disruption of neural cells and pathways [22–28]. But they are not characteristic of vascular disease of any other organ, even in the kidney where high pressure and flow waveforms are known to enter the afferent, and the efferent arteries [4]. Kidney function does decline progressively with age, and to a greater degree than other organs; this is discussed in Chaps. 9, 10, 11, 12, 13, 14, 15, 16, 17, 18, and 19 of this book, and is mentioned later in this chapter.

In this review, we argue that Alzheimer's disease as described by him, is caused by stiffening of major arteries outside the cranium, and is attributable to the sheer magnitude of high pressure and flow pulsations in delicate cerebral microvascular network over many years. Our arguments can be summarised as:

1. Alzheimer was prescient. Senile dementia is not just associated with "senile" arteriosclerosis outside the brain and cranium, but may be indirectly caused by this.
2. The cerebral lesions seen in Alzheimer's disease are a consequence of gross aortic stiffening causing three to four-fold increase in cerebral artery pressure pulsations between age 20–80 years of age, with a lesser increase in pulsatile flow velocity.
3. The root cause of microvascular lesions in Alzheimer's disease is the same as that which contributes to aneurysms in the thoracic aorta and other systemic arteries, to isolated systolic hypertension, and to left ventricular hypertrophy and left ventricular failure in the elderly. Hence the close association between these conditions and Alzheimer's disease.
4. The cause of cerebral vascular lesions is the repetitive pounding of the pulse on the fragile microvascular media causing high tensile stretch and eventual rupture of the media with micro haemorrhages, and with high pulsatile shear stress on the intima, causing cellular detachment and disruption, thrombosis and micro infarction.
5. The high stresses and consequent lesions seen in the brain of patients with Alzheimer's disease are similar to those seen in competitive athletes and boxers (dementia pugilistica) and which are explicable on the basis of repetitive external trauma.
6. As with arteriosclerotic disease and complications of ISH elsewhere, Alzheimer's disease cannot be cured, but can be delayed by use of drugs which appear to improve arterial elasticity through reducing wave reflection into the brain from arterial terminations in the lower part of the body.
7. In Alzheimer's disease, the brain is destroyed internally by the pulse, just as in dementia pugilistica, the brain is "destroyed by the punch" i.e. by repeated external trauma, over many years.

Epidemiology

The present world-wide epidemic in developed and developing countries is of Alzheimer's disease. This affects 5 % of persons over age 60, and 45 % of those over 80 years [27, 28] in the USA. When fully developed, individuals with the condition require expensive commitment of time and resources from family and society, and eventually, institutional care. The condition is destructive to spouses and family, deeply distressing to all, and has no cure.

The condition when fully developed is often associated with frailty and physical decline from co-existing disease or neglect of food and activity. It has been known for centuries and was described by Shakespeare as the last two of the "Seven Ages of Man" where the active wise judge in the fifth age of life slips into ".... the world too wide for his shrunk shank", then to "second childishness and mere oblivion, sans teeth, sans eyes .... sans everything".

Alzheimer's disease develops slowly during later life, and is usually preceded by the subtle symptoms that are so common that they are predictable and taken for granted in business, in the church, in military service, in academic life. These are of cognitive executive and intellectual decline with age. This is the reason for retirement after a busy life irrespective of physical prowess or organic disease. It is the reason for succession cycle planning in the military, in politics, in business and families – in all walks of life. Onset of cognitive decline is insidious and was referred to by William Osler [29] in 1905 to be first apparent as impaired flexibility of thought from the age of around 40 years in his essay on "The Fixed Period", delivered as a valedictory address on his departure from Johns Hopkins in Baltimore to the Regius' Chair in Oxford UK at age 55.

The earlier epidemic of coronary atherosclerosis reached its peak in Western societies around

1968, and has been steadily falling ever since [30–32] as a consequence of risk factor identification and management – of smoking, elevated blood pressure, glucose intolerance, lifestyle. Treatment of established coronary disease has played a lesser part – with anti-platelet drugs, cholesterol lowering agents, revascularisation and better management of cardiac arrest outside hospital, and of risk factors for coronary disease progression, including aggressive treatment of high blood pressure. But just as atherosclerotic disease has been reduced in Western countries, another problem has emerged – an epidemic of cardiac failure in older persons with stiffened aorta and isolated systolic hypertension (ISH) ([33–38], Fig. 25.1b). At least half of these persons do not have ventricular scarring and impaired left ventricular (LV) contractility as cause of failure, but they do have prior ISH as a consequence of aortic stiffening and often have left ventricular hypertrophy [34, 35]. Hypertension appears to be the major risk factor for cardiac failure [33, 34], and to be a consequence of aortic stiffening with age i.e. the cardiomyopathy of overload described by Katz [38]. Symptomatic heart failure is preceded by reduction of exercise capacity which Sir James Mackenzie, father of cardiology in the English speaking world described in 1903 as due to cardiac impairment from aortic stiffening, and to be in evidence from the fourth decade of life ([39], Fig 25.2a). However, in China and Japan, and in other Eastern countries which have been spared from the worst of the atherosclerotic epidemic, the epidemic of dementia appears to be of similar size and severity as that of cardiac failure. Both appear to have the same common source – aging, aortic stiffening and ISH (Fig. 25.2a).

ISH in the elderly has been treated aggressively around the world since the SHEP study was published in 2001 [37] and showed that complications of ISH including heart failure and stroke can be prevented in persons over 60 years of age. If our thesis is correct, age adjusted incidence of dementia would be expected to fall now, 23 years after SHEP was published, and confirmed by similar studies in Europe and China for persons over 60 years. There are suggestions that this is apparent now [6, 40, 41].

In this chapter we pursue the view that Alzheimer's disease is the end result of an aging process that merges into a disease process as the human body comes to outlive the age required by evolutionary processes for propagation of the species. This is the same view pressed elsewhere for ISH and its cause of disease outside the cranium (Fig. 25.2).

Aging: Primary Changes in Cells or Non-cellular Components?

Changes of aging within the body appear to be most marked in its non living components. These non living components are relatively inert and have long half life in the body [4, 42] but they degenerate with age as a consequence of cyclic or periodic stress and comprise elastin in arteries and the skin, hairs of the body, the lens of the eye, cartilage in joints, bones and vertebrae, and are influenced by other physical factors such as the effect of sunlight on the skin. Cells of the body may involute through apoptosis, die, or suffer catastrophic mutation with development of cancer, but most appear to function independently of age and last for long periods, perhaps for life. The germ cells certainly remain normal with age, and with few unusual exceptions, the body of a new baby is not affected by the age of the mother (within the reproductive period) or the father up to his age of even 100 years. We believe it reasonable to progress in this chapter on the principle that aging change of non-living components of the human body is probably responsible for arteriosclerosis, and for the initial extra cranial arterial deterioration which results in Alzheimer's disease [1, 4, 42].

Aging and Cardiovascular Function

The arterial system in young humans is beautifully suited for its functions of cushion and conduit – of receiving spurts of blood from the intermittently-ejecting left ventricle and delivering this in a near-steady stream into the peripheral arterioles and capillaries, according to need [4]. The arterial system is "tuned" to the heart in

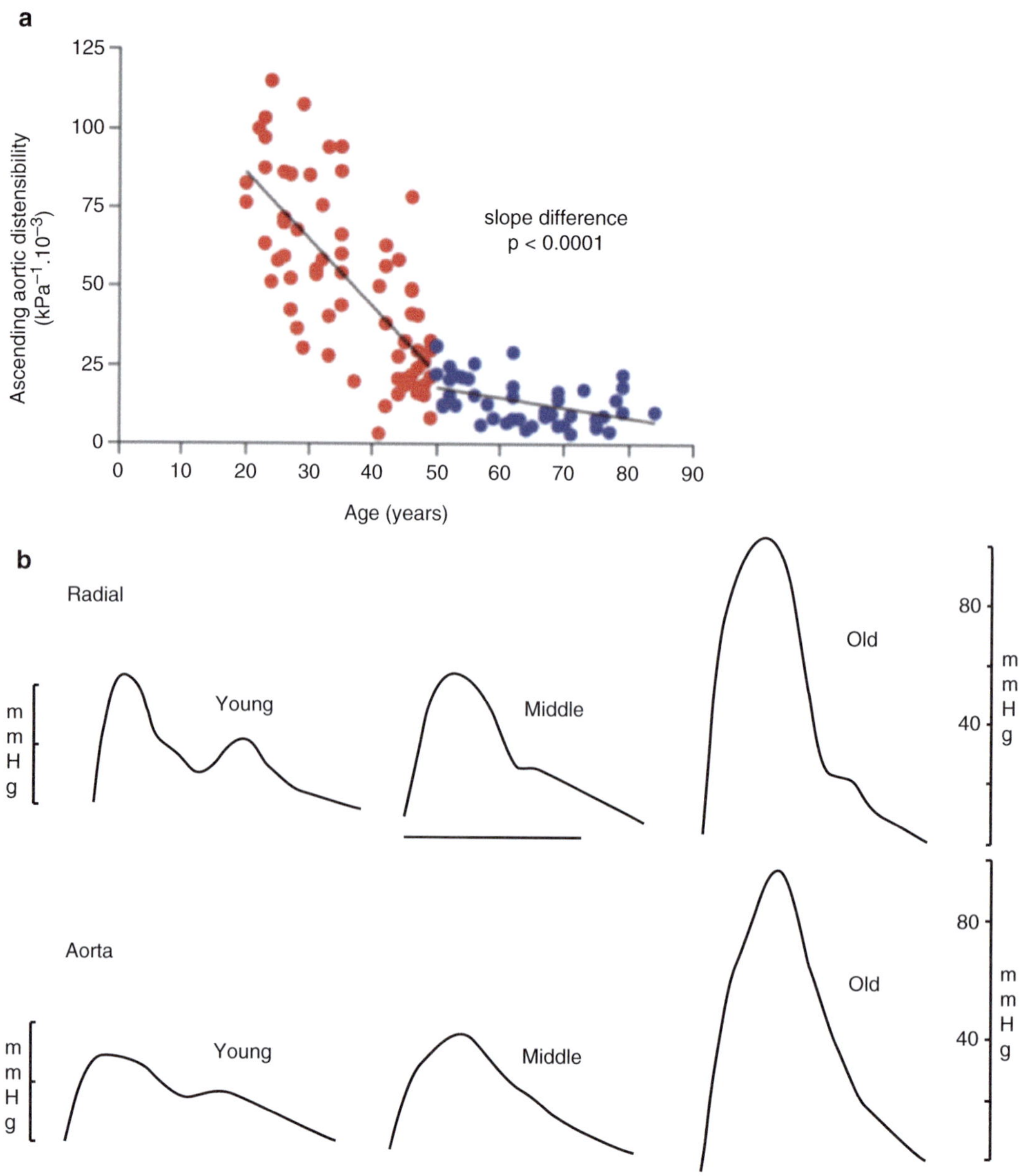

Fig. 25.2 (**a**) Change in ascending aortic distensiblity with age (Reproduced with permission from Ref. [46]). (**b**) Typical pressure waveforms in the arm (*top*) and aorta (*below*) in three women of the same family – 18 year old at *left*, 48 year old (*center*), and 97 year old at *right*. Time calibration 1.0 s (From Ref. [42]). Pulse pressure is increased almost four-fold in the ascending aorta and two-fold in the upper limb

such a way as to present minimal impedance to pulsatile ejection at normal heart rate frequency [4, 42–45]. Such tuning depends on the distensibility of the aorta and on other physical factors [43] especially timing of wave reflection. Tuning is optimal in adolescence [42], but deteriorates with age thereafter as a consequence of fatigue and fracture of elastic fibres in the highly distensible aorta [4, 42]. From around age 40 (Osler's age for beginning senescence [29] and

Mackenzie's age for onset of arteriosclerosis [39], stiffening of the aorta ([4, 42], Fig. 25.2b) leads to progressive detuning such that pulse pressure increases markedly with each beat of the heart to some three time greater than seen in youth [42], and with marked increase in the pulsatile component of pressure and flow into highly perfused organs such as the brain and kidney [18, 45].

These changes with age are underestimated by traditional consideration of brachial sphygmomanometric systolic and diastolic pressures [40], but are revealed by consideration of pulsatile pressure and flow waves in extra cranial arteries such as the aorta, and carotid artery, as well as the intracranial arteries [46–51].

Deterioration in Optimising Features with Age

The principal role of the arterial system is to transmit blood to peripheral tissues according to their need – i.e. to act as a conduit. There is no aging process that impairs conduit flow of blood from the LV to tissues of the body. Conduit flow decrease with age appears to be secondary, and can usually be attributed to atrophy or apoptosis and consequent rarification of the capillary bed of various organs [39]. However cushioning function is markedly impaired by aging, and this can be explained on the basis of fatigue and fracture of elastin fibres in the proximal thoracic aorta, which in youth is considered responsible for 70–80 % of the total arterial buffering function ([4, 18, 42], Fig. 25.3a). In childhood and adolescence, the proximal thoracic aorta expands by approximately 20 % of its total diameter with each beat of the heart. Peripheral arteries such as the brachial, radial, femoral expand by <5 % [52]. Repetitive expansion with each beat of the heart, some 40 million times per year causes change in crystalline structure of non-living elastin fibres, as it does to natural rubber, formed from the sap of trees (Fig. 25.3). The median number of cycles to fracture of such physical materials is determined by the strain (or extent of deformation with each cycle of stress), and the number of cycles. The relationship between strain (S) and number of cycles (N) at the time of fracture can be described as S/N semi-logarithmic curves. Such relationship between S and N for natural rubber is shown in Fig. 25.3b [4]. If this is applied to the elastin in the proximal aorta, fracture would be expected by 30 years of age for the heart beating some 70 times per minute and the aorta expanding by 10–20 % with each beat of the heart [4, 42].

Fracture of elastin fibres can account for the progressive degeneration of the proximal aorta with age. Because the aorta is so "elastic" and pulsates so much, it is subject to earlier degeneration than peripheral arteries which pulsate by <5 %, and would not be expected to show elastin fibre fracture within a life span of 100 years. The fracture of elastin fibres in the aorta does not occur all at once, but progressively, causing the artery to dilate, and to stiffen as stress is transferred to collagenous fibres in the wall. The dilated, stiffened aorta, pulsates far less in later years, and this, rather than catastrophic rupture, is the cause of altered function seen with aging – the increased characteristic impedance, increased pulse wave velocity, increased pulse pressure, and earlier return of reflected waves from peripheral sites. The underlying structural cause is readily apparent in the aortic wall itself – with fractured and frayed elastin fibres, and disorganisation of the orderly architecture of the youthful aorta ([42], Fig. 25.1b).

Progressive stiffening of the thoracic aorta causes other ill-effects on highly perfused vascular beds such as the brain and kidney [18, 22, 48]. These are described below, and are a direct consequence of impaired cushioning function. If pulsations generated by the heart cannot be absorbed by the normal aorta or other arteries and if they are not transmitted through the bed into the central veins and right atrium, they must be absorbed elsewhere in the microvasculature. The most susceptible organs would be those with the highest blood flow and lowest resistance – ie. the brain and kidneys.

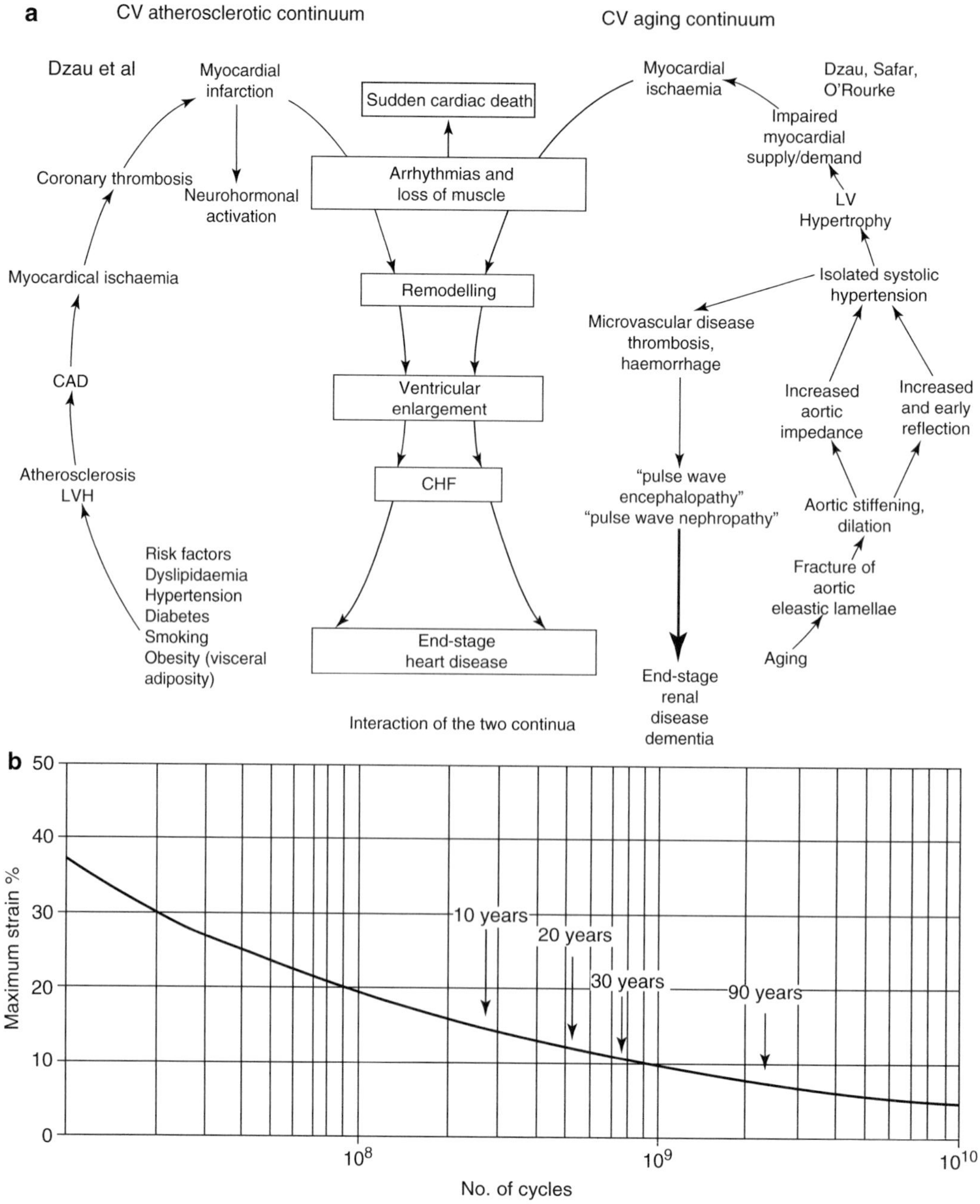

Fig. 25.3 (**a**) The cardiovascular continuum for coronary atherosclerotic disease as proposed by Dzau et al. in 2006 (*left*) and its relationship to the arteriosclerotic aging continuum proposed by O'Rourke, Safar and Dzau in 2010 (Ref. [75]). The former is based on development of end-stage heart disease from atherosclerosis and conventional risk factors, while the latter describes the same end result as a consequence of aging and aortic degeneration. The aging continuum includes development of microvascular disease in brain and kidney, as cause of dementia and end-stage renal disease (Reproduced with permission from Ref. [75]). (**b**) The relationship between pulsatile strain (linear scales, ordinate) and number of pulsatile cycles (abscissa, logarithmic scale) for elastin fibre fracture in human arteries (assuming similarity between aorta and natural rubber). With pulsations of 15 %, fracture will be seen from 10 years (corresponding to 200 million cycles); with pulsation of 10 % at just over 30 years, and for 5 %, well beyond 100 years (From Ref. [42])

Particular Features of the Cerebral Circulation

Blood supply to the brain is through the internal carotid and vertebral arteries. The former enters the cranium through the carotid canal in the skull and the latter through the foramen magnum after traversing canals in cervical vertebrae. The vertebral arteries join to form the basilar artery, then through communicating arteries, with the two carotid arteries to form the circle of Willis, from which arise the right and left anterior, middle, and posterior cerebral vessels. Venous blood leaves the brain parenchymal into the venous sinuses. All coalesce to form the transverse sinuses which become the internal jugular veins as they leave the skull. In the neck, the internal jugular vein is partially collapsed when the subject is upright so that pressure is near atmospheric unless right atrial pressure is elevated from cardiac failure, other disease, or in physiological activities (coughing, straining, swimming).

Blood supply to the brain is high and continuous. Cessation of blood flow causes unconsciousness within seconds and irreversible damage within minutes. The venous flow exiting the skull has relatively low oxygen saturation (around 38 %), whereas arterial blood is nearly 100 % saturated. Blood flow to the brain is high – approximately 0.75 L per minute or around 0.54 L per kg/min (compared to around one eighth of this to the rest of the body at rest (0.07 L/kg/min)). The high rate of perfusion and of oxygen extraction from blood flowing through the brain is a consequence of its high metabolic rate, and this for function of its neural circuitry and the supporting functions of its neuroglia. The high and sustained cerebral mean flow perfusion is achieved by auto regulation – with metabolites contributing to arterial dilation, and with arterial pressure and flow maintained by the carotid and aortic baroreceptors through nervous and hormonal action on the heart and blood vessels in other tissues throughout the body. Sympathetic activity has little influence on calibre of cerebral arteries.

The brain and its blood vessels are contained within the rigid skull which protects the brain from external trauma. The rigid skull can create disordered cerebral perfusion, when the brain is damaged or swollen. These issues are not considered in this paper, but they are extremely important following head injury or stroke. They are considered elsewhere [48–53].

Pressures waves in the ascending aorta are similar to those in the carotid artery, so much so that the carotid pulse is often regarded as a surrogate of the aortic pulse. Pressure waves in the aorta are however quite different from the brachial and radial pulse as a consequence of distortion during transmission down the upper limb. A generalised transfer function can be used to compensate for this upper limb distortion, and so to generate the aortic (or carotid) pulse from that recorded invasively or non-invasively at the wrist [4].

Pressure waves cannot be recorded within the skull unless a catheter is advanced through the carotid or vertebral arteries. What data as are available show that the aortic, carotid, and intracranial pressure waves are normally very similar in amplitude and shape when intracranial pressure is normal (around atmospheric). Flow waves can be recorded by transcranial Doppler techniques in the above named cerebral arteries within the skull, and in the carotid (usually common carotid) artery in the neck. Using the above techniques, we have with Japanese and Chinese colleagues [48–51, 53] measured flow waves and calculated pressure waves at different ages in over 1,000 normal subjects and in over 100 patients with cardiovascular disease.

We have confirmed that amplitude of the pressure pulse in cerebral arteries increases approximately two-fold from that measured in the arm, and around three-fold from that measured in the aorta between age 20 and 80 years of age (Fig. 25.2). We have shown lesser increase (up to 20 %) in the carotid or cerebral artery flow waveforms over this age span. We have shown that both the pressure and flow waveforms are altered in similar fashion, as a consequence of wave reflection from the trunk and lower limbs, and that in older persons, the peak of both pressure and flow waves is created by the reflected wave from the lower body and can be reduced by nitrate therapy [48, 49]. These findings have been supplemented by data obtained acutely in neurological intensive care wards; all support the comments made here on chronic pathophysiology of cerebral vascular lesions. The data we have obtained in normal subjects show that cerebrovascular impedance is normally low, with characteristic impedance modulus approximately 30 % of impedance modulus at zero frequency (resistance) and with calculated reflection coefficient in the bed approximately 40 % [53]. This compares with around 90 % in the femoral vascular bed at rest, and 20 % in the kidney and around 15 % in the lung [4]. Cerebral arteries are shorter than arteries of similar size elsewhere in the body so that as a consequence of very high flow, the smaller arteries, arterioles, capillaries and venules are not protected by upstream vasoconstriction, and hence are exposed to high wall tension and shear stress compared to those elsewhere in the systemic circulation. We have shown that cerebrovascular impedance is not different in males and females and does not change with age in normal subjects.

Pathophysiology of Cerebral Microvascular Lesions

We believe that the above considerations can be linked with the observations of Byrom [16] and subsequently at the US National Institutes of Health by Fry [22, 23]. Byrom viewed pial arteries and arterioles through Lucite windows in the skull of rats during various physical and pharmacological pertubations. The most cogent are the effects of increasing arterial pressure in these vessels. Such elevated pressure (acutely or chronically) could cause incomplete tearing of the wall with serum exuding into the wall or red cells escaping from the lumen into the wall or through the wall. Such pertubations could cause complete rupture of the wall or closure of the lumen. Changes in calibre of the artery were seen to occur apparently spontaneously with extreme narrowing or extreme dilation within the same vascular segment [16]. Local pathology was worse in the regions of dilation, indicating that wall tension, being higher at such sites, was responsible for vascular damage. Damage was associated with later infiltration with leukocytes and macrophages in the process of inflammation and repair, showing features identical to those seen in patients with malignant hypertension [16].

Cullen and colleagues [24] and Stone [25, 26] on the basis of pathology and modelling studies have argued that the lesions and plaques and tangles result from micro bleeds, with escape of blood cells through the wall damaged by repeated high pulsations, with the reparative process not completely removing the heme from broken down red cells, and that the heme induces oligomerisation and deposition of beta amyloid in plaques. When formed in the brain, these plaques and tangles described by Alzheimer are not readily able to be associated with previous cumulative vascular damage over years [24, 25]. We cannot exclude the possibility that the beta amyloid would cause further vascular damage from its presence in the brain. Indeed such a phenomenon could explain the progression of dementia after an amyloid plaque had formed in an elderly person, or a pugilist on his retirement from boxing [26]. However, two recently published trials of anti-amyloid beta antibodies, which can clear amyloid plaque from the brain, have not shown benefit in Alzheimer's disease [54, 55]

Comparison of Brain and Kidney Circulation

The kidneys have lower resistance than the brain and receive even more blood flow than the brain – around 3.7 L/kg/min. Venous efflux from the kidney shows relatively high oxygen saturation, as one would expect, since the kidney's function is to filter blood and reabsorb fluid and electrolytes so as to maintain the constancy of the internal environment. Little of the renal blood flow is required to sustain healthy activity of the renal cells. A whole section of this book (Chaps. 9, 10, 11, 12, 13, 14, 15, 16, 17, 18, and 19) is devoted to normal and abnormal renal function. Here we can just note some similarities and differences between the two organs, brain and kidney under normal and abnormal circumstances, and their blood supply, together with changes with age and intrinsic arterial disease.

Renal function deteriorates at least as much with age as cerebral function, but the kidneys do not show the lesions which correspond to white matter hyperintensities in the brain. This [23, 24] may be due to the marked difference in oxygen content of blood within the kidney and brain, and the probability that hypoxia is more readily induced in the brain than in the kidney.

The kidney shows pressure and flow waves similar to those in the cerebral arteries. Its impedance and resistive index do increase with age [55, 56]. Lesions of fibrinoid necrosis are seen just as in the brain with acute elevation of arterial pressure, and chronic arterial changes with age and hypertension appear to be more extensive. More comparative studies need to be undertaken on this subject.

Clinical Evaluation and Management: The Ideal Approach

The first and greatest clinical implications of the pathophysiological and epidemiological data presented above is that each and every middle-age or older subject with high CV risk and/or evidence of stiffer and thicker large artery should be screened for cognitive function and followed-up for cognitive deterioration. Subjective symptoms and their onset should be recorded, including cognitive, behavioral symptom, and gait problems. Vascular patients should be asked, as part of the routine clinical examination, whether they have recently experienced changes in memory, speed of thinking and acting, or mood, or slowliness or unsteadiness during walking.

In that regard, future clinical guidelines should make clear that cognitive impairment has to be considered and assessed as target-organ damage in hypertensive subjects, though it has been mentioned in the most recent one from European Society of Hypertension [57].

How to assess large artery properties in clinical practice has already been established [58, 59]. So at least three major areas remain to be better investigated and require a more standardized approach to make research findings quickly transferable to clinical practice: (i) neuropsychological characterization of microvascular brain damage; (ii) specific findings on neuroimaging; (iii) effect of pharmacologic treatment on microvascular brain damage.

A major and yet unsolved issue concerns whether there are cognitive domains specifically affected by microvascular brain damage and if they differ from those more commonly detected in age-associated cognitive decline or in Alzheimer's type dementia. Though microvascular brain lesion are commonly detected in subjects with Alzheimer's type dementia [60], it is a general hypothesis that microvascular brain damage electively and predominantly affects executive function, with a slower information processing, impairments in the ability to shift from one task to another, and deficits in the ability to hold and manipulate information (i.e., working memory) [61–63]. Executive functions cannot be explored by Mini Mental State Examination (MMSE), the most widely adopted test for clinical screening of global cognitive function; in fact, its 3-word recall items is scarcely sensitive [64].

Ideally, neuropsychological evaluation should include tests exploring multiple cognitive domains (executive function and activation, language, visuospatial ability, memory) – in addition to neurobehavioural symptoms and mood. Efforts are made to identify whether one brief test can provide useful insight into different domains, anatomical regions, and brain networks [65–68].

Though it is a more specialistic issue, clinicians should be aware of the complexity of the question and of the availability of neuropsychological tests to explore more in depth cognition in patients. Further, working groups of medical and scientific societies should propose a common, minimal, examination in order to detect and follow-up patients on these consequences which may be subtle at their outset and could be unmasked during repetitive examination.

Logic of Prevention

In this chapter we argue that an irreversible problem – degeneration of the elastic properties of the aorta and large arteries – is responsible for microvascular disease in the brain, and for age-related dementia. While aging of arteries will continue as long as the heart beats, there are some reasons for optimism. The favoured drugs for treatment of hypertension (ACEIs, ARBs, CCBs, Renin antagonists, nitrates) have the effect of reducing wave reflection from the trunk and lower limbs and these can offset a major ill effect of large artery stiffening [4, 42, 49]. Use of such drugs can decrease amplitude of pulse pressure and of pulsatile flow in central arteries by up to 50 % [4, 48, Chaps. 41 and 43]. In the PROGRESS trial [69], use of an ACEI/diuretic combination reduced substantially the progression of white matter hyperintensities over a 3 year period, compared to placebo. Studies from England and the US provide evidence that the age adjusted incidence of dementia is declining [40]; this is what we would expect from the basic principles described here on which modern cardiovascular medicine is based [70, Chap. 19].

The studies and considerations presented here provide another reason to physicians, and further motivation to patients for high blood pressure to be recognised and treated from middle age in the majority of the older population with drugs (i.e. those with systolic blood pressure persistently over 140 mmHg by cuff, or 130 mmHg as calculated for central aortic pressure [71], with the conventional drugs which reduce wave reflection. While recent studies encourage reduction in blood pressure to prevent cerebral lesions, older patients with stiffened aorta and known brain lesions may show more rapid memory deterioration if they develop postural hypotension [72]. Such findings support the more moderate views for treatment of elderly persons with hypertension in most recent guidelines [57, 73, 74]. Hope remains in Pandora's Box of cerebral small vessel disease in the elderly, despite negative findings for new drugs designed to clear amyloid beta from the brain [54, 55].

Funding JS was supported by the Sir Zelman Cowen Universities Fund

Declaration JS is Director of CSCM Pty Ltd

References

1. Alzeheimer A. Uber eine eigenartige Erkrankung der Himrinde. Allgemeine Zeitschrift Psychiatrie Psychisch-Gerichtliche Medizin. 1907;64:146–8.
2. Alzheimer A. Uber eigenartige Krankheitsfalle des spateren Alters. Zbl ges Neurol Psychiat. 1911;4:356–85.
3. Osler W. The principles and practice of medicine. 6th ed. New York: Appleton; 1906. p. 848–52.
4. Nichols WW, O'Rourke MF, Vlachopoulos C. McDonald's blood flow in arteries. 6th ed. London: Arnold Hodder; 2011. p. 411–6, 499–6.
5. Kraepelin E. Senile and pre-senile dementias. In: Psychiatrie: ein Lehrbuch fur Studierende und Arzte. Leipzig: Johann Ambrosius Barth; 1910. p. 553–632.
6. Iadecola C. The pathobiology of vascular dementia. Neuron. 2013;80:844–66.
7. Bowler JV. Modern concept of vascular or cognitive dementia. Br Med Bull. 2007;83:291–305.
8. Kang J, Lemaire HG, Unterbeck A, et al. The precursor of Alzheimer's disease amyloid A4 protein resembles a cell surface receptor. Nature. 1987;325:733–6.
9. Glenner GG, Wong CW. Alzheimer's Disease: medical report on the purification and characterisation of a novel cerebrovascular amyloid protein. Biochem Biophys Res Commun. 1984;120:885–90.
10. Ropper M. Two centuries of neurology and psychiatry. N Engl J Med. 2012;367:58–65.
11. Gorelick PB, Scuteri A, Black SE, et al. Vascular contributions to cognitive impairment and dementia: a statement for health care professionals from the American Heart Association/American Stroke Association. Stroke. 2011;42:2671–713.
12. Fischer LCM. Lacunar strokes and infarcts: a review. Neurology. 1982;32:871–6.
13. Pickering G. High blood pressure. London: Churchill; 1968.
14. Russell RW. How does blood pressure cause stroke? Lancet. 1975;2:1283–5.
15. Greenberg SM. Small Vessels, big problems. N Engl J Med. 2006;354:1451–3.
16. Byrom F. The hypertensive vascular crisis – an experimental study. London: Heineman; 1969.
17. Verooij M, Ikram MA, Tanghe HL, et al. Incidental findings on brain MRI in the general population. N Engl J Med. 2007;357:1281–8.
18. O'Rourke MF, Safar ME. Hemodynamic basis for the relationship between aortic stiffening and microvascular disease in brain and kidney: implications for treatment. Hypertension. 2005;46:200–4.

19. Henry-Feugeas MC, de Marco G, Peretti II, et al. Age-related cerebral white matter changes and pulse wave encephalopathy: observations with three dimensional MRI. Magn Reson Imaging. 2005;23:929–37.
20. Bateman GA, Levi CR, Schofield P, et al. Quantitative measurement of cerebral hemodynamics in early vascular dementia and Alzheimer's disease. J Clin Neurosci. 2006;13:563–8.
21. Henry-Feugeas MC, Koskas P. Cerebral vascular aging: extending the concept of pulse wave encephalopathy through capillaries to the cerebral veins. Curr Aging Sci. 2012;5:157–67.
22. Fry D. Acute vascular endothelial changes associated with increased blood velocity gradients. Circ Res. 1968;22:165–97.
23. Fry D. Certain histological and chemical response of the vascular interface to acutely induced mechanical stress in the aorta of the dog. Circ Res. 1969;24:93–108.
24. Cullen KM, Kocsi Z, Stone J. Microvascular pathology in the aging human brain: evidence that senile plaques are sites of microhaemorrhages. Neurobiol Aging. 2006;27:1786–96.
25. Cullen KM, Kocsi Z, Stone J. Pericapillary haem-rich deposits: evidence for microhaemorrhages in aging human cerebral cortex. J Cereb Blood Flow Metab. 2005;25:1656–67.
26. Stone J. What initiates the formation of senile plaques? The origin of Alzheimer-like dementias in capillary haemorrhages. Med Hypotheses. 2008;71:347–59.
27. Stone J, O'Rourke MF. ASMR 2013 abstract. The mechanical cause of age-related dementia: the brain is destroyed by the pulse.
28. Herbert LE, Scherr PA, Bienias JL, Bennett DA, Evans DA. Alzheimer's disease in the US population. Arch Neurol. 2003;60:1119–22.
29. Osler W. "The fixed period". In: Hinohara S, Niki H, editors. Osler's way of life. Durham: Duke University Press; 2001. p. 287–304.
30. Thompson PH, Hobbs MST, Martin CA. The rise and fall of ischemic heart disease in Australia. Aust N Z J Med. 1988;18:327–37.
31. Levy D, Thom T. Death rates from coronary disease – progress and a puzzling paradox (editorial). N Engl J Med. 1998;339:915–6.
32. Levy D, Brink S. A change in heart. New York: Vintage; 2005.
33. Levy D, Kenchaiah S, Larson MG, et al. Long-term trends in the incidence and survival with heart failure. N Engl J Med. 2002;347:1397–402.
34. Levy D, Larson MG, Vasan RS, et al. The progression from hypertension to congestive heart failure. JAMA. 1996;275:1557–62.
35. Redfield MM. Heart failure – an epidemic of uncertain proportions. N Engl J Med. 2002;347:1442–4.
36. Redfield MM, Jacobsen SJ, Burnett JC, et al. Burden of systolic and diastolic ventricular dysfunction in the community: appreciating the scope of the heart failure epidemic. JAMA. 2003;289:194–202.
37. Systolic Hypertension in Elderly Program Cooperative Research Group (SHEP). Prevention of stroke by antihypertensive drug treatment in older persons with isolated systolic hypertension: final results of the Systolic Hypertension in the Elderly Program (SHEP). JAMA. 1991;265:3255–64.
38. Katz AM. Cardiomyopathy of overload. N Engl J Med. 1990;322:100–10.
39. Mackenzie J. The study of the pulse: arterial, venous and hepatic, and of the movement of the heart. Edinburgh: Young J Pentland; 1902.
40. Larson EB, Yaffe K, Langa K, et al. New insights into the dementia epidemic. N Engl J Med. 2013;369:2275–8.
41. Scuteri A, Lakatta E. Bringing prevention in geriatrics evidence from cardiovascular medicine supporting the new challenge. Exp Gerontol. 2013;48:64–8.
42. O'Rourke MF, Hashimoto J. Mechanical factors in arterial aging: a clinical perspective. J Am Coll Cardiol. 2007;50:1–13.
43. Taylor MG. The elastic properties of arteries in relation to the physiological functioning of the arterial system. Gastroenterology. 1967;52:358–63.
44. Milnor WR. Hemodynamics. 2nd ed. Baltimore: Williams & Wilkins; 1989.
45. O'Rourke MF. Commentary on: aortic wavelength as a determinant of the relationship between heart rate and body size in mammals. Am J Physiol. 1981;240:R393–5.
46. Redheuil A, Yu W-C, Wu CO, et al. Reduced ascending aortic strain and distensilibity: earlier manifestations of vascular aging in humans. Hypertension. 2010;55:319–26.
47. Scuteri A, Nilsson PM, Tzourio C, Redon J, Laurent S. Microvascular brain damage with aging and hypertension: pathophysiological consideration and clinical implications. J Hypertens. 2011;29:1469–77.
48. Hirata K, Yaginuma T, O'Rourke MF, Kawakami M. Age-related change in the carotid artery flow and pressure pulses implications to cerebral microvascular disease. Stroke. 2006;37:2552–6.
49. Hirata K, O'Rourke MF. Effect of nitrate on the carotid late systolic flow augmentation – a new strategy against stroke. J Hypertens. 2007;25 Suppl 2:S336–7.
50. Hirata K, O'Rourke M, Momomura S. Flow augmentation index as a risk factor for silent lacunar infarction. J Am Coll Cardiol. 2008;51(Suppl A):A303.
51. Xu TY, Staessen JA, Wei FF, et al. Blood flow pattern in the middle cerebral artery in relation to indices of arterial stiffness in the systemic circulation. Am J Hypertens. 2012;25:319–24.
52. Boutouyrie P, Laurent S, Benetos A, et al. Opposing effects of aging on distal and proximal larger arteries in hypertensives. J Hypertens. 1992;10 Suppl 6:S87–91.

53. Kim MO, Li Y, Wei F, Wang J, O'Rourke M, Avolio A. Influence of wave reflection and lower body arterial properties on cerebral perfusion in apparently normal humans. J Hypertens. 2013;31(e-Suppl A):e23.
54. Salloway S, Sperwing R, Fox N, et al. Two phase 3 trials of Bapineuzumab in mild-to-moderate Alzheimer's disease. N Engl J Med. 2014;370:322–33.
55. Doody RS, Thomas RG, Farlow M, et al. Phase 3 trials of Solanezumab for mild-to-moderate Alzheimer's disease. N Engl J Med. 2014;370:311–21.
56. Hashimoto J, Ito S. Central pulse pressure and aortic stiffness determine renal hemodynamics: Pathophysiological implication of micro albuminuria in hypertension. Hypertension. 2011;58:839–46.
57. Mancia G, Fagard R, Narkiewicz K, Redon J, Zanchetti A, Böhm M, et al. 2013 ESH/ESC Guidelines for the management of arterial hypertension: the Task Force for the management of arterial hypertension of the European Society of Hypertension (ESH) and of the European Society of Cardiology (ESC). J Hypertens. 2013;31:1281–357.
58. Nilsson PM, Boutouyrie P, Cunha P, Kotsis V, Narkiewicz K, Parati G, Rietzschel E, Scuteri A, Laurent S. Early vascular aging in translation: from laboratory investigations to clinical applications in cardiovascular prevention. J Hypertens. 2013;31:1517–26.
59. Laurent S, Cockcroft J, Van Bortel L, Boutouyrie P, Giannattasio C, Hayoz D, Pannier B, Vlachopoulos C, Wilkinson I. Struijker-Boudier H; European Network for Non-invasive Investigation of Large Arteries. Expert consensus document on arterial stiffness: methodological issues and clinical applications. Eur Heart J. 2006;27:2588–605.
60. Esiri MM, Wilcock GK, Morris JH. Neuropathological assessment of the lesions of significance in vascular dementia. J Neurol Neurosurg Psychiatry. 1997;63:749–53.
61. Garrett KD, Browndyke JN, Whelihan W, Paul RH, DiCarlo M, Moser DJ, Cohen RA, Ott BR. The neuropsychological profile of vascular cognitive impairment–no dementia: Comparisons to patients at risk for cerebrovascular disease and vascular dementia. Arch Clin Neuropsychol. 2004;19:745–57.
62. Nyenhuis DL, Gorelick PB, Geenen EJ, Smith CA, Gencheva E, Freels S, DeToledo-Morrell L. The pattern of neuropsychological deficits in vascular cognitive impairment-no dementia (vascular CIND). Clin Neuropsychol. 2004;18:41–9.
63. Troyer AK, Moscovitch M, Winocur G, Alexander MP, Stuss D. Clustering and switching on verbal fluency: the effects of focal frontal- and temporal-lobe lesions. Neuropsychologia. 1998;36:499–504.
64. Hachinski V, Iadecola C, Petersen RC, Breteler MM, Nyenhuis DL, Black SE, Powers WJ, DeCarli C, Merino JG, Kalaria RN, Vinters HV, Holtzman DM, Rosenberg GA, Wallin A, Dichgans M, Marler JR, Leblanc GG. National Institute of Neurological Disorders and Stroke-Canadian Stroke Network vascular cognitive impairment harmonization standards. Stroke. 2006;37:2220–41.
65. Carew TG, Lamar M, Cloud BS, Grossman M, Libon DJ. Impairment in category fluency in ischemic vascular dementia. Neuropsychology. 1997;11:400–12.
66. Lamar MPC, Davis KL, Kaplan E, Libon DJ. Capacity to maintain mental set in dementia. Neuropsychologia. 2002;40:435–45.
67. Wechsler D. WAIS-III administration and scoring manual. New York: The Psychological Corporation; 1997.
68. Kaplan E, Fein D, Morris R, Delis D. The WAIS-Rr as a neuropsychological instrument. San Antonio: Psychological Corporation; 1991.
69. Dufouil C, Chalmers J, Coskun O, et al. Effects of blood pressure lowering on cerebral white matter intensitities in patients with stroke. The PROGRESS Magnetic Resonance Imaging Substudy. Circulation. 2005;112:1644–50.
70. Lee TH. Eugene Braunwald and the rise of modern medicine. Cambridge: Harvard; 2013.
71. Cheng HM, Chuang SY, Sung SH, Yu WC, Pearson A, Lakatta EG, Pan WH, Chen CH. Derivation and validation of diagnostic thresholds for central blood pressure measurements based on long-term cardiovascular risks. J Am Coll Cardiol. 2013;62:1780–7.
72. Scuteri A, Tesauro M, Guglini L, Lauro D, Fini M, de Daniele N. Aortic stiffness and hypotension episodes are associated with impaired cognitive function in older subjects with subjective complements of memory loss. Int J Cardiol. 2013;169:371–7.
73. James PA, Oparil S, Carter BL, Cushman WC, Dennison-Himmelfarb C, Handler J, et al. Evidence-Based Guideline for the Management of High Blood Pressure in Adults: Report From the Panel Members Appointed to the Eighth Joint National Committee (JNC 8). JAMA. 2014;18:2013. doi:10.1001/jama.2013.284427.
74. Bauchner H, Fontanarosa PB, Golub RM. Updated guidelines for management of high blood pressure: recommendations, review, and responsibility. JAMA. 2013. doi:10.1001/jama.2013.284432.
75. O'Rourke MF, Safar ME, Dzau V. The cardiovascular continuum extended: aging effects on the aorta and microvasculature. Vasc Med. 2010;15:461–8.

Arterial Stiffness and Risk in Various Cardiovascular Diseases

26

Charalambos Vlachopoulos,
Dimitrios Terentes-Printzios, Kenji Takazawa,
and Christodoulos Stefanadis

Abstract

Atherosclerotic disease comprises four major areas: coronary artery disease, cerebrovascular disease, peripheral arterial disease, and aortic aneurysm. Investigators have mainly focused on using arterial stiffness and central hemodynamics indices for primary prevention and prediction of risk in patients without cardiovascular disease. Their role in these patients is constantly evolving, and in some cases such as hypertensives and diabetics, their clinical significance has been corroborated by recent guidelines and recommendations. Despite the overwhelming data for their predictive role in primary prevention, secondary prevention prognostic studies are lacking. Especially, data on the role of arterial stiffness in peripheral arterial disease patients, including patients with vasculogenic erectile dysfunction or aortic disease such as aortic aneurysm, Marfan syndrome, and coarctation of the aorta, emerge mostly from cross-sectional studies. Respectively, most prospective predictive studies of arterial stiffness have not used peripheral arterial disease or aortic disease endpoints as an exclusive outcome but preferably as a part of a composite cardiovascular endpoint. This chapter will focus on the link between arterial stiffness and risk of cardiovascular events and organ damage in other cardiovascular diseases such as peripheral arterial and aortic diseases.

Keywords

Cardiovascular disease • Arterial stiffness • Pulse wave velocity • Wave reflection • Peripheral arterial disease • Aortic aneurysm • Marfan syndrome • Coarctation of the aorta • Erectile dysfunction • Prognosis

C. Vlachopoulos, MD, PhD (✉)
D. Terentes-Printzios, MD • C. Stefanadis, MD, PhD
Hypertension and Peripheral Vessels Units,
1st Department of Cardiology,
Athens Medical School, Hippokration Hospital,
114 Vassilissis Sofias Avenue,
Athens 11527, Greece
e-mail: cvlachop@otenet.gr;
dimitristerentes@yahoo.gr; chstefan@med.uoa.gr

K. Takazawa, MD, PhD
Department of Cardiology, Hachioji Medical Center,
Tokyo Medical University, 1163 Tate-Machi,
Hachioji City, Tokyo 193-0998, Japan
e-mail: takazawa@tokyo-med.ac.jp

M.E. Safar et al. (eds.), *Blood Pressure and Arterial Wall Mechanics in Cardiovascular Diseases*,
DOI 10.1007/978-1-4471-5198-2_26,

Abbreviations

AAA Abdominal aortic aneurysm
ABI Ankle–brachial index
ACE Angiotensin-converting enzyme
AIx Augmentation index
ARB Angiotensin receptor blocker
BP Blood pressure
CLI Critical limb ischemia
CV Cardiovascular
ED Erectile dysfunction
LV Left ventricular
PAD Peripheral arterial disease
PDE5i Phosphodiesterase type 5 inhibitors
PWV Pulse wave velocity
TGF-b Transforming growth factor-b

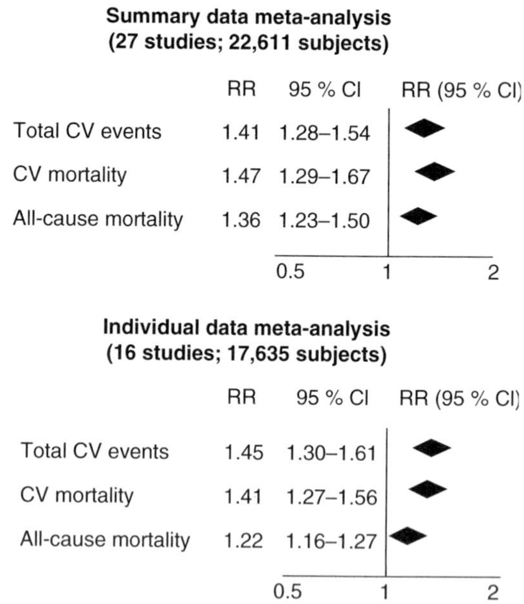

Fig. 26.1 Relative risks and 95 % confidence intervals for a 1-standard deviation increase in aortic pulse wave velocity and clinical events (Reproduced with permission from Vlachopoulos et al. [8])

Introduction

Atherosclerotic disease comprises four major areas: coronary artery disease, cerebrovascular disease, peripheral arterial disease, and aortic aneurysm. The "Cardiovascular Continuum" was described by Dzau and colleagues in 2006 [1] to explain the development over many years of coronary disease with its complications, then end-stage heart failure. William Osler described two forms of arteriosclerosis: "nodular arteriosclerosis" (atherosclerosis), a disease which may be superimposed on arterial aging (his "senile arteriosclerosis"). While the Cardiovascular Continuum put an emphasis on atherosclerosis in prosperous nations, it did not account fully for the problems of aging, which occur in all societies. Aging of the aorta and elastic arteries causes arterial stiffening and leads to the development of cardiac failure and microvascular disease in highly perfused organs such as the brain and kidneys. The term "Vascular Aging Continuum" was recently introduced which dovetails with the late phases of the Cardiovascular Continuum and provides a more comprehensive explanation, especially for vascular diseases in nations with little atherosclerosis [1].

Investigators have mainly focused on using arterial stiffness and central hemodynamics indices for primary prevention and prediction of risk in patients without cardiovascular disease. Their role of these indices is constantly evolving, and in some cases such as hypertensives and diabetics, their clinical significance has been corroborated by recent guidelines and recommendations [2]. A big step in the substantiation of their clinical role was the publication of meta-analyses of prognostic observational studies from published data and individual patient data [3–7] (Fig. 26.1). Despite the overwhelming data for their predictive role in primary prevention, secondary prevention prognostic studies are lacking. Most data stem from high cardiovascular (CV) risk patients such as diabetics with concomitant comorbidities like coronary artery disease, cerebrovascular disease, and to lesser extent peripheral arterial disease. Prognostic studies exclusively on patients with either one of the abovementioned diseases are rare. Especially, data on the role of arterial stiffness in peripheral arterial disease patients, including patients with vasculogenic erectile dysfunction or aortic disease, which is generally depicted as of lower clinical significance to its "rivals" coronary artery disease and cerebrovascular disease, emerge mostly from cross-sectional hypothesis-generating studies. Respectively, most prospective predictive studies of arterial stiffness have not used peripheral arterial or aortic disease endpoints as an exclusive outcome but preferably as a part of a composite cardiovascular event endpoint.

Peripheral Arterial Disease

Peripheral arterial disease (PAD) is an atherosclerotic process that causes stenosis and occlusion of non-cerebral and noncoronary arteries [8]. The definition of PAD is not the same both across studies and across continents, and it was used initially to describe lower extremities PAD. In particular, American guidelines include abdominal aortic aneurysm (AAA), whereas European guidelines discard AAA and incorporate instead extracranial carotid, vertebral, and upper extremity atherosclerotic disease. Both guidelines refer to renal artery and mesenteric atherosclerotic disease. Across this chapter, with the term PAD we will refer to lower extremities PAD.

PAD has an estimated worldwide prevalence of almost 10 %, rising to 15–20 % in people over 70 years of age, and it affects around 27 million people in Europe and North America alone [9]. Only a minority of patients present with classic intermittent claudication, and other symptoms include leg pain with exercise and at rest, leg weakness, and balance problems resulting in falls, all of which can significantly affect functional performance. Critical limb ischemia (CLI)—the most severe manifestation of the disease—can lead to limb loss or even death if not treated promptly.

Ankle–Brachial Index

The ankle–brachial index (ABI) is the ratio of the systolic blood pressure (BP) measured at the ankle to that measured at the brachial artery [10]. Originally described by Winsor in 1950, this index was initially proposed for the noninvasive diagnosis of PAD [10]. Without an obstruction to blood flow, systolic pressure in the ankle is greater than brachial systolic pressure (ABI ≥1.0) because a great amount of reflected waves from the toes merges with the forward wave at the systolic phase of the pressure waveform (due to the small distance between the toes and ankle). As the lumen narrows, systolic pressure beyond the obstruction falls, and a pressure gradient can be measured between sequential segments of each extremity. The fall in peripheral (ankle) systolic pressure lowers the ABI. ABI is also an indicator of atherosclerosis at other vascular sites and can serve as a prognostic marker for cardiovascular events [11] and functional impairment, even in the absence of symptoms of PAD [9]. The postexercise ABI is also predictive of risk [12]. In the case of a normal ABI at rest, the presence of an abnormal ABI after exercise is associated with increased mortality. ABI is a widely used measure of lower extremity atherosclerotic burden given its noninvasive nature, simplicity, and relatively low cost. ABI results should be uniformly reported with noncompressible values defined as greater than 1.40, normal values 1.00–1.40, borderline 0.91–0.99, and abnormal 0.90 or less [12]. The level of ABI also correlates with PAD severity, with a high risk of amputation when the ABI is <0.50. An ABI change >0.15 is generally required to consider worsening of limb perfusion over time or improving after revascularization. The graph of mortality or other cardiovascular outcome by ABI level is a reverse J-shaped curve in which the lowest level of risk (normal) is from 1.11 to 1.40 [11]. One explanation for an increased risk associated with a high ABI is that a high ABI caused by calcified arteries especially in patients with diabetes and chronic kidney disease is associated frequently with occlusive PAD.

PAD and Arterial Stiffness

Vascular dysfunction (arterial stiffness and endothelial dysfunction) is also commonly present in PAD patients [13]. In a large population-based cohort study with over 3,000 elderly subjects, patients with PAD as defined by ABI<0.9 had higher values of carotid–femoral pulse wave velocity (PWV) compared to patients without PAD [14]. Even in case of an alternative clinical definition of PAD based primarily on the history of successful percutaneous interventions, bypass grafting, and/or amputation for PAD, heart–femoral PWV was increased in PAD patients as well [15]. Moreover, brachial–ankle PWV was shown to correlate with both ABI and the angiographically established severity of PAD [16].

The association between ABI and measures of arterial stiffness has been well established in several cross-sectional studies [17] and extends both to patients with and without PAD. In fact, the tight link of PWV with CV outcomes becomes more apparent with the confirmation of a U-shaped association between PWV and ABI, as shown for ABI and CV events [18]. In addition, this association remains largely undiluted even in patients with PAD reflecting a relationship between severity of PAD and arterial stiffness.

Interpretation of arterial stiffness indices should be done with great caution in patients with extremely low ABI and especially CLI. In particular, brachial–ankle PWV due to inherent limitations should be avoided in patients with ABI<0.9. In advanced PAD, a reduced rather than increased aortic PWV may occur, a change that could be attributed to a decline in distending pressures distal to arterial stenoses. Decreases in distending pressures would result in an attenuation of arterial stiffness (a shift to a less steep portion of the exponential vascular pressure–volume relationship) and thus PWV in these distal segments. However, if as a consequence of the presence of stenoses, PWV is reduced in advanced PAD, indices such as central BP and augmentation index (AIx) may remain increased. These observations were substantiated by a recent study [19] in African-Americans with CLI where there was a dissociation of central hemodynamics indices and aortic PWV. Specifically, PWV was lower, whereas AIx and central pulse pressure were higher in participants with CLI compared to controls. It is also possible that blunting of the upstroke of the femoral pressure waveform could lead to late foot detection, overestimation of the carotid–femoral transit time, and underestimation of PWV.

An association between arterial stiffness and exercise performance has also been described in patients with PAD. In a small cross-sectional study with patients who were referred for noninvasive PAD evaluation, measures of arterial stiffness (AIx, pulse pressure, and reflected wave arrival time) were independently associated with shorter walking distance [20]. Almost 1 out of 2 could not complete the exercise protocol, and most had to stop due to either leg discomfort or a combination of leg discomfort and dyspnea. Moreover, brachial–ankle PWV is inversely correlated with functional performance, independent of potential confounders, including ABI [21]. PWV along with undetected PAD was also incriminated for exercise intolerance during a 6 min walk test in patients with chronic obstructive lung disease [22]. Plausible explanation for this association could be the lack of diastolic augmentation, coupled with the increased afterload that may contribute to decreased myocardial perfusion, leading to further supply/demand mismatch and ischemia. Moreover, ventricular–vascular uncoupling with concomitant diastolic dysfunction could amplify poor exercise tolerance, while increased stiffness may suggest microcirculatory dysfunction that leads to impaired perfusion of skeletal muscles during rest and exercise, thereby impairing the performance of skeletal muscles [13]. Finally, increased stiffness is associated with impaired flow volume in lower extremity arteries even in subjects with normal ABI [23].

Arterial Stiffness and PAD in Prognostic Studies

Prospective studies of the association between arterial stiffness and PAD are lacking. Indirect evidence of an association of arterial stiffness indices with future PAD events originate by studies that have included peripheral events in a composite endpoint. However, in a prognostic study in hemodialysis patients that used PAD events as a secondary endpoint, brachial–ankle PWV with its inherent limitations failed to show any predictive role [24]. Likewise, in a study with 520 subjects undergoing coronary angiography

(PAD=42 subjects), none of the central hemodynamics indices such as AIx were associated with the secondary combined endpoint of cerebrovascular and peripheral revascularization [25]. Nevertheless, both studies had small-sized populations and were not designed to investigate future PAD events. On the other hand, some of the patients included in the recent relevant meta-analysis on arterial stiffness included patients with CV disease, where a small part of them had PAD. In fact, in the meta-analysis by Ben-Shlomo et al., PWV in the clinical sample comprising high CV risk patients, including PAD, had similar predictive role to PWV in the general population [3]. However, no studies have been performed exclusively in PAD patients and thus no definitive conclusions can be drawn.

Effects of PAD Treatment on Arterial Stiffness

Finally, few studies have addressed the issue of the use of arterial stiffness as a surrogate endpoint of PAD treatment. Angiotensin-converting enzyme (ACE) inhibitors have been shown to increase walking distance in patients with PAD, and ACE inhibitor-related decreases in arterial stiffness have been suggested as the principal mechanism for improvement in function performance [26]. In particular, in a study of 40 patients with PAD, subjects receiving ramipril 10 mg once daily for 24 weeks experienced a 2.5-fold increase in maximum walking time compared to subjects receiving placebo, while their arterial stiffness parameters improved substantially [26]. Similar results were described in patients with intermittent claudication [27]. Cilostazol, an agent used for relief of intermittent claudication, was also shown to reduce AIx [9]. Comparable results on arterial stiffness seem plausible with other beneficial therapies in PAD patients such as statins and exercise. Finally, promising results are described in PAD patients after percutaneous transluminal angioplasty with improvement in central BP and AIx that translates to improvements in left ventricular (LV) mass and renal dysfunction [28, 29].

Aortic Diseases

Aortic diseases are an important cause of cardiovascular morbidity and mortality. Except when complications are life-threatening, such as acute aortic syndrome (aortic dissection, intramural hematoma, penetrating atherosclerotic ulcer, and aortic rupture), aortic diseases (aortic atherosclerosis and aortic dilatation/aneurysm) are asymptomatic and without abnormalities on physical examination; thus, diagnosis and follow-up depend exclusively on imaging techniques such as ultrasound, computed tomography, and magnetic resonance imaging. Aortic aneurysm is defined as a maximal aortic dimension greater than 3.0 cm or a 50 % increase in size compared with the normal segment proximal to the aneurysm.

Pathophysiology of Aortic Diseases

Central to the pathogenesis of the aneurysm formation is a degenerative process of the media and its elastic components caused by either intrinsic weakness (such as in the Marfan syndrome) or excessive (i.e., hypertension) and/or accumulative (i.e., aging) stress [30]. Ascending aortic aneurysms are mostly caused by medial degeneration, which is characterized by smooth muscle cell necrosis, elastic fiber degeneration, increased deposition of proteoglycans and based on recent data by the presence of inflammatory cell infiltration. Medial degeneration is often seen in patients with inherited connective tissue disorders as the Marfan and the Ehlers–Danlos syndrome but also in patients with bicuspid aortic valve and tricuspid aortic valve stenosis and in elderly patients usually with long-standing hypertension. Preferential weakening of the adventitia and media—rather than an intimal proliferative process, as in atherosclerosis—results in diminished aortic resilience and tensile strength, culminating in aortic wall thinning, dilation, and increased wall stress, all of which may result in rupture [30]. Even though atherosclerosis may be observed in the wall of aneurysms, usually in aneurysms of the descending thoracic and the abdominal aorta, these changes may be a consequence of local turbulent flow as opposed to a cause of aneurysm formation. Furthermore, the extent of systemic atherosclerosis in most cases does not correlate well with the degree of aneurysm formation. However, the presence of detectable atherosclerotic plaques in the aorta indicates the presence of atherosclerotic disease and is a possible source of peripheral embolism while aortic calcifications have shown strong correlation with atherosclerosis and events in other vascular territories [12].

The two critical structural elements in the formation of aortic aneurysms in the aortic wall are elastin and collagen, while matrix metalloproteinases may also play a role by regulating degradation and turnover of extracellular matrix. Elastin provides radial and longitudinal support, enabling the aorta to respond to pulsatile flow while maintaining normal dimensions. Breakdown of elastin alone appears insufficient to cause aneurysmal expansion and rupture. Loss of collagen is an additional contributor, and the relative equilibrium of elastin and collagen deposition, among other factors, may be critical for determining aneurysm formation. Early in aneurysm formation, the aorta compensates for loss of elastin by increasing production of collagen, but as elastin content decreases, collagen (as the major source of tensile strength) is overwhelmed, and aortic expansion occurs. These combined structural alterations promote aortic stiffness that is also amplified by the aging process. In particular, with aging, aortic stiffness due to fragmentation of elastin fibers; deposition of glycosaminoglycans, fibronectin, and collagen; and reduced bioavailability of endothelium-derived nitric oxide is exacerbated [30].

Such remodeling appears to initially protect against rupture, and importantly, failure of such remodeling appears to significantly increase the risk of rupture. According to Laplace's law ($\sigma = P \times r/h$, where P is the pressure in the vessel), wall stress (σ) is higher as the radius (r) of the vessel increases and the wall becomes thinner (h = thickness of the vessel wall); thus, dilatation begets dilatation leading to a vicious circle, with progressively higher rate of aneurysm expansion.

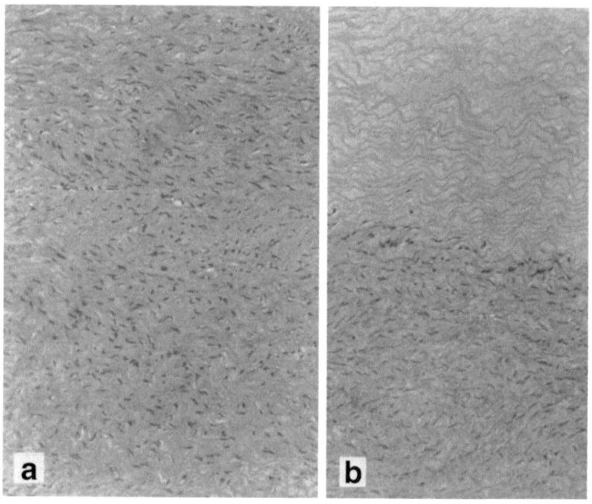

Fig. 26.2 Cross sections of the aortic wall: (**a**) media of an animal with intact vasa vasorum flow. Smooth muscle cells are apparently normal throughout the whole media. (**b**) Media 15 days after vasa vasorum removal. Complete loss of smooth muscle cells is observed in the outer layers of the media (which are nourished by vasa vasorum), whereas smooth muscle cells appear normal in the inner layers. Changes were also observed in elastin fibers in the respective areas (not shown). These changes were accompanied by a decrease in aortic distensibility (Reproduced with permission from Stefanadis et al. [31])

Ultimately, rupture or dissection occurs, unless a reparative process is initiated.

Decreased strength of the inner layer of the aortic wall, increased BP, and high-average wall stress due to increased aortic diameter and decreased wall thickness have been proposed as mechanisms for the development of aortic dissection. High circumferential stress at the inner wall is responsible for the initial tear in the intima leading into the media. Acute aortic syndromes occur when either a tear or an ulcer allows blood to penetrate from the aortic lumen into the media or within rupture of the "vasa vasorum" (Fig. 26.2) within the media [31]; the inflammatory response to blood in the media may lead to aortic dilatation and rupture. Blood penetrates through the tear to the media, and the two layers of the aortic wall (the outer layer and the intimal flap) separate and slide relative to one another producing a false lumen. The vessel is further dilated and the outer wall is thinned due to its separation into two dissected layers; in consequence, it is prone to total rupture. Aortic compliance is further impaired from narrowing of its lumen, and systolic pressure tends to increase favoring progression of dissection.

Aortic Diseases and Arterial Stiffness

The aorta plays an important role in modulating LV performance and arterial function throughout the entire CV system. A comprehensive assessment of aortic and arterial biophysical properties includes (i) evaluation of the aortic pressure–dimension relationship, (ii) arterial stiffness, and (iii) the reflected waves [32].

Arterial stiffness and wave reflection indices have grown substantial attention in patients with aortic dilatation/aneurysm. The reasons are their pathophysiological proximity to the disease, their noninvasive and easy assessment, their well-established predictive role for future events in several disease populations, their alluring potential to predict future expansion or rupture, and their interpretation of treatment effects. Most of the studies were conducted in patients with inherited and developmental aortopathies such as in Marfan syndrome, Ehlers–Danlos syndrome, Loeys–Dietz's syndrome, bicuspid aortic valve diseases, and coarctation of the aorta.

Marfan Syndrome

Marfan syndrome is an autosomal dominant genetic disorder caused by a mutation of the FBN1 gene that encodes fibrillin-1. Fibrillin-1 appears to be a key element in the normal spatial organization of the arterial wall, ensuring adequate loading of elastic components, thereby maintaining physiological arterial stiffness. Fibrillin-1 mutation is associated with increased arterial stiffness [33]. Moreover, changes in the extracellular matrix of elastic tissue have been related to excessive signaling by transforming growth factor-b (TGF-b), with increased proteolytic degradation by serine proteases and matrix metalloproteinases contributing to the phenotypic features of Marfan syndrome including progressive enlargement of the aortic root. Of importance is the finding that central and not peripheral pulse pressure has been found to be a major determinant of ascending aorta diameter [33], thus attesting to the importance of assessing central hemodynamics and stiffness indices. Interestingly, the increase in arterial stiffness is confined to the aorta, with no change in stiffness observed for the carotid, femoral, and radial arteries. A clinical hallmark of Marfan syndrome, and the major cause of morbidity and premature death from this syndrome, is aortic root dilatation and associated aortic regurgitation, dissection, and rupture. The exact mechanisms leading to dilatation are not fully elucidated, but steady and pulsatile stresses are probably important, leading to the mechanical fatigue of abnormal elastic fibers and microdissections. Aortic dilatation probably results from the failure of abnormal elastic fibers to sustain physiological pulsatile stress, by analogy with aging. Consequently, aneurysm growth rate is associated with aortic stiffness in Marfan [34]. In fact, aortic stiffness and wave reflection indices such as augmentation index and probably central BP seem to have an independent predictive value for aortic dilatation, dissection, and rupture in longitudinal follow-up studies of patients with Marfan or Marfan-like syndromes [34–36]. Estimation of aortic biomechanics in Marfan by magnetic resonance imaging is promising for early detection of future complications [32].

Aortic Aneurysms

Aortic aneurysms are also common in the general population with age, male gender, and smoking as essential risk factors and are characterized by location in abdominal and thoracic/thoracoabdominal aortic aneurysms. The aneurysmal dilatation of the abdominal aorta is associated with a significant increase in aortic stiffness, which can be explained by the decreased volume fraction of elastin and smooth muscle cells and increased collagen and ground substance found at the histological examination of the resected aortic specimens [30]. Of importance is the finding that patients with abdominal aortic aneurysm also have increased carotid artery stiffness compared to patients with coronary artery disease, even after adjustment for important risk factors [37]. This supports a causal role of arterial stiffness in a generalized arterial wall disease. Interestingly enough, it has been shown that higher AAA distensibility is positively related to propensity to rupture [38]. Although aneurysms have generally increased stiffness, this may represent a specific phase in the course of some aneurysms during which the wall becomes weaker before rupture.

However, a recent study [39] showed that carotid–femoral PWV may underestimate the degree of aortic stiffness and AIx may overestimate the magnitude of arterial wave reflections in patients with AAA. Aortic PWV is proportional to the square root of aortic stiffness and inversely proportional to the square root of aortic radius with the assumption that there are no significant changes in the vessel cross-sectional area or wall thickness along the arterial segment [30]. The markedly increased radius of the dilated segment of the aorta in patients with AAA apparently violates the assumption and would induce a reduction of aortic PWV. The study [39] showed that indices of arterial stiffness that incorporate also muscular arteries, such as brachial–ankle PWV contrary to carotid–femoral PWV that is mainly associated with elastic arteries, are less likely influenced by the presence of AAA. Specifically, carotid–femoral PWV was significantly lower in patients with AAA than controls without AAA, when brachial–ankle PWV suggested similar degree of arterial stiffness between the two groups. Suggested explanations were that the length of AAA represents only a small fraction of the virtual traveling distance between brachial and ankle arteries and that the irregular vessel wall of AAA along with a potential decrease in BP after the aneurysm could passively decrease aortic PWV. However, in a similar earlier study, Kadoglou et al. showed that carotid–femoral PWV was significantly higher in patients with AAA compared to controls [40]. As for other case–control studies, the matching of the patients with controls is critical and its inherent limitations might explain the diversity of results. As far as indices of wave reflection are concerned, augmentation index seems to be higher in aortic aneurysm (thoracic or abdominal) patients compared to controls [39, 41]; however, it does not seem to be able to discriminate between patients with fast and slow progression of aortic aneurysm in their early phase [42] but rather in their late phase [43]. On the contrary, central BP shows a steady incremental value over peripheral BP in prediction of fast progression, dissection, and rupture of aortic aneurysm [43].

Effects of Treatment of Aortic Diseases on Arterial Stiffness

Aortic dilatation/aneurysm in its initial stages is conservatively managed with medical treatment, unless an acute aortic syndrome occurs that in most cases needs surgical intervention. The mainstream in the pharmacological treatment of aortic dilatation is β-blockade, which retards the rate of dilatation and risk of dissection by reducing wall stress. The benefits of β-adrenoreceptor blockers in this setting are attributable to their ability to reduce (i) peak stress and maximum rate of increase in aortic pressure during systole (dP/dT) through their negative inotropic effect and (ii) the number of cumulating fatiguing pulsations over time through their heart rate slowing effect. The effect of β-blocker therapy on aortic elastic properties is not the same for all agents. While some of them have been shown to improve aortic elastic properties [44], of concern may be the fact that some nonselective β-blocking agents may increase wave reflections [30]. The discrepancy in results seen in studies probably reflects the fact that hemodynamic effects of β-blockers vary with the specific agent. Of particular benefit appear to be β-blockers with vasodilating properties that reduce peak systolic pressure and arterial stress through the reduction in wave reflections.

Experimental studies in an animal model demonstrated that ACE inhibitors and angiotensin receptor blocker (ARB) may prevent or delay the phenotypic expression of Marfan syndrome by antagonizing TGF-b and slowing or even reversing defragmentation of the elastic fibers of the aorta. ACE inhibitors also reduce angiotensin II levels that are associated with medial degeneration contributing to aortic rupture in Marfan syndrome. Promising are the results from ACE inhibitors such as perindopril [45], as well as

ARB such as losartan [46], in reducing aortic dilatation in humans with Marfan syndrome, along with a reduction in aortic PWV independent of BP reduction [45]. Recently, a small short-term (4 weeks) crossover randomized study compared the effects of perindopril, verapamil, and atenolol on arterial stiffness, wave reflection, and aortic dilatation in Marfan syndrome [47]. Despite the slightly favorable effect of perindopril on augmentation index and central BP compared to atenolol, only atenolol induced delayed expansion in the aortic arch and abdominal aorta. No significant changes were noted between drugs in aortic PWV during this short-term study [47].

Several studies have also investigated the effect of interventional management of aortic aneurysm on arterial stiffness. There is compelling evidence that repair of aortic aneurysm either surgically or with the endovascular method causes significant increase in aortic stiffness [39, 48–50]. This increase may reflect the effect of restoration of the uniform cross-sectional area along the abdominal aorta and does not necessarily indicate a real increase in aortic stiffness after intervention. However, this increase after 1 year seems to translate into increase of LV mass, diastolic dysfunction, and ultimately exercise intolerance [49]. Interestingly, in a small pilot study [51], the open surgical repair induced a reduction of stiffness in AAA compared to an increase of the endovascular treatment, which was even higher when endoleaks were present. This may be explained by the fact that the sac, which is fluid-filled, is not pressurized and therefore exhibits greatest wall movement at any given systemic BP. In the case of endoleak after endovascular repair, wall movement is less because the sac is pressurized as compared with the latter situation, implying an increase in stiffness. Integrating this information could partly explain the data from a recent comparison study between open and endovascular repair that showed similar long-term survival despite a perioperative survival advantage with endovascular repair for the first 3 years [52]. Open repair has increased perioperative mortality compared to endovascular treatment. However, the increased aortic stiffness of endovascular repair that associates with future CV events and endoleaks could lead in the long term to increased CV mortality and deaths from aortic ruptures compared to open repair and thus weaken any initial survival advantage [52]. Therefore, it is important to use grafts that do not increase aortic stiffness based on their engineering characteristics and to investigate how this translates in future events.

Coarctation of the Aorta

Hemodynamic Alterations

The important role of arterial stiffness and wave reflections are also prominent in coarctation of the aorta. The clinical features of aortic coarctation are primarily a consequence of altered arterial hemodynamics in the upper part of the body, not of reduced blood flow to the lower part. This is because blood flow to the lower part of the body is maintained at near-normal levels at rest and during exercise through the development of collateral blood flow involving the intercostal, internal mammary, and scapular vessels, which circumvents the stenotic lesion. The pressure waves recorded from the upper part of the body are quite different from the normal. They display a steady rise to a high systolic peak and a near-exponential decay through all diastole. This is due to the following factors [30]:

(i) The site of stricture reflects a great amount of the pulse wave, which otherwise would have traveled until the lower part of the body; thus the reflecting site is transferred closer to the ascending aorta.

(ii) PWV increases as a result of the increase in distending pressure, and thus the pressure waves travel faster within the aorta. In consequence of factors (i) and (ii), the reflected wave returns earlier adding to systole and is enhanced, thus augmenting pressure in the ascending aorta in systole rather than in diastole.

(iii) There is a diminution in size of the arterial segment with cushioning properties; only one third of the total arterial system—the upper part—is able to distend at the ejection of the

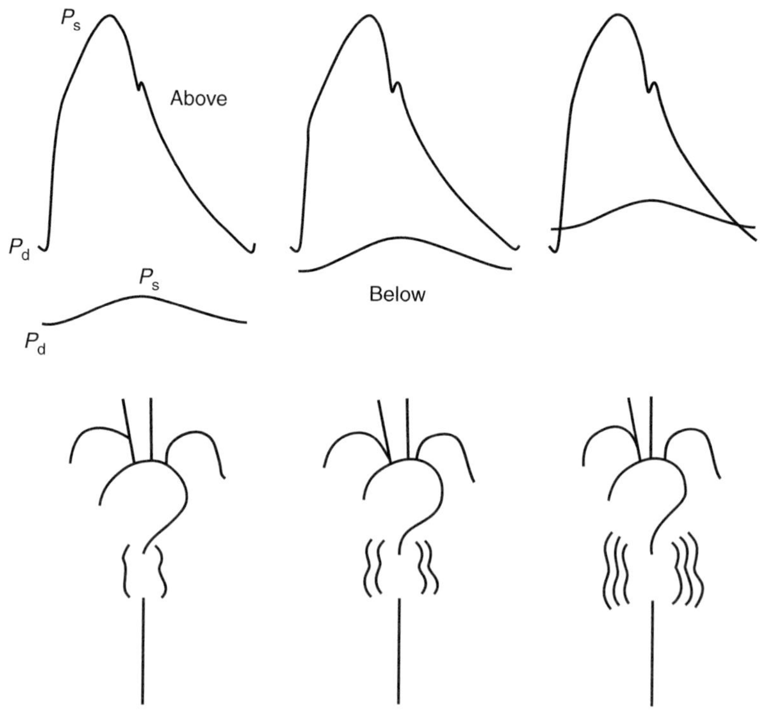

Fig. 26.3 Diagrammatic representation of different degrees of collateral development on arterial pressure waves above and below an obstruction in the descending aorta. When collaterals are poorly developed, both systolic and diastolic pressures are lower beyond the obstruction. When collaterals are well developed, mean pressure is maintained; however, pulse pressure is reduced and diastolic pressure may be higher and systolic pressure reduced beyond the obstruction (Reprinted from O'Rourke [53], with permission)

left ventricle. The collaterals cannot compensate for the altered cushioning function.

The pressure wave in aortic coarctation resembles that recorded in hypertension and arterial degeneration. The main difference between these conditions is that in hypertension and arterial degeneration, the early return of the reflected wave is mainly due to increased PWV; in contrast, in aortic coarctation, the early return of the reflected wave is also due to the smaller distance the pulse and reflected waves have to travel from the aortic valve to the site of stricture and back. During exercise, a dramatic increase in systolic and pulse pressure occurs, which is even greater than the increase seen in patients with essential hypertension. This is mainly due to the reduction of cushioning capacity of the arterial system [30].

If collaterals did not exist, then a dramatic fall in both mean and pulse pressure beyond the obstruction would occur, depending on the degree of lumen narrowing. However, the collaterals are efficient to maintain mean pressure beyond a narrowing to normal levels, usually slightly lower than the mean pressure proximal to the narrowing serving well as substitutes of the aorta as regards its conduit function. On the other hand, pulse pressure is almost always markedly reduced beyond a significant narrowing of the aortic lumen: while diastolic pressure beyond the obstruction remains at the same level or even higher than in the upper body in the presence of well-developed collaterals, systolic pressure is much lower in the arteries beyond the obstruction [53]. The latter is the result of attenuation and delay of the pulse through the long, tortuous and narrow collateral vessels (Fig. 26.3).

III Effects Linked to Pathophysiology

Due to the smaller volume distensibility of the arterial system and the early return of pulse wave, high pulsations are produced in the upper body arteries, which result in systolic hypertension with high pulse pressure. The presence of systolic hypertension from early age accounts for the detrimental effects of aortic coarctation on cardiovascular system, such as LV hypertrophy, intimal thickening, and medial degeneration of the arteries of the upper body, with arteriosclerosis and development of aneurysms located especially in the circle of Willis or within the brain substance itself and atherosclerosis of the coronary arteries. Consequently, main causes of death include heart failure, aortic rupture, aortic dissection, endocarditis, endarteritis, intracerebral hemorrhage, and myocardial infarction [54]. Most of these pathological features are attributable to fatigue of the elastic components of the arterial wall due to the repeated high pulsatile stress over a long period of time and are similar to those seen with aging or long-standing hypertension but occur at a much earlier age. The effect of these hemodynamic and structural changes on arterial function is expressed as decreased distensibility of the proximal aorta, with preservation of the distensibility of the distal aorta. This finding is in contrast with the gradual decline in aortic distensibility from proximal to distal aorta found in normal subjects.

The Effect of Repair on Hypertension

In order to prevent the deleterious effects of aortic coarctation on cardiovascular structure and function, repair of aortic coarctation should be performed in infancy or early childhood [54]. If coarctation escapes early detection, repair should be performed at the time of subsequent diagnosis. In cases with excessive hemodynamic alterations, intervention is performed even in the first months of life. Early repair (which is made usually surgically with end-to-end anastomosis, subclavian flap aortoplasty, bypass graft, or prosthetic patch aortoplasty but also percutaneously with balloon dilatation and stenting of the aorta) is associated with better survival rates; however, some operated patients die prematurely from cardiovascular complications, such as myocardial infarction, sudden death, heart failure, cerebrovascular disease, and ruptured aortic aneurysm. All adult patients with a noninvasive pressure difference >20 mmHg between the upper and lower limbs, regardless of symptoms but with upper limb hypertension, pathological BP response during exercise, or significant LV hypertrophy should have intervention; independent of the pressure gradient, hypertensive patients with ≥50 % aortic narrowing relative to the aortic diameter at the diaphragm level should be considered for intervention [54].

Correction usually reduces arterial pressure in the upper body and results in the restoration of normal femoral pulses and the regression of collaterals and LV hypertrophy. Although preoperative hypertension regresses in most cases postoperatively, it may recur later in life and is related to adverse outcomes [55]. Almost 1 out of 3 patients with repaired coarctation of the aorta developed hypertension in long-term studies. The mechanisms and the risk factors leading to postoperative hypertension are not fully elucidated. Earlier prospective studies suggested that faster repair of the aorta protects from future development of hypertension; however, more recent longer follow-up studies tend to dispute these results. Interestingly, it seems that those who undergo end-to-end anastomosis have lower systolic BP at follow-up than those who undergo subclavian flap repair or patch aortoplasty, while early reports do not show difference in future prevalence between surgical and percutaneous repair [55]. Anatomical causes such as residual stenosis, variations in anatomical shapes of the post-repair aorta, or even presence of prosthetic material may play a role; yet hypertension occurs even in the absence of such anatomical features. The role of sympathetic hyperactivity, renin–aldosterone axis activation, and inflammation has been debated [55]. Altered baroreflex sensitivity, due to precoarctectomy hypertension, plays a major role in reactive hypertension seen in the early postoperative course, and it may also be implicated in late exercise-induced hypertension. However, the main defect leading to late rest and exercise-induced hypertension is the altered structure and function of the arteries in the upper body that remains even after successful repair due to their long-standing high pulsatile stress before the operation (see below "arterial function and structure in relation to repair"). Altered structure leads to altered function, with reduced arterial compliance, which leads to hypertension with high systolic and pulse pressure.

Even in the absence of hypertension at rest, many patients exhibit exercise-induced hypertension.

Similarly to the prevalence of hypertension at rest, about 1 in 3 patients develop exercise-induced hypertension post repair [55]. Exercise-induced hypertension is a predictor of chronic hypertension in the general population. It is possible that the increases in cardiac output, seen with exercise, ejected into a less compliant aorta lead to significant increases in pulse pressure, which normalizes when cardiac output returns to normal. Further aortic remodeling and stiffening induced by continuing low velocity shear stress may lead to changes in baroreceptor sensitivity and progression toward established hypertension. Therefore, recent studies advocate the usefulness of exercise testing as a predictive tool for future hypertension in patients with aortic coarctation repair.

Arterial Function and Structure in Relation to Repair

Altered structure of the wall of arteries in the upper body postoperatively has been demonstrated in experimental animals and includes intima–media proliferation of the aortic arch. These persistent after coarctectomy changes in animals are the same as those seen in coarctectomy specimens in humans or in hypertensive patients, as previously described. This could be translated into inability of coarctectomy to fully reverse the structural changes in the arteries of the upper body induced by increased pulsatile stress.

Several cross-sectional studies on endothelial function and arterial stiffness point to an underlying vascular bed pathology as a cause for the development of hypertension despite early and anatomically successful surgical correction of the aortic coarctation. As regards arterial function, it has been shown that, in patients with coarctation of the aorta, proximal aorta distensibility remains much lower than in normal subjects both shortly and late after successful repair [56]. Furthermore, proximal aorta distensibility remains much lower than the distensibility in the distal aorta. These findings are attributed to structural changes in the proximal aorta. The same changes also account for the increased brachial–radial PWV [57] despite a preserved femoral–dorsalis pedis velocity of pulse wave propagation seen in postcoarctectomy patients. Kenny et al. found a significant (yet moderate) relationship of aortic PWV with baroreceptor reflex sensitivity and ambulatory BP measurements in their post-repair coarctation patients, a relationship that they could not demonstrate for ambulatory BP in their control group [58]. Along these lines, ambulatory arterial stiffness index, an indirect index of arterial stiffness with predictive ability for future CV events [59], was higher in children with repaired coarctation compared to other hypertensive or normotensive children despite no differences in age or BP levels [60].

Another finding in these patients is impaired vascular reactivity of the upper body arteries [57]. Hypertensive postcoarctectomy patients exhibit enhanced vasoconstrictor response to norepinephrine in the arms but normal vascular reactivity of the legs. Hyperemic flow, flow-mediated dilatation, and vasodilatation after administration of nitroglycerin are all impaired in brachial artery but the same is not true for the arteries of the lower limb [57]. Impaired vascular reactivity confined to the upper limb is also observed after exercise-induced hypertension in postcoarctectomy patients compared to controls with similar resting BP [55].

Age at operation is of importance. As discussed earlier, postoperative hypertension is more common in patients with repair at an older age. According to the notion that the longest the high pulsatile stress remains, the greatest the structural and functional abnormalities will be, it was shown that age at intervention is correlated with impaired upper body arterial stiffness. Brili et al. [56] found that age at surgery was inversely correlated to the distensibility index of the aortic arch in postcoarctectomy patients, and de Divitiis et al. found the same correlation with the distensibility of the upper limb arteries [57]. Similarly, in a recent study, Sarkola et al. [61] found more pronounced CV abnormalities (LV mass, adventitial thickness, lumen dimensions, thigh systolic BP, abdominal aorta, carotid and regional stiffness) after aortic coarctation stent implantation compared to surgery that were primarily related to older patient age at the time of intervention for stent implantation. These myocardial abnormalities are apparent even in normotensive patients with repaired aortic coarctation. However, the effect of age on vascular function has been debated [62]. Regarding vascular reactivity, no correlation could be found between age at surgery and vascular reactivity of the upper limb arteries [57]. An explanation is that patients who required surgery in the neonatal period could have a more severe congenital arterial abnormality and might have been exposed to very high BP from birth. Another possible explanation is that early "programming" of vascular reactivity exists during prenatal development or in the first few weeks after birth, as suggests its association with birth weight.

The type of intervention and anatomical variations have been implicated in the development of hypertension. In accordance with studies for hypertension, end-to-end anastomosis is the preferable surgical technique, as it is not associated with impaired vascular function contrary to the subclavian flap repair [63]. Plausible mechanisms are an ongoing regional effect of residual "coarctation" tissue on the upper limb arterial dynamics in subclavian flap repair compared with the fully resected anastomosis approach and earlier reflected waves from the subclavian flap repair site due to subclavian artery's different wall structure or due to a more diffuse scar site that may lead to greater augmentation of central systolic pressure and abnormal arterial compliance through increased mechanical forces. Importantly, elastic properties of the prestenotic aorta of patients with coarctation seem to be impaired primarily, even in neonates, and remain unchanged early after successful operation implying and inborn pathology of the prestenotic aortic vascular bed [64]. Endovascular treatment, on the other hand, does not seem to lead to changes in the inherent vascular pathology, neither acutely nor even in the long term [78,65]. Indeed, initial studies show that stenting is associated with rather increased PWV compared to surgery and with a modest midterm beneficial effect on aortic augmentation index [61, 62, 65]. Reasons for this increased PWV may be related to the mechanical properties of the stent (rigid structure) and to the fact that stent implantation is performed significantly later in life, and it is likely, therefore, that regional BP and age at intervention or at re-intervention may have affected the preductal vascular phenotype. Variations in anatomical shapes also predispose in late hypertension. In particular, angulated Gothic aortic arch is associated with increased systolic wave reflection, as well as increased central aortic stiffness and LV mass index [55]. Importantly, it seems that central pulse pressure is more useful than peripheral BP in identifying patients with recoarctation [66].

Effect of Pharmacological Treatment on Vascular Function

There are a limited number of studies directly comparing the effects between antihypertensive medications on BP control in hypertensive patients with coarctation repair. Moltzer et al. [67] compared the effect of candesartan and metoprolol on BP, large artery stiffness, and neurohormonal response in a small crossover trial and found that metoprolol for 4 weeks was more effective at reducing the mean arterial pressure compared to candesartan. However, there was no effect on aortic PWV with either treatment. On the contrary, we have shown (unpublished data) that both ramipril and candesartan have a beneficial effect on aortic PWV and augmentation index in these patients. In accordance, Brili et al. showed a beneficial effect of ramipril on endothelial function [68]. Such a beneficial effect on endothelial function was shown by the short-term use of statins as well.

Erectile Dysfunction

Vasculogenic erectile dysfunction (ED) may result from impairment of endothelial dependent and/or independent smooth muscle relaxation (i.e., functional vascular ED, early stages), occlusion of the penile arteries by atherosclerosis (i.e., structural vascular ED, late stages), or a combination of these processes [69]. Vasculogenic ED

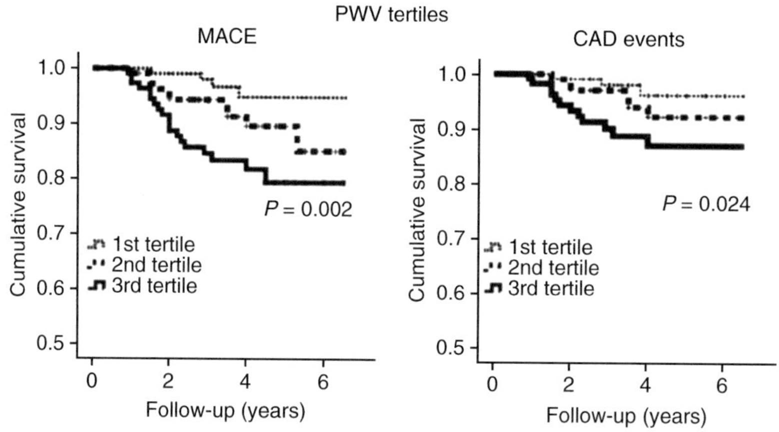

Fig. 26.4 Kaplan–Meier curves for MACE and CAD events by tertile group of carotid–femoral PWV in 376 patients followed for a mean period of 3.4 years. Cutoffs of the tertiles for PWV were 8.0 and 9.2 m/s. *P* values shown were obtained from a long-rank test. *CAD* coronary artery disease, *MACE* major adverse cardiovascular events, *PWV* pulse wave velocity (From Vlachopoulos et al. 7)

or primarily vasculogenic ED (i.e., in cases that the cause of ED is multifactorial along with hormonal disturbances or diabetic neuropathy) should be regarded as harbinger of incident or future CV disease [70]. In fact, ED is associated with a 44 % increase for future CV events and the risk is even higher at younger ages and in intermediate CV risk groups [70].

ED is associated with the presence and extent of subclinical atherosclerosis, including that of the coronary arteries, and precedes the development of clinically evident coronary artery disease (CAD) by a significant amount of time (3–5 years) [71]. Several tests that measure the general atherosclerotic burden (not necessarily obstructive) either in the coronary circulation (i.e., coronary calcium score by electron-beam computed tomography) or in extracoronary vessels (i.e., ankle–brachial index, carotid intima–media thickness) along with functional arterial indices (flow-mediated dilatation) or mixed (functional and structural) arterial indices (aortic stiffness) are also considered surrogate markers of CVD [72]. We have shown that hypertensive patients with ED had higher common carotid intima–media thickness (0.95 vs. 0.83 mm) and carotid–femoral PWV (8.89 vs. 8.11 m/s) and lower flow-mediated dilation of the brachial artery (absolute values of 2.96 vs. 4.07 %) compared to controls [69, 72].

ED carries by itself an independent risk for CV events [89]. It would be extremely clinically useful to identify potential biomarkers that would predict future CV events in the ED population. Pulse pressure, a crude index of arterial stiffness, has also been shown to predict outcome in ED patients [69]. We have recently shown that higher aortic stiffness is associated with increased risk for a major adverse CV event in ED patients (unpublished data) (Fig. 26.4). Aortic PWV improves risk prediction when added to standard risk factors and may represent a valuable biomarker of CV risk prediction in these patients.

While hypogonadism accounts for only 5 % of ED (defined when total testosterone is below 12 nmol/l), approximately one out of three men who see a clinician for ED have testosterone levels that are considered moderately lower than normal. Many studies show a significant association of low testosterone levels with the presence and extent of vasculogenic ED [69]. Low plasma testosterone is associated with increased risk for a CV event in hypertensive patients [73]. Low endogenous androgen concentration improves risk prediction when added to standard risk factors and may represent a valuable biomarker of prediction of cardiovascular disease risk in these patients. We also have shown that testosterone levels are independently associated with aortic stiffening, and this relationship also contributes to the predictive role of aortic stiffness and testosterone for future CV events (unpublished data). The effect of low testosterone concentration on aortic stiffness is emphasized in young men and subjects with higher BP level.

Arterial stiffness can potentially aid in the (i) prediction of the response to an agent and thus determine the therapeutic approach (e.g., choice of drug, dose of drug) and (ii) prediction of the incidence of CV events within the context of ED. Several studies have shown improvement in arterial stiffness and wave reflection indices with phosphodiesterase type 5 inhibitors (PDE5i), implying a possible beneficial CV effect [74, 75]. The application of specific biomarkers for prediction of a change in cardiovascular risk during treatment with "pleiotropic" agents (i.e., PDE5i, statins) represents a major challenge for future studies.

References

1. O'Rourke MF, Safar ME, Dzau V. The cardiovascular continuum extended: aging effects on the aorta and microvasculature. Vasc Med. 2010;15(6):461–8.
2. Mancia G, Fagard R, Narkiewicz K, Redon J, Zanchetti A, Böhm M, et al. 2013 ESH/ESC guidelines for the management of arterial hypertension: the Task Force for the Management of Arterial Hypertension of the European Society of Hypertension (ESH) and of the European Society of Cardiology (ESC). Eur Heart J. 2013;34(28):2159–219.
3. Ben-Shlomo Y, Spears M, Boustred C, May M, Anderson SG, Benjamin EJ, et al. Aortic pulse wave velocity improves cardiovascular event prediction: an individual participant meta-analysis of prospective observational data from 17,635 subjects. J Am Coll Cardiol. 2014;63:636–46.
4. Vlachopoulos C, Aznaouridis K, Terentes-Printzios D, Ioakeimidis N, Stefanadis C. Prediction of cardiovascular events and all-cause mortality with brachial-ankle elasticity index: a systematic review and meta-analysis. Hypertension. 2012;60(2):556–62.
5. Vlachopoulos C, Aznaouridis K, Stefanadis C. Prediction of cardiovascular events and all-cause mortality with arterial stiffness: a systematic review and meta-analysis. J Am Coll Cardiol. 2010;55:1318–27.
6. Vlachopoulos C, Aznaouridis K, O'Rourke MF, Safar ME, Baou K, Stefanadis C. Prediction of cardiovascular events and all-cause mortality with central haemodynamics: a systematic review and meta-analysis. Eur Heart J. 2010;31:1865–71.
7. Vlachopoulos C, Aznaouridis K, Stefanadis C. Aortic stiffness for cardiovascular risk prediction: just measure it, just do it! J Am Coll Cardiol. 2014;63:647–9.
8. Vlachopoulos C, Terentes-Printzios D, Stefanadis C. How to identify subjects with poly-vascular disease? Curr Vasc Pharmacol. 2012;10(6):728–30.
9. Tendera M, Aboyans V, Bartelink ML, Baumgartner I, Clément D, Collet JP, et al. ESC Guidelines on the diagnosis and treatment of peripheral artery diseases: document covering atherosclerotic disease of extracranial carotid and vertebral, mesenteric, renal, upper and lower extremity arteries: the Task Force on the Diagnosis and Treatment of Peripheral Artery Diseases of the European Society of Cardiology (ESC). Eur Heart J. 2011;32(22):2851–906.
10. Aboyans V, Criqui MH, Abraham P, Allison MA, Creager MA, Diehm C, et al. Measurement and interpretation of the ankle-brachial index: a scientific statement from the American Heart Association. Circulation. 2012;126(24):2890–909.
11. Ankle Brachial Index Collaboration, Fowkes FG, Murray GD, Butcher I, Heald CL, Lee RJ, Chambless LE, et al. Ankle brachial index combined with Framingham risk score to predict cardiovascular events and mortality: a meta-analysis. JAMA. 2008;300:197–208.
12. Anderson JL, Halperin JL, Albert NM, Bozkurt B, Brindis RG, Curtis LH, et al. Management of patients with peripheral artery disease (compilation of 2005 and 2011 ACCF/AHA guideline recommendations): a report of the American College of Cardiology Foundation/American Heart Association Task Force on Practice Guidelines. Circulation. 2013;127(13):1425–43.
13. Coutinho T, Rooke TW, Kullo IJ. Arterial dysfunction and functional performance in patients with peripheral artery disease: a review. Vasc Med. 2011;16(3):203–11.
14. van Popele NM, Grobbee DE, Bots ML, Asmar R, Topouchian J, Reneman RS, et al. Association between arterial stiffness and atherosclerosis: the Rotterdam Study. Stroke. 2001;32(2):454–60.
15. Tsuchikura S, Shoji T, Kimoto E, Shinohara K, Hatsuda S, Koyama H, et al. Central versus peripheral arterial stiffness in association with coronary, cerebral and peripheral arterial disease. Atherosclerosis. 2010;211(2):480–5.
16. Xu Y, Wu Y, Li J, Ma W, Guo X, Luo Y, et al. The predictive value of brachial-ankle pulse wave velocity in coronary atherosclerosis and peripheral artery diseases in urban Chinese patients. Hypertens Res. 2008;31(6):1079–85.
17. Coutinho T, Turner ST, Kullo IJ. Aortic pulse wave velocity is associated with measures of subclinical target organ damage. JACC Cardiovasc Imaging. 2011;4(7):754–61.
18. Wohlfahrt P, Palous D, Ingrischová M, Krajcoviechová A, Seidlerová J, Galovcová M, et al. A high ankle-brachial index is associated with increased aortic pulse wave velocity: the Czech post-MONICA study. Eur J Cardiovasc Prev Rehabil. 2011;18(6):790–6.

19. Brand M, Woodiwiss AJ, Michel F, Booysen HL, Veller MG, Norton GR. A mismatch between aortic pulse pressure and pulse wave velocity predicts advanced peripheral arterial disease. Eur J Vasc Endovasc Surg. 2013;46(3):338–46.
20. Brewer LC, Chai HS, Bailey KR, Kullo IJ. Measures of arterial stiffness and wave reflection are associated with walking distance in patients with peripheral arterial disease. Atherosclerosis. 2007;191:384–90.
21. Amoh-Tonto CA, Malik AR, Kondragunta V, Ali Z, Kullo IJ. Brachial-ankle pulse wave velocity is associated with walking distance in patients referred for peripheral arterial disease evaluation. Atherosclerosis. 2009;206(1):173–8.
22. Castagna O, Boussuges A, Nussbaum E, Marqueste L, Brisswalter J. Peripheral arterial disease: an underestimated aetiology of exercise intolerance in chronic obstructive pulmonary disease patients. Eur J Cardiovasc Prev Rehabil. 2008;15(3):270–7.
23. Yoshimura T, Suzuki E, Ito I, Sakaguchi M, Uzu T, Nishio Y, Maegawa H, Morikawa S, Inubushi T, Hisatomi A, Fujimoto K, Takeda J, Kashiwagi A. Impaired peripheral circulation in lower-leg arteries caused by higher arterial stiffness and greater vascular resistance associates with nephropathy in type 2 diabetic patients with normal ankle-brachial indices. Diabetes Res Clin Pract. 2008;80(3):416–23.
24. Tanaka M, Ishii H, Aoyama T, Takahashi H, Toriyama T, Kasuga H, et al. Ankle brachial pressure index but not brachial-ankle pulse wave velocity is a strong predictor of systemic atherosclerotic morbidity and mortality in patients on maintenance hemodialysis. Atherosclerosis. 2011;219(2):643–7.
25. Weber T, O'Rourke MF, Lassnig E, Porodko M, Ammer M, Rammer M, et al. Pulse waveform characteristics predict cardiovascular events and mortality in patients undergoing coronary angiography. J Hypertens. 2010;28(4):797–805.
26. Ahimastos AA, Dart AM, Lawler A, Blombery PA, Kingwell BA. Reduced arterial stiffness may contribute to angiotensin-converting enzyme inhibitor induced improvements in walking time in peripheral arterial disease patients. J Hypertens. 2008;26(5):1037–42.
27. Shahin Y, Cockcroft JR, Chetter IC. Randomized clinical trial of angiotensin-converting enzyme inhibitor, ramipril, in patients with intermittent claudication. Br J Surg. 2013;100(9):1154–63.
28. Eguchi K, Murakami A, Horaguchi T, Kato M, Miyashita H, Kario K. Percutaneous transluminal angioplasty for peripheral artery disease confers cardiorenal protection. J Hum Hypertens. 2014;28(1):51–5.
29. Jacomella V, Shenoy A, Mosimann K, Kohler MK, Amann-Vesti B, Husmann M. The impact of endovascular lower-limb revascularisation on the aortic augmentation index in patients with peripheral arterial disease. Eur J Vasc Endovasc Surg. 2013;45(5):497–501.
30. Nichols WW, O'Rourke MF, Vlachopoulos C. McDonald's blood flow in arteries: theoretical, experimental and clinical principles. 6th ed. London: Hodder Arnold; 2011.
31. Stefanadis CI, Vlachopoulos CV, Karayannacos PE, Boudoulas HK, Stratos CG, Filippides T, et al. Effect of vasa vasorum on structure and function of the aorta in experimental animals. Circulation. 1995;91:2669–78.
32. Evangelista A, Flachskampf FA, Erbel R, Antonini-Canterin F, Vlachopoulos C, Rocchi G, et al. Echocardiography in aortic diseases: EAE recommendations for clinical practice. Eur J Echocardiogr. 2010;11(8):645–58. Erratum in: Eur J Echocardiogr. 2011;12(8):642.
33. Jondeau G, Boutouyrie P, Lacolley P, Laloux B, Dubourg O, Bourdarias JP, et al. Central pulse pressure is a major determinant of ascending aorta dilation in Marfan syndrome. Circulation. 1999;99(20):2677–81.
34. Nollen GJ, Groenink M, Tijssen JG, Van Der Wall EE, Mulder BJ. Aortic stiffness and diameter predict progressive aortic dilatation in patients with Marfan syndrome. Eur Heart J. 2004;25:1146–52.
35. Mortensen K, Baulmann J, Rybczynski M, Sheikhzadeh S, Aydin MA, Treede H, et al. Augmentation index and the evolution of aortic disease in marfan-like syndromes. Am J Hypertens. 2010;23(7):716–24.
36. Mortensen K, Aydin MA, Rybczynski M, Baulmann J, Schahidi NA, Kean G, et al. Augmentation index relates to progression of aortic disease in adults with Marfan syndrome. Am J Hypertens. 2009;22(9):971–9.
37. Dijk JM, van der Graaf Y, Grobbee DE, Banga JD, Bots ML. Increased arterial stiffness is independently related to cerebrovascular disease and aneurysms of the abdominal aorta: the Second Manifestations of Arterial Disease (SMART) Study. Stroke. 2004;35:1642–6.
38. Wilson KA, Lee AJ, Hoskins PR, Fowkes FG, Ruckley CV, Bradbury AW. The relationship between aortic wall distensibility and rupture of infrarenal abdominal aortic aneurysm. J Vasc Surg. 2003;37:112–7.
39. Lee CW, Sung SH, Chen CK, Chen IM, Cheng HM, Yu WC, et al. Measures of carotid-femoral pulse wave velocity and augmentation index are not reliable in patients with abdominal aortic aneurysm. J Hypertens. 2013;31(9):1853–60.
40. Kadoglou NP, Papadakis I, Moulakakis KG, Ikonomidis I, Alepaki M, Moustardas P, et al. Arterial stiffness and novel biomarkers in patients with abdominal aortic aneurysms. Regul Pept. 2012;179(1–3):50–4.
41. Shingu Y, Shiiya N, Ooka T, Tachibana T, Kubota S, Morita S, et al. Augmentation index is elevated in aortic aneurysm and dissection. Ann Thorac Surg. 2009;87(5):1373–7.
42. Ruegg G, Mason RH, Hardinge M, Perkins J, Husmann M, Russi EW, et al. Augmentation index and central aortic blood pressure in patients with abdominal aortic aneurysms. J Hypertens. 2010;28(11):2252–7.
43. Moon J, Lee SH, Ko YG, Jang Y, Shim WH, Choi DH. Central aortic pressure in aortic aneurysm and aortic dissection: a novel prognostic marker. Acta Cardiol. 2010;65(3):303–8.

44. Rios AS, Silber EN, Bavishi N, Varga P, Burton BK, Clark WA, et al. Effect of long-term beta-blockade on aortic root compliance in patients with Marfan syndrome. Am Heart J. 1999;137:1057–61.
45. Ahimastos AA, Aggarwal A, D'Orsa KM, Formosa MF, White AJ, Savarirayan R, et al. Effect of perindopril on large artery stiffness and aortic root diameter in patients with Marfan syndrome: a randomized controlled trial. JAMA. 2007;298(13):1539–47.
46. Groenink M, den Hartog AW, Franken R, Radonic T, de Waard V, Timmermans J, et al. Losartan reduces aortic dilatation rate in adults with Marfan syndrome: a randomized controlled trial. Eur Heart J. 2013;34(45): 3491–500.
47. Williams A, Kenny D, Wilson D, Fagenello G, Nelson M, Dunstan F, et al. Effects of atenolol, perindopril and verapamil on haemodynamic and vascular function in Marfan syndrome - a randomised, double-blind, crossover trial. Eur J Clin Invest. 2012;42(8): 891–9.
48. Kadoglou NP, Moulakakis KG, Papadakis I, Ikonomidis I, Alepaki M, Lekakis J, et al. Changes in aortic pulse wave velocity of patients undergoing endovascular repair of abdominal aortic aneurysms. J Endovasc Ther. 2012;19(5):661–6.
49. Takeda Y, Sakata Y, Ohtani T, Tamaki S, Omori Y, Tsukamoto Y, Aizawa Y, Shimamura K, Shirakawa Y, Kuratani T, Sawa Y, Yamamoto K, Mano T, Komuro I. Endovascular aortic repair increases vascular stiffness and alters cardiac structure and function. Circ J. 2014;78:322–8.
50. Lantelme P, Dzudie A, Milon H, Bricca G, Legedz L, Chevalier JM, et al. Effect of abdominal aortic grafts on aortic stiffness and central hemodynamics. J Hypertens. 2009;27(6):1268–76.
51. Sekhri AR, Lees WR, Adiseshiah M. Measurement of aortic compliance in abdominal aortic aneurysms before and after open and endoluminal repair: preliminary results. J Endovasc Ther. 2004;11(4):472–82.
52. Lederle FA, Freischlag JA, Kyriakides TC, Matsumura JS, Padberg Jr FT, Kohler TR, et al. Long-term comparison of endovascular and open repair of abdominal aortic aneurysm. N Engl J Med. 2012;367(21):1988–97.
53. O'Rourke MF. Arterial function in health and disease. Edinburgh: Churchill Livingstone; 1982.
54. Baumgartner H, Bonhoeffer P, De Groot NM, de Haan F, Deanfield JE, Galie N, et al. ESC Guidelines for the management of grown-up congenital heart disease (new version 2010). Eur Heart J. 2010;31(23):2915–57.
55. Canniffe C, Ou P, Walsh K, Bonnet D, Celermajer D. Hypertension after repair of aortic coarctation–a systematic review. Int J Cardiol. 2013;167(6):2456–61.
56. Brili S, Dernellis J, Aggeli C, Pitsavos C, Hatzos C, Stefanadis C, et al. Aortic elastic properties in patients with repaired coarctation of aorta. Am J Cardiol. 1998;82:1140–3.
57. de Divitiis M, Pilla C, Kattenhorn M, Zadinello M, Donald A, Leeson P, et al. Vascular dysfunction after repair of coarctation of the aorta: impact of early surgery. Circulation. 2001;104 Suppl 1:I165–70.
58. Kenny D, Polson JW, Martin RP, Caputo M, Wilson DG, Cockcroft JR, et al. Relationship of aortic pulse wave velocity and baroreceptor reflex sensitivity to blood pressure control in patients with repaired coarctation of the aorta. Am Heart J. 2011;162(2):398–404.
59. Aznaouridis K, Vlachopoulos C, Protogerou A, Stefanadis C. Ambulatory systolic-diastolic pressure regression index as a predictor of clinical events: a meta-analysis of longitudinal studies. Stroke. 2012; 43(3):733–9.
60. Simonetti GD, VON Vigier RO, Wühl E, Mohaupt MG. Ambulatory arterial stiffness index is increased in hypertensive childhood disease. Pediatr Res. 2008;64(3):303–7.
61. Sarkola T, Redington AN, Slorach C, Hui W, Bradley T, Jaeggi E. Assessment of vascular phenotype using a novel very-high-resolution ultrasound technique in adolescents after aortic coarctation repair and/or stent implantation: relationship to central haemodynamics and left ventricular mass. Heart. 2011;97(21):1788–93.
62. Trojnarska O, Szczepaniak-Chicheł L, Mizia-Stec K, Gabriel M, Bartczak A, Grajek S, et al. Vascular remodeling in adults after coarctation repair: impact of descending aorta stenosis and age at surgery. Clin Res Cardiol. 2011;100(5):447–55.
63. Kenny D, Polson JW, Martin RP, Wilson DG, Caputo M, Cockcroft JR, et al. Surgical approach for aortic coarctation influences arterial compliance and blood pressure control. Ann Thorac Surg. 2010;90(2): 600–4.
64. Vogt M, Kühn A, Baumgartner D, Baumgartner C, Busch R, Kostolny M, et al. Impaired elastic properties of the ascending aorta in newborns before and early after successful coarctation repair: proof of a systemic vascular disease of the prestenotic arteries? Circulation. 2005;111(24):3269–73.
65. Chen SS, Donald AE, Storry C, Halcox JP, Bonhoeffer P, Deanfield JE. Impact of aortic stenting on peripheral vascular function and daytime systolic blood pressure in adult coarctation. Heart. 2008;94(7): 919–24.
66. Szczepaniak-Chicheł L, Trojnarska O, Mizia-Stec K, Gabriel M, Grajek S, Gasior Z, et al. Augmentation of central arterial pressure in adult patients after coarctation repair. Blood Press Monit. 2011;16(1):22–8.
67. Moltzer E, Mattace Raso FU, Karamermer Y, Boersma E, Webb GD, Simoons ML, et al. Comparison of Candesartan versus Metoprolol for treatment of systemic hypertension after repaired aortic coarctation. Am J Cardiol. 2010;105(2):217–22.
68. Brili S, Tousoulis D, Antoniades C, Vasiliadou C, Karali M, Papageorgiou N, et al. Effects of ramipril on endothelial function and the expression of proinflammatory cytokines and adhesion molecules in young normotensive subjects with successfully repaired coarctation of aorta: a randomized cross-over study. J Am Coll Cardiol. 2008;51(7):742–9.
69. Vlachopoulos C, Jackson G, Stefanadis C, Montorsi P. Erectile dysfunction in the cardiovascular patient. Eur Heart J. 2013;34(27):2034–46.

70. Vlachopoulos CV, Terentes-Printzios DG, Ioakeimidis NK, Aznaouridis KA, Stefanadis CI. Prediction of cardiovascular events and all-cause mortality with erectile dysfunction: a systematic review and meta-analysis of cohort studies. Circ Cardiovasc Qual Outcomes. 2013;6(1):99–109.
71. Vlachopoulos C, Rokkas K, Ioakeimidis N, Aggeli C, Michaelides A, Roussakis G, et al. Prevalence of asymptomatic coronary artery disease in men with vasculogenic erectile dysfunction: a prospective angiographic study. Eur Urol. 2005;48:996–1002; discussion 1002–3.
72. Vlachopoulos C, Aznaouridis K, Ioakeimidis N, Rokkas K, Tsekoura D, Vasiliadou C, Stefanadi E, Askitis A, Stefanadis C. Arterial function and intima-media thickness in hypertensive patients with erectile dysfunction. J Hypertens. 2008;26(9):1829–36.
73. Vlachopoulos C, Ioakeimidis N, Terentes-Printzios D, Aznaouridis K, Rokkas K, Aggelis A, et al. Plasma total testosterone and incident cardiovascular events in hypertensive patients. Am J Hypertens. 2013;26(3):373–81.
74. Vlachopoulos C, Hirata K, O'Rourke MF. Effect of sildenafil on arterial stiffness and wave reflection. Vasc Med. 2003;8(4):243–8.
75. Vlachopoulos C, Terentes-Printzios D, Ioakeimidis N, Rokkas K, Samentzas A, Aggelis A, et al. Beneficial effect of vardenafil on aortic stiffness and wave reflections. J Clin Pharmacol. 2012;52(8):1215–21.

27 Large Artery Remodeling and Chronic Kidney Disease

Marie Briet, Michel Delahousse, Gérard London, Stéphane Laurent, and Pierre Boutouyrie

Abstract

In recent years, many studies emphasized the role of arterial remodeling in the development of cardiovascular diseases, and it was shown that stiffening of arteries is associated with increased cardiovascular mortality and morbidity. Moreover, arterial stiffening is linked to decreased glomerular filtration rate, and is predictive of kidney-disease progression and the patient's cardiovascular outcome. Early vascular aging and arterial stiffening are observed with progression of chronic kidney disease (CKD) and in end-stage renal disease (ESRD). This accelerated aging is associated with outward remodeling of large vessels, characterized by increased arterial radius not totally compensated for by artery wall hypertrophy. The mechanisms involved in large artery remodelling associated with CKD are complex including arterial calcification, inflammation, oxidative stress in association with mineral and bone metabolism disorders. Arterial stiffening in CKD and ESRD patients is of multifactorial origin with extensive arterial calcifications representing a major covariate. With aging, arterial stiffening is more pronounced in the aorta than peripheral conduit arteries, leading to the disappearance or inversion of the arterial stiffness gradient and less protection of the microcirculation from high-pressure transmission. Various non-pharmacological or

M. Briet, MD, PhD
Department of Pharmacology,
Centre Hospitalo-Universitaire d'Angers,
Université d'Angers, Angers, France

Lady Davis Institute for Medical Research,
McGill University, Montreal, QC, Canada
e-mail: mariebriet1@free.fr

M. Delahousse, MD, PhD
Department of Nephrology and Transplantation,
Foch Hospital, Suresnes, France
e-mail: delahousse@mac.com

G. London, MD
Department of Nephrology, Hopital Manhes,
Fleury-Mérogis, France
e-mail: glondon@club-internet.fr,
gerard.london@ch-manhes.fr

S. Laurent, MD, PhD (✉) • P. Boutouyrie, MD, PhD
Department of Pharmacology
and Institut National de la Santé et de la Recherche
Médicale U970(Eq7)-PARCC, Hôpital Européen
Georges Pompidou, Assistance Publique-Hôpitaux
de Paris, Université Paris-Descartes, Paris 75015, France
e-mail: stephane.laurent@egp.aphp.fr;
pierre.boutouyrie@egp.aphp.fr

M.E. Safar et al. (eds.), *Blood Pressure and Arterial Wall Mechanics in Cardiovascular Diseases*,
DOI 10.1007/978-1-4471-5198-2_27, © Springer-Verlag London 2014

pharmacological interventions can modestly slow the progression of arterial stiffness, but arterial stiffness is, in part, pressure-dependent and treatments able to stop the process mainly include antihypertensive drugs.

Keywords
Arterial stiffness • Cardiovascular events • Epidemiology • Surrogate end point

Chronic kidney disease (CKD) is associated with severe and frequent cardiovascular (CV) diseases. Clinical and epidemiological studies emphasize the role of large and small artery remodeling as major contributing factors of CV diseases in CKD patients. The specificity of CKD is the exposure to traditional CV risk factors and uremia-linked CV risk factors. Among them, hemodynamic disturbances including hypervolemia and metabolic disorders such as bone and mineral metabolism disorders play a central role in arterial remodeling.

Epidemiology of Chronic Kidney Disease

Chronic kidney disease (CKD) is defined as impaired kidney function or raised proteinuria on two or more occasions at least 3 months apart or abnormal kidney morphology. Current guidelines recommend that kidney function should be assessed by equation, preferentially the CKD-EPI equation (chronic kidney disease epidemiology collaboration) which includes sex, age, serum creatinine concentration and ethnic origin, and proteinuria by the albumin to creatinine ratio. Regarding glomerular filtration rate (GFR) values and proteinuria levels, the new classification of CKD includes 6 categories and 3 categories, respectively (Table 27.1) [1]. Following this definition, CKD affects ≈ 10 % of the population in Europe and North America. Data for the NHANES study emphasizes the growing prevalence of CKD during the last 20 years [2].

Life expectancy is significantly reduced in patients with CKD proportionally to the decrease in GFR. The effect of age on mortality almost disappears at advanced stages meaning that renal failure is the main determinant of mortality in this population [3] (Fig. 27.1). For example, the risk of death of a 40-year-old patient with end-stage renal disease (ESRD) is similar to the risk of death of a 75-year-old subject in the general population [4].

Table 27.1 Chronic kidney disease classification, following the international guidelines KDIGO [1]

Categories, GFR	eGFR, mL/min/1.73 m^2	Categories	Albuminuria mg/g
G1	≥90	A1	<30
G2	60–89	A2	30–300
G3a	45–59	A3	>300
G3b	30–44		
G4	15–29		
G5	<15		

Cardiovascular disease is a major cause of death in patients with end-stage renal disease (ESRD) [5] and also at moderate stages [6]. Even after adjustment for traditional cardiovascular risk factors, an inverse linear relation exists between GFR estimated with the MDRD (Modification of Diet in Renal Disease) formula and cardiovascular events and hospitalizations [6, 7]. It is worth to notice that patients with stage 4 CKD (eGFR between 15 and 30 mL/min/1.73 m^2) are more likely to die from cardiovascular diseases than to progress to ESRD [8]. Data from the ARIC study (the Atherosclerosis Risk in Communities) showed that the risk of heart failure [9], stroke [10], peripheral artery disease [11], coronary heart disease [12], and atrial fibrillation [13] is at least doubled in patients with eGFR below 60 mL/min/1.73 m^2. Despite this high cardiovascular risk, traditional cardiovascular risk factors predict poorly the cardiovascular outcome in patients with CKD. When Framingham

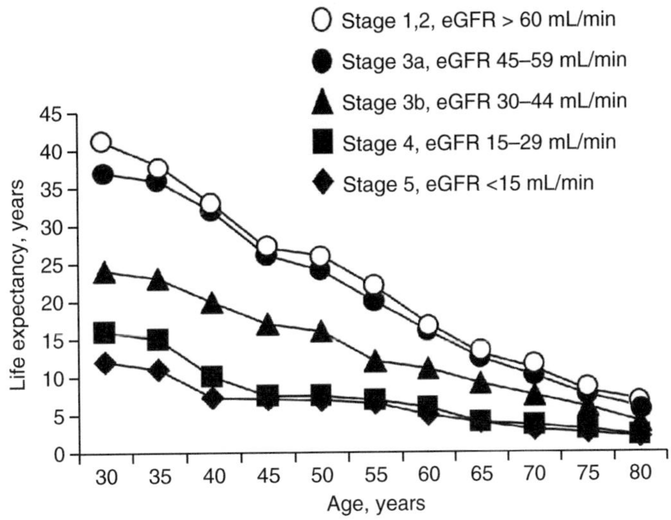

Fig. 27.1 Life expectancy in patients with chronic kidney disease (Adapted with permission from Ref. [3])

equations were used to calculate the cardiovascular risk in patients with CKD from the ARIC and CHS (Cardiovascular Health Study) trials, the prediction of cardiovascular events was very low, predicting only 13.9 and 4.8 % of the 10-year events in men and women, respectively [14]. Part of the specificity of CKD patients comes from the exposure to traditional CV risk factors to uremia-linked CV risk factors, such as anemia, mineral metabolism disorders, inflammation, oxidative stress, asymmetric dimethyl arginine, sympathetic nervous system activation, and uremic toxins [15, 16]. These metabolic abnormalities, in addition to the hemodynamic disturbances including high blood pressure, increased extracellular volume, and sustained activation of the renin-angiotensin system, impact the vascular structure and the cardiovascular prognosis of patients with CKD [15].

Large Artery Remodeling Associated with Chronic Kidney Disease

Hypertrophy and Enlargement

The first observation of an abnormal arterial remodeling in CKD patients was made by Bright in 1843 himself reporting a hypertrophy and enlargement of the arteries in the kidney [17]. Recent development of high-resolution imaging technology helped to improve the characterization of the remodeling of large arteries in CKD patients. In 1990, London et al. were the first to describe an increase in aortic stiffness and an enlargement of the carotid artery in patients with ESRD [18]. In an oversimplified scheme, large artery stiffness or resistance to distension can be defined as the ability of the arteries to accommodate to the stroke volume. During ventricular contraction, part of the stroke volume is forwarded directly to peripheral tissues, and part of this is stored in the aorta. During the diastole, the stored energy recoils the aorta and propels the blood forward into the peripheral tissues ensuring continuous flow [19]. When the stiffness of the aorta is increased, the energy necessary for arterial distension is high, i.e., for a given stroke volume, the pressure increase is high. In this situation the entire stroke volume flows through the arterial system mainly during the systole. As a consequence, the flow is intermittent and the capillary transit time is short, which reduces metabolic exchanges. This oversimplified view is useful; however, it must be modulated toward a more complex and realistic one by reading the dedicated chapters in the present book. This physiological relation between the cardiac work and aortic stiffness has been shown in patients with ESRD. Indeed, aortic stiffness was strongly correlated with left ventricular mass volume in this population [18].

Time Course of the Change in Arterial Stiffness During CKD

As stated earlier, six stages are defined in CKD among the level of eGFR. Changes in arterial geometric and functional properties are not only the prerogative of ESRD patients but appear earlier during the progression of the disease which takes years. By comparison with healthy subjects and hypertensive patients, large artery (aortic and carotid) stiffness is increased in patients with CKD stages 2–5 [20, 21]. During CKD evolution from stage 2 to stage 4, large artery stiffness progression is debated [20, 22–24]. In the NephroTest cohort, the yearly evaluation of arterial parameters in CKD patients stages 2–5 did not show any progression of aortic stiffness [24] (Table 27.2). This observation has been confirmed in another small cohort of CKD patients where aortic stiffness was estimated through brachial-ankle pulse wave velocity [25]. Accordingly, left ventricular mass was stable in CKD patients stages 2–5 in the CRIC (chronic renal insufficiency cohort) study [26]. This may be due to the relative short follow-up period, combined to powerful pathological mechanisms at play during CKD.

At end stage, there is a step increase in arterial stiffness, and a rapid progression of aortic stiffness is observed [27]. The slope of progression of aortic stiffness is almost ten times higher than the one observed in hypertensive patients. The "accelerated aging" in ESRD patients is observed at the level of the aorta and central arteries, whereas arterial stiffness in peripheral muscular arteries remains stable [28] reversing the arterial stiffness gradient between central and peripheral arteries. The stiffness gradient together with arterial branching, changes in arterial diameter, and aortic geometry changes causes partial reflexion of forward pressure waves regulating pressure transmission to the microcirculation. At ESRD, the acceleration in the reduction of the impedance mismatch reduces the buffering capacity to lower pulsatile pressure transmission to the microcirculation.

Table 27.2 Arterial remodeling parameters progression in CKD patients

Parameters	Age- and gender-adjusted slope (unit/year)	*P*
Brachial		
Systolic blood pressure, mmHg	−0.4 ± 0.5	0.45
Diastolic blood pressure, mmHg	−0.7 ± 0.3	0.02
Pulse pressure, mmHg	0.4 ± 0.3	0.22
Central		
Systolic blood pressure, mmHg	−0.5 ± 0.7	0.5
Diastolic blood pressure, mmHg	−0.8 ± 0.3	0.01
Pulse pressure, mmHg	0.47 ± 0.52	0.37
Carotid		
Intima-media thickness, μm	−22 ± 4	<0.0001
Wall cross-sectional area, mm^2	−0.39 ± 0.09	<0.0001
External diameter, mm	0.039 ± 0.014	0.006
Internal diameter, mm	0.083 ± 0.015	<0.0001
Media-to-lumen ratio	−1.1 ± 0.2	<0.0001
Stiffness, m/s	0.28 ± 0.05	<0.0001
Young's elastic modulus, kPa	59.9 ± 9.9	<0.0001
Circumferential wall stress, kPa	2.08 ± 0.43	<0.0001
Aorta		
Aortic pulse wave velocity	0.01 ± 0.04	0.89
Kidney		
Measured GFR, mL/min/1.73 m^2	−1.6 ± 0.3	<0.0001

Adapted with permission from Ref. [24]

Alterations in the Intrinsic Properties of the Arterial Wall During CKD

Besides age, blood pressure is the main determinant of arterial stiffness. At low distending pressure, the tension is borne by the distensible elastin fibers. At high distending pressure, the tension is transferred to the less extensible collagen fibers. For example, in hypertensive patients, most of the reduction in arterial distensibility is due to distending blood pressure level. Indeed, under isobaric conditions, the elastic modulus and distensibility are similar to those observed in normotensive controls age matched [29, 30].

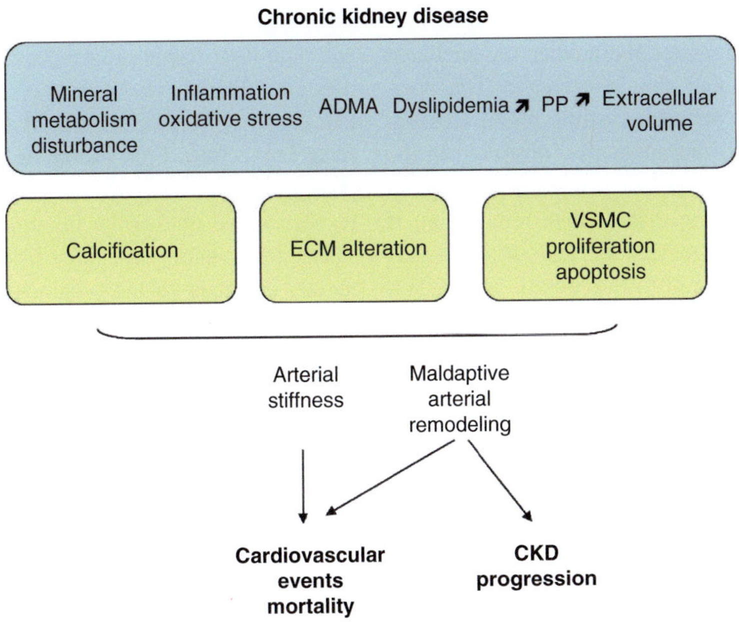

Fig. 27.2 Mechanisms involved in large artery remodeling associated with chronic kidney disease. Patients with CKD are exposed to traditional and nontraditional cardiovascular risk factors including mineral metabolism disturbances, inflammation, oxidative stress, and increased plasma ADMA levels. Altogether, these metabolic and hemodynamic disturbances induce arterial calcification, extracellular matrix remodeling, and vascular smooth muscle cell apoptosis leading to an increase in arterial stiffness and a maladaptive arterial remodeling. Increased arterial stiffness and maladaptive arterial remodeling impact the cardiovascular and renal prognosis of the patients. *ADMA* Asymmetric dimethyl arginine, *PP* Pulse pressure, *ECM* Extracellular matrix, *VSMC* Vascular smooth muscle cells

In ESRD patients, stiffening is associated with an alteration of the intrinsic elastic properties of the arterial wall. Profound alteration of the composition of the arterial wall is observed at ESRD, including fibroelastic intimal thickening, calcification, elastinolysis, inflammation, increased collagen content, and apoptosis of vascular smooth muscle cells [19]. These arterial changes are influenced by classical CV risk factors such as hypertension, age, diabetes, dyslipidemia, genetic, and overweight (Fig. 27.2). However, classical cardiovascular risk factors play a minimal role in the progression of arterial stiffness in ESRD, leaving a place for CKD-related risk factors among them, advanced glycation products [27]. At ESRD, arterial calcification is a determinant of arterial stiffness [31–33], and the acceleration of arterial calcification observed in ESRD is associated with the progression of arterial stiffness [34]. Arterial calcification is a complex process implicating osteogenic differentiation of vascular smooth muscle cells and a crystallization step in the so-called matrix vesicles extruded from viable vascular smooth muscle cells or apoptotic bodies, in addition to a disequilibrium between activators and inhibitors of the calcification (Fig. 27.2) [35–37].

Maladaptive Remodeling of Large Arteries During CKD

The originality of CKD arterial properties concerns the remodeling pattern. Arterial remodeling associated with CKD stages 2–4 is characterized by a paradoxical thinning associated with an enlargement of the diameter leading to an increase in circumferential wall stress [21, 38]. ESRD patients' arterial remodeling is characterized by increased arterial diameters and intima-media thickness; however, the wall-to-lumen ratio is comparable to control subjects [39]. As in earlier CKD stages, the hypertrophic response is not adequate. According to Laplace's

Law, an increase in blood pressure and regardless of the internal arterial diameter, the thickness of the arterial wall should increase. The positive correlation between systolic blood pressure and carotid wall-to-lumen ratio observed in the general population is lost and even reversed in ESRD patients. The maladaptive remodeling is not limited to large vessels, and small vessels are also affected. Wall-to-lumen ratio of resistant arteries isolated from subcutaneous tissues from ESRD patients is similar even lower than the one measured in controls [40]. The defect of wall thickening has also been described at the level of the radial artery in ESRD patients in an experimental situation of increased blood flow caused by arteriovenous fistula surgery. An increase in radial artery diameter was measured at the side of the arteriovenous fistula without increase in radial artery thickness, by comparison with the opposite side. As a consequence, the wall cross-sectional area was unchanged and circumferential wall stress increased [41].

In the longitudinal NephroTest study with yearly evaluation of arterial parameters, the progression of arterial thinning was fast (adjusted slope, -22 ± 4 μm/year; $P<0.0001$) [24] and was the exact opposite of the progression observed in high CV patients (+18 μm) (Table 27.2) [42]. In the PROG-IMT meta-analysis, the intima-media thickness progression in the general population ranges from 0 to 30 μm/year [43]. The carotid internal diameter increased faster than the carotid external diameter leading to a significant decrease in the wall-to-lumen ratio and wall cross-sectional area over time. Brachial and central blood pressures remained stable during follow-up except a moderate decrease in central and peripheral diastolic blood pressure (Table 27.2) [24].

Impact of Large Artery Remodeling and Stiffening on Renal, Cardiovascular, and General Outcomes

In CKD, large artery remodeling and stiffening are linked with general and cardiovascular prognosis as well as with renal disease progression. The kidney perfusion is characterized by low resistances and high flow. Renal resistances in afferent arterioles are relatively low by comparison with resistances in the efferent arterioles in order to maintain renal blood flow. Fluctuations in renal perfusion pressure result in proportional changes in vascular resistance, but glomerular filtration is unchanged. This autoregulatory vascular resistance response is mainly confined to the preglomerular arterioles. As a consequence, glomerular capillary pressures are maintained relatively constant and protected from barotrauma as long as the autoregulatory mechanisms are intact and the BP remains within the autoregulatory range. Conversely, if renal autoregulatory ability is impaired, even modest increases in systemic BP are transmitted to the glomerular capillaries. Two mechanisms are involved in renal autoregulation: (1) rapid myogenic vasoconstriction and (2) tubuloglomerular feedback system. The myogenic response is fast and primarily responsible for protecting against hypertensive injury. In chronic kidney disease, autoregulation response to increase in blood pressure is impaired and represents the predominant mechanism for chronic kidney disease progression [44, 45]. In accordance with these observations, Hashimoto et al. have shown that central pulse pressure and aortic pulse wave velocity were independently associated with the resistive index of the kidney. The latter was associated with proteinuria [46]. From these observations, large artery stiffness and central pulse pressure may be related to CKD progression. In CKD patients, central pulse pressure or aortic stiffness was inconstantly associated with CKD progression or incident ESRD [24, 47, 48]. On the contrary, the outward maladaptive remodeling was an independent determinant of CKD progression and incident ESRD (Fig. 27.3) [24].

In recent years, more than 20 studies have demonstrated that aortic stiffness is an independent predictor of CV events and all-cause mortality, in the various populations including the general population, hypertensive patients, coronary heart disease patients, and diabetes [49]. This was confirmed in a meta-analysis of 17 longitudinal studies that evaluated aortic stiffness and followed 15,877 subjects for a mean of

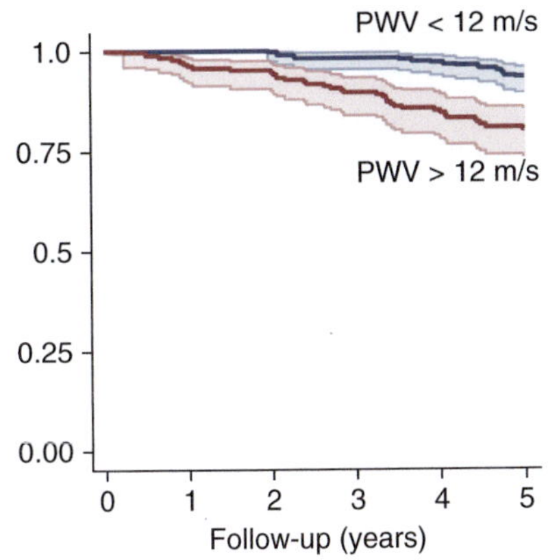

Fig. 27.3 Kaplan-Meier survival curves estimating the overall survival of CKD patients (Adapted from Ref. [51] with permission)

7.7 years. The pooled relative risk for all-cause mortality was 1.90 (95 % confidence interval: 1.61–2.24) [50]. In CKD patients stages 2–4 and ESRD, aortic stiffness was also independently associated with all-cause mortality [51, 52]. Among parameters directly related to large artery stiffness (aortic or carotid stiffness) or indirectly (central pulse pressure, augmentation index), aortic stiffness evaluated through carotid-femoral pulse wave velocity had the strongest correlation with survival in CKD patients stages 2–5 (Fig. 27.3) [51]. In addition, aortic stiffness evaluation improves the prediction of the risk in this population. Indeed, net reclassification improvement based on COX prediction significantly reclassified patients for the risk of all-cause mortality (NRI, 95 % confidence interval, 29 % [2.3–42 %]) [51]. Using competing risk models, carotid-femoral pulse wave velocity was significantly associated with fatal and nonfatal CV events [51]. In CKD stage 5, improvement of aortic stiffness by antihypertensive treatment was associated with a better outcome [53]. This provides strong basis for interventional trials targeting this parameter in ESRD. In CKD stages 2–5, carotid internal diameter enlargement has been associated with overall mortality. The absence of significant association between carotid internal diameter with fatal and nonfatal CV events but the positive and significant association with the competing risk (mortality from non-CV origin) suggests that the remodeling abnormalities may not only be limited to the vascular system but may affect other tissues [51].

Vascular Remodeling Following Kidney Transplantation

Few longitudinal studies have investigated the impact of kidney transplantation on recipient large arteries in the recent years, and conflicting results have been reported. Covic et al. have shown a short-term improvement of aortic stiffness after living-donor kidney transplantation [54], whereas others did not measure any changes 1 year after cadaveric kidney transplantation [55, 56]. With current shortage of organs, the heterogeneity of donor characteristics increases, and this fact must be taken into account when interpreting the impact of kidney transplantation on recipient large arteries. In a prospective cohort including 78 deceased donor kidney recipients with serial PWV measurements, Delahousse et al. have shown that donor age was the main determinant of aortic stiffness change within the first year posttransplantation, independently of any change in blood pressure [57]. In fact, the arterial benefit of kidney transplantation was restricted to recipients of young, "ideal" donor kidneys. By contrast, an increase in aortic stiffness was observed in recipients of the oldest kidneys harvested from so-called extended criteria donors. These observations suggest that removal of uremic "vasculotoxins" by the allograft could play a role in the reduction/progression of aortic stiffness, in addition to undetermined immunologic or non-immunologic factors related to donor age and donor source. Future studies should elucidate the GFR-independent pathophysiological pathways linking donor age and donor source to arterial remodeling and stiffness in renal transplant recipients.

Despite general improvement of indices of arterial function after kidney transplantation, at least in recipients of kidneys harvested from young deceased donors or living donors, cross-sectional studies consistently showed that arterial stiffness remains elevated in kidney recipients compared to normal volunteers or hypertensive patients matched for age, gender, and blood pressure [58, 59]. The potential benefit of kidney transplantation is probably limited by the incomplete restoration of kidney function and offset by the emergence of specific transplantation-related mechanisms responsible for ongoing subclinical arterial damage. Indeed, cross-sectional studies showed an independent association between recipient arterial indices and allograft-related parameters or posttransplant events such as allograft function [58], acute rejection [59], microinflammation [58], new-onset diabetes mellitus after transplantation [60], and hypomagnesemia [61].

Importantly, recent evidences have underlined the effect of components of the immunosuppressive regimen itself on recipient large arteries. Calcineurin inhibitors (CNI) remain the cornerstone of immunosuppression in kidney transplantation. In a prospective randomized study, a CNI-free immunosuppressive regimen based on mTOR inhibitors and MMF was able to prevent conduit artery endothelial dysfunction [62], aortic stiffening, and to improve cardiovascular coupling and central hemodynamics by comparison with cyclosporin A and mycophenolate mofetil [63]. These findings were observed in the context of a decrease in plasma endothelin 1 and oxidative stress markers suggesting that an improvement in endothelial function and oxidative stress balance contributed to the beneficial effect of the CNI-free regimen.

Both aortic stiffness and central wave reflections (augmented pressure) were recently established as strong and independent predictors of fatal and nonfatal cardiovascular events in a large cohort of renal transplant recipients extending the available evidence from the dialysis and hypertensive population to patients with a kidney transplant [64]. Premature CV death with a functioning allograft remains the leading factor in reducing long-term overall graft survival. Taken together, these considerations strongly support a widespread use of carotid-femoral PWV and central pulse pressure in renal transplant recipients in order to stratify the cardiovascular risk more precisely. An important issue will be to determine whether the beneficial impact of CNI-free, mTOR inhibitor-based immunosuppressive regimen on large artery structure and function can be effectively translated into overall graft survival improvement in the all population of patients including older donors, older recipients with high cardiovascular risk, who are now currently considered for renal transplantation.

Mechanisms Involved in Arterial Remodeling in CKD

The mechanisms involved in arterial remodeling in CKD are complex and involve uremia-linked hemodynamic and metabolic disturbance such as high blood pressure, high extracellular volume, mineral metabolism disturbance, inflammation, and oxidative stress. In addition, traditional classical risk factors, for example, diabetes, could also influence arterial remodeling (Fig. 27.2) [65].

Hypertension

Hypertension remains the most important risk factor for CKD progression and premature cardiovascular death [66] and the major determinant, with age, of arterial remodeling. Increased extracellular volume, sustained activation of the renin-angiotensin system, and increased sympathetic tone are the main mechanisms involved in hypertension associated with CKD [15]. Vascular cells can sense and respond mechanical forces generated by pressure and shear stress [67]. Forces are transmitted to the cells by the cytoskeleton and other structural components involved in connections between intra- and extracellular milieus. Mechanotransduction involves these integrated structures such as focal adhesion sites, integrins, cellular junctions, and extracellular matrix. Mechanotransduction initiates transduction cascades, involving among others nuclear factor-kappa B and MAP kinase pathways, leading to functional changes within the cells, growth, and proliferation when stress is increased. Mechanotransduction can be altered by defects in attachment between cells and extracellular matrix [68]. In patients with CKD, chronic increase in circumferential wall stress with progression of disease can be interpreted as a defect in mechanotransduction or in the trophic response to pressure sensing.

Dyslipidemia

Lipid profile evolves during CKD progression. At moderate stages, lipid profile is characterized by an increase in serum total cholesterol and LDL cholesterol, whereas at ESRD serum total cholesterol and LDL cholesterol are usually low [69] but associated with adverse outcome that is the so-called inverse epidemiology. The interpretation of inverse epidemiology is complex and involves both survival bias and confounding variables such as severe concomitant condition. At ESRD, the lipid profile associates high serum triglycerides and very low-density lipoprotein (VLDL), impairment in the clearance of the chylomicrons and their atherogenic remnants, and the presence of small dense LDL and oxidized LDL are described [65]. Observational studies have shown that lipid profile, in particular LDL and HDL cholesterol levels, was an independent determinant of carotid intima-media thickness and aortic stiffness in patients with CKD [70]. However, the AURORA (A Study to Evaluate the Use of Rosuvastatin in Subjects on Regular Hemodialysis) study failed to demonstrate the efficacy of rosuvastatin in CV prevention [71].

Mineral and Bone Metabolism Disorders

Mineral metabolism disorders associated with CKD classically include hyperphosphatemia, hyperparathyroidism, and vitamin D deficiency. Serum phosphate levels have been associated with arterial calcification and a poor cardiovascular and kidney outcome [72]. Phosphate levels are regulated by several hormones including parathyroid hormone (PTH), fibroblast growth factor 23 (FGF-23), klotho, and 1.25 dihydroxy vitamin D. All of these factors are implicated in arterial calcification [73].

FGF-23 has been widely studied the last years and has been associated with poor cardiovascular and kidney outcome in the CRIC study [74]. FGF-23 is a circulating factor, produced by osteoblasts and osteocytes, which exerts its effect binding the FGF receptor in presence of its cofactor klotho. FGF-23 increases urinary phosphate excretion. FGF-23 has been positively associated with aortic calcification in CKD [75]. However, it is complex to disentangle the specific effect of FGF-23 on arterial calcification from its effect on plasma phosphate levels.

Conclusion

CKD progression toward ESRD and kidney transplantation is associated with large artery damage, including arterial stiffening and maladaptive remodeling, which impacts the renal and cardiovascular prognosis of the patients. Kidney transplantation could reverse partially this deleterious arterial remodeling especially in young donors. The mechanisms involved in large artery remodeling associated with CKD are complex including arterial calcification, inflammation, and oxidative stress in association with mineral and bone metabolism disorders.

Disclosures
Marie Briet, none
Michel Delahousse, none
Pierre Boutouyrie, none
Stéphane Laurent, none

References

1. Stevens PE, Levin A, Kidney Disease: Improving Global Outcomes Chronic Kidney Disease Guideline Development Work Group Members. Evaluation and management of chronic kidney disease: synopsis of the kidney disease: improving global outcomes 2012 clinical practice guideline. Ann Intern Med. 2013;158:825–30.
2. Castro AF, Coresh J. CKD surveillance using laboratory data from the population-based National Health and Nutrition Examination Survey (NHANES). Am J Kid Dis. 2009;53:S46–55.
3. Gansevoort RT, et al. Chronic kidney disease and cardiovascular risk: epidemiology, mechanisms, and prevention. Lancet. 2013;382:339–52.
4. Murphy SW, Foley RN, Parfrey PS. Screening and treatment for cardiovascular disease in patients with

chronic renal disease. Am J Kidney Dis. 1998;32: S184–99.
5. Foley RN, Parfrey PS, Sarnak MJ. Clinical epidemiology of cardiovascular disease in chronic renal disease. Am J Kidney Dis. 1998;32:S112–9.
6. Go AS, Chertow GM, Fan D, McCulloch CE, Hsu CY. Chronic kidney disease and the risks of death, cardiovascular events, and hospitalization. N Engl J Med. 2004;351:1296–305.
7. Couser WG, Remuzzi G, Mendis S, Tonelli M. The contribution of chronic kidney disease to the global burden of major noncommunicable diseases. Kidney Int. 2011;80(12):1258–70.
8. Keith DS, Nichols GA, Gullion CM, Brown JB, Smith DH. Longitudinal follow-up and outcomes among a population with chronic kidney disease in a large managed care organization. Arch Intern Med. 2004;164:659–63.
9. Kottgen A, et al. Reduced kidney function as a risk factor for incident heart failure: the atherosclerosis risk in communities (ARIC) study. J Am Soc Nephrol. 2007;18:1307–15.
10. Abramson JL, Jurkovitz CT, Vaccarino V, Weintraub WS, McClellan W. Chronic kidney disease, anemia, and incident stroke in a middle-aged, community-based population: the ARIC Study. Kidney Int. 2003;64:610–5.
11. Wattanakit K, et al. Kidney function and risk of peripheral arterial disease: results from the Atherosclerosis Risk in Communities (ARIC) Study. J Am Soc Nephrol. 2007;18:629–36.
12. Jurkovitz CT, Abramson JL, Vaccarino LV, Weintraub WS, McClellan WM. Association of high serum creatinine and anemia increases the risk of coronary events: results from the prospective community-based atherosclerosis risk in communities (ARIC) study. J Am Soc Nephrol. 2003;14:2919–25.
13. Alonso A, et al. Chronic kidney disease is associated with the incidence of atrial fibrillation: the Atherosclerosis Risk in Communities (ARIC) study. Circulation. 2011;123:2946–53.
14. Weiner DE, et al. The Framingham predictive instrument in chronic kidney disease. J Am Coll Cardiol. 2007;50:217–24.
15. Schiffrin EL, Lipman ML, Mann JF. Chronic kidney disease: effects on the cardiovascular system. Circulation. 2007;116:85–97.
16. Drueke TB, Massy ZA. Chronic kidney disease: medial or intimal calcification in CKD-does it matter? Nat Rev Nephrol. 2011;7:250–1.
17. Toynbee J. On the intimate structure of the human kidney, and on the changes which its several component parts undergo in "Bright's disease". Med Chir Trans. 1846;29:303–26.
18. London GM, et al. Aortic and large artery compliance in end-stage renal failure. Kidney Int. 1990;37: 137–42.
19. Briet M, Boutouyrie P, Laurent S, London GM. Arterial stiffness and pulse pressure in CKD and ESRD. Kidney Int. 2012;82:388–400.
20. Wang MC, Tsai WC, Chen JY, Huang JJ. Stepwise increase in arterial stiffness corresponding with the stages of chronic kidney disease. Am J Kidney Dis. 2005;45:494–501.
21. Briet M, et al. Arterial stiffness and enlargement in mild-to-moderate chronic kidney disease. Kidney Int. 2006;69:350–7.
22. Townsend RR, et al. Aortic PWV in chronic kidney disease: a CRIC ancillary study. Am J Hypertens. 2010;23:282–9.
23. Ford ML, Tomlinson LA, Chapman TP, Rajkumar C, Holt SG. Aortic stiffness is independently associated with rate of renal function decline in chronic kidney disease stages 3 and 4. Hypertension. 2010;55: 1110–5.
24. Briet M, et al. Arterial remodeling associates with CKD progression. J Am Soc Nephrol. 2011;22:967–74.
25. Chen SC, et al. The longitudinal change of arterial stiffness in patients with chronic kidney disease. Am J Med Sci. 2012;343(2):109–13.
26. Bansal N, et al. A longitudinal study of left ventricular function and structure from CKD to ESRD: the CRIC study. Clin J Am Soc Nephrol. 2013;8:355–62.
27. Utescu MS, et al. Determinants of progression of aortic stiffness in hemodialysis patients: a prospective longitudinal study. Hypertension. 2013;62:154–60.
28. Pannier B, Guerin AP, Marchais SJ, Safar ME, London GM. Stiffness of capacitive and conduit arteries: prognostic significance for end-stage renal disease patients. Hypertension. 2005;45:592–6.
29. Hayoz D, et al. Conduit artery compliance and distensibility are not necessarily reduced in hypertension. Hypertension. 1992;20:1–6.
30. Bussy C, Boutouyrie P, Lacolley P, Challande P, Laurent S. Intrinsic stiffness of the carotid arterial wall material in essential hypertensives. Hypertension. 2000;35:1049–54.
31. van Guldener C, Lambert J, Janssen MJ, Donker AJ, Stehouwer CD. Endothelium-dependent vasodilatation and distensibility of large arteries in chronic haemodialysis patients. Nephrol Dial Trans. 1997;12 Suppl 2:14–8.
32. London GM, et al. Arterial media calcification in end-stage renal disease: impact on all-cause and cardiovascular mortality. Nephrol Dial Trans. 2003; 18:1731–40.
33. Raggi P, et al. Association of pulse wave velocity with vascular and valvular calcification in hemodialysis patients. Kidney Int. 2007;71:802–7.
34. Sigrist MK, Taal MW, Bungay P, McIntyre CW. Progressive vascular calcification over 2 years is associated with arterial stiffening and increased mortality in patients with stages 4 and 5 chronic kidney disease. Clin J Am Soc Nephrol. 2007;2:1241–8.
35. Hruska KA, Mathew S, Saab G. Bone morphogenetic proteins in vascular calcification. Circ Res. 2005;97:105–14.
36. Mori K, et al. Association of serum fetuin-A with carotid arterial stiffness. Clin Endocrinol (Oxf). 2007;66:246–50.

37. Gross ML, et al. Calcification of coronary intima and media: immunohistochemistry, backscatter imaging, and x-ray analysis in renal and nonrenal patients. Clin J Am Soc Nephrol. 2007;2:121–34.
38. Hermans MM, et al. Albuminuria, but not estimated glomerular filtration rate, is associated with maladaptive arterial remodeling: the Hoorn Study. J Hypertens. 2008;26:791–7.
39. London GM, et al. Cardiac and arterial interactions in end-stage renal disease. Kidney Int. 1996;50:600–8.
40. Luksha N, et al. Impaired resistance artery function in patients with end-stage renal disease. Clin Sci. 2011;120:525–36.
41. Girerd X, et al. Remodeling of the radial artery in response to a chronic increase in shear stress. Hypertension. 1996;27:799–803.
42. Mack WJ, et al. One-year reduction and longitudinal analysis of carotid intima-media thickness associated with colestipol/niacin therapy. Stroke. 1993;24:1779–83.
43. Lorenz MW, et al. Carotid intima-media thickness progression to predict cardiovascular events in the general population (the PROG-IMT collaborative project): a meta-analysis of individual participant data. Lancet. 2012;379:2053–62.
44. Bidani AK, Polichnowski AJ, Loutzenhiser R, Griffin KA. Renal microvascular dysfunction, hypertension and CKD progression. Curr Opin Nephrol Hypertens. 2013;22:1–9.
45. Bidani AK, Griffin KA, Williamson G, Wang X, Loutzenhiser R. Protective importance of the myogenic response in the renal circulation. Hypertension. 2009;54:393–8.
46. Hashimoto J, Ito S. Central pulse pressure and aortic stiffness determine renal hemodynamics: pathophysiological implication for microalbuminuria in hypertension. Hypertension. 2011;58:839–46.
47. Upadhyay A, et al. Arterial stiffness in mild-to-moderate CKD. J Am Soc Nephrol. 2009;20:2044–53.
48. Gosse P, Coulon P, Papaioannou G, Litalien J, Lemetayer P. Long-term decline in renal function is linked to initial pulse pressure in the essential hypertensive. J Hypertens. 2009;27:1303–8.
49. Laurent S, Mousseaux E, Boutouyrie P. Arterial stiffness as an imaging biomarker: are all pathways equal? Hypertension. 2013;62:10–2.
50. Vlachopoulos C, Aznaouridis K, Stefanadis C. Prediction of cardiovascular events and all-cause mortality with arterial stiffness: a systematic review and meta-analysis. J Am Coll Cardiol. 2010;55:1318–27.
51. Karras A, et al. Large artery stiffening and remodeling are independently associated with all-cause mortality and cardiovascular events in chronic kidney disease. Hypertension. 2012;60:1451–7.
52. Blacher J, et al. Impact of aortic stiffness on survival in end-stage renal disease. Circulation. 1999;99:2434–9.
53. Guerin AP, et al. Impact of aortic stiffness attenuation on survival of patients in end-stage renal failure. Circulation. 2001;103:987–92.
54. Covic A, Goldsmith DJ, Gusbeth-Tatomir P, Buhaescu I, Covic M. Successful renal transplantation decreases aortic stiffness and increases vascular reactivity in dialysis patients. Transplantation. 2003;76:1573–7.
55. Zoungas S, et al. Arterial function after successful renal transplantation. Kidney Int. 2004;65:1882–9.
56. Bachelet-Rousseau C, et al. Evolution of arterial stiffness after kidney transplantation. Nephrol Dial Trans. 2011;26:3386–91.
57. Delahousse M, et al. Aortic stiffness of kidney transplant recipients correlates with donor age. J Am Soc Nephrol. 2008;19:798–805.
58. Verbeke F, Van Biesen W, Peeters P, Van Bortel LM, Vanholder RC. Arterial stiffness and wave reflections in renal transplant recipients. Nephrol Dial Trans. 2007;22:3021–7.
59. Bahous SA, et al. Aortic pulse wave velocity in renal transplant patients. Kidney Int. 2004;66:1486–92.
60. Opazo Saez A, Kos M, Witzke O, Kribben A, Nurnberger J. Effect of new-onset diabetes mellitus on arterial stiffness in renal transplantation. Trans Int. 2008;21:930–5.
61. Van Laecke S, et al. The relation between hypomagnesaemia and vascular stiffness in renal transplant recipients. Nephrol Dial Trans. 2011;26:2362–9.
62. Joannides R, et al. Comparative effects of sirolimus and cyclosporin on conduit arteries endothelial function in kidney recipients. Trans Int. 2010;23:1135–43.
63. Joannides R, et al. Immunosuppressant regimen based on sirolimus decreases aortic stiffness in renal transplant recipients in comparison to cyclosporine. Am J Trans. 2011;11:2414–22.
64. Verbeke F, et al. Aortic stiffness and central wave reflections predict outcome in renal transplant recipients. Hypertension. 2011;58:833–8.
65. Briet M, Burns KD. Chronic kidney disease and vascular remodelling: molecular mechanisms and clinical implications. Clin Sci. 2012;123:399–416.
66. Faqah A, Jafar TH. Control of blood pressure in chronic kidney disease: how low to go. Nephron Clin Pract. 2011;119:c324–31; discussion c331–22.
67. Lehoux S, Tedgui A. Signal transduction of mechanical stresses in the vascular wall. Hypertension. 1998;32:338–45.
68. Loufrani L, et al. Key role of alpha(1)beta(1)-integrin in the activation of PI3-kinase-Akt by flow (shear stress) in resistance arteries. Am J Physiol Heart Circ Physiol. 2008;294:H1906–13.
69. Vaziri ND, Norris K. Lipid disorders and their relevance to outcomes in chronic kidney disease. Blood Purif. 2011;31:189–96.
70. Preston E, Ellis MR, Kulinskaya E, Davies AH, Brown EA. Association between carotid artery intima-media thickness and cardiovascular risk factors in CKD. Am J Kidney Dis. 2005;46:856–62.
71. Fellstrom BC, et al. Rosuvastatin and cardiovascular events in patients undergoing hemodialysis. N Engl J Med. 2009;360:1395–407.

72. Chue CD, et al. Serum phosphate but not pulse wave velocity predicts decline in renal function in patients with early chronic kidney disease. Nephrol Dial Trans. 2011;26:2576–82.
73. Kovesdy CP, Kuchmak O, Lu JL, Kalantar-Zadeh K. Outcomes associated with phosphorus binders in men with non-dialysis-dependent CKD. Am J Kidney Dis. 2010;56:842–51.
74. Scialla JJ, et al. Fibroblast growth factor-23 and cardiovascular events in CKD. J Am Soc Nephrol. 2014;25(2):349–60.
75. Desjardins L, et al. FGF23 is independently associated with vascular calcification but not bone mineral density in patients at various CKD stages. Osteoporos Int. 2012;23(7):2017–25.

28 Arterial Changes in Renal Transplantation

Sola Aoun Bahous, Serge Korjian, Yazan Daaboul, Jacques Blacher, and Michel E. Safar

Abstract

Renal transplantation is the best renal replacement modality for patients with end-stage renal disease in terms of patient survival and quality of life. Despite substantial improvement in recipient outcome, stiffness of the large arterial system and cardiovascular (CV) mortality remain high compared to age- and sex-matched subjects in the general population. In addition to traditional CV risk factors, transplantation-specific parameters emerge and are related to immune interactions, drug specifications, and donor characteristics. Some of these parameters appear to be modulators of risk factors and graft and recipient outcome. Acute rejection, for example, appears as a major and independent determinant of high arterial stiffness in recipients of kidney grafts. Furthermore, past history of CV events, low graft filtration function, and donor age determine long-term patient and graft outcome. Living kidney donors, on the other hand, are normally protected especially that they are carefully selected prior to transplantation. Despite a similar long-term outcome compared to the general population, donors may be at higher risk for stiffening of the large arterial system, especially if they cluster with time, CV comorbidities.

Keywords

Arterial stiffness • Cardiovascular • Donor • End-stage renal disease • Recipient • Transplantation

S. Aoun Bahous, MD, PhD (✉)
Division of Nephrology, Department of Medicine, University Medical Center – Rizk Hospital, May Zahhar Street, Ashrafieh, Beirut 11-3288, Lebanon
e-mail: solabahous@hotmail.com, sola.bahous@lau.edu.lb

S. Korjian, MSc • Y. Daaboul, MSc
Department of Medicine, Gilbert and Rose Marie Chagoury School of Medicine, University Medical Center – Rizk Hospital, May Zahhar Str., Ashafieh, Beirut 11-3288, Lebanon
e-mail: serge.korjian@gmail.com; yazan.daaboul@gmail.com

J. Blacher, MD, PhD • M.E. Safar, MD
Department of Medicine, Paris Descartes University, Assistance Publique des Hôpitaux de Paris, Hôtel-Dieu Hospital, Diagnosis and Therapeutics Center, 1 Place du Parvis Notre- Dame 75004 Paris, France
e-mail: jacques.blacher@htd.aphp.fr; michel.safar@htd.aphp.fr

M.E. Safar et al. (eds.), *Blood Pressure and Arterial Wall Mechanics in Cardiovascular Diseases*, DOI 10.1007/978-1-4471-5198-2_28, © Springer-Verlag London 2014

Introduction and Epidemiologic Background

Kidney transplantation has long been regarded as the most optimal modality of renal replacement therapy in patients with end-stage renal disease (ESRD). Although other forms of renal replacement, such as hemodialysis, help in reducing the complications of ESRD, they do not restore the full functions a normal kidney provides [1, 2]. In addition to being cost-effective, the renal allotransplant has been shown to confer both substantial improvement in the quality of life and increased survival in patients with ESRD when compared with long-term hemodialysis [3]. Studies have persistently demonstrated that patients on hemodialysis have a susceptibility to accelerated vascular disease and increased cardiovascular mortality independently of other risk factors [4]. This further justifies the advantage of preemptive renal transplantation whenever available [5].

The types of renal transplants differ according to the donor-recipient familial relationship, i.e., related or unrelated donor, and according to the graft source, i.e., living, conventional cadaveric, or non-heart-beating donors [6]. Whereas related donors were previously the preferred source of the renal graft due to lower rejection rates, with the advent of novel immunosuppressants, unrelated or emotionally related donors have become an important source of living-donor kidney grafts [7]. Transplants from living donors have risen worldwide in the past decade [8] especially in light of the shortage of cadaveric grafts, with reported rates of up to 39 % of all kidney transplants [9]. By the end of 2004, some 412,000 patients (23 % of patients receiving renal replacement therapy worldwide) were living with a functioning renal graft, and the numbers since have steadily increased [10].

Benefits of Kidney Transplantation

Several studies have shown the noteworthy improvement in overall health and non-health-related quality of life with a functional renal graft. Patients reported improvement in general and mental health, physical and social functioning, and a marked decrease in generalized pain [11]. Although pain associated with the surgery and side effects of the immunosuppressive regimen can have a toll on the quality of life, they tend to diminish significantly after the first post-transplant year [12]. Improvement in the quality of life has also been reported independently of other comorbid conditions and recipient age [12].

But the impact of renal transplantation goes beyond the improvement of the quality of life. It reduces cardiovascular mortality, which would otherwise be tenfold higher when compared to the general population [13]. This is related basically to the restoration of renal function, especially that studies have shown that even a moderate decrease in kidney function can significantly increase all-cause and cardiovascular mortality as well as the number of hospitalizations [14].

Although renal transplantation does not restore the cardiovascular risk to that of the general population, it shrinks the gap when compared to patients maintained on hemodialysis. Mortality from cardiovascular disease is almost halved in transplant patients but still remains at least three to five times higher in comparison to the general population [15]. This may be due in part to the improvement in renal function and the subsequent decrease in the progression of vascular calcifications with improvement of calcium and phosphorus homeostasis and a slower evolution of the accelerated atherosclerosis and ESRD-associated arterial changes [16, 17]. Furthermore, cardiovascular risk factors may be moderated following renal transplantation. Patients frequently have a significant decrease in blood pressure and cholesterol levels [18]. In parallel, it has been documented that an increasing renal transplant vintage strongly correlates with a decrease in death from cardiovascular disease [19]. Conversely, loss of the renal function after transplantation has been shown to be a strong predictor of cardiovascular mortality [20]. Despite the noted benefits of kidney transplantation, death with a functional graft, basically from cardiovascular causes, remains the most important etiology of transplant failure in patients over 55 years of age [21]. This has been attributed to alterations in arterial structure and function with associated decrease in arterial distensibility that likely persists after transplantation.

Evolution of Arterial Stiffness After Transplantation

Several studies have documented increased arterial stiffness in the renal transplant population when compared to the general population. Bahous et al. reported higher aortic pulse wave velocity (PWV) values in the renal transplant population when compared to age-matched healthy controls despite a lower mean blood pressure in the renal transplant group [22]. Similarly, Verbeke et al. demonstrated that central PWV and augmentation index (AIx) values remained higher in transplant recipients compared to healthy controls even after adjustment for confounding factors [23]. Several hypotheses have been provided to explain this discrepancy, including irreversible loss of elastic tissue and medial calcification prior to transplantation, the effect of immunosuppressive treatment [24], and persistent inflammatory changes after transplantation [23].

Despite that fact, renal transplantation does provide a form of arterial protection that can partly be demonstrated by the more substantial arterial stiffness found in patients maintained on other renal replacement modalities. To date, few cross-sectional and cohort studies have studied the short-term effects of transplantation on arterial stiffness. Covic et al. showed that serial measurements of aortic augmentation index in the same population decreased from a mean of 25.1 % while on dialysis to 15.9 % within 3 months after a successful kidney transplantation [25]. In parallel, Zoungas et al. showed a significant decrease of 11 % in peripheral mean arterial pressure (MAP)-adjusted PWV and a 49 % reduction in mean AIx adjusted for heart rate, 1 year after functional transplantation compared to pretransplant levels [26]. In comparison, Bachelet-Rousseau et al. found no difference in the 1-year central PWV evolution despite a decrease in MAP values [27].

The long-term effect of renal transplantation on arterial stiffness has not been studied extensively. In 2011, Strozecki et al. surprisingly found a significant progressive increase in PWV and pulse pressure in a cohort of 61 transplant recipients aged 46 ± 12 years and followed for 24–34 months, with baseline PWV measured within 36 ± 27 months after transplant [28]. Complete data on arterial compliance in late transplant cohorts is still lacking.

Predictors of Arterial Stiffness in Renal Transplant Recipients

Increased arterial stiffness in the transplant population spans beyond the traditional causes of decreased compliance seen in other subjects. Artery structure and function in renal transplant patients are affected by a multitude of factors associated with recipient-related, transplantation-related, and donor-related parameters. A summary of parameters associated with higher arterial stiffness is presented in Table 28.1.

Recipient-Related Predictors of Arterial Stiffness

In contrast to the general population, traditional cardiovascular risk factors are not the only major contributors to increased arterial stiffness in renal transplant recipients. Although age, male gender, and elevated MAP have been shown to be related to increased arterial stiffness in the transplant population in most studies, other traditional risk factors for cardiovascular disease were not as strongly linked [22, 23, 30]. These findings are mirrored in several studies in which traditional cardiovascular risk scores, such as the Framingham Risk Score, were applied to the transplant population. These scores noticeably undervalued the cardiovascular risks in these patients by underestimating the incidence of cardiovascular events [36]. This suggests the importance of other transplantation-specific risk factors

Table 28.1 Individual studies addressing association between arterial stiffness and various parameters

Author and year	Type of study	*N*	Outcome variable	Main findings
Barenbrock et al. 1998 [29]	Cross-sectional	54	Common carotid Distensibility coefficient Common carotid End-diastolic diameter	Lower values associated with: Older age Elevated MAP Elevated iPTH levels Higher values associated with: Older age Elevated serum creatinine
Ferro et al. 2002 [24]	Cross-sectional	250	Augmentation index	Higher values associated with: Female gender Older age Elevated MAP Persistent AV fistula Increased dialysis vintage Cyclosporine
Bahous et al. 2004 [22]	Cross-sectional	106	Aortic PWV	Higher values associated with: Older age Elevated MAP Acute Rejection Smoking
Zoungas et al. 2004 [26]	Cross-sectional	36	Augmentation index	Higher values associated with: Cyclosporine
Kneifel et al. 2006 [30]	Cross-sectional	48	Radial artery stiffness by applanation tonometry	Higher values associated with: Male gender Reduced eGFR Older age of donor
Bahous et al. 2006 [31]	Cross-sectional	101	Aortic PWV	Higher values associated with: Older age Elevated MAP Acute rejection Smoking
Verbeke et al. 2007 [23]	Cross-sectional	200	Aortic PWV	Higher values associated with: Reduced eGFR Elevated CRP
Seckinger et al. 2008 [32]	Randomized controlled trial	39	Aortic PWV	Elevation associated with: Cyclosporine Unchanged with: Everolimus
Delahousse et al. 2008 [33]	Cohort	74	Aortic PWV	Higher values associated with: Older age Elevated MAP Female gender Older donor age
Opazo Saez et al. 2008 [34]	Cross-sectional	318	Aortic PWV	Higher values associated with: Older age Elevated SBP New-onset diabetes mellitus

Table 28.1 (continued)

Author and year	Type of study	*N*	Outcome variable	Main findings
Van Laecke et al. 2011 [35]	Cross-sectional	512	Aortic PWV	Higher values associated with: Older age Elevated MAP Elevated CRP Diabetes mellitus Hypomagnesemia Lower values associated with: Sirolimus

N number of study participants, *MAP* mean arterial pressure, *iPTH* serum levels of parathyroid hormone, *AV* arteriovenous, *PWV* pulse wave velocity, *eGFR* estimated glomerular filtration rate, *CRP* C-reactive protein, *SBP* systolic blood pressure

in addition to the traditional cardiovascular risk factors. Nevertheless, some studies have reported the contribution of certain traditional risk factors on arterial stiffness. Bahous et al. observed that tobacco consumption was independently correlated with higher carotid-femoral PWV and lower graft function [22]. Furthermore, new-onset diabetes following transplantation has also been linked to accelerated arterial stiffening and higher PWV values [34].

An important predictor of aortic calcifications and arterial stiffness in the renal transplant population includes pretransplant dialysis vintage. Several studies have reported an increase in large artery calcification as a function of time on hemodialysis in the ESRD population [4]. This was also highlighted in transplant recipients with increasing prevalence of aortic calcifications in those with greater dialysis vintage prior to transplantation [37]. This proposes that duration of dialysis and the associated arterial calcifications carry through after transplantation. Ferro et al. found that a higher AIx was independently correlated with longer durations on dialysis prior to renal transplantation [24]. Furthermore, mortality rates from cardiovascular events were proportional to the vintage on the transplant waiting list and decreased substantially with earlier referral for transplantation [19].

Many nonclassical risk factors for increased arterial stiffness in renal transplant recipients have been proposed, but substantial evidence is still deficient. Ferro et al. showed that the persistence of an arteriovenous fistula after transplantation was independently associated with an increased AIx [24]. Subclinical inflammation has also been proposed as a mechanism of increase in arterial stiffness possibly accounting for the discrepancy in cardiovascular risk estimation. It has been previously reported that pretransplantation C-reactive protein (CRP) levels are independently correlated with all-cause and cardiovascular mortality [38]. Correspondingly, CRP levels above the median have been associated with a 14 % higher AIx and a 0.9 m/s higher PWV, analogous to approximately a 10-year increase in vascular age [23]. Additionally, hypomagnesemia has also been associated with arterial stiffness in the transplant population. Van Laecke et al. showed PWV to be inversely proportional to magnesium levels particularly in patients aged 55 years or more [35]. Moreover, elevated parathyroid hormone (iPTH) levels have been linked to decreased large artery distensibility [29].

The correlation between other novel parameters, such as fibrinogen, vitamin D, adiponectin and homocysteine, and arterial stiffness has not been thoroughly studied in renal transplant recipients, and knowledge is mostly inferred from studies done on other populations.

Transplantation-Related Predictors of Arterial Stiffness

Although transplant recipients may have relatively normal renal function, their arterial stiffness level remains high compared to their age-matched healthy controls [22]. This may be due to several factors, acquired after transplantation, that aid in the progression of arterial changes. These factors may be related to the transplantation procedure, the immunosuppressive treatment, and/or to the immune status of the recipient.

Cold ischemia time (CIT) in deceased-donor kidney transplants is an important predictor of arterial stiffness and overall graft loss [39]. CIT is defined as the time interval between kidney immersion in the ice solution and removal from ice immediately before transplantation [40]. PWV was found to be lower among patients with cold ischemia time less than 8.3 ± 1.6 h [39]. In contrast, warm ischemia time, defined as the period of circulatory arrest to the kidney graft under normothermic conditions (outside cold perfusion) during both organ retrieval and implantation, has not yet been studied in association with arterial stiffness.

In order to ensure proper engraftment and circumvent imminent rejection, immunosuppressive therapies have been the mainstay in the management of transplant patients. However, these treatments have had their share in the alteration of arterial structure and function in numerous studies. Patients maintained on cyclosporine have been shown to have a higher MAP when compared to patients on other immunosuppressive modalities. A higher AIx was also observed when compared to patients on tacrolimus even after correction for blood pressure [24, 26]. Similarly, when compared to everolimus, cyclosporine was consistently associated with a more elevated PWV after 6 months of therapy [32]. A possible explanation would be the effect of cyclosporine on arterial structure and function, through alteration of endothelial function and decreased nitric oxide production [41]. Furthermore, the hypertensive effect of cyclosporine and its nephrotoxic potential close the loop around an altered vascular status in renal transplant patients. In contrast, Van Laecke et al. demonstrated in a sample of 60 patients that sirolimus immunotherapy was independently associated with a decreased PWV [35]. Little is known about the effect of other novel immunosuppressive medications on arterial compliance.

Although our understanding of the effect of graft function on arterial stiffness is limited due to the small populations studied, one can extrapolate the consequence of glomerular filtration rate (GFR) loss from the chronic kidney disease population. It has been shown that a stepwise increase in arterial stiffness occurs with advancing stages of renal disease [42]. Similarly, certain studies on graft function in transplant recipients have shown PWV and AIx to be higher in renal transplant recipients with a lower eGFR [23, 30]. Another important aspect of graft function linked to altered arterial compliance is graft rejection. Bahous et al. reported that acute renal rejection was associated with increased PWV, independently of serum creatinine, proposing that the mechanism of increased arterial stiffness is not solely related to the decrease in renal function but maybe due to an underlying immune mechanism [22]. Although chronic allograft nephropathy was associated with a decreased graft function and elevation of serum creatinine [43], further studies are still needed to examine the exact contribution of this entity on arterial stiffness.

Donor-Related Predictors of Arterial Stiffness

The impact of donor characteristics on recipient cardiovascular and graft outcome is poorly understood. Recently, many studies have shown that the effect of the donor may be more influential on the recipient than previously thought. It was suggested that donor characteristics affect recipient aortic stiffness, renal outcome, and ultimately cardiovascular mortality despite the significant improvement conferred by transplantation [33].

Conventional donor eligibility criteria required that deceased donors meet standard-criteria-donor (SCD) stratification system, where donors are under 50 years of age and free of cardiovascular disease. However, expanded-criteria-donor (ECD), a novel and more lenient deceased

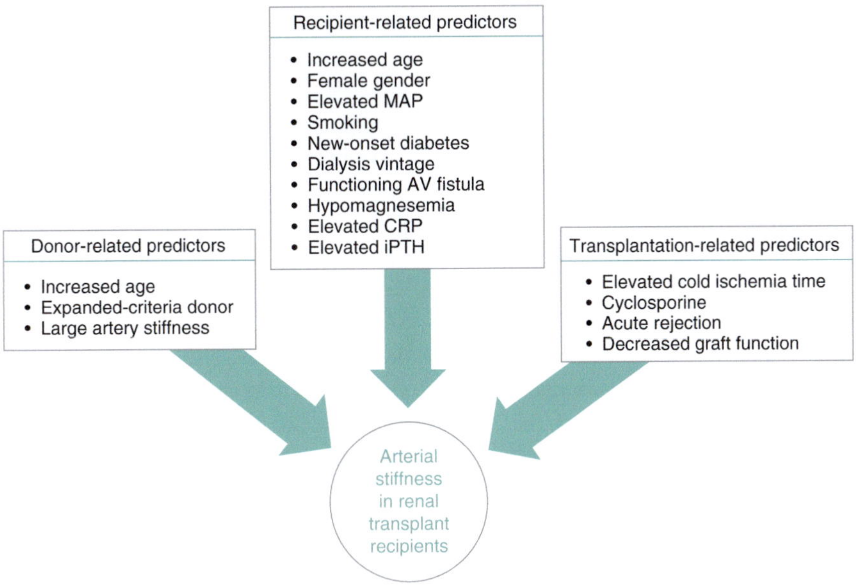

Fig. 28.1 Proposed predictors of increased arterial stiffness in renal transplant recipients. *MAP*, mean arterial pressure; *AV*, arteriovenous; *CRP*, C-reactive protein; *iPTH*, serum levels of parathyroid hormone

donor stratification system established in the early 1990s following the growing demand for renal grafts, has widely replaced the traditional SCD. ECD donor characteristics include age ≥60 years or 50–59 years plus any two of the following parameters: cerebrovascular accidents as cause of death, preexisting hypertension, or serum creatinine prior to kidney removal greater than 1.5 mg/dL or 130 μmol/L [44]. ECD has permitted researchers to study new donor characteristics following its introduction; its use has allowed the reevaluation of the role of the donor kidney in the recipient aortic stiffness and cardiovascular mortality.

In 2008, Delahousse and colleagues studied donor determinants of recipient PWV following a first cadaveric kidney transplantation. Old donor age was an independent determinant of increased recipient PWV only after the third month of transplantation, but not immediately following renal transplantation [33]. At 12 months posttransplantation, the carotid-femoral PWV in recipients of older kidneys (upper tertile of donor age) was >1 m/s higher than those of younger kidneys (lower tertile of donor age). Notably, the association was independent of established important recipient characteristics such as age, gender, blood pressure, dialysis duration, GFR, cardiovascular risk factors, or medications [33].

Further investigation into donor characteristics revealed that donor large artery stiffness is also a predictor of recipient cardiovascular and graft outcome [45]. Donor large artery stiffness, as measured by donor aortic PWV, is associated with the occurrence of adverse recipient outcomes [45].

The effect of donor gender was not clearly studied in relation with arterial stiffness; however, studies including donor gender in the analysis did not show significant correlation [45]. Assessment of the association between recipient arterial stiffness and donor type, whether cadaveric or living, has not yet been described. Despite the high survival rates and the superior graft outcome associated with related and unrelated living kidney donation in comparison to cadaveric donation [7], studies that compare arterial stiffness in living vs. cadaveric donation are still lacking (Fig. 28.1, Table 28.1).

Arterial Stiffness in Donors of Kidney Grafts

Kidney transplantation from living donors follows rigorous donor selection criteria that guarantee donor protection first. The risks to which a donor may be exposed include those related to the pretransplant work-up, the transplantation procedure itself, and to the short- and long-term effect of nephrectomy. Most of the studies addressing donor safety in renal transplantation have confirmed that the incurred risks are minimal and that altruistic kidney donation is safe for the living donor, both on the short and long term [46]. However, other studies have shown that kidney donation predisposes the donor to hemodynamic and/or renal changes without carrying an unjustified risk compared to the general population.

Living donor uninephrectomy is associated with increased blood pressure levels. Despite elevation of blood pressure values, evidence is unclear as to whether the increase in blood pressure is significant enough in normotensive donors to become in the hypertensive range. A meta-analysis by Kasiske and colleagues in 1995 of 48 studies using 3,124 uninephrectomized patients and 1,703 controls showed that uninephrectomy was not associated with hypertension over time despite mild increases in systolic (+2.4 mmHg) and diastolic (+3.1 mmHg) blood pressure values [47]. Following uninephrectomy, studies have illustrated that the incidence of hypertension ranges from 9 to 48 %, using various definitions of hypertension in this specific patient population [48, 49].

In 1987, Torres et al. showed in a cohort of 66 uninephrectomized donors after a 10-year follow-up that 15 % of previously normotensive patients and 38 % of borderline hypertensive donors eventually developed definite hypertension, defined at the time of the study as systolic/diastolic blood pressure values of ≥ 160/95 mmHg [50]. Many mechanisms have been suggested to explain the high blood pressure values, including increased renal reactivity to angiotensin II, renal and glomerular hemodynamic modifications [51], and changes in arterial elasticity after nephrectomy. In contrast, four larger studies with 11–30-year follow-up showed no significant risk of developing hypertension among uninephrectomized donors in comparison to healthy controls [47, 52–54].

Bahous and colleagues showed that arterial pulse wave velocity is significantly increased in donors when compared to healthy controls [31]. Factors associated with increased PWV and pulse pressure (PP) in kidney donors were exclusively of renal origin. Time since kidney donation was positively correlated with PWV, whereas the presence of proteinuria and/or microalbuminuria was linked to higher PP. Compared to the general population, where determinants of aortic PWV are principally age, MAP, and gender, the donor population seems to show additional determining factors related to kidney donation and other cardiovascular risk factors. The authors attribute the increased stiffness and the link between the latter and time since donation to altered renal hemodynamics that occurs after nephrectomy. The decrease in pre-glomerular arteriolar resistance that occurs normally to enhance compensatory hypertrophy allows for augmented transmission of systemic pressure pulsations and may contribute to arterial changes without affecting overall donor outcome and life span [31, 55].

Ultimately, the survival of renal transplant donors has not been shown to be compromised following uninephrectomy. Literature continues to emphasize on the safety of kidney transplantation and the unaffected donor outcome. Nonetheless, further long-term follow-up of donors is still warranted to study the exact relationship between uninephrectomy and arterial structure and function.

Arterial Stiffness as a Predictor of Cardiovascular and Graft Outcome in Recipients

Despite clear improvement in PWV level and cardiovascular outcome following renal transplantation, the risk of cardiovascular events remains higher in the transplant patients compared to their age- and gender-matched subjects in the general population [15, 19, 25, 45]. Large artery stiffness has been shown to be a predictor of cardiovascular outcome in many populations at risk, such those with hypertension and with chronic kidney disease [56, 57].

The measurement of arterial stiffness in recipients and donors has widely gained clinical value as an early independent predictor of cardiovascular function, risk, and mortality in kidney transplant recipients [22, 31, 58–60]. Arterial stiffness level was advanced as a cardiovascular prognostic tool in many studies. In the renal transplant population, elevated arterial stiffness is significantly associated with systolic blood pressure, pulse pressure, and coronary artery disease [60]. Similarly, common carotid distensibility, measured by vessel wall movement using pulsed multigate Doppler system, is a significant independent correlate with cardiovascular events and cardiovascular death when measured 3–6 months after transplantation [61]. The role of recipient arterial stiffness in renal transplant recipients has also been credited in left ventricular systolic pressure, left ventricular hypertrophy, and ventricular oxygen and blood demand, explaining the raised cardiovascular morbidity [61].

Bahous and colleagues studied the role of donor aortic stiffness in graft and cardiovascular outcome in 95 adult kidney transplant recipients by following the doubling of serum creatinine, development of ESRD (eGFR <15 mL/min/1.73 m^2), return to dialysis, development of myocardial infarction, stroke, and occurrence of cardiovascular death [45]. In the study, donor PWV showed borderline significance with the outcome. It was postulated that transplantation transmits donor baseline arterial and renal status to the recipient [45].

Finally, the role of central arterial stiffness as a predictor of outcome in the renal transplant population has been demonstrated in small studies while larger ones are needed to clearly establish its predictive value and suggest early measurement and potential interventions.

Conclusion

There is no doubt that arterial stiffness, an independent marker of cardiovascular outcome, improves in ESRD patients following renal transplantation but may still be inferior to age- and gender-matched individuals in the general population. Arterial stiffness in the renal transplant population was associated with several recipient, transplant, and donor parameters. Despite possible renovascular changes associated with uninephrectomy, the safety of renal transplantation has been highlighted in donors; and kidney donation and transplantation is still considered the most optimal modality of renal replacement therapy for patients with ESRD.

References

1. Krakauer H, Grauman JS, McMullan MR, Creede CC. The recent U.S. experience in the treatment of end-stage renal disease by dialysis and transplantation. N Engl J Med. 1983;308(26):1558–63.
2. Schnuelle P, Lorenz D, Trede M, Van Der Woude FJ. Impact of renal cadaveric transplantation on survival in end-stage renal failure: evidence for reduced mortality risk compared with hemodialysis during long-term follow-up. J Am Soc Nephrol. 1998;9(11):2135–41.
3. Wolfe RA, Ashby VB, Milford EL, Ojo AO, Ettenger RE, Agodoa LY, et al. Comparison of mortality in all patients on dialysis, patients on dialysis awaiting transplantation, and recipients of a first cadaveric transplant. N Engl J Med. 1999;341(23):1725–30.
4. Guérin AP, London GM, Marchais SJ, Metivier F. Arterial stiffening and vascular calcifications in end-stage renal disease. Nephrol Dial Transplant. 2000;15(7):1014–21.
5. Kasiske BL, Snyder JJ, Matas AJ, Ellison MD, Gill JS, Kausz AT. Preemptive kidney transplantation: the advantage and the advantaged. J Am Soc Nephrol. 2002;13(5):1358–64.
6. Nicholson ML, Metcalfe MS, White SA, Waller JR, Doughman TM, Horsburgh T, et al. A comparison of the results of renal transplantation from non–heart-beating, conventional cadaveric, and living donors. Kidney Int. 2000;58(6):2585–91.
7. Terasaki PI, Cecka JM, Gjertson DW, Takemoto S. High survival rates of kidney transplants from spousal and living unrelated donors. N Engl J Med. 1995;333(6):333–6.
8. U.S. Renal Data System (USRDS). Annual data report: atlas of chronic kidney disease and end-stage renal disease in the United States. Am J Kidney Dis. 2013;61(1):e1–480.
9. Horvat LD, Shariff SZ, Garg AX. Donor Nephrectomy Outcomes Research (DONOR) Network. Global trends in the rates of living kidney donation. Kidney Int. 2009;75(10):1088–98.

10. Grassmann A, Gioberge S, Moeller S, Brown G. ESRD patients in 2004: global overview of patient numbers, treatment modalities and associated trends. Nephrol Dial Transplant. 2005;20(12):2587–93.
11. Laupacis A, Keown P, Pus N, Krueger H, Ferguson B, Wong C, et al. A Study of the quality of life and cost-utility of renal transplantation. Kidney Int. 1996;50(1): 235–42.
12. Neipp M, Karavul B, Jackobs S, Meyer zu Vilsendorf A, Richter N, Becker T, et al. Quality of life in adult transplant recipients more than 15 years after kidney transplantation. Transplantation. 2006;81(12):1640–4.
13. Foley RN, Parfrey PS, Sarnak MJ. Clinical epidemiology of cardiovascular disease in chronic renal disease. Am J Kidney Dis. 1998;32(5 Suppl 3):S112–9.
14. Go AS, Chertow GM, Fan D, McCulloch CE, Hsu CY. Chronic kidney disease and the risks of death, cardiovascular events, and hospitalization. N Engl J Med. 2004;351(13):1296–305.
15. Sarnak MJ, Levey AS, Schoolwerth AC, Coresh J, Culleton B, Hamm LL, et al. Kidney disease as a risk factor for development of cardiovascular disease: a statement from the American Heart Association Councils on Kidney in Cardiovascular Disease, High Blood Pressure Research, Clinical Cardiology, and Epidemiology and Prevention. Hypertension. 2003; 42(5):1050–65.
16. Chertow GM, Burke SK, Raggi P, Treat to Goal Working Group. Sevelamer attenuates the progression of coronary and aortic calcification in hemodialysis patients. Kidney Int. 2002;62(1):245–52.
17. Ibels LS, Alfrey AC, Huffer WE, Craswell PW, Anderson JT, Weil R 3rd. Arterial calcification and pathology in uremic patients undergoing dialysis. Am J Med. 1979;66(5):790–6.
18. Pollock CA, Mahony JF, Ong CS, Caterson RJ, Waugh DA, Ibels LS. Hyperlipidemia in renal transplant recipients: Does it matter and can we treat it? Transplant Proc. 1995;27(3):2152–3.
19. Meier-Kriesche HU, Schold JD, Srinivas TR, Reed A, Kaplan B. Kidney transplantation halts cardiovascular disease progression in patients with end-stage renal disease. Am J Transplant. 2004;4(10):1662–8.
20. Meier-Kriesche HU, Baliga R, Kaplan B. Decreased renal function is a strong risk factor for cardiovascular death after renal transplantation. Transplantation. 2003;75(8):1291–5.
21. Lindholm A, Albrechtsen D, Frödin L, Tufveson G, Persson NH, Lundgren G. Ischemic heart disease-major cause of death and graft loss after renal transplantation in Scandinavia. Transplantation. 1995;60(5):451–7.
22. Bahous SA, Stephan A, Barakat W, Blacher J, Asmar R, Safar ME. Aortic pulse wave velocity in renal transplant patients. Kidney Int. 2004;66(4):1486–92.
23. Verbeke F, Van Biesen W, Peeters P, Van Bortel LM, Vanholder RC. Arterial stiffness and wave reflections in renal transplant recipients. Nephrol Dial Transplant. 2007;22(10):3021–7.
24. Ferro CJ, Savage T, Pinder SJ, Tomson CR. Central aortic pressure augmentation in stable renal transplant recipients. Kidney Int. 2002;62(1):166–71.
25. Covic A, Goldsmith DJ, Gusbeth-Tatomir P, Buhaescu I, Covic M. Successful renal transplantation decreases aortic stiffness and increases vascular reactivity in dialysis patients. Transplantation. 2003;76(11):1573–7.
26. Zoungas S, Kerr PG, Chadban S, Muske C, Ristevski S, Atkins RC, et al. Arterial function after successful renal transplantation. Kidney Int. 2004;65(5):1882–9.
27. Bachelet-Rousseau C, Kearney-Schwartz A, Frimat L, Fay R, Kessler M, Benetos A. Evolution of arterial stiffness after kidney transplantation. Nephrol Dial Transplant. 2011;26(10):3386–91.
28. Strozecki P, Adamowicz A, Kozlowski M, Wlodarczyk Z, Manitius J. Progressive arterial stiffening in kidney transplant recipients. Ann Transplant. 2011;16(3):30–5.
29. Barenbrock M, Hausberg M, Kosch M, Kisters K, Hoeks AP, Rahn KH. Effect of hyperparathyroidism on arterial distensibility in renal transplant recipients. Kidney Int. 1998;54(1):210–5.
30. Kneifel M, Scholze A, Burkert A, Offermann G, Rothermund L, Zidek W, et al. Impaired renal allograft function is associated with increased arterial stiffness in renal transplant recipients. Am J Transplant. 2006;6(7):1624–30.
31. Bahous SA, Stephan A, Blacher J, Safar ME. Aortic stiffness, living donors, and renal transplantation. Hypertension. 2006;47(2):216–21.
32. Seckinger J, Sommerer C, Hinkel UP, Hoffmann O, Zeier M, Schwenger V. Switch of immunosuppression from cyclosporine A to everolimus: impact on pulse wave velocity in stable de-novo renal allograft recipients. J Hypertens. 2008;26(11):2213–9.
33. Delahousse M, Chaignon M, Mesnard L, Boutouyrie P, Safar ME, Lebret T, et al. Aortic stiffness of kidney transplant recipients correlates with donor age. J Am Soc Nephrol. 2008;19(4):798–805.
34. Opazo Saez A, Kos M, Witzke O, Kribben A, Nürnberger J. Effect of new-onset diabetes mellitus on arterial stiffness in renal transplantation. Transpl Int. 2008;21(10):930–5.
35. Van Laecke S, Maréchal C, Verbeke F, Peeters P, Van Biesen W, Devuyst O, et al. The relation between hypomagnesaemia and vascular stiffness in renal transplant recipients. Nephrol Dial Transplant. 2011; 26(7):2362–9.
36. Kasiske BL, Chakkera HA, Roel J. Explained and unexplained ischemic heart disease risk after renal transplantation. J Am Soc Nephrol. 2000;11(9): 1735–43.
37. DeLoach SS, Joffe MM, Mai X, Goral S, Rosas SE. Aortic calcification predicts cardiovascular events and all-cause mortality in renal transplantation. Nephrol Dial Transplant. 2009;24(4):1314–9.
38. Varagunam M, Finney H, Trevitt R, Sharples E, McCloskey DJ, Sinnott PJ, et al. Pretransplantation levels of C-reactive protein predict all-cause and

cardiovascular mortality, but not graft outcome, in kidney transplant recipients. Am J Kidney Dis. 2004;43(3):502–7.
39. Strózecki P, Adamowicz A, Kozlowski M, Wlodarczyk Z, Manitius J. Long graft cold ischemia time is associated with increased arterial stiffness in renal transplant recipients. Transplant Proc. 2009;41(9):3580–4.
40. Simforoosh N, Basiri A, Shakhssalim N, Gooran S, Tabibi A, Khoshdel A, et al. Long-term graft function in a randomized clinical trial comparing laparoscopic versus open donor nephrectomy. Exp Clin Transplant. 2012;10(5):428–32.
41. Morris ST, McMurray JJ, Rodger RS, Farmer R, Jardine AG. Endothelial dysfunction in renal transplant recipients maintained on cyclosporine. Kidney Int. 2000;57(3):1100–6.
42. Wang MC, Tsai WC, Chen JY, Huang JJ. Stepwise increase in arterial stiffness corresponding with the stages of chronic kidney disease. Am J Kidney Dis. 2005;45(3):494–501.
43. Nankivell BJ, Borrows RJ, Fung CL, O'Connell PJ, Allen RD, Chapman JR. The natural history of chronic allograft nephropathy. N Engl J Med. 2003;349(24):2326–33.
44. Ojo AO. Expanded criteria donors: process and outcomes. Semin Dial. 2005;18(6):463–8.
45. Bahous SA, Stephan A, Blacher J, Safar ME. Cardiovascular and renal outcome in recipients of kidney grafts from living donors: role of aortic stiffness. Nephrol Dial Transplant. 2012;27(5):2095–100.
46. Davis CL, Delmonico FL. Living-donor kidney transplantation: a review of the current practices for the live donor. J Am Soc Nephrol. 2005;16(7):2098–110.
47. Kasiske BL, Ma JZ, Louis TA, Swan SK. Long-term effects of reduced renal mass in humans. Kidney Int. 1995;48(3):814–9.
48. Fehrman-Ekholm I, Elinder CG, Stenbeck M, Tydén G, Groth CG. Kidney donors live longer. Transplantation. 1997;64(7):976–8.
49. Anderson CF, Velosa JA, Frohnert PP, Torres VE, Offord KP, Vogel JP, et al. The risks of unilateral nephrectomy: status of kidney donors 10 to 20 years postoperatively. Mayo Clin Proc. 1985;60(6):367–74.
50. Torres VE, Offord KP, Anderson CF, Velosa JA, Frohnert PP, Donadio JV Jr, et al. Blood pressure determinants in living-related renal allograft donors and their recipients. Kidney Int. 1987;31(6):1383–90.
51. Guidi E, Cozzi M, Milani S, Spada E. Nephrectomy modifies renal angiotensin II effects in kidney donors. Am J Hypertens. 2008;21(5):592–8.
52. Goldfarb DA, Matin SF, Braun WE, Schreiber MJ, Mastroianni B, Papajcik D, et al. Renal outcome 25 years after donor nephrectomy. J Urol. 2001;166(6):2043–7.
53. Williams SL, Oler J, Jorkasky DK. Long-term renal function in kidney donors: a comparison of donors and their siblings. Ann Intern Med. 1986;105(1):1–8.
54. Ramcharan T, Matas AJ. Long-term (20–37 years) follow-up of living kidney donors. Am J Transplant. 2002;2(10):959–64.
55. Aoun S, Blacher J, Safar ME, Mourad JJ. Diabetes mellitus and renal failure: effects on large artery stiffness. J Hum Hypertens. 2001;15(10):693–700.
56. Blacher J, Asmar R, Djane S, London GM, Safar ME. Aortic pulse wave velocity as a marker of cardiovascular risk in hypertensive patients. Hypertension. 1999;33(5):1111–7.
57. Blacher J, Guerin AP, Pannier B, Marchais SJ, Safar ME, London GM. Impact of aortic stiffness in survival in end-stage renal disease. Circulation. 1999;99(18):2434–9.
58. Guerin AP, Pannier B, Métivier F, Marchais SJ, London GM. Assessment and significance of arterial stiffness in patients with chronic kidney disease. Curr Opin Nephrol Hypertens. 2008;17(6):635–41.
59. Verbeke F, Maréchal C, Van Laecke S, Van Biesen W, Devuyst O, Van Bortel LM, et al. Aortic stiffness and central wave reflections predict outcome in renal transplant recipients. Hypertension. 2011;58(5):833–8.
60. Mitchell A, Opazo Saez A, Kos M, Witzke O, Kribben A, Nürnberger J. Pulse wave velocity predicts mortality in renal transplant patients. Eur J Med Res. 2010;15(10):452–5.
61. Barenbrock M, Kosch M, Jöster E, Kisters K, Rahn KH, Hausberg M. Reduced arterial distensibility is a predictor of cardiovascular disease in patients after renal transplantation. J Hypertens. 2002;20(1):79–84.

Arterial Stiffness, Central Blood Pressure and Coronary Heart Disease

29

Piotr Jankowski, Jacques Blacher, and Thomas Weber

Abstract

Central blood pressure is closer to the heart, coronary and carotid arteries, which are the most important sites of cardiovascular events. The influence of cyclic stretch (owing to cyclic changes in blood pressure) on the arterial wall has been documented at every stage of atherosclerosis development. Apart from mediating atherosclerosis progression and plaque instability, the pulsatile component of blood pressure is the main mechanism leading to plaque rupture and, consequently, to acute coronary syndromes and other vascular complications. A number of studies reported a significant relation between central blood pressure and the extant of coronary atherosclerosis as well as between central blood pressure and cardiovascular risk in patients with coronary heart disease. A lot of attention has been given recently to break the link between pulse pressure and cardiovascular events. Because of the vicious circle consisting of arterial wall stiffness, pulse pressure, and atherosclerosis, the most promising intervention is reduction in arterial stiffness, although increase of the potential benefit requires interventions aiming at all three components of the vicious circle.

Keywords

Blood pressure • Hypertension • Atherosclerosis • Coronary artery disease • Cardiovascular risk • Arterial stiffness • Arterial compliance • Risk factor • Pulse pressure

P. Jankowski, MD, PhD (✉)
I Department of Cardiology and Hypertension, Institute of Cardiology, Jagiellonian University Medical College, 17 Kopernik St, Kraków 31-501, Poland
e-mail: piotrjankowski@interia.pl

J. Blacher, MD, PhD
Department of Medicine, Paris Descartes University, Assistance Publique des Hôpitaux de Paris, Hôtel-Dieu Hospital, Diagnosis and Therapeutics Center, Paris, France
e-mail: jacques.blacher@htd.aphp.fr

T. Weber, MD
Department of Cardiology, Klinikum Wels-Grieskirchen, Grieskirchnerstrasse 42, Wels, 4600, Austria

Paracelsus Medical University, Salzburg, Austria
e-mail: thomas.weber3@liwest.at

M.E. Safar et al. (eds.), *Blood Pressure and Arterial Wall Mechanics in Cardiovascular Diseases*, DOI 10.1007/978-1-4471-5198-2_29,

Introduction

Increased blood pressure (BP) is one of the most important risk factors for cardiovascular (CV) disease. Hypertension is the leading cause of death among women and the second most important cause of death among men [1]. This is a result of the high prevalence of hypertension and a close relationship between BP values and the risk of cardiovascular disease. Increased BP leads to hypertrophy and remodelling of left ventricle and muscular arteries, impairment of endothelial function and finally to the initiation and progression of atherosclerosis. The above alterations, as well as the direct influence of intravascular pressure, increase the frequency of plaque ruptures leading to acute coronary syndromes [2]. Indeed, increasing evidence has been demonstrated that hypertension-initiated abnormal biomechanical stress is strongly associated with CV disease. Reduction of systolic blood pressure (SBP) has explained most of the treatment benefit in outcome trials in which patients with hypertension were studied [3–5]. These results focused attention on factors that influence SBP and pulse pressure (PP) levels in hypertensive individuals, i.e. on the role(s) of increased arterial stiffness and/or wave reflections.

BP is composed of two components: one a steady component, which is approximately equal to mean arterial pressure (MAP), and the other pulsatile (which may be represented by PP). MAP is the product of cardiac output and peripheral resistance, whereas PP is determined by stroke volume, wave reflections and arterial stiffness. The last factor contributes to the "Windkessel" effect, i.e. the ability to transform the cyclic flow coming from the heart into a steady flow at the peripheral level, thereby providing an optimal oxygenation of tissues. MAP and PP are both independent predictors of CV events [6]. While MAP is a predictor of overall event risk (including heart failure and renal insufficiency), PP predominantly predicts atherosclerosis-related complications [2, 7]. It should be, however, underlined that small value of PP may be required for the maintenance of a differentiated and fully functional phenotype of vascular wall cells, as well as for the regulation of migratory properties, proliferation and matrix turnover [8].

One could argue that PP is not an ideal measure representing the pulsatile component of BP as it is quite well correlated with MAP [9]. However, other measures of pulsatile component are also related both to end-organ damage and the extent of coronary atherosclerosis as well as to cardiovascular event risk [10, 11]. Moreover, measures which almost do not correlate with MAP, e.g. fractional pulse pressure (pulsatility), are at least as good predictors of cardiovascular risk as central PP [7].

Blood Pressure and Cardiovascular Risk in Patients with Coronary Heart Disease

High blood pressure is considered as a major cardiovascular risk factor. Data from observational studies involving more than 1 million individuals without pre-existing vascular disease have indicated that the risk of cardiovascular deaths increases progressively with brachial BP [12, 13]. Generally, it is accepted that brachial DBP is a better cardiovascular risk predictor compared to SBP and PP in young patients, in older patients SBP become better predictor compared to DBP and PP, whereas in the elderly PP have the highest predictive value. These relations not necessarily are the same in patients with coronary heart disease. Indeed, in the population of INVEST trial, PP was a weaker predictor of cardiovascular events than SBP, DBP or MAP [14]. Moreover, Protogerou et al. did not find any significant relation between brachial PP and total or cardiovascular mortality in very old (mean age 85 years) subjects with cardiovascular disease [15]. In addition, some studies suggest that this relation in patients with coronary heart disease may be J or U shaped, with higher event rates at very low and very high blood pressure [14–17]. Some studies suggest even lower risk with increasing pulse pressure in patients with cardiovascular disease [18].

Several potential "pathophysiological" mechanisms have been proposed to explain the existence of the above discrepancies. The first explanation is an epiphenomenon of reduced left ventricular function. Indeed, reduced left ventricular stroke volume is related to higher mortality and lower BP values. The latter especially concerns SBP and PP. It is logical that when stroke volume is decreased, the primary wave (often referred to as P1) is lower when aortic walls compliance is not changed. Although wave reflections are a major factor determining aortic pressure augmentation and systolic as well as pulse pressure in patients with normal ejection fraction [10], when ventricular systolic function is impaired, wave reflection does not augment pressure but has a suppressive effect on ventricular ejection and the aortic flow waveform [19, 20]. It means that wave reflection is manifested more as a negative influence on flow than a positive influence on pressure. Therefore, the relation between central PP and prognosis is blunted. The second explanation could be an epiphenomenon of other chronic illness, which increase mortality. Third, low DBP may compromise coronary perfusion during the diastolic phase of the cardiac cycle. Indeed, it was suggested that myocardial revascularization procedures may transform "J" shape into more linear relation, especially when cardiovascular risk – diastolic blood pressure is considered [17]. The fourth explanation could be an epiphenomenon of increased arterial stiffness, a well-known independent marker of vascular disease and increased mortality leading to high PP and low DBP. Finally, the central-to-brachial pressure wave amplification should be taken into account. Indeed, there is increasing evidence that the difference between central and peripheral BP impacts the predictive value of brachial BP. It has been known since several dozen years that BP and the shape of the pulse wave vary throughout the arterial tree [21–23]. Thus, pressure–oscillation amplitude between systole and diastole increases considerably along the aorta. These SBP and PP amplifications are physiological findings, approximating 10–20 mmHg between the thoracic aortic root and the brachial artery in young, healthy subjects [2, 24]. However, this difference is slightly lower in patients with hypertension and, as proven by Safar et al., amounts to 6 – 11 mmHg on average [25]. BP varies also along the aorta. As shown by Temmar et al., SBP amplification along the aorta is about 8.1 mmHg, whereas DBP decreases by about 2.6 mmHg [26]. From mechanistic point of view, the pressure wave amplification is associated with changes in magnitude of each harmonic component of the pressure wave [27]. Although the difference between central and peripheral BP is smaller in older subjects [28] as well as in those with diseases leading to reduced arterial wall compliance (e.g. renal insufficiency, atherosclerosis), the difference still may have clinical significance.

Indeed, central BP is closer to the heart, coronary arteries and carotid arteries, which are the most important sites of CV events [3]. More specifically, aortic, but not brachial, PP has been shown to be independently associated with coronary atherosclerosis in patients undergoing coronary angiography [9, 29, 30]. In 1,109 subjects undergoing coronary angiography followed for 4.5 years, a 10-mmHg aortic PP increase was associated with a 13 % increase of CV events [7]. Moreover, the pulsatile component of central BP was the best predictor of future CV events in this population. In end-stage renal disease patients and in elderly subjects with essential hypertension, central PP was also demonstrated to be an independent predictor of mortality [31]. Central PP was a better predictor of CV events in subjects without overt CV disease at baseline compared with peripheral pressure [32, 33]. Although Mitchell et al. did not find significant association between central PP and CV risk [34], a recently published meta-analysis of five prospective studies showed higher predictive value of central as compared with peripheral PP (although the difference was of borderline significance) [35]. In addition, Wang showed that when central and peripheral SBP are both included into the statistical model, only central SBP remains significantly related to the CV risk [32]. Finally, in a study by Weber at al., who followed 674 patients with normal or only slightly impaired left ventricular systolic function, the hazard ratio of major cardiovascular events related to increase in brachial PP by one standard deviation was (after

Table 29.1 List of studies assessing the predictive value of central BP in coronary patients

Study	*N*	How central pressure was measured	Mean follow-up [years]	Main results
Lu et al. [36]	87	Invasively, fluid-filled system	0.5	The risk of restenosis after PCI increases by 6 % when central PP increases by 1 mmHg
Jankowski et al. [37]	84	Invasively, fluid-filled system	0.7	The risk of restenosis after PCI increases by 72 % when central PP increases by 10 mmHg
Philippe et al. [40]	96	Invasively, fluid-filled system	1	The risk of restenosis after PCI is related to central MAP. No significant relation with central PP
Chirinos et al. [41]	324	Invasively, fluid-filled system	3.2	The risk of death increases by 18 % when central PP increases by 10 mmHg and decreases by 24 % when central DBP increases by 10 mmHg
Jankowski et al. [7]	1,109	Invasively, fluid-filled system	4.6	The risk of CV events increases by 13 % when central PP increases by 10 mmHg; MAP does not influence prognosis
Weber et al. [11]	725	Noninvasively, applanation tonometry	3.8	The risk of CV events increases by 21 % when central PP increases by 10 mmHg; MAP does not influence prognosis

multivariate adjustments) 1.29, whereas hazard ratio related to the increase of central PP was 1.38 [11]. Table 29.1 summarizes the contemporary evidence of the relation between CV risk and central BP in patients with or suspected to have CAD. Clinical models have been recently described suggesting that aortic PP integrates the predictive value of aortic, inflammatory and renal factors [26]. Taken together, these findings demonstrated that central PP was superior to brachial PP for the prediction of CV risk.

As described above several studies have been published assessing the predictive value of central BP in coronary patients (Table 29.1). The first small studies showed the relation between ascending aortic PP and pulsatility and the risk of restenosis after coronary angioplasty [36, 37]. Indeed, it was proved that vascular wall remodelling after balloon angioplasty and arterial wall cell proliferation is significantly related to the cyclic stress of the vascular wall [38]. Kozuma et al. were the first to show the significant relation between tensile stress and plaque growth after coronary angioplasty [39]. However, it seems that stent implantation may diminish the close relation between PP and restenosis, as suggested by the results published by Philippe et al. [40]. Indeed, as stent may carry most of the cyclic tension related to cyclic changes in intra-arterial pressure, these results may be seen as another proof for the role of haemodynamic forces in the development of the "disease" of the vascular walls. Unfortunately, no study investigating the relation between ascending aortic BP and the risk of restenosis in the era of drug-eluting stents has been published so far. Subsequently, Chirinos et al. showed a correlation between central PP and cardiovascular death risk in 324 men with angiographically confirmed coronary atherosclerosis [41]. They also showed higher risk in subjects with lower DBP in the ascending aorta with greater effect in subjects with more severe coronary atherosclerosis. The results of the biggest published study so far were presented in 2008 [7]. This study followed 1,109 patients, of which 83 % had confirmed coronary artery disease, and showed that pulsatile but not steady component of ascending aortic BP is related to cardiovascular risk. In contrast to a number of studies showing the influence of age on the predictive value of brachial PP, age did not influence the predictive value of central PP or pulsatility in this population (Fig. 29.1). Of note the predictive value of central PP was similar in patients with and with-

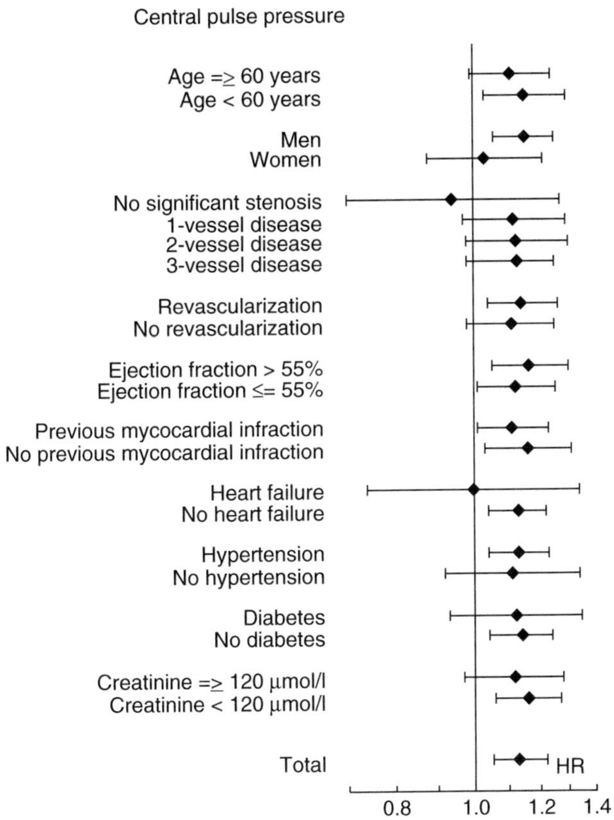

Fig. 29.1 Subgroup analysis of the relationship between central pulse pressure and the risk of the primary end point in 1,109 patients undergoing coronary angiography [7]. Multivariate hazard ratios (*HR*) and 95 % confidence intervals are shown according to a central pulse pressure value increase of 10 mmHg. None of the differences between HRs in the analysed subgroups are significant (all $p = \text{NS}$)

out myocardial infarction in the history. The last study was published by Weber and co-workers who followed 725 patients undergoing coronary angiography including 41.5 % with angiographically confirmed coronary artery disease and once again showed that pulsatile but not steady component of central BP is related to cardiovascular risk [11]. In addition, Weber et al. showed that several other measures of pulsatile haemodynamics are related to the prognosis, among which the backward wave amplitude was the most consistent predictor [11].

Arterial Stiffness and Cardiovascular Risk

Although structural changes related to increased arterial wall stiffness may be quantified pathologically, the clinical evaluation of arterial mechanical properties is more complex, and a complete description of the stress–strain relationship of arteries in vivo is not possible owing to uncertainties arising from non-linear behaviour, viscoelasticity, anisotropy, active tone, residual stresses and tethering [42]. A number of studies have shown that various indices of arterial compliance are related to cardiovascular risk. In the light of the fundamental mechanical principle that pulse waves travel faster in stiffer arteries, PWV measurement is considered the best surrogate to evaluate arterial stiffness, especially in everyday clinical practice. The clinical utility of PWV measurements was recently summarized by Vlachopoulos et al. [43]. The authors calculated that the increase in PWV by 1.0 m/s increases the risk of cardiovascular events by 14 %. This relation is also present in patients with coronary artery disease [44]. Choi et al. showed that the risk of cardiovascular events is increased by 118 % when PWV is higher than 12.5 m/s in patients undergoing coronary angiography [44]. Pressure wave reflections were also shown to be related to end-organ damage and the risk of cardiovascular events in atherosclerotic subjects. Indeed, T. Weber and colleagues in an elegant study showed that backward wave amplitude not only was related to the left ventricular diastolic function parameters, left ventricular hypertrophy, left atrium diameter and GFR but also was independent and the most consistent predictor of the cardiovascular events risk [11].

It is important to understand the mechanism of increased cardiovascular risk in subjects with increased arterial stiffness. The literature suggests several explanations. The first conception underlines that arterial wall stiffness is related to lower DBP and higher SBP in the ascending aorta. Low DBP is related to low perfusion pressure through myocardium and therefore to reduction in coronary perfusion. On the other hand, high SBP increases afterload and oxygen demand of the myocardium and contributes to left ventricular hypertrophy. The net effect is that an increase in arterial stiffness (higher PWV, higher central PP) leads to an imbalance between myocardial oxygen demand and supply, hence ischaemia. This has been proven invasively by Leung and colleagues, who observed a strong inverse relationship between coronary blood flow and PWV/cPP in patients following a coronary intervention [45]. All these effects may increase cardiovascular risk. Second conception underlines that increased stiffness is a symptom of the arterial wall's "disease". Indeed, structural changes contributing to an increase in arterial stiffness include fragmentation of elastin, increased deposition of collagen, arterial calcification, glycation of both elastin and collagen fibres and cross-linking of collagen molecules by advanced glycation end products [46, 47]. In line with this conception, the atherosclerotic plaques develop more easily in the diffusely "diseased" arterial walls leading to coronary and cerebrovascular events. The third conception insists that high arterial stiffness increases the pulsatile component of BP, especially of central BP, which in turn is related to development of atherosclerosis and its complications as well as to damage of microvasculature. Other explanations, including damage of microvasculature leading among others to coronary slow flow [48] as well as to kidney failure [49]

Table 29.2 List of studies assessing the relation between central blood pressure and coronary atherosclerosis

Study	*N*	Main results and conclusions
Nishijima et al. [74]	293	Central PP, but not MAP, is higher in patients with CAD. Central pulsatility correlates with the mean stenosis in the coronary tree
Nakayama et al. [75]	406	The ratio of DBP to MAP, but not the ratio of SBP to MAP, is related to probability of a significant stenosis in the coronary tree
Philippe et al. [40]	99	Only central PP is related to the extent of coronary atherosclerosis
Weber et al. [10]		Central PP is higher in patients with CAD. Augmented pressure correlates with coronary atherosclerosis only in patients at age <60 years
Danchin et al. [76]	280	Central PP is related to the extent of coronary atherosclerosis in men, but not in women
Jankowski et al. [9]	423	Central PP, pulsatility and pulsatility index are related to the number of diseased coronary arteries
Jankowski et al. [77]	445	Central PP and the ratios of central SBP to MAP as well as central DBP to MAP are related to the number of diseased coronary arteries
Jankowski et al. [78]	447	Central PP, pulsatility and pulsatility index are related to the presence of a significant stenosis in coronary tree in women, but not in men
Guray et al. [29]	262	Central PP and pulsatility are related to coronary atherosclerosis in women
Jankowski et al. [79]	375	Central BP-derived indices are not correlated with the extent of coronary atherosclerosis in patients with CAD and impaired left ventricular function
Jankowski et al. [52]	821	The significant relation between pulsatile component of BP and coronary atherosclerosis is present in patients with and without hypertension
Wykrętowicz et al. [30]	201	Central, but not peripheral, pulsatility is related to CAD
Mourad et al. [80]	1,337	Central PP is related to coronary calcification and coronary artery occlusions. Central SBP is related to coronary occlusions

Table 29.2 (continued)

Study	*N*	Main results and conclusions
Pařenica et al. [81]	1,075	Central PP correlates with the number of stenosed coronary arteries
Khoueiry et al. [53]	433	Central PP is higher in patients with stenosis in right compared to left coronary artery
Refiker et al. [82]	245	Central DBP and the extent of coronary atherosclerosis are related to the coronary collateral development

and indirectly to progression of atherosclerosis and its complications, are also possible.

Blood Pressure and Atherosclerosis

Blood vessels are constantly exposed to two kinds of dynamic mechanical forces. One of them is shear stress and the other is the cyclic strain of the vascular wall, which, according to the Laplace's law, is mainly determined by cyclic change of BP [50]. While shear stress affects predominantly endothelial cells, BP changes (and the resulting changes in arterial wall strain) influence all structures of the arterial wall. It is logical to accept that arteries are permanently exposed to a basal stretch, which is related to MAP. MAP is paired to a pulsatile component, owing to the presence of cardiac cycle. Changes in the intramural tension have been recognized as an important factor in the pathogenesis of atherosclerosis [2]. Interestingly, it was suggested that cyclic stretch is a more important factor determining superoxide anion production in the endothelium than shear stress [51].

A number of studies have been published showing the significant relation between central BP and the presence or extent of atherosclerosis in the coronary arteries (Table 29.2). Importantly, the findings that measures such as fractional pulse pressure are related to atherosclerosis suggest that pulsatile component of BP is more closely related to development and progression of atherosclerosis than steady component [9]. Interestingly, the relation between these measures and coronary atherosclerosis tends to be closer in normotensives than in subjects with hypertension [52]. In addition, a recent study showed that PP may be higher in patients with stenosed right coronary artery as compared to those with stenosed left coronary artery, which could suggest that the difference in haemodynamic conditions in right coronary artery and left coronary artery may influence the atherosclerosis development [53]. However, it should be underlined that all these studies were cross-sectional in nature. On the other hand, an in vivo study by Tropea et al. (using an animal model) showed that inhibition of cyclic stretch of the aorta is related to inhibition of the atherosclerotic plaque formation [54]. In the sample studied by Tropea et al., atherogenic diet was not related to the development of atherosclerotic plaque in the absence of cyclic stretch of the arterial wall [54]. Indeed, this report suggests that the arterial wall cyclic stress is an indispensable factor for atherosclerosis development.

Nowadays, the differential effects of steady and pulsatile forces on arterial wall should be considered as obvious, even if several findings have been investigated mainly in vitro. The corresponding in vivo findings remain scarce. Most of them are simply deduced from human epidemiological investigations, indicating that pulsatile stress, as represented by PP, wave reflections and/or arterial stiffness, is a more important predictor of CV risk than steady stress, especially in patients with atherosclerosis [7, 11, 55, 56]. Nevertheless, it should be emphasized that the influence of cyclic stretch on atherosclerosis has been documented on every stage of its development [2]. PP was shown to be an important factor conditioning the infiltration of arterial wall by lipids [57]. Cyclic stretch stimulates the expression of adhesion molecules in the endothelial cells, which facilitates the migration of inflammatory response cells into vascular wall, as well as the production of scavenger receptors, thereby facilitating the transformation of macrophages into foam cells [2, 58]. The activity of metalloproteinases in the atherosclerotic plaque also depends partially on the cyclic stretch of the arterial wall [2]. The influence of vascular wall stretch on migration and proliferation of smooth muscle cells was also documented as well as its

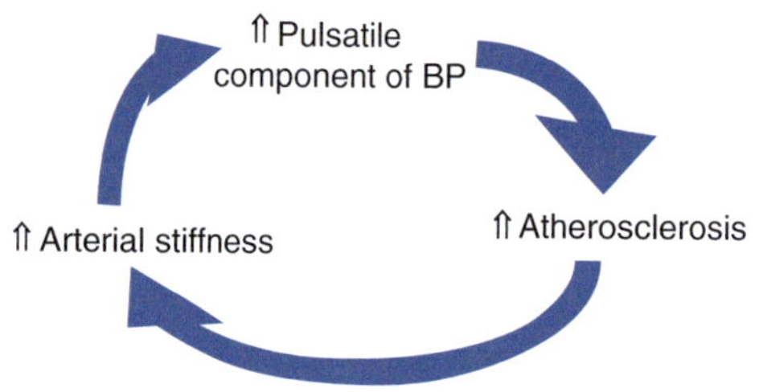

Fig. 29.2 A vicious circle consisting of arterial stiffness, blood pressure and atherosclerosis

impact on the production of glycosaminoglycans by vascular smooth muscle cells [2, 59]. Cyclic stretch causes also plasminogen activator inhibitor-1 (PAI-1) release from endothelial cells [60]. Recently, mechanical strain was proved to induce expression of C-reactive protein in human blood vessels [61]. Finally, apart from mediating atherosclerosis progression and atherosclerotic plaque instability, the pulsatile component of BP is the main mechanism leading to degradation and weakening of the atherosclerotic fibrous cap, plaque rupture and consequently to acute coronary syndromes and other vascular complications. Moreover, Selwaness et al. showed that PP is the strongest determinant of intraplaque haemorrhages [62]. These results are important as intraplaque haemorrhage, besides plaque rupture and plaque erosion, is the main mechanism leading to plaque progression and destabilization and finally to myocardial infarctions, strokes and cardiovascular deaths. The relation between PP and intraplaque haemorrhage can be explained on the basis of damage of microcirculation due to enhanced pulsatile load. Importantly, odds ratios of the presence of intraplaque haemorrhage related to one standard deviation increase in PP and fractional pulse pressure were similar (1.22 and 1.23, respectively), whereas MAP was not related to the presence of haemorrhages. Although it was a cross-sectional study, these findings are another proof that the pulsatile mechanical load that acts on the arterial wall is related to progression of atherosclerosis and its complications, irrespectively of the absolute value of blood pressure [62].

In conclusion, currently there is no doubt as to the existence of a significant relationship between the pulsatile BP component and atherosclerosis. Increased PP may be both the cause and the effect of atherosclerosis: on one hand the presence of the diffuse atherosclerosis may impair elastic properties of the arterial walls [63] (although unstable, lipid-rich plaques do not impair arterial compliance), while reduced large artery compliance enhances the pulsatile component of BP leading to the progression of atherosclerotic plaques. These mechanisms may lead to a vicious circle wherein the pulsatile BP component causes/enhances the progression of atherosclerosis, which in turn, through a reduced arterial compliance and an enhanced wave reflection, augments the pulsatile BP component (Fig. 29.2). According to this concept, a therapeutic interference with this vicious cycle might improve patients' prognosis.

The Beneficial Effects of Interventions Aiming at Improving Survival in CAD Patients

It should be underlined that taking into account the close relation between pulsatile component of BP, arterial stiffness and atherosclerosis, maximizing the benefit requires interventions aiming at all three components of the vicious circle (Fig. 29.2). The recent studies have shown that it is possible to slow the progression of atherosclerosis and to obtain a selective and long-term reduction of brachial and, what is even more important, central SBP and PP by decreasing arterial stiffness and/or wave reflections.

Lifestyle Changes

Lifestyle interventions can reduce arterial stiffness and/or wave reflections. Physical activity is especially effective in reducing arterial wall stiffness [64, 65]. Also low-salt diet improves arterial distensibility by reduction in BP as well as direct effects nondependent on BP changes [66, 67]. Direct beneficial effects of fish oils have been reported by several researchers [68, 69]. Weight loss was also suggested to improve arterial wall compliance [67]. Some researchers have suggested that one of the potential "anti-ageing" benefits of prolonged caloric restriction is a reduction in the rate of increase in arterial stiffness that occurs with age. Of note lifestyle changes reduce cardiovascular risk. It should be, however, underlined that the evidence of beneficial effects of lifestyle interventions (with the exception of cardiac rehabilitation) on arterial wall compliance or central BP in patients with coronary artery disease is scarce.

The Influence of Antihypertensive Drugs on Peripheral and Central BP

Numerous studies have examined the influence of various antihypertensive drugs on central in comparison with brachial BP, including agents which improve survival in patients with cardiovascular disease [70]. The recent consensus document has underlined the clinical consequences of overestimation of the antihypertensive effect of some drug classes and underestimation of BP changes due to the use of other drugs when analysing brachial instead of central BP [71]. The influence of CV drugs on central BP, wave reflections and arterial stiffness is described in detail in other book chapters.

Central Blood Pressure, Coronary Artery Disease and Everyday Clinical Practice

Central wave form assessment might be a useful non-invasive clinical test that stratifies the likelihood of coronary disease and assists in identifying patients who require diagnostic coronary angiography [72]. The recent development of new methods and new devices which allow for quick and (from the physician's point of view) simple measurement of central BP may result in the use of central BP assessment in everyday clinical practice in the near future [73]. However, it should be noted that the usefulness of serial central BP determinations in everyday clinical practice has been never convincingly demonstrated. More data is needed before definitive recommendation about central BP measurements in clinical practice can be done. Especially, better prognosis in patients managed according to central in comparison with peripheral BP should be proved.

Conclusions

Although the differences between central and peripheral blood pressure have been known for decades, the consequences of decision-making based on central rather than peripheral BP have only recently been recognized. Central PP is closer to the heart, coronary and carotid arteries, which are the most important sites of cardiovascular events. The influence of cyclic stretch (owing to cyclic changes in BP) on the arterial wall has been documented at every stage of atherosclerosis development. Apart from mediating atherosclerosis progression and plaque instability, the pulsatile component of BP is the main mechanism leading to plaque rupture and, consequently, to acute coronary syndromes and other vascular complications. A lot of attention has been given recently to break the link between pulse pressure and cardiovascular events. Because of the vicious circle consisting of arterial wall stiffness, pulse pressure and atherosclerosis, the most promising intervention is reduction in arterial stiffness, although increase of the potential benefit requires interventions aiming at all three components of the vicious circle.

References

1. Powles JW, Zatonski W, Vander Hoorn S, Ezzati M. The contribution of leading diseases and risk factors to excess losses of healthy life in Eastern Europe: burden of disease study. BMC Public Health. 2005;5:116.
2. Jankowski P, Bilo G, Kawecka-Jaszcz K. The pulsatile component of BP: its role in the pathogenesis of atherosclerosis. Blood Press. 2007;16:238–45.
3. Nichols WW, O'Rourke MF. McDonald's blood flow in arteries. Theoretical, experimental and clinical principles. 4th ed. London: Edward Arnold; 2006.
4. Black HR. The paradigm has shifted to systolic blood pressure. Hypertension. 1999;34:386–7.

5. Mancia G, Grassi G. Systolic and diastolic blood pressure control in antihypertensive drug trials. J Hypertens. 2002;20:1461–4.
6. Darne B, Girerd X, Safar MF, Cambien F, Guize L. Pulsatile versus steady component of blood pressure: a cross-sectional analysis and a prospective analysis on cardiovascular mortality. Hypertension. 1989;13:392–400.
7. Jankowski P, Kawecka-Jaszcz K, Czarnecka D, Brzozowska-Kiszka M, Styczkiewicz K, Loster M, et al. Pulsatile but not steady component of blood pressure predicts cardiovascular events in coronary patients. Hypertension. 2008;51:848–55.
8. Gambillara V, Thacher T, Silacci P, Stergiopulos N. Effects of reduced cyclic stretch on vascular smooth muscle cell function of pig carotids perfused ex vivo. Am J Hypertens. 2008;21:425–31.
9. Jankowski P, Kawecka-Jaszcz K, Czarnecka D, Brzozowska-Kiszka M, Styczkiewicz K, Styczkiewicz M, et al. Ascending aortic, but not brachial blood pressure-derived indices are related to coronary atherosclerosis. Atherosclerosis. 2004;176:151–5.
10. Weber T, Auer J, O'Rourke MF, Kvas E, Lassnig E, Berent R, et al. Arterial stiffness, wave reflections, and the risk of coronary artery disease. Circulation. 2004;109:184–9.
11. Weber T, Wassertheurer S, Rammer M, Haiden A, Hametner B, Eber B. Wave reflections, assessed with a novel method for pulse wave separation are associated with end-organ damage and clinical outcomes. Hypertension. 2012;60:534–41.
12. Lewington S, Clarke R, Qizilbash N, Peto R, Collins R. Age-specific relevance of usual blood pressure to vascular mortality: a meta-analysis of individual data for one million adults in 61 prospective studies. Lancet. 2002;360:1903–13.
13. Sundström J, Neovius M, Tynelius P, Rasmussen F. Association of blood pressure in late adolescence with subsequent mortality: cohort study of Swedish male conscripts. BMJ. 2011;342:d643.
14. Bangalore S, Messerli FH, Franklin SS, Mancia G, Champion A, Pepine CJ. Pulse pressure and risk of cardiovascular outcomes in patients with hypertension and coronary artery disease: an INternational VErapamil SR-trandolapril STudy (INVEST) analysis. Eur Heart J. 2009;30:1395–401.
15. Protogerou AD, Safar ME, Iaria P, Safar H, Le Dudal K, Filipovsky J, et al. Diastolic blood pressure and mortality in the elderly with cardiovascular disease. Hypertension. 2007;50:172–80.
16. Bangalore S, Messerli FH, Wun CC, Zuckerman AL, DeMicco D, Kostis JB, et al. J-curve revisited: an analysis of blood pressure and cardiovascular events in the Treating to New Targets (TNT) Trial. Eur Heart J. 2010;31:2897–908.
17. Denardo SJ, Messerli FH, Gaxiola E, Aranda Jr JM, Cooper-Dehoff RM, Handberg EM, et al. Coronary revascularization strategy and outcomes according to blood pressure (from the International Verapamil SR-Trandolapril Study [INVEST]). Am J Cardiol. 2010;106:498–503.
18. Schillaci G, Di Luzio S, Coluccini M, Gonzini L, Porcu M, Pozzar F, et al. A low pulse pressure is an independent predictor of mortality in heart failure: data from a large nationwide cardiology database (IN-CHF Registry). Ital Heart J. 2004;5:892–8.
19. Westerhof N, O'Rourke MF. Haemodynamic basis for the development of the left ventricular failure in systolic hypertension and for its logical therapy. J Hypertens. 1995;13:943–52.
20. Weber T, Auer J, Lamm G, O'Rourke MF, Eber B. Arterial stiffness, central blood pressure, and wave reflections in cardiomyopathy – implications for risk stratification. J Card Fail. 2007;13:353–9.
21. Hurthle K. Ueber den Ursprungsort der sekundaren Wellen der Pulscurve. Arch f d ges Physiol. 1890; 47:17.
22. Frank O. Der Puls in den Arterien Ztschr. f Biol. 1905;46:441–53.
23. Wood EH, Fuller J, Clagett OT. Intraluminal pressures recorded simultaneously from different arteries in man (abstract). Am J Physiol. 1951;167:838.
24. O'Rourke MF. Arterial stiffness in hypertension. 1st ed. Amsterdam: Elsevier; 2006. p. 3–20.
25. Safar ME, Blacher J, Protogerou A, Achimastos A. Arterial stiffness and central hemodynamics in treated hypertensive subjects according to brachial BP classification. J Hypertens. 2008;26:130–7.
26. Temmar M, Jankowski P, Peltier M, Mouquet V, Dębicka-Dąbrowska D, Hamida F, et al. Intraaortic pulse pressure amplification in subjects at high coronary risk. Hypertension. 2010;55:327–32.
27. Avolio AP, Van Bortel LM, Boutouyrie P, Cockcroft JR, McEniery CM, Protogerou AD, et al. Role of pulse pressure amplification in arterial hypertension: experts' opinion and review of the data. Hypertension. 2009;54:375–83.
28. Choi CU, Kim EJ, Kim SH, Shin SY, Choi UJ, Kim JW, et al. Differing effects of aging on central and peripheral blood pressures and pulse wave velocity: a direct intraarterial study. J Hypertens. 2010;28: 1252–60.
29. Guray Y, Guray U, Altay H, Cay S, Yilmaz MB, Kisacik HL, et al. Aortic pulse pressure and aortic pulsatility are associated with angiographic coronary artery disease in women. Blood Press. 2005;14: 293–7.
30. Wykretowicz A, Metzler L, Milewska A, Balinski M, Rutkowska A, Adamska K, et al. Noninvasively assessed pulsatility of ascending aortic pressure waveform is associated with the presence of coronary artery narrowing. Heart Vessels. 2008;23:16–9.
31. Safar ME, Blacher J, Pannier B, Guerin A, Marchais S, Guyonvarc'h P, et al. Central pulse pressure and mortality in end-stage renal disease. Hypertension. 2002;39:735–8.
32. Wang KL, Cheng HM, Chuang SY, Spurgeon HA, Ting CT, Lakatta EG, et al. Central or peripheral systolic or pulse pressure: which best relates to target organs and future mortality? J Hypertens. 2009;27: 461–7.

33. Roman MJ, Devereux RB, Kizer JR, Lee ET, Galloway JM, Ali T, et al. Central pressure more strongly relates to vascular disease and outcome than does brachial pressure: the Strong Heart Study. Hypertension. 2007;50:197–203.
34. Mitchell GF, Hwang SJ, Vasan RS, Larson MG, Pencina MJ, Hamburg NM, et al. Arterial stiffness and cardiovascular events: the Framingham Heart Study. Circulation. 2010;121:505–11.
35. Vlachopoulos C, Aznaouridis K, O'Rourke MF, Safar ME, Baou K, Stefanadis C. Prediction of cardiovascular events and all-cause mortality with central haemodynamics: a systematic review and meta-analysis. Eur Heart J. 2010;31:1865–71.
36. Lu TM, Hsu NW, Chen YH, Lee WS, Wu CC, Ding YA, et al. Pulsatility of ascending aorta and restenosis after coronary angioplasty in patients >60 years of age with stable angina pectoris. Am J Cardiol. 2001;88: 964–8.
37. Jankowski P, Kawecka-Jaszcz K, Bryniarski L, Czarnecka D, Zabojszcz M, Styczkiewicz M. Pulse pressure as a predictor of restenosis after percutaneous transluminal coronary angioplasty. Przegl Lek. 2001;58:1025–8.
38. Wentzel JJ, Kloet J, Andhyiswara I, Oomen JAF, Schuurbiers JCH, de Smet BJGL, et al. Shear-stress and wall-stress regulation of vascular remodeling after balloon angioplasty: effect of matrix metalloproteinase inhibition. Circulation. 2001;104:91–6.
39. Kozuma K, Costa MA, Sabate M, Slager CJ, Boersma E, Kay IP, et al. Relationship between tensile stress and plaque growth after balloon angioplasty treated with and without intracoronary betabrachytherapy. Eur Heart J. 2000;24:2063–70.
40. Philippe F, Chemaly E, Blacher J, Mourad JJ, Dibie A, Larrazet F, et al. Aortic pulse pressure and extent of coronary artery disease in percutaneous transluminal coronary angioplasty candidates. Am J Hypertens. 2002;15:672–7.
41. Chirinos JA, Zambrano JP, Chakko S, Veerani A, Schob A, Perez G, et al. Relation between ascending aortic pressures and outcomes in patients with angiographically demonstrated coronary artery disease. Am J Cardiol. 2005;96:645–8.
42. Vito RP, Dixon SA. Blood vessel constitutive models: 1995–2002. Annu Rev Biomed Eng. 2003;5: 413–39.
43. Vlachopoulos C, Aznaouridis K, Stefanadis C. Prediction of cardiovascular events and all-cause mortality with arterial stiffness: a systematic review and meta-analysis. J Am Coll Cardiol. 2010;55: 1318–27.
44. Choi CU, Park EB, Suh SY, Kim JW, Kim EJ, Rha SW, et al. Impact of aortic stiffness on cardiovascular disease in patients with chest pain. Am J Hypertens. 2007;20:1163–9.
45. Leung MCH, Meredith IT, Cameron JD. Aortic stiffness affects the coronary blood flow response to percutaneous coronary intervention. Am J Physiol Heart Circ Physiol. 2006;290:H624–30.
46. Laurent S, Boutouyrie P, Lacolley P. Structural and genetic bases of arterial stiffness. Hypertension. 2005;45:1050–5.
47. Safar ME, Blacher J, Jankowski P. Arterial stiffness, pulse pressure, and cardiovascular disease-is it possible to break the vicious circle? Atherosclerosis. 2011;218:263–71.
48. Guray U, Guray Y, Yilmaz MB, Caldir V, Cay S, Sasmaz H, et al. Aortic pulse pressure and aortic pulsatility in patients with coronary slow flow. Cardiology. 2007;107:233–8.
49. Ishikawa T, Hashimoto J, Morito RH, Hanazawa T, Aikawa T, Hara A, et al. Association of microalbuminuria with brachial-ankle pulse wave velocity: the Ohasama study. Am J Hypertens. 2008;21:413–8.
50. Fuster V, Lewis A. Conner memorial lecture. Mechanisms leading to myocardial infarction: insights from studies of vascular biology. Circulation. 1994;90:2126–46.
51. Thacher TN, Silacci P, Stergiopulos N, da Silva RF. Autonomous effects of shear stress and cyclic circumferential stretch regarding endothelial dysfunction and oxidative stress: an ex vivo arterial model. J Vasc Res. 2009;47:336–45.
52. Jankowski P, Kawecka-Jaszcz K, Czarnecka D. Ascending aortic blood pressure waveform is related to coronary atherosclerosis in hypertensive as well as in normotensive subjects. Blood Press. 2007;16:246–53.
53. Khoueiry G, Azab B, Torbey E, Rafeh NA, Atallah JP, Ahern K, et al. Aortic pulse pressure is associated with the localization of coronary artery disease based on coronary flow lateralization. Am J Hypertens. 2012;25:1055–63.
54. Tropea BI, Schwarzacher SP, Chang A, Asvar C, Huie P, Sibley RK, et al. Reduction of aortic wall motion inhibits hypertension-mediated experimental atherosclerosis. Arterioscler Thromb Vasc Biol. 2000;20: 2127–33.
55. Wang KL, Cheng HM, Sung SH, Chuang SY, Li CH, Spurgeon HA, et al. Wave reflection and arterial stiffness in the prediction of 15-year all-cause and cardiovascular mortalities: a community-based study. Hypertension. 2010;55:799–805.
56. Chirinos JA, Kips JG, Jacobs Jr DR, Brumback L, Duprez DA, Kronmal R, et al. Arterial wave reflections and incident cardiovascular events and heart failure: MESA (Multiethnic Study of Atherosclerosis). J Am Coll Cardiol. 2012;60:2170–7.
57. Kiefer CR, McKenney JB, Trainor JF, Snyder LM. Pulse pressure-driven neutral lipid accumulation and correlative proinflammatory markers of accelerated atherogenesis. Atherosclerosis. 2005;183: 17–24.
58. Sakamoto H, Aikawa M, Hill CC, Weiss D, Taylor WR, Libby P, et al. Biomechanical strain induces class a scavenger receptor expression in human monocyte/macrophages and THP-1 cells. A potential mechanism of increased atherosclerosis in hypertension. Circulation. 2001;104:109–14.

59. Lee RT, Yamamoto C, Feng Y, Potter-Perigo S, Briggs WH, Landschluz KT. Mechanical strain induces specific changes in the synthesis and organization of proteoglycans by vascular smooth muscle cells. J Biol Chem. 2001;276:13847–51.
60. Cheng JJ, Chao YJ, Wung BS, Wang DL. Cyclic strain-induced plasminogen activator inhibitor-1 (PAI-1) release from endothelial cells involves reactive oxygen species. Biochem Biophys Res Commun. 1996;225:100–5.
61. Huang G, Luo C, Gu X, Wu Z, Wang Z, Du Z, et al. Mechanical strain induces expression of C-reactive protein in human blood vessels. J Pharmacol Exp Ther. 2009;330:206–11.
62. Selwaness M, van den Bouwhuijsen QJA, Verwoert GC, Dehghan A, Mattace-Raso FUS, Vernooij M, et al. Blood pressure parameters and carotid intraplaque hemorrhage as measured by magnetic resonance imaging The Rotterdam Study. Hypertension. 2013;61:76–81.
63. Kopeć G, Podolec P, Podolec J, Rubiś P, Zmudka K, Tracz W. Atherosclerosis progression affects the relationship between endothelial function and aortic stiffness. Atherosclerosis. 2009;204:250–4.
64. Collier SR, Kanaley JA, Carhart Jr R, Frechette V, Tobin MM, Hall AK, et al. Effect of 4 weeks of aerobic or resistance exercise training on arterial stiffness, blood flow and blood pressure in pre- and stage-1 hypertensives. J Hum Hypertens. 2008;22: 678–86.
65. Guimarães GV, Ciolac EG, Carvalho VO, D'Avila VM, Bortolotto LA, Bocchi EA. Effects of continuous vs interval exercise training on blood pressure and arterial stiffness in treated hypertension. Hypertens Res. 2010;33:627–32.
66. Avolio AP, Clyde KM, Beard TC, Cooke HM, Ho KK, O'Rourke MF. Improved arterial distensibility in normotensive subjects on a low salt diet. Arteriosclerosis. 1986;6:166–9.
67. Kingwell BA, Cameron JD. Nonpharmacological treatment for increased arterial stiffness and altered wave reflections. In: Safar ME, O'Rourke MF, editors. Arterial stiffness in hypertension. New York: Elsevier; 2006.
68. Yamada T, Strong JP, Ishii T, Ueno T, Koyama M, Wagayama H, et al. Atherosclerosis and omega-3 fatty acids in the populations of a fishing village and a farming village in Japan. Atherosclerosis. 2000;153:469–81.
69. Hamazaki T, Urakaze M, Sawazaki S, Yamazaki K, Taki H, Yano S. Comparison of pulse wave velocity of the aorta between inhabitants of fishing and farming villages in Japan. Atherosclerosis. 1988;73:157–60.
70. Jankowski P, Safar ME, Kawecka-Jaszcz K. How drugs influencing central blood pressure prevent atherosclerosis complications? Curr Pharm Biotechnol. 2012;13:2449–55.
71. Agabiti-Rosei E, Mancia G, O'Rourke MF, Roman MJ, Safar ME, Smulyan H. Central blood pressure measurements and antihypertensive therapy: a consensus document. Hypertension. 2007;50:154–60.
72. Kotecha D, New G, Collins P, Eccleston D, Krum H, Pepper J, et al. Radial artery pulse wave analysis for non-invasive assessment of coronary artery disease. Int J Cardiol. 2013;167:917–24.
73. Weber T, Wassertheurer S, Rammer M, Maurer E, Hametner B, Mayer CC, et al. Validation of a brachial cuff-based method for estimating central systolic blood pressure. Hypertension. 2011;58:825–32.
74. Nishijima T, Nakayama Y, Tsumura K, Yamashita N, Yoshimaru K, Ueda H, et al. Pulsatility of ascending aortic blood pressure waveform is associated with an increased risk of coronary heart disease. Am J Hypertens. 2001;14:469–73.
75. Nakayama Y, Hayashi T, Yoshimaru K, Tsumura K, Ueda H. Low fractional diastolic pressure in the ascending aorta increased the risk of coronary heart disease. J Hum Hypertens. 2002;16:837–41.
76. Danchin N, Benetos A, Lopez-Sublet M, Demicheli T, Safar M, Mourad JJ. Aortic pulse pressure is related to the presence and extent of coronary artery disease in men undergoing diagnostic coronary angiography: a multicenter study. Am J Hypertens. 2004;17:129–33.
77. Jankowski P, Kawecka-Jaszcz K, Bryniarski L, Czarnecka D, Brzozowska-Kiszka M, Pośnik-Urbańska A, et al. Fractional diastolic and systolic pressure in the ascending aorta are related to the extent of coronary artery disease. Am J Hypertens. 2004;17:641–6.
78. Jankowski P, Kawecka-Jaszcz K, Czarnecka D, Bryniarski L. Ascending aortic blood pressure waveform may be related to the risk of coronary artery disease in women, but not in men. J Hum Hypertens. 2004;18:643–8.
79. Jankowski P, Kawecka-Jaszcz K, Czarnecka D, Brzozowska-Kiszka M, Pośnik-Urbańska A, Styczkiewicz K. Ascending aortic blood pressure-derived indices are not correlated with the extent of coronary artery disease in patients with impaired left ventricular function. Atherosclerosis. 2006;184: 370–6.
80. Mourad JJ, Danchin N, Rudnichi A, Lopez-Sublet M, Le Jeune S, Safar ME. Aortic pulse pressure and atherosclerotic structural alterations of coronary arteries. J Hum Hypertens. 2010;24:51–7.
81. Pařenica J, Kala P, Jarkovský J, Poloczek M, Boček O, Jeřábek P, et al. Relationship between high aortic pulse pressure and extension of coronary atherosclerosis in males. Physiol Res. 2011;60:47–53.
82. Ege MR, Zorlu A, Yilmaz MB, Acikgoz S, Tandogan I, Cinar Z. Central diastolic blood pressure is associated with the degree of coronary collateral development. Angiology. 2013;64:546–52.

Part IV

Clinical Involvement: Role of Age, Sex, Inflammatory and Metabolic Alterations

Modifications of Blood Pressure Profiles in the Very Old: Role of Frailty and Comorbidities

30

Athanase Benetos, Sylvie Gautier, and Michel E. Safar

Keywords
Elderly population • Comorbidities • Geriatric medicine • Cardiovascular risk • Alzheimer's disease

The continuously increasing number of elderly people, especially those 80+ years of age, leads into a growing population prone to frailty, multiple comorbidities, and partial loss of autonomy. This is now one of the target populations for geriatric medicine necessitating the development of specific diagnostic and therapeutic approaches [1]. These approaches cannot be derived however from a simple extrapolation of the strategies applied in younger populations or even in elderly robust populations. Thus, assessment of cardiovascular (CV) risk in these subjects represents a major issue. High blood pressure (BP), especially systolic hypertension, is a common condition in the elderly and is considered a major determinant not only of CV morbidity and mortality but also of several other age-related diseases, frailty, and loss of autonomy [2]. Thus, high blood pressure has been related to several age-related diseases such as osteoporosis [3] and Alzheimer's disease [4]. It has also been shown that life expectancy is reduced in middle-aged hypertensives [5, 6].

Therefore, there is no doubt that high blood pressure and high risk of morbidity and mortality go hand in hand. This concept has dominated hypertension epidemiology as well as clinical trials which have shown that in hypertensive subjects, the more important the decrease in systolic or diastolic BP (DBP), the more important the benefits in terms of cardiovascular morbidity and mortality in young, middle-aged, and older populations of both genders [7–10]. Numerous large clinical trials in individuals 65 years or older showed that antihypertensive treatment in older adults is as beneficial as that in younger adults [11]. Thus, large studies such as the Systolic Hypertension in the Elderly Program [12], Swedish Trial in Old Patients [13], Medical Research Council [14], Systolic Hypertension in

A. Benetos, MD, PhD (✉)
Department of Geriatrics, University Hospital of Nancy, Universite De Lorraine, 1, allée du Morvan, Vandoeuvre Les Nancy 54500, France

INSERM U1116,
Université de Lorraine, Nancy, France
e-mail: a.benetos@chu-nancy.fr

S. Gautier, MD
Department of Geriatrics, University Hospital of Nancy, Universite De Lorraine, 1, allée du Morvan, Vandoeuvre Les Nancy 54500, France
e-mail: s.gautier@chu-nancy.fr

M.E. Safar, MD
Department of Medicine, Paris Descartes University, Assistance Publique des Hôpitaux de Paris – Hôtel-Dieu Hospital, Diagnosis and Therapeutics Center, 1 Place du Parvis Notre-Dame, Paris 75004, France
e-mail: michel.safar@htd.apjp.fr

M.E. Safar et al. (eds.), *Blood Pressure and Arterial Wall Mechanics in Cardiovascular Diseases*, DOI 10.1007/978-1-4471-5198-2_30, © Springer-Verlag London 2014

Europe [15], and Systolic Hypertension in China [16] have shown the benefits of reducing BP in elderly subjects. The results of the Hypertension in the Very Elderly (HYVET) study [17] also showed the beneficial effect of antihypertensive treatment in patients 80 years or older.

Although the concept "the lower the blood pressure, the better the prognosis" may be a very appealing message in terms of public health policy, several results especially in the elderly show that this dogma may not always represent the truth. One of the most typical examples is the inverse relationship between DBP and CV risk observed in elderly individuals [18–21]. Furthermore, such an inverse relationship with risk has even been observed with systolic blood pressure (SBP) in very elderly subjects presenting several comorbidities [22, 23]. Actually, although in relatively fit elderly people [7, 17] high SBP is associated with higher morbidity and mortality, no association between high BP and morbidity and mortality was found in very old persons with several comorbidities [22, 24, 25]. Notably, a J-shape or an inverse relationship between BP (both systolic and diastolic) and morbidity/mortality was observed in a subset of studies [26, 27]. Clinical studies in very old persons reported a poor prognosis in those with systolic BP (SBP) <140 mmHg [28, 29]. The J-shape phenomenon associated with excessive diastolic BP reduction in elderly patients has been reported in the Practitioner's Trial on the Efficacy of Antihypertensive Treatment in the Elderly [30] and in some post hoc analyses of large clinical studies, such as the Systolic Hypertension in the Elderly Program [31] and Systolic Hypertension in Europe [32]. In another post hoc analysis of the Systolic Hypertension in the Elderly Program, the greatest benefits in terms of lowering stroke risk were observed in patients with SBP <150 mmHg but not in those with SBP <140 mmHg [33]. Accordingly, excessive reduction of BP in the elderly, particularly in elderly patients with cardiovascular disease, might be harmful because of decreased perfusion of target organs [30].

Hence, the issue that we have attempted to address herein is what does measured BP really means and what are its determinants during the aging process. Actually, as we have developed in a recent review, the demographic, technological, and therapeutic changes over the past 20–30 years make possible now to reconsider the concept of the "role of blood pressure in the cardiovascular risk determination" [34].

The Transition from Diastolic to Systolic and Pulse Pressure (PP) During Aging

The Reasons of Increase in PP with Age

Until the ages of 50–60 years, both SBP and DBP increase with age. Thereafter, in the majority of cases, SBP increases with age disproportionally to DBP. The most common cause for the disruption of the correlation between SBP and DBP (leading to an excessive increase in SBP and PP) is the progressive stiffening of the arterial wall [35, 36]. Indeed, arterial stiffness develops as a consequence of several structural and functional changes of large arteries. Wall hypertrophy, calcium deposits, and changes in the extracellular matrix, such as an increase in collagen and in fibronectin, fragmentation and disorganization of the elastin network, non-enzymatic cross-links, and cell-matrix interactions, are the predominant structural determinants of the decrease in elastic properties and the development of large-artery stiffness [37].

It is important at this juncture to point out that SBP is dependent on left ventricular performance and on the stiffness of the aorta and other large arteries [35]. Thus, peak systolic pressure will be greater if the arterial wall is more rigid. On the other hand, after closure of the aortic valves, arterial pressure gradually falls as blood is drained to peripheral vascular networks. Minimum DBP is determined by the duration of the diastolic interval and the rate at which pressure falls. The rate of fall in pressure is influenced by the rate of outflow, i.e., peripheral resistance, and by viscoelastic arterial properties. At a given vascular resistance, the drop in diastolic pressure will be greater if the rigidity of large arteries is increased. The viscoelastic properties of arterial walls are also a determinant of the speed of propagation of the arterial pressure wave (pulse wave velocity (PWV)) and of the timing of wave reflections. Thus, stiffening of the arteries increases PWV and may be responsible for an earlier return of the reflected waves, which overlaps the incident pressure wave, thus further contributing to the increase in SBP and PP [35, 36]. Moreover, several clinical cross-sectional and longitudinal studies have shown that increases in arterial stiffness with age are not linear, being more pronounced after the age of 55–60 [38, 39], which may in turn explain the more pronounced increase in PP after this age, as reported in the Framingham study [19]. In addition to age, any disease and/or situation that induces an accelerated increase in arterial stiffness will be clinically expressed by an increase in SBP and PP. Diabetes is a typical example of accelerated arterial aging leading to a more noticeable increase in PP with age as compared to nondiabetic patients, due to a more pronounced increase in arterial stiffness [40–42]. In accordance with this concept, increased PP with age is more pronounced in diabetics with initial micro- or macroalbuminuria and retinopathy, suggesting that the progression in arterial aging is more prominent in the presence of target organ damage [42].

The Increasing Impact of Systolic/Pulse Pressure in the Elderly

Taking into account these considerations can better explain why SBP and PP better reflect CVD risk in older subjects, whereas DBP better reflects the risk in younger subjects [20, 43]. Indeed, DBP in young patients is predominantly dependent on peripheral resistance, and, therefore, low DBP reflects low peripheral resistance. In addition, in younger subjects with hyperkinetic circulation, DBP is less variable than SBP, thus better reflecting cardiovascular risk. In older subjects, a low DBP may reflect high arterial stiffness, which is a major manifestation of arterial aging, rather than low peripheral resistance [35, 36]. In this case, low DBP is associated with high SBP and high PP and increased cardiovascular risk. The clinical application of these considerations is that, as clearly stated in the latest guidelines of the JNC, "in persons older than 50 years, SBP is a much more important cardiovascular risk factor than DBP" [8].

Also, in 2003, for the first time, the European recommendations on the management of hypertension [44] have suggested that PP may represent an independent risk factor and that therapeutic studies should henceforth be conducted to assess the benefits of reducing PP in terms of cardiovascular morbidity and mortality, especially among those over 60 years of age [43]. Indeed, since the first study, conduced in 1989, which demonstrated a positive association between PP and target organ damage [45], a large number of clinical studies notably over the past 10 years have shown that increased PP is a strong predictor of coronary disease, incidence of heart failure, and cardiovascular morbidity and mortality, independently of mean BP levels [19, 46–51]. Such observations have been made in a variety of different populations but are apparently more pronounced in diabetics and elderly subjects. Threshold PP risk values have been proposed, notably a value of approximately 65 mmHg [52, 53]. The association between PP and CV mortality has also been observed in elderly patients enrolled in large clinical trials, as shown in a meta-analysis published in 2002 [54], during which seven clinical trials in the elderly were analyzed (EWPHE, HEP, MRC1, MRC2, SHEP, STOP, Syst-Eur). The subjects enrolled in these trials were elderly patients with systolic-diastolic hypertension or isolated systolic hypertension.

The SBP/PP-Related Increase in Cardiovascular Risk: Is It Only a Barometric Phenomenon?

To date, at least three hypotheses can be put forward to explain the association between SBP/PP and CV risk. Actually, these three hypotheses are complementary rather than contradictory:

(a) PP increases arterial cyclic stress: Experimental studies indicate that fatigue and fracture of elastic fibers within the arterial wall are related to both steady-state and pulsatile stress [55, 56]. In vivo, the former is primarily dependent on mean arterial pressure, whereas the latter is related to amplitude of PP and also to heart rate. Therefore, increased PP by itself could be responsible for cardiac and arterial fatigue and subsequent complications such as left ventricular hypertrophy, arterial hypertrophy and dilatation, endothelial damage, and extracellular matrix changes.
(b) Altered ventricular-aortic coupling influences myocardial perfusion by elevating the proportion of coronary flow during the systolic time period [57]. Thus, increased PP and low DBP lead to decreased coronary perfusion, which mainly occurs during the diastolic phase of the cardiac cycle.
(c) PP as an indicator of arterial stiffness: PP is associated with CV risk since it is an indicator of arterial stiffness; therefore, PP is merely an epiphenomenon and not responsible for cardiovascular alterations. This third hypothesis seems to be the main explanation of the relationship between SBP/PP and CV morbidity and mortality. This assumption is based on the fact that the risk related to the PP is mainly observed in the elderly and is due to both high SBP and low DBP [19, 43], reflecting the typical clinical manifestations of arterial aging on the macro- and microcirculation.

The results of epidemiological studies conducted in subjects over 80 years of age also support the view that the association between PP and CV complications is not observed when other than arterial stiffness are the main determinants of PP. In a study involving very elderly institutionalized patients (mean age 87 years.), we found that PP failed to predict cardiovascular mortality. In fact, in this very frail population, low SBP and low PP mainly reflect comorbidities than low arterial stiffness; this explains why in this population aortic PWV, a direct indicator of arterial stiffness, was an independent predictor of cardiovascular mortality [25].

Similar results were also observed in other observational studies in very old, frail patients with absence or even reverse relationships between BP levels and cardiovascular risk [23, 27].

We recently studied this question in the PARTAGE (*P*redictive Values of Blood Pressure and *Art*erial Stiffness in Institutionalized Very *Aged* Population) multicenter study performed in 1,130 frail subjects 80 years or older living in nursing homes [39]. Almost 80 % of the participants were treated for hypertension with a mean 2.2 ± 1.0 drugs, and 63 % of men and 53 % of women treated for hypertension had an SBP <140 mmHg [58]. This contrasts with the much lower frequency (38 % of men, 23 % of women) with SBP <140 mmHg reported for subjects 80 years or older treated for hypertension in a community-living setting [59]. In the PARTAGE study [25], after 2 years, there was a 30 % increase in all-cause mortality in patients ranked in the lowest tertile of SBP (<130 mmHg) compared to the two upper tertiles. These results held after adjusting for several confounders such as age, sex, history of previous cardiovascular disease, index of comorbidity (Charlson), cognitive function (MMSE), and autonomy status (ADL). Thus, a low SBP in very old frail subjects may not simply be a sign of good arterial health. Rather, it might be the expression of malnutrition, heart failure, neurological disorders, and other comorbidities associated with poor prognosis. In fact, at present no study has provided evidence that higher morbidity-mortality rates in elderly patients with very low BP are due to low BP itself or are just a sign of general bad health. It is therefore of particular relevance that participants in the PARTAGE study had several comorbidities and were polymedicated (receiving on average 7.1 different drugs).

Hence, the absence or even the inverse associations between BP levels and CVD risk in the very elderly appears to be linked to several age-related changes as summarized below:

(a) The presence of frequent comorbidities in the very elderly, in particular denutrition, heart failure, and several neurological disorders, reduces BP levels, thereby masking the association between high BP and CVD risk [60].

(b) Exaggeration of BP variability, mainly SBP and PP variability, due to alterations in homeostatic mechanisms. Arterial stiffness, baroreceptor failure, and neurological diseases are responsible for this variability and for the presence of orthostatic or postprandial hypotension [61]. Therefore, SBP and PP recorded during casual measurements may not reflect more permanent SBP and PP levels. Actually, several studies have shown that in the elderly, 24 h ambulatory [62–64] or self-measured [65] BP is a better predictor of cardiovascular risk than clinical BP. Bjorklund et al. [66] showed that PP measured with ABPM has the most powerful prognostic value for cardiovascular morbidity. The Ohasama study [67] also showed that the prediction of stroke was much more precise with self-measurements than with casual clinical measurements, whereas Bobrie et al. [65] have clearly demonstrated in 5,000 treated hypertensive elderly subjects that home measurements but not clinical measurements of BP were able to predict cardiovascular events in these subjects. In the PARTAGE study, we investigated this specific question in the very old institutionalized individuals by comparing the BP levels obtained with standard casual measurements with those recorded following multiple self-measurements. These analyses showed no difference in both BP levels [39] and the predictive value of these BP levels on morbidity and mortality [59]. This result is in contrast with the results observed in community-living more robust elderly persons and shows that the "paradoxical" relationship between BP and events observed in the very old frail subjects cannot be the sole result of BP variability.

(c) Finally, we should mention the relatively frequent overestimation of BP levels in the presence of severe mediacalcosis (pseudohypertension) [68] due to the lack of compressibility of peripheral arteries. However, a recent study has shown that the role of "pseudohypertension" in the elderly has been exaggerated and that what has been perceived as false elevation in brachial BP, as compared with intra-arterial pressure, is the result of discrepancies in office/clinic BP versus home/ambulatory measurements [69]. The authors concluded this interesting analysis on this topic, pointing out that "there are no legitimate elevated BP phenotypes that should be labeled as spurious, artifactual, or as pseudohypertension."

Therefore, we think that the "paradoxical" results observed in old frail individuals are mainly related to the presence of comorbidities and/or conditions that profoundly modify the regulation of blood pressure in these subjects. These data point out the fact that BP measurements are not adequate or even misleading for the evaluation of CVD risk in the very old patients.

Influence of Arterial Aging on the Response to the Antihypertensive Treatment

Beyond this epidemiological evidence, the response to the antihypertensive treatments clearly shows that arterial aging should be taken into account in order to answer a number of questions: *Why is SBP not controlled in the majority of the treated hypertensives? Is there an optimal BP decrease? What is the J-shape curve threshold for DBP, SBP, and PP? Should we be apprehensive of an excessive decrease of the BP in frail patients?*

Failure to Control SBP

It has been suggested that SBP should be under 140 mmHg and that DBP be under 90 mmHg for all treated hypertensive subjects, unless diabetes or target organ damage is present, in which case lower BP levels (<130/85 mmHg) should be targeted [8, 70, 71]. However, this latter statement has been recently questioned by the latest guidelines of the ESC-ESH [2, 72]. Observational studies from several countries have demonstrated that among treated hypertensive individuals, the proportion of those who are well controlled is less than 30 % [73, 74], and a recent survey in the United Kingdom indicated that only 6 % of hypertensive subjects presented BP levels below the limit of 140/90 mmHg [75].

In France, the situation is similar: In a study conducted in a general elderly population (over 60 years of age) in Nancy (Northeast part of France), we found that only 50 % of treated patients were well controlled, i.e., SBP <140 and DBP <90 mmHg [76]. This study showed 2 key results: First, better control rates were observed in women than in men, probably due to a better compliance to the treatment by women. Second, most patients had a well-controlled DBP but still had high SBP levels. Thus, among uncontrolled subjects, 84 % were uncontrolled only for SBP (>140 mmHg) and 14 % for both SBP and DBP (>90 mmHg), while only less than 2 % were controlled for SBP but uncontrolled for DBP. These results are of importance in the prognosis of treated patients, since lack of control of SBP (but not DBP) has been shown to be a major determinant of mortality in treated hypertensives [77].

Several factors can contribute to a poor control of high SBP. Among these, the increasing prevalence of obesity, sedentary life, and high-salt diet can contribute to the resistance to antihypertensive treatment [78]. In addition to these important factors, arterial aging is the main determinant, which could explain current failure in controlling systolic blood pressure. Hence, despite the use of combination therapies, SBP in most patients remains well above the goals determined by international guidelines. However, as we mentioned above, the opposite is observed in very old frail individuals who show much lower BP levels due to the presence of several comorbidities and polymedication [39].

BP Drop with Treatment: The "J-Shape Curve"

Classically, a clinical relevant decrease in BP following antihypertensive treatment signifies a decrease by at least 6–7 mmHg, since this threshold is considered to be associated with a significant decrease in cardiovascular complications [8]. We believe that in order to correctly answer this question, we must follow a different approach: The clinical relevant decrease in BP is the one that results from an improvement in arterial function. In other words, a permanent progressive decrease in DBP and SBP of 10 mmHg in a 50-year-old hypertensive subject with a pretreatment level of 160/100 mmHg can be considered as clinically relevant since it is certainly due to a significant improvement in microcirculation and a decrease in peripheral vascular resistance. On the other hand, the same decrease in DBP but without a decrease in SBP in a 75-year-old diabetic with an initial BP of 175/100 is clearly a bad sign since it reflects the incapacity of the drug to reduce arterial stiffness which is the main determinant of systolic hypertension in this subject. Finally, an abrupt decrease in SBP and DBP from 180/85 to 160/70 in an 80-year-old subject following a combination therapy may be dangerous since it may be an indicator of dehydration and/or a decrease in cardiac output and systolic function due to administered drugs. By contrast, a progressive decrease in SBP by 20 mmHg and DBP by 10 mmHg could be again an indicator of improvement of vascular stiffness and peripheral resistance.

This approach is clearly more complicated than "tell me a number and I'll tell you the risk," but it nonetheless remains the only single possibility to truly answer questions regarding the "J"-shape curve and the clinical relevance and benefits from systolic and/or diastolic BP reduction, especially in the various subgroups of elderly and frail patients.

The "J-curve" describes the relationship between BP and the risk of CV morbidity and mortality. CV risk is high for an elevated BP level and is reduced in parallel with BP reduction until a nadir is reached, below which further BP reduction increases risk [79–81]. Several studies have shown that a J-shape curve exists mainly between DBP and coronary disease especially patients with several CV diseases [79, 80].

Thus, the "J-curve" legitimately brings the motto "the lower, the better" into question and confirms the need for using further diagnostic methods to evaluate arterial hypertension and personalizing the treatment. As mentioned earlier, high PP and isolated systolic hypertension in the elderly are signs of exaggerated vascular aging; thus, these subjects may be considered at high CV risk. Thus, in the presence of large-artery stiffening, antihypertensive treatment can excessively reduce DBP levels and notably protodiastolic pressure, hence contributing to a reduction in coronary flow. Thus, the association between the lowering of BP and the increase in cardiovascular risk recorded in clinical trials most likely results from marked arteriosclerosis and/or a previous unknown coronary artery disease [81].

The question of the J-curve is also of particular interest in the very old subjects. As we mentioned above, the results of the HYVET study [17] showed the beneficial effect of antihypertensive treatment in patients 80 years or older. However, one should always have in mind the design of this study: Actually, this trial was conducted in a highly selected population of fit elderly patients with baseline SBP >160 mmHg and a target SBP <150 mmHg.

Based on these considerations, the 2013 ESC-ESH Guidelines [2] for the management of arterial hypertension stated that "in the elderly, evidence is limited to individuals with initial SBP of >160 mmHg, whose SBP was reduced to values <150 mmHg but not <140 mmHg." Therefore, the recommendation of lowering SBP to <150 mmHg in elderly individuals with SBP >160 mmHg is strongly evidence based. However, at least in elderly individuals 80 years or older, antihypertensive treatment may be considered at SBP >140 mmHg and aimed at values <140 mmHg, if the individuals are fit and treatment is well tolerated [2].

Future Directions

The development in the elderly of several age-related diseases and conditions makes that DBP and even SBP in the very old, may be misleading in the understanding of the underlying arterial state and therefore the evaluation of the cardiovascular risk. As a consequence, no clear recommendation exists regarding target BP in the management of hypertension in very old frail subjects. Moreover, little is known about whether low BP levels (e.g., SBP <130 mmHg) in these individuals in response to therapy increase rather than decrease morbidity and mortality. And then a key question is whether an aggressive lowering of SBP through the use of multiple drugs might be deleterious in very old frail subjects, tipping their delicate balance of survival. Further clinical trials, comparing different therapeutic strategies, will provide critical information to guide physicians how to treat hypertension in these individuals. The knowledge generated by these trials will have major consequences in terms of both individual and public health.

References

1. Tolson D, Morley JE, Rolland Y, Vellas B. Advancing nursing home practice: the International Association of Geriatrics and Gerontology Recommendations. Geriatr Nurs. 2011;32:195–7.
2. Authors/Task Force Members, Mancia G, Fagard R, et al. 2013 ESH/ESC Guidelines for the management of arterial hypertension: the Task Force for the management of arterial hypertension of the European Society of Hypertension (ESH) and of the European Society of Cardiology (ESC). Eur Heart J. 2013;34:2159–219.
3. Alagiakrishnan K, Juby A, Hanley D, Tymchak W, Sclater A. Role of vascular factors in osteoporosis. J Gerontol. 2003;58:362–6.
4. Launer L, Webster Ross G, Petrovitch H, Masaki K, Foley D, White LR, Havlik RJ. Midlife blood pressure and dementia: the Honolulu-Asia aging study. Neurobiol Aging. 2000;21:49–55.
5. Franco OH, Peeters A, Bonneux L, De Laet C. Blood pressure in adulthood and life expectancy with cardiovascular disease in men and women: life course analysis. Hypertension. 2005;46:280–6.
6. Benetos A, Thomas F, Bean KE, Pannier B, Guize L. Role of modifiable risk factors in life expectancy in the elderly. J Hypertens. 2005;23:1803–8.
7. Lewington S, Clarke R, Qizilbash N, Peto R, Collins R, Prospective Studies Collaboration. Age-specific relevance of usual blood pressure to vascular mortality: a meta-analysis of individual data for one million adults in 61 prospective studies. Lancet. 2002;360:1903–13.
8. Chobanian AV, Bakris GL, Black HR, et al. Joint National Committee on Prevention, Detection, Evaluation, and Treatment of High Blood Pressure. National Heart, Lung, and Blood Institute. National High Blood Pressure Education Program Coordinating Committee. Seventh report of the Joint National

Committee on Prevention, Detection, Evaluation, and Treatment of High Blood Pressure. Hypertension. 2003;42:1206–52.
9. Law MR, Morris JK, Wald NJ. Use of blood pressure lowering drugs in the prevention of cardiovascular disease: meta-analysis of 147 randomised trials in the context of expectations from prospective epidemiological studies. BMJ. 2009;338:b1665. doi:10.1136/bmj.b1665.
10. Turnbull F, Neal B, Ninomiya T, Blood Pressure Lowering Treatment Trialists' Collaboration, et al. Effects of different regimens to lower blood pressure on major cardiovascular events in older and younger adults: meta-analysis of randomised trials. BMJ. 2008;336:1121–3.
11. Blood Pressure Lowering Treatment Trialists C, Turnbull F, Neal B, et al. Effects of different regimens to lower blood pressure on major cardiovascular events in older and younger adults: meta-analysis of randomised trials. BMJ. 2008;336:1121–3.
12. Prevention of stroke by antihypertensive drug treatment in older persons with isolated systolic hypertension. Final results of the Systolic Hypertension in the Elderly Program (SHEP). SHEP Cooperative Research Group. JAMA. 1991;265:3255–64.
13. Dahlof B, Lindholm LH, Hansson L, et al. Morbidity and mortality in the Swedish Trial in Old Patients with Hypertension (STOP-Hypertension). Lancet. 1991;338:1281–5.
14. Medical Research Council trial of treatment of hypertension in older adults: principal results. MRC Working Party. BMJ. 1992;304:405–12.
15. Staessen JA, Fagard R, Thijs L, et al. Randomised double-blind comparison of placebo and active treatment for older patients with isolated systolic hypertension. The Systolic Hypertension in Europe (Syst-Eur) Trial Investigators. Lancet. 1997;350:757–64.
16. Liu L, Wang JG, Gong L, et al. Comparison of active treatment and placebo in older Chinese patients with isolated systolic hypertension. Systolic Hypertension in China (Syst-China) Collaborative Group. J Hypertens. 1998;16:1823–9.
17. Beckett NS, Peters R, Fletcher AE, et al. Treatment of hypertension in patients 80 years of age or older. N Engl J Med. 2008;358:1887–98.
18. Benetos A, Zureik M, Morcet J, et al. A decrease in diastolic blood pressure combined with an increase in systolic blood pressure is associated with a higher cardiovascular mortality in men. J Am Coll Cardiol. 2000;35:673–80.
19. Franklin SS, Khan SA, Wong ND, Larson MG, Levy D. Is pulse pressure useful in predicting risk for coronary heart disease ? Circulation. 1999;100:354–60.
20. Khattar RS, Swales JD, Dore C, Senior R, Lahiri A. Effects of aging on the prognostic significance of ambulatory systolic, diastolic and pulse pressure in essential hypertension. Circulation. 2001;104: 783–9.
21. Blacher J, Staessen JA, Girerd X, et al. Pulse pressure not mean pressure determines cardiovascular risk in older hypertensive patients. Arch Intern Med. 2000;160:1085–9.
22. Boshuizen HC, Izaks GJ, van Buuren S, Ligthart GJ. Blood pressure and mortality in elderly people aged 85 and older: community based study. BMJ. 1998;316:1780–4.
23. Satish S, Zhang DD, Goodwin JS. Clinical significance of falling blood pressure among older adults. J Clin Epidemiol. 2001;54:961–7.
24. Meaume S, Benetos A, Henry OF, et al. Aortic pulse wave velocity predicts cardiovascular mortality in subjects >70 years of age. Arterioscler Thromb Vasc Biol. 2001;21:2046–50.
25. Askari M, Kiely DK, Lipsitz LA. Is pulse pressure a predictor of cardiovascular complications in a frail elderly nursing home population? Aging Clin Exp Res. 2004;16:206–11.
26. Oates DJ, Berlowitz DR, Glickman ME, et al. Blood pressure and survival in the oldest old. J Am Geriatr Soc. 2007;55:383–8.
27. Molander L, Lovheim H, Norman T, et al. Lower systolic blood pressure is associated with greater mortality in people aged 85 and older. J Am Geriatr Soc. 2008;56:1853–9.
28. Lagaay AM, van Asperen IA, Hijmans W. The prevalence of morbidity in the oldest old, aged 85 and over: a population-based survey in Leiden, The Netherlands. Arch Gerontol Geriatr. 1992;15:115–31.
29. Rastas S, Pirttila T, Viramo P, et al. Association between blood pressure and survival over 9 years in a general population aged 85 and older. J Am Geriatr Soc. 2006;54:912–8.
30. Ogihara T. Practitioner's trial on the efficacy of antihypertensive treatment in the elderly hypertension (the PATE-hypertension study) in Japan. Am J Hypertens. 2000;13:461–7.
31. Fagard RH, Staessen JA, Thijs L, et al. On-treatment diastolic blood pressure and prognosis in systolic hypertension. Arch Intern Med. 2007;167: 1884–91.
32. Somes GW, Pahor M, Shorr RI, et al. The role of diastolic blood pressure when treating isolated systolic hypertension. Arch Intern Med. 1999;159:2004–9.
33. Perry Jr HM, Davis BR, Price TR, et al. Effect of treating isolated systolic hypertension on the risk of developing various types and subtypes of stroke: the Systolic Hypertension in the Elderly Program (SHEP). JAMA. 2000;284:465–71.
34. Benetos A, Salvi P, Lacolley P. Blood pressure regulation during the aging process: the end of the 'hypertension era'? J Hypertens. 2011;29:646–52.
35. Safar ME, Levy BI, Struijker-Boudier H. Current perspectives on arterial stiffness and pulse pressure in hypertension and cardiovascular disease. Circulation. 2003;107:2864–9.
36. O'Rourke MF, Frolich ED. Pulse pressure: is this a clinically useful risk factor ? Hypertension. 1999;34:372–4.
37. Lakatta E. Arterial and cardiac aging: major shareholders in cardiovascular disease enterprises: part

III: cellular and molecular clues to heart and arterial aging. Circulation. 2003;107:490–7.
38. Benetos A, Adamopoulos C, Bureau JM, et al. Determinants of accelerated progression of arterial stiffness in normotensive subjects and in treated hypertensive subjects over a 6-year period. Circulation. 2002;105:1202–7.
39. Benetos A, Buatois S, Salvi P, et al. Blood pressure and pulse wave velocity values in the institutionalized elderly aged 80 and over: baseline of the PARTAGE Study. J Hypertens. 2010;28:41–50.
40. Ronnback M, Fagerudd J, Forsblom C, Pettersson-Fernholm K, Reunanen A, Groop PH, on behalf of Finnish Diabetic Nephropathy Study Group. Altered age-related blood pressure pattern in type 1 diabetes. Circulation. 2004;110:1076–82.
41. Salomaa V, Riley W, Kark JD, Nardo C, Folsom AR. Non-insulin dependent diabetes mellitus and fasting glucose and insulin concentrations are associated with arterial stiffness indexes. ARIC Study Circulation. 1995;91:1432–43.
42. Schram MT, Kostense PJ, Van Dijk RA, et al. Diabetes, pulse pressure and cardiovascular mortality: the Hoorn Study. J Hypertens. 2002;20:1743–51.
43. Franklin SS, Larson MG, Khan SA, et al. Does the relation of blood pressure to coronary heart disease risk change with aging? Framingham Heart Study Circulation. 2001;103:1245–9.
44. European Society of Hypertension-European Society of Cardiology Guidelines Committee. 2003 European Society of Hypertension–European Society of Cardiology Guidelines Committee. Guidelines for the management of arterial hypertension. J Hypertens. 2003;21:1011–53.
45. Darne B, Girerd X, Safar M, Cambien F, Guize L. Pulsatile versus steady component of blood pressure: a cross-sectional analysis and a prospective analysis on cardiovascular mortality. Hypertension. 1989;13:392–400.
46. Mitchell GF, Moye LA, Braunwald E, et al. for the SAVE Investigators. Sphygmomanometric determined pulse pressure is a powerful independent predictor of recurrent events after myocardial infarction in patients with impaired left ventricular function. Circulation. 1997;96:4254–60.
47. Chae CU, Pfeffer MA, Glynn RJ, Mitchell GF, Taylor JO, Hennekens CH. Increased pulse pressure and risk of heart failure in the elderly. JAMA. 1999;281:634–9.
48. Benetos A, Safar M, Rudnichi A, et al. Pulse pressure, a predictor of long-term cardiovascular mortality. Hypertension. 1997;30:1410–5.
49. Kengne AP, Czernichow S, Huxley R, et al. Blood pressure variables and cardiovascular risk new findings from ADVANCE. Hypertension. 2009;54:399–404.
50. Bangalore S, Messerli FH, Franklin SS, Mancia G, Champion A, Pepine CJ. Pulse pressure and risk of cardiovascular outcomes in patients with hypertension and coronary artery disease: an INternational VErapamil SR-trandolapril Study (INVEST) analysis. Eur Heart J. 2009;30:1395–401.
51. Miura K, Nakagawa H, Ohashi Y, et al. Four blood pressure indexes and the risk of stroke and myocardial infarction in Japanese men and women. A meta-analysis of 16 cohort studies. Circulation. 2009;119:1892–8.
52. Benetos A, Rudnichi A, Safar M, Guize L. Pulse pressure and cardiovascular mortality in normotensive and hypertensive subjects. Hypertension. 1998;32:560–4.
53. de Simone G, Roman MJ, Alderman MH, Galderisi M, de Divitiis O, Devereux RB. Is high pulse pressure a marker of preclinical cardiovascular disease? Hypertension. 2005;45:575–9.
54. Gasowski J, Fagard RH, Staessen JA, et al. INDANA Project Collaborators. Pulsatile blood pressure component as predictor of mortality in hypertension: a meta-analysis of clinical trial control groups. J Hypertens. 2002;20:145–51.
55. Nichols WW, O'Rourke MF. McDonald's blood flow in arteries. Theoretical, experimental and clinical principles. 5th ed. London: Edward Arnold; 2005.
56. Safar ME, Smulyan H. Coronary ischemic disease, arterial stiffness, and pulse pressure. Am J Hypertens. 2004;17:724–6.
57. Kass DA. Ventricular arterial stiffening: integrating the pathophysiology. Hypertension. 2005;46:185–93.
58. Lloyd-Jones DM, Evans JC, Levy D. Hypertension in adults across the age spectrum: current outcomes and control in the community. JAMA. 2005;294:466–72.
59. Benetos A, Gautier S, Labat C, et al. Mortality and cardiovascular events are best predicted by low central/peripheral pulse pressure amplification but not by high blood pressure levels in elderly nursing home subjects: the PARTAGE (Predictive Values of Blood Pressure and Arterial Stiffness in Institutionalized Very Aged Population) study. J Am Coll Cardiol. 2012;60:1503–11.
60. Skoog I, Lernfelt B, Landahl S, et al. 15-year longitudinal study of blood pressure and dementia. Lancet. 1996;347:1141–5.
61. Vanhanen H, Thijs L, Birkenhager W, Bulpitt C, Tilvis R, Sarti C, Tuomilehto J, Staessen JA. Prevalence and persistency of orthostatic blood pressure fall in older patients with isolated systolic hypertension. Syst-Eur Investigators. Hum Hypertens. 1996;10:607–12.
62. Staessen JA, Thijs L, O'Brien ET, et al. Ambulatory pulse pressure as predictor of outcome in older patients with systolic hypertension. Am J Hypertens. 2002;15:835–43.
63. Staessen JA, Thijs L, Fagard R, et al. Predicting cardiovascular risk using conventional vs ambulatory blood pressure in older patients with systolic hypertension. JAMA. 1999;282:539–46.
64. Fagard RH, Staessen JA, Thijs L, et al. Response to antihypertensive therapy in older patients with sustained and nonsustained systolic hypertension. Circulation. 2000;102:1139–44.
65. Bobrie G, Chatellier G, Genes N, Clerson P, Vaur L, Vaisse B, Menard J, Mallion JM. Cardiovascular prognosis of "masked hypertension" detected by

blood pressure self-measurement in elderly treated hypertensive patients. JAMA. 2004;291:1342–9.

66. Björklund K, Lind L, Zethelius B, Berglund L, Lithell H. Prognostic significance of 24-h ambulatory blood pressure characteristics for cardiovascular morbidity in a population of elderly men. J Hypertens. 2004;22:1691–7.
67. Asayama K, Ohkubo T, Kikuya M, Metoki H, Hoshi H, Hashimoto J, Totsune K, Satoh H, Imai Y. Prediction of stroke by self-measurement of blood pressure at home versus casual screening blood pressure measurement in relation to the Joint National Committee 7 classification: the Ohasama study. Stroke. 2004;35:2356–61.
68. Mac Mahon M, Sheahan NF, Colgan MP, Walsh B, Malone J, Coakley D. Arterial closing pressure correlates with diastolic pseudohypertension in the elderly. J Gerontol A Biol Sci Med Sci. 1995;50A:56–8.
69. Franklin SS, Wilkinson IB, McEniery CM. Unusual hypertensive phenotypes: what is their significance? Hypertension. 2012;59:173–8.
70. Clinical practice guidelines: management of adults with essential hypertension- 2005 update – Société française d'hypertension artérielle. Haute Autorité de Santé HAS July 2005. Management of adults with essential hypertension-2005 update-guidelines. J Mal Vasc. 2006;31:16–33.
71. The Task Force for the Management of Arterial Hypertension of the European Society of Hypertension (ESH) and of the European Society of Cardiology (ESC) 2007. Guidelines for the management of arterial hypertension. J Hypertens. 2007;25:1105–87.
72. Mancia G, Laurent S, Agabiti-Rosei E. Reappraisal of European guidelines on hypertension management: a European Society of Hypertension Task Force document. J Hypertens. 2009;27:2121–58.
73. Burt VL, Cutler JA, Higgins M, et al. Trends in the prevalence, awareness, treatment, and control of hypertension in the adult US population: data from the Health Examination Surveys, 1960 to 1991. Hypertension. 1995;26:60–9.
74. Marques-Vidal P, Tuomilehto J. Hypertension awareness, treatment and control in the community: is the "rule of halves" still valid? J Hum Hypertens. 1997;11:213–20.
75. Colhoun HM, Dong W, Poulter NR. Blood pressure screening, management and control in England: results from the health survey for England 1994. J Hypertens. 1998;16:747–52.
76. Perret-Guillaume C, Miget P, Aubry C, Gueguen R, Steyer E, Benetos A. Contrôle de la pression artérielle par le traitement antihypertenseur chez le sujet de plus de 60 ans. Rev Med Interne. 2006;27:285–90.
77. Benetos A, Thomas F, Bean K, Gautier S, Smulyan H, Guize L. Prognostic value of systolic and diastolic pressure in treated hypertensive men. Arch Intern Med. 2002;162:577–81.
78. Chobanian AV. The hypertension paradox – More uncontrolled disease despite improved therapy. N Engl J Med. 2009;361:878–87.
79. Kannel WB, Wilson PWF, Nam BH, D'Agostino RB, Li J. A likely explanation for the J-curve of blood pressure cardiovascular risk. Am J Cardiol. 2004;94:380–4.
80. Messerli FH, Mancia G, Conti CR, et al. Dogma disputed: can aggressively lowering blood pressure in hypertensive patients with coronary artery disease be dangerous? Ann Intern Med. 2006;44:884–93.
81. Messerli FH, Panjrath GS. The J-curve between blood pressure and coronary artery disease or essential hypertension: exactly how essential? J Am Coll Cardiol. 2009;54:1827–34.

Arterial Stiffness and Amplification in the Very Old

31

Athanase Benetos, Ghassan Watfa, Paolo Salvi, and Patrick Lacolley

Abstract

The progressive aging of the population has had a profound impact on the increase in the prevalence and incidence of diseases associated with aging. Arterial aging (as occurs with atherothrombosis, systolic hypertension, heart failure, and vascular dementia) is one of the primary causes of loss of autonomy, morbidity, and mortality in the elderly. Arterial stiffness, expressed as systolic hypertension, is the typical manifestation of arterial aging. In the past, increases in systolic and pulse pressure (PP) were considered part of the aging process and thus did not require therapeutic intervention. However, although arterial stiffening is common, older subjects with increased arterial stiffness have higher cardiovascular morbidity and mortality. It is therefore important to assess arterial stiffness and its consequences in the aging process. Actually, using methods that can analyze the BP curve and/or directly measure arterial elastic properties may represent a very interesting approach to assess the clinical and hemodynamic consequences of the arterial aging.

Keywords

Aging • Arterial stiffness • Aorta • Morbidity • Mortality • Hypertension • Elderly • Cardiovascular • Dementia

A. Benetos, MD, PhD (✉) • G. Watfa, MD, PhD
Department of Geriatrics, University Hospital of Nancy, Universite De Lorraine, 1, allée du Morvan, Vandoeuvre Les Nancy 54500, France

INSERM U1116,
Université de Lorraine, Nancy, France
e-mail: a.benetos@chu-nancy.fr; g.watfa@chu-nancy.fr

P. Salvi, MD, PhD
Department of Cardiology,
IRCCS Istituto Auxologico Italiano,
Via Pellizza da Volpedo41, Milan 20149, Italy
e-mail: psalvio.md@gmail.com

P. Lacolley
Unité INSERM U1116, Université de Lorraine,
Faculté de Médecine, 9 avenue de la foret de Haye,
Vandoeuvre-les-Nancy 54500, France
e-mail: patrick.lacolley@inserm.fr

M.E. Safar et al. (eds.), *Blood Pressure and Arterial Wall Mechanics in Cardiovascular Diseases*,
DOI 10.1007/978-1-4471-5198-2_31, © Springer-Verlag London 2014

Introduction

Aging is accompanied by significant structural changes reflecting a gradual remodeling of the arteries and the heart [1]. This remodeling is characterized by an increase in the size of large arteries and heart cavities as well as a reorganization of the cardiovascular walls: parietal hypertrophy, fragmentation and disruption of arterial elastic fibers, increased collagen content, and nonenzymatic glycation of collagen. These structural alterations lead to an increased stiffness of cardiac and arterial walls. On a functional level, arterial stiffness is responsible for a reduction in distensibility and the amplification of reflected pressure waves from the periphery to the aorta, these two phenomena being responsible for the increase in both systolic blood pressure and pulse pressure [2]. Although arterial stiffening is a common situation, it is now confirmed that older subjects with increased arterial stiffness and elevated systolic and pulse pressure have higher cardiovascular morbidity and mortality [3]. Moreover, we have now solid evidence for the beneficial effects of the treatment of systolic hypertension in the elderly [3] and very recently even in the very elderly, i.e., in subjects over 80 years old [4]. Age-related cardiac dysfunction is dependent on not only intrinsic structural and dynamic changes of the myocardial tissue but also the aforementioned arterial changes responsible for heart-artery mismatching and an increase in cardiac afterload. Hence, large-artery stiffness, notably of the aorta, leads to left ventricular hypertrophy and impaired coronary perfusion. Cardiac fibrosis causes a defect in diastolic expansion of the ventricular walls but also an increase in the risk of arrhythmia. The other consequence of large-artery stiffness is the dysregulation of local tissue efflux, such as in the brain. Arterial stiffness and cardiac fibrosis are both considered to be factors leading to ineffective heart-vessel coupling and thereby increasing cardiovascular risk [5]. These changes are responsible for several cardiovascular diseases in which prevalence dramatically increases with age: heart failure, ischemic disease, and arrhythmias. In addition, age-related arterial changes play an important role in the development of vascular dementia and eventually in degenerative dementias of the Alzheimer's type, even though the relationship between arterial aging and Alzheimer's disease is still poorly understood [6].

Methodological Approaches in Understanding the Effects of Aging on the Arteries: Focus to the Pulse Wave Analysis

Frederick Akbar Mahomed [7, 8], a half-Indian half-British physiologist who lived in Great Britain during the nineteenth century, developed the concept and techniques of pulse waveform analysis. Unfortunately, this approach has been largely ignored for at least two reasons: firstly because Frederick Akbar Mahomed died in 1884 at the very early age of 32 years and secondly, because a few years later, Riva Rocci [9, 10] and Korotkoff [11] introduced the cuff sphygmomanometer, a device much easier to use, although unequivocally yielding less information with regard to arterial function. Over recent years, pulse waveform analyses have experienced somewhat of a revival. Using accurate tonometric recordings at different arterial sites (radial, carotid), analysis of pressure waves by various algorithms [12] is able to estimate ascending aortic waveform. These waveforms are able to provide not only quantitative information regarding central BP levels but also qualitative data relative to the waveforms themselves, thereby enabling to define the elastic properties of the arterial wall as well as the importance and the timing of reflection waves [12, 13]. This analysis is thought to provide a better insight into cardiovascular physiology and disease than brachial blood pressure measured with conventional cuff sphygmomanometers [14, 15].

Moreover, the use of noninvasive tonometry-based devices to record and analyze arterial waveforms [16, 17] now allows to easily obtain pulse waveforms in several arterial segments. These validated noninvasive techniques, used by several research teams, are able to quantify the amplification of pressure by reflected waves and represent a reliable marker of overall arterial health. Several devices allowing to measure the arterial pressure curve through analysis software are currently available [18, 19]. These devices use similar algorithms for the analysis of the pulse waveforms and can provide very significant information about the aging of the arterial system [20].

We develop here the three main analyses of the pulse waveforms used for the evaluation of the arterial aging:

- *Wave reflections and augmentation index (AIx)*
- *Central pulse pressure and central/peripheral pulse pressure amplification (PPA)*
- *Direct arterial stiffness assessment by measuring pulse wave velocity (PWV)*

Pressure Wave Reflections and Augmentation Index (AIx)

At a given location of the arterial bed, the amplitude of the pressure wave corresponds to the difference between systolic peak and the end of the diastolic phase. BP amplification is defined by the elevation of PP from the central aorta toward the periphery and is mainly attributed to the elevation of SBP [12–14, 16, 21]. Pressure wave amplification can be explained by the reflection phenomena of the pulsatile BP wave. Propagation of the BP wave is achieved from the heart to the periphery at a celerity corresponding to the PWV. Depending on the PWV and the distance covered, the reflected wave generated at the periphery will add to the forward BP wave, at a more or less earlier time frame during the cardiac cycle. In the presence of a low PWV, the arrival of the reflected waves at the central arteries will occur later during the diastolic period and therefore will not contribute to increasing systolic and pulse pressure. By contrast in presence of increased aortic PWV and/or arterial lesions inducing proximal (early) reflection sites, retrograde (reflected) waves will arrive earlier, i.e., during the systolic period and therefore will contribute to increasing systolic and pulse pressure. These reflected waves can thus be identified and analyzed when central blood pressure waves are recorded (Fig. 31.1). We can therefore distinguish the initial anterograde systolic wave and the added reflection wave called also augmentation pressure (AuP). The ratio of AuP/PP is called augmentation index (AIx) and represents the % of the reflection waves in the total PP amplitude [13, 16, 22]. AIx increases with age and is higher in women than in men. Several factors codetermine this factor, and although it should theoretically be correlated with the magnitude of the reflected wave, the Asklepios Study has shown that the relationship between wave reflection and AIx is relatively modest, with a correlation coefficient <0.6. Furthermore, the clinical significance of AIx and its relationship with CVD remains controversial, especially in the elderly [21].

Central Blood Pressure and Pulse Pressure Amplification (PPA)

Blood pressure amplification is a phenomenon that is quite stunning for its ingenuity. Merely the fact that, in a mechanical, hydraulic system such as the cardiovascular system, pressure at the periphery is higher than in the center is in itself surprising. Generally, the objective of mechanical devices is to reduce at a minimum the loss of energy when traveling toward the periphery of the system; in the cardiovascular system, by contrast, peripheral BP is actually higher than central BP in the aorta, near the heart pump. One must keep in mind that the heart pump is required in both a permanent and uninterrupted fashion over a very long time, sometimes over a span of 100 years; consequently, the cardiovascular system must therefore implement all of the processes capable of reducing the workload of the heart. Since the aim of cardiovascular system is to distribute oxygen and nutritional elements to organs and peripheral tissues, it is therefore necessary to reduce as much as possible both heart work and peripheral perfusion rate; which is why the ultimate goal is to achieve optimal peripheral perfusion with lowest cardiac effort. The amplification phenomenon also fits in this physiological scheme: the higher the BP amplification, the lower the central BP

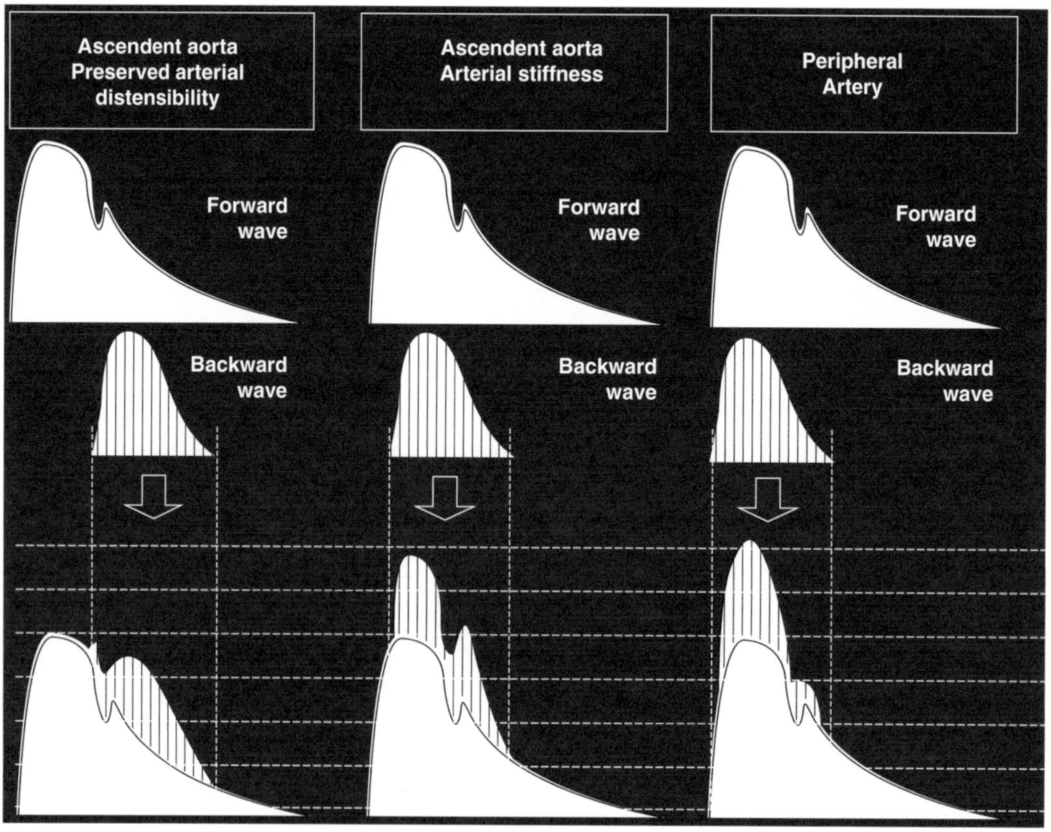

Fig. 31.1 Pulse waveform is determined by interaction between forward wave and backward waves. In the peripheral artery, this interaction occurs earlier due to the close proximity with the reflected sites (*right panel*). In the ascending aorta, in the presence of preserved arterial distensibility (low stiffness), the overlapping between forward and backward waves is prevalently during diastolic phase (*left panel*), and systolic peak is determined only by forward wave. On the contrary, in a situation characterized by high arterial stiffness, the overlapping between forward and backward waves is prevalently during proto-meso-systolic phase (*middle panel*). Thus in the presence of high arterial stiffness, central and peripheral waveforms are similar and the amplification between central and peripheral arteries is very low

and the lower the afterload and hence heart work. BP amplification is in inverse relation to PWV; the faster the return of the reflected wave in the aorta, the earlier the overlapping with the forward wave and thus the lower the difference between peripheral and central BP.

Although the velocity of the transmission of the pulse wave is the main determinant of the early arrival of the reflected waves, other factors such as peripheral artery resistance, arterial tree length, and heart rate are all involved in the magnitude of the amplification.

An important phenomenon that reduces heart work/peripheral perfusion rate is heart rate regulation [13, 14]. It is well known that a lower heart rate reduces heart work, although on the other hand it is also well known that a lower heart rate goes together with lower BP amplification. Thus, the effects of lower heart rate on heart work are both positive (reduction in the number of systolic contractions) and negative (reduction of BP amplification). It is thus necessary to consider both BP amplification and heart rate in the same general context when assessing total heart work.

Clinical Interest of Measuring Central BP and BP Amplification

Theoretically, the assessment of PP amplification requires simultaneous invasive measurements of peripheral and central BP. In clinical practice, however, two methods have been described to estimate central BP: (i) a radial-to-aorta mathematical transformation and (ii) systolic BP in the common carotid artery as a surrogate for the pressure in the ascending aorta. The first method requires measurement of the radial pulse wave by applanation tonometry and its calibration by diastolic and mean BP or diastolic and SBP. The application of the generalized transfer function has been validated to generate central aortic waveforms from the radial pressure wave. The second method uses applanation tonometry to directly record the carotid pulse wave; in this case, calibration is obtained from mean and diastolic BP at the brachial artery. Moreover, it is not necessary to use a generalized transfer function.

The PP amplification (PPA) may be expressed as either brachial minus central PP (mmHg) or as a percent increase: PPA (%) = 100 * (peripheral PP − central PP)/central PP. The Anglo-Cardiff Collaborative Trial has shown that the ratio of brachial/aortic PP varies from 1.7 at less than 20 years of age (meaning that peripheral brachial PP is 70 % higher than central aortic PP) to 1.2 at over 80 years of age (i.e., brachial > aortic PP by only 20 %). When expressed as the absolute change in mmHg, the difference between brachial and central PP varies from 20 to 7 mmHg [12].

The disappearance of aortic-brachial PP amplification, together with an increase in central PP and in PWV, was shown to be significant predictors of all-cause mortality in end-stage renal disease patients undergoing hemodialysis [23]. In addition, the predictive power of PP amplification was superior to peripheral and carotid PP. Recently, our research group has shown that PP amplification rate was strongly associated with both cardiovascular and overall mortality risks, with a hazard ratio of 1.22 (1.12–1.32) and 1.41 (1.14–1.73), respectively [24]. Thus, an increase of 1 SD in PP amplification was associated with a 19 % increase of all-cause mortality and a 30 % increase in cardiovascular mortality. All of these results were independent of any other confounding factors, including pulse rate and drug treatment. The PARTAGE longitudinal analysis in elderly institutionalized frail subjects showed that an increase of 10 % of PPA (corresponding approximately to 1SD) was associated with a decrease of 24 and 17 % of total mortality and major CV events, respectively [25]. Of note, the association between PPA and the endpoints was markedly significant after adjusting for several confounders, including history of CV disease.

These results show that low PPA from central to peripheral arteries strongly predicts mortality and CV adverse effects in middle-aged but also in very old subjects. Assessment of this parameter could help in risk estimation and improve diagnostic and therapeutic strategies in very old, frail, and polymedicated persons.

Some pharmacological clinical studies have shown that the different classes of antihypertensive drugs could have differing effects on central PP despite similar actions on peripheral PP, therefore impacting on amplification [26–28]. These studies suggest that ACEI and/or CCB have more pronounced effects on arterial elastic properties and peripheral resistance than beta blockade with atenolol. However, a major contribution of heart rate in these results cannot be excluded. Indeed, since a lower heart rate leads to a decrease in amplification, the effects observed with the beta blocker atenolol could be explained by the effects of this drug on heart rate [27].

Arterial Stiffness Measured by PWV

Measurement of Pulse Wave Velocity

PWV is the speed with which the pulse wave spreads across an arterial segment [13, 29, 30]. In order to measure this velocity, it is important to record the pressure waves (or blood velocity waves) on two arterial segments and know the distance that separates these two segments. This parameter is inversely proportional to the square root of distensibility of the arteries. The principle of PWV and its relationships with arterial elastic properties was initially described in the nineteenth century [29, 31].

Today, measurement of PWV is based on a noninvasive technique that is both reproducible and easy to achieve. Carotid-femoral PWV is measured using two mechanical sensors: one is placed at the root of the right common carotid artery and the other at the level of the right primitive femoral artery. Both pressure waves are recorded simultaneously, by transcutaneous ultrasonic measurement. PVW is calculated as the time between the onset (foot) of the two pressure waves divided by the distance between both measurement points and based on analysis of ten cardiac cycles. Acquisition and calculation of the PWV are achieved using various dedicated softwares. The Complior system [26, 30] is currently the most widely used device, although other devices are capable of measuring PWV including the SphygmoCor [18] and PulsePen [23, 32, 33] tonometers, already used for analysis of wave reflections. At the present time, PWV is considered to be the most reliable method for measuring arterial stiffness and cardiovascular risk [34].

Interestingly, the observed increase in PWV with age is not linear, being more pronounced after the age of 55–60 [35]. Hence, the annual increase in PWV before the age of 50 is approximately 100 mm/s (i.e., an annual increase of about 1 %) and rises to an annual increase of more than 150 mm/s after the age of 60. Aside from age, several other hemodynamic and biological parameters can accelerate the annual increase in PWV [36, 37]. This age-related increase pertains essentially to aortic PWV, conventionally measured between the carotid and femoral arteries, and much less to PWV measured in peripheral arteries, particularly of the upper and lower limbs [38].

PWV and Cardiovascular Morbidity-Mortality

Over the past few years, PWV has been shown to be a more powerful cardiovascular risk factor than mean arterial pressure, SBP, or PP values [39]. This relationship has been demonstrated not only in the general population but also in subgroups of patients, especially among hypertensive [40, 41] and diabetic patients, coronary patients [42, 43], very old subjects [44], and hemodialysis patients [45–47]. Pulse wave velocity is also considered as a marker of early atherosclerosis [48]. Risk assessment by use of the Framingham equations has indeed allowed to demonstrate that this cardiovascular risk was linearly correlated with the sole measurement of PWV [49]. This is due to the fact that the effects of age are more pronounced on the extracellular matrix, which is abundant in central arteries, and much less in smooth muscle cells, which are more abundant in peripheral arteries. All of the above data have led to the recognition of PWV as an independent factor of cardiovascular risk [40]. The recommendations of the European Societies of Hypertension (ESH) and of Cardiology (ESC) in 2007 [20] recognized for the first time the independent role of PWV in the risk of cardiovascular morbidity and mortality and set the foundations for the clinical use of this parameter for predicting cardiovascular risk in hypertensive patients and ultimately in other patients presenting risk factors. These guidelines have hence proposed that a PWV >12 m/s should be regarded as an abnormally high value and thus associated with increased cardiovascular risk. A large clinical consortium established reference PWV values according to age, gender, and presence of cardiovascular risk factors in various populations [50]. In addition other studies assessed values of PWV in children [51], elderly (>65 years) (85), and very old (>80 years) frail individuals (20). However, PWV values still remain quite variable according to the method used and will therefore require further investigations to clearly define normal threshold values.

PWV and Risk of Dementia and Cognitive Decline

Epidemiological and clinical data have highlighted a link between the vascular component and AD [52]. The involvement of arterial stiffness has been evoked in cognitive impairment, VaD and AD. Previous cross-sectional studies addressing the issue of the relationship between arterial stiffness and cognitive function in a population of elderly subjects reporting memory loss have indicated a significant association between high pulse wave velocity (PWV) values and alterations in cognitive function [53–55].

In a longitudinal study, Scuteri et al. showed that AS, as measured by carotid-femoral PWV (cf PWV), is an independent predictor of longitudinal changes in cognitive function in elderly patients [56]. In a larger cohort of 582 middle-aged patients (54.3 years), PWV was associated with a cognitive decline over a follow-up period of 11 years [57]. However, this association was not found in the Rotterdam study with follow-up of 5 years in 2,767 subjects with mean age of 70.7 ± 6 years [58]. To date, nearly all of the investigative studies have primarily targeted middle-aged and elderly populations, whereas none are currently designed to examine whether arterial stiffness was independently associated with cognitive decline in an institutionalized population over the age of 80 years.

The PARTAGE study showed in a large population of subjects aged 80 and over living in nursing homes that cognitive decline over a period of 1 year [38] was more pronounced in individuals with higher PWV at the beginning of the study. Cognitive decline was assessed by MMSE, and this association with the PWV was beyond the prediction provided by age, education level, blood pressure, and functional status as evaluated by ADL. Interestingly, BP did not show such association with cognitive decline in this population [59].

Arterial stiffness has been shown to be associated with a number of other age-related disorders and diseases indicating that arterial stiffness in the elderly may be a risk factor for developing frailty. Thus, the group of Kohara [60] reported in elderly men that thigh muscle volume as an index for sarcopenia was negatively associated with PWV in men, independently of age and blood pressure. They also observed that the thigh muscle CSA and visceral fat area were significantly and independently associated with arterial stiffness [61].

Some but not all studies also observed associations with others indicating some associations between arterial stiffness and other age-related common alterations and diseases such as osteoporosis [62–64] and risk of falls [65]. Therefore, there is increasing evidence that arterial aging can influence the aging process and contribute to the development of age-related diseases, frailty, and loss of autonomy in the elderly population.

Conclusions

Noninvasive arterial measurements including analysis of central and peripheral arterial waveforms and assessment of PWV can be reliable and easily performed measurements in order to assess arterial aging. For these measurements, there are currently sufficient clinical data showing their association with cardiovascular diseases as well as several other age-related degenerative diseases. There is also the emergence of reference values and beneficial elements of regression by treatment.

References

1. Lakatta EG. Arterial and cardiac aging: major shareholders in cardiovascular disease enterprises: part III: cellular and molecular clues to heart and arterial aging. Circulation. 2003;107:490–7.
2. Safar ME, Smulyan H. Coronary ischemic disease, arterial stiffness, and pulse pressure. Am J Hypertens. 2004;17:724–6.
3. Mancia G, Laurent S, Agabiti-Rosei E, et al. Reappraisal of European guidelines on hypertension management: a European Society of Hypertension Task Force document. J Hypertens. 2009;27:2121–58.
4. Beckett NS, Peters R, Fletcher AE, et al. Treatment of hypertension in patients 80 years of age or older. N Engl J Med. 2008;358:1887–98.
5. Nichols W, O'Rourke MF, McDonald DA. McDonald's blood flow in arteries; theoretical, experimental and principles. 3rd ed. London/Melbourne/Auckland: Arnold E; 1990. p. 77–142, 216–69, 283–89, 398–437.
6. Forette F, Seux ML, Staessen JA, et al. The prevention of dementia with antihypertensive treatment: new evidence from the Systolic Hypertension in Europe (Syst-Eur) study. Arch Intern Med. 2002;162:2046–52.
7. O'Rourke MF. Frederick Akbar Mahomed. Hypertension. 1992;19:212–7.
8. Mahomed F. The physiology and clinical use of the sphygmograph. Med Times Gazette. 1872;62.
9. Riva-Rocci S. Un nuovo sfigmomanometro. Gazzetta Medica di Torino. 1896;50:981–96.
10. Riva-Rocci S. La tecnica della sfigmomanometria. Gazzetta Medica di Torino. 1897;10:181–91.
11. Korotkoff N. On methods of studying blood pressure. St. Petersburg: Bull Imperial Acad Med; 1906. p. 365–7.
12. McEniery CM, Yasmin, Hall IR, et al. Normal vascular aging: differential effects on wave reflection and aortic pulse wave velocity: the Anglo-Cardiff Collaborative Trial (ACCT). J Am Coll Cardiol. 2005;46:1753–60.
13. Nichols WW, O'Rourke MF, McDonald DA. McDonald's blood flow in arteries. Theoretical,

experimental and clinical principles. 5th ed. London: Edward Arnold; 2005.
14. O'Rourke MF, Seward JB. Central arterial pressure and arterial pressure pulse: new views entering the second century after Korotkov. Mayo Clin Proc. 2006;81:1057–68.
15. Benetos A, Salvi P, Lacolley P. Blood pressure regulation during the aging process: the end of the 'hypertension era'? J Hypertens. 2011;29:646–52.
16. Avolio AP, Van Bortel LM, Boutouyrie P, et al. Role of pulse pressure amplification in arterial hypertension: experts' opinion and review of the data. Hypertension. 2009;54:375–83.
17. O'Rourke MF, Gallagher DE. Pulse wave analysis. J Hypertens Suppl. 1996;14:S147–57.
18. Pauca AL, O'Rourke MF, Kon ND. Prospective evaluation of a method for estimating ascending aortic pressure from the radial artery pressure waveform. Hypertension. 2001;38:932–7.
19. Salvi P, Lio G, Labat C, et al. Validation of a new noninvasive portable tonometer for determining arterial pressure wave and pulse wave velocity: the PulsePen device. J Hypertens. 2004;22:2285–93.
20. Mancia G, De Backer G, Dominiczak A, et al. 2007 guidelines for the management of arterial hypertension: the task force for the management of arterial hypertension of the European society of hypertension (ESH) and of the European society of cardiology (ESC). J Hypertens. 2007;25:1105–87.
21. Segers P, Rietzschel ER, De Buyzere ML, et al. Noninvasive (input) impedance, pulse wave velocity, and wave reflection in healthy middle-aged men and women. Hypertension. 2007;49:1248–55.
22. Namasivayam M, McDonnell BJ, McEniery CM, et al. Does wave reflection dominate age-related change in aortic blood pressure across the human life span? Hypertension. 2009;53:979–85.
23. Safar ME, Blacher J, Pannier B, et al. Central pulse pressure and mortality in end-stage renal disease. Hypertension. 2002;39:735–8.
24. Benetos A, Thomas F, Joly L, et al. Pulse pressure amplification a mechanical biomarker of cardiovascular risk. J Am Coll Cardiol. 2010;55:1032–7.
25. Benetos A, Gautier S, Labat C, et al. Mortality and cardiovascular events are best predicted by low central/peripheral pulse pressure amplification but not by high blood pressure levels in elderly nursing home subjects: the PARTAGE (Predictive Values of Blood Pressure and Arterial Stiffness in Institutionalized Very Aged Population) study. J Am Coll Cardiol. 2012;60:1503–11.
26. Asmar RG, London GM, O'Rourke ME, et al. Improvement in blood pressure, arterial stiffness and wave reflections with a very-low-dose perindopril/indapamide combination in hypertensive patient: a comparison with atenolol. Hypertension. 2001;38:922–6.
27. London GM, Asmar RG, O'Rourke MF, et al. Mechanism(s) of selective systolic blood pressure reduction after a low-dose combination of perindopril/indapamide in hypertensive subjects: comparison with atenolol. J Am Coll Cardiol. 2004;43:92–9.
28. Williams B, Lacy PS, Thom SM, et al. Differential impact of blood pressure-lowering drugs on central aortic pressure and clinical outcomes: principal results of the Conduit Artery Function Evaluation (CAFE) study. Circulation. 2006;113:1213–25.
29. Young T. On the functions of heart and arteries (The Croonian Lecture). Phil Trans. 1809;99.
30. Asmar R, Benetos A, Topouchian J, et al. Assessment of arterial distensibility by automatic pulse wave velocity measurement. Validation and clinical application studies. Hypertension. 1995;26:485–90.
31. Bramwell J, Hill AV. Velocity of transmission of the pulse wave. Lancet. 1922;6:891–2.
32. Alecu C, Labat C, Kearney-Schwartz A, et al. Reference values of aortic pulse wave velocity in the elderly. J Hypertens. 2008;26:2207–12.
33. Joly L, Perret-Guillaume C, Kearney-Schwartz A, et al. Pulse wave velocity assessment by external noninvasive devices and phase-contrast magnetic resonance imaging in the obese. Hypertension. 2009;54:421–6.
34. Laurent S, Cockcroft J, Van Bortel L, et al. Expert consensus document on arterial stiffness: methodological issues and clinical applications. Eur Heart J. 2006;27:2588–605.
35. Benetos A, Adamopoulos C, Bureau JM, et al. Determinants of accelerated progression of arterial stiffness in normotensive subjects and in treated hypertensive subjects over a 6-year period. Circulation. 2002;105:1202–7.
36. Safar ME, Thomas F, Blacher J, et al. Metabolic syndrome and age-related progression of aortic stiffness. J Am Coll Cardiol. 2006;47:72–5.
37. Henry RM, Kostense PJ, Spijkerman AM, et al. Arterial stiffness increases with deteriorating glucose tolerance status: the Hoorn Study. Circulation. 2003;107:2089–95.
38. Benetos A, Buatois S, Salvi P, et al. Blood pressure and pulse wave velocity values in the institutionalized elderly aged 80 and over: baseline of the PARTAGE study. J Hypertens. 2010;28:41–50.
39. Willum-Hansen T, Staessen JA, Torp-Pedersen C, et al. Prognostic value of aortic pulse wave velocity as index of arterial stiffness in the general population. Circulation. 2006;113:664–70.
40. Laurent S, Boutouyrie P, Asmar R, et al. Aortic stiffness is an independent predictor of all-cause and cardiovascular mortality in hypertensive patients. Hypertension. 2001;37:1236–41.
41. Laurent S, Katsahian S, Fassot C, et al. Aortic stiffness is an independent predictor of fatal stroke in essential hypertension. Stroke. 2003;34:1203–6.
42. Boutouyrie P, Tropeano AI, Asmar R, et al. Aortic stiffness is an independent predictor of primary coronary events in hypertensive patients: a longitudinal study. Hypertension. 2002;39:10–5.
43. Mattace-Raso FU, van der Cammen TJ, Hofman A, et al. Arterial stiffness and risk of coronary heart dis-

ease and stroke: the Rotterdam Study. Circulation. 2006;113:657–63.
44. Meaume S, Benetos A, Henry OF, et al. Aortic pulse wave velocity predicts cardiovascular mortality in subjects >70 years of age. Arterioscler Thromb Vasc Biol. 2001;21:2046–50.
45. Blacher J, Guerin AP, Pannier B, et al. Impact of aortic stiffness on survival in end-stage renal disease. Circulation. 1999;99:2434–9.
46. Pannier B, Guerin AP, Marchais SJ, et al. Stiffness of capacitive and conduit arteries: prognostic significance for end-stage renal disease patients. Hypertension. 2005;45:592–6.
47. Shoji T, Emoto M, Shinohara K, et al. Diabetes mellitus, aortic stiffness, and cardiovascular mortality in end-stage renal disease. J Am Soc Nephrol. 2001;12:2117–24.
48. Oliver JJ, Webb DJ. Noninvasive assessment of arterial stiffness and risk of atherosclerotic events. Arterioscler Thromb Vasc Biol. 2003;23:554–66.
49. Blacher J, Asmar R, Djane S, et al. Aortic pulse wave velocity as a marker of cardiovascular risk in hypertensive patients. Hypertension. 1999;33:1111–7.
50. Reference Values for Arterial Stiffness' Collaboration. Determinants of pulse wave velocity in healthy people and in the presence of cardiovascular risk factors: 'establishing normal and reference values'. Eur Heart J. 2010;31:2338–50.
51. Reusz GS, Cseprekal O, Temmar M, et al. Reference values of pulse wave velocity in healthy children and teenagers. Hypertension. 2010;56:217–24.
52. Casserly I, Topol E. Convergence of atherosclerosis and Alzheimer's disease: inflammation, cholesterol, and misfolded proteins. Lancet. 2004;363:1139–46.
53. Hanon O, Haulon S, Lenoir H, et al. Relationship between arterial stiffness and cognitive function in elderly subjects with complaints of memory loss. Stroke. 2005;36:2193–7.
54. Kearney-Schwartz A, Rossignol P, Bracard S, et al. Vascular structure and function is correlated to cognitive performance and white matter hyperintensities in older hypertensive patients with subjective memory complaints. Stroke. 2009;40:1229–36.
55. Scuteri A, Brancati AM, Gianni W, et al. Arterial stiffness is an independent risk factor for cognitive impairment in the elderly: a pilot study. J Hypertens. 2005;23:1211–6.
56. Scuteri A, Tesauro M, Appolloni S, et al. Arterial stiffness as an independent predictor of longitudinal changes in cognitive function in the older individual. J Hypertens. 2007;25:1035–40.
57. Waldstein SR, Rice SC, Thayer JF, et al. Pulse pressure and pulse wave velocity are related to cognitive decline in the Baltimore Longitudinal Study of Aging. Hypertension. 2008;51:99–104.
58. Poels MM, van Oijen M, Mattace-Raso FU, et al. Arterial stiffness, cognitive decline, and risk of dementia: the Rotterdam study. Stroke. 2007;38:888–92.
59. Benetos A, Watfa G, Hanon O, et al. Pulse wave velocity is associated with 1-year cognitive decline in the elderly older than 80 years: the PARTAGE study. J Am Med Dir Assoc. 2012;13:239–43.
60. Ochi M, Kohara K, Tabara Y, et al. Arterial stiffness is associated with low thigh muscle mass in middle-aged to elderly men. Atherosclerosis. 2010;212:327–32.
61. Kohara K, Ochi M, Tabara Y, et al. Arterial stiffness in sarcopenic visceral obesity in the elderly: J-SHIPP study. Int J Cardiol. 2012;158:146–8.
62. Seo SK, Cho S, Kim HY, et al. Bone mineral density, arterial stiffness, and coronary atherosclerosis in healthy postmenopausal women. Menopause. 2009;16:937–43.
63. Mangiafico RA, Alagona C, Pennisi P, et al. Increased augmentation index and central aortic blood pressure in osteoporotic postmenopausal women. Osteoporos Int. 2008;19:49–56.
64. Benetos A, Zervoudaki A, Kearney-Schwartz A, et al. Effects of lean and fat mass on bone mineral density and arterial stiffness in elderly men. Osteoporos Int. 2009;20:1385–91.
65. Boddaert J, Tamim H, Verny M, et al. Arterial stiffness is associated with orthostatic hypotension in elderly subjects with history of falls. J Am Geriatr Soc. 2004;52:568–72.

Hypertension in Men and Women: Is It Different?

32

Harold Smulyan and Bruno Pannier

Abstract

This chapter summarizes the extensive and complex literature that describes the many differences in hypertension between men and women. These differences fall into two main groups – physical and hormonal where the menopausal changes with aging in women account for many of the variations. Surprisingly, these many differences have not translated into different guideline recommendations between the sexes for antihypertensive therapy. The last section of the chapter deals with those forms of hypertension that occur only in women, largely related to oral contraceptives and pregnancy.

Keywords

Hypertension • Gender differences • Menopause • Hormonal changes • Estrogen • Antihypertensive therapy • Pre-eclampsia • Oral contraceptives

Introduction

In clinical practice, essential hypertension (HTN) is usually considered as a single disease, independent of gender. But clinical differences in hypertension between men and women were noted as long ago as 1913 by Janeway [1] and repeated by Pickering in 1955 [2]. Hemodynamic differences were described in 1987 by Messerli, who reported a lower systemic vascular resistance (SVR) index and higher cardiac index in young hypertensive women compared to men at the same blood pressure (BP) [3]. The effect of menopause became apparent when this difference in SVR index disappeared over the age of 45. Since that time, evidence has mounted, making it difficult to believe that HTN is the same between the sexes. Some of these gender differences are constant throughout life. But the field is complicated by differences that do change – by aging in men and by both menopause and aging in women. The purpose of this chapter is first, to describe the differences

H. Smulyan, MD (✉)
Cardiology Division, Department of Medicine, Upstate Medical University, 90 Presidential Plaza, Syracuse, NY 13208, USA
e-mail: smulyanh@upstate.edu

B. Pannier, MD
Service de Medecine Interne-Cardiologie, Centre Hospitalier F.H.Manhes, 8 rue Roger Clavier, Fleury Merogis 91700, France
e-mail: brpannier@gmail.com

M.E. Safar et al. (eds.), *Blood Pressure and Arterial Wall Mechanics in Cardiovascular Diseases*, DOI 10.1007/978-1-4471-5198-2_32, © Springer-Verlag London 2014

between the sexes in BP levels and the changing differences in the prevalence of HTN with aging. Then, the multiple and complex mechanisms for these differences will be addressed and related to the effects of aging in men and the interrelated and simultaneous effects of aging and menopause in women. Finally, we describe those forms of HTN that occur in women only.

Gender Differences in Prevalence, Severity and Control

HTN is a common disease. When defined as a systolic BP (SBP) ≥140 mmHg, or a diastolic BP (DBP) ≥90 mmHg, or taking antihypertensive medication, or having been told at least twice by a physician or other health professional that one has HTN, then it is estimated that 1 in 3 adults in the USA have HTN [4]. The 30–45 % estimated prevalence of HTN in Europe is about the same [5]. The overall prevalence of HTN is nearly equal between men and women but under age 45 more men than women are hypertensive. From 45 to 64 years, the percentage of men and women with HTN are similar. However, above age 65 the prevalence is reversed with a higher percentage of hypertensive women than men [4] (Fig. 32.1b). A similar trend is observed for hypertensive control (Fig. 32.1a). One possible explanation is the decreased survival of elderly hypertensive men when compared to women. Another issue is whether menopause alone increases the BP, independent of age. This has been controversial [6], but the weight of evidence from longitudinal, rather than cross sectional studies, supports the independent effect of menopause on BP [7]. There are multiple possible reasons for this effect that will be discussed below.

Even HTN control rates differ between men and women. Data from the Framingham Heart Study of the National Heart Lung and Blood Institute has shown that control of HTN in both men and women was approximately 38 % under the age of 60 [8]. However, control rates for women from 60 to 79 and ≥80 years were only 28 and 23 % respectively, despite treatment rates that were ≈ 64 % across all age groups for both sexes (Fig. 32.1a). There are various explanations for this discrepancy, but none are completely satisfactory. Elderly women may be less aggressively treated, treated with different drug combinations or the increasing obesity of aging in women may play a role. But the most plausible mechanisms lie in the hormonal changes of the menopause that affect the circulation and lead to hypertension in the older female. To this end, it has been well established that in all comers of both sexes, SBP rises steadily with age, while DBP rises until ages 50–55 after which it falls [9]. But when the sexes are analyzed separately, the SBP is lower in women under age 40, but rises more rapidly with aging so that over age 55, the SBP is the same. By contrast, the DBP remains lower in women at all ages. As a result, the pulse pressure (PP), lower in younger women, becomes higher than the PP in men at older ages [10]. This is of considerable importance since a raised PP is more significant than BP alone as a risk factor for cardiovascular disease [11] and helps explain the sharply increasing risk of CV disease among older women.

Fixed Gender Differences

The unchanging gender differences that affect the circulation in hypertension are non-hormonal and largely physical in nature. At all ages, most women are shorter and have a smaller body size than most men. Their smaller body size dictates a lower cardiac output and their shorter stature a faster heart rate. Other things being equal, these two factors result in a smaller stroke volume and a lower SVR at the same BP when women are compared to men. Smaller bodies also have smaller arterial diameters and, at the same BP, females' arterial compliance is lower than those of males.

Shorter stature in women mandates an arterial tree that is also shorter, bringing the arterial reflecting sites of the primary pulse closer to the heart [12]. Since the pulse wave velocity (PWV) is the same, or even faster in older women compared to older men throughout life [10], the forward arterial pressure wave in women reflects

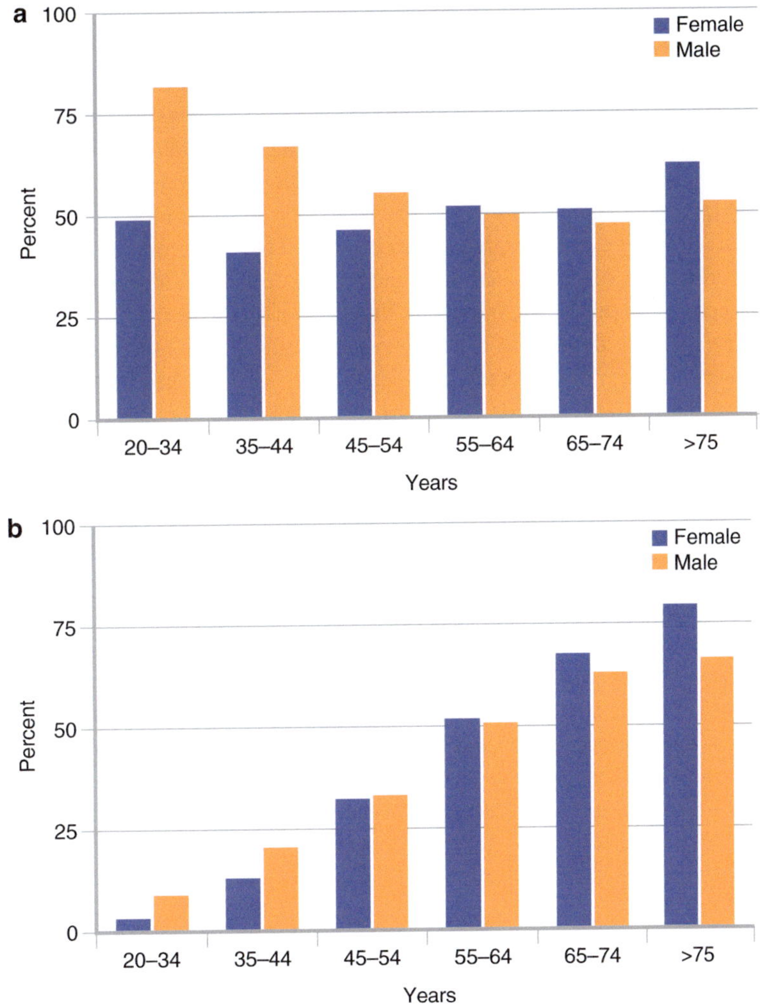

Fig. 32.1 Lack of hypertension control (**a**) and Hypertension prevalence (**b**) in U.S.A. among persons 20 years of age and over. Selected years 1988–1994 through 2005–2008 (Reproduced with permission Engberding and Wenger [75])

off sites closer to the heart than in men and the reflected wave therefore returns to the central aorta earlier in the cardiac cycle. This tends to augment the primary wave in systole, increasing left ventricular (LV) work, rather than augmenting the diastolic wave, where it would support coronary flow. This reduction of pulse amplification is a risk factor by itself [13]. The liability of the shorter arterial tree is partially offset by a faster heart rate since shorter cycle lengths shorten both the systolic and diastolic periods and allow the reflected wave to return to the aorta later in systole or even in early diastole. But the faster heart rate also increases myocardial oxygen demand. These circulatory differences due to stature are life-long and constant throughout the aging process. The circulatory changes of aging that relate to hypertension in men are relatively steady and can be used as a baseline against which the more rapid age-related hormonal changes in women can be compared.

Differences Related to the Menopause

Hormonal Changes

It is well known that the risk of CV disease is lower in pre-menopausal women than men of the same age. This has been attributed to the multiple vascular protective effects of estrogen [14]. The loss of CV protection that develops in women during and after the menopause has been attributed to the associated reduction of sex hormone production and it was only natural to assume that hormonal replacement therapy (HRT) would restore the benefits. When this did not occur [15], it became clear that the entire process was more complex than originally envisioned. The development of other factors in gender related hypertension during the menopause undoubtedly play a role in the failure of HRT to restore pre-menopausal CV risk protection.

Although estrogen or its deficiency cannot be the only factors in male/female hypertensive differences, it is a major player in the control of vascular tone [16]. Estrogen has effects on the multiple vasodilating functions of the endothelium that may be impaired when estrogen becomes deficient. Menopause is associated with a reduction in flow mediated dilation (FMD) in the forearm, attributed to estrogen deficiency [17, 18]. Similarly, post menopausal women (PMW) have been found to have reduced production of the powerful vasodilator, nitric oxide [19]. In an opposing action, PMW have been shown to have increased levels of endothelin, a powerful vasoconstrictor produced by the endothelium [20]. Therefore, hormonal changes, operating through the endothelium, work both to impair vasodilation and augment vasoconstriction in PMW.

Sex steroids influence BP control by means other than their activity on the endothelium. Withdrawal of these hormones are known to stimulate the renin-angiotensin system (RAS) [21] with its known effects on peripheral vasoconstriction and aldosterone production. Also independent of the endothelium is the inhibition of calcium entry into smooth muscle cells by sex hormones, reversed when these hormones are deficient [22]. Salt sensitivity is also well known to increase with the menopause, suggesting another endothelium independent means by which the BP rise can be explained [23].

As described above, estrogen loss activates the RAS system that raises the level of aldosterone, offering an explanation for salt sensitivity. Aldosterone is naturally inhibited by ovarian progesterone and its deficiency during the menopause helps explain the salt sensitivity. In a 2010 review, Boschitsch et al. [24] described the development of two synthetic progesterones, both derivatives of 17 α spironolactone, that have aldosterone inhibiting properties. One, Eplerenone, in the United States is marketed as an aldosterone inhibitor and the other Drospirenone, is sold as a progesterone replacement. Drospirenone is available only in combination with an estrogen as an oral contraceptive (see below) or for the relief of menstrual symptoms. But Drospirenone has been shown to have antihypertensive effects comparable to other commonly used antihypertensive agents [25]. Despite its theoretical appeal, a study of Drospirenone in post-menopausal hypertensive women has not been done nor has an aldosterone antagonist been tested as an antihypertensive agent in PMW.

A role for androgens in post menopausal hypertension has also been proposed [26] but a recent review of this subject concluded that the literature remains unclear on the role of androgens in post-menopausal hypertension [27]. A graphic summary of the many hormonal changes during the menopause and their effects on the BP is displayed in Fig. 32.2.

Other Relevant Differences

Obesity is an established factor in the development of hypertension in both men [28] and women [29]. The prevalence of obesity increases in both men and women as they age but the prevalence of female obesity through the menopausal period may reach as high as 40 %. An independent relationship between body mass index (BMI) and BP has been demonstrated in the SIMONA study [30]. There are multiple mechanisms relating obesity and hypertension during the menopause. These have been summarized [27] and include an association with the metabolic syndrome, insulin resistance, hyperglycemia and dyslipidemia. Even without weight gain, a redistribution of fat to the abdomen, not detected by calculation of the BMI, is significant. Obesity is also associated with an increase in plasma leptin, both of which have been further associated with

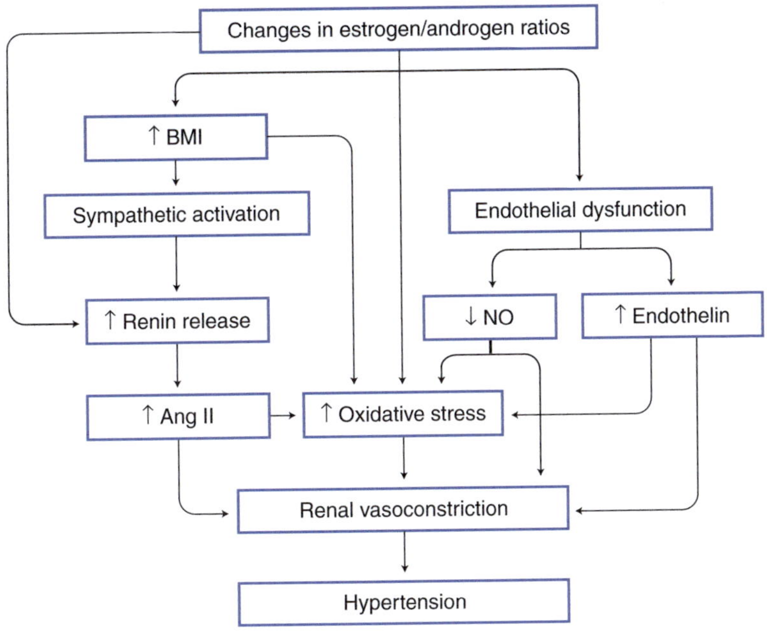

Fig. 32.2 Graphic summary of hormonal changes in postmenopausal women and their influences on blood pressure (Reproduced with permission Coylewright et al. [76])

sympathetic nervous system stimulation, especially that of the renal sympathetic nerves [31, 32]. Interrelationships further complicate matters since the sympathetic stimulation from obesity also activates the RAS system with a resultant increase in renin, angiotensin and aldosterone, all factors that can raise the BP.

The menopause is associated with a rise in C reactive protein (CRP) [33], adipokines [34] and other inflammatory markers independently related to increased CV risk [35]. The rise of inflammatory markers in post-menopausal women has been also related to the abdominal adiposity [34] described above. Although these additional possibilities might have an effect on the development or the effects of hypertension in older women, conclusions from such limited available data must remain speculative.

Hypertension is a polygenetic disorder and numerous polymorphisms have been related to many of the previously described factors in the genesis of high blood pressure during the menopause. The list is long but some of the more recent observations have described polymorphic genetic influences on endothelin converting enzyme – 1 [36], angiotensin converting enzyme 2 [37], the RAS [38], plasminogen activator inhibitor – 1 [39], and leptin [40].

Menopausal Effects on Aortic Stiffness

Finally, increasing aortic stiffness plays a major role in the development of hypertension as the population ages. Male/female differences in the slope relating aortic stiffness to age was noticed as early as 1996 by Karpanou et al. [41] who measured aortic diameters with M-mode echocardiography and brachial arterial pressures using the auscultatory method. The following year, Rajumkar et al. [42] implicated estrogen deficiency as the culprit when they demonstrated that post-menopausal women taking HRT had significantly lower carotid/femoral PWV than untreated women. In women who then discontinued HRT, the PWV velocity rose significantly. In 1999, Stefanidis et al. [43] confirmed the estrogen effect by showing that immediately after IV estrogen administration, aortic distensibility was increased. Similar to the age changes in PP, Waddell et al. [44] in 2001, showed that aortic stiffness was lower in young women than in young men but the reverse was true in an older population (Fig. 32.3). Evidence for the importance of aortic stiffness continued to mount when Zaydun et al. [45] in 2006 showed in 3,149 women, that the slope of the age/PWV (brachial to ankle) was

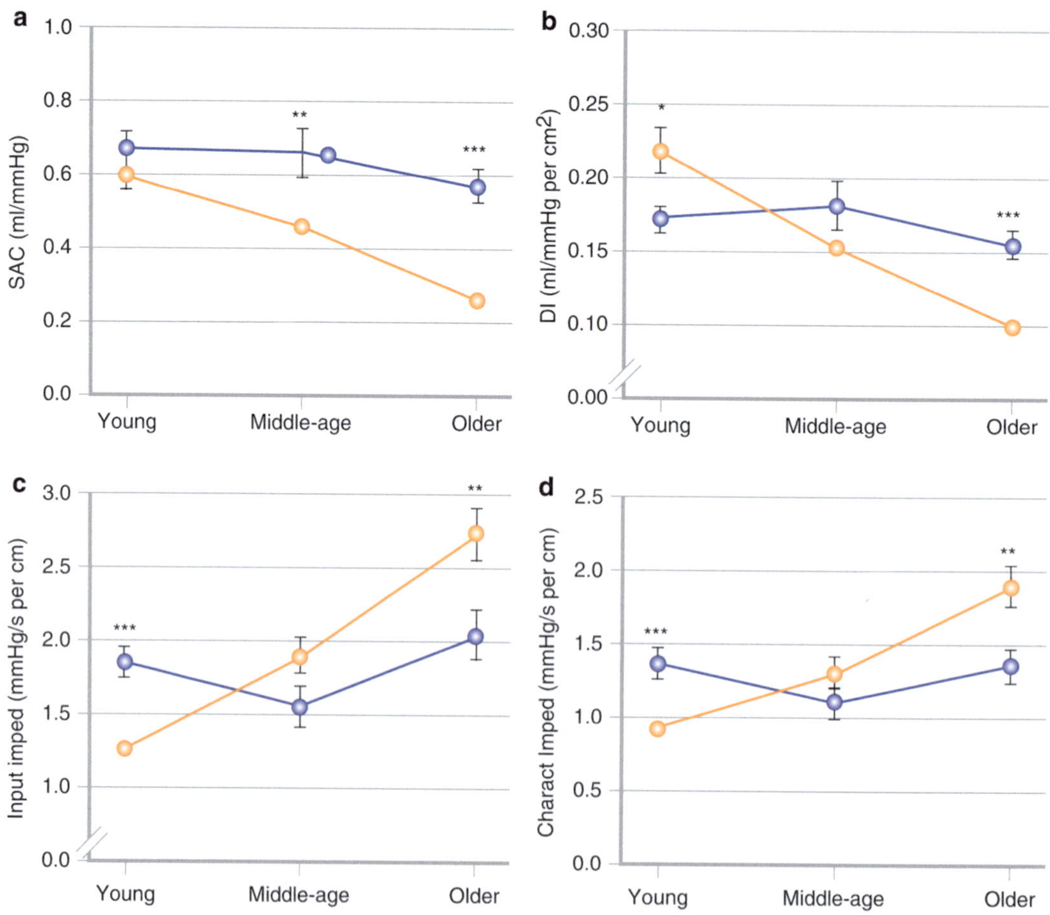

Fig. 32.3 Comparison of (**a**) systemic arterial compliance (*SAC*), (**b**) distensibility index (*DI*), (**c**) aortic input impedance (*Imped*), and (**d**) characteristic impedance (*Charact Imped*) in men (o) and women (•) in the young, middle-age and older populations. Data presented as mean ± SEM. Significant difference between sexes within each age group; * $P<0.05$, ** $P<0.01$, *** $P<0.001$ (Reproduced with permission Waddell et al. [44])

steeper after the menopause and that the stiffest aortas were in women whose menopause was longer than of 6 years duration. This finding was independent of age and of multiple atherosclerotic risk factors. The mechanisms for the effects of estrogen on the aortic wall are many and include changes in the elastin/collagen ratio [46], a decrease in matrix metalloproteinase activity and an increase in aortic vasa vasorum blood flow [47]. This subject has been well reviewed by Rossi et al. in 2011 [47] who concluded that the weight of evidence points to an intrinsically stiffer aorta in women, maintained more compliant by sex hormones in the young. But when hormone deficiency is induced by the menopause, the effects of the basically stiffer female aorta become apparent and help explain the BP gender differences with aging. The importance of aortic stiffness on the blood pressure may be the most significant difference in hypertension between the sexes both in the young and the old.

Gender Differences in Therapy

With this as background, it is not surprising that the superimposition of hypertension later in life, should affect male and female hearts differently. Even after adjusting for age, BMI and DBP in patients with isolated systolic hypertension, women had increased LV wall thickness and mass without chamber enlargement while men had LV dilation and less increase in wall thickness [48]. With regard to therapy, the LIFE study showed that after 1 year of treatment with either a beta blocker or an angiotensin receptor blocker, adjusted LV mass fell more in women than in men for an equivalent reduction in BP [49]. Despite the greater initial reduction in LV mass in women, after 4.8 years of follow-up in the same patients, the prevalence of LVH was still greater in women [50]. Whether these differences would be apparent using other therapeutic agents is unknown.

From the multiple gender differences described above that involve the heart, BP levels, hypertension prevalence, BP control, hormonal and non-hormonal influences on the circulation, it would be reasonable to assume that therapeutic differences would be present as well. The first definitive proof that antihypertensive therapy provided circulatory protection was the United States Veteran Administration trials in 1967 and 1970 in which the patient population was entirely male. Females were included in many large subsequent studies but women were initially under-represented and a comparison of therapeutic benefit between the genders was again not possible. There still has been no single trial designed to answer this question. If present, a demonstrable difference in therapeutic choices would be of considerable importance, since it would halve the therapeutic options that often must be made by trial and error.

In an effort to resolve this question, Gueffier et al. in 1997 [51], published a meta analysis of seven trials in more than 40,000 men and women. In women, there were reductions in CV risks but not in total mortality, while in men both risks and mortality were reduced. The drugs used were primarily thiazide diuretics and beta blockers. The results therefore, cannot be extrapolated to other newer antihypertensive agents. Since then, significant gender differences in the pharmacokinetics among the most frequently used antihypertensive agents have been published [52]. But these differences have not convincingly been translated into routine clinical practice. In 2008, Turnbull et al. [53] reported on a meta-analysis of 31 randomized trials that included 103,268 men and 87,349 women. Achieved BP reductions were comparable for men and women and there was no evidence that men or women obtained different levels of protection from similarly reduced BP's or from any of the antihypertensive agents or groups of agents studied (Fig. 32.4). The regimens reviewed included angiotensin converting enzyme inhibitors, angiotensin receptor blockers, calcium channel blockers, diuretics and beta blockers. Results from a subsequent meta-analysis of 67 randomized trials were similar [54]. Data of this kind have led to guidelines recommending that gender should not be an issue in the selection of antihypertensive agents [5, 55].

Although there are no demonstrable gender differences in efficacy among the various agents, there are clear differences in side effect profiles [56] that could influence decisions in drug selection. Diuretics induce more gout in men but more hyponatremia and hypokalemia in women. Calcium channel blockers produce more edema and angiotensin converting enzyme inhibitors more cough in women than in men. Additionally, angiotensin converting enzyme inhibitors and angiotensin receptor blockers are contraindicated in pregnancy and therefore should be avoided in women who could become pregnant while on antihypertensive therapy.

Hypertension in Women Only

Pregnancy

Major changes in hormones, the neuro-sympathetic system and the consequent hemodynamics occuring early during pregnancy, lead to decreases in BP during the first two trimesters. The BP then rises again to reach the non-pregnant BP values in the third trimester. The early fall in BP relates to a simultaneous decrease in total peripheral resistance, greater in magnitude than the increase in cardiac output [57]. The venous network is also modified during pregnancy with development of new venous channels in the pelvis. Central SBP, calculated from non invasive radial applanation tonometry, decreased

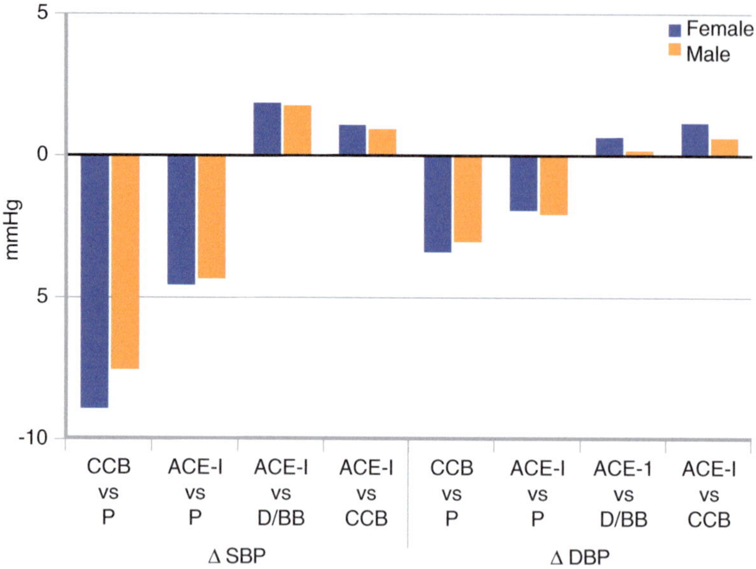

Fig. 32.4 Follow-up blood pressure differences between randomized groups in subgroups of treated women and men. *ACE – 1* ACE Inhibitor, *BP* blood pressure, *CCB* calcium channel blocker, *CV* cardiovascular, *D/BB* diuretic, or **β**-blocker, *P* placebo (Reproduced with permission Engberding and Wenger [75]. Adapted from Turnbull et al. [53])

more than brachial SBP from the first trimester to delivery [58]. Wave reflection, as assessed by the augmentation index (Aix) and adjusted for HR, decreased but PWV adjusted for mean arterial pressure (MAP) was unchanged [59].

Pre-eclampsia, a complex disorder, in part involving dysfunction of the placental endothelium, is characterized by early central hemodynamic alterations. The Aix, at heart rate 75 beats per minute (BPM), is significantly higher than in non-eclamptic controls. This tends to increase the central SBP, important because a higher central pressure, is associated with more severe pre-eclampsia. Similar data has been found in gestational hypertension [60]. The mechanism for increased wave reflection by a change in reflection site(s) is plausible, but a clear explanation is not known.

Polycystic Ovary Syndrome

This complex female endocrinopathy is observed in 3–10 %, but as high as 20 % of child bearing women [61]. Chronic anovulation and polycystic ovarian morphology are associated with multiple disorders such as insulin resistance, hyperandrogenism, obesity, and type 2 diabetes mellitus. With precise measurement of carotid artery geometry (high-resolution wall-tracking system) but using only brachial BP recording, a decrease in carotid artery distensibility was observed. This was associated with a significant increase in SBP [62]. With less accurate conventional vascular echography, the carotid artery intimal medial thickness and forearm FMD were similar to controls as were glycemia, lipid profile, insulin, homeostasis model assessment for insulin resistance and serum markers of inflammation [63]. Finally, central Aix at 75 BPM, increased while the observed increase in central SBP was no longer significant after age adjustment. The observed reduction in circulating vascular progenitor cells was not correlated with hemodynamic parameters [64]. No study has yet defined the hemodynamic abnormality of this syndrome.

Oral Contraceptives

Adverse events from oral contraceptives (OC) include metabolic disorders, weight gain and increase in BP. These major problems are also linked to cardiovascular complications and phlebitis along with potentially lethal pulmonary embolism [65]. Reduction in the dose of estrogen, change in progestin compounds or modification of route of administration have been suggested to reduce these unacceptable events. In the early 90s, a large data source from the Nurse's health study suggested that users of earlier dosages of OC had a significantly increased risk of hypertension (41.5 cases per 10,000 person-years) [66]. More recently, combined oral contraceptive compounds (COC), i.e. with the addition of Drospirenone, have reduced the prevalence of high BP [67, 68]. OC induced hypertension remains an important problem in young women since it may induce vascular damage [69]. Therefore, OC should be offered to hypertensive women only after careful clinical review.

OC steroids have multiple effects on the structure and function of large and small arteries and on the endothelium. In vitro analysis of aortic wall structures has suggested a beneficial role of estrogen and/or progesterone on elastin content, elastin/collagen ratio, and modulation of matrix metalloproteinase 3 [46]. In a large subset of young women (age: 20±3 years), brachial SBP and PP were slightly but significantly increased (average: +2/+1 mmHg). Peripheral resistance was lower while cardiac output (rebreathing technique) was increased in COC users. Central pressures and reflection waves (Aix) were unchanged, but there was a very small but significant increase in aortic stiffness as measured by pulse wave velocity (PWV) [70]. These data should be confirmed because of the small changes, contrary to the experimental data on aortic elastin (see above).

The effect of sex steroids on endothelium dependent vasodilation has been suggested by studies of the normal menstrual cycle. Between early menstrual phase and mid-cycle, measurements of bradykinin or noradrenaline infusion responses were amplified when estrogen levels were increased threefold. However there was no alteration of this response following infusion of the direct vascular muscle cell vasodilator, nitroglycerine (GTN), or the blocker of endothelial nitric oxide (NO) synthase, l-NMMA. These results indicated no estrogenic change in NO-dependent endothelial vasomotion [71]. In summary, menstrual changes in endogenous estrogen contribute to vasomotor changes in small muscular arteries and the arteriolar network.

In a study of forearm vasodilation in 15 young women taking the COC ethynil oestradiol/levonorgestrel, Torgrimson et al. showed no change in endothelial derived vasodilation with the combination, but suggested that the additional progestin compound may have counterbalanced the beneficial role of estrogen alone [72]. When brachial artery diameter was recorded, the same COC showed a decrease in FMD. Similarly, a group of young women treated with medroxyprogesterone alone had a decrease in FMD [73]. In this study, there was no control of endothelium independent vasomotion following GTN, limiting the interpretation of the results. When the COC contained ethinylestradiol and drospirenone, the brachial artery FMD was not altered relative to the GTN effect [74]. In conclusion, OC and recently used low dose COC are associated with small increases in blood pressure in only a small number of individuals. These effects appear more linked to cardiac function and the arteriolar network than to proximal large and middle-size arteries. Although uncommon, the CO induced increase in BP is important and requires that BP be regularly measured in treated patients.

References

1. Janeway TC. A clinical study of hypertensive cardiovascular disease. Arch Intern Med. 1913;12:755–98.
2. Pickering GW. The arterial pressure in the population at large and its relationship to age and prognosis of essential hypertension. In: High blood pressure. London: J. A. Churchill Ltd; 1955. p. 160–1, 301.
3. Messerli FH, Garavaglia GE, Schmieder RE, Sundgaard-Riise K, Nunez BD, Amodeo C. Disparate cardiovascular findings in men and women with essential hypertension. Ann Intern Med. 1987;107:158–61.
4. Go AS, et al. Heart disease and stroke statistics – 2013. Update from the American Heart Association. Circulation. 2013;127:e6–245.
5. Mancia G, et al. ESH/ESC Guidelines for the management of arterial hypertension. The Task force for the management of arterial hypertension of the European Society of Hypertension (ESH) and of the European Society of Cardiology (ESC). J Hypertens. 2013;31:1281–357.
6. Casiglia E, d'Este D, Ginocchio G, Colangeli G, Onesto C, Tramontin P, et al. Lack of influence of menopause on blood pressure and cardiovascular risk profile: a 16-year longitudinal study concerning a cohort of 568 women. J Hypertens. 1996;14:729–36.
7. Staessen JA, Bulpitt CJ, Fagard R, Lijnen P, Amery A. The influence of menopause on blood pressure. J Hum Hypertens. 1989;3:427–33.
8. Lloyd-Jones DM, Evans JC, Levy D. Hypertension in adults across the age spectrum. Current outcomes and control in the community. JAMA. 2005;294:466–72.

9. Franklin SS, Gustin IV W, Wong ND, Larson MG, Weber MA, Kannel WB, et al. Hemodynamic patterns of age-related changes in blood pressure. The Framingham Heart Study. Circulation. 1997;96:308–15.
10. Smulyan H, Asmar RG, Rudnicki A, London GM, Safar ME. Comparative effects of aging in men and women on the properties of the arterial tree. J Am Coll Cardiol. 2001;37:1374–80.
11. Thomas F, Blacher J, Benetos A, Safar ME, Pannier B. Cardiovascular risk as defined in the 2003 European blood pressure classification: the assessment of an additional predictive value of pulse pressure on mortality. J Hypertens. 2008;26:1072–7.
12. Lieber A, Millasseau S, Bourhis L, Blacher J, Protogerou A, Levy B, et al. Aortic wave reflection in women and men. Am J Physiol Heart Circ Physiol. 2010;299:H236–42.
13. Regnault V, Thomas F, Safar ME, Osborne-Pellegrin M, Khalil RA, Pannier B, et al. Sex difference in cardiovascular risk. Role of pulse pressure amplification. J Am Coll Cardiol. 2012;59:1771–7.
14. Xing D, Nozell S, Chen Y-F, Hage F, Oparil S. Estrogen and mechanisms of vascular protection. Arterioscler Thromb Vasc Biol. 2009;29:289–96.
15. Grady D, Herrington D, Bittner V, Blumenthal R, Davidson M, Hlatky M, et al. HERS Research Group. Cardiovascular disease outcomes during 6.8 years of hormone therapy: heart and estrogen/progestin replacement study follow-up (HERS II). JAMA. 2002;288:49–57.
16. Orshal JM, Khalil RA. Gender, sex hormones, and vascular tone. Am J Physiol Regul Integr Comp Physiol. 2004;286:R233–49.
17. Rossi R, Chiurlia E, Nuzzo A, Cioni E, Origliani G, Modena MG. Flow-mediated vasodilation and the risk of developing hypertension in healthy postmenopausal women. J Am Coll Cardiol. 2004;44:1636–40.
18. Taddei S, Agostino V, Lorenzo G, Paola M, Isabella S, Gianpaolo B, et al. Menopause is associated with endothelial dysfunction in women. Hypertension. 1996;28:576–82.
19. Majmudar NG, Robson SC, Ford GA. Effects of the menopause, gender and estrogen replacement therapy on vascular nitric activity. J Clin Endocrinol Metab. 2000;85:1577–83.
20. Ylikorkala O, Orpana A, Puolakka J, Pyorala T, Viinikka L. Postmenopausal hormone replacement decreases plasma levels of endothelin-1. J Clin Endocrinol Metab. 1995;80:3384–7.
21. Yanes LL, Romero DG, Iliescu R, Zhang H, Davis D, Reckelhoff JF. Postmenopausal hypertension. Role of the renin-angiotensin system. Hypertension. 2010;56:359–63.
22. Crews JK, Khalil RA. Gender-specific inhibition of Ca2+entry mechanisms of arterial vasoconstriction by sex hormones. Clin Exp Pharmacol Physiol. 1999;26:707–15.
23. Schulman IH, Aranda P, Raij L, Veronesi M, Aranda FJ, Martin R. Surgical menopause increases salt sensitivity of blood pressure. Hypertension. 2006;47:1168–74.
24. Boschitsch E, Mayerhofer S, Magometschnigg D. Hypertension in women: the role of progesterone and aldosterone. Climacteric. 2010;13:307–13.
25. White W, Hanes V, Chauhan V, Pitt B. Effects of a new hormone therapy, drospirenone and 17-β-estradiol, in postmenopausal women with hypertension. Hypertension. 2006;48:246–53.
26. Reckelhoff JF. Gender differences in the regulation of blood pressure. Hypertension. 2001;37:1199–208.
27. Lima R, Wofford M, Reckelhoff JF. Hypertension in postmenopausal women. Curr Hypertens Rep. 2012;14:254–60.
28. Alvarez GE, Beske SD, Ballard TP, Davy KP. Sympathetic neural activation in visceral obesity. Circulation. 2002;106:2533–6.
29. Britton KA, Pradhan AD, Gaziano JM, Manson JE, Ridker PM, Buring JE, et al. Hemoglobin A1c, body mass index, and the risk of hypertension in women. Am J Hypertens. 2011;24:328–34.
30. Zanchetti A, Facchetti R, Cesana GC, Modena MG, Pirrelli A, Sega R, on behalf of the SIMONA Participants. Menopause-related blood pressure increase and its relationship to age and body mass index: the SIMONA epidemiologic study. J Hypertens. 2005;23:2269–76.
31. Hall JE, da Silva AA, do Carmo JM, Dubinion J, Hamza S, Munusamy S, et al. Obesity-induced hypertension: role of sympathetic nervous system, leptin, and melanocortins. J Biol Chem. 2010;285:17271–6.
32. Mukherjee R, Villarreal D, Reams GP, Freeman RH, Tchoukina I, Spear RM. Leptin as a common link to obesity and hypertension. Drugs of Today. 2005;41:687–95.
33. Kurtz EG, Ridker PM, Rose LM, Cook NR, Everett BM, Buring JE, et al. Oral postmenopausal hormone therapy, C-reactive protein, and cardiovascular outcomes. Menopause. 2011;18:23–9.
34. Lee CG, Carr MC, Murdoch SJ, Mitchell E, Woods NF, Wener MH, et al. Adipokines, inflammation, and visceral adiposity across the menopausal transition: a prospective study. J Clin Endocrinol Metab. 2009;94:1004–110.
35. Rizzo M, Corrado E, Coppola G, Muratori I, Novo G, Novo S. Markers of inflammation are strong predictors of subclinical and clinical atherosclerosis in women with hypertension. Coron Artery Dis. 2009;20:15–20.
36. Funalot B, Courbon D, Brousseau T, Poirier O, Berr C, Cambien F, et al. Genes encoding endothelin-coverting enzyme-1 and endothelin-1 interact to influence blood pressure in women: the EVA study. J Hypertens. 2004;22:739–43.
37. Fan X, Wang Y, Sun K, Zhang W, Yang X, Wang S, et al. Polymorphisms of ACE2 gene are associated with essential hypertension and antihypertensive effects of captopril in women. Clin Pharmacol Ther. 2007;82:187–96.
38. Mansego ML, Redon J, Marin R, Gonzalez-Albert V, Martin-Escudero JC, Fabia MJ, et al. Renin polymor-

phisms and haplotypes are associated with blood pressure levels in postmenopausal women. J Hypertens. 2008;26:230–7.

39. Bjorck HM, Eriksson P, Alehagen U, De Basso R, Ljungberg LU, Persson K, et al. Gender-specific association of the plasminogen activator inhibitor-1 4G/5G polymorphism with central arterial pressure. Am J Hypertens. 2011;24:802–8.
40. Ma D, Feitosa MF, Wilk JB, Laramie JM, Yu K, Leiendecker-Foster C, et al. Leptin is associated with blood pressure and hypertension in women from the National Heart, Lung, and Blood Institute Family Heart Study. Hypertension. 2009;53:473–9.
41. Karapanou EA, Vyssoulis GP, Papakyriakou SA, Toutouza MG, Toutouzas PK. Effects of menopause on aortic root function in hypertensive women. J Am Coll Cardiol. 1996;28:1562–6.
42. Rajkumar C, Kingwell BA, Cameron JD, Waddell T, Mehra R, Christophidis N, et al. Hormonal therapy increases arterial compliance in postmenopausal women. J Am Coll Cardiol. 1997;30:350–6.
43. Stefanadis C, Tsiamis E, Dernellis J, Toutouzas P. Effect of estrogen on aortic function in postmenopausal women. Am J Physiol Heart Circ Physiol. 1999;276:H658–62.
44. Waddell TK, Dart AM, Gatzka CD, Cameron JD, Kingwell BA. Women exhibit a greater age-related increase in proximal aortic stiffness than men. J Hypertens. 2011;19:2205–12.
45. Zaydun G, Tomiyama H, Hashimoto H, Arai T, Koji Y, Yambe M, et al. Menopause is an independent factor augmenting the age-related increase in arterial stiffness in the early postmenopausal phase. Atherosclerosis. 2006;184:137–42.
46. Natoli AK, Medley TL, Ahimastos AA, Drew BG, Thearle DJ, Dilley RJ, et al. Sex steroids modulate human aortic smooth muscle cells matrix protein deposition and matrix metalloproteinase expression. Hypertension. 2005;46:1129–34.
47. Rossi P, Frances Y, Kingwell BA, Ahimastos AA. Gender differences in artery wall biomechanical properties throughout life. J Hypertens. 2011;29:1023–33.
48. Krumholz HM, Larson M, Levy D. Sex differences in cardiac adaptation to isolated systolic hypertension. Am J Cardiol. 1993;72:310–3.
49. Bella JN, Palmieri V, Wachtell K, Liu JE, Gerdts E, Nieminen MS, et al. Sex- related difference in regression of left ventricular hypertrophy with antihypertensive treatment: the LIFE study. J Hum Hypertens. 2004;18:411–6.
50. Gerdts E, Okin PM, de Simone G, Cramariuc D, Wachtell K, Boman K, et al. Gender differences in left ventricular structure and function during antihypertensive treatment. The losartan intervention for endpoint reduction in hypertension study. Hypertension. 2008;51:1109–14.
51. Gueyffier F, Boutitie F, Boissel J-P, Popcock S, Coope J, Cutler J, et al. Effect of antihypertensive drug treatment on cardiovascular outcomes in women and men. A meta-analysis of individual patient data from randomized, controlled trials. Ann Intern Med. 1997;126:761–7.
52. Franconi F, Carru C, Malorni W, Vella S, Mercuro G. The effect of SEX/gender on cardiovascular pharmacology. Curr Pharm Des. 2011;17:1095–107.
53. Turnbull F, Woodward M, Neal B, Barzi F, Ninomiya T, Chalmers J, et al. Do men and women respond differently to blood pressure-lowering treatment? Results of prospectively designed overviews of randomized trials. Eur Heart J. 2008;29:2669–80.
54. Ljungman C, Mortensen L, Kahan T, Manhem K. Treatment of mild to moderate hypertension by gender perspective; a systematic review. J Womens Health (Larchmt). 2009;18:1049–62.
55. Chobanian AV, Bakris GL, Black HR, Cushman WC, Green LA, Izzo JL, et al. Seventh report of the Joint National Committee on Prevention and Detection, Evaluation and Treatment of High Blood Pressure. NIH Publication #04-5230. Hypertension. 2003;42:1206–52.
56. Rosenthal T, Oparil S. Hypertension in women. J Hum Hypertens. 2000;14:691–704.
57. Van Oppen AC, Stigter RH, Bruinse HW. Cardiac output in normal pregnancy: a critical review. Obstet Gynecol. 1996;87:310–8.
58. Fujime M, Tomimatsu T, Okaue Y, Koyama S, Kanagawa T, Taniguchi T, et al. Central aortic blood pressure and augmentation index during normal pregnancy. Hypertens Res. 2012;35:633–8.
59. Mahendru AA, Everett TR, Wilkinson IB, Lees CC, McEniery CM. Maternal cardiovascular changes from pre-pregnancy to very early pregnancy. J Hypertens. 2012;30:2168–72.
60. Khalil A, Jauniaux E, Harrington K. Antihypertensive therapy and central hemodynamics in women with hypertensive disorders in pregnancy. Obstet Gynecol. 2009;113:646–54.
61. Carmina E, Azzizi R. Diagnosis, phenotype, and prevalence of polycystic ovary syndrome. Fertil Steril. 2006;86 Suppl 1:S7–8.
62. Lakhani K, Seifalian AM, Hardiman P. Impaired carotid viscoelastic properties in women with polycystic ovaries. Circulation. 2002;106:81–5.
63. Soares GM, Vieira CS, Martins WP, Franceschini SA, dos Reis RM, de Sa MFS, Ferriani RA. Increased arterial stiffness in nonobese women with polycystic ovary syndrome (PCOS) without comorbidities: one more characteristic inherent to the syndrome? Clin Endocrinol (Oxf). 2009;71:406–11.
64. Dessapt-Baradez C, Reza M, Sivakumar G, Hernandez-Fuentes M, Markakis K, Gnudi L, et al. Circulating vascular progenitor cells and central arterial stiffness in polycystic ovary syndrome. PLoS One. 2011;6(5):1–6.e20317.
65. Shufelt CL, Bairey Merz CN. Contraceptive hormone use and cardiovascular disease. J Am Coll Cardiol. 2009;53:221–31.
66. Chasan-Taber L, Willett WC, Manson JE, Spiegelman D, Hunter DJ, Curhan G, et al. Prospective study of

oral contraceptives and hypertension among women in the United States. Circulation. 1996;94:483–9.
67. Suthipongse W, Taneepanichskul S. An open-label randomized comparative study of oral contraceptives between medications containing 3 mg drospirenone/30 microg ethinylestradiol and 150 microg levonogestrel/30 microg ethinylestradiol in Thai women. Contraception. 2004;69:23–6.
68. Perez-Lopez FR. Clinical experiences with drospirenone: from reproductive to postmenopausal years. Maturitas. 2008;60:78–91.
69. Le-Ha C, Beilin LJ, Burrows S, Huang RC, Oddy WH, Hands B, et al. Oral contraceptive use in girls and alcohol consumption in boys are associated with increased blood pressure in late adolescence. Eur J Prev Cardiol. 2013;20:947–55.
70. Hickson SS, Miles KL, McDonnell BJ, Yasmin, Cockcroft JR, Wilkinson IB, et al; ENIGMA Study Investigators. Use of the oral contraceptive pill is associated with increased large artery stiffness in young women: the ENIGMA study. J Hypertens. 2011;29:1155–9.
71. Chan NN, MacAllister RJ, Colhoun HM, Vallance P, Hingorani AD. Changes in endothelium-dependent vasodilatation and alpha-adrenergic responses in resistance vessels during the menstrual cycle in healthy women. J Clin Endocrinol Metab. 2001;86:2499–504.
72. Torgrimson BN, Meendering JR, Kaplan PF, Minson CT. Endothelial function across an oral contraceptive cycle in women using levonorgestrel and ethinyl estradiol. Am J Physiol Heart Circ Physiol. 2007;292:H2874–80.
73. Lizarelli PM, Martins WP, Vieira CS, Soares GM, Franceschini SA, Ferriani RA, et al. Both a combined oral contraceptive and depot medroxyprogesterone acetate impair endothelial function in young women. Contraception. 2009;79:35–40.
74. Cassiana RG, Giribella NR, Melo RCG, Silva VM, Hong GM, Guerra E, et al. A combined oral contraceptive containing drospirenone changes neither endothelial function nor hemodynamic parameters in healthy Young women: a prospective clinical trial. Contraception. 2012;86:35–41.
75. Engberding N, Wenger NK. Management of hypertension in women. Hypertens Res. 2012;35:251–60.
76. Coylewright M, Reckelhoff JF, Ouyang P. Menopause and hypertension: an age-old debate. Hypertension. 2008;51:952–9.

33 Obesity, Metabolic Syndrome, Diabetes and Smoking

Isabel Ferreira, Roel J.J. van de Laar, and Coen D.A. Stehouwer

Abstract

It is becoming increasingly clear that arterial stiffness may be determined not only by age(ing) and blood pressure, but also by exposure to other cardiovascular risk factors. This chapter reviews the evidence provided by studies adopting an aetiological model of analyses of determinants of arterial stiffness, mainly derived, if available, from prospective designs. Specifically, the following risk factors are examined: the critical axis (central) obesity – metabolic syndrome – (type 2) diabetes, and also smoking. There is convincing evidence, reinforced by recent aetiological prospective studies, that these risk factors, all of which may be preventable, increase arterial stiffness. This may explain, at least in part, the increased cardiovascular disease risk observed in these conditions. However, the molecular basis of greater arterial stiffness associated with these risk factors remains to be fully elucidated. In addition, the prognostic significance of arterial stiffness indices in individuals with these risk factors, and the extent to which intervention on these risk factors improves cardiovascular outcome through beneficial impact on arterial stiffness, is still unclear. Given the high and/or increasing prevalence of these risk factors, these issues constitute an important research agenda.

Keywords

Arterial stiffness • Central obesity • Metabolic syndrome • Diabetes • Smoking • Risk factors • Life course • Ageing

I. Ferreira, PhD (✉)
Department of Clinical Epidemiology and Medical Technology Assessment (KEMTA),
Maastricht University Medical Centre,
P. Debyelaan 25,
Maastricht 6202 AZ, The Netherlands
e-mail: i.ferreira@maastrichtuniversity.nl,
i.ferreira@mumc.nl

R.J.J. van de Laar, MD, PhD
C.D.A. Stehouwer, MD, PhD
Department of Internal Medicine,
Maastricht University Medical Centre,
P.O. Box 5800, Maastricht 6202 AZ, The Netherlands
e-mail: roel.vande.laar@mumc.nl;
cda.stehouwer@mumc.nl

M.E. Safar et al. (eds.), *Blood Pressure and Arterial Wall Mechanics in Cardiovascular Diseases*,
DOI 10.1007/978-1-4471-5198-2_33,

Abbreviations

AGAHLS	Amsterdam Growth and Health Longitudinal Study
AIx	Augmentation index
baPWV	Pulse wave velocity (brachial-ankle)
BMI	Body mass index
BP	Blood pressure
cfPWV	Pulse wave velocity (carotid–femoral)
cIMT	Carotid intima–media thickness
CVD	Cardiovascular disease
CWS	Circumferential wall stress
D	Diameter
EAT	Epicardial adipose tissue
FPG	Fasting plasma glucose
IAD	Inter-adventitial diameter
IGM	Impaired glucose metabolism
IGT	Impaired glucose tolerance
MAP	Mean arterial pressure
MetS	Metabolic syndrome
NGM	Normal glucose metabolism
PP	Pulse pressure
PWV	Pulse wave velocity (aortic)
RF	Risk factor
SAT	Subcutaneous adipose tissue
T1DM	Type 1 diabetes mellitus
T2DM	Type 2 diabetes mellitus
VAT	Visceral adipose tissue

Although arterial stiffness is primarily determined by age(ing) and mean arterial pressure (MAP), exposure to other cardiovascular risk factors (RFs) may contribute as well [1]. Recently, a systematic review suggested that the impact of RFs other than blood pressure (BP) on arterial stiffness was, at best, only modest [2]. However, this conclusion was based on the findings from cross-sectional studies only, most of which adopted predictive rather than aetiological models of analyses.

This raises two important methodological points, that we address below.

I. The Importance of Adopting a Life-course approach to risk factor exposure and their impact on arterial stiffness. To understand the impact of RFs on arterial stiffness (or any other health outcome of interest), a longer period of RF exposure, preferably covering a significant period of an individual's lifetime prior to health outcome, will provide a better insight into their role than when these are assessed at a single time-point as usually seen in cross-sectional studies [1]. For instance, recent analyses from the Framingham Heart Study showed that a construct measure of obese-years (i.e. the product of years lived with obesity by the concomitant level of obesity) was more strongly associated with incident risk of diabetes and cardiovascular and all-cause mortality than the level of body mass index (BMI) or duration of obesity alone [3]. Likewise, exposure to adverse lifestyle and biological RFs early in life, and sustaining such RFs at more adverse levels throughout the course of (young) life, have been linked to higher levels of arterial stiffness in adulthood [1, 4–7].

II. Predictive models are not helpful in understanding aetiology. In the current literature, aetiological and prediction research aims are frequently confused. For example, any RF (*such as central obesity*) that affects BP may thereby affect arterial stiffness because BP is a main determinant of arterial stiffness. As such, the true impact of such RF on arterial stiffness may, in fact, be underestimated in models that adjust for BP (i.e. subtract the indirect impact of the RF on arterial stiffness through BP, or any other intermediate factor(s)). Likewise, when multiple RFs are included in regression models to 'extract' those that are associated with arterial stiffness (often independently of age, sex, and BP, the later assumed to be a confounder and not a mediator), such models will underestimate the impact of any RF in favour of others that may be closer to arterial stiffness in the pathway between RF and arterial stiffness (*e.g. impaired glucose metabolism may mediate a part of the association between central obesity and arterial stiffness; in this case, a predictive model would disclose only glucose, but not central obesity, to be 'significantly' associated with arterial stiffness, often accompanied by the misleading conclusion that central fat is not a determinant of arterial stiffness*). Furthermore, the independent RFs extracted by such predictive models will be highly dependent on the RFs measured/included in the analyses and the level of precision with which they were measured; these aspects are highly variable across studies, thus limiting the comparability of their findings.

For these reasons, we focus, whenever possible, on the evidence provided by prospective studies adopting an aetiological rather than a predictive model of analyses of determinants of arterial stiffness. Specifically, in this chapter, we review the current evidence regarding the critical axis (central) obesity – metabolic syndrome – (type 2) diabetes, and also smoking, as important preventable determinants of arterial stiffness, with emphasis on studies published after earlier reviews [8, 9].

Obesity, Body Fat Distribution/Body Composition and Arterial Stiffness

Increases in arterial stiffness have been proposed as one of the potential pathways through which (central) obesity could lead to cardiovascular disease (CVD) [8, 10]. Many cross-sectional studies have indeed shown that higher levels of body fatness, in particular, a central pattern of fat distribution, are positively associated with arterial stiffness (studies up to 2005 reviewed in [8]). These associations have not been confined to individuals with overweight or obesity, but were seen across the entire range of levels of body mass, and have been shown across all age categories [11, 12], including children and adolescents [13–17] and young [11, 18] and older adults [11, 19, 20]. The increased levels of arterial stiffness observed already among the young suggest that higher levels of central adiposity do not need to be long-lasting to have deleterious effects on the arterial system. Moreover, a greater body of evidence has accumulated in recent years showing that higher levels of central adiposity at young(er) ages are associated with higher arterial stiffness later in life [1, 21] or with steeper stiffness progression [22], likely because central fat tends to track throughout life, thereby leading to increased arterial stiffness due to an accumulated exposure to central obesity-related deleterious factors.

The extent to which *changes in body fat/fat distribution* affect changes in arterial stiffness remains less clear due to a scarcity of longitudinal studies thus far. The detrimental role of excessive body weight was first emphasized by observational studies showing adverse associations of increases in weight with changes in arterial stiffness among young and healthy [23] and overweight middle-aged adults [24] and several small intervention studies, all confined to individuals with obesity or diabetes, showing arterial de-stiffening after weight loss [25–27]. More recent and larger randomized controlled trials confirmed the beneficial effects of weight loss attained by means of diet and/or exercise among nondiabetic overweight/obese individuals with (e.g. the ENCORE study [28]) or without hypertension (e.g. the SAVE trial [29]), supporting the view of an impact of body fat on arterial stiffness independent, at least in part, of related higher BP and metabolic disturbances. However, arterial adaptations related to weight changes do not enable an appreciation of the underlying changes in type of body fat depot (*e.g. visceral vs. subcutaneous*) and/or its distribution (*e.g. central vs. peripheral*) responsible for the effects observed.

In support of a predominant adverse role of abdominal visceral (VAT) rather than subcutaneous adipose tissue (SAT), Orr et al. showed that VAT, but not SAT, was associated with the increases in arterial stiffness resulting from 5 kg weight gain induced by overfeeding nonobese young adult individuals for 6–8 weeks [30]. Despite its small size and highly experimental setting, this was an important proof of concept study. However, recent studies suggest that the adverse effect of central fatness on arterial stiffness (as on metabolic disturbances relating central obesity to poorer cardiovascular outcome) may not only be due to the effects of abdominal VAT but also due to the adverse effects of excessive accumulation of adipose tissue around the epicardium (i.e. epicardial adipose tissue – EAT) [31, 32] and/or in the liver (typical feature of nonalcoholic fatty liver disease) [33, 34]. These studies all had cross-sectional designs [31–34], and thus prospective studies among representative cohorts need to investigate further the interrelations, relative contributions and specific pathobiological mechanisms through which these fat depots may impact on arterial stiffening.

Adopting a model of whole body fat distribution, we had previously shown among apparently healthy young adults from the *Amsterdam Growth and Health Longitudinal Study* (*AGAHLS*) and also among older individuals with different levels of glucose metabolism from the *Hoorn Study* that, in contrast to central fat (i.e. that accumulated in the trunk though without distinctions between SAT, VAT, EAT and/or liver fat), higher levels of peripheral fat mass (i.e. accumulated in the limbs and thus stored mainly subcutaneously) may have an independent favourable impact on arterial stiffness [18, 19]. Recent cross-sectional data from the *Fels Longitudinal Study* confirmed these findings [35]. Indeed, the different lipolytic activity of the two fat regions provides biological support for their opposite effects on arterial stiffness. In addition, these '*dysfunctional*' *vs.* '*functional*' effects of fat could explain why, in general, central fat estimates correlate more strongly with health outcomes than estimates of total body fatness. It is conceivable that adverse changes in body fat distribution may occur with ageing, i.e. increases in central combined with decreases in peripheral fat mass, without being reflected by appreciable changes in total body weight or BMI, though both contributing, additively, to accelerated arterial stiffening. We tested this hypothesis in the *AGAHLS*, in a first longitudinal study to have examined how naturally occurring changes in body fat and its distribution (as assessed by dual x-ray absorptiometry) correlated with changes in arterial stiffness defined by a large set of valid stiffness estimates throughout the arterial tree [36]. The study had three key findings: first, throughout the 6-year longitudinal study, greater levels of trunk fat were adversely whereas greater levels of peripheral fat were favourably associated with carotid and femoral stiffness and cfPWV. These associations likely reflected the more 'chronic' (deleterious) effects of persistent adverse fat distribution over time. Second, increases in trunk fat were adversely whereas increases in peripheral fat were favourably associated with 6-year changes in carotid and aortic, though not femoral, stiffness. These observations suggested a more 'acute' component to the deleterious effects of body fat distribution on arterial stiffness of predominantly elastic arterial segments. Finally, the detrimental effects of *increases* in trunk mass and *decreases* in peripheral fat mass on arterial stiffness were independent of one another and concomitant changes in lean mass and other RFs (including MAP) and were accompanied by only minor increases in body weight. Importantly, we identified a relative prevalent phenotype of change in body fat distribution characterized by increases in trunk but decreases in peripheral fat mass (about one-third of the study population), whose change in BMI levels ranged within the limits assigned to normal weight (Fig. 33.1a), but whose rates of progression in carotid and aortic stiffness were the steepest (Fig. 33.1b, c, respectively). This phenotype of changes in body fat distribution is consistent with the existence of a relative prevalent subgroup of individuals at the population level designated as '*metabolically obese but normal weight*', often characterized by elevated abdominal/visceral adiposity (despite a BMI<25 kg/m^2) and a more atherogenic lipid and/or glucose metabolism profile, and who may be at particular high risk for metabolic and CVD.

Adopting a body composition (i.e. examining also muscle mass in addition to body fat) rather than a body fat/fat distribution-only model has also revealed leg and arm muscle mass as strong independent correlate of arterial stiffness, particularly among the elderly [19, 37–39] but also among young adults [18, 36]. Indeed, as the proportion of older individuals in the population grows, so does the concern about the cardiometabolic consequences of the increasing prevalence of (central) obesity and sarcopenia (i.e. the degenerative loss of skeletal muscle mass and strength associated with ageing), especially when occurring in combination – i.e. *sarcopenic obesity* [40]. How decreases in lean mass may affect arterial stiffness is not clear as the evidence so far has been mainly derived from cross-sectional studies [18, 19, 37–39] and mechanistic studies are lacking. It is possible that the relationship is not causal in the sense that higher muscle mass

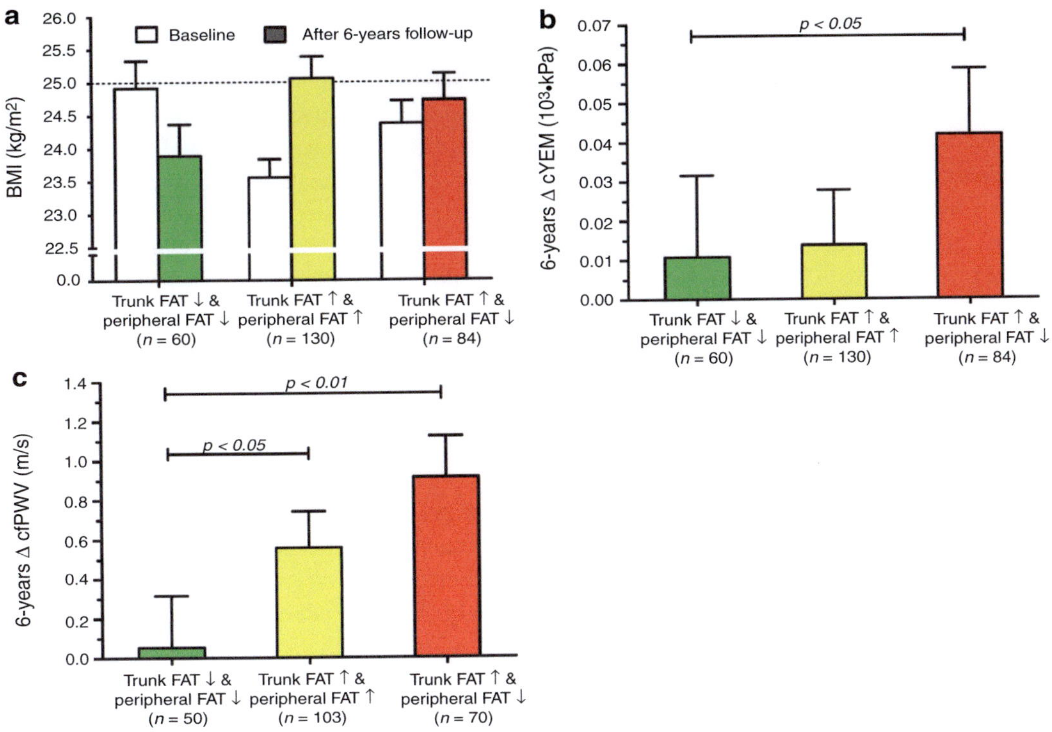

Fig. 33.1 Comparisons across different phenotypes of changes in body fat distribution as observed in a 6-year follow-up from the *Amsterdam Growth and Health Longitudinal Study* of (**a**) body mass index (*BMI*) at baseline and at follow-up, (**b**) changes in carotid Young's elastic modulus (*YEM*) and (**c**) changes in carotid–femoral pulse wave velocity (*cfPWV*). BMI data were adjusted for sex; arterial data were adjusted for sex, body height and changes in mean arterial pressure, lean mass and other biological risk factors. *Error bars* indicate the standard errors of the means. Reproduced from Schouten et al. [36] with permission from the American Society of Nutrition

may be a simple marker of higher (lifelong) physical activity and/or less sedentary levels, better nutrient intake status and/or better glucose uptake/insulin sensitivity, all of which protect against arterial stiffness [4, 6, 9]. Alternatively, it has been suggested that arterial stiffness may promote muscle mass decline/sarcopenia with ageing by reducing limb blood flow and inducing rarefaction and dysfunction in the microcirculation, thereby affecting muscle contraction and ultimately leading to muscle mass rarefaction. This hypothesis was supported by a recent prospective study from the *Health, Aging and Body Composition Study*, showing that older individuals with higher cfPWV at baseline had poorer levels of leg lean mass and sarcopenic index at baseline and over a 6-year follow-up period, independently of age, BMI, BP, diabetes, physical activity, smoking, total fat mass, low-grade inflammation and CVD status [41]. Further longitudinal and intervention studies are needed to clarify the role of muscle mass on arterial stiffening (or vice versa). Nevertheless, the existence of a link between muscle mass and arterial stiffness may have clinical implications by emphasizing the need to ensure that weight loss induced by dietary interventions does not occur at the expense of muscle mass, particularly among the elderly. Inclusion of physical exercise in such interventions may be key in this regard.

Metabolic Syndrome and Arterial Stiffness

A major consequence of central obesity is the clustering of other cardiovascular RFs, such as hypertension, hyperglycaemia and/or insulin resistance and dyslipidaemia, in other words, the metabolic syndrome (MetS). Increased arterial stiffness has been consistently reported in individuals with the MetS or with increasing clustered load or number of traits of the MetS (studies up to 2008 reviewed in [9]). Importantly, such adverse arterial changes have been shown across all ages [42], including young children and adolescents, with [43] or without overt obesity [13, 44], and young [45–47] and older adults [48], including those treated [49] or not for hypertension [50]. The increased arterial stiffness in the MetS thus appears to be caused by subtle metabolic abnormalities, characteristic of prediabetic states, but not necessarily fully developed diabetes.

In support of the reversibility of the adverse effects of the MetS if prevented/targeted early in life, recent analyses of the MetS status in 945 participants from the *Cardiovascular Risk in Young Finns Study* when aged 9–18 years old and again after 21 years of follow-up revealed that children/adolescents with the MetS had higher arterial stiffness in adulthood than those without. Importantly, those who recovered from the MetS between childhood/adolescence and adulthood had lower arterial stiffness in adulthood than those with persistent MetS, such that their levels of PWV were comparable with those who never had the MetS in childhood/adolescence and adulthood [51].

Age-related increases in arterial stiffness seem to be amplified in the presence of the MetS [42, 46], but this evidence was primarily derived from cross-sectional studies. The few prospective cohort studies thus far that have obtained repeated measures of arterial stiffness years apart have shown that individuals with the MetS not only had higher arterial stiffness at baseline but also displayed *steeper* increases in arterial stiffness with ageing as compared with those who did not have the MetS [47, 52–55]. In addition, analyses of the impact of changes in MetS status among young [55] and middle-aged [56] adults showed that those with incident and persistent MetS over the course of time displayed the steepest increases in arterial stiffness than their peers who remained MetS-free throughout time (e.g. Fig. 33.2g). Those who recovered displayed somewhat less steep increases in carotid Young's elastic modulus (YEM) [55] or even comparable increases in baPWV [56] with ageing as those who remained MetS-free throughout. An important observation in one of these studies was that the MetS-related increase in carotid YEM seemed to have preceded structural and local haemodynamic changes consistent with maladaptive carotid remodelling, a process that may explain the increased risk of stroke in individuals with the MetS [55]. Specifically, in the course of time (6-year follow-up between the mean ages of 36 and 42 of the AGAHLS' participants) and in comparison with individuals who remained MetS-free, individuals with persistent MetS displayed significantly steeper increases in carotid intima–media thickness (cIMT), which were accompanied by steeper increases in inter-adventitial (IAD) and lumen diameter (lumen D), but not circumferential wall stress (CWS) which decreased; at baseline, these individuals had already higher IAD, lumen D and CWS, but not cIMT (Fig. 33.2a–f). These findings, observed for the first time in the context of a longitudinal study of not only carotid structural (i.e. cIMT and IAD or lumen D) but also haemodynamic (i.e. CWS) properties with ageing, support the view that increases in cIMT in young adults with the MetS may primarily reflect an adaptive mechanism that attempts to restore local haemodynamic conditions to an equilibrium rather than atherosclerosis *per se*. However, carotid adaptations did not completely restore CWS to levels comparable to those who remained MetS-free throughout time, and, therefore, the patterns of carotid outward remodelling observed under the effects of persistent MetS exposure were maladaptive [55].

Taken together, the longitudinal data reviewed above [47, 51–56] demonstrate *accelerated arterial stiffening and maladaptive remodelling* in the MetS, which may explain, at least in part, the increased cardiovascular risk in these individuals [9]. These findings also emphasize the importance of primary prevention given the observed reversibility of the adverse impact of MetS on arterial structural and functional properties among those individuals who recovered from the MetS. It is important to stress that the association between the MetS and arterial stiffness is not

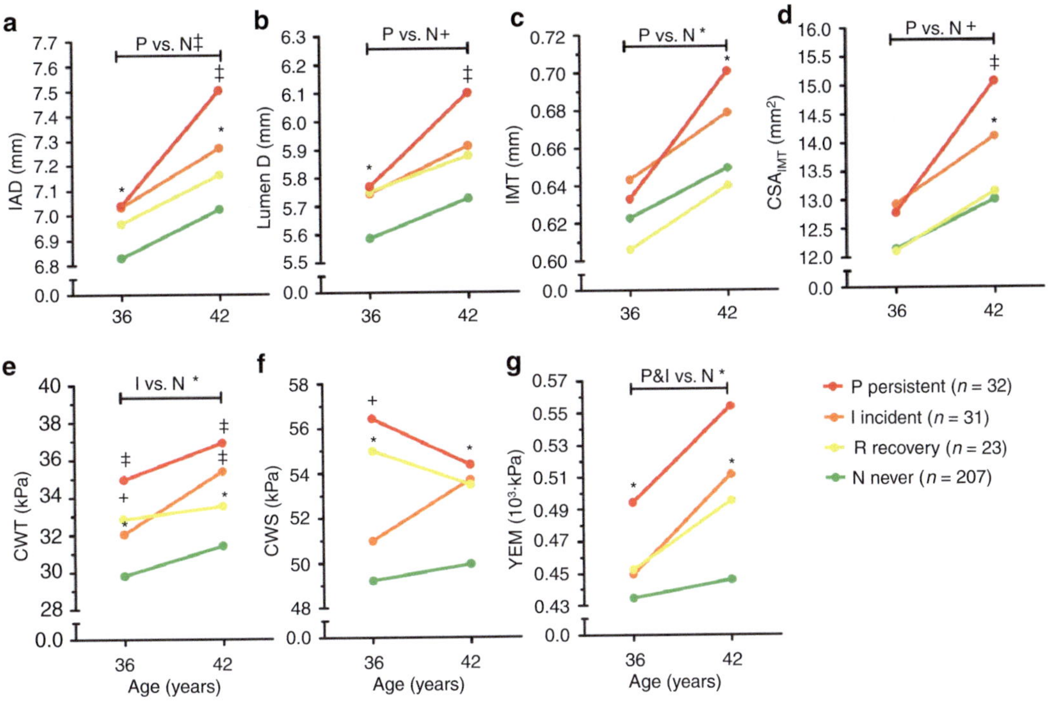

Fig. 33.2 Comparison of trajectories of changes in carotid artery properties by categories of change in metabolic syndrome status as observed in a 6-year follow-up from the *Amsterdam Growth and Health Longitudinal Study*: (**a**) inter-adventitial diameter (*IAD*), (**b**) lumen diameter (*D*), (**c**) intima–media thickness (*IMT*), (**d**) wall cross-sectional area (CSA_{IMT}), (**e**) circumferential wall tension (*CWT*), (**f**) circumferential wall stress (*CWS*) and (**g**) Young's elastic modulus (*YEM*). All data are adjusted for sex, height and (changes in) age, smoking status, alcohol consumption, physical activity, low-density lipoprotein cholesterol and the use of antihypertensive medication. *$P<0.05$, †$P<0.01$, ‡$P<0.001$ (vs. *N* never). Reproduced from Ferreira et al. [55] with permission from Wolters Kluwer Health

only attributed to elevated BP; in addition to (and independently of) BP, (central) obesity and increased glucose levels are traits often associated with arterial stiffness [47, 48, 55], whereas dyslipidaemia (as ascertained by elevated triglycerides and/or decreased HDL cholesterol) has been less or not consistently so. The clustering of central obesity, increased glucose levels and BP appears to be the most prevalent across several populations in the western world [42, 57], and this phenotype is not only associated with the highest arterial stiffness levels [42] but also with the greatest mortality risk [57].

Diabetes and Arterial Stiffness

Increased arterial stiffness may, at least partially, explain the link between diabetes and cardiovascular disease [9]. We have previously reviewed a large body of evidence showing increased arterial stiffness in both type 1 (T1DM) and type 2 (T2DM) diabetes mellitus [9]. These two main forms of diabetes differ in terms of pathophysiology, but the evidence regarding diabetes-related arterial stiffening is overwhelmingly similar. This has been clearly illustrated in the *SEARCH for Diabetes in Youth Study*, a population-based study including 595 10–20-year-olds (90 % with T1DM and 10 % with T2DM), showing increased arterial stiffness (cfPWV or brachial distensibility) in T1DM vs. nondiabetic controls [58] and in T2DM vs. T1DM participants [59]. Of note, increased central adiposity and BP were the common independent determinants of increased arterial stiffness estimates in both youngsters with T1DM or T2DM [59].

In an earlier review [9] we concluded that, in T2DM, arterial stiffening is an early phenomenon because it already occurs in impaired glucose metabolism (IGM) (i.e., impaired fasting glucose (IFG) and/or impaired glucose tolerance (IGT)) or prediabetic states, as also supported by the MetS-arterial stiffness relationships reviewed above. More recent studies have basically confirmed this concept. For example, in a treatment-naïve and mostly 'healthy' population from the ADDITION-Leicester cohort, cfPWV was increased, to a similar extent, in individuals with IFG or IGT as compared with those with normal glucose metabolism (NGM), though 2 h-post-challenge glucose was slightly more strongly associated with cfPWV than fasting plasma glucose (FPG) levels. Moreover, the increased arterial stiffness in subjects with IGM was indistinguishable from that of individuals with newly diagnosed T2DM [60]. On the other hand, in a large cohort study among Chinese individuals who did not have history of hypertension, T2DM or CVD and were free of BP-, glucose- and/or lipid-lowering medication, arterial stiffness increased gradually across NGM, isolated IFG, IGT (including those with both IFG and IGT) and newly diagnosed T2DM individuals in age and sex-adjusted analyses; after adjustments for BP and other traditional cardiovascular RFs, only individuals with IGT and T2DM had greater levels of baPWV than those with NGM [61]. However, in another large study including a random sample of Chinese men and women without known T2DM from the *Guangzhou Biobank Study*, baPWV did not differ significantly between subjects with isolated IFG vs. isolated IGT [62], although it was significantly higher in these individuals vs. those with NGM. In addition, even within the normal range, any increase in FPG is associated with higher baPWV [63]. Taken together, these findings indicate that accelerated arterial stiffening remains a hallmark of increasing impaired glucose metabolism but stress that the sole use of FPG may not be sufficient to identify all individuals who may already be at higher risk and may benefit from timely targeted interventions. It should be noted that the evidence thus far supporting the notion of accelerated arterial ageing has derived exclusively from cross-sectional studies because prospective studies comparing the course of arterial stiffness among individuals with vs. without T2DM (or IGM) are lacking.

We have described that increased arterial stiffness often occurs before the onset of clinically overt micro- or macrovascular disease [9]. Recent studies, particularly those among the young, seem to confirm this [58, 59]. In addition, we have also described that, in both T1DM and T2DM, the presence of microvascular (i.e. (micro)albuminuria and/or retinopathy) and macrovascular complications seems to be accompanied by further increases in arterial stiffness [9]. This was confirmed by recent cross-sectional studies comprising larger groups of patients with T1DM from the *FinnDiane Study* [64] or attending the *Steno Diabetes Center* [65] and with T2DM from the *Taichung Community Health Study* [66]. It remains not completely clear whether increased arterial stiffness is a cause (because greater arterial stiffness is associated with greater pressures in small arteries and capillaries) or a consequence (because microvascular drop-out will increase wave reflection and thus increase stiffness) of microangiopathy or, alternatively, that both phenomena derive from a common antecedent (e.g. endothelial dysfunction or inflammation). A recent observational cohort study demonstrated, for the first time, that aortic stiffness predicted incident albuminuria and decline in renal function (as estimated by glomerular filtration rate), independent of other covariates, in patients with T2DM [67]. Still, the extent to which targeting decreases in arterial stiffness in subjects with (pre)diabetes will ameliorate micro- and macrovascular outcome is not known and needs to be further investigated.

Pathobiological Mechanisms Linking Central Obesity, Metabolic Syndrome and Diabetes to Arterial Stiffening

The adverse association of the critical axis *central obesity – MetS – (pre)diabetes* with arterial stiffness raises important questions about the potential underlying pathological processes. These may include some of the effects central obesity and related insulin resistance are known to exert at the vascular wall level, such as endothelial dysfunction, inflammatory reaction and sympathetic activation. These abnormalities are interrelated and affect vascular tone and stimulate vascular smooth muscle cell proliferation. In addition, changes in the type or structure of elastin and/or collagen in the arterial wall due to hyperglycaemia, particularly the formation of cross-links through nonenzymatic glycosylation of proteins that generate advanced glycation end products, could constitute another mechanism. Several of these putative mediators are likely to increase arterial stiffness. However, currently, we have only fragments of insight regarding the likely myriad of players involved. Teasing apart their (measurable) individual contribution and/or identification of predominant operative pathways may provide key information for tailored interventions aiming at the prevention of arterial stiffening and related cardiovascular *sequelae*. A comprehensive analysis of these issues in the context of a prospective cohort study is still lacking and thus most warranted.

Smoking and Arterial Stiffness

Acute increases in arterial stiffness shortly after smoking have been consistently reported in experimental settings, but the *chronic* effects of smoking on arterial stiffness have been less consistent in earlier studies (those published up to 2005 are reviewed in [8]). The absence of deleterious chronic effects of habitual smoking in earlier studies may have been due to several reasons: first, the cross-sectional designs and self-reported ascertainment of smoking status without verification by biological measures such as salivary or urinary cotinine levels, most often comparing stiffness levels between individuals categorized as current smokers vs. nonsmokers. This may have diluted any differences because the latter could still have included a considerable portion of current smokers (misclassified by socially desirable answers in self-reports) and/or ex-smokers and the former not distinguished by the duration and intensity of smoking. Even when smoking *history* was analysed, for instance, by comparing current, former and never-smokers, such studies were still hampered by the limitations of retrospective assessments, which are more susceptible to misclassification; measures of lifelong exposure to smoking such as pack-years also do not discern duration from intensity. Second, the small study samples and number of smokers included in earlier studies may have limited the power of the analyses. In addition, insufficient account for confounding by other lifestyle RFs, such as physical activity and energy intake (namely, from alcohol consumption), and/or overadjustment for body weight and/or heart rate that may mediate any association between smoking and arterial stiffness could also have blurred and explained, at least in part, the inconsistent findings.

A more recent large study among individuals (18–80 years old) referred for their hypertension status but who had never been treated for it compared the arterial stiffness levels between current ($n=268$), never ($n=150$) and former ($n=136$) smokers and among the latter, investigated the relation of years since smoking cessation with arterial stiffness [68]. Current and ex-smokers for only 1 year had higher cfPWV and augmentation index (AIx) as compared with nonsmokers. Notably, among ex-smokers, the duration of smoking cessation was linearly and favourably associated with cfPWV and AIx, such that after one decade of smoking cessation, cfPWV and AIx levels were estimated to have returned to levels comparable with those who had never smoked [68]. These findings were in agreement with those observed in a younger cohort of apparently healthy adults from *The Bogalusa Heart Study* showing arterial stiffness and systemic vascular resistance after 10 years of smoking cessation that were comparable to never-smokers [69]. Although cross-sectional in nature and dependent on self-reports, these studies supported the view of potential improvement in arterial wall dynamics after long-term smoking cessation. Nevertheless, 'the jury was still out' on the impact of chronic smoking on arterial stiffness in a systematic review published in 2010 as many studies still reported no differences in arterial stiffness between (long-term) smokers and nonsmokers [70].

Recently, in a population-based cohort (*The Northern Ireland Young Heart Project*) with measures of arterial stiffness in young adults whose smoking status was ascertained, prospectively, during adolescence (at the age of 15) and again during young adulthood (between the ages of 20 and 25), we reported that young adults who smoked during adolescence had higher levels of aortoiliac PVW in adulthood despite that such differences were not evident between current vs. nonsmokers in adulthood (Fig. 33.3a) [5]. After cross-tabulation of smoking status in adolescence and adulthood, we observed that persistent smokers, but not starters or quitters, had higher aortoiliac PWV in adulthood than never-smokers (Fig. 33.3b). These findings illustrate the importance of lifelong and prospective RF exposure assessment as a means to better unveil the impact of smoking on arterial stiffness (otherwise missed by cross-sectional ascertainment of current smoking status as simply yes/no or by retrospective assessment of ever smoking). They also support the view of adolescence as a critical period for the initiation of smoking and thus when preventive measures may need to be more aggressive, as most adolescents who smoked persisted doing so in adulthood (80 %). The observation that those who discontinued smoking between adolescence and young adulthood seem to have arterial stiffness comparable to those who never smoked also supported the potential for reversibility of arterial stiffness by quitting smoking.

Another recent large 6-year longitudinal study examining the effects of changes in smoking status and intensity on the rate of progression of arterial stiffness (baPWV) with ageing showed that this was steeper among continuous (heavy) smokers than those who never smoked before and during the follow-up [71]. Notably, rates of arterial stiffening were similar among quitters and never-smokers. In contrast, a 2-year longitudinal study did not show any such beneficial effects of smoking cessation on carotid or femoral stiffness [72]. The small group of quitters and, perhaps more importantly, the short follow-up duration of this study seem to suggest that smoking cessation may need to be sustained for a longer period to be favourably reflected in clinically relevant arterial adaptations. Alternatively, short-term benefits of smoking cessation on arterial stiffness may already be evident among those who were long-term heavy smokers [73], rather than among any former and eventually 'lighter' smokers.

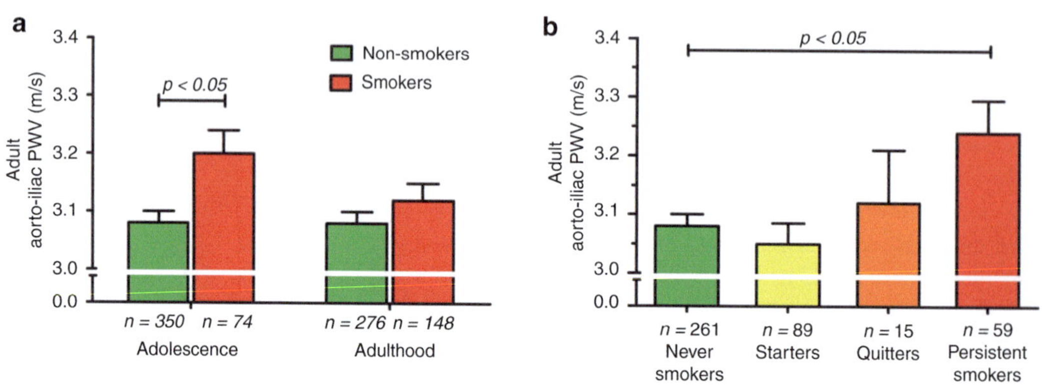

Fig. 33.3 Comparison among young adults from the *Northern Ireland Young Hearts Project* of levels of aortoiliac pulse wave velocity (*PWV*): (**a**) between smokers and nonsmokers in adolescence and in young adulthood (data are adjusted for sex, adult age, body height, social class, mean arterial pressure and other lifestyle variables (i.e. alcohol consumption, energy intake and habitual physical activity)); (**b**) between never-smokers, starters, quitters and persistent smokers (data are adjusted for sex, adult age, body height, social class and mean arterial pressure and changes in other lifestyle variables (i.e. alcohol consumption, energy intake and habitual physical activity)). *Error bars* indicate the standard errors of the means. Reproduced from van de Laar et al. [5] with permission from Wolters Kluwer Health

Pathobiological Mechanisms Linking Smoking to Arterial Stiffening

The underlying pathobiological mechanisms explaining smoking-related arterial stiffening are complex and remain unclear. Traditionally, BP was not seen as a likely culprit because never and ex-smokers tend to have higher BP than smokers, at least as assessed at the brachial artery. However, smokers may have higher central BP [74] and smoking cessation may decrease this and thus central arterial stiffness in particular [75]. Also, because every act of smoking may lead to acute increases in BP, a 20-cigarettes/day smoker may in effect have a higher BP than a nonsmoker during most of the day. Cigarette smoke contains many vasoactive substances of which nicotine and free radicals, but seemingly less so carbon monoxide, are associated with vascular dysfunction; their impact on the vasculature is thought to occur in part through 'downstream' pathways, such as inflammation and endothelial dysfunction. Indeed, nicotine decreases the bioavailability of nitric oxide, downregulates endothelial nitric oxide synthesis, decreases endothelium-dependent vasodilatation and stimulates both adhesion of leukocytes to the endothelial layer and the release of catecholamine. Free-radical-mediated oxidative stress may also explain, to a large extent, smoking-related endothelial dysfunction, inflammation, increased platelet reactivity and reduced fibrinolysis. However, the increased arterial stiffness observed among persistent smokers did not seem to be explained by their higher levels of inflammation and/or endothelial dysfunction [5, 71]. Possibly, sympathetic activation, oxidative stress and production of oxidized LDL may play a more predominant role, but the links explaining the smoking-arterial stiffness relationship still need to be fully unravelled.

Summary

In this chapter, we have reviewed the evidence pertaining to several cardiovascular RFs other than age(ing) and BP as determinants of arterial stiffness, specifically, central obesity, the MetS, diabetes and smoking. Reinforced by recent prospective data, there is convincing evidence that all these RFs increase arterial stiffness, a mechanism that may explain the associated higher CVD risk. There is still relatively few data on the molecular basis of greater arterial stiffness associated with these RFs, the prognostic significance of arterial stiffness indices in individuals with these RFs and the extent to which intervention on these RFs improves cardiovascular outcome through beneficial impact on arterial stiffness. Given the high and increasing prevalence of these RFs, particularly obesity, the MetS and diabetes, these issues constitute an important research agenda.

References

1. Ferreira I, van de Laar RJ, Prins MH, Twisk JW, Stehouwer CD. Carotid stiffness in young adults: a life-course analysis of its early determinants: the Amsterdam Growth and Health Longitudinal Study. Hypertension. 2012;59(1):54–61.
2. Cecelja M, Chowienczyk P. Dissociation of aortic pulse wave velocity with risk factors for cardiovascular disease other than hypertension: a systematic review. Hypertension. 2009;54(6):1328–36.
3. Abdullah A, Wolfe R, Mannan H, Stoelwinder JU, Stevenson C, Peeters A. Epidemiologic merit of obese-years, the combination of degree and duration of obesity. Am J Epidemiol. 2012;176(2):99–107.
4. van de Laar RJ, Ferreira I, van Mechelen W, Prins MH, Twisk JW, Stehouwer CD. Lifetime vigorous but not light-to-moderate habitual physical activity impacts favorably on carotid stiffness in young adults: the Amsterdam Growth and Health Longitudinal Study. Hypertension. 2010;55(1):33–9.
5. van de Laar RJ, Stehouwer CD, Boreham CA, Murray LM, Schalkwijk CG, Prins MH, et al. Continuing smoking between adolescence and young adulthood is associated with higher arterial stiffness in young adults: the Northern Ireland Young Hearts Project. J Hypertens. 2011;29(11):2201–9.
6. van de Laar RJ, Stehouwer CD, van Bussel BC, te Velde SJ, Prins MH, Twisk JW, et al. Lower lifetime dietary fiber intake is associated with carotid artery stiffness: the Amsterdam Growth and Health Longitudinal Study. Am J Clin Nutr. 2012;96(1): 14–23.
7. Aatola H, Hutri-Kahonen N, Juonala M, Viikari JS, Hulkkonen J, Laitinen T, et al. Lifetime risk factors and arterial pulse wave velocity in adulthood: the

Cardiovascular Risk in Young Finns Study. Hypertension. 2010;55(3):806–11.
8. Stehouwer CD, Ferreira I. Diabetes, lipids and other cardiovascular risk factors. In: Safar ME, O'Rourke MF, editors. Arterial stiffness in hypertension, Handbook of Hypertension, vol. 23. Amsterdam: Elsevier; 2006. p. 427–56.
9. Stehouwer CD, Henry RM, Ferreira I. Arterial stiffness in diabetes and the metabolic syndrome: a pathway to cardiovascular disease. Diabetologia. 2008;51(4):527–39.
10. Seals DR, Gates PE. Stiffening our resolve against adult weight gain. Hypertension. 2005;45(2):175–7.
11. Wildman RP, Mackey RH, Bostom A, Thompson T, Sutton-Tyrrell K. Measures of obesity are associated with vascular stiffness in young and older adults. Hypertension. 2003;42(4):468–73.
12. Scuteri A, Orru M, Morrell CH, Tarasov K, Schlessinger D, Uda M, et al. Associations of large artery structure and function with adiposity: effects of age, gender, and hypertension. The SardiNIA Study. Atherosclerosis. 2012;221(1):189–97.
13. Whincup PH, Gilg JA, Donald AE, Katterhorn M, Oliver C, Cook DG, et al. Arterial distensibility in adolescents: the influence of adiposity, the metabolic syndrome, and classic risk factors. Circulation. 2005;112(12):1789–97.
14. Geerts CC, Evelein AM, Bots ML, van der Ent CK, Grobbee DE, Uiterwaal CS. Body fat distribution and early arterial changes in healthy 5-year-old children. Ann Med. 2012;44(4):350–9.
15. Sakuragi S, Abhayaratna K, Gravenmaker KJ, O'Reilly C, Srikusalanukul W, Budge MM, et al. Influence of adiposity and physical activity on arterial stiffness in healthy children: the lifestyle of our kids study. Hypertension. 2009;53(4):611–6.
16. Urbina EM, Kimball TR, Khoury PR, Daniels SR, Dolan LM. Increased arterial stiffness is found in adolescents with obesity or obesity-related type 2 diabetes mellitus. J Hypertens. 2010;28(8):1692–8.
17. Aggoun Y, Farpour-Lambert NJ, Marchand LM, Golay E, Maggio AB, Beghetti M. Impaired endothelial and smooth muscle functions and arterial stiffness appear before puberty in obese children and are associated with elevated ambulatory blood pressure. Eur Heart J. 2008;29(6):792–9.
18. Ferreira I, Snijder MB, Twisk JW, van Mechelen W, Kemper HC, Seidell JC, et al. Central fat mass versus peripheral fat and lean mass: opposite (adverse versus favorable) associations with arterial stiffness? The Amsterdam Growth and Health Longitudinal Study. J Clin Endocrinol Metab. 2004;89(6):2632–9.
19. Snijder MB, Henry RM, Visser M, Dekker JM, Seidell JC, Ferreira I, et al. Regional body composition as a determinant of arterial stiffness in the elderly: the Hoorn Study. J Hypertens. 2004;22(12):2339–47.
20. Sutton-Tyrrell K, Newman A, Simonsick EM, Havlik R, Pahor M, Lakatta E, et al. Aortic stiffness is associated with visceral adiposity in older adults enrolled in the study of health, aging, and body composition. Hypertension. 2001;38(3):429–33.
21. Johansen NB, Vistisen D, Brunner EJ, Tabak AG, Shipley MJ, Wilkinson IB, et al. Determinants of aortic stiffness: 16-year follow-up of the Whitehall II study. PLoS One. 2012;7(5):e37165.
22. Birru MS, Matthews KA, Thurston RC, Brooks MM, Ibrahim S, Barinas-Mitchell E, et al. African-American ethnicity and cardiovascular risk factors are related to aortic pulse-wave velocity progression. Am J Hypertens. 2011;24(7):809–15.
23. Wildman RP, Farhat GN, Patel AS, Mackey RH, Brockwell S, Thompson T, et al. Weight change is associated with change in arterial stiffness among healthy young adults. Hypertension. 2005;45(2):187–92.
24. Yamada J, Tomiyama H, Matsumoto C, Yoshida M, Koji Y, Shiina K, et al. Overweight body mass index classification modifies arterial stiffening associated with weight gain in healthy middle-aged Japanese men. Hypertens Res. 2008;31(6):1087–92.
25. Rider OJ, Tayal U, Francis JM, Ali MK, Robinson MR, Byrne JP, et al. The effect of obesity and weight loss on aortic pulse wave velocity as assessed by magnetic resonance imaging. Obesity (Silver Spring). 2010;18(12):2311–6.
26. Barinas-Mitchell E, Kuller LH, Sutton-Tyrrell K, Hegazi R, Harper P, Mancino J, et al. Effect of weight loss and nutritional intervention on arterial stiffness in type 2 diabetes. Diabetes Care. 2006;29(10):2218–22.
27. Dengo AL, Dennis EA, Orr JS, Marinik EL, Ehrlich E, Davy BM, et al. Arterial destiffening with weight loss in overweight and obese middle-aged and older adults. Hypertension. 2010;55(4):855–61.
28. Blumenthal JA, Babyak MA, Hinderliter A, Watkins LL, Craighead L, Lin PH, et al. Effects of the DASH diet alone and in combination with exercise and weight loss on blood pressure and cardiovascular biomarkers in men and women with high blood pressure: the ENCORE study. Arch Intern Med. 2010;170(2):126–35.
29. Cooper JN, Buchanich JM, Youk A, Brooks MM, Barinas-Mitchell E, Conroy MB, et al. Reductions in arterial stiffness with weight loss in overweight and obese young adults: potential mechanisms. Atherosclerosis. 2012;223(2):485–90.
30. Orr JS, Gentile CL, Davy BM, Davy KP. Large artery stiffening with weight gain in humans: role of visceral fat accumulation. Hypertension. 2008;51(6):1519–24.
31. Kim BJ, Kim BS, Kang JH. Echocardiographic epicardial fat thickness is associated with arterial stiffness. Int J Cardiol. 2013;167(5):2234–8.
32. Natale F, Tedesco MA, Mocerino R, de Simone V, Di Marco GM, Aronne L, et al. Visceral adiposity and arterial stiffness: echocardiographic epicardial fat thickness reflects, better than waist circumference, carotid arterial stiffness in a large population of hypertensives. Eur J Echocardiogr. 2009;10(4):549–55.
33. Huang Y, Bi Y, Xu M, Ma Z, Xu Y, Wang T, et al. Nonalcoholic fatty liver disease is associated with atherosclerosis in middle-aged and elderly Chinese. Arterioscler Thromb Vasc Biol. 2012;32(9):2321–6.

34. Salvi P, Ruffini R, Agnoletti D, Magnani E, Pagliarani G, Comandini G, et al. Increased arterial stiffness in nonalcoholic fatty liver disease: the Cardio-GOOSE study. J Hypertens. 2010;28(8):1699–707.
35. Lee M, Choh AC, Demerath EW, Towne B, Siervogel RM, Czerwinski SA. Associations between trunk, leg and total body adiposity with arterial stiffness. Am J Hypertens. 2012;25(10):1131–7.
36. Schouten F, Twisk JW, de Boer MR, Stehouwer CD, Serne EH, Smulders YM, et al. Increases in central fat mass and decreases in peripheral fat mass are associated with accelerated arterial stiffening in healthy adults: the Amsterdam Growth and Health Longitudinal Study. Am J Clin Nutr. 2011;94(1):40–8.
37. Ochi M, Kohara K, Tabara Y, Kido T, Uetani E, Ochi N, et al. Arterial stiffness is associated with low thigh muscle mass in middle-aged to elderly men. Atherosclerosis. 2010;212(1):327–32.
38. Kim TN, Park MS, Lim KI, Yang SJ, Yoo HJ, Kang HJ, et al. Skeletal muscle mass to visceral fat area ratio is associated with metabolic syndrome and arterial stiffness: the Korean Sarcopenic Obesity Study (KSOS). Diabetes Res Clin Pract. 2011;93(2):285–91.
39. Kohara K, Ochi M, Tabara Y, Nagai T, Igase M, Miki T. Arterial stiffness in sarcopenic visceral obesity in the elderly: J-SHIPP study. Int J Cardiol. 2012;158(1):146–8.
40. Prado CM, Wells JC, Smith SR, Stephan BC, Siervo M. Sarcopenic obesity: A Critical appraisal of the current evidence. Clin Nutr. 2012;31(5):583–601.
41. Abbatecola AM, Chiodini P, Gallo C, Lakatta E, Sutton-Tyrrell K, Tylavsky FA, et al. Pulse wave velocity is associated with muscle mass decline: Health ABC study. Age (Dordr). 2012;34(2):469–78.
42. Scuteri A, Najjar SS, Orru M, Usala G, Piras MG, Ferrucci L, et al. The central arterial burden of the metabolic syndrome is similar in men and women: the SardiNIA study. Eur Heart J. 2010;31(5):602–13.
43. Iannuzzi A, Licenziati MR, Acampora C, Renis M, Agrusta M, Romano L, et al. Carotid artery stiffness in obese children with the metabolic syndrome. Am J Cardiol. 2006;97(4):528–31.
44. Pandit D, Chiplonkar S, Khadilkar A, Kinare A, Khadilkar V. Efficacy of a continuous metabolic syndrome score in Indian children for detecting subclinical atherosclerotic risk. Int J Obes (Lond). 2011;35(10):1318–24.
45. Ferreira I, Henry RM, Twisk JW, van Mechelen W, Kemper HC, Stehouwer CD. The metabolic syndrome, cardiopulmonary fitness, and subcutaneous trunk fat as independent determinants of arterial stiffness: the Amsterdam Growth and Health Longitudinal Study. Arch Intern Med. 2005;165(8):875–82.
46. Li S, Chen W, Srinivasan SR, Berenson GS. Influence of metabolic syndrome on arterial stiffness and its age-related change in young adults: the Bogalusa Heart Study. Atherosclerosis. 2005;180(2):349–54.
47. Koskinen J, Magnussen CG, Viikari JS, Kahonen M, Laitinen T, Hutri-Kahonen N, et al. Effect of age, gender and cardiovascular risk factors on carotid distensibility during 6-year follow-up. The Cardiovascular Risk in Young Finns study. Atherosclerosis. 2012;224(2):474–9.
48. Della-Morte D, Gardener H, Denaro F, Boden-Albala B, Elkind MS, Paik MC, et al. Metabolic syndrome increases carotid artery stiffness: the Northern Manhattan Study. Int J Stroke. 2010;5(3):138–44.
49. Protogerou AD, Blacher J, Aslangul E, Le Jeunne C, Lekakis J, Mavrikakis M, et al. Gender influence on metabolic syndrome's effects on arterial stiffness and pressure wave reflections in treated hypertensive subjects. Atherosclerosis. 2007;193(1):151–8.
50. Schillaci G, Pirro M, Vaudo G, Mannarino MR, Savarese G, Pucci G, et al. Metabolic syndrome is associated with aortic stiffness in untreated essential hypertension. Hypertension. 2005;45(6):1078–82.
51. Koivistoinen T, Hutri-Kahonen N, Juonala M, Aatola H, Koobi T, Lehtimaki T, et al. Metabolic syndrome in childhood and increased arterial stiffness in adulthood: the Cardiovascular Risk In Young Finns Study. Ann Med. 2011;43(4):312–9.
52. Nakanishi N, Suzuki K, Tatara K. Clustered features of the metabolic syndrome and the risk for increased aortic pulse wave velocity in middle-aged Japanese men. Angiology. 2003;54(5):551–9.
53. Safar ME, Thomas F, Blacher J, Nzietchueng R, Bureau JM, Pannier B, et al. Metabolic syndrome and age-related progression of aortic stiffness. J Am Coll Cardiol. 2006;47(1):72–5.
54. Li CI, Kardia SL, Liu CS, Lin WY, Lin CH, Lee YD, et al. Metabolic syndrome is associated with change in subclinical arterial stiffness: a community-based Taichung Community Health Study. BMC Public Health. 2011;11:808.
55. Ferreira I, Beijers HJ, Schouten F, Smulders YM, Twisk JW, Stehouwer CD. Clustering of metabolic syndrome traits is associated with maladaptive carotid remodeling and stiffening: a 6-year longitudinal study. Hypertension. 2012;60(2):542–9.
56. Tomiyama H, Hirayama Y, Hashimoto H, Yambe M, Yamada J, Koji Y, et al. The effects of changes in the metabolic syndrome detection status on arterial stiffening: a prospective study. Hypertens Res. 2006;29(9):673–8.
57. Guize L, Thomas F, Pannier B, Bean K, Jego B, Benetos A. All-cause mortality associated with specific combinations of the metabolic syndrome according to recent definitions. Diabetes Care. 2007;30(9):2381–7.
58. Urbina EM, Wadwa RP, Davis C, Snively BM, Dolan LM, Daniels SR, et al. Prevalence of increased arterial stiffness in children with type 1 diabetes mellitus differs by measurement site and sex: the SEARCH for Diabetes in Youth Study. J Pediatr. 2010;156(5):731–7, 7.e1.
59. Wadwa RP, Urbina EM, Anderson AM, Hamman RF, Dolan LM, Rodriguez BL, et al. Measures of arterial stiffness in youth with type 1 and type 2 diabetes: the SEARCH for Diabetes in Youth Study. Diabetes Care. 2010;33(4):881–6.
60. Webb DR, Khunti K, Silverman R, Gray LJ, Srinivasan B, Lacy PS, et al. Impact of metabolic indices on central artery stiffness: independent association

of insulin resistance and glucose with aortic pulse wave velocity. Diabetologia. 2010;53(6):1190–8.

61. Li CH, Wu JS, Yang YC, Shih CC, Lu FH, Chang CJ. Increased arterial stiffness in subjects with impaired glucose tolerance and newly diagnosed diabetes but not isolated impaired fasting glucose. J Clin Endocrinol Metab. 2012;97(4):E658–62.
62. Xu L, Jiang CQ, Lam TH, Cheng KK, Yue XJ, Lin JM, et al. Impact of impaired fasting glucose and impaired glucose tolerance on arterial stiffness in an older Chinese population: the Guangzhou Biobank Cohort Study-CVD. Metabolism. 2010;59(3):367–72.
63. Shin JY, Lee HR, Lee DC. Increased arterial stiffness in healthy subjects with high-normal glucose levels and in subjects with pre-diabetes. Cardiovasc Diabetol. 2011;10:30.
64. Gordin D, Waden J, Forsblom C, Thorn LM, Rosengard-Barlund M, Heikkila O, et al. Arterial stiffness and vascular complications in patients with type 1 diabetes: the Finnish Diabetic Nephropathy (FinnDiane) Study. Ann Med. 2012;44(2):196–204.
65. Theilade S, Lajer M, Persson F, Joergensen C, Rossing P. Arterial stiffness is associated with cardiovascular, renal, retinal, and autonomic disease in type 1 diabetes. Diabetes Care. 2013;36(3):715–21.
66. Liu CS, Pi-Sunyer FX, Li CI, Davidson LE, Li TC, Chen W, et al. Albuminuria is strongly associated with arterial stiffness, especially in diabetic or hypertensive subjects – a population-based study (Taichung Community Health Study, TCHS). Atherosclerosis. 2010;211(1):315–21.
67. Bouchi R, Babazono T, Mugishima M, Yoshida N, Nyumura I, Toya K, et al. Arterial stiffness is associated with incident albuminuria and decreased glomerular filtration rate in type 2 diabetic patients. Diabetes Care. 2011;34(12):2570–5.
68. Jatoi NA, Jerrard-Dunne P, Feely J, Mahmud A. Impact of smoking and smoking cessation on arterial stiffness and aortic wave reflection in hypertension. Hypertension. 2007;49(5):981–5.
69. Li H, Srinivasan SR, Berenson GS. Comparison of the measures of pulsatile arterial function between asymptomatic younger adult smokers and former smokers: the Bogalusa Heart Study. Am J Hypertens. 2006;19(9):897–901.
70. Doonan RJ, Hausvater A, Scallan C, Mikhailidis DP, Pilote L, Daskalopoulou SS. The effect of smoking on arterial stiffness. Hypertens Res. 2010;33(5):398–410.
71. Tomiyama H, Hashimoto H, Tanaka H, Matsumoto C, Odaira M, Yamada J, et al. Continuous smoking and progression of arterial stiffening: a prospective study. J Am Coll Cardiol. 2010;55(18):1979–87.
72. van den Berkmortel FW, Wollersheim H, van Langen H, Smilde TJ, den Arend J, Thien T. Two years of smoking cessation does not reduce arterial wall thickness and stiffness. Neth J Med. 2004;62(7):235–41.
73. Polonia J, Barbosa L, Silva JA, Rosas M. Improvement of aortic reflection wave responses 6 months after stopping smoking: a prospective study. Blood Press Monit. 2009;14(2):69–75.
74. Tabara Y, Takahashi Y, Setoh K, Muro S, Kawaguchi T, Terao C, et al. Increased aortic wave reflection and smaller pulse pressure amplification in smokers and passive smokers confirmed by urinary cotinine levels: the Nagahama Study. Int J Cardiol. 2013;168(3):2673–7.
75. Takami T, Saito Y. Effects of smoking cessation on central blood pressure and arterial stiffness. Vasc Health Risk Manag. 2011;7:633–8.

Glucose, Insulin and Potential Strategies of Vascular Stiffening

34

Guanghong Jia, Annayya R. Aroor, Gerald A. Meininger, and James R. Sowers

Abstract

Hyperglycemia and hyperinsulinemia which are independent risk factors for vascular stiffening and diabetic vasculopathy are present in most patients with Type 2 diabetes mellitus. In this review we discuss these factors which promote vascular stiffness. We also discuss the roles of renin- angiotensin II -aldosterone (RAAS) activation, obesity, hypertension, dyslipidemia and insulin resistance, features which often present in the CardioRenal metabolic syndrome. Here, we provide new insights in the pathogenesis of vascular stiffening induced by RAAS, including the dysfunction of vascular smooth muscle cells and endothelial cells; inflammation, oxidation stress, as well as alterations in collagen and elastin. We also introduce a novel concept where both β1-integrin and α-smooth muscle actin are likely major players in the increased vascular stiffening as ascertained by atomic force microscopy technology. We explore therapies such as estrogens aimed at vascular de-stiffening which may improve vascular function in patients. This review highlights recent evidence supporting the role of RAAS and insulin resistance in the development of vascular stiffening in diabetic patients.

G. Jia, PhD • A.R. Aroor, MD, PhD
Research Service Harry S Truman Memorial Veterans Hospital, Research Service, 800 Hospital Dr, Columbia, MO 65212, USA

Division of Endocrinology and Metabolism, Department of Medicine, University of Missouri School of Medicine, Columbia, MO 65212, USA
e-mail: jiag@health.missouri.edu; Aroora@health.missouri.edu

G.A. Meininger, PhD
Dalton Cardiovascular Research Center, University of Missouri School of Medicine, 134 Research Park Drive, Columbia, MO 65211, USA

Department of Medical Pharmacology and Physiology, University of Missouri School of Medicine, MA415 Medical Sciences Building, One Hospital Drive, Columbia, MO 65212, USA
e-mail: meiningerg@missouri.edu

J.R. Sowers, MD (✉)
Division of Endocrinology and Metabolism, Department of Medicine, University of Missouri School of Medicine, Columbia, MO 65212, USA

Research Service Harry S Truman Memorial Veterans Hospital, 800 Hospital Dr, Columbia, MO 65201, USA

Department of Medical Pharmacology and Physiology, University of Missouri School of Medicine, MA415 Medical Sciences Building, One Hospital Drive, Columbia, MO 65212, USA

Dalton Cardiovascular Research Center, University of Missouri School of Medicine, 134 Research Park Drive, Columbia, MO 65211, USA
e-mail: sowersj@health.missouri.edu

M.E. Safar et al. (eds.), *Blood Pressure and Arterial Wall Mechanics in Cardiovascular Diseases*, DOI 10.1007/978-1-4471-5198-2_34, © Springer-Verlag London 2014

Keywords
Cardiorenal • Hyperglycemia • Insulin resistance • Vascular stiffening • Vascular smooth muscle cells • Endothelial cells • Angiotensin II • Aldosterone • Inflammation • Oxidative stress

Introduction

Increased vascular stiffness and associated lower vascular elasticity is a major contributor to hypertension and cardiovascular disease (CVD) [1–3]. Obesity, diabetes, hypertension, kidney disease, and aging are conditions that predispose to vascular stiffening [1–11]. Measurements of arterial stiffness include central pulse pressure/stroke volume index, pulse wave velocity (PWV), total arterial compliance, pulse pressure amplification, and augmentation index. Increasingly, these measurements, especially PWV, are used in assessing overall CVD risk in various populations [1–11]. Accordingly, heart contraction generates a PWV that travels through the circulation. The stiffness of the arteries affects the speed of travel or velocity of this PWV. Typical values of PWV in the aorta range from approximately 5 m/s to >15 m/s [1]. A fixed threshold value (12 m/s) was proposed as arterial stiffness in the 2007 European Society of Hypertension (ESH)/European Society of Cardiology (ESC) hypertension guidelines based on published epidemiological studies [3]. When the vasculature stiffens, the PWV increase is then reflected in the heart at the end of systole instead of diastole and causes augmentation of systolic blood pressure and pulse pressure, and therefore hypertension and increased cardiac afterload [2].

Epidemiological studies demonstrate that hyperglycemia and hyperinsulinemia/insulin resistance are independent risk factors for vascular stiffening and other elements of diabetic vasculopathy. Previous studies from diabetic patients have reported that a higher PWV is associated with increased arterial stiffness or lower arterial compliance compared with non-diabetic controls, and that increased plasma insulin correlates with the increase in stiffness and decreased compliance of the arteries [3–7]. A cross-sectional study of the relation of arterial stiffness indexes with glucose tolerance and serum insulin from a biracial sample of 4,701 men and women aged 45–64 at risk for atherosclerosis showed that persons with borderline abnormal glucose intolerance or noninsulin-dependent diabetes mellitus (NIDDM) had stiffer arteries than their counterparts with normal glucose tolerance and decreased elasticity was independent of artery wall thickness [8]. It was suggested that the integrative effects of elevated glucose, insulin, and triglycerides may have a considerable impact on arterial stiffness and play an important role in the early pathophysiology of macrovascular disease in patients with type 2 diabetes [8]. Vascular stiffening has been observed in all age groups of individuals with the cardiorenal metabolic syndrome (CRS) and those with clinical diabetes, including children. Indeed, these obese children prematurely manifest signs of vascular stiffening [9]. In individuals 40 years and older, multiple logistic and linear regression analyses from a total of 2,188 individuals demonstrated that arterial stiffness was independently associated with insulin resistance in middle-aged adults [10]. In elderly people without diabetes mellitus, the Rotterdam study found that impaired fasting glucose was associated with increased arterial stiffness [11]. Therefore, a deeper understanding of the mechanisms of vascular stiffening in obesity, hyperglycemia and hyperinsulinemia has great clinical significance. In the present review, we will focus on recent studies examining the pathophysiological processes by which vascular stiffening contributes to CVD, as well as the contemporary understanding of potential therapeutic strategies.

Endothelial Dysfunction in Vascular Stiffening

The endothelium is a critical component to vascular homeostasis, actively responding to biochemical and physical stimuli through the release of a diverse set of vasoactive substances [12]. The term "endothelial dysfunction" refers to a maladapted endothelial phenotype characterized by reduced nitric oxide (NO) bioavailability, increased oxidative stress, elevated expression of pro-inflammatory and pro-thrombotic factors, and reduced endothelial derived vasodilation [13]. It has been proposed that endothelial dysfunction is one of the first steps toward overt vascular stiffening.

Hyperglycemia is a contributor to endothelial dysfunction and is an early predictor of CVD, particularly coronary artery disease and stroke [14]. Studies have shown that elevated glucose concentration may activate the tissue renin–angiotensin system (RAS) and this plays an important role in the pathogenesis of the vascular complications of diabetes [15, 16]. *In vivo* exposure of healthy human subjects to an acute glucose load leads to attenuated endothelium-dependent vascular relaxation [17]. This impaired endothelial relaxation is associated with increased oxidative stress, adhesion molecule expression, vascular permeability, and plasma levels of plasminogen activator inhibitor-1 [17]. *In vitro*, both high glucose and angiotensin II (Ang II) induced a progressive increase in Ang II receptor type 1 receptor 1 (AT-1R) expression on the cultured human endothelial cells (EC). Furthermore, high glucose enhanced Ang II-mediated peroxisome proliferation-activated receptor-γ inactivation and expression of pro-inflammatory adhesion molecules via signaling through the AT-1R [18]. With chronic exposure to elevated plasma glucose, the resulting glucotoxicity may stimulate mitogen activated protein kinase (MAPK) thus increasing the secretion of inflammatory cytokines and inhibiting phosphatidylinositol 3-kinase (PI3K)/protein kinase B (Akt) signaling leading to reduced NO production and endothelial dysfunction.

Insulin resistance and resulting hyperinsulinemia are frequently present in obesity, hypertension, coronary artery disease, dyslipidemias, the CRS and type 2 diabetes [19]. Insulin metabolic signaling is an important contributor to normal vascular function and homeostasis. In this regard, insulin stimulates production of the vasodilator NO via activation of insulin receptor substrate (IRS)-1/PI3K signaling in endothelial cells. In contrast, insulin stimulates production of the vasoconstrictor endothelin-1 (ET-1) via a MAPK-dependent signaling pathway [20]. Indeed, endothelial insulin resistance is typically accompanied by reduced PI3K-NO pathway and heightened MAPK-ET-1 pathway [21]. Our recent studies have explored the signaling pathways by which enhanced tissue RAS contributed insulin resistance in cardiovascular tissue. To this point, Ang II increased serine phosphorylation of IRS-1 and inhibited the insulin-stimulated phosphorylation of endothelial nitric oxide synthase (eNOS) through activation of S6 kinase (S6K) signaling pathway. An inhibitor of rapamycin (mTOR) attenuated the Ang II-stimulated phosphorylation of p70S6K and IRS-1 and blocked the ability of Ang II to impair insulin-stimulated phosphorylation of eNOS and NO dependent -arteriole vasodilation. From these results, we conclude that activation of mTOR/p70S6K by Ang II in vascular endothelium may contribute to the impairment of insulin-stimulated vasodilation through phosphorylation of IRS-1 [22]. Recent data also suggests that increased mineralocorticoid signaling receptor (MR) is associated with insulin resistance. Thus, enhanced renin-Ang II-aldosterone (RAAS) activation may represent a link between obesity, hypertension, dyslipidemia and insulin resistance, features present in the CRS [23]. Studies have demonstrated a relationship between MR activation and decreased insulin sensitivity in animal models and humans. For example, patients with primary hyperaldosteronism were found to have insulin resistance suggesting the contribution of MR signaling to insulin resistance [24]. Spironolactone, a blocker of the MR, has been shown to decrease local inflammation and vascular stiffness in rodent models of hypertension and insulin resistance [25, 26]. These observations suggest that inhibition of MR might be a beneficial therapeutic approach for preventing vascular stiffening in diet-induced obesity and insulin resistance [26]. AT-1R- and MR-mediated insulin resistance and endothelial dysfunction appear to be fertile areas to explore in investigating the pathogenesis of vascular stiffening (Fig. 34.1). Further recent evidence has demonstrated a link between aldosterone and endothelial dystfunction [27].

Aldosterone was shown to increase epithelial Na+ channel expression on the endothelial cell surface that correlated with increased cortical stiffness of the cytoskeleton in endothelial cells. Of potential importance is that the increased in endothelial cell stiffness was associated with a reduced release of NO. Thus, this could provide yet another putative link that would contribute to increased vascular resistance and arterial wall stiffness.

Vascular Smooth Muscle Cell Dysfunction in Vascular Stiffening

Vascular smooth muscle cells (VSMCs) are the predominant cell type found in the arterial wall and are essential for the structural and functional integrity of the vessel. VSMCs are also a target of insulin action and are affected by insulin resistance as discussed for endothelial cells. VSMC insulin resistance and associated functional abnormalities are involved in the vascular stiffening [20]. Insulin induced vasodilation in VSMCs is mediated by metabolic signaling which includes IRS-1/h PI3K and cyclic guanosine monophosphate (cGMP) signaling pathways. This signaling leads to a reduction of free intracellular calcium and reductions in calcium sensitivity [28]. Thus, insulin resistance in VSMCs impairs vascular vasodilation. Indeed, studies from the obese Zucker insulin resistant rat have shown that VSMCs from these rats manifested greater concentrations of reactive oxygen species and impaired activation of the NO/cGMP/PKG pathway with when compared to VSMC from the lean, insulin-sensitive Zucker rats [28]. Our recent data also showed excessive serine phosphorylation of IRS-1 as a key mechanism underlying cellular insulin resistance in VSMCs. Furthermore, after treatment with aldosterone, VSMCs show increased activation of p70 S6K1 signaling pathway, increased proteosomal degradation of IRS-1 and attenuated insulin-induced Akt phosphorylation [20]. These observations provide a biochemical basis for insulin resistance in VSMCs in the development of vascular stiffening (Fig. 34.1).

Vascular calcification in patients with diabetes mellitus and end stage renal disease is strongly associated with vascular stiffening and CVD [29]. We have known that VSMCs can differentiate from a quiescent, contractile phenotype to a proliferative, synthetic phenotype following arterial injury and in atherosclerotic diseases [30]. Indeed, VSMCs are capable of osteoblast transdifferentiation in calcifying arteries [29]. Many factors, such as hyperinsulinemia and oxidative stress, contribute to the development of vascular calcification [31, 32]. Epidemiological data have shown that higher insulin levels in diabetes can independently predicate arterial calcification [33]. The mechanisms of insulin involved in arterial calcification in these clinical settings are still controversial. Furthermore, it has been demonstrated that insulin enhanced the calcification of VSMCs *in vitro* [34]. In this regard, insulin promotes alkaline phosphatase activity, osteocalcin expression and the formation of mineralized nodules in VSMCs by increased receptor expression of NF-κB ligand (RANKL) through Erk 1/2 activation [31]. However, *others* suggested that insulin attenuated VSMC calcification induced by high phosphate conditions [35]. These contradictory results may be explained by different cell types or different experimental conditions.

There is evidence that RAS activation plays an important role in the pathogenesis of vascular calcification. In the course of RAS-induced vascular inflammation, Ang II binds to the AT-1R to induce oxidative stress, mainly mediated by NAD(P)H oxidase. Increased reactive oxygen species (ROS) production leads to the activation of redox-sensitive pro-inflammatory transcription factors, such as NF-κB and transcription factor runt-related transcription factor 2 (Runx2), and further results in the phenotypic switch of VSMCs into osteoblast-like cells [36]. It has been reported that Ang II exacerbated vascular calcification through activation of the transcription factors, Runx2 and NF-κB, regulation of matrix gla protein, and inflammatory cytokine expression in human VSMCs [37]. Thus, advancements in our understanding of the cellular and molecular mechanisms by which Ang II and hyperinsulinemia promote vascular

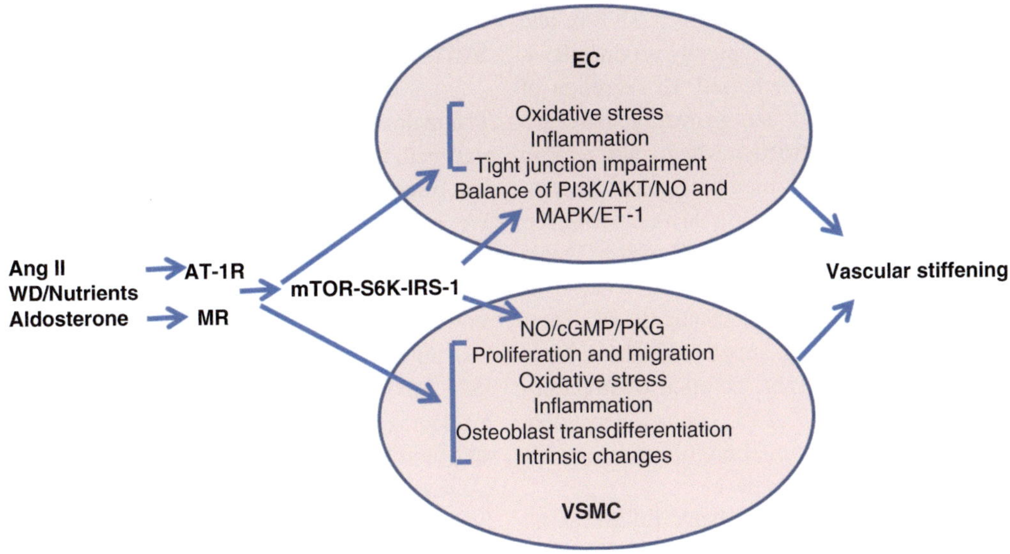

Fig. 34.1 Mechanisms of arterial stiffness in vascular cells. Activation of AT-1R and MR lend to out of balance in PI3KAKT/NO and MAPK/ET-1 signaling pathways on EC and subsequently impair the NO/cGMP/PKG signaling pathway in VSMCs through phosphorylation of mTOR-S6K-IRS-1 signal. Meanwhile, Activation of AT-1R and MR directly increase oxidative stress and inflammation on both EC and VSMC. Furthermore, Activation of AT-1R and MR induce the tight junction impairment on EC and SMC intrinsic changes and osteoblast transdifferention, respectively. *AT-1R* Ang II receptor 1, *MR* Mineralocorticoid receptor, *mTOR* rapamycin, *S6K* S6 kinase, *IRS-1* insulin receptor substrate -1, *PI3K* phosphatidylinositol 3-kinase (*PI3K*), *AKT* protein kinase B, *NO* nitric oxide, *MAPK* active mitogen activated protein kinase, *ET-1* endothelin-1, *cGMP* cyclic guanosine monophosphate, *PKG* cGMP-dependent protein kinase

calcification should provide a viable target for anti-vascular stiffening strategy.

Inflammation and Oxidation Stress in Vascular Stiffening

Vascular stiffness is increased in patients with systemic lupus erythematous, rheumatoid arthritis, and inflammatory bowel disease [38–41]. An epidemiological study has investigated the associations among endothelial biomarkers of inflammation such as p-selectin, thrombomodulin, intercellular adhesion molecules 1, cytokine C-reactive protein (CRP), serum amyloid A, interleukin 6 (IL-6), IL-8, tumor necrosis factor-α (TNF-α), and intercellular adhesion molecule 1 (ICAM-1) in 293 healthy adults over a 6 year period. This study elucidated biomarkers of endothelial dysfunction and association of cytokine inflammation with greater arterial stiffness [42]. CRP has been reported to be an independent predictor of adverse CVD events and is strongly associated with inflammation in the progression of arterial stiffness and endothelial dysfunction [43]. Consequently, endothelial dysfunction may result in increased expression of pro-inflammatory cytokines and cell adhesion molecules. It is likely that the increased vascular inflammation will impair endothelial mediated vasodilation and promote vascular fibrosis, which will subsequently lead to increases in arterial stiffness [44]. Meanwhile, inflammatory cytokines can promote leukocyte infiltration and activate VSMCs, which in turn, increase the expression and activity of matrix metalloproteinases (MMPs) that contribute to arterial stiffening [45].

Recently, it has been recognized that the adaptive immune system is important in the genesis of vascular stiffening. Specifically, T lymphocytes, a population of immune cells, have been identified in the artery walls. Activated T cells can be subtyped according to their cytokine profile.

T helper (Th) 1 cells secrete IL-2, TNF-ß, and IFN-γ, whereas Th2 cells typically produce IL-4, -5, -6, and -10 [46]. Increased Th secretion of cytokines, chemokines, and growth factors leads to an inflammatory process which may lead to fragmentation of elastic membranes and destruction of cell-protective matrix layers. However, $CD4^+CD25^+Foxp3^+$ Regulatory T cells (Tregs) can protect the pro-inflammatory activation of vascular cells. Several mechanisms of Treg-mediated inflammatory suppression have been proposed, including Treg secretion of immunosuppressive cytokines, cell contact–dependent suppression, and functional modification or killing of activated protein C [47].

Many factors that have been linked to an increased prevalence of vascular stiffening are associated with elevated oxidative stress, including diabetes mellitus, hypertension, and hypercholesterolemia [48]. Oxidant induced cellular injury may be a fundamental causal pathway leading directly or indirectly to loss of elasticity in the arterial wall. Excess oxidant burden alters DNA transcription leading to cellular proliferation and interruption of numerous redox sensitive signaling pathways that influence arterial remodeling [49]. The generation of ROS is required for normal cell signaling and physiological responses. Some of our studies confirmed a critical role for increased AT-1R and signaling MR in conjunction with an altered redox-mediating impaired endothelial, cardiac and renal function in the CRS [50]. Recently, it was shown that prolonged exposure to increased mitochondrial oxidative stress, decreased aortic compliance and induced cardiac dysfunction [51]. Specifically, the data elucidated the significance of lifelong superoxide dismutase 2 deficiency on the phenotype, function, and molecular signaling pathways in aortic SMCs. These results further show how oxidative stress promotes aortic stiffening by inducing vascular wall remodeling, intrinsic changes in SMC stiffness, and aortic SMC apoptosis [51]. The link between oxidative stress and arterial stiffness offers new clues to identify vascular dysfunction and may allow for development of novel targeted therapeutic interventions.

Collagen and Elastin in Vascular Stiffening

The major structural components within the arterial wall, collagen and elastin, also play important roles in the development of arterial stiffness. We have reported that alterations of collagen and elastin fibers are involved in arterial stiffening which is associated with the aging process and disease states such as hypertension, diabetes, atherosclerosis, and chronic renal failure [52]. Indeed, vascular stiffening is characterized by decreased turnover of collagen and elastin, and increased advanced glycation end-products (AGEs) and extracellular matrix (ECM) cross-links. Elastic fibers undergo lysis and disorganization subsequent to their replacement by collagen and other matrix components. These events cause the loss of elasticity and induce stiffening [53]. Studies have investigated the susceptibility of elastin to glycation and subsequent changes in its physicochemical properties [54]. It was found that purified elastin and collagen-elastin preparation from the porcine thoracic aorta rapidly incorporated glucose and ribose. Glycation of the charged lysine and arginine side-chain residues was associated with the appearance of the AGEs [54]. Thus, AGEs enhance collagen content and induce changes in mechanical properties of the conjunctive tissue by conferring a high resistance to enzymatic proteolysis, decreasing their rate of degradation, increasing the production of extracellular matrix, and creating the cross-linking of the extracellular proteins [55]. It is also highly likely that these changes alter VSMC and EC adhesion to these extracellular matrix proteins that would have an additional set of functional implications.

In the context of vascular stiffening, MMPs are involved in the regulation of the structural integrity of the ECM. When the vessel wall is exposed to immunological stress, inflammatory cells like polymorphonuclear neutrophils (PMNs) and macrophages, produce a variety of MMPs (MMP-1, -7, -8, -13) as well as elastase. MMPs degrade the ECM by affecting the production of weaker collagen and frayed elastin fibers [56]. The activity of these enzymes is regulated by augmented gene expression, post-translational activation of cleavage of pro-MMPs, and interaction among MMPs, plasmin, thrombin and ROS [57]. Recently, it was reported that in the arterial vasculature from chronic kidney disease patients, the presence of diabetes markedly up-regulated MMP-2 and -9, a process strongly associated with elastic fiber degradation, arterial stiffening, and calcification. The increase in MMPs in diabetic vessels was also accompanied by a pronounced generation of angiostatin, and the reduction of microvascular density was associated with impaired vasorelaxation [58]. These data confirm that MMPs are up-regulated in the arterial vasculature of chronic kidney disease patients with diabetes compared with those without diabetes.

In addition to the ECM, it has recently been demonstrated that intrinsic changes in the mechanical properties of VSMCs contribute to vascular stiffening. In a mature blood vessel, VSMC exhibit a "contractile" or differentiated phenotype characterized by the expression of contractile markers specific to smooth muscle, such as smooth muscle myosin heavy chain, smooth muscle α-actin, h-caldesmon, and calponin, which are important for the regulation of contraction [59]. Upon injury, such as after angioplasty or stimulation with growth factors, VSMCs differentiate into a "synthetic" phenotype, as demonstrated by an increased rate of proliferation, migration, and synthesis of extracellular matrix components. This differentiated phenotype plays a major pathophysiological role in the development of vascular stiffening, atherosclerosis, and hypertension [60]. Recent work from the Meininger group has demonstrated that VSMC isolated from aged monkeys had an elastic modulus that was approximately three times greater than that observed in younger cells. In addition, aged monkey VSMC contained more actin and had increased integrin expression. Their studies also demonstrated unique dynamic differences in VSMC stiffness visible as oscillations in VSMC cortical membrane stiffness [61, 62]. These data support the novel concept that increased vascular stiffness is attributed not only to changes in ECM but also to intrinsic changes in VSMCs.

Assessment Methods for Vascular Stiffening

Noninvasive measurement of arterial stiffness usually falls into three categories: analysis of pulse transit time, wave contour of the arterial pulse, direct measurement of arterial geometry and pressure that correspond to regional, systemic, and local determination of stiffness, and modern cell and tissue technologies (Table 34.1). Aortic PWV, widely regarded as the gold standard measure of arterial stiffness today, is less sensitive to cardiac function and thus may provide a better estimate of aortic stiffness [1]. In a practical sense, PWV is measured by obtaining a recording of the arterial pulse wave at a proximal artery such as the common carotid, as well as a distal vessel such as the femoral. These two vessels are widely used because they are relatively superficial, permitting accurate identification and ease in using a tonometer [63]. Briefly, carotid–femoral PWV is usually measured with subjects in the supine position. After five minutes of rest, blood pressure is measured twice using an automatic blood pressure recorder. The time delay between the feet of simultaneously recorded pulse waves in the carotid artery and the femoral artery is measured using an automatic device. The distance traveled by the pulse wave is measured between the sternal notch and the femoral artery using a tape measure. Aortic PWV is calculated as the ratio of the distance traveled by the pulse wave and the foot-to-foot time delay and is expressed in meters per second [2]. However, this gold standard measure of stiffness has limitations. The distance traveled is not straightforward. As an advancing pressure wave travels up the brachiocephalic and carotid arteries, it also travels around the aortic arch. This parallel transmission complicates assessment of the carotid-femoral transit distance [64]. The PWV is also influenced by intravascular pressure as high pressure, per se, increases PWV. Other noninvasive measurement methods for vascular stiffening are included in Table 34.1.

Vascular biology has been revolutionized by current developments in new technologies. As an important example, atomic force microscopy

Table 34.1 Methods of measuring vascular stiffening

Category	Method	Advantage	Limitation
Pulse transit time	Pulse wave velocity	Most reliable measurement regarded as the present gold standard measure of arterial stiffness	Location and blood pressure dependent
Wave contour of the arterial pulse	Wave form analysis	Reliable and direct measurement	
	Augmentation Indexes	Simple and easy to use	Affected by heart rate, stroke volume and vasomotor tone
	Pulse pressure	Simple and straight forward measurement	Confounded by heart rate, stroke volume and the pattern of ventricular ejection
	Magnetic resonance imaging	Anatomic and functional characterization of vascular wall	Requirement of skilled operator and expensive equipment
	Flow- mediated dilation	Reliable measurement of endothelial dysfunction	Variability of the technical method
	Atomic force microscopy	Details at macro- and nano-scale	
	Vessel rings	Reliable and easy method	*Ex vivo* studies
	Vascular tissue engineering	*Ex vivo* vascular scaffolds	

(AFM) has proven to be a powerful investigative tool for working with live cells and tissues at the macro- scale and with single molecules at the nano-scale. This approach has been used for real-time monitoring of VSMC stiffness and adhesion [65]. They operate the AFM using a nano-indentation protocol to measure VSMC stiffness by using silicon nitride cantilevers. For combined AFM and fluorescent imaging, VSMCs are fluorescently labeled with Alexa 568-phalloidin and recorded with an integrated AFM-confocal microscope system. AFM probes bio-conjugated with fibronectin are also used to assess β1-integrin binding and cell adhesion to the ECM. These studies have applied this advanced technique and provided a novel concept in the single living VSMC that both β1-integrin and α-smooth muscle actin are likely major players in the increased stiffness of VSMCs [62].

Potential Therapies in Vascular Stiffening

Current evidence indicates that lifestyle modifications, in particular aerobic exercise and sodium restriction, appear to be clinically efficacious therapeutic interventions for preventing and treating arterial stiffening in patients with metabolic syndrome [66]. However, the most powerful therapy to reduce arterial stiffness is vigorous treatment of hypertension with pharmacological agents, such as diuretics, β-blockers, Ang II receptor antagonists, and calcium channel antagonists. Because anti-hypertensive drugs are primarily designed to reduce peripheral resistance, they may not alter the pathological process of arterial stiffening itself or electively reduce systolic blood pressure [67]. The current view is that blockers of the RAAS system are particularly efficacious in vascular stiffening with diabetes since increased RAAS signaling is a potent pro-fibrotic stimulus, and the turnover of the ECM in the arterial wall translates into changes in mechanical properties of the vessel [68]. Numerous small-scale interventional studies have looked into the possibility of using anti-inflammatory treatments in the prevention of vascular stiffness. But until now, only antibodies against TNF-α have been shown to improve arterial stiffness in patients with different chronic inflammatory diseases [69]. In addition, statins and other cholesterol-reducing agents have shown to have beneficial effects on wave reflection and aortic stiffness reduction because of the properties in anti-inflammatory and up-regulation of endothelial nitric oxide synthase expression [69]. Drugs targeting glycemic control have also been shown to improve arterial stiffness [68]. Recently, a new drug called an AGE cross-link breaker has been shown to reduce arterial stiffness and subsequently reduce the pulsatile blood pressure component without influencing mean arterial pressure [70]. Further, α-Aminoguanidine, a first-line compound for breaking AGE deposits, has been shown to reduce myocardial and arterial stiffness [68]. The newest investigational compound is alagebrium that has been reported to reduce aortic stiffness and intra-aortic pulse pressure through breaking collagen crosslinks in hypertensive dogs. Unfortunately AGE cross-link breakers may induce dilatation of the aorta and therefore limit their use in clinical practice [70].

Estrogens, the major female sex hormones, are suggested to protect against development of the metabolic syndrome and the prevalence of obesity, insulin resistance, and type 2 diabetes increases in post-menopausal woman [71]. It has been observed that vascular stiffening may benefit from sex hormone therapy [68]. Sex differences in vascular function have been demonstrated in the aorta, coronary, mesenteric, and renal arteries [72]. Our previous data have reported that there were important sex-related differences in the prevalence of obesity, type 2 diabetes mellitus and cardiovascular disease [73]. Indeed, women are thought to be protected against CVD by estrogen during their reproductive years. Nonetheless, the impact and the mechanisms that link sex hormone therapy to vascular stiffening remain to be fully elucidated.

Summary

Vascular stiffening is a useful risk biomarker and is an independent predictor for the complication related to hyperglycemia and hyperinsulinemia. Elucidation of mechanisms leading to the pathophsiological alterations in vascular will aid in more specifically targeted therapeutic interventions because currently available cardiovascular medications fall short at reducing the vascular stiffness. In the future, prospective studies analyzing the effects of medications on vascular stiffness may provide insights to novel strategies to prevent or reduce this pathological process and reduce CVD.

Acknowledgements Studies in the Sowers and Meininger laboratories are supported by NIH grant (NIH P01HL095486) to G.A. Meininger and NIH (R01 HL73101-01A and R01 HL107910-01) and the Veterans Affairs Merit System (0018) for J.R. Sowers. The authors which to thank Brenda Hunter for editing this chapter.

References

1. Luft FC. Molecular mechanisms of arterial stiffness: new insights. J Am Soc Hypertens. 2012;6:436–8.
2. Wang X, Keith Jr JC, Struthers AD, Feuerstein GZ. Assessment of arterial stiffness, a translational medicine biomarker system for evaluation of vascular risk. Cardiovasc Ther. 2008;26:214–23.
3. The Reference Values for Arterial Stiffness' Collaboration. Determinants of pulse wave velocity in healthy people and in the presence of cardiovascular risk factors: 'establishing normal and reference values'. Eur Heart J. 2010;31:2338–50.
4. Lo CS, Relf IRN, Myers KA, Wahlquist ML. Doppler ultrasound recognition of preclinical changes in arterial wall in diabetic subjects: compliance and pulse-wave damping. Diabetes Care. 1986;9:27–31.
5. Wahlquist ML, Lo CS, Myers KE, Simpson RW, Simpson JM. Putative determinants of arterial wall compliance in NIDDM. Diabetes Care. 1988;11:787–90.
6. Lehmann EO, Gosling RG, Söuksen PH. Arterial wall compliance in diabetes. Diabet Med. 1992;9:114–9.
7. Neutel JM, Smith DHG, Graettinger WF, Weber MA. Dependency of arterial compliance on circulating neuroendocrine and metabolic factors in normal subjects. Am J Cardiol. 1992;69:1340–4.
8. Salomaa V, Riley W, Kark JD, Nardo C, Folsom AR. Non-insulin-dependent diabetes mellitus and fasting glucose and insulin concentrations are associated with arterial stiffness indexes. The ARIC Study Atherosclerosis Risk in Communities Study. Circulation. 1995;91:1432–43.
9. Tounian P, Aggoun Y, Dubern B, Varille V, Guy-Grand B, Sidi D, Girardet JP, Bonnet D. Presence of increased stiffness of the common carotid artery and endothelial dysfunction in severely obese children: a prospective study. Lancet. 2001;27(358):1400–4.
10. Ho CT, Lin CC, Hsu HS, Liu CS, Davidson LE, Li TC, Li CI, Lin WY. Arterial stiffness is strongly associated with insulin resistance in Chinese–a population-based study (Taichung Community Health Study, TCHS). J Atheroscler Thromb. 2011;18:122–30.
11. van Popele NM, Elizabeth Hak A, Mattace-Raso FU, Bots ML, van der Kuip DA, Reneman RS, Hoeks AP, Hofman A, Grobbee DE, Witteman JC. Impaired fasting glucose is associated with increased arterial stiffness in elderly people without diabetes mellitus: the Rotterdam Study. J Am Geriatr Soc. 2006;54:397–404.

12. Siekmeier R, Grammer T, März W. Roles of oxidants, nitric oxide, and asymmetric dimethylarginine in endothelial function. J Cardiovasc Pharmacol Ther. 2008;13:279–97.
13. Muniyappa R, Sowers JR. Endothelial insulin and IGF-1 receptors: when yes means NO. Diabetes. 2012;61:2225–7.
14. Vaccari CS, Lerakis S, Hammoud R, Khan BV. Mechanisms of benefit of angiotensin receptor blockers in coronary atherosclerosis. Am J Med Sci. 2008;336:270–7.
15. Daemen MJ, Lombardi DM, Bosman FT, Schwartz SM. Angiotensin II induces smooth muscle cell proliferation in the normal and injured rat arterial wall. Circ Res. 1991;68:450–6.
16. Sodhi CP, Kanwar YS, Sahai A. Hypoxia and high glucose upregulate AT1 receptor expression and potentiate ANG II-induced proliferation in VSM cells. Am J Physiol Heart Circ Physiol. 2003;284:H846–52.
17. Reusch JE, Wang CC. Cardiovascular disease in diabetes: where does glucose fit in? J Clin Endocrinol Metab. 2011;96:2367–76.
18. Min Q, Bai YT, Jia G, Wu J, Xiang JZ. High glucose enhances angiotensin-II-mediated peroxisome proliferation-activated receptor-gamma inactivation in human coronary artery endothelial cells. Exp Mol Pathol. 2010;88:133–7.
19. Shanik MH, Xu Y, Skrha J, Dankner R, Zick Y, Roth J. Insulin resistance and hyperinsulinemia: is hyperinsulinemia the cart or the horse? Diabetes Care. 2008;31:S262–8.
20. Bender SB, McGraw AP, Jaffe IZ, Sowers JR. Mineralocorticoid receptor-mediated vascular insulin resistance: an early contributor to diabetes-related vascular disease? Diabetes. 2013;62:313–9.
21. Rask-Madsen C, Kahn CR. Tissue-specific insulin signaling, metabolic syndrome, and cardiovascular disease. Arterioscler Thromb Vasc Biol. 2012;32:2052–9.
22. Kim JA, Jang HJ, Martinez-Lemus LA, Sowers JR. Activation of mTOR/p70S6 kinase by ANG II inhibits insulin-stimulated endothelial nitric oxide synthase and vasodilation. Am J Physiol Endocrinol Metab. 2012;302:E201–8.
23. Garg R, Adler GK. Role of mineralocorticoid receptor in insulin resistance. Curr Opin Endocrinol Diabetes Obes. 2012;19:168–75.
24. Underwood PC, Adler GK. The renin angiotensin aldosterone system and insulin resistance in humans. Curr Hypertens Rep. 2013;15:59–70.
25. Wada T, Kenmochi H, Miyashita Y, Sasaki M, Ojima M, Sasahara M, Koya D, Tsuneki H, Sasaoka T. Spironolactone improves glucose and lipid metabolism by ameliorating hepatic steatosis and inflammation and suppressing enhanced gluconeogenesis induced by high-fat and high-fructose diet. Endocrinology. 2010;151:2040–9.
26. Benetos A, et al. Prevention of aortic fibrosis by spironolactone in spontaneously hypertensive rats. Arterioscl Thom Vas Biol. 1997;17:1152–6.
27. Jeggle P, Callies C, Tarjus A, Fassot C, Fels J, Oberleithner H, Jaisser F, Kusche-Vihrog K. Epithelial sodium channel stiffens the vascular endothelium in vitro and in liddle mice. Hypertension. 2013;61(5):1053–9.
28. Doronzo G, Russo I, Mattiello L, Anfossi G, Bosia A, Trovati M. Insulin activates vascular endothelial growth factor in vascular smooth muscle cells: influence of nitric oxide and of insulin resistance. Eur J Clin Invest. 2004;34:664–73.
29. Johnson RC, Leopold JA, Loscalzo J. Vascular calcification: pathobiological mechanisms and clinical implications. Circ Res. 2006;99:1044–59.
30. Speer MY, Yang HY, Brabb T, Leaf E, Look A, Lin WL, Frutkin A, Dichek D, Giachelli CM. Smooth muscle cells give rise to osteochondrogenic precursors and chondrocytes in calcifying arteries. Circ Res. 2009;104:733–41.
31. Yuan LQ, Zhu JH, Wang HW, Liang QH, Xie H, Wu XP, Zhou H, Cui RR, Sheng ZF, Zhou HD, Zhu X, Liu GY, Liu YS, Liao EY. RANKL is a downstream mediator for insulin-induced osteoblastic differentiation of vascular smooth muscle cells. PLoS One. 2011;6:e29037.
32. Byon CH, Javed A, Dai Q, Kappes JC, Clemens TL, Darley-Usmar VM, McDonald JM, Chen Y. Oxidative stress induces vascular calcification through modulation of the osteogenic transcription factor Runx2 by AKT signaling. J Biol Chem. 2008;283:15319–27.
33. Blaha MJ, DeFilippis AP, Rivera JJ, Budoff MJ, Blankstein R, Agatston A, Szklo M, Lakoski SG, Bertoni AG, Kronmal RA, Blumenthal RS, Nasir K. The relationship between insulin resistance and incidence and progression of coronary artery calcification: the Multi-Ethnic Study of Atherosclerosis (MESA). Diabetes Care. 2011;34:749–51.
34. Olesen P, Nguyen K, Wogensen L, Ledet T, Rasmussen LM. Calcification of human vascular smooth muscle cells: associations with osteoprotegerin expression and acceleration by high-dose insulin. Am J Physiol Heart Circ Physiol. 2007;292:H1058–64.
35. Wang CC, Sorribas V, Sharma G, Levi M, Draznin B. Insulin attenuates vascular smooth muscle calcification but increases vascular smooth muscle cell phosphate transport. Atherosclerosis. 2007;195:e65–75.
36. Schiffrin EL, Lipman ML, Mann JF. Chronic kidney disease: effects on the cardiovascular system. Circulation. 2007;116:85–97.
37. Jia G, Stormont RM, Gangahar DM, Agrawal DK. Role of matrix Gla protein in angiotensin II-induced exacerbation of vascular calcification. Am J Physiol Heart Circ Physiol. 2012;303:H523–32.
38. Barnes JN, Nualnim N, Sugawara J, Sommerlad SM, Renzi CP, Tanaka H. Arterial stiffening, wave reflection, and inflammation in habitually exercising systemic lupus erythematosus patients. Am J Hypertens. 2011;24:1194–200.
39. Mäki-Petäjä KM, Elkhawad M, Cheriyan J, Joshi FR, Ostör AJ, Hall FC, Rudd JH, Wilkinson IB. Anti-tumor necrosis factor-α therapy reduces aortic

inflammation and stiffness in patients with rheumatoid arthritis. Circulation. 2012;126:2473–80.
40. Zanoli L, Cannavò M, Rastelli S, Di Pino L, Monte I, Di Gangi M, Boutouyrie P, Inserra G, Laurent S, Castellino P. Arterial stiffness is increased in patients with inflammatory bowel disease. J Hypertens. 2012;30:1775–81.
41. Kals J, Kampus P, Kals M, Pulges A, Teesalu R, Zilmer K, Kullisaar T, Salum T, Eha J, Zilmer M. Inflammation and oxidative stress are associated differently with endothelial function and arterial stiffness in healthy subjects and in patients with atherosclerosis. Scand J Clin Lab Invest. 2008;68:594–601.
42. van Bussel BC, Schouten F, Henry RM, Schalkwijk CG, de Boer MR, Ferreira I, Smulders YM, Twisk JW, Stehouwer CD. Endothelial dysfunction and low-grade inflammation are associated with greater arterial stiffness over a 6-year period. Hypertension. 2011;58:588–95.
43. Woodard GA, Mehta VG, Mackey RH, Tepper P, Kelsey SF, Newman AB, Sutton-Tyrrell K. C-reactive protein is associated with aortic stiffness in a cohort of African American and white women transitioning through menopause. Menopause. 2011;18:1291–7.
44. Park S, Lakatta EG. Role of inflammation in the pathogenesis of arterial stiffness. Yonsei Med J. 2012;53:258–61.
45. Cooper JN, Tepper P, Barinas-Mitchell E, Woodard GA, Sutton-Tyrrell K. Serum aldosterone is associated with inflammation and aortic stiffness in normotensive overweight and obese young adults. Clin Exp Hypertens. 2012;34:63–70.
46. Ait-Oufella H, Salomon BL, Potteaux S, Robertson AK, Gourdy P, Zoll J, Merval R, Esposito B, Cohen JL, Fisson S, Flavell RA, Hansson GK, Klatzmann D, Tedgui A, Mallat Z. Natural regulatory T cells control the development of atherosclerosis in mice. Nat Med. 2006;12:178–80.
47. He S, Li M, Ma X, Lin J, Li D. CD4+CD25+Foxp3+ regulatory T cells protect the proinflammatory activation of human umbilical vein endothelial cells. Arterioscler Thromb Vasc Biol. 2010;30:2621–30.
48. Wykretowicz A, Adamska K, Krauze T, Guzik P, Szczepanik A, Rutkowska A, Wysoki H. The plasma concentration of advanced oxidation protein products and arterial stiffness in apparently healthy adults. Free Radic Res. 2007;41:645–9.
49. Patel RS, Al Mheid I, Morris AA, Ahmed Y, Kavtaradze N, Ali S, Dabhadkar K, Brigham K, Hooper WC, Alexander RW, Jones DP, Quyyumi AA. Oxidative stress is associated with impaired arterial elasticity. Atherosclerosis. 2011;218:90–5.
50. Whaley-Connell A, Sowers JR. Oxidative stress in the cardiorenal metabolic syndrome. Curr Hypertens Rep. 2012;14:360–5.
51. Zhou RH, Vendrov AE, Tchivilev I, Niu XL, Molnar KC, Rojas M, Carter JD, Tong H, Stouffer GA, Madamanchi NR, Runge MS. Mitochondrial oxidative stress in aortic stiffening with age: the role of smooth muscle cell function. Arterioscler Thromb Vasc Biol. 2012;32:745–55.
52. Winer N, Sowers JR. Diabetes and arterial stiffening. Adv Cardiol. 2007;44:245–51.
53. Sell DR, Monnier VM. Molecular basis of arterial stiffening: role of glycation - a mini-review. Gerontology. 2012;58:227–37.
54. Winlove CP, Parker KH, Avery NC, Bailey AJ. Interactions of elastin and aorta with sugars in vitro and their effects on biochemical and physical properties. Diabetologia. 1996;39:1131–9.
55. Corman B, Duriez M, Poitevin P, Heudes D, Bruneval P, Tedgui A, Levy BI. Aminoguanidine prevents age-related arterial stiffening and cardiac hypertrophy. Proc Natl Acad Sci U S A. 1998;95:1301–6.
56. Shirwany NA, Zou MH. Arterial stiffness: a brief review. Acta Pharmacol Sin. 2010;31:1267–76.
57. Dollery CM, McEwan JR, Henney AM. Matrix metalloproteinases and cardiovascular disease. Circ Res. 1995;77:863–8.
58. Chung AW, Yang HH, Sigrist MK, Brin G, Chum E, Gourlay WA, Levin A. Matrix metalloproteinase-2 and -9 exacerbate arterial stiffening and angiogenesis in diabetes and chronic kidney disease. Cardiovasc Res. 2009;84:494–504.
59. Rzucidlo EM, Martin KA, Powell RJ. Regulation of vascular smooth muscle cell differentiation. J Vasc Surg. 2007;45(Suppl A):A25–32.
60. Rzucidlo EM. Signaling pathways regulating vascular smooth muscle cell differentiation. Vascular. 2009;17 Suppl 1:S15–20.
61. Zhu Y, Qiu H, Trzeciakowski JP, Sun Z, Li Z, Hong Z, Hill MA, Hunter WC, Vatner DE, Vatner SF, Meininger GA. Temporal analysis of vascular smooth muscle cell elasticity and adhesion reveals oscillation waveforms that differ with aging. Aging Cell. 2012;11:741–50.
62. Qiu H, Zhu Y, Sun Z, Trzeciakowski JP, Gansner M, Depre C, Resuello RR, Natividad FF, Hunter WC, Genin GM, Elson EL, Vatner DE, Meininger GA, Vatner SF. Short communication: vascular smooth muscle cell stiffness as a mechanism for increased aortic stiffness with aging. Circ Res. 2010;107:615–9.
63. Poels MM, Zaccai K, Verwoert GC, Vernooij MW, Hofman A, van der Lugt A, Witteman JC, Breteler MM, Mattace-Raso FU, Ikram MA. Arterial stiffness and cerebral small vessel disease: the Rotterdam Scan Study. Stroke. 2012;43:2637–42.
64. Mitchell GF. Arterial stiffness and wave reflection: biomarkers of cardiovascular risk. Artery Res. 2009;3:56–64.
65. Hong Z, Sun Z, Li Z, Mesquitta WT, Trzeciakowski JP, Meininger GA. Coordination of fibronectin adhesion with contraction and relaxation in microvascular smooth muscle. Cardiovasc Res. 2012;96:73–80.
66. Tanaka H, Safar ME. Influence of lifestyle modification on arterial stiffness and wave reflections. Am J Hypertens. 2005;18:137–44.

67. Soro-Paavonen A, Forbes JM. Novel therapeutics for diabetic micro- and macrovascular complications. Curr Med Chem. 2006;13:1777–88.
68. Boutouyrie P, Lacolley P, Briet M, Regnault V, Stanton A, Laurent S, Mahmud A. Pharmacological modulation of arterial stiffness. Drugs. 2011;71:1689–701.
69. Mäki-Petäjä KM, Wilkinson IB. Anti-inflammatory drugs and statins for arterial stiffness reduction. Curr Pharm Des. 2009;15:290–303.
70. Safar ME, Blacher J, Jankowski P. Arterial stiffness, pulse pressure, and cardiovascular disease-is it possible to break the vicious circle? Atherosclerosis. 2011;218:263–71.
71. Pettersson US, Waldén TB, Carlsson PO, Jansson L, Phillipson M. Female mice are protected against high-fat diet induced metabolic syndrome and increase the regulatory T cell population in adipose tissue. PLoS One. 2012;7:e46057.
72. Ma Y, Qiao X, Falone AE, Reslan OM, Sheppard SJ, Khalil RA. Gender-specific reduction in contraction is associated with increased estrogen receptor expression in single vascular smooth muscle cells of female rat. Cell Physiol Biochem. 2010;26:457–70.
73. Manrique C, Lastra G, Habibi J, Mugerfeld I, Garro M, Sowers JR. Loss of estrogen receptor α signaling leads to insulin resistance and obesity in young and adult female mice. Cardiorenal Med. 2012;2:200–10.

Arterial Stiffness in Chronic Inflammation

35

Kaisa M. Mäki-Petäjä, Carmel M. McEniery, Stanley S. Franklin, and Ian B. Wilkinson

Abstract

A strong body of evidence demonstrates that inflammation plays an important role in arterial stiffening. This chapter explores the relationship between inflammation and arterial stiffness and explains possible mechanisms by which inflammation could lead to arterial stiffening. Also, recent studies, which have investigated the effect of anti-inflammatory drugs for arterial stiffness reduction, will be discussed.

Keywords

Inflammation • Arterial stiffness • Pulse wave velocity • Vascular inflammation • Anti-inflammatory therapy • Rheumatoid arthritis • Chronic inflammatory disease

Abbreviations

AIx	Augmentation index
aPWV	Aortic pulse wave velocity
BH_4	Tetrahydrobiopterin
BP	Blood pressure
COPD	Chronic obstructive pulmonary disease
CRP	C-reactive protein
CVD	Cardiovascular disease
ECM	Extra cellular matrix
ENOS	Endothelial nitric oxide synthase
F-FDG	18F-fluoro-deoxyglucose
GAG	Glycosaminoglycan
HA	Hyaluronan
IL-6	Interleukin-6
INOS	Inducible nitric oxide synthase
MAP	Mean arterial pressure
MMP	Matrix metalloproteinase
MPO	Myeloperoxidase

K.M. Mäki-Petäjä, PhD, BSc (✉) • C.M. McEniery, PhD
I.B. Wilkinson, FRCP, DM, BM BCh
Clinical Pharmacology Unit,
University of Cambridge,
Addenbrooke's Hospital,
Box 110, Hills Road, Cambridge, CB2 0QQ, UK
e-mail: km391@medschl.cam.ac.uk;
cmm41@cam.ac.uk; ibw20@cam.ac.uk

S.S. Franklin, MD, FACO, FAHA, FASN
Preventive Cardiology Program,
Division of Cardiology, Department of Medicine,
C240 Medical Sciences, University
of California, Irvine, Spague Hall 112,
Irvine, CA 92697, USA
e-mail: ssfranklinmd@earthlink.net

M.E. Safar et al. (eds.), *Blood Pressure and Arterial Wall Mechanics in Cardiovascular Diseases*,
DOI 10.1007/978-1-4471-5198-2_35,

NO	Nitric oxide
O_2^-	Superoxide
PET	Positron emission tomography
PG	Proteoglycan
PMR	Polymyalgia rheumatica
PWV	Pulse wave velocity
RA	Rheumatoid arthritis
ROS	Reactive oxygen species
SLE	Systemic lupus erythematosus
TNF-α	Tumour necrosis factor- alpha
VSMC	Vascular smooth muscle cell

Introduction

Inflammation is a key element in atheroma formation, playing a pivotal role in the initiation, progression and propagation of the disease [1]. Circulating levels of several cytokines including interleukin-6 and tumour necrosis factor-α (TNF-α) are elevated in subjects with atherosclerosis, and correlate with disease burden. Levels of the acute phase reactant C-reactive protein (CRP) also predict the risk of future cardiovascular events both in subjects with known cardiovascular disease (CVD) [2], and in apparently healthy individuals [3]. Moreover, the incidence of CVD is increased in patients with chronic systemic inflammatory diseases such as rheumatoid arthritis (RA) [4, 5], systemic lupus erythematosus (SLE) [6], psoriasis [7], chronic obstructive pulmonary disease (COPD) [8], and polymyalglia rheuamatica (PMR) [9]. As the inflammatory process of RA resembles the one seen in atherosclerosis, both diseases involving activation of macrophages, T-cells, especially CD4+CD28- and B-cells as well as increased expression of adhesion molecules and increased circulating levels of TNF-α and CRP [10], RA is a useful "model" in which to investigate the relationship between systemic inflammation and CVD. The mechanism by which inflammation leads to increased CV risk remains unknown. Inflammation could lead to an increase of cardiovascular risk by accelerating the atherosclerosis process, destabilizing plaques, via endothelial dysfunction, via premature stiffening of the large arteries or direct vascular inflammation.

This chapter aims to explore the relationship between inflammation and arterial stiffness and to explain possible mechanisms by which inflammation could lead to arterial stiffening. Also, recent studies, which have investigated the effect of anti-inflammatory drugs for arterial stiffness reduction, will be discussed.

Arterial Stiffness

The importance of arterial stiffness has been recognized for many centuries, and recent outcome data from various patient groups demonstrate that arterial stiffness is a powerful, independent predictor of cardiovascular disease [11]. Aortic stiffening leads to increase in systolic blood pressure (BP) and a fall in diastolic BP and, therefore, to a widening of pulse pressure. This increases left ventricular after load and oxygen demand, whilst decreasing coronary blood flow. Increased pulse pressure also raises the risk of stroke and damages capillaries e.g. in renal circulation. Arterial stiffening may also directly accelerate the atherosclerotic process due to changes in shear stress and vascular remodelling [12].

Arterial stiffness is regulated by numerous factors. Traditionally, mean arterial pressure and structural changes in the components of arterial wall were thought to be main determinants of arterial stiffness. With ageing, the neat arrangement of the elastin fibers within the media is lost and the elastin fibers become thinner and fragmented, and the stiffer collagen fibers become the load bearing ones [13]. Additionally, the loss of elastin fibers is associated with an increase in stiffer collagen fibers within the media, and arterial calcification. Moreover, the balance between the elastin synthesis and breakdown, by the matrix metalloproteinases contributes towards the arterial stiffening [12]. It is now recognized that arterial stiffness is also regulated by the smooth muscle tone, and that endothelium derived mediators, such as NO and endothelin-1, contribute to the functional regulation of arterial stiffness [14, 15]. It has also become apparent that inflammation has an important role in the stiffening of the large arteries [16], possibly via changes in the composition of the arterial wall due to inflammatory cell infiltration or via endothelial dysfunction [16, 17].

Clinical Evidence for Inflammation-Induced Arterial Stiffening

Epidemiological data from numerous outcome studies demonstrate the importance of inflammation in CVD [18]. A study in healthy individuals indicated an association between arterial stiffness and serum levels of CRP [19] and showed that aortic and brachial pulse wave velocity (PWV) and augmentation index (AIx) were independently related to the levels of inflammation, suggesting that inflammation plays a role in the regulation of arterial stiffening [19]. Most recently, data from the Caerphilly Prospective Study showed that both current CRP, and CRP at the beginning of the 20-year follow-up were strongly associated with aortic pulse wave velocity (aPWV) [16]. However, study by Schumacher et al. looking at three single nucleotide polymorphisms in the CRP gene found no relationship between any of the CRP genotypes and aortic pulse wave velocity despite different CRP levels, suggesting that CRP is a simply a marker of vascular damage/inflammation, not the causal molecule [20]. Furthermore, a large genome-wide association study by Elliott et al. concluded that the lack of concordance between the effect on coronary heart disease risk of CRP genotypes and CRP levels argues against a causal association of CRP with coronary heart disease [21].

Further information about the causality between inflammation and arterial stiffness can be gained by answering the following questions; (1) does inflammation cause arterial stiffening? (2) does a reduction in inflammation improve arterial stiffness?

Does Inflammation Cause Arterial Stiffening?

One approach to answer this question is to take a cohort of healthy individuals and induce an inflammatory response and observe the changes in arterial stiffness parameters. Such an experimental model of acute inflammation can be developed using *Salmonella typhi* vaccination. In healthy individuals this leads to an increase in aPWV 8 h post-vaccination, which is preventable by pre-treatment with aspirin [22] or simvastatin [23]. However, the effect on aPWV is very modest and a better way to study the role of inflammation in arterial stiffening may be to study patients with an existing inflammatory condition, such as RA and to reduce inflammation.

RA and other chronic inflammatory diseases represents ideal model to study effect of inflammation on arterial stiffness as they are associated with increased CV mortality [4, 6, 8, 9, 24], independently of traditional CV risk factors [5]. Numerous studies have demonstrated that RA [25, 26] and other inflammatory conditions, such as vasculitis [27], lupus [26], human immunodeficiency virus infection [28], COPD [29], inflammatory bowel disease [30], psoriasis [31], polymyalgia rheumatica [32] are associated with aortic stiffening. Moreover, arterial stiffness correlates, independently of blood pressure, age and gender, with the degree of active inflammation [25], suggesting that inflammation could be a potential target for drug therapy for arterial stiffness reduction.

Does a Reduction in Inflammation Improve Arterial Stiffness?

Anti-inflammatory Drugs

Although, many studies have looked at the effect of anti-inflammatory drugs on arterial stiffness, these studies have been relatively small and some conventionally used anti-inflammatory drugs may actually increase CV risk. Corticosteroids cause dyslipidaemia, hypertension, impaired glucose tolerance, and imbalances in thrombosis and fibrinolysis [33]. Methotrexate use can lead to hyperhomocysteinaemia, which is an independent predictor of CV events, although this problem can be overcome by concomitant supplementation of folic acid [34]. Selective COX-2 inhibitors and also non-selective NSAIDs increase mortality and CV events in numerous patients groups due to an inbalance of thromboxane A2 and prostacyclin [35]. However, these drugs also have an ameliorating effect on the vasculature by the reduction of inflammation and hence oxidative stress.

Corticosteroids has also been shown to have beneficial effect on arterial stiffness; a study by Pieringer et al. demonstrated a reduction in AIx in patients with PMR; from 28±9 to 25±10 %, P=0.006 [36]. Recently, Schillaci et al. demonstrated in patients with PMR that treatment with prednisolone reduced aPWV (from 11.8±3 to 10.5±3 m/s, P=0.015), and AIx (from 34±7 to 29±8 %, P=0.01). Notably these changes were independent of BP and heart rate changes and the change in aPWV correlated with change in plasma CRP (r=0.40, P=0.037) [32]. The results of these studies are contradicted by a study by Wong et al. who found that anti-inflammatory therapy with COX inhibitors; indomethacin and rofecoxib, did not improve endothelial function or reduce arterial stiffening [37]. However, this could be explained by the reduction of prostacyclin production, a powerful vasodilator, by COX inhibitors.

New immunomodulatory drugs represent better pharmacological tool to investigate the role of inflammation on stiffness as they are much more specific anti-inflammatory agents. Mäki-Petäjä et al. demonstrated in patients with RA, that anti-TNF-α therapy reduced aPWV (from 8.82±2.04 to 7.68±1.56 m/s, P<0.001) and, concomitantly, normalised endothelial function [25]. More recently, these findings have been confirmed in a larger cohort of patients with inflammatory arthropathies. Angel et al. demonstrated that aPWV was reduced in the group of patients receiving anti-TNF-α therapy, but not in a control group (−0.50±0.78 *versus* 0.05±0.54 m/s; P=0.002) [38]. On the contrary, van Doornum et al. and more recently, Pieringer et al., Mathieu et al. reported that anti-TNF-α-therapy did not reduce arterial stiffness in patients with chronic inflammatory conditions [39–41]. However, two of the studies assessed arterial stiffness by measuring AIx rather than aPWV. AIx may not be the most appropriate parameter to measure arterial stiffness in this particular cohort, since AIx is a composite measure of stiffness and probably more representative of wave reflection and peripheral vascular resistance. In patients with a high baseline inflammation, a reduction in inflammation could lead to a subsequent peripheral vasoconstriction, which would lead to increased impedance mis-match at the point of reflection and therefore the net effect on AIx would remain unchanged, despite a reduction in a wave speed (PWV). This notion was confirmed in the study by Vlachopoulos et al. where the experimentally induced inflammation led to an increase of aPWV, but a reduction of wave reflections (AIx) [22].

Only very few studies have investigated the effect of anti-inflammatory drugs on arterial stiffness in healthy individuals. Vlachopoulos et al. used *Salmonella typhi* vaccination to induce acute inflammation healthy subjects [22]. Interestingly, they demonstrated that there was no change in aPWV following the vaccination in those subjects that were randomised to receive aspirin pre-treatment, whereas aPWV significantly increased in the placebo group. Using the same model of acute inflammation, Wallace et al. similarly demonstrated that pre-treatment with Simvastatin also prevents inflammation-induced aortic stiffening [23].

Anti-lipideamic Drugs

Recently, numerous studies have reported so called “pleiotropic effects” of HMG-CoA reductase inhibitors (statins) use. These include improvement of endothelial function, increased nitric oxide bioavailability, antioxidant and anti-inflammatory effects as well a proposed role as an immunomodulator. Therefore it comes as no surprise that numerous studies have investigated statins as a means to reduce arterial stiffness [42].

Tomochika et al. was the first to show in late 1990’s that arterial stiffness can be reduced with a strict cholesterol-lowering therapy with pravastatin and probucol and diet [43]. A year later, Muramatsu et al. demonstrated in with hypercholesterolemia, that those patients who had 15 % or more reduction in total cholesterol following the pravastatin therapy also had a significant decrease in pulse wave velocity and total peripheral resistance [44]. Since these first two studies in the 1990's, several groups have studied the effect of different statins on arterial stiffness in numerous different cohorts, such as patients with hypercholesterolaemia, hypertension, CVD, chronic kidney disease, diabetes, RA and obesity and demonstrated that statins have favourable effect on arterial stiffness parameters [42]. However, CAFE-LLA study, a substudy of ASCOT, which was designed to assess the impact of lipid-lowering therapy with atorvastatin 10 mg versus placebo on central aortic pressures and hemodynamics, found no effect on central blood pressure or Aix, but no information about baseline CRP or whether CRP was reduced is available [45].

How Does Inflammation Lead to Arterial Stiffening- Potential Mechanisms?

Endothelial Dysfunction

Endothelial function can regulate arterial stiffness via changes in smooth muscle tone. Both basal and stimulated nitric oxide (NO) production can regulate muscular artery distensibility. There is also an inverse correlation between endothelial function, as measured by flow mediated dilatation response, and aPWV, which appears independent of potential confounding factors, including age and mean arterial pressure (MAP) [46]. Furthermore, local arterial distensibility is reduced by blockade of endogenous NO synthesis with the NO synthase inhibitor NG-monomethyl-L-arginine (LNMMA) in human iliac artery [14]. However, the role of nitric oxide in regulating stiffness of more elastic thoracic aorta, remains controversial, and may not be as important as regulation of muscular artery stiffness.

The association between acute and chronic inflammation and endothelial dysfunction has been demonstrated in numerous studies [47]. However, the mechanisms behind this are incompletely understood. One possibility is that certain cytokines induce expression of inducible nitric oxide synthase (iNOS) leading to a production reactive oxygen species (ROS) and subsequent uncoupling of endothelial NOS (eNOS) and reduction in nitric oxide (NO) production [48]. Moreover, acute phase protein CRP may also decrease eNOS expression and thus reduce NO bioavailability directly [49]. Production of myeloperoxidase (MPO) is another potential key mediator in inflammation-induced endothelial dysfunction. MPO is released for activated neutrophils during inflammation. MPO can catalytically consume NO, thus reducing NO bioavailability. Furthermore, MPO has the unique ability to produce hypochlorous acid and subsequently lead to uncoupling of eNOS [50], oxidation tetrabiopterin (BH_4) [51] and again further superoxide (O_2^-) production. Tetrahydrobiopterin (BH_4), a naturally occurring essential co-factor for eNOS is thought to play an important role. Recent, *in vitro* studies, suggest that activation of iNOS may lead to endothelial dysfunction by depleting the bioavailability of BH_4 from eNOS and subsequently uncouple eNOS, resulting to production of superoxide (O_2^-) rather than NO [52]. When O_2^- reacts with NO *in vivo*, peroxynitrite is formed, leading to oxidation of BH_4 and a reduction in the allosteric stability of eNOS, further uncoupling of eNOS. Furthermore, increased levels of adhesion molecules may damage the endothelial cells and lead to altered endothelial function [53], activation of neutrophils by anti-neutrophil cytoplasm antibodies within the vascular lumen may contribute to endothelial cell injury [54] or oxidation of LDL promoted by inflammation may lead to direct endothelial cell toxicity [55] and disturbed eNOS function.

Increased Synthesis of Matrix Metalloproteinases

Another mechanism, which could be responsible arterial stiffening during inflammation, is an accelerated elastin breakdown by matrix metalloproteinases (MMP). MMP synthesis is induced by CRP and the release of MMPs from the leukocytes can degrade elastin within the media. Yasmin et al. demonstrated in 677 subjects, that MMP-9 levels are independently associated with aortic stiffness [56]. In a further study, Yasmin et al. have demonstrated that aortic stiffness and elastase activity are influenced by MMP-9 gene polymorphisms, suggesting that the genetic variation in this protein may have a causal role in the process of large artery stiffening [57]. Although, elastin degradation may play important role in arterial stiffness over long periods of time, it is unlike to explain the more acute changes seen and also to explain how anti-inflammatory therapies are able to reduce stiffness. After all very little, if any, elastin is synthesised beyond the first year of life [58].

Calcification

Calcification is another potential mechanism behind inflammation-induced arterial stiffness. Several mediators of inflammation such as oxidation, carbonyl stress, C-reactive protein, and cytokines may directly stimulate vascular calcification [59]. This can lead to a phenotypic transformation of vascular smooth muscle cells, which increases bioapatite formation and therefore calcification as well as a transformation of vascular smooth muscle cells to osteoblast-like cells. Also, fetuin-A, an endogenous inhibitor of vascular calcification, is downregulated during inflammation and recently it has been demonstrated that fetuin-A is an independent risk factor for progressive arterial stiffness [60] in patients with chronic kidney disease. A study in children on dialysis, demonstrated that fetuin-A, and another physiological inhibitor of calcification osteoprotegerin are associated with increased aortic stiffness and calcification [61].

Smooth Muscle Proliferation and Changes in the Composition of Extracellular Matrix

The inflammatory response initiates an accumulation of leukocytes into the vascular endothelium. This can lead to a complex cascade of vascular smooth muscle cell (VSMC) activation, migration and proliferation. Activated VSMC can synthesise and secrete biologically active mediators such as endothelin, angiotensin II, cytokines, proteases, collagen and proteoglycans that regulate contraction, relaxation, inflammation, proliferation, apoptosis and matrix alterations [62] and can therefore subsequently lead to arterial stiffening. Alternatively, inflammation can alter the extracellular matrix (ECM).

ECM is a complex collection of fibrous proteins and glycoproteins, which are embedded in a hydrated ground substance of proteoglycans (PG), proteins with glycosaminoglycan (GAG) chain attached to them [63]. PGs have numerous specific roles within the vascular extracellular matrix, such as hydration, filtration, and regulation of various cellular activities as well as inflammatory processes [64]. During atherosclerosis and inflammation arterial GAGs within the intima accumulate, and inflammatory cytokines have capacity to alter GAGs in both quantitatively and qualitatively manner [65]. In intermediate and advanced atherosclerotic lesions, GAGs: decorin, versican, biglycan and hyaluronan (HA) are upregulated and alterations in HA metabolism, distribution, function has been documented in many diseases, e.g. RA & other inflammatory conditions and vascular disease [66]. Tissue enriched with hyaluronan tends to trap water and swell, forming a viscous hydrate gel which allows ECM to resist compression forces [66], i.e. making the wall stiffer. Also, overproduction of HA in the aorta results in stiffening of the arterial wall by thinning of elastic lamellae in animal models [67]. *In vitro* findings indicate that upregulation of hydrating GAGs lead to an increased water content of the vessel wall. This has been confirmed in a recent *in vivo* experiment using MRI with a gadolinium-based contrast, which indicated that in patients with CVD, inflammation causes increase in water content in the arterial wall, which correlated with histological markers of inflammation [68]. Although changes in the amount of hydrating GAGs in ECM can alter stiffness *in vitro*, to date there are no published *in vivo* data available in humans.

Direct Vascular Inflammation

Aortic stiffness in chronic inflammatory conditions may, at least in RA, be driven by direct vascular inflammation. Although the prevalence

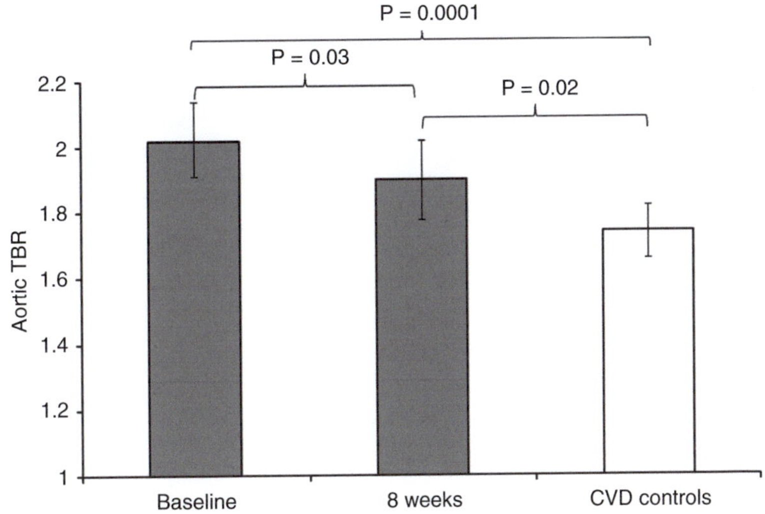

Fig. 35.1 The effect of anti-TNF-α therapy on ^{18}F-FDG uptake. Tissue to background ratio (*TBR*) in the whole aorta. *Bars* represent means and 95 % confidence intervals of means. n = 17 RA subjects and n = 34 age-matched controls with stable CVD (From Mäki-Petäjä et al. [73])

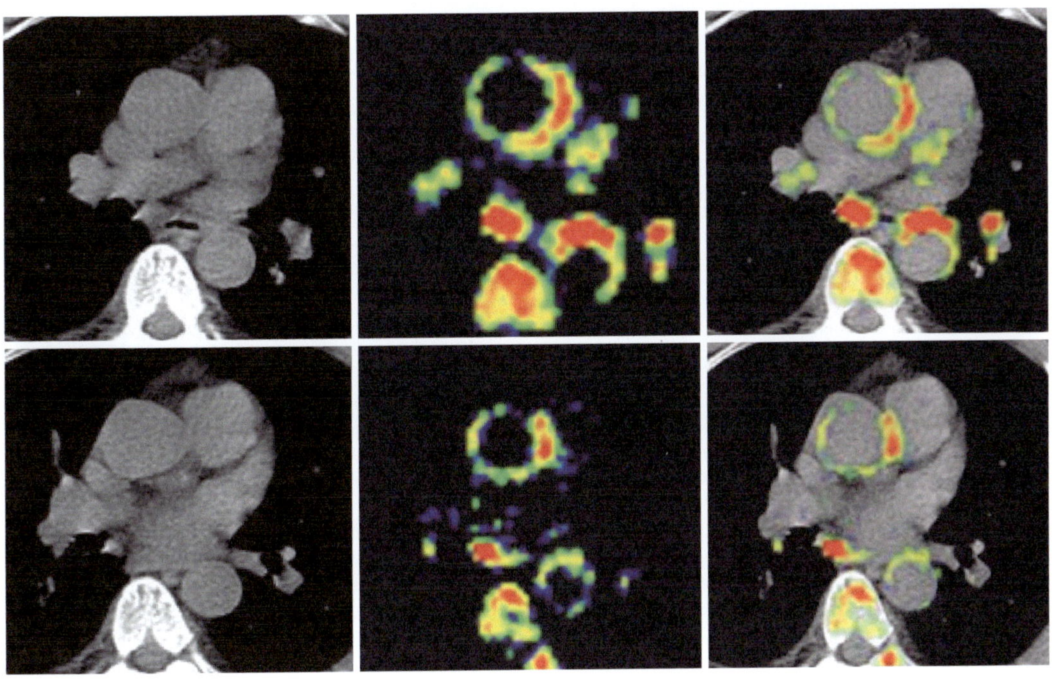

Fig. 35.2 Typical ^{18}F-FDG PET/CT images before and after anti-TNF-α therapy. Axial images of ascending and descending aorta from a typical RA patient. *Left to right*: CT, ^{18}F-FDG PET and fused PET/CT images. Baseline images are shown on the *top row* and after intervention on the *bottom row* (From Mäki-Petäjä et al. [73])

of clinical vasculitis in RA is low [69], the results of an autopsy series [70] and histological studies [71] suggest that sub-clinical vasculitis in RA is may be relatively common. However, it is rarely recognised or focused on in the clinical practice due to limited diagnostic opportunities [72]. A recent study in patients with severe RA, but without clinically manifest CVD, demonstrated increased aortic inflammation using, 18F-FDG PET/CT imaging, in comparison to subjects with established, stable CVD [73]. Additionally, the study demonstrated, leads to a reduction in inflammation along the whole aorta (Figs. 35.1 and 35.2), as well as in its most diseased segment following anti-TNF-α therapy, and that the reduction in aortic inflammation correlates with the reduction in aortic stiffness. Interestingly, RA patients exhibited generalised increase in aortic inflammation, rather than punctuate uptake, suggesting that RA patients exhibit a sub-clinical vasculitis, rather than increased atherosclerosis, which could provide a mechanism for the increased CVD risk seen in RA [74].

Conclusion

A strong body of evidence demonstrates that inflammation plays an important role in arterial stiffening. There are number of potential mechanisms which may explain this association including endothelial dysfunction and subsequent change in smooth muscle tone, smooth muscle proliferation and activation, changes in the composition of the extracellular matrix, and direct vascular inflammation. At present it is unclear which of these possible mechanisms is responsible, and therefore further studies are required to understand inflammation-induced arterial stiffening.

References

1. Libby P. Inflammation in atherosclerosis. Nature. 2002;420(6917):868–74.
2. Liuzzo G, Biasucci LM, Gallimore JR, Grillo RL, Rebuzzi AG, Pepys MB, et al. The prognostic value of C-reactive protein and serum amyloid a protein in severe unstable angina. N Engl J Med. 1994;331(7):417–24.
3. Ridker PM, Rifai N, Rose L, Buring JE, Cook NR. Comparison of C-reactive protein and low-density lipoprotein cholesterol levels in the prediction of first cardiovascular events. N Engl J Med. 2002;347(20):1557–65.
4. Wolfe F, Mitchell DM, Sibley JT, Fries JF, Bloch DA, Williams CA, et al. The mortality of rheumatoid arthritis. Arthritis Rheum. 1994;37(4):481–94.
5. del Rincon ID, Williams K, Stern MP, Freeman GL, Escalante A. High incidence of cardiovascular events in a rheumatoid arthritis cohort not explained by traditional cardiac risk factors. Arthritis Rheum. 2001;44(12):2737–45.
6. Knight JS, Kaplan MJ. Cardiovascular disease in lupus: insights and updates. Curr Opin Rheumatol. 2013;25(5):597–605.
7. Samarasekera EJ, Neilson JM, Warren RB, Parnham J, Smith CH. Incidence of cardiovascular disease in individuals with psoriasis: a systematic review and meta-analysis. J Invest Dermatol. 2013;133(10):2340–6.
8. Sin DD, Man SF. Chronic obstructive pulmonary disease as a risk factor for cardiovascular morbidity and mortality. Proc Am Thorac Soc. 2005;2(1):8–11.
9. Hancock AT, Mallen CD, Belcher J, Hider SL. Association between polymyalgia rheumatica and vascular disease: a systematic review. Arthrit Care Res (Hoboken). 2012;64(9):1301–5.
10. Pasceri V, Yeh ET. A tale of two diseases: atherosclerosis and rheumatoid arthritis. Circulation. 1999;100(21):2124–6.
11. Vlachopoulos C, Aznaouridis K, Stefanadis C. Prediction of cardiovascular events and all-cause mortality with arterial stiffness: a systematic review and meta-analysis. J Am Coll Cardiol. 2010;55(13):1318–27.
12. Zieman SJ, Melenovsky V, Kass DA. Mechanisms, pathophysiology, and therapy of arterial stiffness. Arterioscler Thromb Vasc Biol. 2005;25(5):932–43.
13. O'Rourke MF, Nichols WW. Aortic diameter, aortic stiffness, and wave reflection increase with age and isolated systolic hypertension. Hypertension. 2005;45(4):652–8.
14. Schmitt M, Avolio A, Qasem A, McEniery CM, Butlin M, Wilkinson IB, et al. Basal NO locally modulates human iliac artery function in vivo. Hypertension. 2005;46(1):227–31.
15. McEniery CM, Wallace S, Mackenzie IS, McDonnell B, Yasmin, Newby DE, et al. Endothelial function is associated with pulse pressure, pulse wave velocity, and augmentation index in healthy humans. Hypertension. 2006;48(4):602–8.
16. McEniery CM, Spratt M, Munnery M, Yarnell J, Lowe GD, Rumley A, et al. An analysis of prospective risk factors for aortic stiffness in men: 20-year follow-up from the Caerphilly prospective study. Hypertension. 2010;56(1):36–43.
17. Laurent S, Cockcroft J, Van Bortel L, Boutouyrie P, Giannattasio C, Hayoz D, et al. Expert consensus document on arterial stiffness: methodological issues and clinical applications. Eur Heart J. 2006;27(21):2588–605.
18. Currie CJ, Poole CD, Conway P. Evaluation of the association between the first observation and the longitudinal change in C-reactive protein, and all-cause mortality. Heart. 2008;94(4):457–62.
19. Yasmin, McEniery CM, Wallace S, Mackenzie IS, Cockcroft JR, Wilkinson IB. C-reactive protein is associated with arterial stiffness in apparently healthy individuals. Arterioscl Throm Vas Biol. 2004;24(5):969–74.
20. Schumacher W, Cockcroft J, Timpson NJ, McEniery CM, Gallacher J, Rumley A, et al. Association between C-reactive protein genotype, circulating levels, and aortic pulse wave velocity. Hypertension. 2009;53(2):150–7.
21. Elliott P, Chambers JC, Zhang W, Clarke R, Hopewell JC, Peden JF, et al. Genetic Loci associated with C-reactive protein levels and risk of coronary heart disease. JAMA. 2009;302(1):37–48.
22. Vlachopoulos C, Dima I, Aznaouridis K, Vasiliadou C, Ioakeimidis N, Aggeli C, et al. Acute systemic

inflammation increases arterial stiffness and decreases wave reflections in healthy individuals. Circulation. 2005;112(14):2193–200.
23. Wallace SM, Maki-Petaja KM, Cheriyan J, Davidson EH, Cherry L, McEniery CM, et al. Simvastatin prevents inflammation-induced aortic stiffening and endothelial dysfunction. Br J Clin Pharmacol. 2010;70(6):799–806.
24. Wallberg-Jonsson S, Johansson H, Ohman ML, Rantapaa-Dahlqvist S. Extent of inflammation predicts cardiovascular disease and overall mortality in seropositive rheumatoid arthritis. A retrospective cohort study from disease onset. J Rheum. 1999;26(12):2562–71.
25. Maki-Petaja KM, Hall FC, Booth AD, Wallace SM, Yasmin, Bearcroft PW, et al. Rheumatoid arthritis is associated with increased aortic pulse-wave velocity, which is reduced by anti-tumor necrosis factor-alpha therapy. Circulation. 2006;114(11):1185–92.
26. Roman MJ, Devereux RB, Schwartz JE, Lockshin MD, Paget SA, Davis A, et al. Arterial stiffness in chronic inflammatory diseases. Hypertension. 2005; 46:1–6.
27. Booth AD, Wallace S, Yasmin, Jayne DR, Brown J. Inflammation and arterial stiffness in systemic vasculitis: a model of vascular inflammation. Arthritis Rheum. 2004;50(2):581–8.
28. Schillaci G, De Socio GV, Pucci G, Mannarino MR, Helou J, Pirro M, et al. Aortic stiffness in untreated adult patients with human immunodeficiency virus infection. Hypertension. 2008;52(2):308–13.
29. Sabit R, Bolton CE, Edwards PH, Pettit RJ, Evans WD, McEniery CM, et al. Arterial stiffness and osteoporosis in chronic obstructive pulmonary disease. Am J Respir Crit Care Med. 2007;175(12):1259–65.
30. Zanoli L, Cannavo M, Rastelli S, Di PL, Monte I, Di GM, et al. Arterial stiffness is increased in patients with inflammatory bowel disease. J Hypertens. 2012;30(9):1775–81.
31. Yiu KH, Yeung CK, Chan HT, Wong RM, Tam S, Lam KF, et al. Increased arterial stiffness in patients with psoriasis is associated with active systemic inflammation. Br J Dermatol. 2011;164(3):514–20.
32. Schillaci G, Bartoloni E, Pucci G, Pirro M, Settimi L, Alunno A, et al. Aortic stiffness is increased in polymyalgia rheumatica and improves after steroid treatment. Ann Rheum Dis. 2012;71(7):1151–6.
33. Maxwell SR, Moots RJ, Kendall MJ. Corticosteroids: do they damage the cardiovascular system? Postgrad Med J. 1994;70(830):863–70.
34. Slot O. Changes in plasma homocysteine in arthritis patients starting treatment with low-dose methotrexate subsequently supplemented with folic acid. Scand J Rheumatol. 2001;30(5):305–7.
35. Gislason GH, Jacobsen S, Rasmussen JN, Rasmussen S, Buch P, Friberg J, et al. Risk of death or reinfarction associated with the use of selective cyclooxygenase-2 inhibitors and nonselective nonsteroidal antiinflammatory drugs after acute myocardial infarction. Circulation. 2006;113(25):2906–13.
36. Pieringer H, Stuby U, Hargassner S, Biesenbach G. Treatment with corticosteroids reduces arterial stiffness in patients with polymyalgia rheumatica as measured with pulse wave analysis. Ann Rheum Dis. 2008;67(2):279.
37. Wong M, Jiang BY, McNeill K, Farish S, Kirkham B, Chowienczyk P. Effects of selective and non-selective cyclo-oxygenase inhibition on endothelial function in patients with rheumatoid arthritis. Scand J Rheumatol. 2007;36(4):265–9.
38. Angel K, Provan SA, Gulseth HL, Mowinckel P, Kvien TK, Atar D. Tumor necrosis factor-alpha antagonists improve aortic stiffness in patients with inflammatory arthropathies: a controlled study. Hypertension. 2010;55(2):333–8.
39. Doornum SV, McColl G, Wicks IP. Tumour necrosis factor antagonists improve disease activity but not arterial stiffness in rheumatoid arthritis. Rheumatology (Oxford). 2005;44:1428–32.
40. Pieringer H, Stuby U, Pohanka E, Biesenbach G. Augmentation index in patients with rheumatoid arthritis and ankylosing spondylitis treated with infliximab. Clin Rheumatol. 2010;29(7):723–7.
41. Mathieu S, Pereira B, Couderc M, Rabois E, Dubost JJ, Soubrier M. No significant changes in arterial stiffness in patients with ankylosing spondylitis after tumour necrosis factor alpha blockade treatment for 6 and 12 months. Rheumatology (Oxford). 2013;52(1):204–9.
42. Maki-Petaja KM, Wilkinson IB. Anti-inflammatory drugs and statins for arterial stiffness reduction. Curr Pharm Des. 2009;15(3):290–303.
43. Tomochika Y, Okuda F, Tanaka N, Wasaki Y, Tokisawa I, Aoyagi S, et al. Improvement of atherosclerosis and stiffness of the thoracic descending aorta with cholesterol-lowering therapies in familial hypercholesterolemia. Arterioscler Thromb Vasc Biol. 1996;16(8):955–62.
44. Muramatsu J, Kobayashi A, Hasegawa N, Yokouchi S. Hemodynamic changes associated with reduction in total cholesterol by treatment with the HMG-CoA reductase inhibitor pravastatin. Atherosclerosis. 1997;130(1–2):179–82.
45. Williams B, Lacy PS, Cruickshank JK, Collier D, Hughes AD, Stanton A, et al. Impact of statin therapy on central aortic pressures and hemodynamics: principal results of the Conduit Artery Function Evaluation-Lipid-Lowering Arm (CAFE-LLA) Study. Circulation. 2009;119(1):53–61.
46. Wallace SM, Yasmin, McEniery CM, Maki-Petaja KM, Booth AD, Cockcroft JR, et al. Isolated systolic hypertension is characterized by increased aortic stiffness and endothelial dysfunction. Hypertension. 2007;50(1):228–33.
47. Hingorani AD, Cross J, Kharbanda RK, Mullen MJ, Bhagat K, Taylor M, et al. Acute systemic inflammation impairs endothelium-dependent dilatation in humans. Circulation. 2000;102(9):994–9.
48. Gunnett CA, Lund DD, McDowell AK, Faraci FM, Heistad DD. Mechanisms of inducible nitric oxide

synthase-mediated vascular dysfunction. Arterioscler Thromb Vasc Biol. 2005;25(8):1617–22.
49. Fichtlscherer S, Breuer S, Schachinger V, Dimmeler S, Zeiher AM. C-reactive protein levels determine systemic nitric oxide bioavailability in patients with coronary artery disease. Eur Heart J. 2004;25(16):1412–8.
50. Xu J, Xie Z, Reece R, Pimental D, Zou MH. Uncoupling of endothelial nitric oxidase synthase by hypochlorous acid: role of NAD(P)H oxidase-derived superoxide and peroxynitrite. Arterioscler Thromb Vasc Biol. 2006;26(12):2688–95.
51. Laursen JB, Somers M, Kurz S, McCann L, Warnholtz A, Freeman BA, et al. Endothelial regulation of vasomotion in apoE-deficient mice: implications for interactions between peroxynitrite and tetrahydrobiopterin. Circulation. 2001;103(9):1282–8.
52. Kinoshita H, Tsutsui M, Milstien S, Katusic ZS. Tetrahydrobiopterin, nitric oxide and regulation of cerebral arterial tone. Prog Neurobiol. 1997; 52(4):295–302.
53. Wallberg-Jonsson S, Cvetkovic JT, Sundqvist KG, Lefvert AK, Rantapaa-Dahlqvist S. Activation of the immune system and inflammatory activity in relation to markers of atherothrombotic disease and atherosclerosis in rheumatoid arthritis. J Rheumatol. 2002;29(5):875–82.
54. Savage CO, Pottinger BE, Gaskin G, Pusey CD, Pearson JD. Autoantibodies developing to myeloperoxidase and proteinase 3 in systemic vasculitis stimulate neutrophil cytotoxicity toward cultured endothelial cells. Am J Pathol. 1992;141(2):335–42.
55. Morel DW, Hessler JR, Chisolm GM. Low density lipoprotein cytotoxicity induced by free radical peroxidation of lipid. J Lipid Res. 1983;24(8):1070–6.
56. Yasmin, Wallace S, McEniery CM, Dakham Z, Pusalkar P, Maki-Petaja K, et al. Matrix metalloproteinase-9 (MMP-9), MMP-2, and serum elastase activity are associated with systolic hypertension and arterial stiffness. Arterioscler Thromb Vasc Biol. 2005;25(2):372.
57. Yasmin, McEniery CM, O'Shaughnessy KM, Harnett P, Arshad A, Wallace S, et al. Variation in the human matrix metalloproteinase-9 gene is associated with arterial stiffness in healthy individuals. Arterioscler Thromb Vasc Biol. 2006;26(8):1799–805.
58. Martyn CN, Greenwald SE. Impaired synthesis of elastin in walls of aorta and large conduit arteries during early development as an initiating event in pathogenesis of systemic hypertension. Lancet. 1997;350(9082):953–5.
59. Moe SM, Chen NX. Inflammation and vascular calcification. Blood Purif. 2005;23(1):64–71.
60. Ford ML, Tomlinson LA, Smith ER, Rajkumar C, Holt SG. Fetuin-A is an independent determinant of change of aortic stiffness over 1 year in non-diabetic patients with CKD stages 3 and 4. Nephrol Dial Transplant. 2010;25(6):1853–8.
61. Shroff RC, Shah V, Hiorns MP, Schoppet M, Hofbauer LC, Hawa G, et al. The circulating calcification inhibitors, fetuin-A and osteoprotegerin, but not matrix Gla protein, are associated with vascular stiffness and calcification in children on dialysis. Nephrol Dial Transplant. 2008;23(10):3263–71.
62. Dzau VJ, Braun-Dullaeus RC, Sedding DG. Vascular proliferation and atherosclerosis: new perspectives and therapeutic strategies. Nat Med. 2002;8(11):1249–56.
63. Raines EW. The extracellular matrix can regulate vascular cell migration, proliferation, and survival: relationships to vascular disease. Int J Exp Pathol. 2000;81(3):173–82.
64. Jacob MP. Extracellular matrix remodeling and matrix metalloproteinases in the vascular wall during aging and in pathological conditions. Biomed Pharmacother. 2003;57(5–6):195–202.
65. Kaji T, Hiraga S, Yamamoto C, Sakamoto M, Nakashima Y, Sueishi K, et al. Tumor necrosis factor alpha-induced alteration of glycosaminoglycans in cultured vascular smooth-muscle cells. Biochim Biophys Acta. 1993;1176(1–2):20–6.
66. Toole BP, Wight TN, Tammi MI. Hyaluronan-cell interactions in cancer and vascular disease. J Biol Chem. 2002;277(7):4593–6.
67. Chai S, Chai Q, Danielsen CC, Hjorth P, Nyengaard JR, Ledet T, et al. Overexpression of hyaluronan in the tunica media promotes the development of atherosclerosis. Circ Res. 2005;96(5):583–91.
68. Li D, Fayad ZA, Bluemke DA. Can contrast-enhanced cardiac magnetic resonance assess inflammation of the coronary wall? JACC Cardiovasc Imaging. 2009;2(5):589–91.
69. Watts RA, Mooney J, Lane SE, Scott DG. Rheumatoid vasculitis: becoming extinct? Rheumatology (Oxford). 2004;43(7):920–3.
70. Gravallese EM, Corson JM, Coblyn JS, Pinkus GS, Weinblatt ME. Rheumatoid aortitis: a rarely recognized but clinically significant entity. Medicine (Baltimore). 1989;68(2):95–106.
71. Hollan I, Prayson R, Saatvedt K, Almdahl SM, Nossent HC, Mikkelsen K, et al. Inflammatory cell infiltrates in vessels with different susceptibility to atherosclerosis in rheumatic and non-rheumatic patients: a controlled study of biopsy specimens obtained at coronary artery surgery. Circ J. 2008;72(12):1986–92.
72. Hollan I, Meroni PL, Ahearn JM, Cohen Tervaert JW, Curran S, Goodyear CS, et al. Cardiovascular disease in autoimmune rheumatic diseases. Autoimmun Rev. 2013;12(10):1004–15. Ref Type: Journal (Full).
73. Maki-Petaja KM, Elkhawad M, Cheriyan J, Joshi FR, Ostor AJK, Hall FC, et al. Anti-tumor factor-α therapy reduces aortic inflammation and stiffness in patients with rheumatoid arthritis. Circulation. 2012;126(21):2473–80. Ref Type: Journal (Full).
74. Fayad ZA, Greenberg JD, Bucerius J. Subclinical vasculitis as a potential mechanism to explain the heightened cardiovascular risk in rheumatoid arthritis. Circulation. 2012;126(21):2449–51.

Part V

Stratifications of Cardiovascular Risk and Therapeutic Consequences on Arterial Stiffness and Wave Reflections

36 Outcome-Driven Thresholds for Pulse Pressure on Office and Out-of-the-Office Blood Pressure Measurement

Yumei Gu, Lucas S. Aparicio, Yanping Liu, Kei Asayama, Tine W. Hansen, Teemu J. Niiranen, José Boggia, Lutgarde Thijs, and Jan A. Staessen

Abstract

Longitudinal studies demonstrated that the risk of cardiovascular disease increased with pulse pressure (PP). However, PP remains an elusive cardiovascular risk factor with findings being inconsistent between studies. The 2013 ESH/ESC guideline proposed that PP is useful in stratification and

Y. Gu, MD, PhD • Y. Liu, MD, PhD • L. Thijs, MSC
Studies Coordinating Centre, Division of Hypertension and Cardiovascular Rehabilitation, Department of Cardiovascular Sciences, University of Leuven, Leuven, Belgium
e-mail: yumei.gu@med.kuleuven.be; yanping.liu@med.kuleuven.be; lutgarde.thijs@med.kuleuven.be

L.S. Aparicio, MD, DDS
Internal Medicine – Hypertension Section, Hospital Italiano De Buenos Aires, Juan D. Peron 4190, Buenos Aires C1199ABD, Argentina
e-mail: lucas.aparicio@hospitalitaliano.org.ar

K. Asayama, MD, PhD
Studies Coordinating Centre, Division of Hypertension and Cardiovascular Rehabilitation, Department of Cardiovascular Sciences, University of Leuven, Leuven, Belgium

Department of Planning for Drug Development and Clinical Evaluation, Tohoku University Graduate School of Pharmaceutical Sciences, 6-3 Aramaki-Aza-Aoba, Aoba-ku, Sendai 980-8578, Japan

Department of Hygiene and Public Health, Teikyo University School of Medicine, 2-11-1 Kaga, Itabashi-ku, Tokyo 173-8605, Japan
e-mail: kei@asayama.org

T.W. Hansen, MD, PhD
Department of Complications, Steno Diabetes Center, Niels Steensens Vej 2-4, Gentofte 2820, Denmark
e-mail: twih@steno.dk

T.J. Niiranen, MD, PhD
Department of Chronic Disease Prevention, National Institute for Health and Welfare, Peltolantie 3, Turku 20720, Finland

Department of Medicine, Turku University Hospital, PO Box 52, Turku 20521, Finland
e-mail: teemu.niiranen@thl.fi

J. Boggia, MD, PhD
Centro de Nefrología and Departamento de Fisiopatología, Hospital de Clínicas, Dr Manuel Quintela, Av Italia 2870, Piso 15, ala oeste, Of 13, Montevideo 11600, Uruguay
e-mail: ppboggia@gmail.com, jboggia@hc.edu.uy

J.A. Staessen, MD, PhD (✉)
Studies Coordinating Centre, Division of Hypertension and Cardiovascular Rehabilitation, Department of Cardiovascular Sciences, University of Leuven, Kapucijnenvoer 35, Block D, 7001 BE-3000, Leuven, Belgium

Department of Epidemiology, Maastricht University, Peter Debyeplein 1, 616, Maastricht 6200, The Netherlands
e-mail: jan.staessen@med.kuleuven.be, jan.staessen@maastrichtuniversity.nl

M.E. Safar et al. (eds.), *Blood Pressure and Arterial Wall Mechanics in Cardiovascular Diseases*, DOI 10.1007/978-1-4471-5198-2_36, © Springer-Verlag London 2014

suggested 60 mmHg as threshold, moving it up to by 10 mmHg compared with the 2007 guideline without providing any justification. Published thresholds of PP are based on office blood pressure measurement and often on arbitrary categorical analyses. In the International Database on Ambulatory blood pressure in relation to Cardiovascular Outcomes (IDACO) and in the International Database on Home blood pressure in relation to Cardiovascular Outcome (IDHOCO), we determined outcome-driven thresholds for PP based on ambulatory or home blood pressure measurement, respectively. The main findings are that below age 60 PP does not refine risk stratification, whereas in older people the thresholds were 64 and 76 mmHg for the ambulatory and home PP, respectively. However, PP provided little added predictive value over and beyond classical risk factors.

Keywords

Pulse pressure • Thresholds • Blood pressure measurement • Epidemiology • Cardiovascular diseases

Introduction

Pulse pressure (PP), the difference between systolic and diastolic blood pressure, depends on left ventricular ejection, the elasticity of the central arteries, and the timing and intensity of the backward wave originating at reflection sites in the peripheral circulation. PP widens in the elderly, because with advancing age systolic blood pressure continues to rise, whereas the age-related increase in diastolic blood pressure levels off or even reverses in the fifth decade of life [1] (Fig. 36.1).

PP as a Cardiovascular Risk Factor

Previous cohort studies found that peripheral PP, as measured by conventional sphygmomanometry, was an independent risk in patients with hypertension [2–5], coronary heart disease [2], or severe renal dysfunction [6, 7] or in populations [8–13]. However, other studies [14–16] were contradictory in that cardiovascular risk was not associated with PP. Several limitations of previous studies likely contributed to the contradictory findings in the literature. They mostly used the office blood pressure measurement or only recorded fatal endpoints [6, 7, 9, 11–15] or applied recruitment criteria confined to high-risk patients [2–5, 7, 15], a narrow age range [9, 13], or elderly [5, 12] or reported that the association of outcome and PP was present only in diabetic [11] or treated hypertensive patients [4].

Studies in Patients

In the International Verapamil SR-Trandolapril Study (INVEST), Bangalore and colleagues [2] analyzed 22,576 hypertensive patients with coronary artery disease. The relation between the incidence and multivariable-adjusted hazard ratio (HR) for all-cause mortality, nonfatal myocardial infarction, and nonfatal stroke with PP during follow-up was J- or U-shaped [2]. With adjustments applied for baseline covariables, both the linear and quadratic terms of PP were significant ($p<0.0001$) [2]. The nadir was at 54 mmHg with 95 % confidence interval (CI) derived by bootstrapping ranging from 42 to 60 mmHg [2]. The relation of stroke with PP was linear [2].

Greenberg and colleagues [4] analyzed 2,939 hypertensive patients from 33 to 87 years old, enrolled in the Epidemiologic Follow-up Study (NHEFS) of the First National Health and Nutrition Examination Survey (NHANES I). For cardiovascular mortality, the HRs associated with

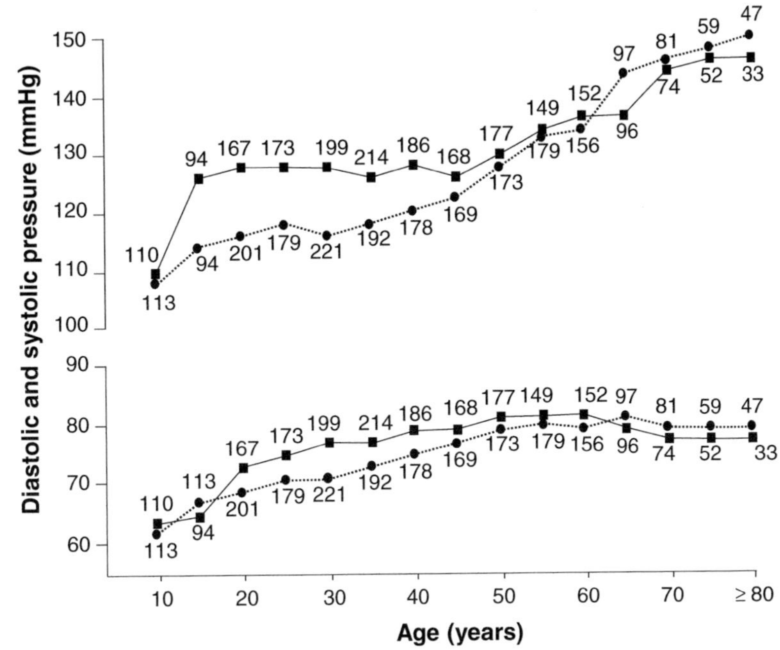

Fig. 36.1 Systolic and diastolic blood pressures in 5-year age classes in a representative sample (n=4,202) of the population of five Belgian districts. In each subject, five blood pressure readings were obtained at each of two separate home visits. The five blood pressure readings from the second home visit were averaged for this presentation. For each sex and age group, the number of subjects contributing to the mean is given. ■, men (n=2,044); ●, women (n=2,158) (Reproduced with permission from Ref. [1])

a 10-mmHg increment in PP were 1.16 (CI, 1.08–1.25) and 1.12 (CI, 0.99–1.26) in treated and untreated hypertensive patients, respectively [4]. In the Systolic Hypertension in the Elderly Program (SHEP), Domanski and colleagues [5] demonstrated for a 10-mmHg increase in PP that the risk of all-cause mortality and of fatal stroke increased by 16 and 11 %, respectively.

Several studies investigated the risk of renal function associated with PP [6, 7]. Liu and colleagues [7] studied 153 patients (mean age, 54.5 ± 14.2 years) with end-stage renal disease on peritoneal dialysis. PP was measured monthly for 3 months. The Kaplan-Meier survival estimates showed a significantly higher total mortality associated with increasing tertiles of PP (p<0.05) [7]. These findings were consistent in the analysis adjusted for systolic or diastolic blood pressure [7].

Studies in Populations

In 2001, the Framingham investigators [8] reported that with increasing age, there was a gradual shift from diastolic blood pressure to systolic blood pressure and then to PP as predictors of coronary heart disease. In 1989, Darne and colleagues [13] evaluated the risk associated with PP and mean arterial pressure, while addressing the collinearity between these two predictive variables. Darne and colleagues [13] used principal components analysis of systolic and diastolic blood pressure to generate a pulsatile and a steady component index of arterial pressure. The pulsatile component index was positively correlated with PP and the steady component index with mean arterial pressure, but in statistical terms the two new indices were completely unrelated [13]. In 18,336 men and 9,351 women, aged 40–69 years and followed for an average of 9.5 years, the investigators demonstrated that the steady component index of blood pressure was a strong predictor of all types of cardiovascular death in both sexes [13]. In contrast, the pulsatile component index was unrelated to prognosis in men, but in women it was positively and independently correlated with death from coronary heart disease and inversely with stroke mortality [13]. However, the latter relations in women were based only on 15 deaths from myocardial infarction and 22 from stroke [13].

Along similar lines, Benetos and colleagues [9] recruited 19,083 French men, aged 40–69 years at baseline and captured them in follow-up for 19.5 years. A wide PP was an independent and significant predictor of all cause (odds ratio for 10-mmHg increase in younger participants vs. in older participants, 1.28 vs. 1.19; $p<0.05$), total cardiovascular (1.36 vs. 1.24; $p<0.05$), and, especially, coronary mortality (1.40 vs. 1.20; $p<0.05$) [9]. In 1981, the National Institute on Aging initiated its epidemiologic studies of the elderly people [12], Glynn and colleagues followed 9,431 participants aged 65–102 years for 10.6 years. In sex- and age-adjusted survival analysis, both elevated systolic blood pressure over 160 mmHg and low diastolic blood pressure below 70 mmHg independently predicted total (relative risk, 1.39 for systolic and 1.27 for diastolic; CI, 1.26–1.53 and 1.16–1.38) and cardiovascular mortality (1.59 for systolic and 1.38 for diastolic; CI, 1.39–1.81 and 1.22–1.55, $p<0.001$) [12]. Pulse pressure correlated strongly with systolic pressure ($r=0.82$)[12] confirming the issue of collinearity first raised by Darne and colleagues [13]. The investigators reported that PP was a slightly stronger predictor of both total (relative risk, 1.34; CI, 1.23–1.46) and cardiovascular mortality (relative risk, 1.57; CI, 1.39–1.77) [12].

In the Hoorn study, Schram and colleagues [11] followed 2,484 people including 208 type-2 diabetic patients for 8.8 years. PP was associated with cardiovascular mortality among the diabetic, but not among the nondiabetic individuals [adjusted relative risk (CI) per 10 mmHg increase, 1.27 (1.00–1.61) and 0.98 (0.85–1.13), p interaction$=0.07$] [11]. Further adjustment for other risk factors gave similar results [11]. The association, at baseline, between age and PP was dependent on the presence of diabetes (p interaction$=0.03$) and on the mean arterial pressure (p interaction<0.001) [11]. That is, there was a stronger association when diabetes was present and when mean arterial pressure was higher [11].

IDACO Study

To define outcome-driven thresholds for ambulatory PP, we did a subject-level meta-analysis of 9,938 people recruited from 11 populations and enrolled in the IDACO [17]. Because of the Framingham results [18] and the lower age boundary in several randomized clinical trials on antihypertensive treatment in the elderly [19], we stratified our analyses by 60 years of age. Exploratory analyses demonstrated that the association of endpoints with 24-h PP was not always log-linear. To account for this nonlinear association, we applied the deviation from mean coding [20] to compute HRs in tenths of the 24-h PP distribution. This approach expresses the risk in each tenth relative to the overall risk in the whole study population and allows computing CIs for the HRs in all tenths without definition of an arbitrary reference group. HRs relating endpoints to mean arterial pressure expressed the risk associated with a 1-SD increase in the level. We applied the generalized R^2 statistic to assess the risks additionally explained by 24-h PP over and beyond mean arterial pressure and other covariables [21]. In an attempt to refine the level of PP that was associated with significantly increased risk, we did a stepwise analysis. We calculated HRs for 1-mmHg increments in PP for thresholds ranging from the 10th to the 90th percentile. These HRs expressed the risk in participants whose PP exceeded the cutoff point versus average risk. We plotted these HRs and their 95 % confidence limits versus the increasing cutoff points with the goal to determine at which level the lower confidence limit of the HRs crossed unity.

Among 6,028 younger participants (<60 years), median follow-up was 12.1 years. Over 68,853 person-years, 228 participants died and 221 experienced a fatal or nonfatal cardiovascular complication. Only in the highest tenth of the PP distribution (threshold, ≥55.6 mmHg; mean, 60.1 mmHg) the risk of the composite cardiovascular endpoint was elevated (HR, 1.58; CI, 1.11–2.25; $p=0.011$) with a similar trend for cardiac endpoints (HR, 1.52; CI, 0.99–2.33; $p=0.056$). Otherwise, the risks across tenths of the PP distribution did not deviate from average ($p\geq0.058$). For stroke, Cox models across tenths of the PP distribution did not converge, because of the low number of events ($n=63$). While calculating the thresholds of 24-h PP levels that stepwise increased by 1-mmHg from the 10th to the 90th percentile, for all endpoints under study, the lower boundary of the confidence interval of the successive HRs did not cross unity.

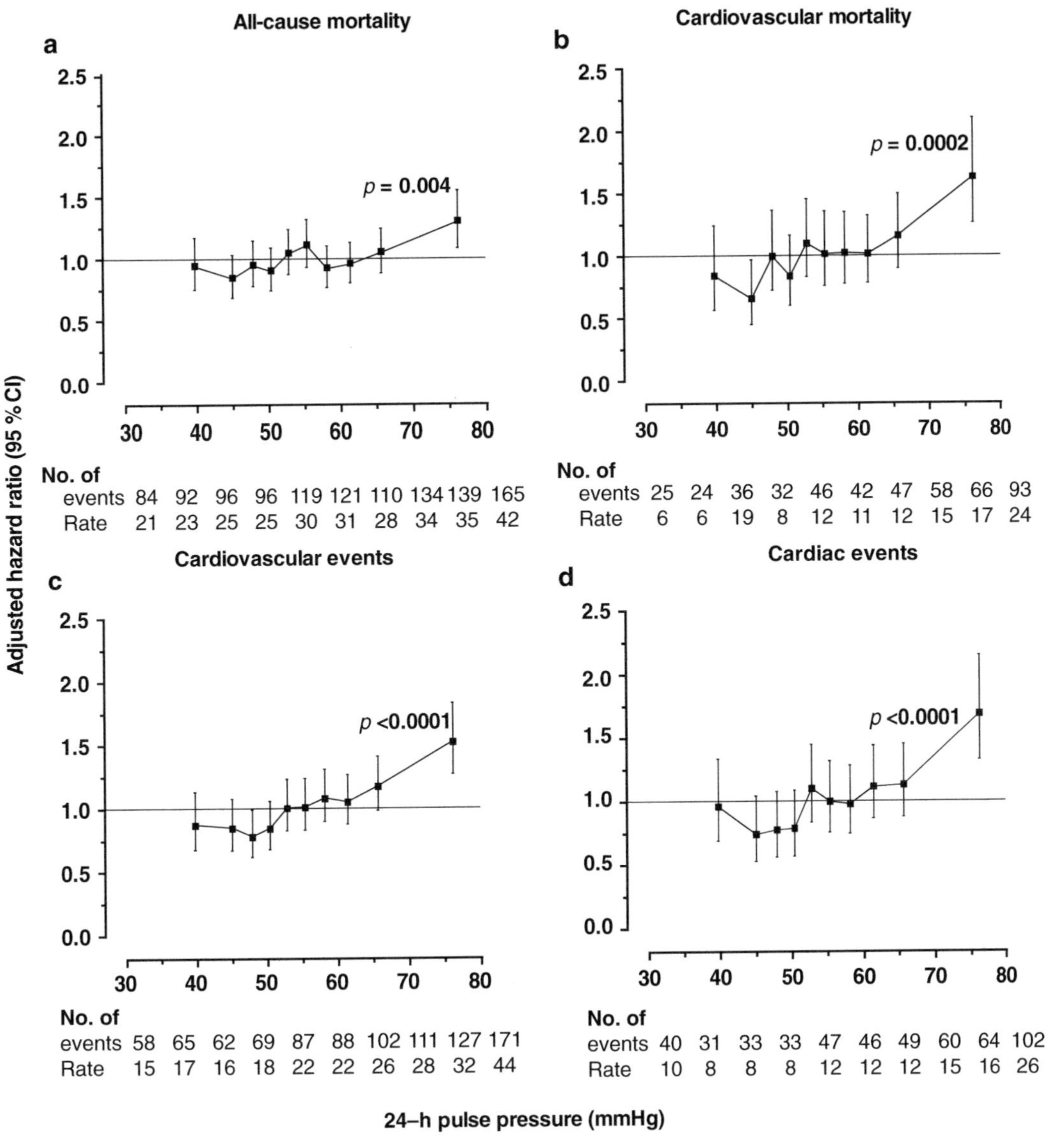

Fig. 36.2 Hazard ratios in tenths of the distribution of 24-h pulse pressure in 3,910 older participants. Hazard ratios for total (**a**) and cardiovascular (**b**) mortality and for cardiovascular (**c**) and cardiac (**d**) events express the risk in each tenth compared with average risk. The hazard ratios were adjusted for cohort, sex, age, 24-h mean arterial pressure, 24-h heart rate, body mass index, smoking and drinking, serum cholesterol, history of cardiovascular disease and diabetes, and antihypertensive drug treatment. *Vertical bars* denote 95 % confidence intervals. For each tenth, the number of events and unadjusted incidence rates (in percent) are given. The p value refers to the significance of the hazard ratio in the top tenth of the 24-h pulse pressure distribution (Reproduced with permission from Ref. [17])

Among 3,910 older participants (≥60 years), median follow-up was 10.7 years. Over 39,923 person-years, 1,160 participants died and 940 experienced a fatal or nonfatal cardiovascular complication. The risk of any death, cardiovascular mortality, a composite cardiovascular endpoint, or a cardiac event was consistently elevated in the top tenth of the PP distribution (threshold, ≥68.8 mmHg; mean, 76.1 mmHg, Fig. 36.2). The HRs were 1.30, 1.62, 1.52, and 1.69, respectively (Fig. 36.2). The HR for stroke in the top tenth of the PP distribution was 1.40 ($p=0.028$). Otherwise, the risks across tenths of the PP distribution did not deviate from average. The R^2

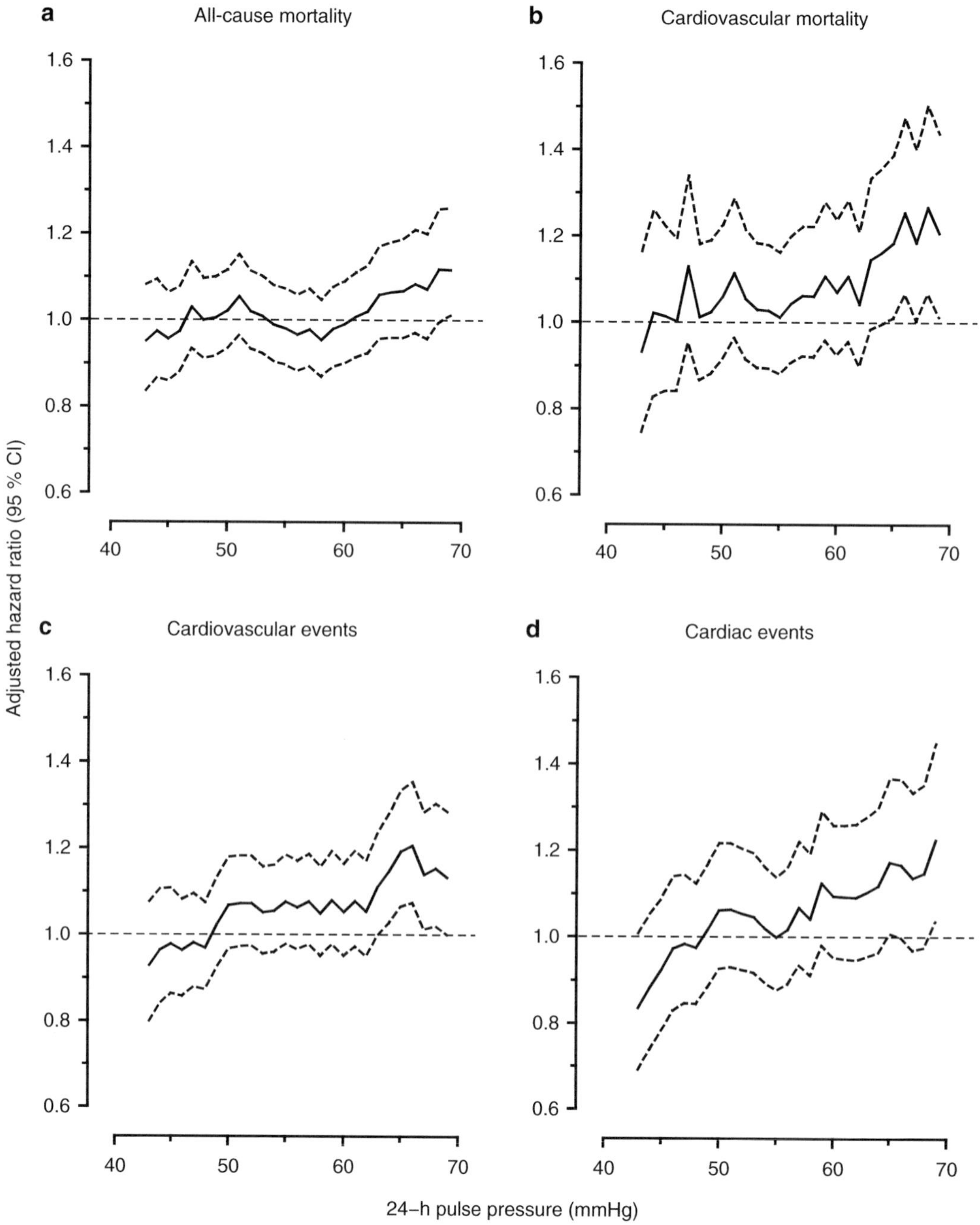

Fig. 36.3 Hazard ratios according to 24-h pulse pressure levels ranging from the 10th to the 90th percentile in 3,910 older participants. Hazard ratios for total (**a**) and cardiovascular (**b**) mortality and for cardiovascular (**c**) and cardiac (**d**) events express the risk at each level of pulse pressure compared with average risk. Solid and dotted lines denote the point estimates and the 95 % confidence intervals, respectively. The hazard ratios were adjusted as in Fig. 36.2 (Reproduced with permission from Ref. [17])

statistics for adding a design variable coding for the top tenth of the 24-h PP distribution to Cox models including all other covariables were 0.10 and 0.12 % for total and cardiovascular mortality and 0.27, 0.21, and 0.09 % for the composite cardiovascular endpoint, all cardiac events, and stroke, respectively. For most endpoints under study (Fig. 36.3) with the exception of stroke, the lower boundary of the confidence interval of the successive HRs crossed the reference line at levels ranging from 64 mmHg (composite cardiovascular endpoint) to 69 mmHg (total mortality and cardiac events).

IDHOCO Study

We analyzed the IDHOCO data [22] following the same methods as described above for IDACO. Among 3,285 younger subjects, median follow-up was 8.3 years. Over 32,671 person-years of follow-up, 149 participants died and 161 experienced a fatal or nonfatal cardiovascular complication. The cause of death was cardiovascular in 41 participants. The association between outcome and PP did not deviate significantly from log-linearity ($p \geq 0.092$). Table 36.1 shows the standardized HRs associated with home mean blood pressure and home PP. With adjustments applied for cohort, sex, age, body mass index, smoking and drinking, serum cholesterol, home pulse rate, history of cardiovascular disease, diabetes mellitus, and antihypertensive treatment, the home PP significantly predicted all outcomes, except fatal and nonfatal stroke. After further adjustment for mean arterial pressure, PP only predicted total and cardiovascular mortality (Table 36.1). The low number of events precluded an analysis by tenths of the PP distribution in younger participants.

Among 3,185 older subjects, median follow-up was 8.2 years (5th to 95th percentile interval, 7.2–16.8 years). Over 26,655 person-years of follow-up, 663 participants died and 555 experienced a fatal or nonfatal cardiovascular complication. The cause of death was cardiovascular in 253 participants. Considering fully adjusted models, the home PP predicted all of the endpoints ($p \leq 0.044$), except fatal combined with nonfatal cardiac events ($p = 0.052$) and stroke ($p = 0.083$). The generalized R^2 statistic for adding home PP as predictor of outcome over and beyond mean arterial pressure was ≤0.20 %.

Figure 36.4 shows the multivariable-adjusted HRs for outcomes in the top tenth of the distribution of home PP versus the average risk in all of the elderly. The HRs reached statistical significance in the upper tenths for total mortality, cardiovascular mortality, all cardiovascular events, all cardiac events, and all coronary events. The risk of stroke in the upper tenth did not exceed the average risk among all elderly. PP in the ninth and top tenth of the distribution of home PP averaged 71.3 mmHg (range, 67.8–75.9 mmHg) and 84.9 mmHg (range, 76.0–125.8 mmHg).

Interpretation of IDACO and IDHOCO Studies

The Seventh Report of the Joint National Committee on Prevention, Detection, Evaluation, and Treatment of High Blood Pressure [23] proposed that PP is only marginally stronger than systolic blood pressure for risk stratification in individuals over age 60 and that under age 60, PP is not predictive. According to the 2007 European guideline [24], PP is a derived measure, which combines the imprecision of the original systolic and diastolic measurements. The 2007 guideline stated that, although levels of 50–55 mmHg have been suggested [24], no practical cutoff values separating PP normality from abnormality is available. The 2013 European guideline increased this threshold to 60 mmHg without any justification [25]. The IDACO analyses [17] established that below age 60, a 24-h PP level of about 60 mmHg might be associated with increased risk, but that a safe threshold could not be established. Among the elderly participants, a 24-h PP of about 76 mmHg was definitely associated with higher risk, and levels below 64 mmHg were probably safe. Using intra-arterial monitoring, Khattar and colleagues [26] observed that survival rates were highest below age 60, if the 24-h PP was less than 70, and highest among elderly participants with a 24-h PP of 70 mmHg or more. To our knowledge, only one study published by Khattar [26] proposed an outcome-driven threshold for 24-h PP. However, this article does not include any justification why 70 mmHg was chosen as threshold in a dichotomized analysis. The results rested on an unadjusted Kaplan-Meier survival function analysis, and the study population consisted of patients with essential hypertension, in whom treatment had been withdrawn for 8 weeks [26]. All other proposals for PP thresholds relied on conventional blood pressure measurement. In analyses adjusted but not stratified for age, two studies [3, 10] derived a threshold from the 66th percentile of the PP

Table 36.1 Standardized hazard ratios relating outcomes to home pulse pressure by age group

		Age <60 years			Age ≥60 years		
		N° events	Hazard ratios			Hazard ratios	
Endpoint	Model		Mean pressure	Pulse pressure	N° events	Mean pressure	Pulse pressure
Mortality							
All causes	A	149	1.24 (1.01–1.51)[a]	1.28 (1.08–1.52)[b]	663	1.04 (0.95–1.13)	1.14 (1.05–1.25)[b]
	FA		1.08 (0.86–1.37)	1.24 (1.01–1.51)[a]		0.96 (0.86–1.06)	1.17 (1.06–1.30)[b]
Cardiovascular	A	41	1.44 (0.98–2.10)	1.56 (1.15–2.11)[b]	253	1.08 (0.94–1.24)	1.22 (1.07–1.40)[b]
	FA		1.15 (0.75–1.77)	1.47 (1.03–2.10)[a]		0.96 (0.82–1.14)	1.25 (1.06–1.47)[b]
Fatal plus nonfatal events							
All cardiovascular	A	161	1.50 (1.24–1.80)[d]	1.34 (1.15–1.56)[d]	555	1.26 (1.15–1.38)[d]	1.25 (1.14–1.36)[d]
	FA		1.35 (1.09–1.68)[b]	1.18 (0.98–1.41)		1.18 (1.06–1.32)[b]	1.14 (1.02–1.27)[a]
Cardiac	A	90	1.66 (1.31–2.10)[d]	1.38 (1.15–1.66)[c]	246	1.01 (0.88–1.16)	1.12 (0.98–1.27)
	FA		1.50 (1.12–2.00)[b]	1.15 (0.92–1.45)		0.91 (0.77–1.09)	1.18 (1.00–1.39)
Coronary	A	76	1.54 (1.20–2.00)[c]	1.26 (1.03–1.55)[a]	175	1.03 (0.87–1.21)	1.15 (0.99–1.34)
	FA		1.49 (1.08–2.06)[a]	1.05 (0.81–1.35)		0.90 (0.73–1.11)	1.22 (1.00–1.49)[a]
Stroke	A	73	1.25 (0.94–1.68)	1.31 (1.01–1.71)[a]	320	1.51 (1.34–1.70)[d]	1.37 (1.21–1.56)[d]
	FA		1.13 (0.82–1.56)	1.25 (0.94–1.68)		1.42 (1.23–1.63)[d]	1.14 (0.98–1.32)

Reproduced with permission from Ref. [22]

Hazard ratios, presented with 95 % confidence interval, express the risk associated with a 1-SD (11.7 and 11.2 mmHg in subjects <60 and ≥60 years, respectively) increase in mean home blood pressure or a 1-SD (8.8 and 13.4 mmHg) increase in home PP. All models were stratified for cohort and adjusted for sex, age, body mass index, smoking and drinking, serum cholesterol, home pulse rate, diabetes mellitus, history of cardiovascular disease, and antihypertensive treatment. Adjusted models (A) include either the mean blood pressure or pulse pressure, while fully adjusted models (FA) include both mean blood pressure and PP in addition to the aforementioned covariates

Significance of the hazard ratios: [a]$p<0.05$, [b]$p<0.01$, [c]$p<0.001$, and [d]$p<0.0001$

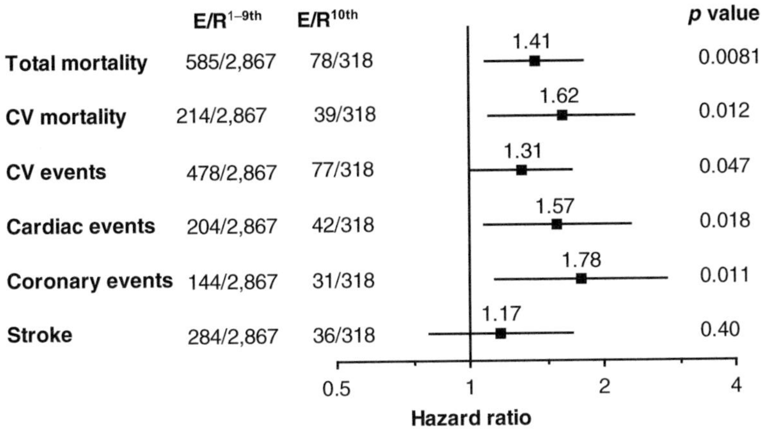

Fig. 36.4 Multivariable-adjusted hazard ratios for outcomes in relation to home pulse pressure in 3,185 older participants (≥60 years). The hazard ratios, presented with 95 % confidence interval, express the risk in the top tenth compared with the average risk in the participants. Home pulse pressure threshold delineating the top tenth was ≥76.0 mmHg and the corresponding mean level in the top tenth was 84.9 mmHg, respectively. All models were adjusted for cohort, sex, age, body mass index, smoking and drinking, serum cholesterol, home pulse rate, home mean blood pressure, diabetes mellitus, history of cardiovascular disease, and antihypertensive treatment. *P* values are for the risk in the top tenth relative to the overall risk in the whole study population. CV denotes cardiovascular. E/R1–9 and E/R10 indicate the number of events and participants at risk below the 90th percentile of the pulse pressure distribution and in the top tenth, respectively (Reproduced with permission from Ref. [22])

distribution. Madhavan and colleagues [3] proposed 63 mmHg based on the incidence of myocardial infarction in 2,207 hypertensive patients aged 55 years, and Borghi and colleagues [10] suggested 67 mmHg based on the incidence of cardiovascular disease among 2,939 Italian participants (14–84 years). Asmar and colleagues [27] derived a threshold of 65 mmHg from the mean PP plus 2 SDs in 61,724 French people (16–90 years). The IDHOCO analyses [22] established that below age 60, total and cardiovascular mortality were log-linearly associated with home PP, but that due to the small number of events, no outcome-driven threshold could be established. In the elderly, home PP predicted all endpoints with the exception of stroke, but the refinement of prognostication over and beyond traditional risk factors and the steady component of blood pressure was small. Among elderly, the threshold delineating increased risk of death is around 68 mmHg and for fatal combined with non-fatal cardiovascular events 76 mmHg.

Conclusions

After review of the available literature, we did a subject-level meta-analysis to derive outcome-driven thresholds for PP based on 24-h ambulatory monitoring or self-measured blood pressure measured at home. All results are generalizable because they originate from 14 randomly recruited population samples, representing 13 countries and three continents. Below age 60, irrespective of measurement methods, PP does not add to risk stratification. Starting from 60 years onward, higher PP conferred increased cardiovascular risk. However, while accounting for all covariables, have a PP in the top tenth of the distribution contributed less than 0.3 % to the overall risk among the elderly. The proposed thresholds are 64 mmHg or higher for 24-h PP and 76 mmHg for the home PP. These observations could inform guidelines and be of help to clinicians in diagnosing and managing patients.

References

1. Staessen J, Amery A, Fagard R. Editorial review. Isolated systolic hypertension. J Hypertens. 1990;8: 393–405.
2. Bangalore S, Messerli FH, Franklin SS, Mancia G, Champion A, Pepine CJ. Pulse pressure and risk of cardiovascular outcomes in patients with hypertension

and coronary artery disease: an INternational VErapamil SR-trandolapril STudy (INVEST) analysis. Eur Heart J. 2009;30:1395–401.
3. Madhaven S, Ooi WL, Cohen H, Alderman MH. Relation of pulse pressure and blood pressure reduction to the incidence of myocardial infarction. Hypertension. 1994;23:395–401.
4. Greenberg J. Antihypertensive treatment alters the predictive strength of pulse pressure and other blood pressure measures. Am J Hypertens. 2005;18:1033–9.
5. Domanski MJ, Davis BR, Pfeffer MA, Kastantin M, Mitchell GF. Isolated systolic hypertension: prognostic information provided by pulse pressure. Hypertension. 1999;34:375–80.
6. Amar J, Vernier I, Rossignol E, Bongard V, Arnaud C, Conte JJ, Salvador M, Chamontin B. Nocturnal blood pressure and 24–hour pulse pressure are potent indicators of mortality in hemodialysis patients. Kidney Int. 2000;57:2485–91.
7. Liu JH, Chen CC, Wang SM, Chou CY, Liu YL, Kuo HL, Lin HH, Wang IK, Yang YF, Huang CC. Association between pulse pressure and 30-month all-cause mortality in peritoneal dialysis patients. Am J Hypertens. 2008;21:1318–23.
8. Franklin SS, Larson MG, Khan SA, Wong ND, Leip EP, Kannel WB, Levy D. Does the relation of blood pressure to coronary heart disease change with aging? The Framingham Heart Study. Circulation. 2001;103: 1245–9.
9. Benetos A, Safar M, Rudnichi A, Smulyan H, Richard JL, Ducimetieère P, Guize L. Pulse pressure: a predictor of long-term cardiovascular mortality in a French male population. Hypertension. 1997;30:1410–5.
10. Borghi C, Dormi A, Ambrosioni E, Gaddi A, on behalf of the Brisighella Heart Study working party. Relative role of systolic, diastolic and pulse pressure as risk factors for cardiovascular events in the Brisighella Heart Study. J Hypertens. 2002;20:1737–42.
11. Schram MT, Kostense PJ, van Dijk RA, Dekker JM, Nijpels G, Bouter LM, Heine RJ, Stehouwer CD. Diabetes, pulse pressure and cardiovascular mortality: the Hoorn Study. J Hypertens. 2002;20:1743–51.
12. Glynn RJ, Chae CU, Guralnik JM, Taylor JO, Hennekens CH. Pulse pressure and mortality in older people. Arch Intern Med. 2000;160:2765–72.
13. Darne B, Girerd X, Safar M, Cambien F, Guize L. Pulsatile versus steady component of blood pressure: a cross-sectional analysis and a prospective analysis on cardiovascular mortality. Hypertension. 1989;13:392–400.
14. Lewington S, Clarke R, Qizilbash N, Peto R, Collins R, Prospective Studies Collaboration. Age-specific relevance of usual blood pressure to vascular mortality: a meta-analysis of individual data for one million adults in 61 prospective studies. Lancet. 2002;360: 1903–13.
15. Domanski M, Mitchell G, Pfeffer M, Neaton JD, Norman J, Svendsen K, Grimm R, Cohen J, Stamler J, MRFIT Research Group. Pulse pressure and cardiovascular disease-related mortality. JAMA. 2002;287:2677–83.
16. Miura K, Dyer AR, Greenland P, Daviglus ML, Hill MA, Liu K, Garside DB, Stamler J, Chicago Heart Association. Pulse pressure compared with other blood pressure indexes in the prediction of 25-year cardiovascular and all-cause mortality rates: The Chicago Heart Association Detection Project in Industry Study. Hypertension. 2001;38:232–7.
17. Gu YM, Thijs L, Asayama K, Boggia J, Hansen TW, Liu YP, Ohkubo T, Bjorklund-Bodegård K, Jeppesen J, Dolan E, Torp-Pedersen C, Kuznetsova T, Stolarz-Skrzypek K, Tikhonoff V, Malyutina S, Casiglia E, Nikitin Y, Lind L, Sandoya E, Kawecka-Jaszcz K, Imai Y, Mena LJ, Wang J, O'Brien E, Verhamme P, Filipovsky J, Maestre GE, Staessen JA, on behalf of the International Database on Ambulatory blood pressure monitoring in relation to Cardiovascular Outcomes (IDACO) investigators. Outcome-driven thresholds for ambulatory pulse pressure in 9938 participants recruited from 11 populations. Hypertension. 2014;63:229–37.
18. Franklin SS, Gustin 4th W, Wong ND, Larson MG, Weber LA, Kannel WB, Levy D. Hemodynamic patterns of age-related changes in blood pressure. The Framingham Heart Study. Circulation. 1997;96:308–15.
19. Staessen JA, Thijs L, Fagard R, O'Brien ET, Clement D, de Leeuw PW, Mancia G, Nachev C, Palatini P, Parati G, Tuomilehto J, Webster J. Predicting cardiovascular risk using conventional vs ambulatory blood pressure in older patients with systolic hypertension. Systolic hypertension in Europe trial investigators. JAMA. 1999;282:539–46.
20. Hosmer Jr DW, Leleshow S. Applied logistic regression. New York: Wiley; 1989. p. 47–56.
21. Gillespie BW. Use of generalized R-squared in Cox regression. https://apha.confex.com/apha/134am/techprogram/paper_135906.htm. APHA scientific session and event listing. 2006. Accessed 15 Dec 2013.
22. Aparicio LS, Thijs L, Asayama K, Barochiner J, Boggia J, Gu YM, Cuffaro PE, Liu YP, Niiranen TJ, Ohkubo T, Johansson JK, Kikuya M, Hozawa A, Tsuji I, Imai Y, Sandoya E, Waisman GD, Staessen JA, on behalf of the International Database on HOme blood pressure in relation to Cardiovascular Outcome (IDHOCO) Investigators. Reference frame for home pulse pressure based on cardiovascular risk in 6470 subjects from 5 populations. Hypertension Res. 2014. Mar 20. doi: 10.1038/hr.2014.45.
23. Chobanian AV, Bakris GL, Black HR, Cushman WC, Green LA, Izzo Jr JL, Jones DW, Materson BJ, Oparil S, Wright Jr JT, Roccella EJ, Joint National Committee on Prevention, Detection, Evaluation, and Treatment of High Blood Pressure; National Heart, Lung, and Blood Institute; National High Blood Pressure Education Program Coordinating Committee. Seventh report of the Joint National Committee on Prevention, Detection, Evaluation, and Treatment of High Blood Pressure. Hypertension. 2003;42:1206–52.
24. Mancia G, De Backer G, Dominiczak A, Cifkova R, Fagard R, Germano G, Grassi G, Heagerty AM, Kjeldsen SE, Laurent S, Narkiewicz K, Ruilope L, Rynkiewicz A, Schmieder RE, Struijker-Boudier HA,

Zanchetti A, Vahanian A, Camm J, De Caterina R, Dean V, Dickstein K, Filippatos G, Funck-Brentano C, Hellemans I, Kristensen SD, McGregor K, Sechtem U, Silber S, Tendera M, Widimsky P, Zamorano JL, Erdine S, Kiowski W, Agabiti-Rosei E, Ambrosioni E, Lindholm LH, Manolis A, Nilsson PM, Redon J, Struijker-Boudier HA, Viigimaa M, Adamopoulos S, Bertomeu V, Clement D, Farsang C, Gaita D, Lip G, Mallion JM, Manolis AJ, O'Brien E, Ponikowski P, Ruschitzka F, Tamargo J, van Zwieten P, Waeber B, Williams B. 2007 guidelines for the management of arterial hypertension: The Task Force for the Management of Arterial Hypertension of the European Society of Hypertension (ESH) and of the European Society of Cardiology (ESC). Eur Heart J. 2007;28:1462–536.

25. Mancia G, Fagard R, Narkiewicz K, Redon J, Zanchetti A, Bohm M, Christiaens T, Cifkova R, De Backer G, Dominiczak A, Galderisi M, Grobbee DE, Jaarsma T, Kirchhof P, Kjeldsen SE, Laurent S, Manolis AJ, Nilsson PM, Ruilope LM, Schmieder RE, Sirnes PA, Sleight P, Viigimaa M, Waeber B, Zannad F. 2013 ESH/ESC guidelines for the management of arterial hypertension: the Task Force for the Management of Arterial Hypertension of the European Society of Hypertension (ESH) and of the European Society of Cardiology (ESC). Eur Heart J. 2013;34:2159–219.
26. Khattar RS, Swales JD, Dore C, Senior R, Lahiri A. Effect of aging on the prognostic significance of ambulatory systolic, diastolic, and pulse pressure in essential hypertension. Circulation. 2001;104:783–9.
27. Asmar R, Vol S, Brisac AM, Tichet J, Topouchian J. Reference values for clinic pulse pressure in a nonselected population. Am J Hypertens. 2001;14:415–8.

37 Properties of Central Arteries in Populations of Different Ethnicity: Ethnicity and Central Arteries

Augustine Nonso Odili, Yumei Gu, and Jan A. Staessen

Abstract

Recent studies have established a strong and independent association between central haemodynamics of central arteries and cardiovascular morbidity and mortality. Evaluation of indices of central arterial stiffness will thus improve cardiovascular risk assessment. While age modifies the structure of the aorta and as such contributes significantly to the changes in the central haemodynamics, other known cardiovascular risk factors as well as genetic factors modulate these age-dependent changes. Interracial variations in cardiovascular risk factors and genetic composition are responsible for the differences in properties of the central arteries across different ethnic populations. Establishing operational threshold for distinguishing normal and abnormal values among different ethnic populations is essential for making clinical decisions.

Keywords

Central haemodynamics • Thresholds • Blood pressure measurement • Ethnic populations • Cardiovascular risk factors

A.N. Odili, MD
Department of Internal Medicine, Faculty of Clinical Sciences, College of Health Sciences, University of Abuja, Gwagwalada, Abuja, Nigeria

Research Unit Hypertension and Cardiovascular Epidemiology, KU leuven Department of Cardiovascular Science, Studies Coordinating Centre, University of Leuven, Leuven, Belgium
e-mail: odilimercy@yahoo.com

Y. Gu, MD, PhD
Research Unit Hypertension and Cardiovascular Epidemiology, KU leuven Department of Cardiovascular Science, Studies Coordinating Centre, University of Leuven, Leuven, Belgium
e-mail: yumei.gu@med.kuleuven.be

J.A. Staessen, MD, PhD (✉)
Research Unit Hypertension and Cardiovascular Epidemiology, KU leuven Department of Cardiovascular Science, Studies Coordinating Centre, University of Leuven, Leuven, Belgium

Department of Cardiovascular Sciences, UZ Leuven Campus Sint Rafael, University of Leuven, Kapucijnenvoer 35, 7001, BE-3000 Leuven, Belgium

Department of Epidemiology, Maastricht University, Peter Debyeplein 1, 616, Maastricht 6200, The Netherlands

Research Unit Hypertension and Cardiovascular Epidemiology, Department of Cardiovascular Sciences, Studies Coordinating Centre, University of Leuven, Kapucijnenvoer 35, Block D, 7001, BE-3000 Leuven, Belgium
e-mail: jan.staessen@med.kuleuven.be, jan.staessen@maastrichtuniversity.nl

M.E. Safar et al. (eds.), *Blood Pressure and Arterial Wall Mechanics in Cardiovascular Diseases*, DOI 10.1007/978-1-4471-5198-2_37, © Springer-Verlag London 2014

Introduction

Among all properties of the central arteries, arterial stiffness has proven to be the most useful in cardiovascular risk assessment. Wall stiffness of the central arteries (aorta and carotid arteries) is dependent on the contribution of two major support proteins—collagen and elastin. Ageing leads to reduction in quantities of elastin and overproduction of abnormal collagen thus resulting in vascular stiffness. Other conditions including genetic factors and known cardiovascular risk factors such as hypertension, diabetes, hypercholesterolaemia and cigarette smoking work synergistically to accelerate the age-related vascular stiffness. Properties of large arteries vary across different ethnic populations. Differences in environmental risk factors, gene-gene and gene-environment interaction, linkage disequilibrium structure, expression of target variants and presence of allelic heterogeneity across different ethnic populations are some of the factors responsible for interracial variations in large artery properties.

Reference Values of Central Haemodynamics of Central Arteries Derived in Caucasian, Asian and African Populations

Carotid-femoral pulse wave velocity (PWV), aortic pulse pressure (cPP) and aortic augmentation index (Aix) are the major parameters used in assessing the central arterial stiffness. The use of non-standardised techniques to measure central haemodynamics makes comparison across different populations rather imprecise. Three studies designed for establishment of reference values based on distribution of cPP and Aix among Caucasians [1], Asians [2] and Africans [3] however deployed the SphygmoCor device. In all the three studies, the radial arterial waveform was recorded at the dominant arm with applanation tonometry using a high-fidelity micrometre interfaced with a laptop computer running the SphygmoCor software (AtCor Medical, West Ryde, New South Wales, Australia). From the radial signal, the SphygmoCor software calculates the aortic pulse wave by means of a validated and population-based generalised transfer function [4–6]. Aortic augmentation index (Aix) is the difference between the second and first systolic peaks given as a percentage.

The study among Caucasians [1] included 870 subjects randomly recruited from three European countries of Belgium, Poland and Czech Republic under the framework of European Project on Genes in Hypertension. Five hundred and thirty four of these subjects had no cardiovascular disease and were thus included in the analysis to generate the reference value. The investigators reported that before age 40, men had higher central PP and lower central Aix than women. After age 40, gender difference in central PP disappears. The proposed threshold based on the upper 95th prediction band of the curvilinear relationship between the central arterial haemodynamics and age is shown in Table 37.1.

Table 37.1 Central haemodynamics measured with SphygmoCor in three ethnic populations

	20			30			40			50			60		
Age	As	Ca	AF	As	Ca	AF	As	Ca	AF	As	Ca	AF	As	Ca	AF
Central PP (mmHg)															
Men	47	37	–	46	38	–	48	40	–	51	43	–	59	47	–
Women	40	36	–	42	38	–	46	40	–	52	42	–	58	46	–
Both	–	–	–	–	–	50	–	–	54	–	–	58	–	–	62
Central Aix (%)															
Men	22	10	–	32	22	–	40	30	–	48	37	–	54	41	–
Women	25	17	–	37	29	–	46	37	–	53	44	–	58	48	–
Both	–	–	–	–	–	40	–	–	46	–	–	52			52

As Asians derived from a random sample of participants from 14 villages in the Jingning County, a rural area 500 km south of Shanghai [2], *Ca* Caucasians derived from randomly recruited nuclear families of Caucasian extraction in Hechtel-Eksel, Belgium; Cracow, Poland; and Pilsen, the Czech Republic [1], *Af* Africans random sample of South Africans of Nguni and Sotho chiefdoms living in the metropolitan area of Johannesburg [3]. "–" Sex-specific or combined data not provided by the authors

Using the same methodological approach, Li and colleagues [2] recruited 1,486 Chinese from 14 villages in the Jingning County, a rural area 500 km south of Shanghai. The proposed limit of normality in this Asian cohort was 8 mmHg and 10 % higher than the cPP and Aix values reported among Caucasians (Table 37.1). Shubari and colleagues [3] analysed data from a random sample of 347 Africans of South African origin recruited under the framework of African Project on Genes in Hypertension. The mean age of this cohort which included 77 men and 108 women was 33.5 years. Both central Aix and PP increased with increasing age with the 95th prediction bands at 30 years of age approximated to 50 mmHg for PP and 40 % for Aix. For each decade that age differs from 30 years, the authors proposed an adjustment by approximately 4.0 mmHg and 6 % for central PP and Aix, respectively (Table 37.1).

Comparing the three studies that employed the SphygmoCor to measure arterial stiffness in Caucasians, Asians and Africans, one can conclude that the central arteries of Africans are stiffer than that of Asians and Caucasians. This observation is supported by an earlier finding among the blacks in the United States of America recruited in the Atherosclerosis Risk in Community (ARIC) [7] study. Din-Dzietham and colleagues [7] analysed a subsample of ARIC cohort from the Forsyth County, North Carolina, which included 278 blacks out of the 2,727 participants. They calculated the β carotid index, a measure of carotid stiffness from an echo-tracked systolic and diastolic common carotid diameter [8, 9]. After adjustment for selected cardiovascular risk factors, the mean β index was 9 % higher for African Americans (mean ± SEM, 11.3 + 0.3) than the whites (mean ± SEM, 10.3 + 0.1).

The measurement of PWV is generally accepted as the gold standard for assessing arterial stiffness because a large body of evidence has demonstrated a clear association between PWV and cardiovascular outcome in different patient groups [10–13] as well as in general population [14]. Reference values for PWV in different ethnic populations have not been established due to lack of standardisation of methodology for PWV assessment. The 2013 ESH/ESC guidelines [15] proposed a fixed value of 10 m/s without taking into account multiple factors affecting PWV.

Table 37.2 Age-specific normal values of PWV among normotensive Caucasians

Age category (years)	PWV (m/s) Mean ± 2SD	Median (10–90 pct)
<30	6.2 (4.7–7.6)	6.1 (5.3–7.1)
30–39	6.5 (3.8–9.2)	6.4 (5.2–8.0)
40–49	7.2 (4.6–9.8)	6.9 (5.9–8.6)
50–59	8.3 (4.5–12.1)	8.1 (6.3–10.0)
60–69	10.3 (5.5–15.0)	9.7 (7.9–13.1)
≥70	10.9 (5.5–16.3)	10.6 (8.0–14.6)

Reproduced with permission from The Reference Values for Arterial Stiffness' Collaboration [16]

SD standard deviation, *10 pct* the lower limit of 10th percentile, *90 pct* the lower limit of 90th percentile

The Reference Values for Arterial Stiffness' Collaboration [16] gathered data from 16,867 subjects and patients from 13 different centres across eight European countries in which PWV was measured. They aimed to establish normal values of carotid to femoral PWV in a population with no CVD risk factor and reference value in a population with various degrees of CVD risk factors. They included studies that used various techniques to measure the PWV. Although data on ethnicity was not presented, the authors stated that non-Caucasian individuals were in the minority. They proposed a threshold value that is dependent on age and blood pressure as shown in Table 37.2 and Fig. 37.1

In an attempt to circumvent the imprecision inherent in pooling studies that deployed various methodological approaches to measurement of PWV, Khoshdel and colleagues [17] did a meta-analysis to estimate an age-specific reference values for PWV by including 25 studies in which carotid-femoral pulse wave was measured using Complior (Colson, Paris, France). The total patient/subject population of 8,167 were categorised into normal ($n = 2{,}008$), moderate ($n = 5{,}978$) and high ($n = 180$) cardiovascular risk groups. Individual level data were simulated for each group. They plotted an age-adjusted normal curve for PWV, and using the 95th percentile as the threshold, they showed that 10.94, 11.86 and 13.18 m/s for 20, 40 and 60 years, respectively, have a construct validity to identify medium- and high-risk cardiovascular groups accurately.

Willium-Hansen et al. [14] studied a random sample of 1,678 Caucasians of Danish origin

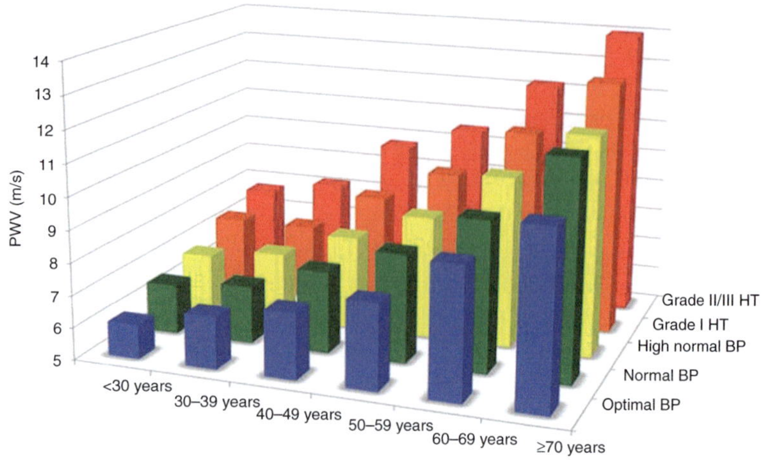

Fig. 37.1 Reference values for pulse wave velocity (*PWV*): mean values according to age and blood pressure (*BP*) categories (11,092 subjects). *HT* hypertension (Reproduced with permission from The Reference Values for Arterial Stiffness' Collaboration [16])

aged 40–70 years. They measured their PWV at baseline using two piezoelectric pressure transducers (Hellige GmbH) to record the arterial wave simultaneously at the left common carotid and femoral arteries. PWV was the distance between the two transducers measured on the body surface divided by the transit time determined manually by the foot-to-foot velocity method [18]. The cohort was followed up for a median period of 9.4 years for all-cause mortality, cardiovascular mortality and fatal and nonfatal coronary events. Subjects whose PWV were above 10 m/s at baseline had a relative hazard ratio that was above unity for composite cardiovascular events.

Age Dependence of Central Haemodynamics in Caucasian and Asian Populations

The aorta undergoes many structural and functional changes as part of the normal ageing process: its length increases and becomes more tortuous; the lumen dilates with an increase in the intimal surface area; and the walls become more stiff leading to an increase in pulse wave velocity. These age-dependent changes in the aorta have been adduced to alterations in content and architectural structure of elastin and collagen. First, the concentration of elastin decreases due to increase in other components such as collagen while maintaining the elastin content [19, 20]. Second, histidinoalanine, a senescent elastin and collagen cross-linking residue, increases markedly with ageing. Histidinoalanine amino acids can form cross-links between neighbouring acidic proteins and elastin, between acidic proteins and collagen and between the acidic protein molecules themselves [21]. Repeated pulsatile wall strain experienced by the aorta during each cardiac cycle throughout an individual's lifetime is said to cause a fragmentation of elastin fibres. Age not only increases the amount of collagen on the aortic wall; it also increases the cross-linking of collagen fibres sequel to age-dependent increase in histidinoalanine and advanced glycation products. The advanced glycation products formed from glycation and oxidising reaction between sugar and protein in amino acids of protein molecules form bridges between collages fibres.

The prevalence of hypertension and atherosclerosis, the two major clinico-pathological conditions that affect arterial structure and function, increases with ageing and thus accelerates the age-dependent arterial wall changes [22–24]. Prevalence, pathophysiological mechanisms and clinical manifestation of both hypertension and atherosclerosis vary among different racial groups. In addition, elastin and collagen composition in different segments of the aortic wall differ across different ethnic populations.

In the Anglo-Cardiff Collaborative trial, McEniery and colleagues tested the hypothesis that age-related changes in Aix are more prominent in younger subjects, whereas changes in large artery stiffness per se were more prominent in older subjects. They recruited 4,001 healthy (normotensive, not diabetic, no renal or cardiovascular disease, total cholesterol <6.5 mmol/l) subjects selected from the local general practice lists and open-access cardiovascular risk assessment clinics across East Anglia and Wales. Ninety two percent of the subjects were Caucasians, 4 % Asian, 2 % Far Eastern and 2 % Afro-Caribbean. They reported that both Aix and PWV increase with age; however, the relationship is non-linear in that for Aix, greater increases are seen in individuals less than 50 years, while the age-dependent increment in PWV is steeper in older individuals. They concluded that Aix is a more sensitive maker of arterial stiffness in the young, while PWV is a better measure in the elderly.

The findings among Asians [2] and Caucasians [1] and the Framingham cohort [25] are all consistent with a curvilinear relationship between central haemodynamics and age. While the systolic pressure increases continuously throughout life, the diastolic pressure levels off or even declines after the age of 55 years. Expectedly, the PP in the elderly will be higher than in the young subjects. The steeper increase in the PP (denominator for computation of Aix) in older subjects might result in the less increase or even decrease of Aix in the elderly.

Conclusion and Research Perspectives

Age is the main determinant of aorta stiffness across all ethnic populations. Reference values for central arterial properties should be age specific and not fixed for all age groups. Non-standardisation of methodological approach to assessment of parameters of central aorta makes it difficult to compare studies carried out among different populations. Available data however indicate that people of African origin tend to have higher values of central haemodynamic parameters when compared to their Asian and Caucasian counterparts.

The higher values of both Aix and cPP reported among African and Asian populations suggest a possibility of a shared pathophysiological mechanism between arterial stiffness and keloid, a disease that affects highly pigmented skin commonly seen among black Africans and Asians. It appears as a thick scar tissue that invades the normal skin, produced by deposition of excessive amount of collagen produced over prolonged periods. Over the years, there has been an increasing interest in the relationship of keloids to hypertension [26–28]. Dustan and colleagues [26] provided a strong support for the hypothesis that the black/white differences in severity of hypertension reflect a specific response to vascular smooth muscle cells to growth factors reminiscent of skin fibroblast whose abnormal growth factor production and responsiveness are expressed as keloids in blacks. This hypothesis should be extended to the study of central arterial properties. Gene expression studies that will investigate collagen synthesis in keloid formation and collagen deposition in ageing artery or atherosclerotic arterial changes may give insight into the pathophysiological mechanisms underlying arterial stiffness.

Racial differences in response to anti-hypertensive agents are well documented in the literature. While attention has been focused on ethnic variations in response to different classes of anti-hypertensive agents as determined by peripheral blood pressure, the possible variations on central PP, PWV and Aix are less studied. There is a need to explore the differential effects of anti-hypertensive agents on different parts of the arterial tree across the ethnic lines.

Targeting the structural causes of arterial stiffening such as AGE (Advanced Glycated End-product) linked collagen with experimental agents such as aminoguanidine and pyridoxamine is a potential therapeutic option for reducing arterial stiffness. Additionally, novel therapeutic agents that will affect or modify the tumour growth factor β, a central player in development of fibrosis, will likely provide a needed solution that has eluded scientists looking for solution to arterial stiffness.

References

1. Wojciechowska W, Staessen JA, Nawrot T, Cwynar M, Seidlerova J, Stolarz K, et al. Reference values in white Europeans for the arterial pulse wave recorded by means of the SphygmoCor device. Hypertens Res. 2006;29:475–83.
2. Li Y, Staessen JA, Li LH, Huang QF, Lu L, Wang JG. Reference values for the arterial pulse wave in Chinese. Am J Hypertens. 2008;21:668–73.
3. Shiburi CP, Staessen JA, Maseko M, Wojciechowska W, Thijs L, Van Bortel LM, et al. Reference values for SphygmoCor measurements in South Africans of African ancestry. Am J Hypertens. 2006;19:40–6.
4. Chen CH, Ting CT, Nussbacher A, Nevo E, Kass DA, Pak P, et al. Validation of carotid artery tonometry as a means of estimating augmentation index of ascending aortic pressure. Hypertension. 1996;27:168–75.
5. Chen CH, Nevo E, Fetics B, Pak PH, Yin FC, Maughan WL, et al. Estimation of central aortic pressure waveform by mathematical transformation of radial tonometry pressure. Validation of generalized transfer function. Circulation. 1997;95:1827–36.
6. Pauca AL, O'Rourke MF, Kon ND. Prospective evaluation of a method for estimating ascending aortic pressure from the radial artery pressure waveform. Hypertension. 2001;38:932–7.
7. Din-Dzietham R, Couper D, Evans G, Arnett DK, Jones DW. Arterial stiffness is greater in African Americans than in whites: evidence from the Forsyth County, North Carolina, ARIC cohort. Am J Hypertens. 2004;17:304–13.
8. Riley WA, Evans GW, Sharrett AR, Burke GL, Barnes RW. Variation of common carotid artery elasticity with intimal-medial thickness: the ARIC Study. Atherosclerosis Risk in Communities. Ultrasound Med Biol. 1997;23:157–64.
9. Kawasaki T, Sasayama S, Yagi S, Asakawa T, Hirai T. Non-invasive assessment of the age related changes in stiffness of major branches of the human arteries. Cardiovasc Res. 1987;21:678–87.
10. Blacher J, Guerin AP, Pannier B, Marchais SJ, Safar ME, London GM. Impact of aortic stiffness on survival in end-stage renal disease. Circulation. 1999;99:2434–9.
11. Cruickshank K, Riste L, Anderson SG, Wright JS, Dunn G, Gosling RG. Aortic pulse-wave velocity and its relationship to mortality in diabetes and glucose intolerance: an integrated index of vascular function? Circulation. 2002;106:2085–90.
12. Choi CU, Park EB, Suh SY, Kim JW, Kim EJ, Rha SW, et al. Impact of aortic stiffness on cardiovascular disease in patients with chest pain: assessment with direct intra-arterial measurement. Am J Hypertens. 2007;20:1163–9.
13. Ben-Shlomo Y, Spears M, Boustred C, May M, Anderson SG, Benjamin EJ, et al. Aortic pulse wave velocity improves cardiovascular event prediction: an individual participant meta-analysis of prospective observational data from 17,635 subjects. J Am Coll Cardiol. 2014;63(7):636–46.
14. Willum-Hansen T, Staessen JA, Torp-Pedersen C, Rasmussen S, Thijs L, Ibsen H, et al. Prognostic value of aortic pulse wave velocity as index of arterial stiffness in the general population. Circulation. 2006;113:664–70.
15. Mancia G, Fagard R, Narkiewicz K, Redon J, Zanchetti A, Bohm M, et al. 2013 ESH/ESC guidelines for the management of arterial hypertension: the Task Force for the Management of Arterial Hypertension of the European Society of Hypertension (ESH) and of the European Society of Cardiology (ESC). Eur Heart J. 2013;34:2159–219.
16. The Reference Values for Arterial Stiffness' Collaboration. Determinants of pulse wave velocity in healthy people and in the presence of cardiovascular risk factors: 'establishing normal and reference values'. Eur Heart J. 2010;31:2338–50.
17. Khoshdel AR, Thakkinstian A, Carney SL, Attia J. Estimation of an age-specific reference interval for pulse wave velocity: a meta-analysis. J Hypertens. 2006;24:1231–7.
18. Asmar R, Benetos A, Topouchian J, Laurent P, Pannier B, Brisac AM, et al. Assessment of arterial distensibility by automatic pulse wave velocity measurement. Validation and clinical application studies. Hypertension. 1995;26:485–90.
19. Sans M, Moragas A. Mathematical morphologic analysis of the aortic medial structure. Biomechanical implications. Anal Quant Cytol Histol. 1993;15:93–100.
20. Tsamis A, Krawiec JT, Vorp DA. Elastin and collagen fibre microstructure of the human aorta in ageing and disease: a review. J R Soc Interface. 2013;10:20121004.
21. Fujimoto D. Aging and cross-linking in human aorta. Biochem Biophys Res Commun. 1982;109:1264–9.
22. Avolio AP, Deng FQ, Li WQ, Luo YF, Huang ZD, Xing LF, et al. Effects of aging on arterial distensibility in populations with high and low prevalence of hypertension: comparison between urban and rural communities in China. Circulation. 1985;71:202–10.
23. Virmani R, Avolio AP, Mergner WJ, Robinowitz M, Herderick EE, Cornhill JF, et al. Effect of aging on aortic morphology in populations with high and low prevalence of hypertension and atherosclerosis. Comparison between occidental and Chinese communities. Am J Pathol. 1991;139:1119–29.
24. O'Rourke MF. Arterial function in health and disease. London: Churchill Livingstone; 1982.
25. Mitchell GF, Parise H, Benjamin EJ, Larson MG, Keyes MJ, Vita JA, et al. Changes in arterial stiffness and wave reflection with advancing age in healthy men and women: the Framingham Heart Study. Hypertension. 2004;43:1239–45.
26. Dustan HP. Does keloid pathogenesis hold the key to understanding black/white differences in hypertension severity? Hypertension. 1995;26:858–62.
27. Woolery-Lloyd H, Berman B. A controlled cohort study examining the onset of hypertension in black patients with keloids. Eur J Dermatol. 2002;12:581–2.
28. Snyder AL, Zmuda JM, Thompson PD. Keloid associated with hypertension. Lancet. 1996;347:465–6.

Changing Concepts on the Role of Blood Pressure Reduction in Stroke Prevention with the Focus on β-Blocking Agents

38

Ji-Guang Wang, Feng-Hua Ding, Li-Hua Li, and Yan Li

Abstract

In a recent meta-analysis, we investigated effects of β-blockers versus other classes of antihypertensive drugs on central hemodynamic measurements and explored the impact of heart rate on central hemodynamics and the risk of stroke. The pooled estimates of nine randomized controlled trials ($n=754$) showed that β-blockers were less efficacious in reducing central augmentation index (cAI) than all the other classes of antihypertensive drugs (8.6 %, $P<0.001$) and less efficacious in reducing central systolic blood pressure (cSBP) than angiotensin-converting enzyme inhibitors (7.7 mmHg, $P=0.02$) and angiotensin receptor blockers (3.6 mmHg, $P=0.005$) but not calcium channel blockers or diuretics ($P\geq0.50$). In a meta-regression analysis of these 9 trials, the baseline-adjusted difference in heart rate between randomized groups was significantly associated with cAI (7.0 % increase for each 10 beats/min decrease in heart rate, $P=0.02$), which was associated with cSBP (1.2 mmHg increase for each 1 % increase in cAI, $P=0.009$). In 5 outcome trials, the pooled odds ratio of stroke was 1.23 ($P<0.001$), which would be accounted for by the difference in cSBP derived from the above meta-regression analysis. These meta-analyses and meta-regression analyses have demonstrated that β-blockers by slowing the heart rate may increase cAI and in turn may decrease cSBP less than other classes of antihypertensive drugs. This mechanism might account for the less reduction in the risk of stroke by

J.-G. Wang, MD, PhD (✉)
Centre for Epidemiological Studies and Clinical Trials, The Shanghai Institute of Hypertension, Ruijin Hospital, Shanghai Jiaotong University School of Medicine, Ruijin 2nd Road 197, Shanghai 200025, China
e-mail: jiguangw@gmail.com

F.-H. Ding, MD, PhD
Centre for Epidemiological Studies and Clinical Trials, The Shanghai Institute of Hypertension, Ruijin Hospital, Shanghai Jiaotong University School of Medicine, Ruijin 2nd Road 197, Shanghai 200025, China

Department of Cardiology, Ruijin Hospital, Shanghai Jiatong University School of Medicine, Ruijin 2nd Road 197, Shanghai 200025, China
e-mail: ruijindfh@126.com

L.-H. Li, MD • Y. Li, MD, PhD
Centre for Epidemiological Studies and Clinical Trials, The Shanghai Institute of Hypertension, Ruijin Hospital, Shanghai Jiaotong University School of Medicine, Ruijin 2nd Road 197, Shanghai 200025, China
e-mail: lilihuayncn@163.com; liyanshcn@yahoo.com

M.E. Safar et al. (eds.), *Blood Pressure and Arterial Wall Mechanics in Cardiovascular Diseases*, DOI 10.1007/978-1-4471-5198-2_38,

β-blockers in hypertension. These findings suggest that central hemodynamics should be measured in the diagnosis and therapeutic monitoring of hypertension, especially when a β-blocker is used.

Keywords
β-blockers • Central systolic blood pressure • Central augmentation index • Heart rate • Stroke • Meta-analysis

Introduction

Hypertension is one of the most powerful risk factors for cardiovascular disease [1]. Antihypertensive treatment, by lowering blood pressure, may substantially reduce the risk of cardiovascular complications, particularly stroke, regardless of the hypertension subtype [2, 3]. Most of the current national [4, 5] or international [6] hypertension guidelines recommend the use of five classes of antihypertensive drugs, i.e., angiotensin-converting enzyme (ACE) inhibitors, angiotensin receptor blockers (ARB), β-blockers, calcium channel blockers (CCB), and thiazide diuretics, as initial and maintenance therapy. However, several randomized controlled trials [7–10] and subsequent meta-analyses [11, 12] repeatedly demonstrated that β-blockers were less efficacious in the prevention of stroke in hypertensive patients. This phenomenon was not observed in other trials [13–17] or in a much larger meta-analysis, in which trials in congestive heart failure were also included [18].

Stroke is known to be directly related to blood pressure. Between-group differences in brachial blood pressure might explain the results of some [8, 9] but not all of these trials [10]. In our previous meta-analysis [19], the higher risk of stroke on β-blockers versus the CCB diltiazem in the Nordic Diltiazem (NORDIL) trial could not be explained by the between-group systolic blood pressure difference, which was on average 3 mmHg in favor of the β-blocker group [10].

The Conduit Artery Function Evaluation (CAFE) substudy of the Anglo-Scandinavian Cardiac Outcomes Trial (ASCOT) suggested that blood pressure in the central aorta might be an explanation, because the β-blocker atenolol-based antihypertensive regimen was less efficacious in reducing central systolic blood pressure (4.3 mmHg) than the CCB amlodipine-based regimen [20]. This difference in central systolic blood pressure could largely be explained by the heart rate slowing effect of atenolol [21]. Slowing the heart rate will increase central augmentation index and in turn detract blood pressure lowering effect of β-blockers in the central aorta. This mechanism might explain the inferior protective effect of β-blockade against stroke.

In a recent overview article [22], we performed meta-analysis of randomized controlled trials that compared β-blockers with other classes of antihypertensive drugs in reducing central systolic blood pressure and augmentation index and then explored in a meta-regression analysis to what extent the difference in heart rate may account for the difference in central systolic blood pressure and augmentation index and investigated in a meta-analysis of outcome trials the odds ratios of stroke in relation to heart rate. In this chapter, we summarize the major findings of these meta-analyses and meta-regression analyses and discuss the clinical implications of these findings for the prevention of cardiovascular complications, particularly stroke.

Effects of β-Blockers Versus Other Antihypertensive Drugs on Central Hemodynamics

For meta-analysis, we searched randomized controlled trials that compared β-blockers with other classes of antihypertensive drugs in reducing central systolic blood pressure and augmentation index and identified 11 trials [20, 23–32] published between 2001 and 2011. We excluded 2 trials, because central hemodynamics was not measured at baseline [20] or because the combination of perindopril and indapamide was compared with the atenolol monotherapy [32].

Among the 9 trials remaining in the meta-analysis, 6 had a crossover design [23–28], and 3 had a parallel design [29–31]. The number of comparator drugs was 4 in 2 trials [24, 25], 3 in 1 trial [30], and 1 in 6 trials [23, 26–29, 31]. The β-blocker was atenolol [23, 25, 27–31] in 7 trials and bisoprolol [24, 26] in 2 trials. The SphygmoCor system (AtCor Medical, Sydney, Australia) was used in all trials.

Our meta-analysis was based on the summary statistics reported in the literature [22]. For brachial and central blood pressure, central augmentation index, and heart rate, we extracted for the β-blocker and control groups separately means and standard deviations at baseline and during follow-up and if available in the published report also changes during follow-up. Although in 2 trials [27, 31] central augmentation index was reported after adjustment to a standard heart rate of 75 beats per minute, unadjusted central augmentation index was extracted from all trials and used in the analysis. Within each trial, the control group consisted of patients on ACE inhibitors, ARBs, CCBs, diuretics, or α-blockers. We calculated the absolute difference in the mean change from baseline to the end of follow-up between β-blockers and control groups for each comparison within each trial and computed the standard error (SE) of the difference as described previously [19, 33]. We used a random effects model, which incorporates a within-study and an additive between-study component of variance, to calculate the pooled effect for each grouping of trials from the point estimate for each separate trial [33]. Heterogeneity of effect sizes was checked across trials using the I-squared test [34].

The nine trials in the meta-analysis included 754 randomly assigned patients and compared two different β-blockers (atenolol [23, 25, 27–31] and bisoprolol [24, 26]) with ACE inhibitors ($n=140$) [23–27, 30], ARBs ($n=429$) [28, 29, 31], CCBs ($n=76$) [24, 25, 30], diuretics ($n=75$) [24, 25, 30], or an α-blocker ($n=30$) [24].

For central systolic blood pressure, β-blockers were less efficacious than ACE inhibitors (7.7 mmHg, $P=0.02$) and ARBs (3.7 mmHg, $P=0.005$), while no significant difference was observed in the comparisons versus CCBs ($P=0.50$), diuretics ($P=0.89$), or an α-blocker ($P=0.54$, Fig. 38.1). Overall, a random effects model demonstrated that β-blockers were

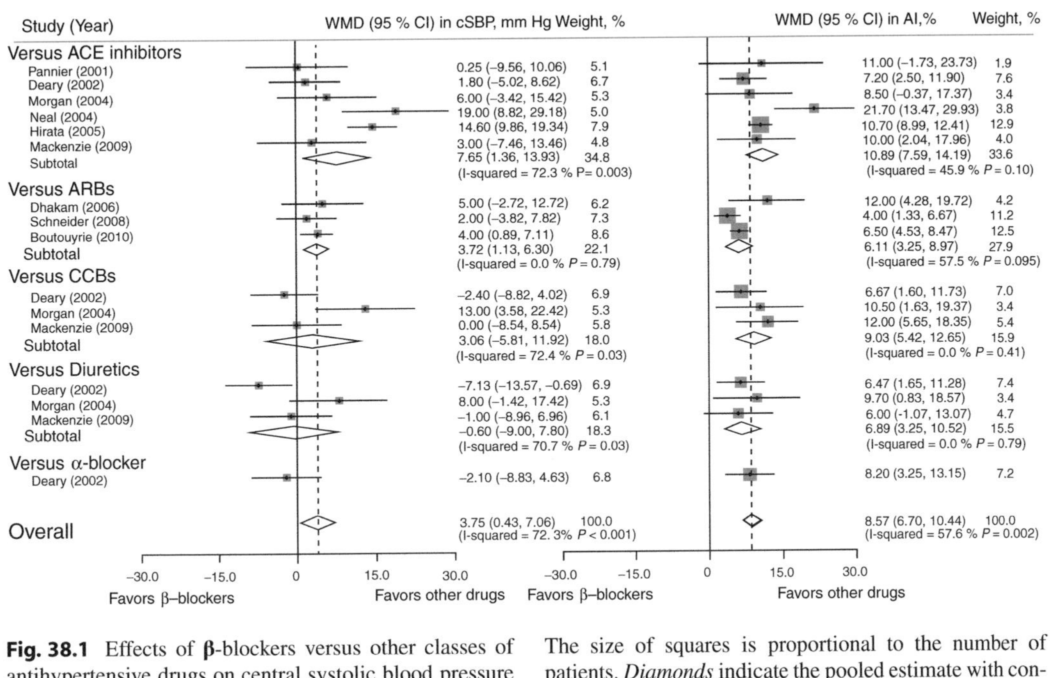

Fig. 38.1 Effects of β-blockers versus other classes of antihypertensive drugs on central systolic blood pressure (*left panel*) and central augmentation index (*right panel*). *Squares* indicate the point estimate of individual trials, and the *horizontal lines* indicate 95 % confidence intervals. The size of squares is proportional to the number of patients. *Diamonds* indicate the pooled estimate with confidence intervals. *WMD* weighted mean difference, *AI* central augmentation index (Reproduced with permission from Ding et al. [22])

significantly less efficacious than other classes of antihypertensive drugs by 3.8 mmHg (95 % CI, 0.4–7.0, $P=0.03$). There was significant ($P\leq0.03$) heterogeneity for all grouping comparisons except for ARBs ($P=0.79$) [22].

For central augmentation index, β-blockers were less efficacious than all the other classes of antihypertensive drugs ($P\leq0.001$), without significant heterogeneity for the comparisons versus each specific drug class ($P\geq0.095$, Fig. 38.1). Overall, a random effects model demonstrated that β-blockers were significantly less efficacious than the other classes of antihypertensive drugs by 8.6 % (95 % CI, 6.7–10.4, $P<0.001$), with significant heterogeneity across the comparator drug classes ($P=0.002$) [22].

We performed sensitivity analyses after exclusion of trials on bisoprolol or each specific comparator drug class, such as ACE inhibitor, ARB, etc. In these sensitivity analyses, our findings did not materially change except for the results on central systolic blood pressure after exclusion of the comparison versus ACE inhibitors. Indeed, after exclusion of the comparisons versus ACE inhibitors in 6 trials [16–20, 24], a random effects model demonstrated that the overall difference between β-blockers and ARBs, CCBs, diuretics, or an α-blocker in reducing central systolic blood pressure was not statistically different ($P=0.35$) [22].

We tested for publication bias visually by the funnel plot and statistically by the Begg's test [35]. Publication bias was not apparent in the funnel plot and was not statistically significant in terms of either central systolic blood pressure ($P=0.21$) or augmentation index ($P=0.15$) [22].

Our meta-analysis [22] extends the results of a recent narrative review on the effects of various antihypertensive drugs on pressure amplification [36] and a meta-analysis on the effect of ACE inhibitors versus other antihypertensive drugs on central augmentation index [37]. In the narrative review, the authors drew conclusions mainly based on the count of positive, neutral, or negative studies for diuretics (4 trials), β-blockers (4 trials), ACE inhibitors (11 trials), ARBs (4 trials), and CCBs (3 trials) [36]. The authors concluded that the evidence was compelling for β-blockers and ACE inhibitors that respectively decreased and increased pressure amplifications, and more evidence would be required for the other three classes of antihypertensive drugs. These conclusions are to some extent consistent with the results of our study on central systolic blood pressure. β-blockers and ACE inhibitors were in the two extremes and the others in between. However, it is noteworthy that the nonsignificant results might be attributable to the smaller number of observations in the comparison versus CCBs and to the neutral effect of diuretics on pressure amplifications. In the meta-analysis of trials on ACE inhibitors and central augmentation index, the only significant association was observed between ACE inhibitors and β-blockers [37]. In our meta-analysis, β-blockers were significantly less efficacious than all the other classes of drugs [22]. This observation suggests that there is a consistent mechanism that β-blockade increases central augmentation index by slowing the heart rate.

Meta-regression Analysis on Central Hemodynamics and Heart Rate

Also in a random effects model, we performed meta-regression analyses to correlate central systolic blood pressure and augmentation index with the baseline-adjusted differences in heart rate between randomized groups [22]. The regression line was weighted by the inverse of the within-study and between-study variance.

In meta-regression, the baseline-adjusted differences in central augmentation index between randomized groups were significantly associated with the baseline-adjusted between-group differences in heart rate (adjusted R [2]=0.296, $P=0.02$, Fig. 38.2). Each 10 beats per minute decrease in heart rate was associated with 7.0 % (95 % CI, 1.1–12.9 %) less reduction in central augmentation index. A similar meta-regression analysis on central systolic blood pressure revealed a significant association with the baseline-adjusted between-group differences in central augmentation index (adjusted R [2]=0.457,

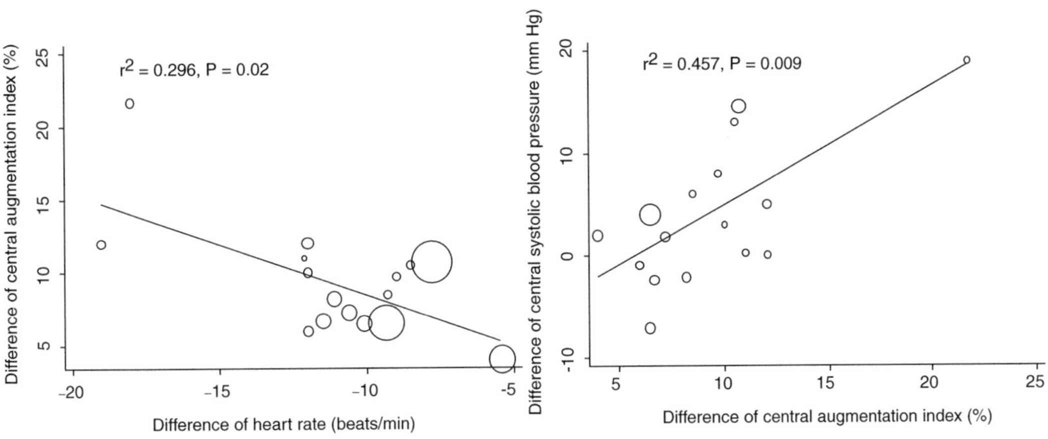

Fig. 38.2 Meta-regression analysis on the baseline-adjusted differences in central augmentation index with heart rate (*left panel*) and central systolic blood pressure with central augmentation index (*right panel*). The size of the *circles* was proportional to the number of patients. The regression line was weighted by the inverse of the within-study and additive between-study variance (Reproduced with permission from Ding et al. [22])

$P=0.009$, Fig. 38.2). Each 1 % increase in central augmentation index was associated with 1.2 mmHg (95 % CI, 0.3–2.0 mmHg) higher central systolic blood pressure. The association between the baseline-adjusted differences in central systolic blood pressure and the differences in heart rate did not reach statistical significance (adjusted *R* [2]=0.054, $P=0.76$) [22].

Our meta-regression analysis [22] can be compared with the mechanistic analysis of the ASCOT-CAFE trial that compared the β-blocker atenolol-based regimen with the CCB amlodipine-based regimen [20, 21]. The main finding of this analysis was that each 10 beats per minute reduction in heart rate was associated with 4.9 % and 3.0 mmHg increase in central augmentation index and central systolic blood pressure. However, when the reduction of heart rate was analyzed, heart rate explained 34 and 5 % of variability of central augmentation index and central systolic blood pressure, respectively. We also found in our meta-regression that the contribution of heart rate to central augmentation index was substantially greater than to central systolic blood pressure (29.6 % vs. 5.4 %). The latter measurement can be significantly influenced by any efficacious antihypertensive therapy in addition to wave reflections as measured by the augmentation index.

Meta-regression Analysis on Odds Ratios of Stroke and Heart Rate

For meta-analysis, we searched outcome trials that compared β-blockers with other classes of antihypertensive drugs in hypertensive patients and had a follow-up for at least 2 years and a sample size of at least 100 patients. We identified 11 trials [8–10, 13–17, 38–40] published between 1980 and 2011. We excluded 6 trials that did not report heart rate (or pulse rate) during follow-up ($n=5$) [10, 14, 17, 38, 39] or did not clearly define the control treatment ($n=1$) [15]. All of the 5 remaining trials included a single comparison of a β-blocker with an angiotensin receptor blocker (ARB, Losartan Intervention For Endpoint [LIFE] [9]), dihydropyridine (ASCOT [8] and European Lacidipine Study on Atherosclerosis [ELSA] [40]) or nondihydropyridine (INternational VErapamil-trandolapril STudy [INVEST] [16]) CCBs or a diuretic (Heart Attack Primary Prevention in HYpertension [HAPPHY] [13]).

We extracted fatal and nonfatal stroke (excluding transient ischemic attacks) from the published reports and accepted the definitions of stroke as given by the investigators. We computed odds ratios in stratified 2×2 contingency

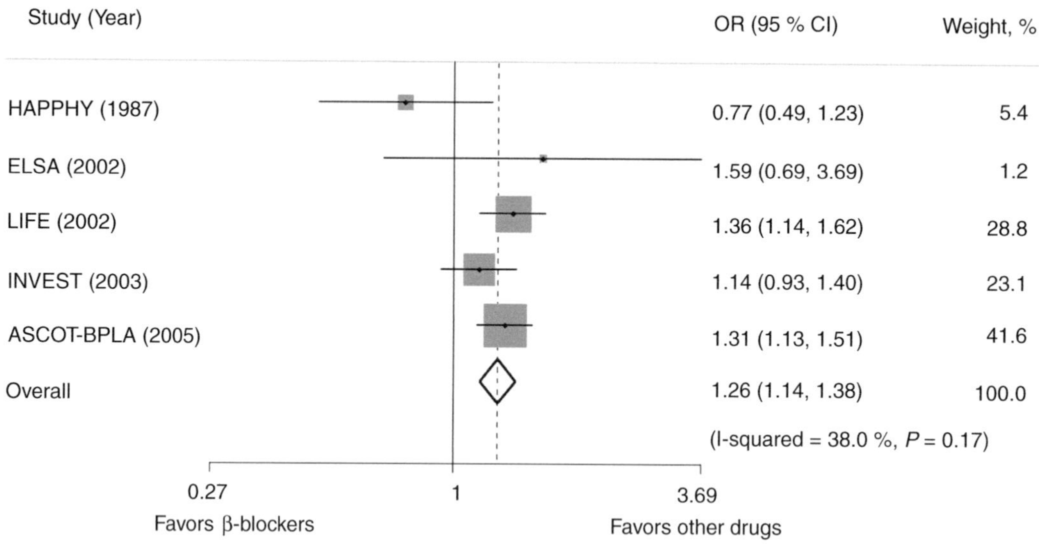

Fig. 38.3 Effects of β-blockers versus other classes of antihypertensive drugs on stroke. Acronyms of trials are explained in the text. For further information, see Fig. 38.1 (Reproduced with permission from Ding et al. [22])

tables. We checked the heterogeneity of odds ratios also by the I-squared statistic [34]. We also applied a random effects model to compute pooled estimates. We evaluated dependency of odds ratios of stroke on blood pressure by comparing the pooled odds ratio with the odds ratio corresponding to the between-group difference in systolic blood pressure according to our previous meta-regression analysis [19, 41].

The five eligible trials included 59,929 randomized patients [8, 9, 13, 16, 40]. The odds ratios of stroke in these 5 trials were not significantly heterogeneous (I [2]=38 %, P=0.17). The pooled estimate of odds ratios was 1.23 (95 % CI, 1.08–1.42, P<0.001, Fig. 38.3). Overall, the baseline-adjusted mean difference in heart rate between randomized groups was 7.4 beats per minute. According to the above meta-regression analysis, this difference in heart rate was associated with 5.1 % of central augmentation index and in turn 5.9 mmHg of central systolic blood pressure. According to our previous meta-regression analysis [19], which was based on brachial systolic blood pressure, this 5.9 mmHg derived difference in central systolic blood pressure should have a 1.47 (95 % CI, 1.22–1.64) odds ratio of stroke, which did not significantly deviate from the pooled estimate of the observed odds ratios (P=0.08) [22].

According to our meta-analysis and meta-regression analysis [22], it is clear that by slowing the heart rate β-blockers may substantially increase central augmentation index and, to a much less extent, in turn also slightly increase or decrease central systolic blood pressure. However, whether this mechanism can explain the outcome results of β-blockers versus other antihypertensive drugs remains controversial [42, 43]. We attempted to address this question using a meta-regression analysis approach. However, there were too few trials that reported sufficient data, such as treatment-induced changes in heart rate. Our interpretation had to rely on the between-group mean differences in central systolic blood pressure derived from heart rate and central augmentation index. According to our previous meta-regression analysis of outcome trials in hypertension, which was based on brachial systolic blood pressure, 1 mmHg of brachial systolic blood pressure difference may contribute to approximately 10 % of changes in the risk of stroke [19] but apparently is unable to explain 26 % of less stroke reduction by β-blockers. However, 5.9 mmHg derived difference in central systolic blood pressure could well account for the odds ratio of 1.26. Although until now, there is no study specifically quantifying the association between central systolic blood pressure and stroke [44], and central systolic blood pressure should not be less, if not more, influencing on stroke risk than its brachial counterpart [45]. Nonetheless, it is difficult to understand why the less reduction in central systolic blood pressure by β-blockade does not offset the coronary benefit.

Conclusions and Implications

The main finding of our meta-analyses and meta-regression analyses was that the efficacy of β-blockade was less than antihypertensive treatment of other mechanisms in reducing central augmentation index and less than ACE inhibitors and ARBs in reducing central systolic blood pressure, mainly because of its intrinsic heart rate-slowing effect. This mechanism might explain the inferior effect of β-blockers on stroke prevention.

Nonetheless, our findings cannot be directly extrapolated to other β-blockers, such as nebivolol and carvedilol, which have vasodilating effect in the peripheral circulation and less heart rate-slowing effect in the heart. Our finding should also be cautiously extrapolated to instruments other than the SphygmoCor device that was used in all trials included in the present meta-analysis. The built-in algorithm of the SphygmoCor device for the estimation of the augmentation index is frequency dependent and thus at different heart rate may give different results of the augmentation index. The present meta-analysis may therefore overestimate the association between the changes in heart rate and the changes in the augmentation index.

Despite these limitations, our overview is conclusive that β-blockade is less efficacious than other classes of antihypertensive drugs in reducing central augmentation and to a less extent in reducing systolic blood pressure. The heart rate slowing effect of β-blockade may largely account for its less reduction in central augmentation and to some extent also for its less reduction in central systolic blood pressure and in the risk of stroke. Our study is not intended to suppress the use of β-blockers in the management of hypertension. The intention is for the proper use of β-blockers. For instance, if a β-blocker is used in controlling hypertension, central hemodynamics should be measured. Otherwise, a more stringent target level of brachial blood pressure might have to be adopted.

While we accept in the management of hypertension ambulatory blood pressure that measures blood pressure variability with time and/or locations and conditions of measurement, we should readily accept central hemodynamics that measures blood pressure variability with arterial sites. With current technology, measurement of central hemodynamics has become feasible in clinical practice and can even be done simultaneously with the brachial blood pressure [46]. It is therefore imperative to build operational thresholds for central augmentation index or blood pressure in the diagnosis and therapeutic monitoring of hypertension on the basis of prospective observational studies [47] and randomized controlled trials.

References

1. Staessen JA, Wang JG, Bianchi G, Birkenhäger WH. Essential hypertension. Lancet. 2003;361:1629–41.
2. Collins R, Peto R, MacMahon S, Hebert P, Fiebach NH, Eberlein KA, Godwin J, Qizilbash N, Taylor JO, Hennekens CH. Blood pressure, stroke, and coronary heart disease. Part 2, Short-term reductions in blood pressure: overview of randomised drug trials in their epidemiological context. Lancet. 1990;335:827–38.
3. Staessen JA, Gąsowski J, Wang JG, Thijs L, Den Hond E, Boissel J, Coope J, Ekbom T, Gueyffier F, Liu L, Kerlikowske K, Pocock S, Fagard RH. Risks of untreated and treated isolated systolic hypertension in the elderly: meta-analysis of outcome trials. Lancet. 2000;355:865–72.
4. Liu LS, Writing Group of 2010 Chinese Guidelines for the Management of Hypertension. 2010 Chinese guidelines for the management of hypertension. Zhonghua Xin Xue Guan Bing Za Zhi. 2011;39:579–615.
5. Ogihara T, Kikuchi K, Matsuoka H, Fujita T, Higaki J, Horiuchi M, Imai Y, Imaizumi T, Ito S, Iwao H, Kario K, Kawano Y, Kim-Mitsuyama S, Kimura G, Matsubara H, Matsuura H, Naruse M, Saito I, Shimada K, Shimamoto K, Suzuki H, Takishita S, Tanahashi N, Tsuchihashi T, Uchiyama M, Ueda S, Ueshima H, Umemura S, Ishimitsu T, Rakugi H, Japanese Society of Hypertension Committee. The Japanese Society of Hypertension Guidelines for the Management of Hypertension (JSH 2009). Hypertens Res. 2009;32:3–107.

6. Mancia G, Fagard R, Narkiewicz K, Redón J, Zanchetti A, Böhm M, Christiaens T, Cifkova R, De Backer G, Dominiczak A, Galderisi M, Grobbee DE, Jaarsma T, Kirchhof P, Kjeldsen SE, Laurent S, Manolis AJ, Nilsson PM, Ruilope LM, Schmieder RE, Sirnes PA, Sleight P, Viigimaa M, Waeber B, Zannad F, Task Force for the management of arterial hypertension of the European Society of Hypertension (ESH) and of the European Society of Cardiology (ESC). 2013 ESH/ESC Guidelines for the management of arterial hypertension. J Hypertens. 2013;31: 1281–357.
7. Medical Research Council Working Party. MRC trial of treatment of mild hypertension: principal results. Br Med J (Clin Res Ed). 1985;291:97–104.
8. Dahlof B, Sever PS, Poulter NR, Wedel H, Beevers DG, Caulfield M, Collins R, Kjeldsen SE, Kristinsson A, McInnes GT, Mehlsen J, Nieminen M, O'Brien E, Ostergren J. Prevention of cardiovascular events with an antihypertensive regimen of amlodipine adding perindopril as required versus atenolol adding bendroflumethiazide as required, in the Anglo-Scandinavian Cardiac Outcomes Trial-Blood Pressure Lowering Arm (ASCOT-BPLA): a multicentre randomised controlled trial. Lancet. 2005;366:895–906.
9. Dahlof B, Devereux RB, Kjeldsen SE, Julius S, Beevers G, de Faire U, Fyhrquist F, Ibsen H, Kristiansson K, Lederballe-Pedersen O, Lindholm LH, Nieminen MS, Omvik P, Oparil S, Wedel H. Cardiovascular morbidity and mortality in the Losartan Intervention For Endpoint reduction in hypertension study (LIFE): a randomised trial against atenolol. Lancet. 2002;359:995–1003.
10. Hansson L, Hedner T, Lund-Johansen P, Kjeldsen SE, Lindholm LH, Syvertsen JO, Lanke J, de Faire U, Dahlof B, Karlberg BE. Randomised trial of effects of calcium antagonists compared with diuretics and beta-blockers on cardiovascular morbidity and mortality in hypertension: the Nordic Diltiazem (NORDIL) study. Lancet. 2000;356:359–65.
11. Messerli FH, Grossman E, Goldbourt U. Are beta-blockers efficacious as first-line therapy for hypertension in the elderly? A systematic review. JAMA. 1998;279:1903–7.
12. Lindholm LH, Carlberg B, Samuelsson O. Should beta blockers remain first choice in the treatment of primary hypertension? A meta-analysis. Lancet. 2005;366:1545–53.
13. Wilhelmsen L, Berglund G, Elmfeldt D, Fitzsimons T, Holzgreve H, Hosie J, Hornkvist PE, Pennert K, Tuomilehto J, Wedel H. Beta-blockers versus diuretics in hypertensive men: main results from the HAPPHY trial. J Hypertens. 1987;5:561–72.
14. Hansson L, Lindholm LH, Ekbom T, Dahlof B, Lanke J, Schersten B, Wester PO, Hedner T, de Faire U. Randomised trial of old and new antihypertensive drugs in elderly patients: cardiovascular mortality and morbidity the Swedish Trial in Old Patients with Hypertension-2 study. Lancet. 1999;354:1751–6.
15. The IPPPSH Collaborative group. Cardiovascular risk and risk factors in a randomized trial of treatment based on the beta-blocker oxprenolol: the International Prospective Primary Prevention Study in Hypertension (IPPPSH). J Hypertens. 1985;3:379–92.
16. Pepine CJ, Handberg EM, Cooper-DeHoff RM, Marks RG, Kowey P, Messerli FH, Mancia G, Cangiano JL, Garcia-Barreto D, Keltai M, Erdine S, Bristol HA, Kolb HR, Bakris GL, Cohen JD, Parmley WW. A calcium antagonist vs a non-calcium antagonist hypertension treatment strategy for patients with coronary artery disease. The International Verapamil-Trandolapril Study (INVEST): a randomized controlled trial. JAMA. 2003;290:2805–16.
17. UK Prospective Diabetes Study Group. Efficacy of atenolol and captopril in reducing risk of macrovascular and microvascular complications in type 2 diabetes: UKPDS 39. BMJ. 1998;317:713–20.
18. Law MR, Morris JK, Wald NJ. Use of blood pressure lowering drugs in the prevention of cardiovascular disease: meta-analysis of 147 randomised trials in the context of expectations from prospective epidemiological studies. BMJ. 2009;338:b1665.
19. Staessen JA, Wang JG, Thijs L. Cardiovascular protection and blood pressure reduction: a meta-analysis. Lancet. 2001;358:1305–15.
20. Williams B, Lacy PS, Thom SM, Cruickshank K, Stanton A, Collier D, Hughes AD, Thurston H, O'Rourke M. Differential impact of blood pressure-lowering drugs on central aortic pressure and clinical outcomes: principal results of the Conduit Artery Function Evaluation (CAFE) study. Circulation. 2006; 113:1213–25.
21. Williams B, Lacy PS. Impact of heart rate on central aortic pressures and hemodynamics: analysis from the CAFE (Conduit Artery Function Evaluation) study: CAFE-Heart Rate. J Am Coll Cardiol. 2009;54: 705–13.
22. Ding FH, Li Y, Li LH, Wang JG. Impact of heart rate on central hemodynamics and stroke: a meta-analysis of β-blocker trials. Am J Hypertens. 2013;26: 118–25.
23. Pannier BM, Guerin AP, Marchais SJ, London GM. Different aortic reflection wave responses following long-term angiotensin-converting enzyme inhibition and beta-blocker in essential hypertension. Clin Exp Pharmacol Physiol. 2001;28:1074–7.
24. Deary AJ, Schumann AL, Murfet H, Haydock S, Foo RS, Brown MJ. Influence of drugs and gender on the arterial pulse wave and natriuretic peptide secretion in untreated patients with essential hypertension. Clin Sci (Lond). 2002;103:493–9.
25. Morgan T, Lauri J, Bertram D, Anderson A. Effect of different antihypertensive drug classes on central aortic pressure. Am J Hypertens. 2004;17:118–23.
26. Neal DA, Brown MJ, Wilkinson IB, Byrne CD, Alexander GJ. Hemodynamic effects of amlodipine, bisoprolol, and lisinopril in hypertensive patients after liver transplantation. Transplantation. 2004;77: 748–50.

27. Hirata K, Vlachopoulos C, Adji A, O'Rourke MF. Benefits from angiotensin-converting enzyme inhibitor 'beyond blood pressure lowering': beyond blood pressure or beyond the brachial artery. J Hypertens. 2005;23:551–6.
28. Dhakam Z, McEniery CM, Yasmin, Cockcroft JR, Brown MJ, Wilkinson IB. Atenolol and eprosartan: differential effects on central blood pressure and aortic pulse wave velocity. Am J Hypertens. 2006;19:214–9.
29. Schneider MP, Delles C, Klingbeil AU, Ludwig M, Kolloch RE, Krekler M, Stumpe KO, Schmieder RE. Effect of angiotensin receptor blockade on central haemodynamics in essential hypertension: results of a randomised trial. J Renin Angiotensin Aldosterone Syst. 2008;9:49–56.
30. Mackenzie IS, McEniery CM, Dhakam Z, Brown MJ, Cockcroft JR, Wilkinson IB. Comparison of the effects of antihypertensive agents on central blood pressure and arterial stiffness in isolated systolic hypertension. Hypertension. 2009;54:409–13.
31. Boutouyrie P, Achouba A, Trunet P, Laurent S. Amlodipine-valsartan combination decreases central systolic blood pressure more effectively than the amlodipine-atenolol combination: the EXPLOR study. Hypertension. 2010;55:1314–22.
32. London GM, Asmar RG, O'Rourke MF, Safar ME. Mechanism(s) of selective systolic blood pressure reduction after a low-dose combination of perindopril/indapamide in hypertensive subjects: comparison with atenolol. J Am Coll Cardiol. 2004;43:92–9.
33. Dickersin K, Berlin JA. Meta-analysis: state-of-the-science. Epidemiol Rev. 1992;14:154–76.
34. Higgins JP, Thompson SG. Quantifying heterogeneity in a meta-analysis. Stat Med. 2002;21:1539–58.
35. Begg CB, Mazumdar M. Operating characteristics of a rank correlation test for publication bias. Biometrics. 1994;50:1088–101.
36. Protogerou AD, Stergiou GS, Vlachopoulos C, Blacher J, Achimastos A. The effect of antihypertensive drugs on central blood pressure beyond peripheral blood pressure. Part II: Evidence for specific class-effects of antihypertensive drugs on pressure amplification. Curr Pharm Des. 2009;15:272–89.
37. Shahin Y, Khan JA, Chetter I. Angiotensin converting enzyme inhibitors effect on arterial stiffness and wave reflections: A meta-analysis and meta-regression of randomised controlled trials. Atherosclerosis. 2012;221:18–33.
38. MRC Working Party. Medical Research Council trial of treatment of hypertension in older adults: principal results. BMJ. 1992;304:405–12.
39. Black HR, Elliott WJ, Grandits G, Grambsch P, Lucente T, White WB, Neaton JD, Grimm Jr RH, Hansson L, Lacourciere Y, Muller J, Sleight P, Weber MA, Williams G, Wittes J, Zanchetti A, Anders RJ. Principal results of the Controlled Onset Verapamil Investigation of Cardiovascular End Points (CONVINCE) trial. JAMA. 2003;289:2073–82.
40. Zanchetti A, Bond MG, Hennig M, Neiss A, Mancia G, Dal Palu C, Hansson L, Magnani B, Rahn KH, Reid JL, Rodicio J, Safar M, Eckes L, Rizzini P. Calcium antagonist lacidipine slows down progression of asymptomatic carotid atherosclerosis: principal results of the European Lacidipine Study on Atherosclerosis (ELSA), a randomized, double-blind, long-term trial. Circulation. 2002;106:2422–7.
41. Staessen JA, Wang JG, Thijs L. Cardiovascular prevention and blood pressure reduction: a quantitative overview updated until 1 March 2003. J Hypertens. 2003;21:1055–76.
42. Epstein BJ, Anderson S. Discordant effects of beta-blockade on central aortic systolic and brachial systolic blood pressure: considerations beyond the cuff. Pharmacotherapy. 2007;27:1322–33.
43. Elliott WJ, Childers WK. Should beta blockers no longer be considered first-line therapy for the treatment of essential hypertension without comorbidities. Curr Cardiol Rep. 2011;13:507–16.
44. Agabiti-Rosei E, Mancia G, O'Rourke MF, Roman MJ, Safar ME, Smulyan H, Wang JG, Wilkinson IB, Williams B, Vlachopoulos C. Central blood pressure measurements and antihypertensive therapy: a consensus document. Hypertension. 2007;50:154–60.
45. Hashimoto J, Imai Y, O'Rourke MF. Indices of pulse wave analysis are better predictors of left ventricular mass reduction than cuff pressure. Am J Hypertens. 2007;20:378–84.
46. Cheng HM, Sung SH, Shih YT, Chuang SY, Yu WC, Chen CH. Measurement of central aortic pulse pressure: noninvasive brachial cuff-based estimation by a transfer function vs. a novel pulse wave analysis method. Am J Hypertens. 2012;25:1162–9.
47. Cheng HM, Chuang SY, Sung SH, Yu WC, Pearson A, Lakatta EG, Pan WH, Chen CH. Derivation and validation of diagnostic thresholds for central blood pressure measurements based on long-term cardiovascular risks. J Am Coll Cardiol. 2013;62:1780–7.

39 Decreasing Arterial Stiffness and/or Wave Reflections Independently of Mean Arterial Pressure: Effect of Antihypertensive Drugs (Part 1)

Hélène Beaussier, Stéphane Laurent, and Pierre Boutouyrie

Abstract

Change in arterial stiffness with drugs is a major end point in clinical trials, although evidence for arterial stiffness as a therapeutic target still needs to be confirmed. Drugs which affect arterial stiffness include antihypertensive drugs, mostly blockers of the renin–angiotensin–aldosterone system. Other drugs will be addressed in Chap. 40. Whether the reduction in arterial stiffness after antihypertensive treatment is only due to the blood pressure (BP) lowering which unloads the stiff components of the arterial wall such as collagen, or additional BP-independent effects are involved, has been largely debated. Currently, an increasing body of evidence, including theoretical aspects of arterial mechanics, long-term observational studies in humans and recent meta-analyses of double-blind, randomized, controlled trials, suggests that only part of aortic stiffness could be reduced through the normalization of BP by pharmacological treatment, and further reduction of aortic stiffness would require arterial structural changes, including reduction in collagen density and rearrangement of the wall materials. Mechanistic pharmacological studies are required to demonstrate that novel pharmacological classes have true "de-stiffening" properties.

Keywords

Antihypertensive drugs • De-stiffening drugs • Arterial stiffness • Wave reflection • Lipid-lowering drugs • Antidiabetic drugs • Cross-link breakers

H. Beaussier
Clinical Research Unit and Pharmacy, Fondation Hôpital Saint Joseph, Paris, France

Hopital Europeen Georges Pompidou, Assistance Publique Hôpitaux de Paris, Université Paris Descartes, Paris, France

S. Laurent • P. Boutouyrie (✉)
Department of Pharmacology and Institut National de la Santé et de la Recherche Médicale U970(Eq7)-PARCC, Hôpital Européen Georges Pompidou, Assistance Publique-Hôpitaux de Paris, Université Paris-Descartes, 20, rue Leblanc, 75015 Paris, France
e-mail: stephane.laurent@egp.aphp.fr; pierre.boutouyrie@egp.aphp.fr

M.E. Safar et al. (eds.), *Blood Pressure and Arterial Wall Mechanics in Cardiovascular Diseases*, DOI 10.1007/978-1-4471-5198-2_39, © Springer-Verlag London 2014

Arterial stiffness has emerged as an important marker of cardiovascular risk. More than 20 independent studies have shown that carotid to femoral pulse wave velocity (PWV) predicted cardiovascular outcome independently of major classical cardiovascular risk factors in different populations [1, 2] and can be modified by certain drug groups [3]. This simple, non-invasive measurement was recently included in official guidelines, and while reference values have been published, its implementation in clinical practice as a surrogate marker awaits evidence to suggest that this modification is associated with a better clinical outcome.

Since extensive reviews of the literature have been recently published [3–5], the objective of the present article is to present an overview of published evidence for the effect of cardiovascular drugs on arterial stiffness and/or wave reflection, with particular emphasis on drugs' impact independently of mean blood pressure (MBP) in hypertension. Since the topic is very wide, we chose to address it in two chapters, this chapter dealing with antihypertensive drugs and Chap. 40 dealing with drugs not directly influencing blood pressure. For this chapter, we searched the Cochrane library, MEDLINE and EMBASE, from January 1993 to October 2013. We used the search terms "arterial stiffness" OR "arterial compliance" AND either "hypertension/pharmacology" OR "hypertension/therapy". Although we selected publications in the past 20 years, we did not exclude commonly referenced and highly regarded old publications. We included review articles to provide a more comprehensive overview than can be included in our report. We also searched www.clinicaltrials.gov to determine which clinical trials have been (or are currently) performed with novel molecules.

Theoretical Aspects

Theoretical aspects are precisely described in Chaps. 1 and 5. We will thus only stress on the relevant points for this chapter.

Arterial stiffness depends on different parameters. First is the composition of the arterial wall; distensible material is represented by elastin and stiff material by collagen, although the various components of the extracellular matrix also play a role, through their own elastic modulus and interactions with smooth muscle cells (SMCs). Smooth muscle cells play an important role in arterial stiffness, depending not only on their contractile status but also on phenotype dedifferentiation in some disease, and thus secretory activity. When relaxed, their contribution to arterial stiffness is modest, but when contracted, they behave as a stiff material linking fibrous components [6]. Elastin fibres are under permanent load, whereas collagen fibres are curled and progressively recruited as the arterial wall is stretched. This explains why arterial stiffness increases with blood pressure. This is of the utmost importance because antihypertensive drugs may improve arterial stiffness passively, solely by decreasing blood pressure and without changing arterial wall properties. This fact complicates the demonstration of a true pleiotropic effect of de-stiffening drugs. It is therefore mandatory to systematically adjust for changes in blood pressure before interpreting the modification in arterial stiffness. This also implies that the changes in blood pressure may affect arterial stiffness differently depending on whether they are acute or chronic. Indeed, blood pressure, especially its pulsatile component, is one of the strongest growth signals for the arterial wall [7], and chronic changes in blood pressure are most likely to induce changes in arterial wall properties. Furthermore, ageing needs to be taken into account during long-term trials (>1 year). In terms of arterial stiffness, the arterial tree is heterogeneous; the large arteries close to the heart are the most elastic as they contain large amounts of elastin, fewer collagen and SMCs. As we go more distally, medium-size peripheral arteries such as the radial artery become stiffer [8]. Therefore, when studying arterial stiffness, it is important to specify which site is studied, although the aorta (through CF-PWV) and the common carotid artery (CCA) are overwhelmingly used in clinical studies. In the present article, the term arterial stiffness corresponds to the aortic and/or carotid sites if not otherwise specified.

It is important to note that this paper is only referring to valid measures of arterial stiffness such as listed in the consensus paper [9].

Animal Studies

Exploration of the effects of treatment on arterial stiffness necessitates the use of models associated with changes in arterial stiffness, mostly hypertension, such as spontaneous hypertension, secondary hypertension and hypertension induced by surgical, pharmacological and transgenic means (see Chap. 6). These different experimental models indeed confirm the role of extracellular matrix (ECM) and muscular tone as essential targets for treatment. They also enhance the necessity of acting at the multiple interactions existing between SMCs and ECM [10].

Pharmacological Interventions on Arterial Stiffness in Humans

Influence of Antihypertensive Drugs

Antihypertensive medications have the best potential to improve arterial stiffness because they passively improve it by reducing blood pressure and may have further long-term effect on remodelling on small [11] and large arteries [12]. Blood pressure lowering produces a shift to the more compliant segment of compliance–pressure curve and may also modify attachments of VSMC to extracellular matrix (see Chap. 6). Antihypertensive therapy may also have direct effects on the large arteries, particularly calcium channel blockers (CCBs), angiotensin-converting enzyme inhibitors (ACEIs), angiotensin receptor blockers (ARBs), mineralocorticoid receptor blockers and nitrates. The changes that occur may depend on the agent and dose used, the degree to which blood pressure is lowered and the duration of treatment and the vascular bed examined. In addition, the mechanisms may differ: for instance, nitrates mainly increase compliance by vasodilatation, whereas ACEIs and CCBs may decrease stiffness (elastic modulus) without affecting arterial diameter [13].

Table 39.1 Comparison of the effect on pulse wave velocity (PWV) and wave reflection by various antihypertensive drug classes

Drug class	PWW	Wave reflection
ACE inhibitors	↘	↘↘
Angiotensin receptor blockers	↘	↘↘
Aldosterone antagonists	⇔	↘
Thiazides	⇔	⇔
Calcium channel blocker: dihydropyridines	↘	↘↘
Calcium channel blockers: verapamil	↘	↘
Alpha-blockers	⇔	↘↘
Beta-blockers: non-vasodilating	↘	↗
Beta-blockers: vasodilating	↘	↘
Nitrates	⇔	↘

Numerous studies have been published on the effect of antihypertensive drugs on arterial stiffness and are summarized in Table 39.1. Recent reviews [3–5] underline important differences between the effects of various classes of antihypertensive drugs. The general view is that drugs antagonizing the renin–angiotensin system (RAS) are superior in reducing arterial stiffness compared with the other classes; however, the evidence is scarce [14]. This may be as the RAS system is a potent pro-fibrotic system. The turnover of the extracellular matrix in the arterial wall translates into changes in mechanical properties of the vessel, although the three-dimensional organization of extracellular matrix components, and their interaction with SMC, is more important than the absolute content of distensible or stiff material to explain arterial stiffness [10]. Until now, no drug is capable of directly targeting extracellular matrix turnover. ARBs [15] and mineralocorticoid receptor blockers [16] exert direct effects on conduit blood vessels resulting in decreased stiffness. Some of these effects are related to the ability of ACEIs, ARBs, CCBs and mineralocorticoid receptor blockers to exert antifibrotic actions, usually as a result of downregulation of expression of transforming growth factor-β (TGF-beta). This leads to decreased activation of SMADs that are transcription factors that mediate the action of TGF-beta on collagen synthesis and consequently reduced vascular stiffness as less collagen is deposited in the media of large vessels.

At the same time, similar changes in small arteries contribute to reduce impedance and wave reflection, having a positive effect on augmentation of pulse pressure (PP) in the proximal aorta.

ACE inhibitors were the first class extensively studied. Benetos et al. [17] demonstrated a favourable decrease in the CF-PWV after both acute (3 h after first dose) and chronic administration (after 15 days) of ramipril. Other studies have shown similar findings with different drugs within the same class [14, 18, 19] for full references). The mechanism is thought to imply a virtuous circle with reduction of the wave reflection and augmentation index with subsequent lowering of PP and SBP, in parallel with direct reduction of fibrosis of the wall, all resulting in regression of large arteries and LV remodelling [20].

The role of angiotensin II receptor blockers on arterial stiffness is not yet clear, given the small number of studies including limited sample sizes. A substudy of the ONTARGET trial evaluated the effects on arterial stiffness of telmisartan alone or in combination with ramipril on arterial stiffness; however, no true quantification of the effect according to treatment arms was provided [21, 22]. The EXPLOR trial showed that although central SBP and PP were decreased to a larger extent by an ARB (valsartan) added to a CCB (amlodipine) than by a non-vasodilating beta-blocker (atenolol) added to a CCB (amlodipine), PWV was decreased similarly by both drugs. Recently, the promising compound 21, a selective non-peptide angiotensin II type 2 receptor agonist, has been tested in an animal model and was showed to improve arterial stiffness, without any change in blood pressure, suggesting that part of the positive effect of ARBs might be mediated by overstimulation of AT2 receptors [23]. A recent study compared the effects of aliskiren (150–300 mg/daily) or ramipril (5–10 mg/daily) for 12 weeks on arterial stiffness and endothelial function. Both drugs had similar effects on blood pressure and PWV. Aliskiren induced a greater AIx reduction than ramipril [24].

Because most of published clinical trials were of limited size, we performed a meta-analysis of double-blind, randomized, controlled trials [25]

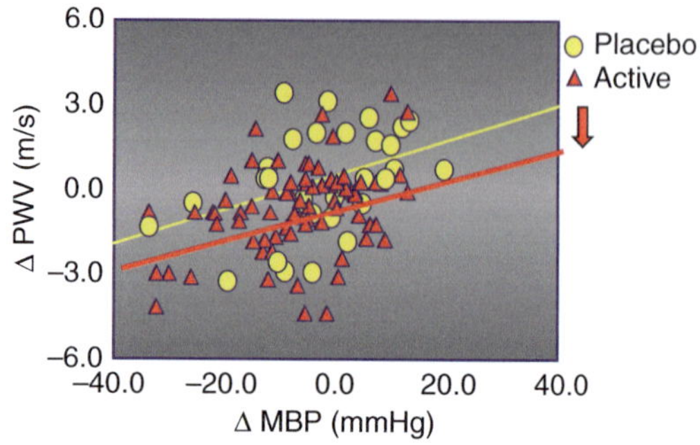

Fig. 39.1 Changes in pulse wave velocity related to changes in mean blood pressure. The downward shift between the two regression lines, indicated by the *arrow*, shows the pressure-independent reduction in pulse wave velocity (Redrawn from Ref. [25])

comparing different antihypertensive drugs and/or placebo in both the short and long term. In this study, we correlated changes in PWV with changes in blood pressure while adjusting for the initial value of PWV. We showed that active treatment was associated with a reduction in arterial stiffness compared with placebo (Fig. 39.1). Furthermore, PWV was reduced to a greater extent after long-term antihypertensive treatment than in the short-term, and changes in PWV were dependent on MBP and PP changes, not on heart rate. In long-term trials, ACE inhibitors were more potent than calcium antagonists, beta-blockers and diuretics, independently of changes in blood pressure (Fig. 39.2). One important limitation of this study was that the study patients were those recruited for clinical trials and therefore did not represent the general hypertensive population. Furthermore, duration of trials was too short to assess very long-term changes in PWV.

We thus performed an observational prospective study under conditions of routine clinical practice, comprising 97 patients with treated essential hypertension with well-controlled blood pressure who had more than two measurements of aortic stiffness [26]. We showed that the reduction in PWV (from 14.2 to 11.0 m/s; $p<0.0001$) over 5.4 years follow-up was associated with a significant reduction in central SBP and central PP, contrasting with a smaller change in brachial SBP and no change in brachial PP. The reduction in PWV was independent of the reduction in MBP, whereas

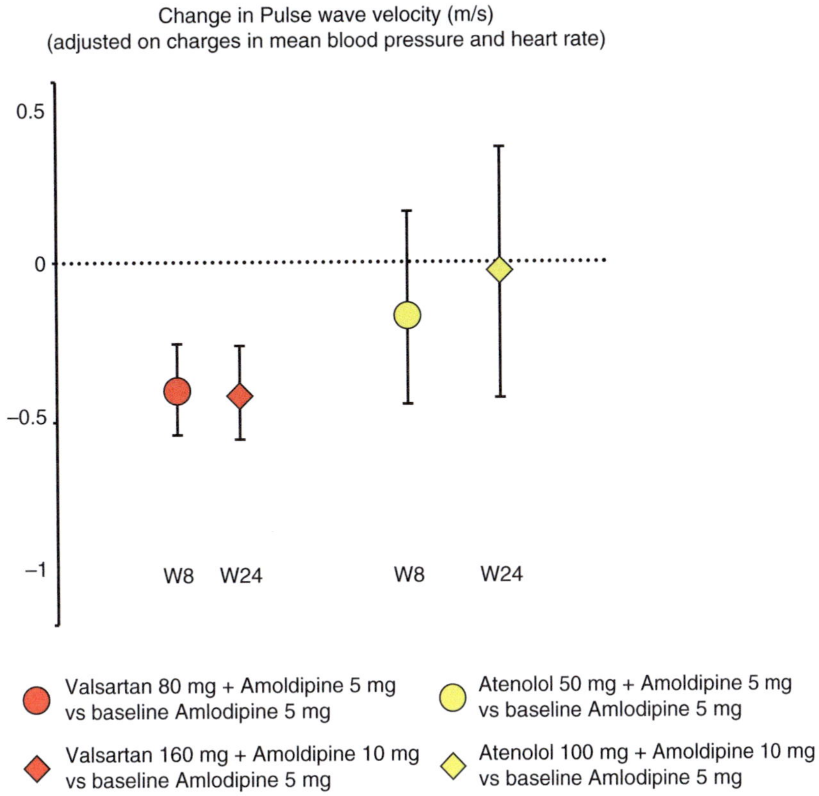

Fig. 39.2 Changes in pulse wave velocity during the EXPLOR trial, after adjustment on mean blood pressure and heart rate. This picture shows that atenolol did not induce changes in pulse wave velocity independently of blood pressure and heart rate changes, whereas valsartan induced significant decrease of pulse wave velocity (Redrawn from Ref.[49])

the reduction in central PP was largely explained by the reduction in PWV. These results suggest that a large and sustained decrease in aortic stiffness can be obtained in treated hypertensive patients in routine clinical practice. These changes most likely represent a delayed response to the long-term normalization of BP and cardiovascular risk factors, through arterial remodelling.

A recent meta-analysis [14] was conducted to investigate the effect of ACEI on large arteries in comparison to placebo and to other antihypertensive agents. In 5 trials including 469 patients, treatment with ACEIs ($n=227$) versus placebo ($n=216$) significantly reduced PWV (−1.69 m/s [−2.05, −1.33], $p<0.00001$). In 9 trials (378 patients), treatment with ACEIs ($n=178$) did not reduce PWV more than other antihypertensive drugs (ARBs, CCBs, beta-blockers, diuretics and a combination of ACEI and ARB) ($n=220$) (mean difference −0.19 m/s, [−0.59, 0.21], $p=0.36$). ACEI reduced AIx more than placebo (−3.8 % [−9.0, −1.6], $p=0.0006$). Treatment with ACEIs significantly reduced AIx when compared with other antihypertensive drugs (−1.84 %, [−3, −0.68], $p=0.002$); however, this effect was only significant when compared with beta-blockers. In this meta-analysis, changes in PWV were not associated with changes in blood pressure. The authors stressed on the lack of adequately powered trial [14].

Blockers of the RAS system are particularly efficacious in patients with diabetes mellitus [27, 28], and here, high dosage [29], complete blockade and significant reduction in blood pressure [30] are mandatory to improve arterial stiffness in these patients. Multifactorial intervention is probably the best way to improve arterial stiffness in patients with diabetes mellitus; however, the clinical evidence for this is relatively limited [31].

The capacity of a given drug to reverse aortic stiffening independently of changes in BP should theoretically be dose dependent. However, only one dose was tested in most studies. A major argument in favour of a BP-independent reduction in

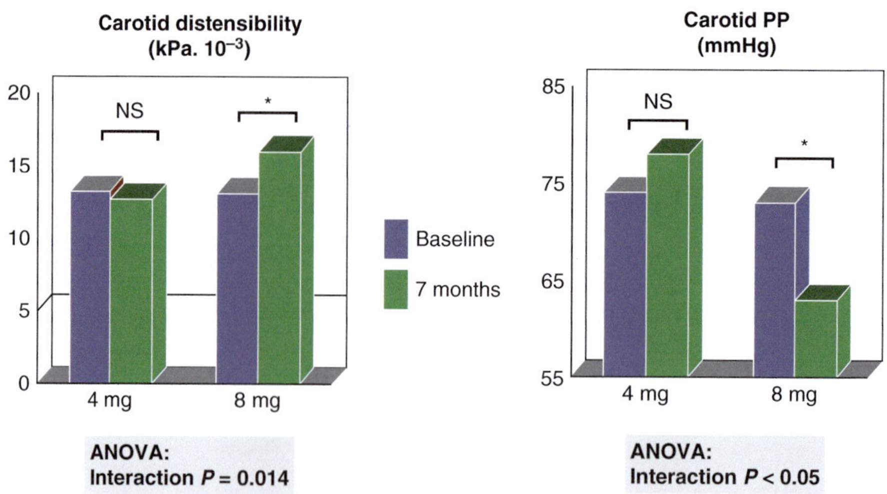

Fig. 39.3 Additional effect of high-dose ACE inhibitor perindopril 8 mg compared to 4 mg on carotid distensibility and central pressure (Redrawn from Ref. [29])

aortic stiffness by a RAAS blocker would come from the demonstration of a dose-dependent reduction in aortic stiffness for a given MBP reduction. We tested whether a large dose of ACE inhibitor perindopril (8 mg) was superior than the usual dose (4 mg) at decreasing arterial stiffness in a population of hypertensive diabetic patients [29]. We were able to show that carotid stiffness decreased with the 8 mg and not with the 4 mg dose, whereas blood pressure remained identical (Fig. 39.3). These two studies demonstrate that the BP-independent changes in arterial stiffness could be obtained with most antihypertensive drugs, but particularly with RAS antagonists, and that they are enhanced by larger doses and long-term treatment. These results probably reflect the slow turnover rate of extracellular matrix, the long time constant of arterial remodelling and the necessity to act on tissue systems to influence changes in arterial stiffness beyond blood pressure.

The effects of CCB on central pressure and stiffness are detailed in Chap. 42. The largest study to investigate the effect of calcium channel blockers on PP is the Conduit Artery Function Evaluation (CAFE) study [32], which examined the impact of two different blood pressure-lowering regimens (atenolol ± thiazide vs. amlodipine ± perindopril) on derived central aortic pressures and haemodynamic status in 2,073 participants with hypertension and at least three additional risk factors. Central aortic PP was significantly lower with amlodipine ± perindopril compared with atenolol ± thiazide-based therapy when brachial PP was identical (see Chap. 42). As previously mentioned, this could be predominantly determined by the beta-blocker effects on heart rate and stroke volume. No differences were seen for PWV in the small subgroup ($n = 114$) who had CF-PWV measurements [32].

Matsui et al. conducted a prospective, randomized, open-label, blinded end point study (J-CORE study) aimed to compare the effects of CCBs or diuretics when used in combination with ARBs on aortic systolic blood pressure (BP) and brachial ambulatory systolic BP. These data showed that the combination of olmesartan (20 mg) and azelnidipine (16 mg) had a more beneficial effect on central systolic BP and arterial stiffness than the combination of olmesartan (20 mg) and hydrochlorothiazide (12.5 mg) [33]. We showed from the EXPLOR trial that despite the presence of amlodipine, the differential effect between the ARB (valsartan) and beta-blocker (atenolol) could still be observed on central BP [22]. However, the effect of both compounds on PWV was similar.

The role of sodium load on large arteries is developed elsewhere (Chap. 13). In elderly individuals with hypertension, sodium restriction rapidly reduces large artery stiffness [34]. Thus, it seemed reasonable to expect that thiazide diuretics would decrease aPWV. Diuretics did not have any beneficial effect on arterial stiffness or wave reflection in most studies [33, 35–40], despite that all classes of antihypertensive drugs might potentially reduce aortic PWV (aPWV) indirectly by lowering MAP, the distending pressure in elastic tubes [41]. In a comparative study, Mahmud and Feely [40] showed that the reduction in aPWV was significantly larger with an aldosterone receptor antagonist than with a thiazide diuretic even after adjusting for the reduction in MAP [40]. Matsui et al. showed from the J-CORE study data that the less performing group received hydrochlorothiazide. They observed that the change in plasma aldosterone was significantly and positively associated with the change in aPWV in patients treated with hydrochlorothiazide. These findings suggest that hyperaldosteronism in response to volume depletion may exert deleterious effect on arterial stiffness and partly explain why thiazide diuretics have little effect on large artery stiffness [42].

A special attention should be put on beta-blockers. Beta-blockers decrease both heart rate and blood pressure. Because non-vasodilating beta-blockers induce a certain level of vasoconstriction, they have a potential to increase wave reflections. The Regression of Arterial Stiffness in a Controlled Double-Blind Study (REASON) compared perindopril (2 mg/day) plus indapamide (0.625 mg/day) versus atenolol (50 mg/day) alone for 12 months in hypertensive subjects. At 1 year, brachial and central SBP reduction achieved with combination therapy of ACEI plus diuretic was greater than that with beta-blocker alone or even ACEI alone. This effect was translated into greater structural changes of arterial stiffness more pronounced in central than in peripheral arteries [43]. Higher CF-PWV was closely correlated with higher SBP as a marker of more resistant hypertension requiring greater antihypertensive doses. In other words, increased arterial stiffening might be the reason of poor SBP response to drug treatment [44]. In most clinical trials in hypertensive patients, the reduction in MBP after beta-blockers is sufficient to reduce PWV, despite a possible direct pro-fibrotic effect of beta-blockers on the arterial wall, as stated by animal studies. Thus, an important finding comes from the BBEST study [45], during which celiprolol, a beta-1 antagonist with beta-2 agonist properties, administered for 4 years in patients with Ehlers–Danlos disease, increased the stiffness of the carotid wall material (elastic modulus), compared to placebo. This effect was unmasked because BP was not lowered. Various pharmacological mechanisms are possible, to explain such a pro-stiffening effect of beta-blockers. They include the stimulation of beta-2 adrenergic receptors, which is associated with activation of TGF-beta and overstimulation of TGF-beta receptor, and an unopposed alpha-adrenergic stimulation by displacement of endogenous agonist from beta-receptors and baroreflex stimulation, which is also associated with activation of TGF-beta.

Non-vasodilating beta-blockers such as atenolol have been shown to be less efficacious than vasodilating drugs such as calcium antagonists, RAS blockers [32, 22, 43] and vasodilating beta-blockers in reducing wave reflection and central pressures [46–48] although arterial stiffness may be reduced to the same extent with all these drug groups. In the recent meta-analysis of antihypertensive drugs [25], the beta-blocker bisoprolol was almost as effective as other drugs at lowering aortic stiffness. The most commonly quoted explanation is that the reduction in arterial stiffness is due to the reduction in heart rate because of viscoelastic properties of the arterial wall (counterbalancing the lack of intrinsic improvement of arterial stiffness) [32]. At the same time, reduced heart rate leads to increased wave reflection resulting in a lower reduction in aortic versus brachial systolic pressure and reduced PP amplification. The peripheral vasoconstriction associated with atenolol may be an additional mechanism responsible for a negative effect on wave reflection.

We recently reanalyzed the EXPLOR data to study the changes in PWV in relation with the changes in blood pressure, heart rate and major covariates. We showed that although reductions in mean BP and PWV were not significantly different between groups, the determinants of the reduction in PWV differed between both treatment arms. Half of the decrease in PWV in response to valsartan was not explained by the reduction in MBP and HR. By contrast, in the atenolol group, the decrease in PWV in response to atenolol was fully explained by the reduction in MBP and HR [49]. Finally, Casey et al. recently suggested that beta-adrenergic receptor sensitivity in the peripheral vasculature differs between sexes, women been oversensitive to the increased wave reflection [50], and the same team showed that the negative effects (i.e. increased aortic wave reflection) of non-selective beta-adrenergic blockade are less pronounced in postmenopausal than in young women [51].

By contrast to non-vasodilating beta-blockers, vasodilating beta-blockers may exert less deleterious effects on central BP. Indeed, nebivolol, which is a selective beta-1 blocker with nitric oxide potentiating vasodilatory effect, has been shown to slightly decrease the augmentation index, when compared with atenolol [42]. Whether this would result in less aortic stiffening and more favourable outcomes remains to be determined. This aspect is developed elsewhere (Chap. 40).

Nitric Oxide Donors

Nitric oxide is a powerful vasodilator and has been shown to improve arterial stiffness and central pressure without altering peripheral pressure [52–55]. NO dilates more the large arteries than the small one, opposite to other vasodilators; they also improve wave reflection and decrease specifically central systolic pressure [56]. However, clinical use of nitrates for treating hypertensive patients in the long term is limited by their short duration of action; the tolerance event tachyphylaxia; and their side effects, such as headache. Different compounds are currently tested, which are supposed to overcome these caveats.

Pharmacological Perspectives

A recent and exhaustive review [57] described several novel cell-signalling pathways and pathophysiological mechanisms that emerged in the past few years, providing new pharmacological targets to treat hypertension and by extension new potential reflections to improve arterial stiffness and/or wave reflections. For instance, two new pharmacological strategies could bring out mechanisms of interest. The first mechanism described [57] dual vasopeptidase inhibitors. Besides angiotensin-converting enzyme, two other zinc metalloproteinases neprilysin (also called neutral endopeptidase) and endothelin-converting enzyme are pharmacological targets for hypertension [58]. Combined inhibition of these three enzymes aimed not only to improve blood pressure control in patients with hypertension, particularly those with resistant hypertension, but also to reduce target organ damage through enhanced antiproliferative, anti-fibrotic and anti-inflammatory effects [59]. Although several dual or triple neprilysin and angiotensin-converting enzyme inhibitors (i.e. vasopeptidase inhibitors) were developed [60], only a few reached the clinical development stage because of side effects. Combined neprilysin and endothelin-converting enzyme inhibitors have clear synergistic profiles [61] which might be of great interest for de-stiffening arteries.

A second class of combined drugs are dual-acting angiotensin receptor neprilysin inhibitors [57]. LCZ696 (Novartis Pharmaceuticals), a first-in-class inhibitor of dual-acting angiotensin II type 1 receptor and neprilysin inhibitors [62]. Again, these compounds have great interest in terms of de-stiffening potential.

Despite the efficacy of antihypertensive drugs at reducing and controlling blood pressure, no intervention has been shown to normalize arterial stiffness [63, 64]. Multifactorial interventions might be needed [26] controlling for blood pressure, other risk factors (see Chap. 40) and improvement in lifestyle (see Chap. 43), in order to reverse and eventually normalize arterial stiffness. The effect of drugs not designed to lower blood pressure on arterial stiffness will be developed in Chap. 40. It remains that arterial stiffness as to prove its value as a true surrogate in clinical trials. The only evidence yet comes from one small study performed in patients with end-stage renal disease [64]. It was shown here that following the same protocol for reducing blood pressure yielded protection only in patients who showed an improvement in arterial stiffness, not in those who did not improve. This hypothesis is being tested on a larger scale in hypertensive subjects in the SPARTE trial [65], and we eagerly await the results which could potentially have a profound effect on medical practice.

References

1. Vlachopoulos C, Aznaouridis K, Stefanadis C. Prediction of cardiovascular events and all-cause mortality with arterial stiffness: a systematic review and meta-analysis. J Am Coll Cardiol. 2010;55:1318–27.
2. Ben-Shlomo Y, Spears M, Boustred C, May M, Anderson SG, Benjamin EJ, Boutouyrie P, Cameron J, Chen CH, Cruickshank JK, Hwang SJ, Lakatta EG, Laurent S, Maldonado J, Mitchell GF, Najjar SS, Newman AB, Ohishi M, Pannier B, Pereira T, Vasan RS, Shokawa T, Sutton-Tyrell K, Verbeke F, Wang KL, Webb DJ, Hansen TW, Zoungas S, McEniery CM, Cockcroft JR, Wilkinson IB. Aortic pulse wave velocity improves cardiovascular event prediction: an individual participant meta-analysis of prospective observational data from 17,635 subjects. J Am Coll Cardiol. 2014;63(7):636–46.
3. Boutouyrie P, Lacolley P, Briet M, Regnault V, Stanton A, Laurent S, Mahmud A. Pharmacological modulation of arterial stiffness. Drugs. 2011;71:1689–701.
4. Protogerou AD, Papaioannou TG, Lekakis JP, Blacher J, Safar ME. The effect of antihypertensive drugs on central blood pressure beyond peripheral blood pressure. Part i: (patho)-physiology, rationale and perspective on pulse pressure amplification. Curr Pharm Des. 2009;15:267–71.
5. Protogerou AD, Stergiou GS, Vlachopoulos C, Blacher J, Achimastos A. The effect of antihypertensive drugs on central blood pressure beyond peripheral blood pressure. Part ii: Evidence for specific class-effects of antihypertensive drugs on pressure amplification. Curr Pharm Des. 2009;15:272–89.
6. Galmiche G, Labat C, Mericskay M, Aissa KA, Blanc J, Retailleau K, Bourhim M, Coletti D, Loufrani L, Gao-Li J, Feil R, Challande P, Henrion D, Decaux JF, Regnault V, Lacolley P, Li Z. Inactivation of serum response factor contributes to decrease vascular muscular tone and arterial stiffness in mice. Circ Res. 2013;112:1035–45.
7. Boutouyrie P, Bussy C, Lacolley P, Girerd X, Laloux B, Laurent S. Association between local pulse pressure, mean blood pressure, and large-artery remodeling. Circulation. 1999;100:1387–93.
8. Boutouyrie P, Laurent S, Benetos A, Girerd XJ, Hoeks AP, Safar ME. Opposing effects of ageing on distal and proximal large arteries in hypertensives. J Hypertens Suppl. 1992;10:S87–91.
9. Laurent S, Cockcroft J, Van Bortel L, Boutouyrie P, Giannattasio C, Hayoz D, Pannier B, Vlachopoulos C, Wilkinson I, Struijker-Boudier H. Expert consensus document on arterial stiffness: methodological issues and clinical applications. Eur Heart J. 2006;27:2588–605.
10. Laurent S, Boutouyrie P, Lacolley P. Structural and genetic bases of arterial stiffness. Hypertension. 2005;45:1050–5.
11. Schiffrin EL. Circulatory therapeutics: use of antihypertensive agents and their effects on the vasculature. J Cell Mol Med. 2010;14:1018–29.
12. Boutouyrie P, Bussy C, Hayoz D, Hengstler J, Dartois N, Laloux B, Brunner H, Laurent S. Local pulse pressure and regression of arterial wall hypertrophy during long-term antihypertensive treatment. Circulation. 2000;101:2601–6.
13. Van Bortel LM, Kool MJ, Boudier HA, Struijker Boudier HA. Effects of antihypertensive agents on local arterial distensibility and compliance. Hypertension. 1995;26:531–4.
14. Shahin Y, Khan JA, Chetter I. Angiotensin converting enzyme inhibitors effect on arterial stiffness and wave reflections: a meta-analysis and meta-regression of randomised controlled trials. Atherosclerosis. 2012;221:18–33.
15. Benetos A, Gautier S, Lafleche A, Topouchian J, Frangin G, Girerd X, Sissmann J, Safar ME. Blockade of angiotensin ii type 1 receptors: effect on carotid and radial artery structure and function in hypertensive humans. J Vasc Res. 2000;37:8–15; discussion 68–70.
16. Davies J, Gavin A, Band M, Morris A, Struthers A. Spironolactone reduces brachial pulse wave velocity and piiinp levels in hypertensive diabetic patients. Br J Clin Pharmacol. 2005;59:520–3.
17. Benetos A, Vasmant D, Thiery P, Safar M. Effects of ramipril on arterial hemodynamics. J Cardiovasc Pharmacol. 1991;18 Suppl 2:S153–6.
18. Heesen WF, Beltman FW, Smit AJ, May JF, de Graeff PA, Muntinga JH, Havinga TK, Schuurman FH, van der Veur E, Meyboom-de Jong B, Lie KI. Reversal of pathophysiologic changes with long-term lisinopril treatment in isolated systolic hypertension. J Cardiovasc Pharmacol. 2001;37:512–21.
19. Mitchell GF, Dunlap ME, Warnica W, Ducharme A, Arnold JM, Tardif JC, Solomon SD, Domanski MJ, Jablonski KA, Rice MM, Pfeffer MA, Prevention of Events With Angiotensin-Converting Enzyme Inhibition I. Long-term trandolapril treatment is associated with reduced aortic stiffness: the prevention of events with angiotensin-converting enzyme inhibition hemodynamic substudy. Hypertension. 2007;49:1271–7.
20. O'Rourke MF, Safar ME, Dzau V. The cardiovascular continuum extended: aging effects on the aorta and microvasculature. Vasc Med. 2010;15:461–8.
21. Topouchian J, El Feghali R, Pannier B, Wang S, Zhao F, Smetana K, Teo K, Asmar R. Arterial stiffness and pharmacological interventions–the transcend arterial stiffness substudy (trans study). Vasc Health Risk Manag. 2007;3:381–7.

22. Boutouyrie P, Achouba A, Trunet P, Laurent S. Amlodipine-valsartan combination decreases central systolic blood pressure more effectively than the amlodipine-atenolol combination: the explor study. Hypertension. 2010;55:1314–22.
23. Paulis L, Becker ST, Lucht K, Schwengel K, Slavic S, Kaschina E, Thone-Reineke C, Dahlof B, Baulmann J, Unger T, Steckelings UM. Direct angiotensin ii type 2 receptor stimulation in nomega-nitro-l-arginine-methyl ester-induced hypertension: the effect on pulse wave velocity and aortic remodeling. Hypertension. 2012;59:485–92.
24. Virdis A, Ghiadoni L, Qasem AA, Lorenzini G, Duranti E, Cartoni G, Bruno RM, Bernini G, Taddei S. Effect of aliskiren treatment on endothelium-dependent vasodilation and aortic stiffness in essential hypertensive patients. Eur Heart J. 2012;33:1530–8.
25. Ong KT, Delerme S, Pannier B, Safar ME, Benetos A, Laurent S, Boutouyrie P. Aortic stiffness is reduced beyond blood pressure lowering by short-term and long-term antihypertensive treatment: a meta-analysis of individual data in 294 patients. J Hypertens. 2011;29(6):1034–42.
26. Ait-Oufella H, Collin C, Bozec E, Laloux B, Ong KT, Dufouil C, Boutouyrie P, Laurent S. Long-term reduction in aortic stiffness: a 5.3-year follow-up in routine clinical practice. J Hypertens. 2010;28:2336–41.
27. Asmar R. Effect of telmisartan on arterial distensibility and central blood pressure in patients with mild to moderate hypertension and type 2 diabetes mellitus. J Renin Angiotensin Aldosterone Syst. 2001;2 Suppl 2:S8–11.
28. Karalliedde J, Smith A, DeAngelis L, Mirenda V, Kandra A, Botha J, Ferber P, Viberti G. Valsartan improves arterial stiffness in type 2 diabetes independently of blood pressure lowering. Hypertension. 2008;51:1617–23.
29. Tropeano AI, Boutouyrie P, Pannier B, Joannides R, Balkestein E, Katsahian S, Laloux B, Thuillez C, Struijker-Boudier H, Laurent S. Brachial pressure-independent reduction in carotid stiffness after long-term angiotensin-converting enzyme inhibition in diabetic hypertensives. Hypertension. 2006;48:80–6.
30. Spoelstra-de Man AM, van Ittersum FJ, Schram MT, Kamp O, van Dijk RA, Ijzerman RG, Twisk JW, Brouwer CB, Stehouwer CD. Aggressive antihypertensive strategies based on hydrochlorothiazide, candesartan or lisinopril decrease left ventricular mass and improve arterial compliance in patients with type ii diabetes mellitus and hypertension. J Hum Hypertens. 2006;20:599–611.
31. Jensen-Urstad KJ, Reichard PG, Rosfors JS, Lindblad LE, Jensen-Urstad MT. Early atherosclerosis is retarded by improved long-term blood glucose control in patients with iddm. Diabetes. 1996;45:1253–8.
32. Williams B, Lacy PS, Thom SM, Cruickshank K, Stanton A, Collier D, Hughes AD, Thurston H, O'Rourke M. Differential impact of blood pressure-lowering drugs on central aortic pressure and clinical outcomes: principal results of the conduit artery function evaluation (cafe) study. Circulation. 2006;113:1213–25.
33. Matsui Y, Eguchi K, O'Rourke MF, Ishikawa J, Miyashita H, Shimada K, Kario K. Differential effects between a calcium channel blocker and a diuretic when used in combination with angiotensin ii receptor blocker on central aortic pressure in hypertensive patients. Hypertension. 2009;54:716–23.
34. Gates PE, Tanaka H, Hiatt WR, Seals DR. Dietary sodium restriction rapidly improves large elastic artery compliance in older adults with systolic hypertension. Hypertension. 2004;44:35–41.
35. Asmar RG, Benetos A, Chaouche-Teyara K, Raveau-Landon CM, Safar ME. Comparison of effects of felodipine versus hydrochlorothiazide on arterial diameter and pulse-wave velocity in essential hypertension. Am J Cardiol. 1993;72:794–8.
36. Benetos A, Lafleche A, Asmar R, Gautier S, Safar A, Safar ME. Arterial stiffness, hydrochlorothiazide and converting enzyme inhibition in essential hypertension. J Hum Hypertens. 1996;10:77–82.
37. Ishimitsu T, Numabe A, Masuda T, Akabane T, Okamura A, Minami J, Matsuoka H. Angiotensin-ii receptor antagonist combined with calcium channel blocker or diuretic for essential hypertension. Hypertens Res. 2009;32:962–8.
38. Kool MJ, Lustermans FA, Breed JG, Struyker Boudier HA, Hoeks AP, Reneman RS, Van Bortel LM. The influence of perindopril and the diuretic combination amiloride + hydrochlorothiazide on the vessel wall properties of large arteries in hypertensive patients. J Hypertens. 1995;13:839–48.
39. Mahmud A, Feely J. Effect of angiotensin ii receptor blockade on arterial stiffness: beyond blood pressure reduction. Am J Hypertens. 2002;15:1092–5.
40. Mahmud A, Feely J. Aldosterone-to-renin ratio, arterial stiffness, and the response to aldosterone antagonism in essential hypertension. Am J Hypertens. 2005;18:50–5.
41. Safar ME. Can antihypertensive treatment reverse large-artery stiffening? Curr Hypertens Rep. 2010;12:47–51.
42. Matsui Y, Eguchi K, O'Rourke MF, Ishikawa J, Shimada K, Kario K. Association between aldosterone induced by antihypertensive medication and arterial stiffness reduction: the j-core study. Atherosclerosis. 2011;215:184–8.
43. London GM, Asmar RG, O'Rourke MF, Safar ME. Mechanism(s) of selective systolic blood pressure reduction after a low-dose combination of perindopril/indapamide in hypertensive subjects: comparison with atenolol. J Am Coll Cardiol. 2004;43:92–9.
44. Protogerou A, Blacher J, Stergiou GS, Achimastos A, Safar ME. Blood pressure response under chronic antihypertensive drug therapy: the role of aortic stiffness in the reason (preterax in regression of arterial stiffness in a controlled double-blind) study. J Am Coll Cardiol. 2009;53:445–51.
45. Ong KT, Perdu J, De BJ, Bozec E, Collignon P, Emmerich J, Fauret al, Fiessinger JN, Germain DP, Georgesco G, Hulot JS, De PA, Plauchu H,

Jeunemaitre X, Laurent S, Boutouyrie P. Effect of celiprolol on prevention of cardiovascular events in vascular ehlers-danlos syndrome: a prospective randomised, open, blinded-endpoints trial. Lancet. 2010;376:1476–84.
46. Dhakam Z, Yasmin, McEniery CM, Burton T, Brown MJ, Wilkinson IB. A comparison of atenolol and nebivolol in isolated systolic hypertension. J Hypertens. 2008;26:351–6.
47. Mahmud A, Feely J. Beta-blockers reduce aortic stiffness in hypertension but nebivolol, not atenolol, reduces wave reflection. Am J Hypertens. 2008;21:663–7.
48. McEniery CM, Schmitt M, Qasem A, Webb DJ, Avolio AP, Wilkinson IB, Cockcroft JR. Nebivolol increases arterial distensibility in vivo. Hypertension. 2004;44:305–10.
49. Boutouyrie P, Beaussier H, Achouba A, Laurent S. Destiffening effect of valsartan and atenolol: influence of heart rate and blood pressure. J Hypertens. 2014;32(1):108–14.
50. Casey DP, Curry TB, Joyner MJ, Charkoudian N, Hart EC. Acute beta-adrenergic blockade increases aortic wave reflection in young men and women: differing mechanisms between sexes. Hypertension. 2012;59:145–50.
51. Casey DP, Curry TB, Charkoudian N, Joyner MJ, Hart EC. The effects of acute beta-adrenergic blockade on aortic wave reflection in postmenopausal women. Am J Hypertens. 2013;26:503–10.
52. Westling H, Jansson L, Jonson B, Nilsen R. Vasoactive drugs and elastic properties of human arteries in vivo, with special reference to the action of nitroglycerine. Eur Heart J. 1984;5:609–16.
53. Laurent S, Arcaro G, Benetos A, Lafleche A, Hoeks A, Safar M. Mechanism of nitrate-induced improvement on arterial compliance depends on vascular territory. J Cardiovasc Pharmacol. 1992;19:641–9.
54. Kool MJ, Spek JJ, Struyker Boudier HA, Hoeks AP, Reneman RS, van Herwaarden RH, Van Bortel LM. Acute and subacute effects of nicorandil and isosorbide dinitrate on vessel wall properties of large arteries and hemodynamics in healthy volunteers. Cardiovasc Drugs Ther. 1995;9:331–7.
55. Van Bortel LM, Spek JJ, Balkestein EJ, Sardina M, Struijker Boudier HA. Is it possible to develop drugs that act more selectively on large arteries? J Hypertens. 1999;17:701–5.
56. Fok H, Jiang B, Clapp B, Chowienczyk P. Regulation of vascular tone and pulse wave velocity in human muscular conduit arteries: selective effects of nitric oxide donors to dilate muscular arteries relative to resistance vessels. Hypertension. 2012;60:1220–5.
57. Laurent S, Schlaich M, Esler M. New drugs, procedures, and devices for hypertension. Lancet. 2012;380:591–600.
58. Corti R, Burnett Jr JC, Rouleau JL, Ruschitzka F, Luscher TF. Vasopeptidase inhibitors: a new therapeutic concept in cardiovascular disease? Circulation. 2001;104:1856–62.
59. Dive V, Chang CF, Yiotakis A, Sturrock ED. Inhibition of zinc metallopeptidases in cardiovascular disease–from unity to trinity, or duality? Curr Pharm Des. 2009;15:3606–21.
60. Daull P, Jeng AY, Battistini B. Towards triple vasopeptidase inhibitors for the treatment of cardiovascular diseases. J Cardiovasc Pharmacol. 2007;50:247–56.
61. Kalk P, Sharkovska Y, Kashina E, von Websky K, Relle K, Pfab T, Alter M, Guillaume P, Provost D, Hoffmann K, Fischer Y, Hocher B. Endothelin-converting enzyme/neutral endopeptidase inhibitor slv338 prevents hypertensive cardiac remodeling in a blood pressure-independent manner. Hypertension. 2011;57:755–63.
62. Gu J, Noe A, Chandra P, Al-Fayoumi S, Ligueros-Saylan M, Sarangapani R, Maahs S, Ksander G, Rigel DF, Jeng AY, Lin TH, Zheng W, Dole WP. Pharmacokinetics and pharmacodynamics of lcz696, a novel dual-acting angiotensin receptor-neprilysin inhibitor (arni). J Clin Pharmacol. 2010;50:401–14.
63. Arcaro G, Laurent S, Jondeau G, Hoeks AP, Safar ME. Stiffness of the common carotid artery in treated hypertensive patients. J Hypertens. 1991;9:947–54.
64. Guerin AP, Blacher J, Pannier B, Marchais SJ, Safar ME, London GM. Impact of aortic stiffness attenuation on survival of patients in end-stage renal failure. Circulation. 2001;103:987–92.
65. Laurent S, Briet M, Boutouyrie P. Arterial stiffness as surrogate end point: needed clinical trials. Hypertension. 2012;60:518–22.

40 Decreasing Arterial Stiffness and/or Wave Reflections Independently of Mean Arterial Pressure: Effect of Non-antihypertensive Drugs (Part 2)

Héléne Beaussier, Stéphane Laurent, and Pierre Boutouyrie

Abstract

Change in arterial stiffness with drugs is a major endpoint in clinical trials, although evidence for arterial stiffness as a therapeutic target still needs to be confirmed. Although antihypertensive drugs have been the most studied (as developed in Chap. 39), other drug classes have also been assessed, including hormone replacement therapy, lipid-lowering drugs, some antidiabetic agents, and anti-inflammatory drugs. For these drugs which do not directly affect blood pressure, the mechanism by necessity includes direct effect on the arterial wall and the extracellular matrix. We also present some recent evidence of completely different pathways such as interaction with the lamin A pathway which have demonstrated true "destiffening" properties.

Keywords

Antihypertensive drugs • Destiffening drugs • Arterial stiffness • Wave reflection • Lipid-lowering drugs • Antidiabetic drugs • Cross-link breakers

Arterial stiffness has emerged as an important marker of cardiovascular risk. More than 20 independent studies have shown that carotid to femoral pulse wave velocity (PWV) predicted cardiovascular outcome independently of major classical cardiovascular risk factors in different populations [1, 2] and can be modified by certain drug groups [3]. This simple, noninvasive measurement was recently included in official guidelines, and while reference values have been published, its implementation in clinical practice as a surrogate marker awaits evidence to suggest that this modification is associated with a better clinical outcome.

We have developed in the previous chapter the influence of antihypertensive drugs on arterial stiffness, which was the most obvious since passive decrease in blood pressure is accompanied by a decrease in arterial stiffness. However, for most antihypertensive classes, a

H. Beaussier
Clinical Research Unit and Pharmacy, Fondation Hôpital Saint Joseph, Paris, France

Hopital Europeen Georges Pompidou, Assistance Publique Hôpitaux de Paris, Université Paris Descartes, Paris, France

S. Laurent • P. Boutouyrie (✉)
Department of Pharmacology and Institut National de la Santé et de la Recherche Médicale U970(Eq7)-PARCC, Hôpital Européen Georges Pompidou, Assistance Publique-Hôpitaux de Paris, Université Paris-Descartes, 20, rue Leblanc, 75015 Paris, France
e-mail: stephane.laurent@egp.aphp.fr; pierre.boutouyrie@egp.aphp.fr

M.E. Safar et al. (eds.), *Blood Pressure and Arterial Wall Mechanics in Cardiovascular Diseases*,
DOI 10.1007/978-1-4471-5198-2_40, © Springer-Verlag London 2014

true, pressure-independent effect of drug treatment has been demonstrated, especially during long-term treatments. The objective of this chapter is to investigate whether non-antihypertensive drugs might influence arterial stiffness in different clinical situations and in a concluding part (common to the previous chapter and this), which are the different options in the future to develop new approaches directly targeted on the arterial wall. The modalities of data search were similar to Chap. 39, adding one of the following terms: "lipid-lowering drug," "antiplatelet drug," "antidiabetic drug," "nitric oxide donors," "hormone replacement therapy," or "drug treatment." We also searched www.clinicaltrials.gov to determine which clinical trials have been (or are currently) performed with novel molecules.

The Effect of Pharmacological Interventions Not Related to Blood Pressure on Arterial Stiffness in Humans

Lipid-Lowering Drugs

Statins are the most potent drug group to reduce LDL cholesterol, and these drugs have several effects beyond LDL cholesterol lowering which might improve arterial stiffness. The effect of statins may also be more important in the context of inflammation. Wicks et al. found that atorvastatin reduced aortic stiffness in patients with rheumatoid arthritis [4]. More recently, Wallace et al. showed that simvastatin reduced inflammation-induced aortic stiffening, through a lipid reduction mechanism [5]. Atorvastatin prevented the age-associated increase in aortic stiffness in patients with no dialyzed chronic kidney disease [6]. It has been recently shown that low-dose atorvastatin induced reductions in aortic PWV and showed significant associations with changes in AIx(75), central aortic systolic blood pressure, and PP in patients with mild hypertension and hypercholesterolemia [7]. Atorvastatin could also improve arterial stiffness by reducing oxidative stress levels in elderly hypertensive patients [8]. So did pravastatin in patients with mild to moderate CKD [9].

However, the role of statins in arterial stiffness remains controversial. Some studies have not shown important improvements in aortic hemodynamics [10]. Nevertheless, a few small randomized placebo-controlled studies, in different populations, have shown that statins decrease the inflammatory marker levels in addition to having favorable effects on aortic distensibility [11–13]. In addition, rosuvastatin has been shown to reduce 3-nitrotyrosine levels (a marker of peroxynitrite-mediated oxidative stress) and to decrease aortic PWV. Interestingly, reduction of plasma cholesterol was the only independent predictor of reduced arterial stiffness in patients with primary hypercholesterolemia after rosuvastatin therapy [14]. A systematic review of published trials was performed and identified 9 trials with 471 participants [15]. These trials were heterogeneous regarding the populations studied and techniques employed. When aortic PWV was studied, only 2 of 4 trials showed improvement with statins. When peripheral arterial stiffness was studied, 4 out of 5 trials were positive. This may reflect a publication bias or a true effect of statins, preferentially destiffening medium-size arteries than the aorta. The effect of statin treatment on the long term has never been studied.

Antidiabetic Drugs

Type 2 diabetes mellitus is associated with increased arterial stiffness [16]. The difference between diabetics and nondiabetic patients is 1.5–2 m/s for aortic PWV, which corresponds to over 20 years of age. The origin of increased arterial stiffness is multifactorial and includes co-segregation with other cardiovascular risk factors (including genetics), increased sympathetic tone, increased sensitivity to the renin-angiotensin system, and the effect of advanced glycation end products (AGE) [17]. These compounds result from the nonenzymatic glycation of proteins, especially collagen, establishing progressive cross-links between collagen fibers and stiffening the arterial wall.

Advanced glycation end products (AGE) correspond to nonenzymatic glycation of proteins and are associated with increased arterial stiffness in hypertension [18], but mostly in the presence of diabetes since AGE deposits are enhanced by chronic hyperglycemia, the deposits occur continuously, earlier if diabetes is not well controlled [19]. Drugs reversing AGE deposits are good candidate as destiffening drugs. Alpha-amino guanidine, a first-line compound breaking AGE deposit, has been shown to reduce myocardial and arterial stiffness [20] (see [19] for review). One compound, thiazolium derivative alagebrium (Synvista Therapeutics, ALT 711) which breaks collagen cross-links, has been extensively studied in phase I and II studies showing good safety and tolerability profile [21]. In hypertensive diabetics, aortic stiffness and endothelial function were improved independently of any change in blood pressure [22, 23].

Drugs targeting glycemic control have also been shown to improve arterial stiffness. Although metformin has been shown to reduce arterial stiffness [24], the most studied class is glitazones. Several papers have shown that these compounds could decrease aortic stiffness [25] (together with intima media thickness), better than other drugs, and that this effect could be proportional to the increase in adiponectin in diabetics [26] and hypertensives [27]. Because of the safety profile of this class of antidiabetic drugs, this favorable effect on arterial stiffness did not translate into clinical benefit. A recent study demonstrated that sitagliptin, a novel antidiabetic class, but not glibenclamide, showed a significant beneficial effect on BMI and triglyceride levels. However, arterial stiffness, blood pressure, oxidative stress, and inflammatory status were not significantly affected by adding sitagliptin or glibenclamide to metformin-treated type 2 diabetes patients [28]. The new class of sodium glucose transport inhibitors (such as dapagliflozin) have a high probability of inducing changes in arterial stiffness because by increasing elimination of glucose in the urine, they also induce sodium excretion and mild decrease in blood pressure [29]. This class of drug might then cumulate the beneficial effects of glucose reduction and blood pressure reduction.

Anti-inflammatory Drugs

Chronic inflammation is associated with increased arterial stiffness, either severe inflammation such as seen in rheumatoid arthritis (RA) [30, 31] or chronic low-grade inflammation as seen in patients with inflammatory bowel disease [32] or advanced forms of atherosclerosis. Anti-inflammatory drugs have a potential to improve arterial stiffness [33]. Several drugs have been tested, but up to now, only antibodies against TNF-alpha have been shown to improve arterial stiffness, independently of any change in blood pressure, in patients with different chronic inflammation diseases [34, 35]. Maki-Petaja et al. also demonstrated recently that antitumor necrosis factor-alpha therapy reduces aortic inflammation in patients with RA, and this effect correlates with the decrease in aortic stiffness (from 9.09+/−1.77 to 8.63+/−1.42 m/s, $P=0.04$). These results suggested that RA patients exhibit a subclinical vasculitis, which provides a mechanism for the increased cardiovascular disease risk seen in RA [36]. However, not all trials were positive [37, 38]. Nonsteroidal anti-inflammatory drugs have not been tested in arterial stiffness. As mentioned above, statins exhibit destiffening properties only in the presence of inflammation [4, 5, 15].

Hormone Replacement Therapy (HRT)

Women are thought to be protected against cardiovascular diseases by their hormonal status during their reproductive years. This view led to several trials of HRT with arterial stiffness as outcome. Since the seminal observation of decreased arterial stiffness in patients with HRT [39], more than 80 papers were produced (Medline search). Thirteen publications concerned randomized controlled trials (see [3] for full references). Out of these publications, 7 were negative. Among positive trials (showing improvement), one concerned raloxifene, a potent selective estrogen receptor modulator (SERM), one studied small cerebral arteries, and two studied hormone replacement therapy on arteries with MRI. Negative results were observed with all modalities of HRT: estrogen alone, combination, oral, or transdermal. The effect of estrogens might be modulated by the endothelium since Moreau et al. recently studied the effect of tetrahydrobiopterin (BH(4)), a critical cofactor for endothelial nitric oxide synthase to produce nitric oxide that improved endothelial function and arterial stiffness in estrogen-deficient postmenopausal women, not in premenopausal females [40].

Antiplatelet Drugs

This aspect will be developed elsewhere (Chap. 32). Although platelets have the potential to modify vascular tone after aggregation and several reports have shown relations between aggregation and arterial stiffness [41], classical drugs such as aspirin or clopidogrel have not shown substantial effects on the arterial wall properties. The only evidence for action of aspirin has been observed in an acute inflammation study, for preventing inflammation-associated increase in aortic stiffness [42].

Pharmacological Perspectives

It is known that chronic obstructive pulmonary disease (COPD) is associated with increased arterial stiffness which may in part explain the cardiovascular morbidity observed in the disease. Prior studies suggest that fluticasone propionate/salmeterol may improve cardiovascular outcomes in COPD, and a recent study showed that fluticasone propionate/salmeterol does not reduce aPWV in all patients with moderate to severe COPD, but may have effects in those with elevated arterial stiffness. But additional studies are required to determine if aPWV could serve as a surrogate for cardiovascular events in COPD [43].

Large artery structure and function are significantly impaired in renal transplant recipient (RTR) which contributes to their high cardiovascular morbidity (see Chap. 26) and could be altered by erythropoietin. However, Bartels et al. compared effects of erythropoiesis-stimulating agents' therapy on large artery stiffness and endothelial function in RTR with chronic allograft dysfunction and renal anemia randomized to a group receiving darbepoetin alfa and a control group. They showed that therapy with darbepoetin alfa during 8 months did not significantly impact parameters of large artery stiffness and endothelial function in RTR. These data suggest that therapy with erythropoietin does not deteriorate arterial stiffness and endothelial function in RTR [44].

Future Issues

We have not yet identified a novel molecular determinant or a new signaling pathway mainly because arterial stiffness is a multifactorial phenotype. In the quest for new biological pathways contributing to arterial stiffness, genes identified by genome-wide association using powerful SNP technology should bring new impetus to treatment hypothesis generating [45].

Numerous papers have shown that selected alimentary compound can improve arterial stiffness (see Chap. 43). Recently, dietary nitrate that elevated nitrite levels approximately 1.5-fold caused substantial reductions in systolic (approximately 12 mmHg) and diastolic blood pressures and PWV which might support the concept of dietary nitrate supplementation as an effective, but simple and inexpensive, antihypertensive strategy [46]. It is unclear whether these alimentary compounds might have synergistic or additive effects among themselves and/or in combination with drugs and whether they confer protection against cardiovascular disease. Several recent published papers showed positive results (see review by Kingwell in Chap. 43). It should be possible to target the arterial wall and the turnover of extracellular matrix in the future for pharmacological intervention. Many pathways are only identified as determinants of early vascular aging or aging pathways [47]. Drugs could be designed to reduce arterial stiffness or accelerated stiffening with time. For instance, the farnesyl transferase pathway, implied in the severe genetic disease Hutchinson-Gilford progeria, and farnesyl transferase inhibitors have been shown to reduce arterial stiffness (Fig. 40.1) in this rare disease [48, 49]. The telomere length and the potential use of telomerase inhibitors [50] are also promising (see Chap. 8). What is more probable is that arterial stiffness will constitute a new target for already available drugs during multifactorial intervention trials, aiming at correcting target organ damage, in the present case large artery stiffness. Whether destiffening drugs have purely positive effects is pure speculation. Indeed, threads are also expected. Stiffness is also important for resistance of vessels to rupture (although brittleness may have different determinants from

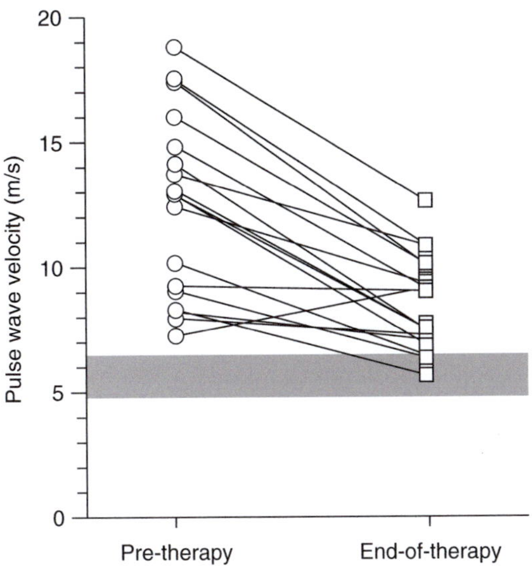

Fig. 40.1 Effect of 24-month course of lonafarnib, a farnesyl transferase inhibitor on carotid to femoral pulse wave velocity in patients with Hutchinson-Gilford progeria syndrome (Reproduced with permission of Ref. [49])

stiffness), and inappropriate arterial distensibility may lead to propensity for dilatation and rupture. Plaque stability could also be compromised by reduction of fibrosis at the level of vulnerable plaques. This may explain the unexpected results of the ROADMAP trial [51] where a potent antifibrotic compound, olmesartan, increased cardiovascular mortality despite a positive effect on albuminuria. On the contrary, we recently showed in patients with vascular Ehlers-Danlos syndrome, a condition associated with cutaneous and arterial fragility, that celiprolol, a beta1 antagonist with beta2 partial agonist properties, conferred an important protection against arterial dissection and rupture together with increased arterial stiffness [52], suggesting that stiffer arteries were also more resistant (Fig. 40.2). There are also concerns about aging pathway inhibition and promotion of cancer. All these points must be considered in the development of destiffening drugs.

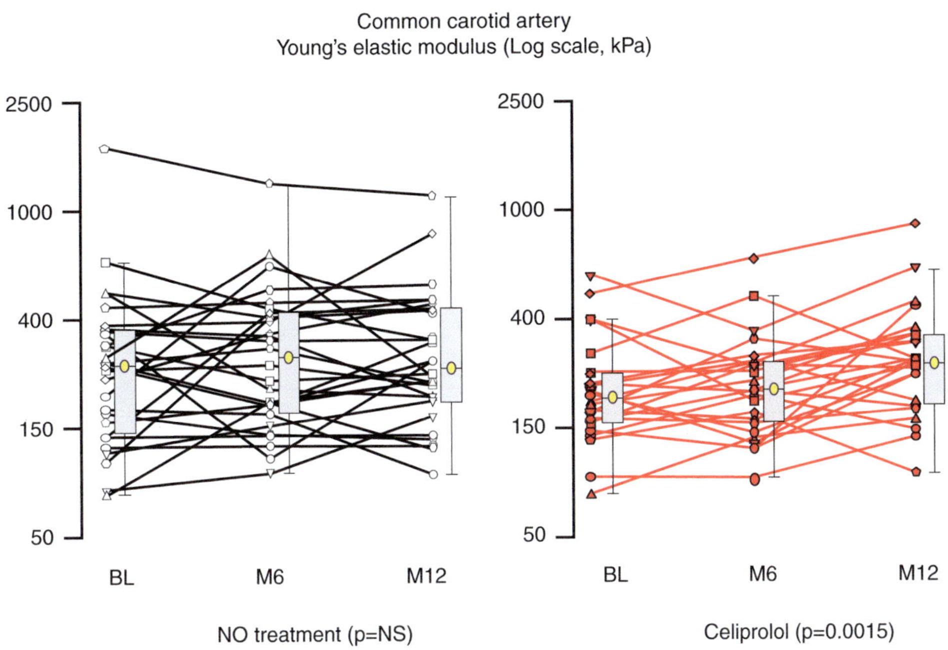

Fig. 40.2 Annual rate of change in carotid stiffness following celiprolol treatment in patients with vascular Ehlers-Danlos syndrome (Adapted from Ref. [52]). Data are represented between baseline, months 6 and 12, because of significant crossing over to treatment in the untreated group. Young's elastic modulus is log transformed. *Boxes and whiskers* represent the median (*dot*), 25th and 75th percentile (*box*), and adjacent values (*whiskers*, median-1.5*IRQ and median+1.5*IRQ). Points falling out of the whiskers are outliers

References

1. Vlachopoulos C, Aznaouridis K, Stefanadis C. Prediction of cardiovascular events and all-cause mortality with arterial stiffness: a systematic review and meta-analysis. J Am Coll Cardiol. 2010;55:1318–27.
2. Ben-Shlomo Y, Spears M, Boustred C, May M, Anderson SG, Benjamin EJ, Boutouyrie P, Cameron J, Chen CH, Cruickshank JK, Hwang SJ, Lakatta EG, Laurent S, Maldonado J, Mitchell GF, Najjar SS, Newman AB, Ohishi M, Pannier B, Pereira T, Vasan RS, Shokawa T, Sutton-Tyrell K, Verbeke F, Wang KL, Webb DJ, Hansen TW, Zoungas S, McEniery CM, Cockcroft JR, Wilkinson IB. Aortic pulse wave velocity improves cardiovascular event prediction: an individual participant meta-analysis of prospective observational data from 17,635 subjects. J Am Coll Cardiol. 2014;63(7):636–46.
3. Boutouyrie P, Lacolley P, Briet M, Regnault V, Stanton A, Laurent S, Mahmud A. Pharmacological modulation of arterial stiffness. Drugs. 2011;71: 1689–701.
4. Van DS, McColl G, Wicks IP. Atorvastatin reduces arterial stiffness in patients with rheumatoid arthritis. Ann Rheum Dis. 2004;63:1571–5.
5. Wallace SM, Maki-Petaja KM, Cheriyan J, Davidson EH, Cherry L, McEniery CM, Sattar N, Wilkinson IB, Kharbanda RK. Simvastatin prevents inflammation-induced aortic stiffening and endothelial dysfunction. Br J Clin Pharmacol. 2010;70:799–806.
6. Fassett RG, Robertson IK, Ball MJ, Geraghty DP, Sharman JE, Coombes JS. Effects of atorvastatin on arterial stiffness in chronic kidney disease: a randomised controlled trial. J Atheroscler Thromb. 2010;17:235–41.
7. Kanaki AI, Sarafidis PA, Georgianos PI, Kanavos K, Tziolas IM, Zebekakis PE, Lasaridis AN. Effects of low-dose atorvastatin on arterial stiffness and central aortic pressure augmentation in patients with hypertension and hypercholesterolemia. Am J Hypertens. 2013;26:608–16.
8. Wang J, Xu J, Zhou C, Zhang Y, Xu D, Guo Y, Yang Z. Improvement of arterial stiffness by reducing oxidative stress damage in elderly hypertensive patients after 6 months of atorvastatin therapy. J Clin Hypertens. 2012;14:245–9.
9. Veringa SJ, Nanayakkara PW, van Ittersum FJ, Vegting IL, van Guldener C, Smulders YM, ter Wee PM, Stehouwer CD. Effect of a treatment strategy consisting of pravastatin, vitamin e, and homocysteine lowering on arterial compliance and distensibility in patients with mild-to-moderate chronic kidney disease. Clin Nephrol. 2012;78:263–72.
10. Williams B, Lacy PS, Cruickshank JK, Collier D, Hughes AD, Stanton A, Thom S, Thurston H, Cafe, Investigators A. Impact of statin therapy on central aortic pressures and hemodynamics: principal results of the conduit artery function evaluation-lipid-lowering arm (cafe-lla) study. Circulation. 2009;119:53–61.
11. Shige H, Dart A, Nestel P. Simvastatin improves arterial compliance in the lower limb but not in the aorta. Atherosclerosis. 2001;155:245–50.
12. Kontopoulos AG, Athyros VG, Pehlivanidis AN, Demitriadis DS, Papageorgiou AA, Boudoulas H. Long-term treatment effect of atorvastatin on aortic stiffness in hypercholesterolaemic patients. Curr Med Res Opin. 2003;19:22–7.
13. Ichihara A, Hayashi M, Ryuzaki M, Handa M, Furukawa T, Saruta T. Fluvastatin prevents development of arterial stiffness in haemodialysis patients with type 2 diabetes mellitus. Nephrol Dial Transplant. 2002;17:1513–7.
14. Pirro M, Schillaci G, Mannarino MR, Savarese G, Vaudo G, Siepi D, Paltriccia R, Mannarino E. Effects of rosuvastatin on 3-nitrotyrosine and aortic stiffness in hypercholesterolemia. Nutr Metab Cardiovasc Dis. 2007;17:436–41.
15. Rizos EC, Agouridis AP, Elisaf MS. The effect of statin therapy on arterial stiffness by measuring pulse wave velocity: a systematic review. Curr Vasc Pharmacol. 2010;8:638–44.
16. Kool MJ, Lambert J, Stehouwer CD, Hoeks AP, Struijker Boudier HA, Van Bortel LM. Vessel wall properties of large arteries in uncomplicated iddm. Diabetes Care. 1995;18:618–24.
17. Stehouwer CD, Henry RM, Ferreira I. Arterial stiffness in diabetes and the metabolic syndrome: a pathway to cardiovascular disease. Diabetologia. 2008;51:527–39.
18. McNulty M, Mahmud A, Feely J. Advanced glycation end-products and arterial stiffness in hypertension. Am J Hypertens. 2007;20:242–7.
19. Aronson D. Cross-linking of glycated collagen in the pathogenesis of arterial and myocardial stiffening of aging and diabetes. J Hypertens. 2003;21:3–12.
20. Wolffenbuttel BH, Boulanger CM, Crijns FR, Huijberts MS, Poitevin P, Swennen GN, Vasan S, Egan JJ, Ulrich P, Cerami A, Levy BI. Breakers of advanced glycation end products restore large artery properties in experimental diabetes. Proc Natl Acad Sci U S A. 1998;95:4630–4.
21. Susic D, Varagic J, Ahn J, Frohlich ED. Crosslink breakers: a new approach to cardiovascular therapy. Curr Opin Cardiol. 2004;19:336–40.
22. Kass DA, Shapiro EP, Kawaguchi M, Capriotti AR, Scuteri A, deGroof RC, Lakatta EG. Improved arterial compliance by a novel advanced glycation end-product crosslink breaker. Circulation. 2001;104:1464–70.
23. Zieman SJ, Melenovsky V, Clattenburg L, Corretti MC, Capriotti A, Gerstenblith G, Kass DA. Advanced glycation endproduct crosslink breaker (alagebrium) improves endothelial function in patients with isolated systolic hypertension. J Hypertens. 2007;25:577–83.
24. Agarwal N, Rice SP, Bolusani H, Luzio SD, Dunseath G, Ludgate M, Rees DA. Metformin reduces arterial stiffness and improves endothelial function in young women with polycystic ovary syndrome: a randomized, placebo-controlled, crossover trial. J Clin Endocrinol Metab. 2010;95:722–30.

25. Yu J, Jin N, Wang G, Zhang F, Mao J, Wang X. Peroxisome proliferator-activated receptor gamma agonist improves arterial stiffness in patients with type 2 diabetes mellitus and coronary artery disease. Metabolism. 2007;56:1396–401.
26. Nakamura T, Matsuda T, Kawagoe Y, Ogawa H, Takahashi Y, Sekizuka K, Koide H. Effect of pioglitazone on carotid intima-media thickness and arterial stiffness in type 2 diabetic nephropathy patients. Metabolism. 2004;53:1382–6.
27. Mahmud A, Feely J. Adiponectin and arterial stiffness. Am J Hypertens. 2005;18:1543–8.
28. Koren S, Shemesh-Bar L, Tirosh A, Peleg RK, Berman S, Hamad RA, Vinker S, Golik A, Efrati S. The effect of sitagliptin versus glibenclamide on arterial stiffness, blood pressure, lipids, and inflammation in type 2 diabetes mellitus patients. Diabetes Technol Ther. 2012;14:561–7.
29. Vasilakou D, Karagiannis T, Athanasiadou E, Mainou M, Liakos A, Bekiari E, Sarigianni M, Matthews DR, Tsapas A. Sodium-glucose cotransporter 2 inhibitors for type 2 diabetes: a systematic review and meta-analysis. Ann Intern Med. 2013;159:262–74.
30. Amar J, Ruidavets JB, Sollier CB, Bongard V, Boccalon H, Chamontin B, Drouet L, Ferrieres J. Relationship between c reactive protein and pulse pressure is not mediated by atherosclerosis or aortic stiffness. J Hypertens. 2004;22:349–55.
31. Maki-Petaja KM, Hall FC, Booth AD, Wallace SM, Yasmin, Bearcroft PW, Harish S, Furlong A, McEniery CM, Brown J, Wilkinson IB. Rheumatoid arthritis is associated with increased aortic pulse-wave velocity, which is reduced by anti-tumor necrosis factor-alpha therapy. Circulation. 2006;114:1185–92.
32. Zanoli L, Cannavo M, Rastelli S, Di Pino L, Monte I, Di Gangi M, Boutouyrie P, Inserra G, Laurent S, Castellino P. Arterial stiffness is increased in patients with inflammatory bowel disease. J Hypertens. 2012;30:1775–81.
33. Maki-Petaja KM, Wilkinson IB. Anti-inflammatory drugs and statins for arterial stiffness reduction. Curr Pharm Des. 2009;15:290–303.
34. Wong M, Oakley SP, Young L, Jiang BY, Wierzbicki A, Panayi G, Chowienczyk P, Kirkham B. Infliximab improves vascular stiffness in patients with rheumatoid arthritis. Ann Rheum Dis. 2009;68:1277–84.
35. Angel K, Provan SA, Gulseth HL, Mowinckel P, Kvien TK, Atar D. Tumor necrosis factor-alpha antagonists improve aortic stiffness in patients with inflammatory arthropathies: a controlled study. Hypertension. 2010;55:333–8.
36. Maki-Petaja KM, Elkhawad M, Cheriyan J, Joshi FR, Ostor AJ, Hall FC, Rudd JH, Wilkinson IB. Anti-tumor necrosis factor-alpha therapy reduces aortic inflammation and stiffness in patients with rheumatoid arthritis. Circulation. 2012;126:2473–80.
37. Van DS, McColl G, Wicks IP. Tumour necrosis factor antagonists improve disease activity but not arterial stiffness in rheumatoid arthritis. Rheumatology (Oxford). 2005;44:1428–32.
38. Capkin E, Karkucak M, Kiris A, Durmus I, Karaman K, Karaca A, Tosun M, Ayar A. Anti-tnf-alpha therapy may not improve arterial stiffness in patients with as: a 24-week follow-up. Rheumatology. 2012;51:910–4.
39. Rajkumar C, Kingwell BA, Cameron JD, Waddell T, Mehra R, Christophidis N, Komesaroff PA, McGrath B, Jennings GL, Sudhir K, Dart AM. Hormonal therapy increases arterial compliance in postmenopausal women. J Am Coll Cardiol. 1997;30:350–6.
40. Moreau KL, Meditz A, Deane KD, Kohrt WM. Tetrahydrobiopterin improves endothelial function and decreases arterial stiffness in estrogen-deficient postmenopausal women. Am J Physiol Heart Circ Physiol. 2012;302:H1211–8.
41. Wilkinson IB, Megson IL, MacCallum H, Sogo N, Cockcroft JR, Webb DJ. Oral vitamin c reduces arterial stiffness and platelet aggregation in humans. J Cardiovasc Pharmacol. 1999;34:690–3.
42. Vlachopoulos C, Dima I, Aznaouridis K, Vasiliadou C, Ioakeimidis N, Aggeli C, Toutouza M, Stefanadis C. Acute systemic inflammation increases arterial stiffness and decreases wave reflections in healthy individuals. Circulation. 2005;112:2193–200.
43. Dransfield MT, Cockcroft JR, Townsend RR, Coxson HO, Sharma SS, Rubin DB, Emmett AH, Cicale MJ, Crater GD, Martinez FJ. Effect of fluticasone propionate/salmeterol on arterial stiffness in patients with copd. Respir Med. 2011;105:1322–30.
44. Bartels V, Hillebrand U, Kosch M, Hausberg M, Kisters K, Di Marco GS, Reiermann S, Pavenstaedt H, Lang D. Influence of erythropoietin on arterial stiffness and endothelial function in renal transplant recipients. Am J Nephrol. 2012;36:355–61.
45. Mitchell GF, Verwoert GC, Tarasov KV, Isaacs A, Smith AV, Yasmin, Rietzschel ER, Tanaka T, Liu Y, Parsa A, Najjar SS, O'Shaughnessy KM, Sigurdsson S, De Buyzere ML, Larson MG, Sie MP, Andrews JS, Post WS, Mattace-Raso FU, McEniery CM, Eiriksdottir G, Segers P, Vasan RS, van Rijn MJ, Howard TD, McArdle PF, Dehghan A, Jewell ES, Newhouse SJ, Bekaert S, Hamburg NM, Newman AB, Hofman A, Scuteri A, De Bacquer D, Ikram MA, Psaty BM, Fuchsberger C, Olden M, Wain LV, Elliott P, Smith NL, Felix JF, Erdmann J, Vita JA, Sutton-Tyrrell K, Sijbrands EJ, Sanna S, Launer LJ, De Meyer T, Johnson AD, Schut AF, Herrington DM, Rivadeneira F, Uda M, Wilkinson IB, Aspelund T, Gillebert TC, Van Bortel L, Benjamin EJ, Oostra BA, Ding J, Gibson Q, Uitterlinden AG, Abecasis GR, Cockcroft JR, Gudnason V, De Backer GG, Ferrucci L, Harris TB, Shuldiner AR, van Duijn CM, Levy D, Lakatta EG, Witteman JC. Common genetic variation in the 3′-bcl11b gene desert is associated with carotid-femoral pulse wave velocity and excess cardiovascular disease risk: the aortagen consortium. Circ Cardiovasc Genet. 2012;5:81–90.

46. Ghosh SM, Kapil V, Fuentes-Calvo I, Bubb KJ, Pearl V, Milsom AB, Khambata R, Maleki-Toyserkani S, Yousuf M, Benjamin N, Webb AJ, Caulfield MJ, Hobbs AJ, Ahluwalia A. Enhanced vasodilator activity of nitrite in hypertension: critical role for erythrocytic xanthine oxidoreductase and translational potential. Hypertension. 2013;61:1091–102.
47. Nilsson PM, Boutouyrie P, Laurent S. Vascular aging: a tale of eva and adam in cardiovascular risk assessment and prevention. Hypertension. 2009;54:3–10.
48. Gerhard-Herman M, Smoot LB, Wake N, Kieran MW, Kleinman ME, Miller DT, Schwartzman A, Giobbie-Hurder A, Neuberg D, Gordon LB. Mechanisms of premature vascular aging in children with hutchinson-gilford progeria syndrome. Hypertension. 2011; 59:92–7.
49. Gordon LB, Kleinman ME, Miller DT, Neuberg DS, Giobbie-Hurder A, Gerhard-Herman M, Smoot LB, Gordon CM, Cleveland R, Snyder BD, Fligor B, Bishop WR, Statkevich P, Regen A, Sonis A, Riley S, Ploski C, Correia A, Quinn N, Ullrich NJ, Nazarian A, Liang MG, Huh SY, Schwartzman A, Kieran MW. Clinical trial of a farnesyltransferase inhibitor in children with hutchinson-gilford progeria syndrome. Proc Natl Acad Sci U S A. 2012;109:16666–71.
50. Nawrot TS, Staessen JA, Holvoet P, Struijker-Boudier HA, Schiffers P, Van Bortel LM, Fagard RH, Gardner JP, Kimura M, Aviv A. Telomere length and its associations with oxidized-ldl, carotid artery distensibility and smoking. Front Biosci (Elite Ed). 2010;2: 1164–8.
51. Haller H, Ito S, Izzo Jr JL, Januszewicz A, Katayama S, Menne J, Mimran A, Rabelink TJ, Ritz E, Ruilope LM, Rump LC, Viberti G. Olmesartan for the delay or prevention of microalbuminuria in type 2 diabetes. N Engl J Med. 2011;364:907–17.
52. Ong KT, Perdu J, De BJ, Bozec E, Collignon P, Emmerich J, Fauret al, Fiessinger JN, Germain DP, Georgesco G, Hulot JS, De PA, Plauchu H, Jeunemaitre X, Laurent S, Boutouyrie P. Effect of celiprolol on prevention of cardiovascular events in vascular ehlers-danlos syndrome: a prospective randomised, open, blinded-endpoints trial. Lancet. 2010;376:1476–84.

41 Blood Pressure Variability: Measurements, Influential Factors, Prognosis and Therapy

Yi Zhang, Davide Agnoletti, Alexandra Yannoutsos, Michel E. Safar, and Jacques Blacher

Abstract

It was reported that, in addition to blood pressure (BP) level, BP variability could also provide prognostic value of target organ damage, cardiovascular and all-cause mortality. Therefore, evaluation of patients' BP variability could potentially offer guiding information on their clinical therapy. BP variability could be assessed by calculating standard deviation, coefficient of variation and other parameters of BP readings from 24-h ambulatory BP monitor, known as short-term BP variability. More recently, an emerging BP variability can be derived from regular home and office BP recordings for 1 week or several months, known as long-term BP variability. Although the cause and meaning of fluctuated BP was not well elucidated, several factors, including age, mean BP, heart rate variability and arterial stiffness, may influence patients' BP variability. Most clinical investigations indicated a significant prognostic value of either short- or long-term BP variability, with regards to target organ damage, cardiovascular events and mortality, but controversy exists in this field, especially its incremental prognostic value in addition to BP level. Till now, there is no solid evidence indicating any effective agent in terms of BP variability reduction, but some clinical studies favor CCB in reducing both short- and long-term BP variability. Further studies are warranted to investigate the standardized evaluation of patients' BP variation, its cause and added prognostic significance, as well as effective treatment.

Y. Zhang, MD, PhD
Department of Cardiology, Shanghai Tenth People's Hospital, Tongji University School of Medicine, Middle Yanchang Road 301, Shanghai 200072, China
e-mail: yizshcn@gmail.com

D. Agnoletti, MD, PhD • A. Yannoutsos, MD
Diagnosis and Therapeutic Center, Hôtel-Dieu Hospital, Assistance Publique des Hôpitaux de Paris, Paris Descartes University, 1, Place du Parvis Notre-Dame, 75181 Paris, France
e-mail: davide_agnoletti@hotmail.com; alexyanne2504@yahoo.fr

M.E. Safar, MD • J. Blacher, MD, PhD (✉)
Department of Medicine, Diagnosis and Therapeutic Center, Hôtel-Dieu Hospital, Assistance Publique des Hôpitaux de Paris, Paris Descartes University, 1, Place du Parvis Notre-Dame, 75181 Paris, France
e-mail: michel.safar@htd.apjp.fr; jacques.blacher@htd.aphp.fr

M.E. Safar et al. (eds.), *Blood Pressure and Arterial Wall Mechanics in Cardiovascular Diseases*, DOI 10.1007/978-1-4471-5198-2_41,

Keywords

Blood pressure variability • Visit-to-visit blood pressure variability • 24-h ambulatory blood pressure monitor • Cardiovascular events • Mortality • Antihypertensive treatment

Ambulatory blood pressure (BP) was proved to be superior to conventional BP in predicting CV events and mortality by solid evidence [1, 2], but some clinical investigations indicated that, independent of BP level, BP variability also provided significant but modest prognostic information. Short-term BP variability derived from 24-hour (24 h) ambulatory BP monitor (ABPM) has previously dominated in this field, but since 2010, as Rothwell et al. proposed a long-term BP variability based on regular office BP measurements, the novel visit-to-visit BP variability was extensively investigated. This chapter summarizes current knowledge on both short- and long-term BP variability, involving its methodology, influential factors, prognostic significance and therapy.

Methodology of Blood Pressure Variability Measurement

From a practical point of view, BP variability can be derived from either 24 h ABPM or regular BP measurement in clinic or at home. There are also many different methods and formula for the calculation of patients' BP variability. In this section, we would like to only focus on several classical methodologies in this field.

Calculation of BP Variability by 24-h ABPM

Intra-individual Standard Deviation and Coefficient of Variation

The most simple assessment of patient' BP variability is to calculate the standard deviation (SD) and coefficient of variation of all the valid readings from the 24 h ABPM [3], as following formulas. Amount of BP readings actually depends on the defined time intervals between measurements. For instance, 96 readings would be available with a 15-min interval throughout the whole day, but 48 readings with a 30-min setting.

$$\mathrm{SD} = \sqrt{\sum_{k=1}^{n}\left(BP_k - \overline{BP}\right)^2 / (n-1)}$$

$$\mathrm{CV} = SD / \overline{BP}$$

where k ranges from 1 to n, BP_k is one BP measurement, $\overline{BP}$ is mean BP, and n is the number of BP readings in 24 h.

Time-Weighted Intra-individual Standard Deviation

In routine clinical practice of 24 h ABPM, measurement setting was sometimes defined with an interval of 15–30-min in the daytime and of 30–60-min in the nighttime. Furthermore, not each measurement could be correctly recorded, and measurement errors occurred. In this case, sometimes devices would retry to record BP 5-min later, and if fail again, there would be a missing value at this recording time. From a statistical point of view, with different measurement intervals in a 24 h recording, each BP reading did not contribute evenly to the mean BP, so time need to be weighted. A formula is available to calculate the time-weighted SD of BP as follows.

$$\text{Time}-\text{weighted SD} = \sqrt{\sum_{k=1}^{n}\left[w_k \times \left(BP_k - \overline{BP}\right)^2\right] / (n-1) / \sum_{k=1}^{n} w_k}$$

where w is the corresponding time interval.

Time-Weighted Intra-individual Standard Deviation in Daytime, Nighttime and 24-h

To avoid the contribution of nocturnal BP dipping in physiological condition, daytime and

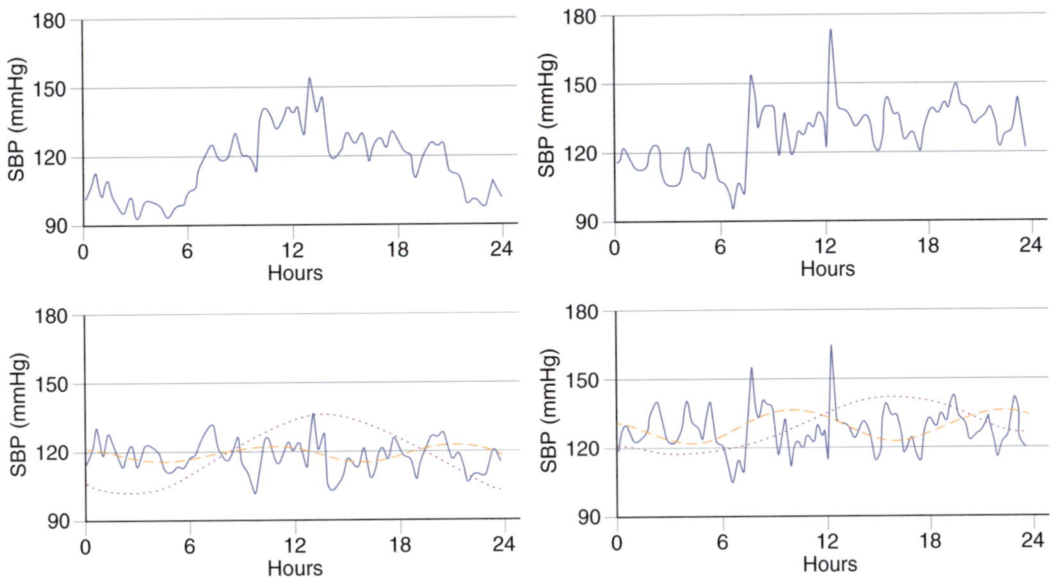

Fig. 41.1 The *top panels* show 24-h SBP tracing, whereas the *bottom panels* show the first component (*dotted lines*), second cyclic (*dashed lines*), and residual SBP variability (*continuous lines*) as derived from Fourier analysis. Data were from two different subjects (Adapted from Mancia et al. [6], with permission)

nighttime are normally defined as from 6:00 to 22:00 and from 22:00 to next 6:00, respectively, or defined by the reported time awake and asleep [4], and time-weighted intra-individual SD is calculated by the above-mentioned formula in daytime and nighttime, separately. 24-h BP variability is then calculated by the following formula.

$$24-\text{h SD} = (DaytimeSD \times AT) + (NighttimeSD \times ST)/(AT + ST)$$

where AT and ST stand for awake and sleeping time in hours.

Individual Residual Variability by the Fourier Spectral Analysis

Since BP variability can be largely (over 95 %) attributed to two cyclic components, namely circadian rhythm and diet-related effect, the fast Fourier transform spectral analysis was applied to identify and then rule out these cyclic components, in order to obtain patients' residual BP variability [5, 6]. There are three steps for this process. Firstly, individual BP readings were averaged to obtain the circadian BP profile of a group as a whole, and the Fourier spectral analysis was applied to identify the cyclic components that accounted for most of BP variations. Secondly, the two above-mentioned cyclic components were tested to fit the circadian BP profile in each subject. Lastly, individual residual BP variability, as variability unexplained by the cyclic components, was identified by calculating the sum squared of the difference between the observed and the fitted profile of BP in each subject. Figure 41.1 shows two examples of patients' residual BP variability by the Fourier spectral analysis.

Reading-to-Reading BP Variability

In order to better elucidate patients' reading-to-reading difference in 24 h ABPM, two novel SD-independent methodologies were invented, namely successive variation (SV) [7] and average real variability (ARV) [8, 9]. From a mathematical point of view, both SV and ARV can reflect patients' real BP variability by considering each difference between consecutive BP readings, and its superiority to SD-dependent

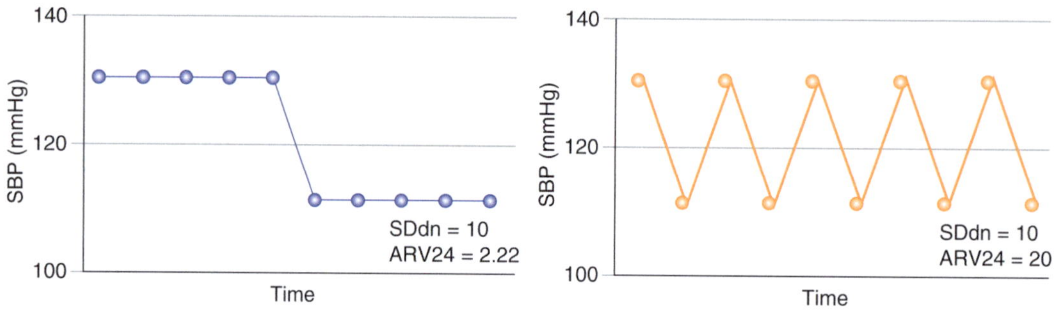

Fig. 41.2 In some cases with distinct blood pressure signals, SD can be the same, whereas ARV24 is not (Adapted from Hansen et al. [9], with permission)

indexes, in some cases as shown in Fig. 41.2, are considerable. SV and ARV can be calculated by the following formula.

$$SV = \sqrt{\frac{1}{\sum w}\sum_{k=1}^{n} w \times \left(BP_k - BP_{k-1}\right)^2}$$

$$ARV = \frac{1}{\sum w}\sum_{k=1}^{n} w \times \left|BP_k - BP_{k-1}\right|$$

where k ranges from 1 to n, w is the time interval between BP_{k-1} and BP_k, and n is the number of BP readings in 24 h.

Calculation of BP Variability by Office BP Measurements

Visit-to-Visit BP Variability

In 2010, an emerging BP variability, so called visit-to-visit BP variability, was derived from the re-analysis of several large-scale clinical trials [10, 11]. Instead of readings from ABPM, mean office BP readings at each visit, normally with an interval of 4–6 months, were applied to calculate patients' long-term BP variability. Similarly, SD, CV, SV and ARV of these readings can be calculated with the above-mentioned formula, but it is recommended to have BP readings from at least 7 visits.

Several investigations indicated that long-term visit-to-visit BP variability was independent of seasonal and weekly variation, with an acceptable reproducibility [12, 13]. However, other investigators argued that this long-term BP variability were loosely associated with classical short-term BP variability derived from 24 h ABPM, with the squared correlation coefficients (r^2) ranging from 0.02 to 0.06 [14, 15]. In this case, definition and calculation of this long-term BP variability are still needed to be investigated in the future.

Influential Factors of Blood Pressure Variability

Theoretically, BP variability may be influenced by many factors, such as seasonal change, mental and physical stress, hormone secretion, baroreceptor's sensitivity, vasoactive substance, etc. In literature, Schutte et al. reported that, age, gender, systolic BP level, body mass index, history of peripheral arterial disease and use of β-blocker were significant correlates of systolic BP variability [16]. Similarly, we reported that, in the X-CELLENT study, the major determinants of BP variability included age, mean BP and the corresponding heart rate variability, in the daytime, nighttime, 24-h and ARV setting [17]. On the other hand, Muntner et al. indicated the significant influential factors of visit-to-visit BP variability, including age, gender, history of myocardial infarction, BP level and the use of angiotensin converting enzyme inhibitor (ACEI), in 956 participants from the NHANES III survey [18]. Moreover, Ohira et al. reported that, in a Japanese cohort, habitual alcohol intake was positively associated with enlarged day-night BP difference and increased daytime BP variability in diastolic BP, but not in systolic BP [19]. In theory, patients with obstructive sleep apnea syndrome (OSAS) may have a fluctuated sympathetic activity at night, and consequently a greater nighttime BP variation. However, three case control studies with small sample sizes only indicated a significant association of OSAS or its severity with less non-dipping pattern of circadian BP variation [20], elevated nighttime BP [21], and 24-h BP variability [22]. In this respect, further clinical investigations are warranted to explore the association of OSAS with nocturnal BP fluctuation and consequent complications. Lastly and most importantly, increased arterial stiffness, indicated by elevated pulse wave velocity, would theoretically be a cause of augmented BP variability. This association was recently proved in a Japanese diabetic cohort [23], but with a brachial-to-ankle pulse wave velocity and home BP variability. In this respect, further studies are warranted to investigate this interesting relationship, but also the real cause of elevated BP variability, to help a better understanding of this multifaceted phenomenon.

Prognosis of Blood Pressure Variability

Target Organ Damage

Table 41.1 shows major investigations on the association of target organ damage with BP variability. Most studies indicated a significant association, except for the ELSA study, in which Mancia et al. [14] and Giannattasia et al. [30] reported that BP variability, assessed by SD of systolic BP either in visit-to-visit or in 24 h ambulatory setting, failed to significantly correlated to carotid artery wall thickness or distensibility, after adjustment for mean BP and other CV risk factors. It is noteworthy that, using a special calculation of 24 h rate of systolic BP variation, Zakopoulos and colleagues reported a constant and significant association between 24 h rate of systolic BP variation and four target organ damages, namely carotid IMT [27, 28], large coronary plaque [31], left ventricular mass [5] and impaired renal function [39], with adjustment for mean BP and other CV risk factors. Secondly, some investigators indicated that SD of nighttime systolic BP yielded a more pronounced predictive value of target organ damage, as compared to daytime systolic BP [24, 31, 36]. Lastly, it was observed that much more evidences were accumulated in literature with regards to an association of BP variability with carotid IMT and stroke, but it remained unclear whether BP variability was superior in predicting stroke and carotid thickness, as compared to other target organ damages. In this respect, a systematic clinical investigation or a meta-analysis, with taking all established target organ damages into account, is warranted to compare their association with BP variation, which would help to have a better understanding of BP variability, from a pathophysiologic viewpoint.

CV and All-Cause Mortality

As shown in Table 41.2, clinical studies on association of CV events and mortality with BP variability were summarized. Three investigations failed to indicate a significant relationship. Pringle et al. reported that, in the 744 elderly hypertensives of the Syst-Eur study, SD of systolic BP failed to predict patients' CV mortality [36], and Pierdomenico et al. indicated that, in two separate hypertensive cohorts, patients with the highest quartile of SD of systolic BP did not present a higher CV risk, as compared with the lowest quartile, after adjustment for mean BP and other CV risk factors [46, 47]. In 2012 participants from the PAMELA study, Mancia et al. reported that, with adjustment of mean BP, age and gender, SD of systolic and diastolic BP was not identified as a significant predictor of CV and all-cause mortality, but the calculated residual diastolic BP variation could significantly predict CV and all-cause mortality with similar adjustment [6]. To sum up, when SD or ARV of BP, but not its quartiles as proposed by Pierdomenico,

Table 41.1 Major investigations on association of target organ damage with blood pressure variability

	Participants (mean age, years)	BPV measurements	TOD measurements	Adjustment	Sign
Sander and Klingelhöfer [24]	216 normotensives + 208 hypertensives (68.0)	Nighttime SBP SD	Carotid IMT	Age, mean BP, smoking	+
Sander et al. [25]	286 CV patients (68.0)	SBP SD	Carotid IMT and progress	Age, mean BP, smoking	+
Moncia et al. (ELSA) [26]	1,662 hypertensives (56.2 ± 7.7)	SBP/PP SD	Carotid IMT	Age, mean BP, 24 h HR SD	+
Zakopoulos et al. [27]	280 normotensives + 234 hypertensives (53.0)	24 h rate of SBP variation	Carotid IMT	Age, gender, smoking, cholesterol	+
Stamatelopoulos et al. [28]	241 normotensives + 232 hypertensives (55.0)	24 h rate of SBP variation	Carotid IMT	Age, gender, 24 h HR, BMI	+
Nagai et al. [29]	201 high-risk elderly (79.9 ± 6.4)	DBP CV	Carotid IMT	Age, mean BP, smoking, cholesterol, treatment	+
Mancia et al. (ELSA) [14]	1,264 hypertensives (55.8 ± 7.4)	SBP VVV	Carotid IMT	Age, mean BP, gender, smoking, DM, cholesterol, treatment	–
Giannattasio et al. (ELSA) [30]	124 hypertensives (56.3)	SBP SD	Carotid artery distensibility	Age, mean BP	–
Shimbo et al. (MESA) [31]	2,640 subjects (60.0)	SBP VVV	Aortic distensibility	Age, mean BP, gender, CV risk factors, treatment	+
Hata et al. (ADVANCE) [32]	8,811 diabetes (66 ± 6)	SBP VVV	Macrovascular and microvascular events	Age, mean BP, gender, smoking, alcohol, BMI, DM duration, HR, cholesterol, treatment	+
Manios et al. [33]	162 normotensives (61.0)	24 h rate of SBP variation	Coronary artery lesion	Mean BP, smoking, DM, cholesterol	+
Iwata et al. [34]	795 subjects (71 ± 9)	Nighttime SBP SD	Coronary plaque	Age, mean BP, gender, smoking, DM, cholesterol, treatment	+
Kukla et al. [35]	118 subjects (70.0)	SBP SD	Lacunar infarction	Age, mean BP, hypertension	+
Pringle et al. (Syst-Eur) [36]	744 elderly hypertensives (69.5)	Nighttime SBP SD	Stroke	Age, mean BP, gender	+
Rothwell et al. [11] (TIA/ASCOT-BPLA)	2,006 patients after TIA (60.3 ± 9.1)	SBP VVV	Stroke	Mean BP	+
	2,011 hypertensives	SBP VVV	Stroke + coronary events	Mean BP	+
Shimbo et al. [37]	58,228 postmenopausal women (50–79)	SBP VVV	Stoke	Age, mean BP, race, smoking, BMI, other CV risk	+

Table 41.1 (continued)

	Participants (mean age, years)	BPV measurements	TOD measurements	Adjustment	Sign
Sega et al. [5]	1,648 subjects (48.2 ± 13.1)	Residual SBP/DBP BPV	LVMI	Age, mean BP, gender	+
Zakopoulos et al. [38]	365 normotensive + 185 whitecoat + 448 uncomplicated hypertensives (53.4 ± 12.9)	24 h rate of SBP variation	LVM	Age, mean BP, gender, HR, BMI, BP dipping	+
Manios et al. [39]	803 hypertensives (54.6 ± 13.0)	24 h rate of SBP variation	Impaired renal function	Age, mean BP, gender	+
Okada et al. [40]	422 diabetes (65.8 ± 9.1)	SBP CV	Log UAE	HbA1c, mean BP, UC, ACEI/ARB	+
Okada et al. [41]	354 diabetes (65.5 ± 9.3)	SBP CV	Development of albuminuria	mean BP, cholesterol	+
Leoncini et al. [42]	169 untreated hypertensives (47.1 ± 9.5)	SBP SD/ARV	Number of organ damage	Age	+

+/– indicates significant/non-significant association of target organ damage with BP variability
BP blood pressure, *SBP* systolic blood pressure, *PP* pulse pressure, *BPV* blood pressure variability, *TOD* target organ damage, *Sig* significance, *SD* standard deviation, *IMT* intema-media thickness, *HR* heart rate, *BMI* body mass index, *VVV* visit-to-visit variability, *DM* diabetes mellitus, *CV* cardiovascular, *LVM* left ventricular mass, *UAE* urinary albumin excretion, *UC* uric acid, *ACEI* ageniotensin converting enzyme inhibitor, *ARB* ageniotensin receptor blocker, *ARV* average real variability

was considered, most studies in Table 41.2 validated a significant prognostic value of patients' BP variability derived from 24 h ABPM. However, it is also noteworthy that, as proposed by Hansen et al. in an international survey composed of 8,938 participants from 11 populations, independent of 24 h mean BP, ARV of BP only provided about 1 % additional prognostic value [9]. In this respect, the effectiveness analysis of 24 h BP variability measurement, with regard to death prediction, need to be re-assessed.

Visit-to-Visit Blood Pressure Variability

Since Rothwell et al. reported the significant and independent prognostic value of a long-term BP variability, so-called visit-to-visit BP variability in 2010 [11], this novel parameter was extensively investigated in clinical studies. For instance, Mancia et al. [14] and Shimbo et al. [31] reported a significant association of carotid IMT and aortic distensibility with visit-to-visit BP variability, respectively, in their recent publications. Meanwhile, after Rothwell's report on the significant relationship between stroke and visit-to-visit BP variability in the TIA and ASCOT-BPLA studies [11], Shimbo et al. also indicated that, in 58,228 postmenopausal women, visit-to-visit systolic BP variability was significantly and independently associated with stroke, after adjustment for mean BP and other CV risk factors [37]. On the other hand, it is controversial for the role of visit-to-visit BP variability in the death prediction. Schutte et al. reported that, in a general population, systolic BP variability, in the visit-to-visit setting, failed to predict CV and all-cause mortality [16], and Mancia et al. also indicated a similar result with regards to CV events in a hypertensive cohort [14]. However, Muntner et al. Poortvliet et al. and Rossignol et al., in the NHANES [18], PROSPER [51] and FOSIDIAL [52] studies, respectively, indicated a significant prognostic value of visit-to-visit BP variability. It is of note that Kikuya et al. and Asayama et al. in the Ohasama study [49, 55] and Hsieh et al. in the Finn-Home study all reported a significant and

Table 41.2 Major investigations on association of mortality and events with blood pressure variability

	Participants (mean age, years)	BPV measurements	Events and mortality	Adjustment	Sign
Kikuya et al. (Ohasama) [43]	1,542 subjects	SBP SD	CV mortality	Age, mean BP, gender, smoking, DM, obesity, HR, cholesterol, CV diseases, treatment	+
Pringle et al. (Syst-Eur) [36]	744 elderly hypertensives (69.5)	SBP SD	CV mortality	Age, mean BP, gender	–
Bjorklund et al. [44]	872 elderly subjects (>70)	Daytime SBP SD	CV mortality	Smoking, DM, BMI, cholesterol, treatment	+
ETO et al. [45]	106 elderly hypertensives (73.9 ± 8.1)	Higher vs lower SBP SD	CV events	Age, mean BP, gender, smoking, DM, obesity, cholesterol, CV diseases	+
Pierdomenico et al. [46]	1,088 uncomplicated mild hypertensives	Higher vs lower SBP SD	CV events	Age, mean BP, smoking, cholesterol	–
Pierdomenico et al. [47]	1,472 treated hypertensives	Higher vs lower SBP SD	CV events	Age, mean BP, smoking, cholesterol, DM, LVM	–
Verdecchia et al. [48]	2,649 untreated hypertensives (51.2 ± 12.0)	Nighttime SBP SD	Cardiac events	Age, gender, smoking, cholesterol, DM, LVH	+
Mancia et al. (PAMELA) [6]	2,012 subjects (49.3 ± 13.4)	SBP/DBP SD residual DBP BPV	CV and all-cause mortality CV and all-cause mortality	Age, mean BP, gender	– +
Kikuya et al. (Ohasama) [49]	2,455 subjects (59.4 ± 12.3)	Home SBP SD/CV	CV and all-cause mortality	Age, mean BP, gender, smoking, DM, obesity, HR, alcohol, cholesterol, CV diseases, treatment	+
Eguchi et al. [50]	300 uncomplicated diabetes (67.8 ± 9.6)	Nighttime SBP/DBP SD	CV events	Age, gender, smoking, BMI, creatinine	+
Hansen et al. [9]	8,938 subjects (53.0)	SBP/DBP SD SBP/DBP ARV	CV and all-cause mortality Mortality + CV events + stroke	Age, mean BP, gender, smoking, DM, BMI, HR, alcohol, cholesterol, CV diseases, treatment	+ +
Muntner et al. (NHANES) [18]	956 subjects (47.4 ± 17.7)	SBP VVV	All-cause mortality	Age, mean BP, gender, MI, treatment	+
Schutte et al. [16]	2,944 subjects (44.9)	SBP/DBP SD/ARV SBP/DBP VVV	CV and all-cause mortality CV and all-cause mortality	Age, mean BP, gender, smoking, HR, BMI, glucose, cholesterol, CV diseases, treatment	– –
Mancia et al. (ELSA) [14]	1,264 hypertensives (55.8 ± 7.4)	SBP VVV	CV events	Age, mean BP, gender, smoking, DM, cholesterol, treatment	–

Poortvliet et al. [51] (PROSPER)	1,808 elderly hypertensives (75.2 ± 3.3)	SBP/DBP/PP VVV	Vascular and total mortality	Age, mean BP, gender, smoking, BMI, cholesterol, CV diseases, treatment	+
Rossignol et al. [52] (FOSIDIAL)	397 patients with hemodialysis + LVH (67)	SBP VVV	CV mortality	Age, stroke, PAD, CAD, DM, LVM	+
Hsieh et al. [53]	2,161 diabetic patients (63.5 ± 11.9)	SBP/DBP/PP VVV	CV and all-cause mortality	Age, mean BP, gender, BMI, glucose, HbA1C, cholesterol, creatinine, estimated GFR	+
Johansson et al. [54] (Finn-Home)	1,866 subjects (66.4 ± 8.5)	Daytime home SBP SD	All-cause mortality	Age, mean BP, gender, smoking, DM, BMI, HR, alcohol, cholesterol, CV diseases, treatment	+
Asayama et al. [55] (Ohasama)	2,421 subjects (58.6)	Home SBP SD	All-cause mortality	Age, mean BP, gender, smoking, DM, BMI, HR, alcohol, cholesterol, CV diseases	+
Hastie et al. [56]	14,522 hypertensives (50)	SBP VVV (ARV)	CV and all-cause mortality	Age, mean BP, gender, smoking, alcohol, BMI, cholesterol, CV diseases, estimated GFR	+
Mallamaci et al. [57]	1,618 patients with 2–5 stage CKD (64 ± 12)	SBP VVV	CV events and mortality	Age, mean BP, gender, smoking, DM, BMI, cholesterol, CV diseases, treatment, estimated GFR	+

+/– indicates significant/non-significant association of events and mortality with BP variability

BP blood pressure, *SBP* systolic blood pressure, *DBP* diastolic blood pressure, *PP* pulse pressure, *BPV* blood pressure variability, *Sig* significance, *SD* standard deviation, *HR* heart rate, *BMI* body mass index, *VVV* visit-to-visit variability, *DM* diabetes mellitus, *CV* cardiovascular, *LVM* left ventricular mass, *LVH* left ventricular hypertrophy, *ARV* average real variability, *MI* myocardial infarction, *PAD* peripheral artery disease, *CAD* coronary artery disease, *GFR* glomerular filtration rate independent prognostic value of day-by-day BP variability derived from home BP measurements, which undoubtedly casted another prospective topic in this field.

Effects of Antihypertensive Agents on Blood Pressure Variability

Short-Term Blood Pressure Variability

Although effect of various antihypertensive agents on BP reduction was extensively proved in numerous randomized clinical trials since 1980s, evidences of their influence on BP variability were very limited. In a randomized clinical trial, Floras et al. indicated that β-adrenoceptor antagonists significantly reduced patients' daytime systolic BP but did not change its SD, and consequently increased patients' coefficient of variation in systolic BP [58]. Mancia et al. also reported in 236 mild hypertensives that angiotensin ACEI or calcium channel blocker (CCB), with a 4–8 weeks therapy, significantly but modestly decreased patients' daytime SD of BP, which was proportional or less than proportional to the reduction in mean BP, resulting in no change or an increase in coefficient of variation in BP [59]. Later, Mancia and colleagues also reported that, in 1,523 hypertensive patients, SD of systolic and diastolic BP was reduced significantly and progressively by 4-year therapy of lacidipine or atenolol, but their coefficient of variation remained unchanged after treatment [60]. Similarly, in the Syst-Eur study, active treatment (nitrendipine in 86 % of participants) caused a significant reduction in SD of both daytime and nighttime BP, but without influence on coefficient of variation [36]. In 100 untreated hypertensives, it was reported that, after a follow-up of 12 months, amlodipine, but not valsartan, could significantly reduce SD of daytime systolic BP derived from 24 h ABPM [61]. Lastly, in the X-CELLENT study, a randomized, double-blinded and placebo-controlled clinical trial, we reported that, after a 3-month treatment, amlodipine and indapamide sustained release (SR), but not candesartan, could significantly reduce patients' systolic BP variability, in daytime, nighttime, 24-h and ARV settings [17]. All those above-mentioned clinical investigations indicated a superiority of CCB in lowering patients' BP variability derived from 24 h ABPM, as so-called short-term BP variability.

Long-Term Blood Pressure Variability

In 2010, a novel visit-to-visit BP variability, also termed as long-term BP variability, was firstly proposed by Rothwell and his colleagues, which was proven as an important indicator of stroke and other CV events and mortality. In ASCOT-BPLA study, visit-to-visit BP variability was greater in patients randomized to atenolol treatment arm than in the amlodipine group, with the latter having fewer CV events [11]. Second, by reviewing data from comparison of atenolol, diuretics or placebo treatment, a significant association of visit-to-visit BP variability with subsequent stroke was detected in atenolol treatment group [62]. Third, in a post-hot analysis of 389 clinical trials, Webb et al. reported a 19 % reduction in visit-to-visit BP variability with CCB and a 13 % with non-loop diuretics, but 8 % increase with ACEI, 16 % increase with angiotensin receptor blocker (ARB) and 17 % increase with β-adrenoreceptor antagonists, with CCB exhibiting the greatest reduction (24 %) as compared with placebo [63]. Moreover, Webb et al. also recently reported that impact of β-adrenoreceptor antagonists on augmentation in BP variability and impact of CCB on BP variability reduction were both dose-dependent [64]. However, those above-mentioned findings should also be cautiously interpreted within the context of their limitations. Firstly, as criticized by Zanchetti [65] and Mancia [66], all those findings were derived from post-hoc analysis of reviewing previous clinical trials. Secondly and more importantly, although intra-individual visit-to-visit BP variability (SD of an individual's BP measured from visit to visit) was scientifically sound as a reliable surrogate of long-term BP variability, inter-individual BP variability (SD of BP in a group of patients in those clinical trials) was actually calculated instead and analyzed in all Rothwell's post-poc analysis. Authors may argue that the two variabilities were strongly (about 50 %) correlated, but with different meaning, they were definitely not identical or replaceable. In this respect, clinical investigations in the prospective setting and with intra-individual calculation are undoubtedly warranted.

Non-pharmacotherapy on Blood Pressure Variability

Many studies indicated an essential role of automatic nervous system (ANS) in BP variability and its reduction, and the increased BP variability was partly attributable to sympathetic overdrive [67, 68]. Recently, catheter-based renal sympathetic denervation (RSD) emerged as a prospective treatment option for patients with resistant hypertension, which is to ablate both afferent and efferent sympathetic nerve in the adventitial of both renal arteries [69, 70]. Considering its significant influence on sympathetic tone, this procedure, in theory, would have an impact on patient's BP variability. In a small interventional study of 11 resistant hypertensives, patients' SD of systolic BP was significantly reduced 6 months after RSD [71]. The effect of this prospective procedure on BP variability and subsequent CV events and mortality needs to be explored by future investigations.

Perspective

Although the cause and exact meaning of BP fluctuation have not been fully understood, several factors, including age, mean BP, heart rate variability and arterial stiffness, may influence patients' BP variation. A large body of evidence has shown a significant association of short- and long-term BP variability with target organ damage, CV events and CV and all-cause mortality, but controversy exists in this field, especially its incremental prognostic value in addition to BP level. Till now, there is no solid evidence indicating any effective agent in terms of BP variability reduction, but some clinical studies are in favor of CCB in reducing both short- and long-term BP variability.

The unknown is still much greater than the known in this field. There are several critical issues need to be addressed for future investigations. First, best estimate of BP variability, calculated by a standardized procedure, either in short- or long-term setting, needs to be fixed, as well as its reference value. Second, with this standardized BP variation, specific cause and meaning of BP variability need to be explored, especially from a pathophysiologic point of view, as well as an effectiveness analysis on its additional prognostic significance in prospective studies. Third, from a therapeutic viewpoint, since BP variability is ultimately supposed to guide clinical treatment, effect of BP variability lowering therapy needs to be conducted in well-designed randomized clinical trials with head-to-head comparison of different antihypertensive agents, especially CCB and diuretics. Forth, limited data are available in the prognostic value of day-by-day BP variability derived from regular home BP measurements. It is obviously prospective to apply standardized home BP variability as a reliable and effective estimate of patients' BP variation, because it is much more convenient and practical than visit-to-visit BP variability. Lastly, a non-invasive device (Mobil-O-Graph NG, Germany) was recently validated by invasive method to record patients' 24 h ambulatory brachial and central BP simultaneously [72], by which the 24-h profile of human's central BP can be explored, as well as central BP variability. Difference and potential superiority of central to brachial BP variability remain unknown and further studies are undoubtedly warranted.

References

1. Staessen JA, Thijs L, Fagard R, O'Brien ET, Clement D, de Leeuw PW, et al. Predicting cardiovascular risk using conventional vs ambulatory blood pressure in older patients with systolic hypertension. Systolic Hypertension in Europe Trial Investigators. JAMA. 1999;282:539–46.
2. Dolan E, Stanton A, Thijs L, Hinedi K, Atkins N, McClory S, et al. Superiority of ambulatory over clinic blood pressure measurement in predicting mortality: the Dublin outcome study. Hypertension. 2005;46:156–61.

3. Mancia G, Ferrari A, Gregorini L, Parati G, Pomidossi G, Bertinieri G, et al. Blood pressure and heart rate variabilities in normotensive and hypertensive human beings. Circ Res. 1983;53:96–104.
4. Bilo G, Giglio A, Styczkiewicz K, Caldara G, Maronati A, Kawecka-Jaszcz K, et al. A new method for assessing 24-h blood pressure variability after excluding the contribution of nocturnal blood pressure fall. J Hypertens. 2007;25:2058–66.
5. Sega R, Corrao G, Bombelli M, Beltrame L, Facchetti R, Grassi G, et al. Blood pressure variability and organ damage in a general population: results from the PAMELA study (Pressioni Arteriose Monitorate E Loro Associazioni). Hypertension. 2002;39:710–4.
6. Mancia G, Bombelli M, Facchetti R, Madotto F, Corrao G, Trevano FQ, et al. Long-term prognostic value of blood pressure variability in the general population: results of the Pressioni Arteriose Monitorate e Loro Associazioni Study. Hypertension. 2007;49:1265–70.
7. Mena L, Pintos S, Queipo NV, Aizpúrua JA, Maestre G, Sulbarán T. A reliable index for the prognostic significance of blood pressure variability. J Hypertens. 2005;23:505–11.
8. Yong M, Diener HC, Kaste M, Mau J. Characteristics of blood pressure profiles as predictors of long-term outcome after acute ischemic stroke. Stroke. 2005;36:2619–25.
9. Hansen TW, Thijs L, Li Y, Boggia J, Kikuya M, Björklund-Bodegård K, et al. Prognostic value of reading-to-reading blood pressure variability over 24 hours in 8938 subjects from 11 populations. Hypertension. 2010;55:1049–57.
10. Rothwell PM, Howard SC, Dolan E, O'Brien E, Dobson JE, Dahlöf B, et al. Prognostic significance of visit-to-visit variability, maximum systolic blood pressure, and episodic hypertension. Lancet. 2010; 375:895–905.
11. Rothwell PM. Limitations of the usual blood pressure hypothesis and importance of variability, instability, and episodic hypertension. Lancet. 2010;375:938–48.
12. Howard SC, Rothwell PM. Reproducibility of measures of visit-to-visit variability in blood pressure after transient ischaemic attack or minor stroke. Cerebrovasc Dis. 2009;28:331–40.
13. Muntner P, Joyce C, Levitan EB, Holt E, Shimbo D, Webber LS, et al. Reproducibility of visit-to-visit variability of blood pressure measured as part of routine clinical care. J Hypertens. 2011;29:2332–8.
14. Mancia G, Facchetti R, Parati G, Zanchetti A. Visit-to-visit blood pressure variability in the European Lacidipine Study on Atherosclerosis: methodological aspects and effects of antihypertensive treatment. J Hypertens. 2012;30:1241–51.
15. Muntner P, Shimbo D, Diaz KM, Newman J, Sloan RP, Schwartz JE. Low correlation between visit-to-visit variability and 24-h variability of blood pressure. Hypertens Res. 2013;36(11):940–6.
16. Schutte R, Thijs L, Liu YP, Asayama K, Jin Y, Odili A, et al. Within-subject blood pressure level–not variability–predicts fatal and nonfatal outcomes in a general population. Hypertension. 2012;60:1138–47.
17. Zhang Y, Agnoletti D, Safar ME, Blacher J. Effect of antihypertensive agents on blood pressure variability: the Natrilix SR versus candesartan and amlodipine in the reduction of systolic blood pressure in hypertensive patients (X-CELLENT) study. Hypertension. 2011;58:155–60.
18. Muntner P, Shimbo D, Tonelli M, Reynolds K, Arnett DK, Oparil S. The relationship between visit-to-visit variability in systolic blood pressure and all-cause mortality in the general population: findings from NHANES III, 1988 to 1994. Hypertension. 2011; 57(2):160–6.
19. Ohira T, Tanigawa T, Tabata M, Imano H, Kitamura A, Kiyama M, et al. Effects of habitual alcohol intake on ambulatory blood pressure, heart rate, and its variability among Japanese men. Hypertension. 2009;53:13–9.
20. Noda A, Okada T, Hayashi H, Yasuma F, Yokota M. 24-hour ambulatory blood pressure variability in obstructive sleep apnea syndrome. Chest. 1993;103: 1343–7.
21. Nagata K, Osada N, Shimazaki M, Kida K, Yoneyama K, Tsuchiya A, et al. Diurnal blood pressure variation in patients with sleep apnea syndrome. Hypertens Res. 2008;31:185–91.
22. Kallianos A, Trakada G, Papaioannou T, Nikolopouloss I, Mitrakou A, Manios E, et al. Glucose and arterial blood pressure variability in obstructive sleep apnea syndrome. Eur Rev Med Pharmacol Sci. 2013;17:1932–7.
23. Fukui M, Ushigome E, Tanaka M, Hamaguchi M, Tanaka T, Atsuta H, et al. Home blood pressure variability on one occasion is a novel factor associated with arterial stiffness in patients with type 2 diabetes. Hypertens Res. 2013;36:219–25.
24. Sander D, Klingelhöfer J. Diurnal systolic blood pressure variability is the strongest predictor of early carotid atherosclerosis. Neurology. 1996;47:500–7.
25. Sander D, Kukla C, Klingelhöfer J, Winbeck K, Conrad B. Relationship between circadian blood pressure patterns and progression of early carotid atherosclerosis: a 3-year follow-up study. Circulation. 2000;102: 1536–41.
26. Mancia G, Parati G, Hennig M, Flatau B, Omboni S, Glavina F, et al. Relation between blood pressure variability and carotid artery damage in hypertension: baseline data from the European Lacidipine Study on Atherosclerosis (ELSA). J Hypertens. 2001;19:1981–9.
27. Zakopoulos NA, Tsivgoulis G, Barlas G, Papamichael C, Spengos K, Manios E, et al. Time rate of blood pressure variation is associated with increased common carotid artery intima-media thickness. Hypertension. 2005;45:505–12.
28. Stamatelopoulos KS, Manios E, Barlas G, Koroboki E, Zacharoulis A, Tsivgoulis G, et al. Time rate of blood pressure variation is superior to central hemodynamics as an associate of carotid intima-media thickness. J Hypertens. 2010;28:51–8.

29. Nagai M, Hoshide S, Ishikawa J, Shimada K, Kario K. Visit-to-visit blood pressure variations: new independent determinants for carotid artery measures in the elderly at high risk of cardiovascular disease. J Am Soc Hypertens. 2011;5:184–92.
30. Giannattasio C, Failla M, Hennig M, Hollweck R, Laurent S, Mallion JM, et al. Different relation between 24-h blood pressure and distensibility at different peripheral arteries. Data from the European Lacidipine Study on Atherosclerosis (ELSA). J Hypertens. 2005; 23:557–62.
31. Shimbo D, Shea S, McClelland RL, Viera AJ, Mann D, Newman J, et al. Association of aortic distensibility and arterial elasticity with long-term visit-to-visit blood pressure variability: the Multi-Ethnic Study of Atherosclerosis (MESA). Am J Hypertens. 2013;26: 896–902.
32. Hata J, Arima H, Rothwell PM, Woodward M, Zoungas S, Anderson C, et al. Effects of visit-to-visit variability in systolic blood pressure on macrovascular and microvascular complications in patients with Type 2 diabetes mellitus: the ADVANCE trial. Circulation. 2013;128:1325–34.
33. Manios E, Stamatelopoulos K, Tsivgoulis G, Barlas G, Koroboki E, Tsagalis G, et al. Time rate of blood pressure variation: a new factor associated with coronary atherosclerosis. J Hypertens. 2011; 29:1109–14.
34. Iwata S, Jin Z, Schwartz JE, Homma S, Elkind MS, Rundek T, et al. Relationship between ambulatory blood pressure and aortic arch atherosclerosis. Atherosclerosis. 2012;221:427–31.
35. Kukla C, Sander D, Schwarze J, Wittich I, Klingelhöfer J. Changes of circadian blood pressure patterns are associated with the occurence of lucunar infarction. Arch Neurol. 1998;55:683–8.
36. Pringle E, Phillips C, Thijs L, Davidson C, Staessen JA, de Leeuw PW, et al. Systolic blood pressure variability as a risk factor for stroke and cardiovascular mortality in the elderly hypertensive population. J Hypertens. 2003;21:2251–7.
37. Shimbo D, Newman JD, Aragaki AK, LaMonte MJ, Bavry AA, Allison M, et al. Association between annual visit-to-visit blood pressure variability and stroke in postmenopausal women: data from the Women's Health Initiative. Hypertension. 2012;60:625–30.
38. Zakopoulos NA, Tsivgoulis G, Barlas G, Spengos K, Manios E, et al. Impact of the time rate of blood pressure variation on left ventricular mass. J Hypertens. 2006;24:2071–7.
39. Manios E, Tsagalis G, Tsivgoulis G, Barlas G, Koroboki E, Michas F, et al. Time rate of blood pressure variation is association with impaired renal function in hypertensive patients. J Hypertens. 2009;27: 2244–8.
40. Okada H, Fukui M, Tanaka M, Inada S, Mineoka Y, Nakanishi N, et al. Visit-to-visit variability in systolic blood pressure is correlated with diabetic nephropathy and atherosclerosis in patients with type 2 diabetes. Atherosclerosis. 2012;220:155–9.
41. Okada H, Fukui M, Tanaka M, Matsumoto S, Mineoka Y, Nakanishi N, et al. Visit-to-visit blood pressure variability is a novel risk factor for the development and progression of diabetic nephropathy in patients with type 2 diabetes. Diabetes Care. 2013;36: 1908–12.
42. Leoncini G, Viazzi F, Storace G, Deferrari G, Pontremoli R. Blood pressure variability and multiple organ damage in primary hypertension. J Hum Hypertens. 2013;27(11):663–70.
43. Kikuya M, Hozawa A, Ohokubo T, Tsuji I, Michimata M, Matsubara M, et al. Prognosis significance of blood pressure and heart rate variabilities: the Ohasama study. Hypertension. 2000;36:901–6.
44. Björklund K, Lind L, Zethelius B, Berglund L, Lithell H. Prognostic significance of 24-h ambulatory blood pressure characteristics for cardiovascular morbidity in a population of elderly men. J Hypertens. 2004;22:1691–7.
45. Eto M, Toba K, Akishita M, Kozaki K, Watanabe T, Kim S, et al. Impact of blood pressure variability on cardiovascular events in elderly patients with hypertension. Hypertens Res. 2005;28:1–7.
46. Pierdomenico SD, Lapenna D, Bucci A, Manente BM, Mancini M, Cuccurullo F, et al. Blood pressure variability and prognosis in uncomplicated mild hypertension. Am Heart J. 2005;149:934–8.
47. Pierdomenico SD, Lapenna D, Di Tommaso R, Di Carlo S, Esposito AL, Di Mascio R, et al. Blood pressure variability and cardiovascular risk in treated hypertensive patients. Am J Hypertens. 2006;19:991–7.
48. Verdecchia P, Angeli F, Gattobigio R, Rapicetta C, Reboldi G. Impact of blood pressure variability on cardiac and cerebrovascular complications in hypertension. Am J Hypertens. 2007;20:154–61.
49. Kikuya M, Ohkubo T, Metoki H, Asayama K, Hara A, Obara T, Inoue R, et al. Day-by-day variability of blood pressure and heart rate at home as a novel predictor of prognosis: the Ohasama study. Hypertension. 2008;52:1045–50.
50. Eguchi K, Ishikawa J, Hoshide S, Pickering TG, Schwartz JE, Shimada K, et al. Night time blood pressure variability is a strong predictor for cardiovascular events in patients with type 2 diabetes. Am J Hypertens. 2009;22:46–51.
51. Poortvliet RK, Ford I, Lloyd SM, Sattar N, Mooijaart SP, de Craen AJ, Westendorp RG, et al. Blood pressure variability and cardiovascular risk in the PROspective Study of Prevastatin in the Elderly at Risk (PROSPER). PLoS One. 2012;7:e52438.
52. Rossignol P, Cridlig J, Lehert P, Kessler M, Zannad F. Visit-to-visit blood pressure variability is a strong predictor of cardiovascular events in hemodialysis: insights from FOSIDIAL. Hypertension. 2012;60:339–46.
53. Hsieh YT, Tu ST, Cho TJ, Chang SJ, Chen JF, Hsieh MC. Visit-to-visit variability in blood pressure strongly predicts all-cause mortality in patients with type 2 diabetes: a 5·5-year prospective analysis. Eur J Clin Invest. 2012;42:245–53.
54. Johansson JK, Niiranen TJ, Puukka PJ, Jula AM. Prognostic value of the variability in home-

measured blood pressure and heart rate: the Finn-Home Study. Hypertension. 2012;59:212–8.
55. Asayama K, Kikuya M, Schutte R, Thijs L, Hosaka M, Satoh M, et al. Home blood pressure variability as cardiovascular risk factor in the population of Ohasama. Hypertension. 2013;61:61–9.
56. Hastie CE, Jeemon P, Coleman H, McCallum L, Patel R, et al. Long-term and ultra long-term blood pressure variability during follow-up and mortality in 14 522 patients with hypertension. Hypertension. 2013;62: 698–705.
57. Mallamaci F, Minutolo R, Leonardis D, D'Arrigo G, Tripepi G, Rapisarda F, et al. Long-term visit-to-visit office blood pressure variability increases the risk of adverse cardiovascular outcomes in patients with chronic kidney disease. Kidney Int. 2013;84:381–9.
58. Floras JS, Hassan MO, Jones JV, Osikowska BA, Sever PS, et al. Factors influencing blood pressure and heart rate variability in hypertensive humans. Hypertension. 1988;11:273–81.
59. Mancia G, Omboni S, Ravogli A, Parati G, Zanchetti A. Ambulatory blood pressure monitoring in the evaluation of antihypertensive treatment: additional information from a large data base. Blood Press. 1995;4: 148–56.
60. Mancia G, Parati G, Bilo G, Maronati A, Omboni S, Baurecht H, et al. Assessment of long-term antihypertensive treatment by clinic and ambulatory blood pressure: data from the European Lacidipine Study on Atherosclerosis. European Lacidipine Study on Atherosclerosis. J Hypertens. 2007;25:1087–94.
61. Ichihara A, Kaneshiro Y, Takemitsu T, Sakoda M. Effects of amlodipine and valsartan on vascular damage and ambulatory blood pressure in untreated hypertensive patients. J Hum Hypertens. 2006;20:787–94.
62. Rothwell PM, Howard SC, Dolan E, O'Brien E, Dobson JE, Dahlöf B, et al. Effects of beta blockers and calcium-channel blockers on within-individual variability in blood pressure and risk of stroke. Lancet Neurol. 2010;9:469–80.
63. Webb AJ, Fischer U, Mehta Z, Rothwell PM. Effects of antihypertensive-drug class on interindividual variation in blood pressure and risk of stroke: a systematic review and meta-analysis. Lancet. 2010;375:906–15.
64. Webb AJ, Rothwell PM. Effect of dose and combination of antihypertensives on interindividual blood pressure variability: a systematic review. Stroke. 2011;42: 2860–5.
65. Zanchetti A. Wars, war games, and dead bodies on the battlefield: variations on the theme of blood pressure variability. Stroke. 2011;42:2722–4.
66. Mancia G. Short- and long-term blood pressure variability: present and future. Hypertension. 2012;60: 512–7.
67. Narkiewicz K, Winnicki M, Schroeder K, Phillips BG, Kato M, Cwalina E, et al. Relationship between muscle sympathetic nerve activity and diurnal blood pressure profile. Hypertension. 2002;39:168–72.
68. Zhang Y, Agnoletti D, Blacher J, Safar ME. Blood pressure variability in relation to autonomic nervous system dysregulation: the X-CELLENT study. Hypertens Res. 2012;35:399–403.
69. Krum H, Schlaich M, Whitbourn R, Sobotka PA, Sadowski J, Bartus K, et al. Catheter-based renal sympathetic denervation for resistant hypertension: a multicentre safety and proof-of-principle cohort study. Lancet. 2009;373:1275–81.
70. Mahfoud F, Schlaich M, Kindermann I, Ukena C, Cremers B, Brandt MC, et al. Effect of renal sympathetic denervation on glucose metabolism in patients with resistant hypertension: a pilot study. Circulation. 2011;123:1940–6.
71. Zuern CS, Rizas KD, Eick C, Stoleriu C, Bunk L, Barthel P, et al. Effects of renal sympathetic denervation on 24-hour blood pressure variability. Front Physiol. 2012;3:134.
72. Weber T, Wassertheurer S, Rammer M, Maurer E, Hametner B, Mayer CC, et al. Validation of a brachial cuff-based method for estimating central systolic blood pressure. Hypertension. 2011;58:825–32.

Nitrate: The Ideal Drug Action for Isolated Systolic Hypertension in Elderly?

42

Xiong J. Jiang and Michael F. O'Rourke

Abstract

Nitrates such as nitroglycerine and isosorbide mononitrate are unique drugs, and at least in theory ideal for treating Isolated Systolic Hypertension in the Elderly (ISHE). Early wave reflection from aortic stiffening increases late systolic pressure in the ascending aorta and left ventricle, and is the cause of ISHE, but diastolic pressure and mean pressure are normal. Nitrates decrease or abolish wave reflection from peripheral arterioles, "trapping" this within the peripheral arterial networks (Yaginuma et al. Cardiovasc Res 20:153–160, 1986).

While having the most favourable of all mechanisms for treatment of angina pectoris and ISHE, nitrates have disadvantages over conventional modern anti-anginal and antihypertensive drugs, and so are usually used in conjunction with other drugs.

The purpose of this chapter is to describe the actions of nitrates, the properties that make them useful, and those which can detract from their use in clinical medicine. All have been clarified by modern concepts of aortic elasticity, arteriolar resistance, wave reflection, and pressure pulse wave analysis. Surprisingly, few if any of the mechanistic concepts are considered in contemporary journals and textbooks.

Keywords

Nitrates • Systolic hypertension • Central aortic pressure • Wave reflection • Tolerance

X.J. Jiang, MD
Department of Cardiology, Hypertension Centre,
Fuwai Hospital, Cardiovascular Institute,
Chinese Academy of Medical Sciences,
National Centre for Cardiovascular Diseases,
Peking Union Medical College, 167 Beilishi Rd,
Xicheng sitrict, Beijing 100037, China
e-mail: jxj103@hotmail.com

M.F. O'Rourke, MD, DSc (✉)
Department of Cardiovascular and Hypertension,
St. Vincent's Clinic, University of New South Wales,
Victor Chang Cardiac Research Institute, Suite 810
St. Vincent Clinic, 438 Victoria Street, Darlinghurst,
Sydney, NSW 2010, Australia
e-mail: m.orourke@unsw.edu.au

M.E. Safar et al. (eds.), *Blood Pressure and Arterial Wall Mechanics in Cardiovascular Diseases*,
DOI 10.1007/978-1-4471-5198-2_42, © Springer-Verlag London 2014

Nitrates in Clinical Practice

Nitrates were introduced as anti-anginal agents in the late nineteenth century, and immediately taken up as the basis of therapy for this condition. Nitrates were administered by inhalation (amyl nitrate) or by topical application under the tongue. The first paper on clinical use of glyceryl trinitrate [1] showed a typical effect on the sphygmogram, recorded from the radial artery. This we can now interpret as showing reduction in wave reflection from peripheral sites [2, 3]. During the twentieth century, nitroglycerine remained the mainstay for treatment of angina, but its mode of action remained a mystery [4]. It was effective in relieving anginal pain without reducing brachial systolic or diastolic pressure. It did not appear to reduce peripheral resistance, so that its effect was considered due to reduction in venous tone, causing reduced venous return to the heart. This together with dilation of coronary arteries [5] appeared to explain therapeutic effects, which by the beginning of the twenty-first century included relief of acute cardiac failure as well, again, attributed to reduction in venous return and left ventricular preload [6]. Studies on central and peripheral pressures have clarified the action of nitrates on cardiovascular properties. These are discussed in detail later, but are still not recognised in major recent clinical papers on nitrates [7] or in textbooks.

Problems with Clinical Use of Nitrates

Nitrates are volatile, hence tablets and other preparations only remain effective for a short period of time. They are not readily or uniformly absorbed from the gastrointestinal tract, so that older oral preparations did not prove reliable in action. Nitrates dilate muscular arteries and readily induce headache, and flushing. The drugs can precipitate migraine, and can in excessive dose induce syncope. Therapeutic doses of glyceryl trinitrate (0.4–0.6 mg) per tablet often need be divided into halves or quarters in order to obtain therapeutic response without headache. One tiny glyceryl trinitrate tablet provides over 10 min as much as the smallest available (5 mg) nitrate patch delivers over 1 h [8]. The smallest available patch (5 mg) often has to be cut into a half or even one quarter in order to provide therapeutic effect without headache.

Another major problem with nitrate is tolerance – loss of drug action as a consequence of continuing exposure. This is a reason for using nitroglycerine patch over a continuous 12–14 h period when angina pain is most likely to occur, or blood pressure is likely to be highest, or cardiac failure most in evidence, then removing the patch for a 10–12 h period before reapplying the patch on the following day. Our most recent work confirms tolerance, showing from studies of central pulse pressure or augmentation that this is reduced by around 35 % during constant exposure after 6 days; this however is not sufficiently great as to render the dose ineffective [9].

The last major problem with nitrate is the difficulty in measuring its action through the effect on arterial pressure [10–13]. This is described below, where benefits of measuring central aortic pressure are emphasised.

The major problem with nitrates remains headache; this can usually be prevented without compromising drug action by reduction in dose. Present formulations often contain too much of the drug for too many of the patients on whom it is used.

Actions of Nitrates

Yaginuma et al. [1] in 1986 studied the effects of sublingual nitroglycerine on ascending aortic impedance, determined from use of high frequency pressure manometer and electromagnetic flow waveforms at cardiac catheterisation. They were able to show that nitroglycerine reduced wave reflection markedly without significant effect on peripheral resistance (impedance at zero frequency) or on aortic characteristic impedance (a measure of aortic stiffness, and closely related to aortic pulse wave velocity). Yaginuma et al. [1] explained the findings to indicate an action of vasodilation on muscular conduit arteries throughout the body which was systematically greater at a branch in the daughter than in parent arteries. This action confirmed the findings of Feldman et al. [5] on differential effects of nitroglycerine on arteries of different size in the heart, and the minimal effects of the drug on arterioles (measured as peripheral resistance) and on the aorta itself, measured as aortic characteristic impedance. It was in keeping with Womersley's calculation on wave reflection under different conditions at arterial branches [14]. These studies showed that impedance is usually almost perfectly matched at arterial branches by the area ratio of two daughter to one parent artery, and wave reflection is minimal whereas if the area ratio is reduced (daughter ÷ parent), wave reflection is increased and if the ratio is increased, wave reflection is decreased. This is the simple explanation given by Yaginuma et al. [1], but this can be enhanced by an arterial dilator such as nitroglycerine which relaxes muscular tone in the daughter branches, so transferring stress from collagenous to elastic elements in the wall and rendering the dilated daughter arteries more distensible [3, 15]. Change in both diameter and distensibility serve to decrease impedance in vessels beyond a branch, so reducing reflection returning from the arterioles, and "trapping" this reflection in the peripheral arterioles. Such action is readily apparent in Fig. 42.1.

The study by Yaginuma with nitroglycerine on ascending aorta impedance confirmed studies on other arterial dilating and antihypertensive drugs. These drugs however, usually showed reduction in peripheral resistance, attributable to a substantial effect on arterioles and peripheral resistance [1, 3, 15] and relatively less effect on wave reflection.

Yaginuma's studies were pursued by Kelly who was a pioneer of arterial tonometry for non-invasive measurement of central arterial pressure [16, 17]. Kelly et al. [10] showed that the reduction in central aortic pressure induced by nitrate was not apparent as a similar reduction in brachial or radial pressure measured either invasively by catheter or non-invasively by cuff or applanation tonometry [11]. He explained this on the basis that peak of the central wave in older adults was due to wave reflection, whereas the radial peak was not, since reflection in the brachial or radial pulse was manifest as a secondary shoulder in late systole (Fig. 42.1). This established how the benefit of nitrate reduction in wave reflection was seen in reduction of systolic aortic and left ven-

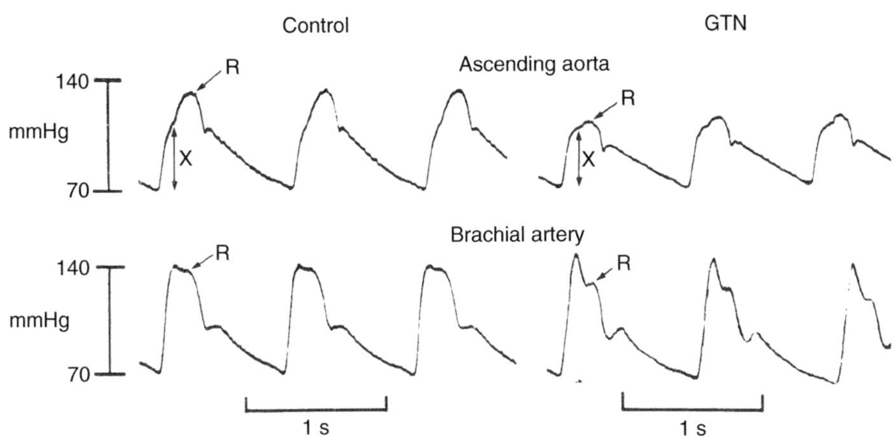

Fig. 42.1 Pressure waves measured invasively in the ascending aorta and brachial artery at cardiac catheterisation, before (*left*) and after (*right*) administration of 0.5 mg nitroglycerine sublingually in a human adult. Nitroglycerine caused little change in brachial systolic pressure, since the initial peak of the wave (caused directly by ventricular ejection and indicated by the *vertical bar marked by X*) was higher than the late systolic reflected wave (*R*). In the ascending aorta, the second late systolic peak caused by wave reflection was higher than the initial peak. When this was reduced by nitroglycerine, systolic peak pressure was reduced by almost 20 mmHg (Reproduced with permission from Kelly et al. [10])

tricular pressure but not in brachial or radial pressure. This finding was promptly confirmed by Fitchett in Montreal [13] and Takazawa et al. in Tokyo [12]. These studies more than any others drew early attention to central aortic pressure as superior to brachial cuff pressure for assessment of drug effect, and led on to the REASON [18], CAFE [19] and J-CORE [20] studies in showing superior value of arterial vasodilating drugs in treatment of hypertension. All are summarised in books *Arterial Vasodilation: Mechanism and Therapy* (by O'Rourke, Safar, Dzau [3]) and successive editions of *McDonald's Blood Flow in Arteries* [15].

The hemodynamic studies of central pressure and flow showed another predicted effect of nitrates in reduction of wave reflection. In older adults with systolic heart failure, wave reflection can have a predominant effect in reducing late systolic flow, rather than causing augmentation of late systolic pressure [21, 22]. With administration of nitrate, such patients usually show increase in stroke volume rather than reduction in pressure augmentation [15, 22]. This is also apparent in Doppler and especially MRI ascending aortic waveforms [23–25].

Maurice McGregor of Montreal [4] was one of the first to draw attention to the unique action of nitrates in clinical practice. This stimulated the work of Fitchett and Kelly in Montreal and Toronto [26] and preceded that of Yaginuma et al. [1]. McGregor [4] noted the strong pulsation of tissue especially the pulse of the finger as well as of arteries such as the radial and superficial temporal (which was linked to headache), and correctly attributed this to selective dilation of tiny peripheral arteries [27, 28]. This was confirmed by plethysmographic studies at the forearm and finger tip (now widely used as photoplethysmography) as well as through ultrasound of individual larger arteries [15]. Administration of nitrate was shown to cause marked increase in diameter of arteries such as the radial without corresponding change in amplitude of the pressure waveform [4, 15]. Changes were attributable to relaxation of smooth muscle in the arterial wall. This smooth muscle acts as though in series with stiff collagenous elements in the wall, but in parallel with elastin fibres [15]. Relaxation of smooth muscle in the wall transferred stress to the more extensible elastin fibres, so that the small muscular arteries dilated, and became more distensible at the same time. Arteries throughout the body dilate passively with greater distending pressure, such as with elevation of arterial pressure, but become progressively more stiff as they dilate; the action of nitrates causes an opposite, paradoxical effect: i.e. dilation with less stiffness [15].

The effect of nitrates is of dilation and reduced stiffness of muscular arteries throughout the whole body. The overall effect is manifest as reduction in wave reflection, and this is best measured from change in the pulse waveform – as noted by Murrell 130 years ago [2, 3], and foreshadowed by McGregor over 30 years ago [4].

Use of Central Pulse Pressure to Study Nitrate Action

Invasive and Non-invasive Studies

From simultaneous measure of central aortic and radial pressure waveforms in patients under intensive care prior to cardiopulmonary bypass, Pauca et al. [29] were able to demonstrate the dramatic effect of glyceryl-trinitrate in reducing or abolishing augmentation of late systolic pressure through reduction of wave reflection (Fig. 42.2) in a series of 50 patients. This occurred despite the drug having no demonstrable effect in the low doses administered on the initial pressure wave generated by ventricular ejection. Such findings could not be explained on the basis of reduction in venous return from venodilatation, but were readily explicable on the basis of reduction in wave reflection from peripheral (arteriolar) sites. Pauca's analysis of the same recordings of radial/aorta pressure waves in a larger patient group [30] was used to test the then new SphygmoCor method for generation of central aortic pressure waveforms from the radial pulse. This showed strong relationship between the aortic pulse, synthesised from the radial pulse with the simultaneously recorded directly measured

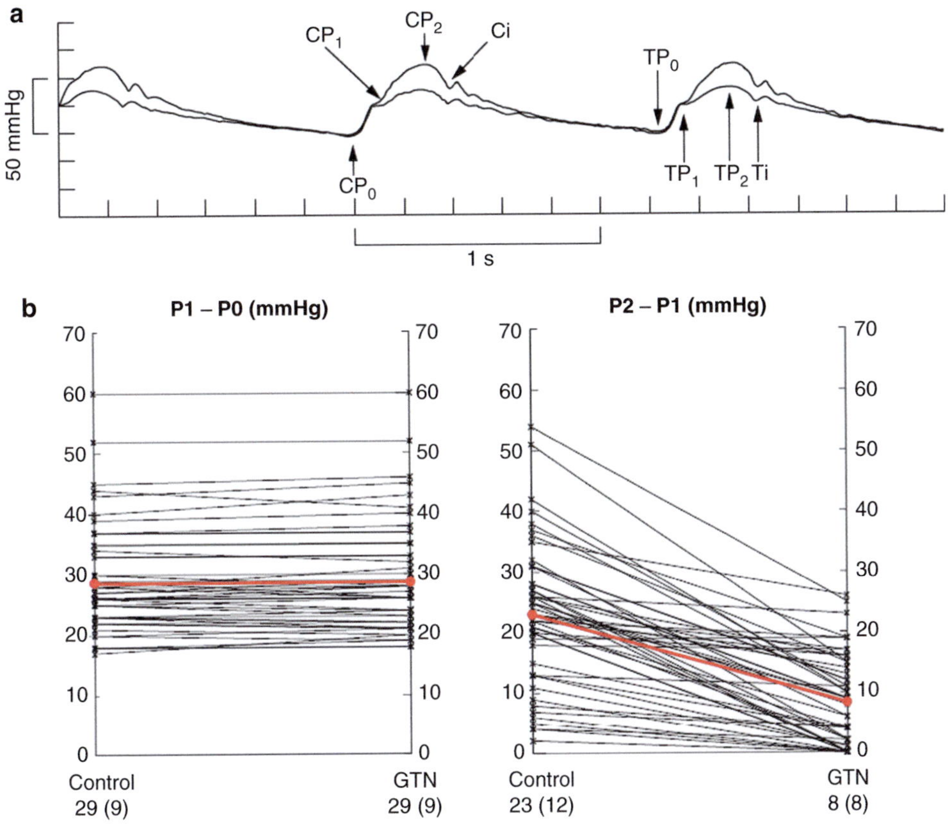

Fig. 42.2 (**a**) Invasively recorded ascending aortic pressure waves in a patient with regular (paced) heart rate, before (*top trace*) and after (*bottom trace*) infusion of nitroglycerine (6 mg/kg/min) prior to initiation of cardiopulmonary bypass. Effects of the drug are readily apparent on the reflected component of the wave. *CP0* central pressure in diastole, *CP1* initial impulse generated by ventricular systole, *CP2* peak of reflected wave and of systolic pressure, *Ci* central pressure at the incisura (ie. at aortic valve closure), *TP0* foot of initial wave (t=0), *TP1* time of initial peak (usually about 100 ms), *TP2* time to reflected wave peak, *T1* time to incisura (aortic valve closure). (**b**) Ascending aortic pressure waves in 50 patients, taken prior to cardiopulmonary bypass. *Left*: Change of initial wave peak (P0 – P1) from control to steady state with nitrate infusion (29±9 mmHg) before and after nitroglycerine. *Right*: Change in augmented pressure (P2 – P1) before and after nitroglycerine (23±12 mmHg) to 8±8 mmHg) (Reproduced with permission from Pauca et al. [29])

aortic pressure waveform [8]. This work was largely responsible for acceptance of the SphygmoCor method by the US Food and Drug Administration (FDA) for generation of the aortic pressure waveform from the radial pressure, recorded invasively (US FDA K002742) or non-invasively (US FDA K0012487) and calibrated to brachial cuff pressure.

Those responsible for development of the Sphygmocor process, were surprised by the correspondence of synthesised with measured aortic waveforms, particularly after nitroglycerine, in view of its known effect on muscular arteries in the upper limb which link the ascending aorta to the radial artery. They were called on by FDA examiners to compare the transfer function used in Sphygmocor with that seen at the peak effect of nitrate action, using the Pauca data. This was done, and did show blunting of the transfer function compared to that originally described. The degree of "blunting" did not interfere with use of Sphygmocor during vasodilatation challenge such as use of nitrate [30]. Satisfaction on this issue provided a non-invasive method to obtain information which would not have been possible except from direct aortic pressure measurement

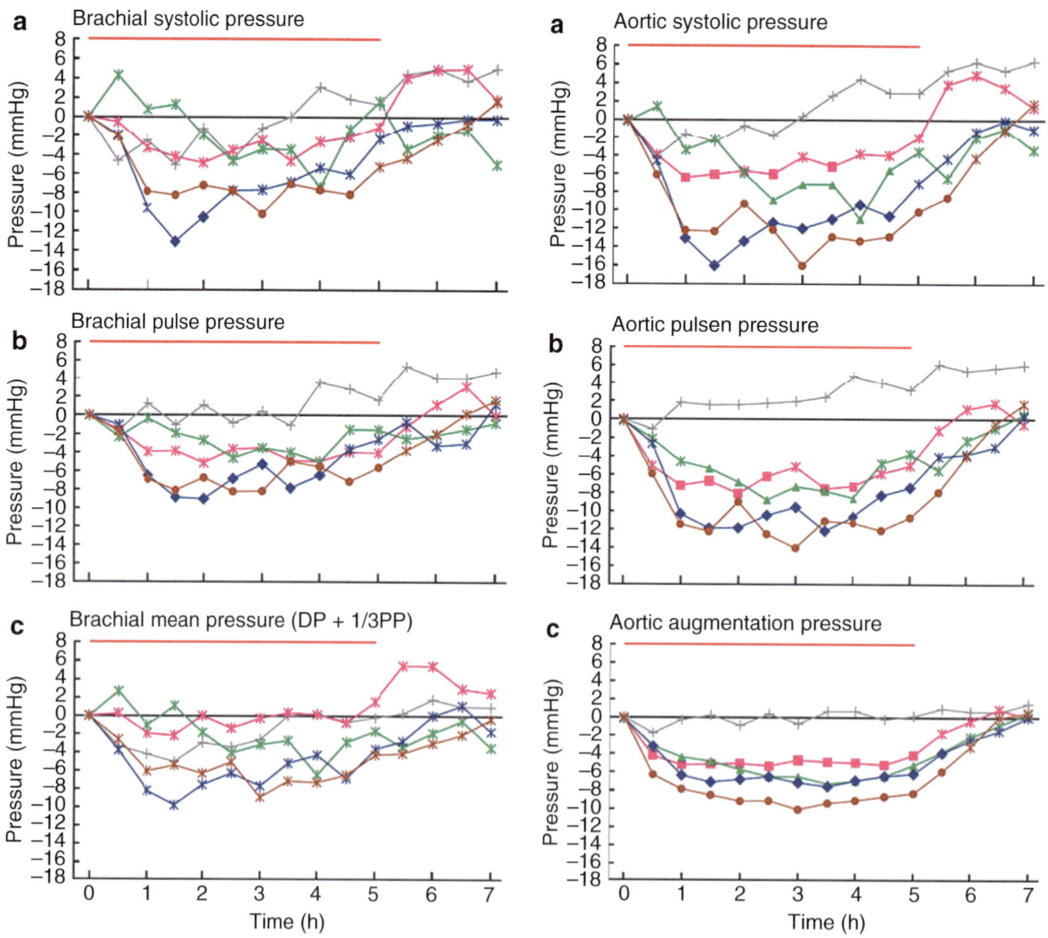

Fig. 42.3 Analysis of change in radial (*left*) and aortic (*right*) pressure waves determined non-invasively by SphygmoCor over 24 h after application of nitroglycerine patch. *Left panels*: radial systolic (*top*), pulse (*centre*) and mean (*bottom*) pressures taken from integration of the radial pressure wave. *Right panels*: aortic systolic (*top*), pulse (*centre*) and augmentation (*bottom*) pressures. *Colours*: *grey* inactive patch, *pink* 0.104 mg/h, *green* 0.208 mg/h, *blue* 0.416 mg/h, *brown* 0.625 mg/h. *Small symbols* indicate not significant, *large solid symbols* p<0.01. Change in mean pressure was relatively small, and only seen with higher doses. Change in augmented pressure as clearly dose dependent, and significant with all doses over the entire dosing rate. No significant change in radial systolic or pulse pressure for the lower doses. Significant change in aortic systolic and pulse pressure for all doses (Reproduced with permission from Jiang et al. [8])

[30], or by taking the tonometric measurement of the carotid pressure wave as a surrogate of the aortic pressure pulse [17, 31].

Non-invasive Studies: Dose Dependent Effects

Dose ranging studies were concluded on 46 volunteers (patients awaiting electrophysiological studies at Fu Wai hospital, Beijing) [8]. Subjects were randomly assigned to different doses of nitroglycerine patch (2.5–20 mg/24 h) over 24 h each with one day without therapy in between. Results are shown in Fig. 42.3, which shows effects on brachial cuff pressures and on central pressure indices. In general, there was little apparent effect on nitrate on brachial systolic, diastolic or mean pressures, but definite effect on central systolic and pulse pressure, together with

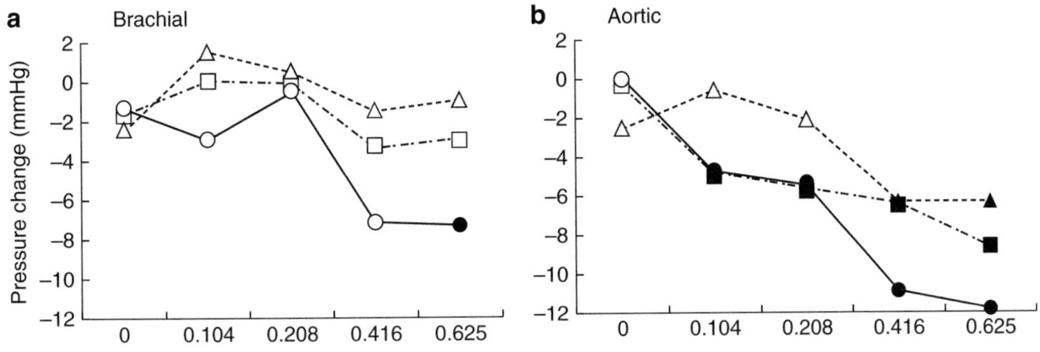

Fig. 42.4 Averaged change between 0.5 and 5 h as a function of nitrate doses. (**a**) Brachial systolic (*open circles*), diastolic (*open squares*) and mean (*open triangles*) pressures. (**b**) Aortic systolic (*open circles*), augmented (*open squares*) and mean (*open triangles*) pressures integrated from aortic pressure wave. Closed symbols represent $p<0.01$ for brachial pressures, $p<0.001$ for aortic pressures. For brachial systolic pressure, significant change only seen in the highest dose 0.625 mg/h. Significant change in aortic systolic and augmented pressure for all doses, only at dose >0.416 mg/h for aortic mean pressure (Reproduced with permission from Jiang et al. [8])

substantial effect on augmentation and augmentation index, even with the lowest dose of nitroglycerine (2.5 mg/24 h, approximately 0.1 mg/h). Findings confirmed the view that nitroglycerine in low dosage reduces wave reflection, and thereby reduces pressure wave augmentation, together with aortic systolic and pulse pressure, with this effect not apparent from measures of brachial pressure.

From the study we were able to gauge the effects of nitroglycerine on arteriolar calibre and on venous return – the former from reduction in mean pressure, and the latter from reduction in ejection duration. To be completely confident of our views we would have had to measure cardiac output at the same time. This was not done. However, amplitude of the aortic pressure wave from foot to first systolic shoulder is an indirect index of stroke volume and this was not altered by the administration of nitroglycerine (Fig. 42.2). Duration of ejection is also related to stroke volume and this was decreased at high doses of nitroglycerine. We believe that venodilation was largely responsible for this, but it was only seen at high doses in these subjects with normal ventricular function (Fig. 42.3).

These data confirmed our previous views – that very small doses of nitroglycerine have clinically significant effects on muscular conduit arteries. These effects remain at higher doses, but are not linearly increased (Fig. 42.4). Higher doses of nitroglycerine can cause arteriolar dilation and venodilation. The study confirmed our view that the main effect of nitroglycerine is seen at low doses of the drug, and is caused by reduction in wave reflection and on left ventricular afterload.

Non-invasive Study: Effects of Phosphodiesterase 5 (PDE5) Inhibitors

Phosphodiesterase 5 inhibitors act by delaying breakdown of cyclic GMP which is generated by nitric oxide from nitrates. They are widely used in men for treatment of erectile dysfunction, but they do have the effect of increasing action of nitroglycerine, and so of inducing headache and syncope when used together.

We have investigated this drug interaction by studying effects of nitroglycerine patch application in subjects to whom sildenafil or tadalafil had been administered [32]. Findings were of (approximate) doubling of nitrate effect from use of the PDE5 drug. There were no surprises. Findings supported the view that use of the two drugs together is not absolutely contra-indicated, but can be warranted if a sufficiently small dose of nitroglycerine is used, and/or if the drug interaction can be monitored through measurement of central aortic pressure.

Nitrates and Nitric Oxide

The pharmacological action of nitrates are attributable to their conversion to nitric oxide (NO) in the body. Nitric oxide has been identified by Louis Ignarro [33] as the 'endothelially-derived relaxing factor" which has a tonic effect on smooth muscle in blood vessels throughout the body, and helping maintain their normal function. Nitrates can thus be seen as mimicking a normal regulatory function in the body, and so as a unique drug for use when endothelial function is compromised, as it is when endothelium is damaged as by denudation, or when the pathway from endothelial cell (where NO is produced) to site of action (medial smooth muscle cell) is abnormally thickened or diseased – as in the presence of atherosclerosis, or hyperplasia. NO is a volatile gas which is quickly degraded in such passage. NO is also the neurotransmitter of the parasymphathetic nerve supply to penile arteries [34], causing their vasodilation with penile turgidity and erection. Nitrates have no direct effect on erectile dysfunction, probably because the amount of NO released from the orally or transdermally administered drug in the penis is small, compared to that generated through activation by excitation of the penile nerve endings.

Endothelial Function

Study of vascular endothelial properties has led to major advances in drug therapy over the last 40 years, and to Nobel Prizes in 2 years – the first to Vane in 1982 [35] for the discovery of prostaglandins and related biologically related substances, and the second to Furchgott, Murad and Ignarro in 1998 for their work on endothelially-derived relaxing factor as a signalling agent in the endothelium and media of blood vessels. The best summaries of work are the Nobel Prize addresses of these men, posted on the Nobel Prize website [35–38]. Arising from the first cycle of endothelial function study were drugs such as tissue plasminogen activator, used widely now for dissolution of coronary thromboses and treatment of evolving myocardial infarction [39], and for dissolution of cerebral thromboses in evolving non-hemorrhagic stroke [40]. From the later work arose PDE5 inhibitors drugs such as sildenafil and tadalafil for treatment of erectile dysfunction in men [41], and for pulmonary hypertension [42].

Ignarro's contribution [33, 34, 38] was identification of NO as the endothelially-derived relaxing factor which is produced continually by the vascular endothelium, and which diffuses across from endothelial cells lining the blood vessel to the medial coat where it has a tonic effect, causing relaxation of smooth muscle though generation of cyclic GMP. Ignarro explained that clinical problems can result from defective formation of NO in vascular endothelial cells (as when endothelium has been denuded) or when the pathway from site of origin in endothelial cell to site of action in the medial muscle cell has been blocked by disease such as atherosclerosis or intimal hyperplasia. He and others showed that nitrate drugs have their direct action by the breakdown with release of NO in the media and other tissues [38]. The efficacy and unique action of nitrates to which we have previously referred can be attributed to their taking over an action in the body which sustains vascular potency and reactivity, and which is impaired in older persons, and in the presence of endothelial disease such as diabetes and atherosclerosis.

Conclusion

There are few drugs as efficacious in clinical practice as nitroglycerine and the nitrates. There are few drugs that have been used for such a long time (over 130 years). There are few drugs about which so little is known [43]. There are few drugs with actions so well suited for use in ISHE.

Problems in understanding nitrate action stem from their predominant clinical effect of reducing wave reflection. This major therapeutic action is seen in older persons in whom early wave reflection is responsible for boosting (augmenting) pressure in late systole [15, 44], and so inducing ill-effects on the left ventricle (with increased load, hypertrophy, myocardial ischemia, failure) on the large arteries [15], and on the small arteries of the brain and kidneys [44, 45]. The problems in understanding arise from the reduction in wave reflection which alters the relationship between systolic pressure in the aorta, left ventricle and brain, and systolic pressure in the brachial artery, where effects of a drug are traditionally measured [44, 45]. Beneficial effects of nitrates in older persons with early wave reflection (from a stiffened aorta) are not apparent from measurement of cuff brachial arterial pressure, and can only be gauged from measurement of central aortic pressure [10–15]. Ironically, the clue to understanding is contained in the radial pressure tracings recorded in Murrell's 1879s paper, which show evidence of marked reduction in wave reflection.

The most recent papers on nitrate tolerance and nitrate action [7, 43] and virtually all major textbooks (with the exception of Hurst's The Heart) make no mention of wave reflection and its ill-effects on the elderly, nor nitrate action from brachial pressure. One expects this field to expand, and for nitrates to be used more widely, and more confidently, and for analogs with better absorption, less tolerance, and longer duration of action to emerge, when the clue in Murrell's (1879) pulse waveforms is applied [2], and the limits of the cuff sphygmomanometer (introduced in 1896) and of brachial blood pressure are fully recognised [15].

References

1. Yaginuma T, Avolio AP, O'Rourke MF, et al. Effect of glyceryl trinitrate on peripheral arteries alters left ventricular hydraulic load in man. Cardiovasc Res. 1986;20:153–60.
2. Murrell W. Nitroglycerin as a remedy for angina pectoris. Lancet. 1879;80:80–1, 113–5, 51–2, 225–7.
3. O'Rourke MF, Safar ME, Dzau V. Arterial vasodilatation: mechanism and therapy. Philadelphia: Lea and Febiger; 1993. p. 220–3.
4. McGregor M. The nitrates and myocardial ischemia. Circulation. 1982;66:689–92.
5. Feldman RL, Pepine CJ, Conti CR. Magnitude of dilation of large and small coronary arteries by nitroglycerin. Circulation. 1981;64:324–33.
6. Cohn JN, Johnson G, Ziesche S, et al. A comparison of enalapril with hydralazine-isosorbide dinitrate in the treatment of chronic congestive heart failure. N Engl J Med. 1991;325:303–10.
7. Gupta D, Georgiopoulou VV, Kalogeropoulos AP, et al. Nitrate therapy for heart failure. J Am Coll Card Heart Fail. 2013;1:183–91.
8. Jiang XJ, O'Rourke MF, Jin W, et al. Quantification of glyceryl trinitrate effect through analysis of the synthesised ascending aortic pressure waveform. Heart. 2002;88:143–8.
9. Ji W, Jiang X, Liu Y, et al. Pulse wave analysis may be feasible to monitor development of nitrate tolerance. Int J Cardiol 2011;152(S1):S71.
10. Kelly RP, Gibbs HH, O'Rourke MF, et al. Nitroglycerin has more favourable effects on left ventricular afterload than apparent from measurement of pressure in a peripheral artery. Eur Heart J. 1990;11:138–44.
11. Kelly RP, Gibbs H, Morgan J, et al. Brachial artery pressure measurements underestimate beneficial effects of nitroglycerin on left ventricular afterload. J Am Coll Cardiol. 1989;13(2):231A.
12. Takazawa K, Tanaka N, Takeda K, et al. Underestimation of vasodilator effects of nitroglycerin by upper limb blood pressure. Hypertension. 1995;26:520–3.
13. Simkus GJ, Fitchett DH. Radial arterial pressure measurements may be a poor guide to the beneficial effects of nitroprusside on left ventricular systolic pressure in congestive heart failure. Am J Cardiol. 1990;66:323–6.
14. Womersley JR. Oscillatory flow in arteries: the reflection of the pulse wave at junctions and rigid inserts in the arterial system. Phys Med Biol. 1958;2: 313–23.
15. Nichols WW, O'Rourke MF, Vlachopoulos C. McDonald's blood flow in arteries. 6th ed. London: Hodder Arnold; 2011.
16. Kelly R, Hayward C, Ganis J, et al. Non-invasive registration of the arterial pressure pulse waveform using high fidelity applanation tonometry. J Vasc Med Biol. 1989;1:142–9.
17. Kelly R, Karamanoglu M, Gibbs H, et al. Non-invasive carotid pressure wave registration as an indicator of ascending aortic pressure. J Vasc Med Biol. 1989;1:241–7.
18. London GM, Asmar RG, O'Rourke MF, REASON Project Investigators, et al. Mechanism(s) of selective systolic blood pressure reduction after a low-dose combination of perindopril/indapamide in hypertensive subjects: comparison with atenolol. J Am Coll Cardiol. 2004;43:92–9.
19. Williams B, Lacy PS, Thom SM, et al. Differential impact of blood pressure-lowering drugs on central aortic pressure and clinical outcomes. Circulation. 2006;113:1213–25.

20. Matsui Y, Eguchi K, O'Rourke MF, et al. Differential effects between a calcium channel blocker and a diuretic when used in combination with angiotensin II receptor blocker on central aortic pressure in hypertensive patients. Hypertension. 2009;54:716–23.
21. Westerhof N, O'Rourke MF. Haemodynamic basis for the development of left ventricular failure in systolic hypertension and for its logical therapy. J Hypertens. 1995;13:943–52.
22. Uebaba K, O'Rourke MF, Sindone AP, et al. Arterial pulse wave analysis for the assessment of cardiac failure: value of non-invasive applanation tonometry of radial artery. Jpn J Appl Physiol. 2002;32:147–57.
23. Carroll JD, Shroff S, Wirth P, et al. Arterial mechanical properties in dilated cardiomyopathy: aging and the response to nitroprusside. J Clin Invest. 1991;87:1002–9.
24. Miyashita H, Ikeda U, Tsuruya Y, et al. Noninvasive evaluation of the influence of aortic wave reflection on left ventricular ejection during auxotonic contraction. Heart Vessels. 1994;9:30–9.
25. Bensalah MZ, Bollache E, Kachenoura N, et al. Geometry is a major determinant of flow reversal in proximal aorta. Am J Physiol Heart Circ Physiol 2014;306:H1408–16.
26. Kelly R, Fitchett D. Noninvasive determination of aortic input impedance and external left ventricular power output: a validation and repeatability study of a new technique. J Am Coll Cardiol. 1992;20:952–63.
27. Safar ME. Antihypertensive effects of nitrates in chronic human hypertension. J Appl Cardiol. 1990;5:69–81.
28. Fitchett DH, Simkus GJ, Beaudry JP, et al. Reflected pressure waves in the ascending aorta: effect of glyceryl trinitrate. Cardiovasc Res. 1988;22:494–500.
29. Pauca AL, Kon ND, O'Rourke MF. Benefit of glyceryl trinitrate on arterial stiffness is directly due to effects on peripheral arteries. Heart. 2005;91:1428–32.
30. Pauca AL, O'Rourke MF, Kon ND. Prospective evaluation of a method for estimating ascending aortic pressure from the radial artery pressure waveform. Hypertension. 2001;38:932–7.
31. Kelly R, Daley J, Avolio A, et al. Arterial dilation and reduced wave reflection: benefit of dilevanol in hypertension. Hypertension. 1989;14:14–21.
32. O'Rourke MF, Nichols WW. Potential for use of pulse wave analysis in determining the interaction between sildenafil and glyceryl trinitrate. Clin Cardiol. 2002;25: 295–9.
33. Ignarro LJ, Byrns RE, Buga GM, et al. Endothelium derived relaxing factor from pulmonary artery and vein possesses pharmacologic and chemical properties identical to those of nitric oxide radical. Circ Res. 1987;61:866–79.
34. Ignarro LJ, Napoli C, Loscalzo J. Nitric oxide donors and cardiovascular agents modulating the bioactivity of nitric oxide: an overview. Circ Res. 2002;90:21–8.
35. Vane JR. Adventures and excursions in bioassay: the stepping stones to prostacyclin. 1982. www.nobelprize.org/nobel_prizes/medicine/laureates/1982/vane-lecture.html.
36. Furchgott RF. Endothelium-derived relaxing factor: discovery, early studies, and identification as nitric oxide. 1998. www.nobelprize.org/nobel_prizes/medicine/laureates/1998/furchgott-lecture.html.
37. Ignarro LJ. Nitric oxide: a unique endogenous signaling molecule in vascular biology. 1998. www.nobelprize.org/nobel_prizes/medicine/laureates/1998/ignarro-lecture.html.
38. Murad F. Discovery of some of the biological effects of nitric oxide and its role in cell signaling. 1998. www.nobelprize.org/nobel_prizes/medicine/laureates/1998/murad-lecture.html.
39. Cannon CP, McCabe CH, Gibson M, TIMI 10A Investigators, et al. TNK-tissue plasminogen activator in acute myocardial infarction results of the Thrombolysis in Myocardial Infarction (TIMI) 10A dose-ranging trial. Circulation. 1997;95:351–6.
40. Del Zoppo GJ, Poeck K, Pessin MS, et al. Recombinant tissue plasminogen activator in acute thrombotic and embolic stroke. Ann Neurol. 1992;32: 78–86.
41. Goldstein I, Lue TF, Padma-Nathan H, et al. Oral sildenafil in the treatment of erectile dysfunction. Sildenafil Study Group. N Engl J Med. 1998;338:1397–404.
42. Galie N, Ghofrani HA, Torbicki A, Sildenafil Use in Pulmonary Arterial Hypertension (SUPER) Study Group, et al. Sildenafil citrate Therapy for pulmonary arterial hypertension. N Engl J Med. 2005;353:2148–57.
43. Münzel T, Daiber A, Gori T. More answers to the still unresolved question of nitrate tolerance. Eur Heart J. 2013;34:2666–73.
44. O'Rourke MF, Hashimoto J. Mechanical factors in arterial aging. J Am Coll Cardiol. 2007;50:1–13.
45. O'Rourke MF, Safar ME. Relationship between aortic stiffening and microvascular disease in brain and kidney: cause and logic of therapy. Hypertension. 2005;46:200–4.

43 De-stiffening Strategy, Sodium Balance, and Blockade of the Renin–Angiotensin System

Athanase D. Protogerou, Michel E. Safar, Gerard E. Plante, and Jacques Blacher

Abstract

Arterial stiffening, especially of the large elastic arteries, is a fundamental vascular aging trait, which is, however, accelerated in the presence of genetic and environmental factors. It is an early marker of subclinical arterial disease but also a well-established biomarker of clinical cardiovascular disease events and cardiovascular disease mortality. Preventive strategies on the basis of aortic stiffness have been proposed. Efficient de-stiffening strategies are thus of major importance, but specific tools are currently lacking. Sodium balance and blockade of the renin–angiotensin system are among the most important ones, since disturbed homeostasis of these two systems contributes significantly to accelerated arterial stiffening. In this chapter we will present both classical and novel or hypothetical key issues related to the effect of the two systems on the arterial wall and its components. We will also discuss the current treatment strategies that involve (1) the sodium balance, (2) the blockade of the renin–angiotensin system, and (3) their combination. We conclude that the correct sodium balance (either with dietary restriction or the prudent use of diuretics) and mostly the blockade of the renin–angiotensin system are still the

A.D. Protogerou, MD, PhD (✉)
Cardiovascular Research Laboratory and Hypertension Center, First Department of Propedeutic and Internal Medicine, "Laiko" Hospital, Medical School, National and Kapodistrian University of Athens, 17 Ag. Thoma str, Athens 117 25, Greece
e-mail: aprotog@med.uoa.gr

M.E. Safar, MD • J. Blacher, MD, PhD
Department of Medicine, Diagnosis and Therapeutics Center, Hôtel-Dieu Hospital, Assistance Publique des Hôpitaux de Paris, Paris Descartes University, 1, Place du Parvis Notre-Dame, 75181 Paris, France
e-mail: michel.safar@htd.apjp.fr; jacques.blacher@htd.aphp.fr

G.E. Plante
Institut de Pharmacologie, Universitye de Sherbrooke, 3001, 12 eme avenue Nord, J1H5N4 Sherbrooke, QC, Canada
e-mail: gerard.e.plante.@usherbrooke.ca

M.E. Safar et al. (eds.), *Blood Pressure and Arterial Wall Mechanics in Cardiovascular Diseases*, DOI 10.1007/978-1-4471-5198-2_43, © Springer-Verlag London 2014

cornerstones of an effective de-stiffening strategy. However, in the light of novel evidence regarding (1) the potential harmful effect of extreme sodium depletion on the arterial wall and the cardiovascular disease; (2) the modulating role of age, gender, race, inflammation, and impaired metabolism; as well as (3) the gradual emergence of other de-stiffening tools, such as calcium channel blockade and allopurinol, a careful individualized de-stiffening strategy on the basis of sodium balance, in combination with the renin–angiotensin system blockade, appears to be the currently available optimal strategy.

Keywords

Sodium balance • Salt restriction diet • Diuretics • Renin–angiotensin system blockade • Arterial stiffness

Introduction

Large artery rigidity develops in a variety of disorders, in addition to the so-called physiological senescence of the vascular system [1]. Arterial hypertension [1, 2], diabetes mellitus [3] with or without dyslipidemia, chronic renal failure [4], and other systemic diseases have been recognized to be associated with conduit artery rigidity. It is now well established that increased arterial stiffness is associated with elevated cardiovascular mortality and overall mortality in most of these morbid conditions [5]. In some of them, arterial rigidity has even been identified before the classical features of disease development: elevated blood pressure (BP) and blood sugar in hypertensive [6] and diabetic subjects [3], respectively. For these reasons, arterial de-stiffening is a major clinical target in contemporary clinical practice. Acute blood pressure reduction with drug treatment or other strategies is associated with a reduction in several biomarkers that describe the arterial stiffening. However, this is mostly attributed to functional changes due to the decreased distending pressure within the arterial lumen, rather than to structural changes in the arterial wall components. The actual de-stiffening process is a long-term process that includes specific molecular changes taking place within the arterial wall.

Almost half a century ago, the renin–angiotensin system has been shown to play a central role in the physiopathology of arterial hypertension [7], but it is often activated in other comorbidities and especially in insulin resistance states [8]. The identification of the two major angiotensin vascular receptors (AT1R and AT2R) made possible to examine the respective direct and indirect actions of the peptide on the structural and functional components of blood vessels. It has been also well described that sodium balance is important not only for the BP control but also for preserving the arterial function. High dietary sodium intake has adverse effects on the arterial wall [9, 10], often independent of BP effects [11, 12]. The role of the renin–angiotensin system in regulating sodium balance is cardinal, but there is also a close interplay between sodium balance treatment strategies and the blockade of the renin–angiotensin system. As shown by Brunner et al. [13], the plasma renin activity within the physiological levels correlates inversely with the amount of sodium intake in both normotensive and hypertensive individuals. In other words, for any given level of sodium intake, the level of angiotensin fluctuates between the normal limits in order to maintain normal pressure and sodium balance [14]; in this case the pressure elevation to inappropriate levels depends on the circulating intra-arterial fluid volume [14].

In the present chapter we describe several aspects of the de-stiffening process. We focus in the blockade of the renin–angiotensin system on arterial vessels and emphasize the role of sodium balance and some important aspects of the clinical management of renin–angiotensin inhibition.

Blockade of the Renin–Angiotensin System and the Hypertensive Arterial Wall: Old and New Aspects

The structure of large arteries includes the following components: (1) the endothelial cells; (2) the vascular smooth muscle (VSM) cells distributed in three different orientations (circular, oblique, longitudinal); (3) the collagen and elastin fibers; (4) other interstitial environment macromolecules (proteoglycans, fibronectins, integrins, and others) immersed in extracellular fluid, the composition of which is regulated by the local cell populations [15] and the autonomic nerve endings [16]; and (5) the luminal to adventitial microcirculation, i.e., the vasa vasorum. The endothelial cell basement membranes, as well as the highly specialized proteins involved in cell–cell communication between the barrier and the contractile cellular populations, are involved and responsible for intimate relationships within the large artery wall [17].

Each of these parts of the arterial wall may be sensitive to stimulation and blockade of the renin–angiotensin system as well as subjected to modulation by local sodium concentration. Some of these classical as well as some novel aspects are detailed below.

The Old and New Role of Endothelial Cells and the Renin–Angiotensin System

Several experimental studies, performed in renovascular as well as in spontaneous hypertension rats [18–21], have shown that blockade of the renin–angiotensin system increases carotid arterial compliance and distensibility. The finding occurs both under acute and chronic blockades and is observed even in isobaric conditions. The presence of the endothelium is a prerequisite to obtain this effect, as shown in the early 1990s by Levy at al. [22]. Both in untreated normotensive and hypertensive animals, de-endothelialization is associated with an increase of carotid diameter and stiffness [18, 19]. Blockade of the renin–angiotensin system has no effect in such conditions, but the effect is restored in the presence of the endothelium. Such results strongly suggest that, in normotensive and hypertensive animals, (1) the resting carotid diameter in isobaric conditions results from the balance between the respective influence of vasodilating (nitric oxide (NO) and others) and vasoconstrictive (catecholamines, angiotensin II) agents and (2) the blockade of the renin–angiotensin system is responsible for an enhancement of NO bioavailability and/or release [18, 19].

The recently described new role of the endothelial cells involves the endothelial glycocalyx, a network of membrane-bound proteoglycans and glycoproteins covering the endothelium luminally, which although described almost 40 years ago just recently re-attracted the researchers' attention. Data suggest that it is modulated by the renin–angiotensin system, as well as by sodium balance. In the presence of aldosterone and increased extracellular sodium concentration, the endothelial glycocalyx shrinks and becomes stiffer [23]. As a result, sodium overload causes a reduction of the heparan sulfate residue, the endothelial glycocalyx gets destabilized and collapses, and sodium overload shifts the endothelial cells from a sodium release into a sodium-absorbing state. Spironolactone prevents these changes [23]. Thus, the endothelial glycocalyx serves as an effective buffer barrier for sodium; when damaged in the presence of aldosterone, it facilitates sodium entry into the endothelial cells. These observations by the group of Oberleithner et al. provided one more link in the pathway between endothelial dysfunction, arterial hypertension, and increased sodium intake [23].

Under angiotensin blockade, numerous other components of the arterial wall may also interfere, such as the vasa vasorum, the smooth muscle cells, the vascular collagen, and the interstitium.

The Effect on VSM

Studies looking at the contractile response of the VSM cells clearly indicate the expected dose-response constriction induced by angiotensin II, suggesting a predominant net effect on VSM. However, the response profile differs in the aorta, the mesenteric artery, as well as in vein samples measured in vitro, and the phenomenon varies greatly with age in normal rats [24]. However, in most studies in which the response of VSM cells to vasoactive compounds was examined, the classical helicoidal strips of vascular tissue preparation have been utilized. This approach does not allow the evaluation of the different smooth muscle subpopulations. In particular, the eventual contribution of circular subtype of smooth muscle cells to large artery rigidity has not yet been extensively examined [25]. These cells, obtained from spontaneously hypertensive rats, do contract in a prolonged, sustained, and dose-related manner, when thoracic aortic ring preparations are stimulated with bradykinin, as opposed with control tissues obtained from Wistar-Kyoto rats. Surprisingly, the results obtained in already-hypertensive animals (8 and 12 weeks of age) are also documented in rats before elevation of BP (4-week-old). The response is completely and selectively blocked by HOE140, a B2-bradykinin receptor blocker. In contrast, angiotensin II- and phenylephrine-induced contractions are identical in both groups of rats [25]. Further data suggest that the regulation of the arterial distensibility by the angiotensin-converting enzyme inhibition involves the stimulation of B2-bradykinin receptor [26]. The pathophysiological and clinical significance of these results remains to be further explored, but requires some reference to the potential role of bradykinin-related effects of angiotensin-converting enzyme inhibitors, as opposed to AT_1 receptor blockade and their consequence on changes of arterial stiffness. Of note, the role of bradykinin signaling is further implicated in the regulation (decrease) of sodium reabsorption at the level of the aldosterone-sensitive distal nephron – especially under conditions of elevated sodium intake – thus contributing to the natriuretic and antihypertensive effect of the angiotensin-converting enzyme inhibition [27].

Fibers and Interstitial Macromolecular Components

Under chronic blockade of the renin–angiotensin system, two different structural changes may be identified [18–21]. First, the cross-sectional area of the vessel wall is reduced, in parallel with BP reduction. Second, independently of BP changes, a reduction of carotid and aortic collagen content is observed, in association with an increase in distensibility. Such findings, already observed in cell cultures, seem to be exclusively related to angiotensin II blockade of AT1R receptors and do not involve the role of bradykinin. Moreover, in vivo and ex vivo human studies have shown that angiotensin-converting enzyme inhibition increased arterial elasticity, decreased collagen deposition by 50 %, and increased elastin and fibrilin-1 deposition by more than threefold and that the latter effect was mediated via increased fibrillin-1 gene expression [28]; on the other hand, both the gene and protein expressions of metalloproteinases were reduced [28]. An important finding is that collagen reduction is observed only in the presence of normal, but not high-sodium, diet. It is worth noting that high salt intake alone is associated with an increase in the thickness of the arterial wall, a huge development of extracellular matrix, and an increase of vascular stiffness [20, 21]. Furthermore, in the presence of high-sodium diet, carotid and aortic arterial fibronectin is constantly increased. The association of fibronectin with increased specific integrins induces a further enhancement of the attachments between the VSM and the collagen, thus preventing any reduction of arterial stiffness. It is also noticeable that, at the endothelium level, gap junctions also play a role in intercellular coordination. Connexins 37 and 40, as opposed to connexin 30, are highly sensitive to the AT1R blockade by candesartan [17]. The endothelium-derived hyperpolarizing factor might also play an additional role of messenger between the various cellular populations [29]. Just recently, it was shown in animal models that a genetic polymorphism of connexin 40 enhances the sensitivity to intraluminal pressure and increases arterial stiffness by preventing endothelium-derived hyperpolarization during myogenic constriction; thus a new link between the renin–angiotensin system and arterial stiffening is further starting to be elucidated [30].

The interstitial macromolecular composition of large conduit arteries has been extensively examined with respect to different subtypes of collagen. The recent ex vivo studies performed in the normal rabbit thoracic aorta have revealed that elastic fibers of the internal and external laminae are differently oriented in relation to the normal direction of blood flow under stable nonpulsatile flow conditions [31]. For instance, the internal elastic lamina is oriented against the flow direction, as opposed to the parallel orientation of elastic fibers in the external layer [32]. It is possible that the different distribution of stress and strain parameters along the thoracic and abdominal aortic segments, as observed in a normal pig experimental model, could be associated with various orientation profiles according to the local particularities of some interstitial macromolecular components [33]. An interesting aspect is provided by studies on glycosaminoglycans (GAGs), which seem to play a significant role on large artery compliance in the spontaneously hypertensive rat model subjected to a high-sodium diet [33]. The physical characteristics of GAGs, in particular their polyanionic and hydrophilic properties, suggest complex interactions between sodium, renin–angiotensin system, and arterial wall mechanics [34]. Independently of the elastin to collagen ratio, high-sodium diet is associated with low-isobaric systemic compliance together with low-hyaluron content within the carotid and aortic wall. An opposite effect is observed under administration of the diuretic indapamide [33]. Other observations have shown the additional effect of angiotensin II and high-sodium intake on GAGs sulfate incorporation [35]. The results raise the potential opposite, but not necessarily negative and/or deleterious effects, of angiotensin II on the arterial wall, with enhanced smooth muscle contraction and increased elasticity and compliance through changes in GAGs absorbing capacity. It is worthy to note that the impact of conductance artery destruction of swollen GAGs by hyaluronidase was also found to be associated with significant reduction in the measured thickness of the arterial wall obtained in normal mice. The corresponding media/lumen ratio was decreased because of the hyaluronidase-induced effect on media thickness. In such experiments, the calculated changes in arterial stiffness varied clearly in the direction of increased rigidity [35].

Vasa Vasorum

The microcirculatory network of the large conduit arteries (the vasa vasorum) is responsible for approximately two-thirds of the entire vascular wall nutrition [36]. Because the lymphatic circulation is poorly developed in large arteries [37], and because adventitial microcirculation disturbances develop in various systemic vascular disorders, accumulation of foreign molecules transiting from the lumen to the adventitia may interfere with critical muscular and interstitial functions taking place in the media [38]. Unfavorable events for the arterial wall may therefore occur, including alteration in compliance, matrix calcification, and atherogenesis [39]. The vasa vasorum contains receptors for potent vasoactive autacoids and hormones, including angiotensin, bradykinin, and endothelin. In young spontaneously hypertensive rats, a moderately high-salt diet leads to blood vessel hypertrophy and hypertension, and this is possibly mediated by angiotensin II within the vasa vasorum [40].

Additional structural and functional characteristics that could be responsible for increased large artery rigidity must also be carefully examined in relation to the renin–angiotensin system. Hyperuricemia has recently been reevaluated as a potential source of vascular damage in hypertensive subjects [41]. A large number of clinical observations indicate that hyperuricemia now represents a significant cardiovascular risk factor, more important in female than in male populations. Using a uricase inhibitor to reproduce a rat model of hyperuricemia, Johnson and coworkers [42] were able to show a direct toxic effect of uric acid on different renal vascular segments, from the interlobar to arciform, interlobular, and even afferent arterioles. These blood vessels in vivo exposed to hyperuricemia develop a clear hypertrophy of the media. More recent data showed that uric acid concentration is an independent predictor of arterial stiffness, particularly in women [43, 44]. Of note, experimental increase in uric acid was associated with increased plasma renin activity, plasma aldosterone, and urine K to Na ratio [45]. Structural changes are prevented by reducing serum uric acid levels, either by synthesis inhibition, using allopurinol, or by increasing urinary uric acid excretion with probenecid. These findings were verified by more recent studies that showed significant improvement in arterial and heart function and structure after treatment with allopurinol [46]. The question raised by the eventual vasculotoxic actions of uric acid could represent a central axis in terms of hypertensive target organ damage. Obesity, type I and type II diabetes mellitus, and serum lipid abnormalities are all associated with hyperuricemia [47, 48]. Interestingly, the antagonist of the angiotensin II AT1R receptor, losartan, is able to reduce hyperuricemia. However, to our knowledge, there is no interventional study showing that the reduction of uric acid is associated with the reduction of cardiovascular events.

Blockade of the Renin–Angiotensin System and Clinical Management of Large Artery Stiffness

Theoretically, the clinical management of arterial hypertension should start with measures able to identify early detection of the arterial dysfunction/remodeling [49]. The development of methods capable of picking up early large artery stiffening rigidity, such as increased pulse wave velocity or disturbed wave reflections [50], is now well documented in elderly patients with isolated systolic hypertension [51] and in young subjects with positive family history, with or without borderline hypertension [52], and now represents interesting opportunities. Lifestyle modification, such as physical exercise performed by normal male and female subjects, has been shown to produce changes in arterial stiffness, even before hypertension develops [53], and thus represents a recommended prevention strategy.

Several randomized and double-blind studies have shown that, with pharmacological agents modulating the renin–angiotensin–aldosterone system, three major changes in large arteries may be observed in the long term: (1) large artery stiffness can be reduced independently of BP changes (see reviews in references [18, 54–56]), (2) carotid and aortic wave reflections are constantly delayed and/or attenuated [55], and mostly (3) systolic and pulse pressure (PP) are reduced more in central than in peripheral arteries [57, 58]. Indeed, a recent extensive review of the available literature showed that in 10 out of the 15 reviewed studies, the blockade of the renin–angiotensin system resulted in an increase in PP amplification, mostly due to reduced wave reflections but also due to reduction in arterial stiffness [59]. The related available data regarding the inhibition of the angiotensin-converting enzyme are particularly abundant [59] and recently replicated in a meta-analysis and meta-regression analysis [60]. The latter meta-analysis provided more evidence on the role of renin–angiotensin system blockade. The angiotensin-converting enzyme inhibition significantly improved arterial stiffness and wave reflections compared to placebo. While the reduction in pressure wave reflections was mediated by BP reduction, on the contrary the improvement in arterial rigidity was independent from pressure reduction [60]. The same conclusion reached another meta-analysis suggesting that pulse wave velocity after angiotensin-converting enzyme inhibition decreases independently from BP reduction in both short-term and long-term (>4 months) follow-up [61]. Conclusions regarding the comparison of angiotensin-converting enzyme inhibition vs. the angiotensin II blockade, and the role of bradykinin, cannot be drawn due to the lack of sufficient data [60, 61].

Sodium Balance Strategies and Clinical Management of Large Artery Stiffness

Control of the external and/or internal sodium balance can be achieved by non-pharmacological dietary measures, as well as by pharmacological treatment, such as the thiazide or thiazide-like diuretics which are capable of maintaining the external sodium homeostasis through renal actions (aldosterone antagonists are specifically studied in a separate chapter of this book). We have previously proposed the hypothesis that in the middle age, thiazide diuretics do not reduce isobaric arterial stiffness, probably as a conse-

Table 43.1 Arterial changes following hydrochlorothiazide vs. felodipine in subjects with essential hypertension of middle age [62]

	Baseline	Felodipine	HCTZ	Felodipine vs. HCTZ
Systolic blood pressure (mmHg)	162 ± 12	140 ± 17	150 ± 13	<0.02
Diastolic blood pressure (mmHg)	96 ± 9	85 ± 9	89 ± 9	<0.05
CF-PWV (m/s)	10.9 ± 2.0	9.2 ± 1.8	10.1 ± 2	<0.005
FT-PWV (m/s)	12.8 ± 1.7	11.1 ± 1.9	12.2 ± 1.7	<0.005
CR-PWV (m/s)	11.7 ± 1.9	10.0 ± 2	11.8 ± 1.8	<0.005
Brachial arterial diameter (cm)	0.437 ± 0.06	0.449 ± 0.06	0.431 ± 0.05	<0.05
Brachial vascular resistance (dyne s/cm^4)	104 ± 40	72 ± 30	92 ± 46	0.05
Brachial artery compliance (dyne/cnrr/10^7)	1.13 ± 0.48	1.71 ± 0.83	1.19 ± 0.57	0.005

PWV pulse wave velocity, *CF* carotid femoral, *FT* foot tibial, *CR* carotid radial

quence of the associated extreme activation of the renin–angiotensin system secondary to salt and water depletion (Table 43.1) [62]. In the elderly subjects, diuretics might be able to reduce arterial stiffness because the response of the renin–angiotensin system is attenuated [19, 20]. In old populations, diuretics are indeed very efficient to reduce selectively systolic BP and PP [2, 19, 20, 54]; yet, the presence of increased salt sensitivity in the elderly and the ability of diuretics to reduce BP and stiffness are expected to be also modulated by the degree of lost functional nephrons. The overall published data on the basis of monotherapy with thiazide or thiazide-like diuretics have shown conflicting results regarding their ability to reduce arterial stiffness (both positive [63, 64] and negative data exist [65–67]). These conflicting data can be related to the different methodologies, to the duration of treatment, and mainly to the existing differences between diuretics. It might also be related with the hypothesis of extreme sodium depletion of the arterial wall due to diuretic drug treatment.

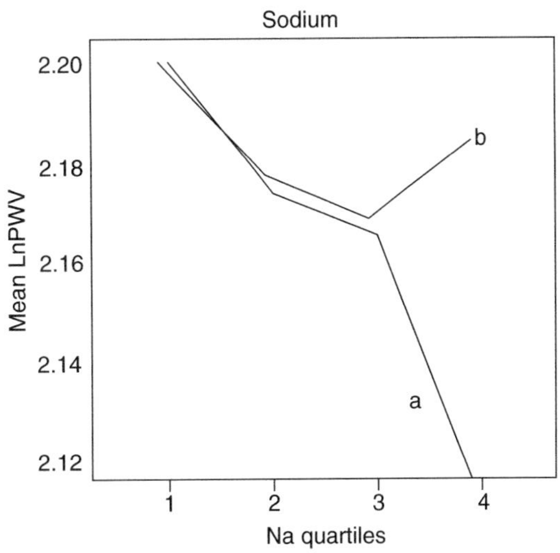

Fig. 43.1 Relationship of sodium intake grouped by quartiles with arterial stiffness, assessed by pulse wave velocity (*PWV*) and expressed as lnPWV. *Line a* unadjusted; *line b* adjusted for age, gender, smoking status, ethanol intake, total energy intake, systolic 24 h blood pressure, antihypertensive medications, antidiabetic medications, and lipid-lowering drugs (Reprinted from [68] with permission from Elsevier)

On the other hand, it was just recently shown in a randomized crossover study that in a population with mean age 62 years the dietary sodium restriction strategies (low sodium (1,200 mg/day) compared to normal sodium intake (3,600 mg/day)) [10] reversed endothelial function (at the level of both the micro- and macrocirculation), as well as arterial stiffness (assessed by PP). This effect was mediated by improved oxidative status, and the effect on the arterial wall was independent from pressure reduction. Moreover, the same group [9], almost a decade ago, showed in a similar experiment that in older adults (age >64 years) both office and ambulatory systolic BP as well as carotid stiffness were significantly and progressively reduced over a period of 4 weeks in the low sodium state but not in the normal sodium state. Most importantly, in line with the hypothesis of extreme sodium depletion and the activation of the renin–angiotensin system, a J-curve association between sodium intake and pulse wave velocity was described (Fig. 43.1) [68]. This observation also strengthens the proposed hypothesis regarding the presence of a J-curve association between dietary sodium and cardiovascular disease [69], which has been supported by several recent findings from epidemiologic studies [70], meta-analysis [71], and clinical trials [72].

Finally evidence regarding the role of race and genetic predisposition exists; it was recently shown that a modest reduction in salt intake, approximately the amount of the current public health recommendations, leads to reduction in BP and urinary albumin/creatinine ratio in whites, blacks, and Asians, but the decrease in pulse wave velocity was significant only in blacks [73]. All the above data suggest that a balanced and judiciously individualized dietary sodium restriction or drug-induced reduction strategy may be more appropriate.

Combination of Sodium Balance Strategies and Blockade of the Renin–Angiotensin System and Clinical Management of Large Artery Stiffness

The combination of pharmacological treatment involving both diuretics and renin–angiotensin blockade is a well-established strategy for the effective reduction of systolic BP and PP. There are also convincing evidences regarding the ability of this combination to reduce efficiently central hemodynamics including aortic stiffness, wave reflections, and aortic BP [74]. The potential superiority of the angiotensin-converting enzyme inhibition over other classical antihypertensive drugs is difficult to be established due to the lack of well-designed studies; however, there are related evidences both for central stiffness and mostly for pressure wave reflections (augmentation index) [60]. Similarly, there are no sufficient data to conclude regarding the superiority of the combined effect of diuretics/angiotensin-converting enzyme inhibition over other combination treatments [60]. Moreover, there are no data regarding the effect of the combination of dietary sodium restriction with angiotensin-converting enzyme inhibition on arterial stiffness.

However a recent study suggested that a more modern combination including blockade of the renin–angiotensin system (AT2R blockade) and calcium channel blockade may have a better impact on central arterial properties, including both aortic stiffness and BP vs. the classical combination with diuretics [75]. These data are in line with the outcome of the Accomplish clinical trial in nonobese individuals [76] which demonstrated greater capacity of the combination of angiotensin-converting enzyme inhibition with amlodipine, rather than with hydrochlorothiazide, in reducing cardiovascular events in patients with hypertension who were at high risk for such events.

The newly raised hypothesis [77] that patients with high on-treatment plasma renin activity (PRA) levels die sooner of cardiovascular events because they are excessively sodium volume depleted challenges the uncritical use of the diuretics/renin–angiotensin system blockade combination since it can induce such high PRA levels which is evidence of sodium depletion [77]. However, this critical question remains largely unanswered and requires specifically design trials with different dosages of treatment regiments. Other important issues which need to be addressed in order to further elucidate this topic include the matter of optimal timing of treatment strategies, e.g., before the development of irreversible arterial stiffening or the establishment of renal damage. In the same line of thinking, not only body mass as previously discussed but also aging and race may be an important modulator of the optimal de-stiffening strategy, particularly since differences exist in terms of salt sensitivity. Last but not least, the impact of dietary intake of nutrients beyond sodium, such as potassium, has to be taken into account in future studies.

Conclusion

In the present chapter we examined classical and novel key issues related to the effect of the sodium balance and of the renin–angiotensin system blockade and showed that they both interact and affect most components of the arterial wall. We did not discuss other specific de-stiffening strategies that involve inflammation or metabolism since it will be discussed in other chapters. We focused on the current treatment strategies that involve (1) the sodium balance, (2) the blockade of the renin–angiotensin system, and (3) their combination. We conclude that the correct sodium balance (with either dietary restriction or prudent use of diuretics) and mostly the blockade of the renin–angiotensin system are still the cornerstones of an effective de-stiffening strategy. However, in the light of novel evidence regarding (1) the potential harmful effect of extreme sodium depletion on the arterial wall and the cardiovascular disease; (2) the modulating role of age, gender, race, inflammation, and impaired metabolism; as well as (3) the gradual emergence of other de-stiffening tools, such as calcium channel blockade and allopurinol, a careful individualized de-stiffening strategy on the basis of sodium balance in combination with the renin–angiotensin system blockade appears to be the currently available optimal strategy.

References

1. Benetos A, Laurent S, Hoeks AP, Boutouyrie P, Safar ME. Arterial alterations with aging and high blood pressure. A noninvasive study of carotid and femoral artery. Arterioscler Thromb. 1993;13:90–7.
2. Benetos A, Asmar R, Gautier S, Salvi P, Safar ME. Heterogeneity of the arterial tree in essential hypertension: a noninvasive study of the terminal aorta and the common carotid artery. J Hum Hypertens. 1994;8:501–7.
3. Plante GE, Alfred J, Chakir M. The blood vessel, linchpin of diabetic lesions. Metabolism. 1999;48:406–9.
4. Amar J, Chamontin B, Vernier I, Lenfant V, Conte J, Salvador M. Arterial blood pressure changes, circadian rhythm and arterial elasticity in hemodialysed patients. Arch Mal Coeur Vaiss. 1994;87:921–4.
5. Vlachopoulos C, Aznaouridis K, Stefanadis C. Prediction of cardiovascular events and all-cause mortality with arterial stiffness: a systematic review and meta-analysis. J Am Coll Cardiol. 2010;55:1318–27.
6. Girerd X, Chanudet X, Larroque P, Clement R, Laloux B, Safar ME. Early arterial modifications in young patients with borderline hypertension. J Hypertens Suppl. 1989;7 Suppl 1:S45–7.
7. Vane JR. The history of inhibitors of angiotensin converting enzyme. In: D' Orleans-Juste P, Plante GE, editors. ACE inhibitors. Basel/Boston: Birkhauser Verlag; 2001. p. 1–10.
8. Zhou MS, Schulman IH, Zeng Q. Link between the renin-angiotensin system and insulin resistance: implications for cardiovascular disease. Vasc Med. 2012;17:330–41.
9. Gates PE, Tanaka H, Hiatt WR, Seals DR. Dietary sodium restriction rapidly improves large elastic artery compliance in older adults with systolic hypertension. Hypertension. 2004;44:35–41.
10. Jablonski KL, Racine ML, Geolfos CJ, Gates PE, Chonchol M, McQueen MB, Seals DR. Dietary sodium restriction reverses vascular endothelial dysfunction in middle-aged/older adults with moderately elevated systolic blood pressure. J Am Coll Cardiol. 2013;61:335–43.
11. Frohlich ED. The salt conundrum: a hypothesis. Hypertension. 2007;50:161–6.
12. Dickinson KM, Clifton PM, Keogh JB. Endothelial function is impaired after a high-salt meal in healthy subjects. Am J Clin Nutr. 2011;93:500–5.
13. Brunner HR, Larahg JH, Baer L, et al. Essential hypertension: renin and aldosterone, heart attack and stroke. N Engl J Med. 1972;286:41–449.
14. DeClue JW, Guyton AC, Cowley Jr AW, et al. Subpressor angiotensin infusion, renal sodium handling, and salt-induced hypertension in the dog. Circ Res. 1978;43:503–12.
15. Comper WD, Laurent TC. Physiological function of connective tissue polysaccharides. Physiol Rev. 1978;58:255–315.
16. Siche JP, Chevallier M, Tremel F, De Gaudemaris R, Boutelant S, Comparat V, et al. Baroreflex sensitivity and vascular involvement in hypertension. Arch Mal Coeur Vaiss. 1995;88:1243–6.
17. Ko YS, Coppen SR, Dupont E, Rotherv S, Severs NJ. Regional differentiation of desmin, connexin 43, and connexin 45 expression patterns in rat aortic smooth muscle. Arterioscler Thromb Vasc Biol. 2001;21:355–64.
18. Safar ME, Van Bortel L, Struijker-Boudier H. Resistance and conduit arteries following converting enzyme inhibition in hypertension. Vasc Res. 1997;81:67–81.
19. Safar ME, Struijker Boudier HA], Van Bortel MAB, London GM. Arterial structure and function and blockade of the renin-angiotensin system in hypertension. In: D'Orleans-Juste P, Plante GE, editors. ACE inhibitors. Basel/Boston: Birkhauser Verlag; 2001. p. 81–128.
20. Safar ME, Thuillez CH, Richard V, Benetos A. Pressure-independent contribution of sodium to large artery structure and function in hypertension. Cardiovasc Res. 2000;46:269–76.
21. Safar ME, Benetos A. Factors influencing arterial stiffness in systolic hypertension in the elderly: role of sodium and the renin-angiotensin system. Am J Hypertens. 2003;16:249–58.
22. Levy BI, Benessiano J, Poitevin P, Safar ME. Endothelium-dependent mechanical properties of the carotid artery in WKY and SHR. Role of

angiotensin converting enzyme inhibition. Circ Res. 1990;66:321–8.
23. Oberleithner H, Peters W, Kusche-Vihrog K, Korte S, Schillers H, Kliche K, Oberleithner K. Salt overload damages the glycocalyx sodium barrier of vascular endothelium. Pflugers Arch. 2011;462:519–28.
24. Mulvany MJ, Aalkjaer C. Structure and function of small arteries. Physiol Rev. 1990;70:921–61.
25. Et-Taouil K, Regoli D, Plante GE. A bradykinin B,-receptor dependent smooth muscle event precedes elevation of blood pressure in the spontaneously hypertensive rats. Hypertens. 2004;22 Suppl 2:S200.
26. Aartsen WM, Hilgers HRP, Schiffers PMH, Daemen MJAP, De May JGR, Smits JFM. Changes in vascular distensibility during angiotensin converting enzyme inhibition involve bradykinin type 2 receptors. J Vasc Res. 2004;41:18–27.
27. Mamenko M, Zaiki O, Doris PA, Pochynyuk O. Salt-dependent inhibition of epithelial Na channel-mediated sodium reabsorption in the aldosterone–sensitive distal nephron by bradykinin. Hypertension. 2012;60:1234–41.
28. Ahimastos A, Natoli AK, Lawler A, Blombery PA, Kingwell BA. Ramipril reduces large artery stiffness in peripheral arterial disease and promotes elastogenic remodeling in cell culture. Hypertension. 2005;45:94-1194-1199.
29. Mombouli JV, Bissiriou I, Agboton VD, Vanhoutte PM. Bioassay of endothelium-derived hyperpolarizing factor. Biochem Bioplys Res Commun. 1996;221:484–8.
30. Chaston DJ, Baillie BK, Courjaret RJ, Heisler JM, Lau KA, Machca K, Nicholson BJ, Asthon A, Matthaei KI, Hill CE. Polymorphisms in endothelial connexin 40 enhances sensitivity to intraluminal pressure and increased arterial stiffness. Arterioscler Thromb Vasc Biol. 2013;33:962–70.
31. Farand P, Garon A, Plante GE. Modelisation et etude de la structure, de la rigidite et de la permeabilite des gros troncs arteriels. Arch Mal Coeur Vaiss. 2004;97 Suppl 4:42–6.
32. Womersley JR. Oscillatory flow in arteries: the reflection of the pulse wave at junctions and rigid inserts in the arterial system. Phys Med Biol. 1958;2:213–23.
33. Et-Taouil K, Schiavi P, Levy BI, Plante GE. Sodium intake, large artery stiffness and proteoglycans in the SHR. Hypertension. 2001;38:1172–6.
34. Titze J, Shakibaei M, Schafflhuber M, Schulze-Tanzil G, Porst M, Schwind KH, et al. Glycosaminoglycan polymerization may enable osmotically inactive Na+ storage in the skin. Am J Physiol Heart Circ Physiol. 2004;287(1):H203–8.
35. Intengan HD, Schiffrin EL. Structure and mechanical properties of resistance arteries in hypertension. Role of adhesion molecules and extracellular matrix determinants. Hypertension. 2000;36:312–8.
36. Heistad DD, Marcus ML, Law EG, Armstrong ML, Ehrhardt JC, Abboud FM. Regulation of blood flow to the aortic media in dogs. J Clin Invest. 1978;62:133–40.
37. Simionescu N. Cellular aspects of transcapillary exchanges. Physiol Rev. 1983;63:1536–617.
38. Belmin J, Corrnan B, Merval R, Tedgui A. Age-related changes in endothelial permeability and distribution volume of albumin in rat aorta. Am J Physiol. 1993;264:H679–85.
39. Scotland R, Vallance P, Ahluwalia A. Endothelin alters the reactivity of vasa vasorum: mechanisms and implications for conduit vessel physiology and pathophysiology. Br J Pharmacol. 1999;128:1229–34.
40. Gould AB, Goodman SA. Effect of a renin-system inhibitor on blood-vessel adaptation in spontaneously hypertensive rats. J Hypertens Suppl. 1987;5:S53–8.
41. Johnson RJ, Feig D, Herrera-Acosta J, Kang DH. Resurrection of uric acid as a causal risk factor in essential hypertension. Hypertension. 2005;45:18–20.
42. Kang DH, Nakagawa T, Feng L, Watanabe S, Han L, Mazzali M, et al. A role for uric acid in the progression of renal disease. J Am Soc Nephrol. 2002;13:2888–97.
43. Bian S, Guo H, Ye P, Luo L, Wu H, Xiao W. Serum uric Acid level and diverse impacts on regional arterial stiffness and wave reflection. Iran J Public Health. 2012;41:33–41.
44. Ishizaka N, Ishizaka Y, Toda E, Hashimoto H, Nagai R, Yamakado M. Higher serum uric acid is associated with increased arterial stiffness in Japanese individuals. Atherosclerosis. 2007;192:131–7.
45. Eräranta A, Kurra V, Tahvanainen AM, Vehmas TI, Kööbi P, Lakkisto P, Tikkanen I, Niemelä OJ, Mustonen JT, Pörsti IH. Oxonic acid-induced hyperuricemia elevates plasma aldosterone in experimental renal insufficiency. J Hypertens. 2008;26:1661–8.
46. Rekhraj S, Gandy SJ, Szwejkowski BR, Nadir MA, Noman A, Houston JG, Lang CC, George J, Struthers AD. High-dose allopurinol reduces left ventricular mass in patients with ischemic heart disease. J Am Coll Cardiol. 2013;61:926–32.
47. Plante GE, Durivage J, Lemieux G. Renal excretion of hydrogen in primary gout. Metabolism. 1968;17:377–82.
48. Gutman AB, Yu TF. Gout: a derangement of purine metabolism. Adv Intern Med. 1952;5:227–302.
49. Plante GE, Bissonnette M, Sirois MG, Regoli D, Sirois P. Renal permeability alteration precedes hypertension and involves bradykinin in the spontaneously hypertensive rat. J Clin Invest. 1992;89:2030–4.
50. Kawasaki T, Sasayama S, Yagi SI, Asakawa T, Hirai T. Non-invasive assessment of age related changes in stiffness of the human arteries. Cardiovasc Res. 1987;21:678–87.
51. Simon AC, Levenson JA, Bouthier JA, Safar ME, Avolio AO. Evidence of early degenerative changes in large arteries in human essential hypertension. Hypertension. 1985;7(5):675–80.
52. Lantelme P, Milon H, Gharib C, Gayet C, Fortrat JO. White coat effect and reactivity to stress: cardiovascular and autonomic nervous system responses. Hypertension. 1998;31(4):1021–9.
53. Siche JP, Mansour P, De Gaudemaris R, Mallion JM. Arterial compliance during exercise in hypertensive and normal subjects of the same age. Arch Mal Coeur Vaiss. 1989;82(7):1077–82.

54. Van Bortel LM, Struijker-Boudier HA, Safar ME. Pulse pressure, arterial stiffness, and drug treatment of hypertension. Hypertension. 2001;38:914–21.
55. Lacourciere Y, Beliveau R, Conter HS, Burgess ED, Lepage S, Pesant Y, et al. Effects of perindopril on elastic and structural properties of large arteries in essential hypertension. Can J Cardiol. 2004;20:795–9.
56. London GM, Asmar RG, O'Rourke MF, Safar ME, REASON Project Investigators. Mechanism(s) of selective systolic blood pressure reduction after a low-dose combination of perindopril/indapamide in hypertensive subjects: comparison with atenolol. J Am Coll Cardiol. 2004;43:92–9.
57. Hirata K, Vlachopoulos C, Adji A, O'Rourke MF. Benefits from angiotensin-converting enzyme inhibitor 'beyond blood pressure lowering': beyond blood pressure or beyond the brachial artery. J Hypertens. 2005;23:5551–6.
58. Mitchell GF, Izzo JL, Lacourciere Y, Ouellet JP, Neutel J, Qian C, et al. Omapatrilat reduces pulse pressure and proximal aortic stiffness in patients with systolic hypertension. Results of the conduit hemodynamics of omapatrilat international research study. Circulation. 2002;105:2955–61.
59. Protogerou AD, Stergiou GS, Vlachopoulos C, Blacher J, Achimastos A. The effect of antihypertensive drugs on central blood pressure beyond peripheral blood pressure. Part II: Evidence for specific class-effects of antihypertensive drugs on pressure amplification. Curr Pharm Des. 2009;15:245–53.
60. Shahin Y, Khan JA, Chetter I. Angiotensin converting enzyme inhibitors effect on arterial stiffness and wave reflections: a meta-analysis and meta-regression of randomized controlled trials. Atherosclerosis. 2012;221:18–33.
61. Ong KT, Delerme S, Pannier B, Safar ME, Benetos A, Laurent S, Boutouyrie P. Aortic stiffness is reduced beyond blood pressure lowering by short term and long term antihypertensive treatment: a meta-analysis of individual data in 294 patients. J Hypertens. 2011;29:1034–42.
62. Asmar R, Benetos A, Chaouche-Teyara K, Raveau-Landon C, Safar M. Comparison of effects of felodipine versus hydrochlorothiazide on arterial diameter and pulse-wave velocity in essential hypertension. Am J Cardiol. 1993;72:794–8.
63. Bénétos A, Laflèche A, Asmar R, Gautier S, Safar A, Safar ME. Arterial stiffness, hydrochlorothiazide and converting enzyme inhibition in essential hypertension. J Hum Hypertens. 1996;10:77–82.
64. Spoelstra-de Man AM, van Ittersum FJ, Schram MT, Kamp O, van Dijk RA, Ijzerman RG, Twisk JW, Brouwer CB, Stehouwer CD. Aggressive antihypertensive strategies based on hydrochlorothiazide, candesartan or lisinopril decrease left ventricular mass and improve arterial compliance in patients with type II diabetes mellitus and hypertension. J Hum Hypertens. 2006;20:599–611.
65. Mahmud A, Feely J. Effect of angiotensin ii receptor blockade on arterial stiffness: beyond blood pressure reduction. Am J Hypertens. 2002;15:1092–5.
66. Mackenzie IS, McEniery CM, Dhakam Z, Brown MJ, Cockcroft JR, Wilkinson IB. Comparison of the effects of antihypertensive agents on central blood pressure and arterial stiffness in isolated systolic hypertension. Hypertension. 2009;54: 409–13.
67. Agnoletti D, Zhang Y, Borghi C, Blacher J, Safar ME. Effects of antihypertensive drugs on central blood pressure in humans: a preliminary observation. Am J Hypertens. 2013;26:1045–52.
68. García-Ortiz L, Recio-Rodríguez JI, Rodríguez-Sánchez E, Patino-Alonso MC, Agudo-Conde C, Rodríguez-Martín C, Castaño-Sánchez C, Runkle I, Gómez-Marcos MA. Sodium and potassium intake present a J-shaped relationship with arterial stiffness and carotid intima-media thickness. Atherosclerosis. 2012;225:497–503.
69. Alderman MH. Presidential address: 21st scientific meeting of international hypertension: dietary sodium and cardiovascular disease: the "J"-shaped relation. J Hypertens. 2011;75:903–7.
70. Cohen H, Hailpern S, Fang J, et al. Sodium intake and mortality in the NHANES II follow-up study. Am J Med. 2006;1191:275e14.
71. Taylor RS, Ashton KE, Moxham T, et al. Reduced dietary salt for the prevention of cardiovascular disease: a meta-analysis of randomized controlled trials (Cochrane review). Am J Hypertens. 2011;24: 843–53.
72. O'Donnell MJ, Yusuf S, Mente A, et al. Urinary sodium and potassium excretion and risk of cardiovascular events. JAMA. 2011;306:2229–38.
73. He FJ, Marciniak M, Visagie E, Markandu ND, Anand V, Dalton RN, MacGregor GA. Salt reduction on blood pressure, urinary albumin, and pulse wave velocity in white, black, and asian mild hypertensives. Hypertension. 2009;54:482.
74. Asmar RG, London GM, O'Rourke ME, Safar ME, REASON Project Coordinators and Investigators. Improvement in blood pressure, arterial stiffness and wave reflections with a very-low-dose perindopril/indapamide combination in hypertensive patient: a comparison with atenolol. Hypertension. 2001;38:922–6.
75. Matsui Y, Eguchi K, O'Rourke MF, Ishikawa J, Miyashita H, Shimada K, Kario K. Differential effects between a calcium channel blocker and a diuretic when used in combination with angiotensin II receptor blocker on central aortic pressure in hypertensive patients. Hypertension. 2009;54:716–23.
76. Weber MA, Jamerson K, Bakris GL, Wier MR, ZAppe D, Zhang Y, Dalhof B, Velazquez EJ, Pitt B. Effects of body size and hypertension treatments on cardiovascular events rates: subanalysis of the ACCOMPLISH randomized controlled trial. Lancet. 2013;381:537–45.
77. Sealey JE, Alderman MH, Furberg CD, Laragh JH. Renin-angiotensin system blockers may create more risk than reward for sodium-depleted cardiovascular patients with high plasma renin levels. Am J Hypertens. 2013;26:727–38.

Long-Term Effects of Calcium Channel Blockers on Central and Peripheral Arteries

44

Yoshio Matsui and Michael F. O'Rourke

Abstract

Calcium channel blockers (CCBs) are reported to be more effective in reducing cerebrovascular events than other antihypertensive drugs in hypertensive patients. Large artery stiffness could be partly reduced through the reduction of the distending pressure and arterial structural changes by long-term treatment with CCBs. Because CCBs reduce the magnitude of wave reflection by attenuating the vascular tone of peripheral muscular arteries, CCBs cause a greater fall in the central aortic pressure than did β-blockers or diuretics, despite no difference in peripheral (brachial) pressure. The de-stiffening of the large arteries and the dilation of peripheral muscular arteries by CCBs might be underlying mechanisms of the significant reductions in central pressure and blood pressure variability, thus reducing carotid atherosclerosis, cerebral arteriosclerotic damage, and cerebrovascular events in hypertensive patients.

Keywords

Arteriosclerosis • Augmentation index • Blood pressure variability • Calcium channel blockers • Central aortic pressure • Large artery stiffness • Muscular arteries • Pulse wave velocity • Wave reflection

Introduction

Several large clinical trials have shown that dihydropyridine (DHP)-calcium channel blockers (CCBs) are as effective in reducing brachial blood pressure (BP) and cardiovascular events as other classes of antihypertensive drugs when administered as monotherapy or part of combination therapy in both low- and high-risk hypertensive patients [1–6]. In particular, DHP-CCBs were reported to reduce the risk of stroke in comparison to angiotensin-converting enzyme inhibitors

Y. Matsui, MD, PhD (✉)
Division of Cardiovascular Medicine, Department of Medicine, Jichi Medical University School of Medicine, 3311-1 Yakushiji, Shimotsuke, Tochigi 329-0498, Japan

Department of Internal Medicine, Iwakuni Medical Center, 3-6-12 Muronoki, Iwakuni, Yamaguchi 740-0021, Japan
e-mail: yoshio@jichi.ac.jp

M.F. O'Rourke, MD, DSc
Department of Cardiovascular and Hypertension, St Vincent's Clinic, University of New South Wales, Victor Chang Cardiac Research Institute, Suite 810 St Vincent Clinic, 438 Victoria Street, Darlinghurst, Sydney, NSW 2010, Australia
e-mail: m.orourke@unsw.edu.au

M.E. Safar et al. (eds.), *Blood Pressure and Arterial Wall Mechanics in Cardiovascular Diseases*, DOI 10.1007/978-1-4471-5198-2_44, © Springer-Verlag London 2014

(ACE-Is) [7]. DHP-CCBs also have been shown in large clinical trials to reduce morbidity and mortality in patients with isolated systolic hypertension (ISH), a condition in which wide pulse pressure (PP) and early wave reflection result from excessive large artery stiffness [1].

These clinical trials suggest that DHP-CCBs may have vasculo-protective actions beyond simply lowering brachial BP. The therapeutic benefits of DHP-CCBs on arteries consist of two major effects: the effects due to sustained BP lowering and the direct effects of CCBs on the arterial wall. Arteries are of three types: the large central, predominantly elastic conduit arteries, including aorta and carotid arteries, the smaller peripheral muscular conduit arteries, such as the brachial, radial and femoral arteries; and the smallest pre-arteriolar arteries, which are entirely muscular. The therapeutic target of CCBs in these arteries would be the elastic properties of the muscular arteries, which are modified by smooth muscle tone, resulting in more distensible arteries with their vasodilation.

This chapter focuses on the long-term effects of DHP-CCBs on the properties of central elastic arteries and those of peripheral muscular arteries in hypertensive patients. Long-term studies (>12 weeks) are more meaningful because hypertension is a chronic disease and acute effects may not predict chronic efficacy because of counter-regulatory mechanism (i.e. the activation of the renin–angiotensin and/or sympathetic nervous systems).

CCB and Large Artery Stiffness

Part of large artery stiffness could be reduced through the reduction of the distending pressure by CCBs, and further reduction of arterial stiffness would require arterial structural changes obtained through long-lasting BP normalization [8]. The effects of CCBs on the large artery stiffness are determined by their actions on endothelial function, smooth muscle cells proliferation, collagen/elastin ratio, extracellular matrix composition, oxidative stress, inflammation, and baroreflex mechanism. It has not been unequivocally shown that long-term drug administration of CCBs can modify these wall components at the site of proximal elastic large arteries. A decreased nitric oxide production from endothelium is involved in the development of structural alterations in large elastic arteries, including changes in the mechanical properties [9]. It is generally known that DHP-CCBs improve vascular endothelial dysfunction; therefore, the NO-mediated effects of DHP-CCBs might theoretically lead to a reversal of endothelial dysfunction and to a decrease of large artery stiffness.

At present, the gold standard for evaluating large artery stiffness in clinical practice is the aortic pulse wave velocity (PWV), assessed by carotid-femoral PWV. Because aortic PWV was shown to be an independent predictor of cardiovascular mortality in hypertensive patients [10], large arterial stiffness assessed by measuring aortic PWV is increasingly recognized as a surrogate endpoint of cardiovascular risk during antihypertensive treatment. After 12 weeks' treatment, felodipine reduced aortic PWV more than a thiazide diuretic, despite of similar brachial BP reductions [11]. One year of treatment with nitrendipine decreased significantly aortic PWV, similarly to the effects of ACE-I, in hypertensives with end-stage renal disease [12]. After 24 weeks' treatment, both amlodipine and eplerenone significantly reduced aortic PWV from baseline [13]. After 12 months' treatment, both amlodipine and valsartan significantly reduced the brachial-ankle PWV (baPWV), which reflect a stiffness of the large- to- middle-sized arteries, to a similar degree in hypertensives [14]. Similarly, 38 weeks' treatment, both amlodipine and valsartan significantly reduced aortic PWV in hypertensive postmenopausal women to a similar degree [15]. During 24 weeks of antihypertensive combination treatment, the addition of azelnidipine to olmesartan reduced the aortic PWV more than the addition of thiazide diuretic to olmesartan [16].

On the other hand, there are several studies reporting the negative effects of CCBs on the aortic PWV despite their BP lowering effects. After 6 months' treatment, amlodipine did not significantly reduce the aortic PWV, while quinapril did [17]. After 6 months' treatment, barnidipine had no significant effects on the local measures of large artery stiffness [18]. These are considered to be unsuitable measures of arterial stiffness and not associated with cardiovascular events [19] when allowance is not made for amplification of the pulse between central (carotid or aorta) and brachial arteries. In elderly hypertensives with ISH, 12 weeks' treatment of lercanidipine did not reduce the aortic PWV, despite the reduction in brachial BP [20]. After 12 weeks' treatment, slow release nifedipine coat-core did not reduce the baPWV, while valsartan did [21]. In diabetic hypertensives, 24 weeks' treatment of amlodipine reduced the aortic PWV, but this reduction was lower than valsartan/diuretic combination treatment [22]. Long-term (2.5 year) treatment with amlodipine significantly reduced the baPWV, but this effect was inferior to candesartan [23]. Thus, in contrast to the beneficial effects of ACE-Is or angiotensin II receptor blockers (ARBs) on the aortic PWV, there is no clear agreement on the effect of DHP-CCBs on large artery stiffness.

During 24 weeks' treatment, cilnidipine caused a significantly greater reduction in baPWV than amlodipine, at doses where both drugs had similar brachial BP reductions [24]. Recently, 24 weeks' treatment of olmesartan/azelnidipine combination achieved greater reductions in baPWV and heart rate (HR) than did olmesartan/amlodipine combination [25]. Nifedipine and amlodipine increased the HR [21, 22, 25]. Interestingly, PWV was well reduced in patients with greater hypotensive response without any tachycardia even in a group treated with nifedipine [21]. All these findings suggest that sympathetic activation might be related to the large artery stiffening. Thus, nifedipine and amlodipine could limit an improvement of arterial stiffness if they would induce sympathetic activation. On the other hand, cilnidipine and azelnidipine deceased the HR due to their inhibition of increased sympathetic nervous activity [16, 24, 25]. Because it was also shown that the decreased HR itself was associated with improvement in aortic PWV [16], the HR-lowering effects of cilnidipine and azelnidipine through their sympathetic inhibition may be, in part, responsible for the greater effects on the large artery stiffness. A clinical study has demonstrated that cilnidipine and azelnidipine leads to reduced activation of the renin-angiotensin-aldosterone system, and thereby reduced production of aldosterone, compared to the other L-type CCBs [26, 27]. The significant association between aldosterone induced by antihypertensive medication and the aortic stiffness change was reported in hypertensive patients [28]. Therefore, the reduced increase of aldosterone by cilnidipine and azelnidipine might also have been partly involved in the mechanism of their marked reduction of PWV.

CCB and Carotid Atherosclerosis

A meta-analysis of randomized controlled trials revealed that DHP-CCBs reduce the risk of stroke in comparison to other antihypertensive drugs [7]. Another meta-analysis of randomized controlled trials supporting this specific protection against stroke by CCBs suggested their greater effectiveness in the prevention of carotid intima-media thickening (IMT) than other antihypertensive drugs [29]. The PREVENT study reported that the 36 months' treatment of amlodipine had a significant suppressive effect on the progression of carotid IMT in patients with coronary artery disease, while this treatment did not appear to prevent the progression of moderate or advanced coronary artery stenoses [30]. This discrepancy may be explained by the BP-lowering action of amlodipine: reduction in wall stress may have different effects on the large central arteries and smaller coronary arteries. In the ELSA study, a randomized, double-blind trial in 2,334 hypertensives, 4 years' antihypertensive treatment with lacidipine slowed down progression of carotid atherosclerosis significantly more than atenolol [31]. The greater efficacy of lacidipine on carotid IMT progression and number of plaques per patient, despite a smaller ambulatory BP reduction, suggests an anti-atherosclerotic action of lacidipine independent of its antihypertensive action. This anti-atherosclerotic process of DHP-CCBs may be involved with their improvement of endothelial function, anti-inflammation effects, anti-oxidant effects, and anti-proliferation effects on vascular smooth muscle cells.

CCB and Peripheral Muscular Arteries

DHP-CCBs reversibly inhibit calcium entry into vascular smooth muscle cells by binding to L-type voltage-sensitive calcium channels. This decreases intracellular calcium concentrations, resulting in smooth muscle cell relaxation. There is firm evidence that CCBs can markedly reduce the magnitude of wave reflections by their effect on peripheral muscular arteries, and thereby decrease the augmentation index (AIx) and augmentation pressure of the central arteries [12, 16, 18, 20, 22, 32–37] (Fig. 44.1). Although large artery stiffness may not be a readily modifiable risk factor, independent of BP change, muscular artery stiffness is a modifiable risk factor, and is held responsible for the strong effects of nitroglycerine in reducing wave reflection [38]. The manifestation of change in muscular artery stiffness is the reduction in amplitude of wave reflection. Why and how do CCBs decrease muscular artery stiffness, and how does this reduce wave reflection? These mechanisms might be explained as follows; smooth muscle in muscular arteries behaves as though in series with collagenous fibers and in parallel with elastic fibers. Hence, contraction of smooth muscle in the arterial wall makes it both narrower and stiffer, and increases wave reflection. Relaxation of smooth muscle by CCBs transfers stresses from collagenous to elastic fibers, dilates the muscular artery, and makes it less stiff, resulting in decrease in wave reflection [38]. In a study using nitroglycerine, Yaginuma et al. demonstrated that the combination of dilation and decreased stiffness of the muscular conduit arteries causes reduction in wave reflection [38]. Yaginuma et al. also pointed out that progressively larger effects of the drug on smaller than large muscular arteries can enhance reduction in wave reflection [38].

Hypertensive remodeling of small resistance arteries is characterized by the increased wall/lumen ratio of arterioles, which represent the principal sites of vascular resistance and also the origin of most of the wave reflections [39]. Schiffrin et al. reported that the long-term treatment with CCB amlodipine caused the regression of the arterial hypertrophy due to structural changes in the peripheral arterial network, that is, decreased wall/lumen ratio of small resistance arteries [40]. This modification with CCB might contribute to decrease of reflection coefficients, thus lowering the amplitude of wave reflections [39]. Thus, CCBs have predominant effects on the muscular arteries from reduction in early wave reflection back in to the central elastic arteries and heart (Figs. 44.1 and 44.2).

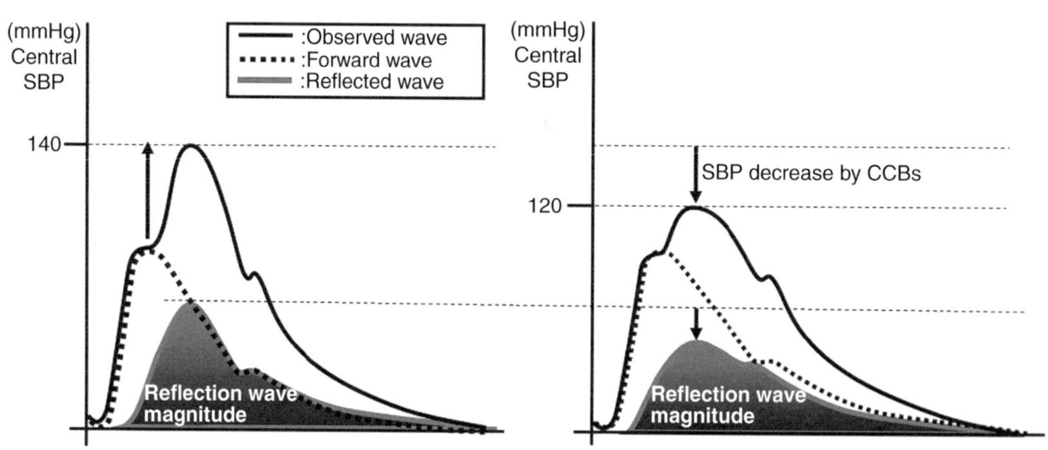

Fig. 44.1 The main hemodynamic mechanism of the central BP-lowering effect of the dihydropiridine calcium channel blockers (*CCBs*): reduction of the magnitude of the reflected wave

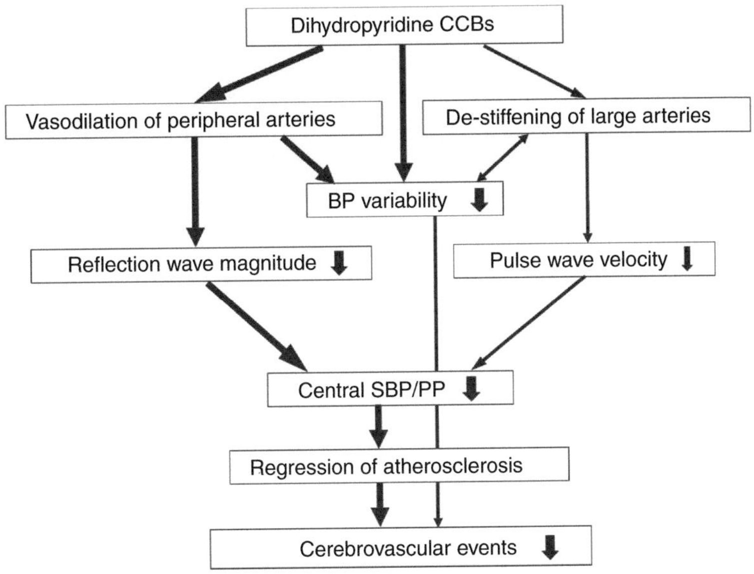

Fig. 44.2 The mechanisms of the reduction of cerebrovascular events by dihydropiridine calcium channel blockers (*CCBs*)

CCB and Central Aortic Pressure

Recent studies using validated methods have reported that non-invasively determined central systolic BP (SBP)/PP more strongly relates to the extent of target organ damage and future cardiovascular events than peripheral (brachial) BP [34, 41, 42]. The ASCOT-CAFÉ study demonstrated that central BP-lowering by antihypertensive medication contributes to an improvement of cardiovascular outcomes beyond those achieved by brachial BP-lowering [34]. This has led to the suggestion that central BP rather than brachial BP should be a therapeutic target for cardiovascular risk reduction in hypertensive patients.

Although there was no difference in the change of brachial SBP/PP among the various antihypertensive drug classes, CCBs caused a greater fall in the central SBP/PP than did β-blockers or thiazide diuretics [16, 20, 32–37]. This discrepancy can be explained by the differences of changes in the magnitude of wave reflections, but not the large artery stiffness between these drugs, because the reduction of wave reflection from conduit arteries effectively reduces the central SBP but does not necessarily change the peripheral SBP [18, 20, 22, 34, 36] (Figs. 44.1 and 44.2). Studies of nitrates at cardiac catheterization have shown marked reduction in wave reflection and in aortic systolic pressure without significant change in aortic stiffness [38]. Such beneficial effects were also confirmed at cardiac catheterization with acute administration of CCB nifedipine [43]. In this study [43], there was no significant change in pulmonary vascular impedance with nifedipine, while there was a clear change in the systemic vascular impedance (Fig. 44.3). The characteristic impedance fell by 22 %, but this change did not reach the level of statistical significance. The decrease in aortic SBP/PP by nifedipine can be mainly explained on the basis of the decrease in the amplitude of the reflected wave, not solely by the change in mean arterial pressure and characteristic impedance [43].

The J-CORE study examined the effects of CCB azelnidipine versus a thiazide diuretic (hydrochlorothiazide) in combination with the same ARB (olmesartan) on central pressure [16]. The extent of reduction in central SBP was significantly greater in the ARB/CCB group, whereas the difference in the reduction in brachial SBP between the two groups was not significant. The aortic PWV and AIx adjusted for HR in the ARB/CCB group decreased more than those in the ARB/diuretic group. In addition, this study provided evidence on the mechanism of reduction of central SBP/PP by CCB, namely by

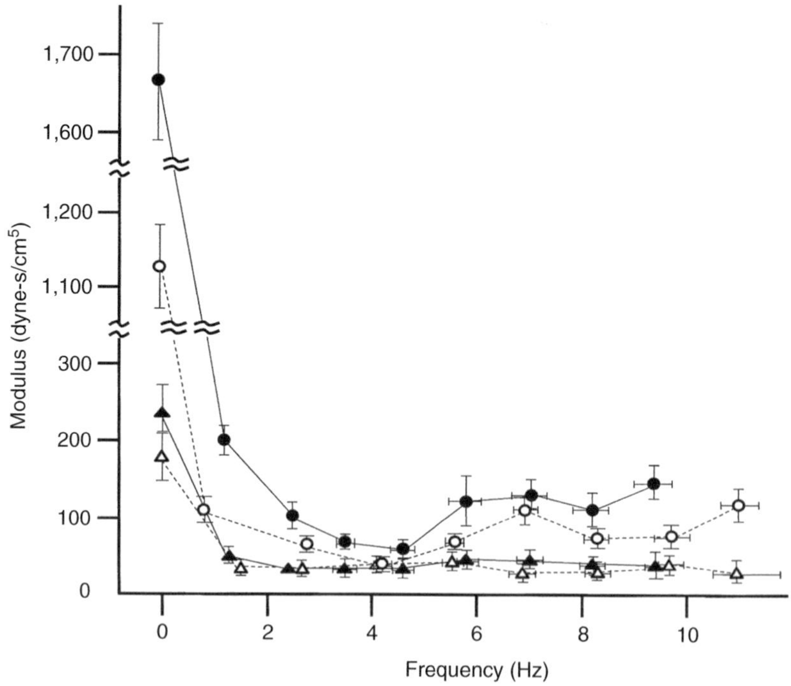

Fig. 44.3 Modulus of impedance in the ascending aorta (*circles*) and main pulmonary artery (*triangles*) before (*closed circles/triangles, solid lines*) and after (*open circles/triangles, dashed lines*) administration of nifedipine. *Bars* ± SD (From Noda et al. [43])

reducing AIx and PWV. Reduction of magnitude of pressure wave reflections is the first important mechanism of central SBP reduction by CCB (Fig. 44.1). Second mechanism is that the reflection wave arrival time may have been delayed because of changes in aortic PWV. Although HR was decreased in the azelnidipine arm, thus favoring an earlier timing of wave reflections in systole, AIx was reduced. This may be explained partly by the prolonged time of return of the reflected wave because of lower PWV. In the ACCOMPLISH trial [5], the benefit of peripheral arterial vasodilation with an ACE-I/CCB combination for survival was greater than would be expected from analysis of brachial cuff pressure measurements. This can be explained on the basis of greater SBP/PP reduction in central aorta [16].

CCB and BP Variability

Recent evidence has been provided that independently of mean BP levels, increased short-, mid-, and long-term BP variability (BPV) are associated with the severity of target organ damage, and with an increased risk of cardiovascular events and mortality [44–46]. It was reported that CCBs could lower short-term BPV as assessed by ambulatory BP monitoring [47], mid-term BPV as assessed by day-by-day home BPV [48], and long-term BPV as assessed by visit-to-visit office BPV [49]. The greater reduction in BPVs among subjects treated with CCBs may be best explained by their more profound effects on the relaxation of peripheral muscular arteries, mainly by attenuating the myogenic response of vascular smooth muscle cells [50] (Fig. 44.2). On the other hand, the J-CORE study reported that the reduction of aortic PWV was independently associated with the reduction in home BPV in subjects with CCB treatment [48]. Cross-sectional studies have demonstrated that all term BPVs were significantly associated with large artery stiffness [48, 51, 52]. However, it remains to be clarified whether a reduction in BPV by CCB could contribute to an improvement in arterial stiffness [14], or if the CCB-induced reduction in arterial stiffness would lead to reduced BPV [48] (Fig. 44.2). Use of well tolerated, long acting CCBs may be responsible for lower BPVs, through their success in decreasing large artery stiffness.

Conclusion

It has been recognized that the mechanisms of the anti-arteriosclerotic effects mediated by DHP-CCBs are mainly caused be their sustained peripheral BP lowering actions; however, recent trials suggest that long-term treatment with CCBs may have beneficial effects beyond the reduction of peripheral (brachial) mean arterial pressure. The de-stiffening of the large arteries and the dilation of peripheral muscular arteries by CCBs might be underlying mechanisms of the significant reductions in central SBP/PP and BPV, each of which was reported to be an independent predictor of cerebrovascular events [34, 44–46]. Thus, these processes could provide a key to understanding why CCBs appear more effective than other antihypertensive drugs for reducing carotid atherosclerosis, cerebral arteriosclerotic damage, and cerebrovascular events in hypertensive patients (Fig. 44.2).

References

1. Staessen JA, Fagard R, Thijs L, Celis H, Arabidze GG, Birkenhäger WH, Bulpitt CJ, de Leeuw PW, Dollery CT, Fletcher AE, Forette F, Leonetti G, Nachev C, O'Brien ET, Rosenfeld J, Rodicio JL, Tuomilehto J, Zanchetti A. Randomised double-blind comparison of placebo and active treatment for older patients with isolated systolic hypertension. The Systolic Hypertension in Europe (Syst-Eur) Trial Investigators. Lancet. 1997;350:757–64.
2. ALLHAT Officers and Coordinators for the ALLHAT Collaborative Research Group. Major outcomes in high-risk hypertensive patients randomized to angiotensin-converting enzyme inhibitor or calcium channel blocker vs diuretic: the Antihypertensive and Lipid-Lowering Treatment to Prevent Heart Attack Trial (ALLHAT). JAMA. 2002;288:2981–97.
3. Julius S, Kjeldsen SE, Weber M, Brunner HR, Ekman S, Hansson L, Hua T, Laragh J, McInnes GT, Mitchell L, Plat F, Schork A, Smith B, Zanchetti A, VALUE trial group. Outcomes in hypertensive patients at high cardiovascular risk treated with regimens based on valsartan or amlodipine: the VALUE randomised trial. Lancet. 2004;363:2022–31.
4. Dahlöf B, Sever PS, Poulter NR, Wedel H, Beevers DG, Caulfield M, Collins R, Kjeldsen SE, Kristinsson A, McInnes GT, Mehlsen J, Nieminen M, O'Brien E, Ostergren J, ASCOT Investigators. Prevention of cardiovascular events with an antihypertensive regimen of amlodipine adding perindopril as required versus atenolol adding bendroflumethiazide as required, in the Anglo-Scandinavian Cardiac Outcomes Trial-Blood Pressure Lowering Arm (ASCOT-BPLA): a multicentre randomized controlled trial. Lancet. 2005;366:895–906.
5. Jamerson K, Weber MA, Bakris GL, Dahlöf B, Pitt B, Shi V, Hester A, Gupte J, Gatlin M, Velazquez EJ, ACCOMPLISH Trial Investigators. Benazepril plus amlodipine or hydrochlorothiazide for hypertension in high-risk patients. N Engl J Med. 2008;359: 2417–28.
6. Ogihara T, Nakao K, Fukui T, Fukiyama K, Ueshima K, Oba K, Sato T, Saruta T, Candesartan Antihypertensive Survival Evaluation in Japan Trial Group. Effects of candesartan compared with amlodipine in hypertensive patients with high cardiovascular risks: candesartan antihypertensive survival evaluation in Japan trial. Hypertension. 2008;51: 393–8.
7. Costanzo P, Perrone-Filardi P, Petretta M, Marciano C, Vassallo E, Gargiulo P, Paolillo S, Petretta A, Chiariello M. Calcium channel blockers and cardiovascular outcomes: a meta-analysis of 175,634 patients. J Hypertens. 2009;27:1136–51.
8. Ong KT, Delerme S, Pannier B, Safar ME, Benetos A, Laurent S, Boutouyrie P, investigators. Aortic stiffness is reduced beyond blood pressure lowering by short-term and long-term antihypertensive treatment: a meta-analysis of individual data in 294 patients. J Hypertens. 2011;29:1034–42.
9. Wilkinson IB, Qasem A, McEniery CM, Webb DJ, Avolio AP, Cockcroft JR. Nitric oxide regulates local arterial distensibility in vivo. Circulation. 2002;105: 213–7.
10. Laurent S, Boutouyrie P, Asmar R, Gautier I, Laloux B, Guize L, Ducimetiere P, Benetos A. Aortic stiffness is an independent predictor of all-cause and cardiovascular mortality in hypertensive patients. Hypertension. 2001;37:1236–41.
11. Asmar RG, Benetos A, Chaouche-Teyara K, Raveau-Landon CM, Safar ME. Comparison of effects of felodipine versus hydrochlorothiazide on arterial diameter and pulse-wave velocity in essential hypertension. Am J Cardiol. 1993;72:794–8.
12. London GM, Pannier B, Guerin AP, Marchais SJ, Safar ME, Cuche JL. Cardiac hypertrophy, aortic compliance, peripheral resistance, and wave reflection in end-stage renal disease. Comparative effects of ACE inhibition and calcium channel blockade. Circulation. 1994;90:2786–96.
13. White WB, Duprez D, St Hillaire R, Krause S, Roniker B, Kuse-Hamilton J, Weber MA. Effects of the selective aldosterone blocker eplerenone versus the calcium antagonist amlodipine in systolic hypertension. Hypertension. 2003;41:1021–6.
14. Ichihara A, Kaneshiro Y, Takemitsu T, Sakoda M. Effects of amlodipine and valsartan on vascular damage and ambulatory blood pressure in untreated hypertensive patients. J Hum Hypertens. 2006;20: 787–94.

15. Hayoz D, Zappe DH, Meyer MA, Baek I, Kandra A, Joly MP, Mazzolai L, Haesler E, Periard D. Changes in aortic pulse wave velocity in hypertensive postmenopausal women: comparison between a calcium channel blocker vs angiotensin receptor blocker regimen. J Clin Hypertens (Greenwich). 2012;14:773–8.
16. Matsui Y, Eguchi K, O'Rourke MF, Ishikawa J, Miyashita H, Shimada K, Kario K. Differential effects between a calcium channel blocker and a diuretic when used in combination with angiotensin II receptor blocker on central aortic pressure in hypertensive patients. Hypertension. 2009;54:716–23.
17. Rajzer M, Klocek M, Kawecka-Jaszcz K. Effect of amlodipine, quinapril, and losartan on pulse wave velocity and plasma collagen markers in patients with mild-to-moderate arterial hypertension. Am J Hypertens. 2003;16:439–44.
18. Palombo C, Malshi E, Morizzo C, Rakebrandt F, Corretti V, Santini F, Fraser AG, Kozakova M. Arterial wave reflection during antihypertensive therapy with barnidipine: a 6-month, open-label study using an integrated cardiovascular ultrasound approach in patients with newly diagnosed hypertension. Clin Ther. 2009;31:2873–85.
19. Laurent S, Cockcroft J, Van Bortel L, Boutouyrie P, Giannattasio C, Hayoz D, Pannier B, Vlachopoulos C, Wilkinson I, Struijker-Boudier H, European Network for Non-invasive Investigation of Large Arteries. Expert consensus document on arterial stiffness: methodological issues and clinical applications. Eur Heart J. 2006;27:2588–605.
20. Mackenzie IS, McEniery CM, Dhakam Z, Brown MJ, Cockcroft JR, Wilkinson IB. Comparison of the effects of antihypertensive agents on central blood pressure and arterial stiffness in isolated systolic hypertension. Hypertension. 2009;54:409–13.
21. Munakata M, Nagasaki A, Nunokawa T, Sakuma T, Kato H, Yoshinaga K, Toyota T. Effects of valsartan and nifedipine coat-core on systemic arterial stiffness in hypertensive patients. Am J Hypertens. 2004;17:1050–5.
22. Karalliedde J, Smith A, DeAngelis L, Mirenda V, Kandra A, Botha J, Ferber P, Viberti G. Valsartan improves arterial stiffness in type 2 diabetes independently of blood pressure lowering. Hypertension. 2008;51:1617–23.
23. Tomiyama H, Yoshida M, Yamada J, Matsumoto C, Odaira M, Shiina K, Yamashina A. Arterial-cardiac destiffening following long-term antihypertensive treatment. Am J Hypertens. 2011;24:1080–6.
24. Morimoto S, Yano Y, Maki K, Iwasaka T. Renal and vascular protective effects of cilnidipine in patients with essential hypertension. J Hypertens. 2007;25:2178–83.
25. Takami T, Saito Y. Effects of Azelnidipine plus OlmesaRTAn versus amlodipine plus olmesartan on central blood pressure and left ventricular mass index: the AORTA study. Vasc Health Risk Manag. 2011;7:383–90.
26. Konoshita T, Makino Y, Kimura T, Fujii M, Wakahara S, Arakawa K, Inoki I, Nakamura H, Miyamori I, Genomic Disease Outcome Consortium Study Investigators. A new-generation N/L-type calcium channel blocker leads to less activation of the renin-angiotensin system compared with conventional L type calcium channel blocker. J Hypertens. 2010;28:2156–60.
27. Kondo T, Goto R, Sonoda K, Yasuda T, Ono K, Takaki Y, Yatsuda R, Miyamura N, Araki E. Plasma renin activity and aldosterone concentration are not altered by the novel calcium channel antagonist, azelnidipine, in hypertensive patients. Intern Med. 2010;49:637–43.
28. Matsui Y, Eguchi K, O'Rourke MF, Ishikawa J, Shimada K, Kario K. Association between aldosterone induced by antihypertensive medication and arterial stiffness reduction: the J-CORE study. Atherosclerosis. 2011;215:184–8.
29. Wang JG, Staessen JA, Li Y, Van Bortel LM, Nawrot T, Fagard R, Messerli FH, Safar M. Carotid intima-media thickness and antihypertensive treatment: a meta-analysis of randomized controlled trials. Stroke. 2006;37:1933–40.
30. Pitt B, Byington RP, Furberg CD, Hunninghake DB, Mancini GB, Miller ME, Riley W. Effect of amlodipine on the progression of atherosclerosis and the occurrence of clinical events. PREVENT Investigators. Circulation. 2000;102:1503–10.
31. Zanchetti A, Bond MG, Hennig M, Neiss A, Mancia G, Dal Palù C, Hansson L, Magnani B, Rahn KH, Reid JL, Rodicio J, Safar M, Eckes L, Rizzini P, European Lacidipine Study on Atherosclerosis investigators. Calcium antagonist lacidipine slows down progression of asymptomatic carotid atherosclerosis: principal results of the European Lacidipine Study on Atherosclerosis (ELSA), a randomized, double-blind, long-term trial. Circulation. 2002;106:2422–7.
32. Deary AJ, Schumann AL, Murfet H, Haydock S, Foo RS, Brown MJ. Influence of drugs and gender on the arterial pulse wave and natriuretic peptide secretion in untreated patients with essential hypertension. Clin Sci (Lond). 2002;103:493–9.
33. Morgan T, Lauri J, Bertram D, Anderson A. Effect of different antihypertensive drug classes on central aortic pressure. Am J Hypertens. 2004;17:118–23.
34. Williams B, Lacy PS, Thom SM, Cruickshank K, Stanton A, Collier D, Hughes AD, Thurston H, O'Rourke M, CAFE Investigators; Anglo-Scandinavian Cardiac Outcomes Trial Investigators; CAFE Steering Committee and Writing Committee. Differential impact of blood pressure-lowering drugs on central aortic pressure and clinical outcomes: principal results of the Conduit Artery Function Evaluation (CAFE) study. Circulation. 2006;113:1213–25.
35. Miyashita H, Aizawa A, Hashimoto J, Hirooka Y, Imai Y, Kawano Y, Kohara K, Sunagawa K, Suzuki H, Tabara Y, Takazawa K, Takenaka T, Yasuda H, Shimada K. Cross-sectional characterization of all classes of antihypertensives in terms of central blood pressure in Japanese hypertensive patients. Am J Hypertens. 2010;23:260–8.
36. Boutouyrie P, Achouba A, Trunet P, Laurent S, EXPLOR Trialist Group. Amlodipine-valsartan combination decreases central systolic blood pressure more effectively than the amlodipine-atenolol combination: the EXPLOR study. Hypertension. 2010;55:1314–22.

37. Doi M, Miyoshi T, Hirohata S, Kamikawa S, Usui S, Kaji Y, Sakane K, Ogawa H, Ninomiya Y, Kusachi S. Combination therapy of calcium channel blocker and angiotensin II receptor blocker reduces augmentation index in hypertensive patients. Am J Med Sci. 2010;339:433–9.
38. Yaginuma T, Avolio A, O'Rourke M, Nichols W, Morgan JJ, Roy P, Baron D, Branson J, Feneley M. Effect of glyceryl trinitrate on peripheral arteries alters left ventricular hydraulic load in man. Cardiovasc Res. 1986;20:153–60.
39. Safar ME, Rizzoni D, Blacher J, Muiesan ML, Agabiti-Rosei E. Macro and microvasculature in hypertension: therapeutic aspects. J Hum Hypertens. 2008;22:590–5.
40. Schiffrin EL, Pu Q, Park JB. Effect of amlodipine compared to atenolol on small arteries of previously untreated essential hypertensive patients. Am J Hypertens. 2002; 15:105–10.
41. Roman MJ, Devereux RB, Kizer JR, Lee ET, Galloway JM, Ali T, Umans JG, Howard BV. Central pressure more strongly relates to vascular disease and outcome than does brachial pressure: the Strong Heart Study. Hypertension. 2007;50:197–203.
42. Wang KL, Cheng HM, Chuang SY, Spurgeon HA, Ting CT, Lakatta EG, Yin FC, Chou P, Chen CH. Central or peripheral systolic or pulse pressure: which best relates to target organs and future mortality? J Hypertens. 2009;27:461–7.
43. Noda T, Yaginuma T, O'Rourke MF, Hosoda S. Effects of nifedipine on systemic and pulmonary vascular impedance in subjects undergoing cardiac catheterization. Hypertens Res. 2006;29:505–13.
44. Kikuya M, Hozawa A, Ohokubo T, Tsuji I, Michimata M, Matsubara M, Ota M, Nagai K, Araki T, Satoh H, Ito S, Hisamichi S, Imai Y. Prognostic significance of blood pressure and heart rate variabilities: the Ohasama study. Hypertension. 2000;36:901–6.
45. Kikuya M, Ohkubo T, Metoki H, Asayama K, Hara A, Obara T, Inoue R, Hoshi H, Hashimoto J, Totsune K, Satoh H, Imai Y. Day-by-day variability of blood pressure and heart rate at home as a novel predictor of prognosis: the Ohasama study. Hypertension. 2008; 52:1045–50.
46. Rothwell PM, Howard SC, Dolan E, O'Brien E, Dobson JE, Dahlöf B, Sever PS, Poulter NR. Prognostic significance of visit-to-visit variability, maximum systolic blood pressure, and episodic hypertension. Lancet. 2010;375:895–905.
47. Zhang Y, Agnoletti D, Safar ME, Blacher J. Effect of antihypertensive agents on blood pressure variability: the Natrilix SR versus candesartan and amlodipine in the reduction of systolic blood pressure in hypertensive patients (X-CELLENT) study. Hypertension. 2011;58:155–60.
48. Matsui Y, O'Rourke MF, Hoshide S, Ishikawa J, Shimada K, Kario K. Combined effect of angiotensin II receptor blocker and either a calcium channel blocker or diuretic on day-by-day variability of home blood pressure: the Japan Combined Treatment With Olmesartan and a Calcium-Channel Blocker Versus Olmesartan and Diuretics Randomized Efficacy Study. Hypertension. 2012;59:1132–8.
49. Rothwell PM, Howard SC, Dolan E, O'Brien E, Dobson JE, Dahlöf B, Poulter NR, Sever PS, ASCOT-BPLA and MRC Trial Investigators. Effects of beta blockers and calcium-channel blockers on within-individual variability in blood pressure and risk of stroke. Lancet Neurol. 2010;9:469–80.
50. Julien C. Pharmacological attenuation of blood pressure variability. Acta Pharmacol Sin. 2005;26: 1288–9.
51. Nagai M, Hoshide S, Ishikawa J, Shimada K, Kario K. Visit-to-visit blood pressure variations: new independent determinants for carotid artery measures in the elderly at high risk of cardiovascular disease. J Am Soc Hypertens. 2011;5:184–92.
52. Schillaci G, Bilo G, Pucci G, Laurent S, Macquin-Mavier I, Boutouyrie P, Battista F, Settimi L, Desamericq G, Dolbeau G, Faini A, Salvi P, Mannarino E, Parati G. Relationship between short-term blood pressure variability and large-artery stiffness in human hypertension: findings from 2 large databases. Hypertension. 2012;60:369–77.

Exercise Training for the Modification of Arterial Stiffness and Wave Reflections

45

Julian W. Sacre and Bronwyn A. Kingwell

Abstract

Clinically significant modulating effects of lifestyle factors on both age- and disease-related arterial stiffening – particularly those relating to habitual physical activity – are widely recognised. Consequently, exercise training may represent an important strategy in the non-pharmacological treatment of arterial stiffening and related complications – often apparent even at an early stage of the cardiometabolic disease continuum. Observational and interventional data relevant to this context are reviewed in the current chapter.

Arterial de-stiffening certainly appears achievable with aerobic exercise in young adults, and may even begin at a lower volume threshold than current exercise guidelines. However, the response in older individuals and those with cardiovascular risk factors appears highly variable. Where short-term training adaptations are evident (weeks to months), these probably reflect functional mechanisms related to blood pressure-lowering. Intrinsic changes in arterial wall structure are difficult to assess in humans, but may be possible when exercise is commenced in young adulthood and performed continually throughout the life course. Resistance training promotes arterial stiffening at high intensities, but may otherwise have a neutral or beneficial effect – particularly in combination with aerobic exercise.

Keywords

Aerobic Exercise • Aortic Stiffness • Arteriosclerosis • Exercise • Pulse Wave Analysis • Pulse Wave Velocity • Resistance Training • Vascular Stiffness

Introduction

Stiffening of the large conduit arteries is inherent to the ageing process and compounded by a number of cardiometabolic diseases. It constitutes the main cause of isolated systolic hypertension, with additional salient contributions to cardiac

J.W. Sacre, BScApp, PhD
B.A. Kingwell, BSc, PhD (✉)
Metabolic and Vascular Physiology, Baker IDI Heart and Diabetes Institute, 75 Commercial Road, Melbourne, VIC 3004, Australia
e-mail: julian.sacre@bakeridi.edu.au; bronwyn.kingwell@bakeridi.edu.au

M.E. Safar et al. (eds.), *Blood Pressure and Arterial Wall Mechanics in Cardiovascular Diseases*, DOI 10.1007/978-1-4471-5198-2_45, © Springer-Verlag London 2014

dysfunction and remodelling [1]. However, it is clear that several aspects of lifestyle – particularly physical activity – can modulate the rate of both age- and disease-related changes in arterial biomechanical properties [2–5]. It therefore follows that exercise training represents a valid target for intervention to reduce the rate of arterial stiffening and associated complications. This chapter builds on an earlier edition of this publication [6] in focussing on the efficacy of exercise interventions to reduce large artery stiffening throughout the life course and in certain clinical contexts, drawing on both observational and intervention data.

The studies discussed have applied a variety of methodologies to assess arterial biomechanical and/or wave reflection properties, each associated with its own advantages, limitations and assumptions [7, 8]. These have been discussed earlier in this volume and include systemic measures of whole body arterial compliance using Windkessel (capacitance) models, as well as measures of local compliance using 2D echocardiography and magnetic resonance imaging (β index), regional methods such as pulse wave velocity (PWV) and indices of wave reflection including peripheral (e.g. radial) and central (carotid or derived ascending aortic) augmentation index (AIx), which rely on distributive models [1]. As in the previous version of this chapter [6], no distinction will be made based on the parameter reported in original works. For the present purpose it is adequate to consider increased arterial stiffness, however assessed, as being a disadvantageous state compared with more compliant, less stiff arteries.

Aerobic Exercise

Observational Studies in Healthy Individuals

The prospect of aerobic exercise preventing – or even reversing – the increased arterial stiffness of ageing and disease is founded on a strong body of observational data. Early studies using magnetic resonance imaging to characterise total and regional aortic compliance observed their marked augmentation in athletes – hypothesised to be an adaptive mechanism to accommodate high cardiac output and prevent extreme blood pressure (BP) elevation during exercise [9]. Greater arterial compliance and more favourable wave reflection status in endurance athletes compared with the recreationally active or sedentary controls has since been supported by a number of investigators [10, 11].

Importantly, arterial adaptations with aerobic exercise do not appear to be limited to a highly trained state. Correlations of higher peak oxygen uptake (VO_{2peak}) with lower aortic PWV/central AIx are apparent in more sedentary individuals ($<3\times20$ min exercise per week) [12]. Cross-sectional studies in both men [13] and women [14] have demonstrated substantive attenuation of age-related central artery stiffening in those who are physically active. Indeed, differences in carotid arterial compliance between older (~65 years old) vs. younger sedentary men (~30 years old) were almost twice those observed in similarly aged men who engaged in regular, vigorous aerobic exercise [13]. Similar findings apply to aortic PWV in post- vs. pre-menopausal women (~60 vs. 30 years old) [14].

A question that naturally arises from these data pertains to the importance of exercise dose (including frequency, intensity and duration of activity). In a Japanese study of older individuals who wore a pedometer/accelerometer over 1 year, aortic PWV was inversely correlated with both daily step count and time spent in activities at an intensity >3 metabolic equivalents (METs; i.e. moderate-vigorous intensity). However, no additional benefit was apparent once daily activity of 6,600 steps or 16 min of exercise at >3 METs was exceeded [15]. Notably, this exercise volume is less than is advocated by public health guidelines (30 min on most days of the week). With respect to exercise intensity, moderate and vigorous activity appear to be stronger correlates of central artery stiffness compared with light intensity activity [16, 17]. This dovetails well with the lower arterial stiffness of aerobically trained athletes and raises the prospect of greater efficacy from exercise interventions targeting gains in cardiorespiratory fitness (e.g. high intensity and/or interval training). It has also been reported that arterial stiffness is inversely associated with both "sports-related" physical activity (questionnaire-based) and cardiorespiratory fitness in young adults, but the latter relationship is stronger [18].

Finally, it should be acknowledged that the inverse association of physical activity with arterial stiffness may be moderated or even reversed at the most extreme levels of aerobic exercise. In studies of ultra-endurance athletes and marathon runners, central AIx was shown to be similar [19] and aortic PWV elevated [20] compared with recreationally-active controls.

Intervention Studies in Healthy Individuals

Young Adults

Consistent with observational data, exercise training studies indicate that the threshold for benefit from aerobic exercise (i.e. in relation to arterial adaptations) may be relatively low. The first intervention trial [21] (moderate intensity cycling 3 × 30 min/week) demonstrated that post-training systemic arterial compliance and aortic β-stiffness index in previously sedentary males (18–32 years) reached levels akin to elite athletes [22] within as little as 4 weeks. More recently, just six consecutive days of moderate intensity cycling (2 h/day) showed reductions in aortic and peripheral (femoral-ankle) PWV [23]. Notably, the magnitude of change in aortic PWV over this short time frame (−0.5 m/s) was as high as has been observed during interventions lasting weeks-months. Indeed, a 0.3 m/s reduction in aortic PWV was reported in similarly aged (mean 25 years) sedentary males following an 8-week cycling program (3–4 days/week for 60 min; moderate intensity) [24]. Exercise intensity may also be important. A 16-week randomised controlled trial (RCT) in young women with a family history of hypertension demonstrated greater efficacy for aortic PWV reduction with interval training (2 min/1 min bouts at 50–60 %/80–90 % of VO_{2peak}, respectively) compared with equal-volume continuous moderate intensity walking/running exercise (60–70 % of VO_{2peak}) [25].

Middle-Aged and Older Adults

In middle-aged/older adults (mean age 50–64 years), uncontrolled intervention studies have also reported improvements in systemic [26] and local (carotid) arterial compliance [13, 16, 27, 28], carotid β-stiffness index [13, 16, 27], and aortic PWV [28] with walking/running or cycling interventions lasting between 12 and 26 weeks (moderate-vigorous intensity). Although these findings provide proof-of-concept, RCT evidence for aerobic exercise in middle-aged and older adults is equivocal. Three RCTs have evaluated responses of arterial stiffness to 8-week combined walking/cycling programs (60–75 % peak heart rate [HR]) in postmenopausal women (mean age 58–60 years). Although one study demonstrated improvements in carotid artery compliance and β-stiffness index [29], another reported mixed effects on these endpoints [30]. In the most recent trial [31], no changes in aortic PWV or AIx were observed. Thus, the responsiveness of some arterial properties to aerobic exercise training may be diminished with ageing, although it is important to acknowledge that this conclusion is based on only a small number of controlled studies.

Mechanisms

Direct effects on the vasculature are purported to fill large parts of the "risk factor gap" between physical activity and improved cardiovascular outcomes [32], and these may reflect both functional and structural adaptations in the arterial wall.

Functional Pathways

Aerobic exercise may promote arterial de-stiffening via smooth muscle cell relaxation – an outcome of improvements in one or both of endothelial function and reduced sympathetic

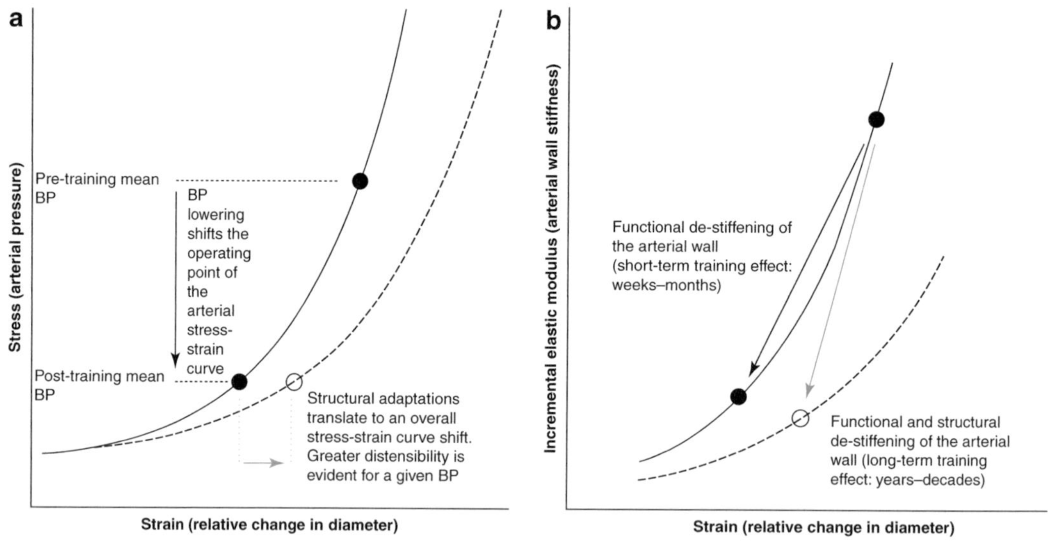

Fig. 45.1 Theoretical mechanical representation of the functional and structural basis for arterial de-stiffening with exercise. Panel (**a**) displays the arterial stress-strain relationship, while Panel (**b**) displays the corresponding elastic modulus as a function of strain (where elastic modulus is the ratio of stress/strain and reflects 'intrinsic' arterial stiffness). Exercise-mediated blood pressure (*BP*) lowering unloads the arterial wall and shifts the operating point of the non-linear stress-strain curve to a flatter section. Thus, the elastic modulus may be reduced even if intrinsic wall properties do not change ("functional" de-stiffening). In the event that aerobic exercise does alter wall properties (i.e. structural change) – as demonstrated in animal studies [37–39] – the entire stress-strain curve is flattened. Thus, the elastic modulus may be reduced at any given strain. The curves displayed are based in part on previously published figures [39, 40]

activity/vasoconstrictor tone. The former is widely recognised to occur with aerobic exercise independent of cardiovascular risk factors [32] and largely reflects local shear stress-mediated augmentation of nitric-oxide and other endothelium-derived vasodilators [33]. Aside from sympathetic withdrawal, the autonomic nervous system may adapt by enhancement of baroreflex sensitivity [34], although it is unclear whether this actively contributes to – or is a favourable consequence of – changes in arterial compliance.

Structural Pathways

Structural determinants of arterial stiffness relate mainly to arterial wall scaffolding proteins [2]. Put simply, a lower ratio of elastin-to-collagen fibres typifies a stiffened artery [8]. Animal studies give some indication that this is modifiable by aerobic exercise based on a relative increase in aortic elastin [35] and reduction in collagen in exercised vs. sedentary rats [36]. These exercise-induced compositional changes affect the intrinsic arterial wall properties to increase the slope of the diameter-pressure relationship [37–39].

Functional vs. Structural Pathways in Exercise-Mediated Arterial De-stiffening

Theoretical mechanical representations of functional vs. structural changes with exercise are depicted in Fig. 45.1. Exercise-mediated reduction in mean BP (related to functional pathways) shifts the operating point of the non-linear stress-strain curve [40] (largely responsible for the BP-dependence of many arterial stiffness and wave reflection parameters) [7]. Importantly, this manifests in reduced stiffness (by the incremental elastic modulus; ratio of stress/strain) even if underlying structural adaptations in the arterial wall are absent. In contrast, structural pathways linking exercise with elevated compliance would manifest as an overall curve shift.

Whether the basis of arterial stiffness modification by aerobic exercise is mainly functional or structural remains unanswered. There is a pervasive view that since exercise trials report positive outcomes from interventions lasting days-to-weeks – a length of time considered insufficient to realise meaningful changes in scaffolding proteins – that functional adaptations must be predominant [2, 5]. Stronger associations of cardiorespiratory fitness with stiffness of muscular arterial segments compared with the more proximal elastic segments also fits with this contention [18]. Alternately, this may simply reflect that shifts in the aortic stress-strain curve [37–39] are more difficult to detect in humans compared with trained rats. Theoretical pressure-volume relationships (based on compliance calculations at different points of the diastolic pressure waveform) were favourably altered within 4 weeks in the first exercise trial examining arterial stiffness [21]. This provides some evidence that the arteries of young adults (18–32 years) may be amenable to structural changes. More recent studies using a novel index of aortic stiffness derived from stroke volume and central pressure waveform measurements – the "Modelflow aortic age" – have shed new light on this issue in older persons. The Modelflow aortic age method uses aortic impedance estimation, which is theoretically not influenced by ambient blood pressure and therefore provides an index of structural aspects of aortic stiffness [41, 42]. Notably, Masters athletes were shown to have a "younger" aortic age (40 years) than their chronologic age (68 years), whereas matched, sedentary controls showed equivalency of aortic and chronologic ages [42]. However, in further determining whether this index was "trainable" in older, sedentary individuals (mean 71 years for both chronologic and aortic age), the same investigators found that the aortic age did not get "younger" following 12-months of intensive aerobic training (up to 200 min/week; sufficient to elicit a rise in VO_{2peak} of 19 %) [42]. Despite this, improvements in stroke volume, HR, effective arterial elastance, peripheral vascular resistance and systemic arterial compliance were observed to such extents that they were comparable with the Masters athletes. Collectively, these data (displayed in Fig. 45.2) are consistent with the notion that adverse structural changes in the arterial wall are not *reversible* with aerobic exercise in older individuals, although BP-dependent markers of arterial stiffness may improve on account of favourable haemodynamic and functional adaptations. However, aerobic exercise performed across the life span may have a beneficial *preventative* effect in slowing age-related structural changes [42].

Intervention Studies in Individuals with Cardiovascular Risk Factors

In addition to the functional and structural pathways described above, arterial stiffness may be reduced in consort with both traditional and novel cardiovascular risk factors.

Hypertension

Aerobic exercise remains a cornerstone of lifestyle modification recommendations for individuals with hypertension due to its well-established BP-lowering effects. Indeed, a meta-analysis of training data involving >3,000 individuals demonstrated that reductions in systolic and diastolic BP are greater in hypertensive (−6.9/−4.9 mmHg) vs. normotensive (−2.4/−1.6 mmHg) individuals [43]. The mechanistic basis for the antihypertensive effects of aerobic exercise is certainly multifactorial, though many postulated mechanisms share reduced arterial stiffness as an endpoint [44]. Of course, any change in arterial stiffness or wave reflection may simply reflect the BP-dependence of these markers [7], as highlighted in Fig. 45.1. From available controlled trials, lowering of BP may be a prerequisite for beneficial effects on arterial properties, albeit without necessarily correlating. Guimaraes et al. [45] compared 16 weeks of high intensity interval (2 min/1 min bouts at 50 %/80 % of HR reserve, respectively) vs. continuous moderate intensity treadmill training (60 % of HR reserve) in patients with pharmacologically controlled hypertension. Despite BP lowering of a similar extent in each training group, concurrent reduction in aortic PWV was observed only in patients who performed high-intensity interval training. More recently, carotid artery compliance (but not central AIx or femoral-ankle PWV) was shown to improve in pre-/stage 1 systolic hypertension with 12 weeks swimming training (mostly vigorous intensity) – a change that was not associated

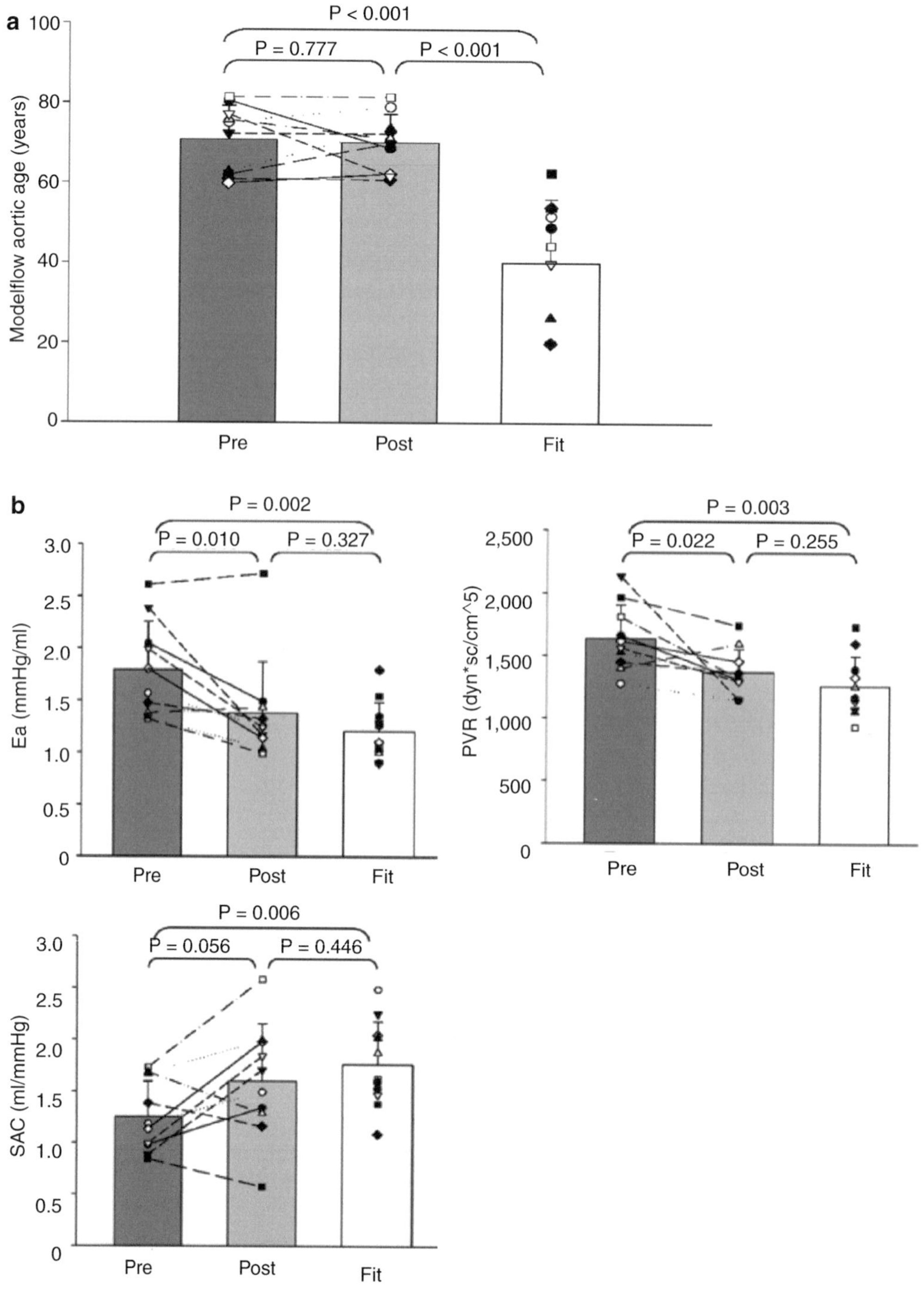

with concurrent BP reduction [34]. Cycling [46] and walking [47] interventions of similar duration and intensity failed to improve aortic PWV or other arterial properties; notably, these interventions also failed to lower BP. In three 12-week RCTs of low-moderate intensity training programs in hypertensive individuals (directed by blood lactate targets; 2.0–2.5 mmol/L during thrice weekly 30 min sessions), changes in large artery compliance were not detected by radial pulse wave analysis despite significant reductions in ambulatory BP [44, 48, 49].

Overweight/Obesity

There is an independent, positive association between adiposity and elevated arterial stiffness [50]. Short-term, weight-neutral training studies in healthy individuals provide proof-of-concept that arterial de-stiffening is possible in the absence of weight loss [21]. This is important to recognise given volumes of exercise recommended for the general population may be inadequate to achieve weight loss of a clinically significant magnitude (particularly in the absence of co-interventions targeting energy intake) [51]. Given a paucity of studies, it remains uncertain whether aerobic exercise (either weight-neutral or with accompanying weight loss) modifies arterial properties in overweight or obese individuals. In one study of obese men and women aged 39–60 years, short-term exercise training *without* weight loss (10 consecutive days of treadmill walking for 60 min; 70–75 % VO_{2peak}) was found to be ineffective for PWV reduction (both aortic and peripheral [i.e. femoral-ankle]) [52]. In contrast, a longer intervention of 12 weeks (3 days/week walking/running for 40–60 min; light-vigorous intensity) elicited improvements in carotid artery compliance and β-stiffness index in the context of modest (3.7 %), but statistically significant weight loss in overweight/obese men (mean age of 50 years) [53]. These findings from two small and uncontrolled studies should not be interpreted to indicate that weight loss is a prerequisite for positive outcomes from exercise training in this setting; indeed, the divergence may have reflected BP lowering of greater magnitude in the latter trial, or any of multiple differences in study design (e.g. duration of intervention, endpoints). Clearly, larger controlled studies are required to inform whether the stiffened arteries of overweight/obese individuals are responsive to aerobic exercise independently of weight loss.

Type 2 Diabetes

The metabolic milieu of type 2 diabetes, which may include insulin resistance, hyperglycaemia and hyperinsulinaemia, independently promotes arterial stiffening via mechanisms such as local renin-angiotensin-aldosterone system activation, endothelial dysfunction, and advanced glycation end-product accumulation [2]. As exercise training is known to reverse hyperglycaemia and insulin resistance to an extent equivalent to anti-diabetic pharmacotherapy [54], there are important addi-

Fig. 45.2 The data show changes in vascular properties before ("Pre") and after ("Post") a 12-month exercise training intervention in previously sedentary, healthy, older individuals and in reference to a group of similarly aged Masters athletes ("Fit" group). Panel (**a**) displays data for the "Modelflow aortic age". This method uses aortic impedance estimation in generating an index of stiffness that – in being independent of BP – theoretically reflects intrinsic aortic structural properties [41, 42]. Panel (**b**) displays data for more conventional measures: effective arterial elastance (*Ea*), peripheral vascular resistance (*PVR*) and systemic arterial compliance (*SAC*) (all BP-dependent and influenced by both functional and structural factors). Exercise training by the previously sedentary – sufficient to realise a large increment in peak oxygen uptake (19 %) – improved Ea, PVR and SAC to such an extent that they achieved values similar to those observed in Masters athletes [42]. However, although the "younger" Modelflow aortic age of Masters athletes indicated that this index may also be responsive to exercise, it was unchanged in the previously sedentary by 12 months training. Collectively, the data support that age-related intrinsic arterial structural changes can be attenuated by aerobic exercise, but may be irreversible in older individuals once established. Functional pathways by which exercise may reduce arterial stiffness appear to remain intact (Panel **a** and **b** figures are reproduced from Ref. [42] with permission of The American Physiological Society).

tional pathways in this population by which arterial properties may be positively affected. This concept was supported in a 3-week cohort study of low-moderate intensity walking/cycling (23 individuals with type 2 diabetes), in which improvements in β-stiffness index (carotid and femoral arteries) were significantly associated with the extent of concurrent improvement in insulin sensitivity (based on euglycemic-hyperinsulinemic clamp) [55]. Unchanged BP, HbA_{1c} and anthropometrics over this short-term intervention supported that insulin sensitisation constituted the primary driver of these arterial adaptations (i.e. via functional mechanisms such as improved endothelium-dependent vasodilation). A subsequent controlled study in individuals with type 2 diabetes and multiple cardiovascular risk factors found that 3 months of vigorous walking/cycling training reduced both aortic and arm PWVs [56]. Unfortunately, insulin resistance was not measured in this study, but since changes in BP and glycaemic control (fasting glucose) were only borderline significant and weight loss was not achieved, the findings collectively supported that arterial changes may reflect other metabolic factors and/or direct vascular effects.

Notwithstanding these positive results, a 2012 RCT of aerobic exercise – larger than both former studies – found no change in brachial-ankle PWV with a 12-week moderate intensity walking program (300 min/week) in women with type 2 diabetes (mean age of 54 years) [57]. This was despite significant weight loss and reductions in both BP and HbA_{1c}. The negative finding may reflect reliance on a non-specific arterial stiffness marker (i.e. composite of aortic and peripheral PWV), but nevertheless highlights a need for additional data in this population.

Kidney Disease

Progressive decline in renal function is independently associated with increased arterial stiffness and wave reflections [58]. These represent important targets for therapy given mortality in end-stage kidney disease is strongly predicted by aortic stiffness [59]. Three studies have evaluated aerobic exercise for this purpose in haemodialysis patients. Central AIx improved in a small, uncontrolled study (n = 11) after 3 months light-moderate treadmill/cycling training (120 min/week) – a benefit that was lost following 3 months of de-training [60]. More compelling evidence of benefit for arterial properties lies with a crossover trial of intra-dialytic exercise in 19 patients, which resulted in aortic PWV reduction after 3 months of cycling training even though BP did not change (self-guided intensity; ≥90 min/week) [61]. Unfortunately, these findings were not replicated in a more recent study – a multicentre, 6-month RCT that evaluated intra-dialytic and home-based exercise programs [62]. Neither exercise intervention (both of moderate intensity; 45–65 min/week) altered aortic PWV, AIx or related parameters relative to usual care, though retrospective power calculations demonstrated inadequacy of the sample size (n = 15–16 per group) for these endpoints. In predialysis patients with chronic kidney disease, aerobic exercise has been evaluated in one RCT – a pilot study of light-vigorous intensity exercise (median 43.4 min/week). Compared with controls, AIx was significantly lower in the exercise training group after 12 months (despite no change in body mass, BP or other confounders) [63].

Given mixed, but promising findings from this series of small studies in kidney disease patients, larger trials powered for arterial stiffness endpoints are awaited with interest.

Resistance Training

Resistance training is associated with health benefits independent of aerobic exercise and is recommended for many sub-populations characterised by stiffened arteries, including elderly and cardiometabolic disease populations. Despite long-held concerns that it promotes arterial stiffening – first highlighted by Bertovic et al. [64] – it is now apparent that adverse effects may be restricted to high-intensity training that is not performed in conjunction with aerobic exercise.

Miyachi [65] identified an overall 10.7 % increase in arterial stiffness (by PWV or carotid β-stiffness index) in a meta-analysis that considered eight RCTs (n = 193) up to April 2011.

However, sub-analyses revealed that this was limited to high-intensity training (>70 % of 1 repetition-maximum), which is consistent with the notion that repeated exposures to marked BP elevation (up to 480/350 mmHg has been recorded during a resistance exercise set) [66] are largely responsible for adverse stiffening effects [65]. Chronically increased vasoconstriction – secondary to raised sympathetic activity – is also implicated [65] even though resistance training is usually associated with a fall in resting BP [67].

Importantly, training at a mild-to-moderate intensity, as recommended by the American Heart Association [67], does not appear to elicit adverse effects [65]. Indeed, a study not included in Miyachi's meta-analysis reported that brachial-ankle PWV and endothelial function were *improved* following resistance training performed at 50 % of 1 repetition-maximum and with short 30-s breaks between sets [68]. This style of training – similar to a 'circuit' style – can introduce an aerobic component while still facilitating gains in strength and muscle function. Performance of rhythmic/continuous movements may also help to avoid breath-holding/Valsalva manoeuvre-induced BP elevations, which are typical of high intensity or isometric loading [66, 67]. Readers are referred to the American Heart Association guidelines for additional details regarding safe prescription of resistance training in the clinical setting [67].

Another important consideration is that resistance training should only ever complement – and not replace – aerobic exercise [67]. Combined aerobic/resistance training has been shown to either improve [69, 70], or have no effect on arterial properties [71, 72].

Conclusions

In line with trends in the broader research field of therapy for large artery structure and function, studies of exercise training have burgeoned since an earlier iteration of this chapter published in 2006 [6]. However, a number of important limitations prevail in the literature and must be acknowledged. Firstly, many published intervention studies (typically small) have investigated changes in arterial stiffness or wave reflection as secondary endpoints without specific *a priori* power calculations. In addition, the plethora of arterial stiffness/wave reflection markers featured in the literature make it difficult to synthesise data and compare studies.

Notwithstanding these drawbacks, a number of conclusions can be drawn. With respect to aerobic exercise, observational data are convincing for a protective effect against age-related arterial stiffening. In contrast, intervention studies are less positive and offer conflicting evidence regarding efficacy for shorter-term improvement (i.e. up to 12 months) – particularly regarding the potential for reversibility of arterial stiffening that is well-advanced (i.e. by ageing or the presence of cardiovascular risk factors). Where improvements in arterial stiffness or wave reflection are observed after a training period, this may often be attributable to concurrent functional or haemodynamic changes. Nevertheless, structural adaptations are evident in trained animals and more recent data indicate that they are also possible in humans when exercise is commenced before older adulthood and high cardiorespiratory fitness is maintained. Resistance exercises performed dynamically and at a low-moderate intensity are unlikely to promote the arterial stiffening observed in individuals trained at a high intensity and may even be beneficial (though further study is required, particularly in the context of heightened cardiovascular risk).

Of course, even if exercise training demonstrates potential for *efficacy* in relation to arterial de-stiffening, translation to clinical *effectiveness* will always be limited to some extent by poor adherence. Moreover, even if exercise training interventions are implemented successfully and positive changes in arterial properties realised, it is unclear whether this extends to improved outcomes over the life course. However, this may never be known given the difficulties associated with undertaking such large-scale and long-term lifestyle intervention trials. In the absence of this information, the value of exercise interventions to favourably modify arterial stiffness and wave reflections should consider their well-established links to cardiovascular sequelae, the prevention of which is clearly an outcome worth targeting.

References

1. Dart AM, Kingwell BA. Pulse pressure–a review of mechanisms and clinical relevance. J Am Coll Cardiol. 2001;37(4):975–84.
2. Zieman SJ, Melenovsky V, Kass DA. Mechanisms, pathophysiology, and therapy of arterial stiffness. Arterioscler Thromb Vasc Biol. 2005;25(5):932–43.
3. Vlachopoulos C, Alexopoulos N, Stefanadis C. Lifestyle modification and arterial stiffness and wave reflections: a more natural way to prolong arterial health. Artery Res. 2006;1(Supplement 1):S15–22.
4. Seals DR, Desouza CA, Donato AJ, Tanaka H. Habitual exercise and arterial aging. J Appl Physiol. 2008;105(4):1323–32.
5. Gates PE, Seals DR. Decline in large elastic artery compliance with age: a therapeutic target for habitual exercise. Br J Sports Med. 2006;40(11):897–9.
6. Kingwell BA, Jennings GL, Cameron JD. Non-pharmacological treatment for increased arterial stiffness and altered wave reflections. In: Safar ME, O'Rourke MF, editors. Arterial stiffness in hypertension. United Kingdom: Elsevier; 2006. p. 567–80.
7. O'Rourke MF, Hashimoto J. Arterial stiffness: a modifiable cardiovascular risk factor? J Cardiopulm Rehabil Prev. 2008;28(4):225–37.
8. Laurent S, Cockcroft J, Van Bortel L, Boutouyrie P, Giannattasio C, Hayoz D, et al. Expert consensus document on arterial stiffness: methodological issues and clinical applications. Eur Heart J. 2006;27(21):2588–605.
9. Mohiaddin RH, Underwood SR, Bogren HG, Firmin DN, Klipstein RH, Rees RS, et al. Regional aortic compliance studied by magnetic resonance imaging: the effects of age, training, and coronary artery disease. Br Heart J. 1989;62(2):90–6.
10. Edwards DG, Lang JT. Augmentation index and systolic load are lower in competitive endurance athletes. Am J Hypertens. 2005;18(5 Pt 1):679–83.
11. D'Andrea A, Cocchia R, Riegler L, Salerno G, Scarafile R, Citro R, et al. Aortic stiffness and distensibility in top-level athletes. J Am Soc Echocardiogr. 2012;25(5):561–7.
12. Vaitkevicius PV, Fleg JL, Engel JH, O'Connor FC, Wright JG, Lakatta LE, et al. Effects of age and aerobic capacity on arterial stiffness in healthy adults. Circulation. 1993;88(4 Pt 1):1456–62.
13. Tanaka H, Dinenno FA, Monahan KD, Clevenger CM, DeSouza CA, Seals DR. Aging, habitual exercise, and dynamic arterial compliance. Circulation. 2000;102(11):1270–5.
14. Tanaka H, DeSouza CA, Seals DR. Absence of age-related increase in central arterial stiffness in physically active women. Arterioscler Thromb Vasc Biol. 1998;18(1):127–32.
15. Aoyagi Y, Park H, Kakiyama T, Park S, Yoshiuchi K, Shephard RJ. Yearlong physical activity and regional stiffness of arteries in older adults: the Nakanojo Study. Eur J Appl Physiol. 2010;109(3):455–64.
16. Sugawara J, Otsuki T, Tanabe T, Hayashi K, Maeda S, Matsuda M. Physical activity duration, intensity, and arterial stiffening in postmenopausal women. Am J Hypertens. 2006;19(10):1032–6.
17. van de Laar RJ, Ferreira I, van Mechelen W, Prins MH, Twisk JW, Stehouwer CD. Lifetime vigorous but not light-to-moderate habitual physical activity impacts favorably on carotid stiffness in young adults: the amsterdam growth and health longitudinal study. Hypertension. 2010;55(1):33–9.
18. Boreham CA, Ferreira I, Twisk JW, Gallagher AM, Savage MJ, Murray LJ. Cardiorespiratory fitness, physical activity, and arterial stiffness: the Northern Ireland Young Hearts Project. Hypertension. 2004;44(5):721–6.
19. Knez WL, Sharman JE, Jenkins DG, Coombes JS. Central hemodynamics in ultra-endurance athletes. J Sci Med Sport. 2008;11(4):390–5.
20. Vlachopoulos C, Kardara D, Anastasakis A, Baou K, Terentes-Printzios D, Tousoulis D, et al. Arterial stiffness and wave reflections in marathon runners. Am J Hypertens. 2010;23(9):974–9.
21. Cameron JD, Dart AM. Exercise training increases total systemic arterial compliance in humans. Am J Physiol. 1994;266(2 Pt 2):H693–701.
22. Kingwell BA, Cameron JD, Gillies KJ, Jennings GL, Dart AM. Arterial compliance may influence baroreflex function in athletes and hypertensives. Am J Physiol. 1995;268(1 Pt 2):H411–8.
23. Currie KD, Thomas SG, Goodman JM. Effects of short-term endurance exercise training on vascular function in young males. Eur J Appl Physiol. 2009;107(2):211–8.
24. Kakiyama T, Sugawara J, Murakami H, Maeda S, Kuno S, Matsuda M. Effects of short-term endurance training on aortic distensibility in young males. Med Sci Sports Exerc. 2005;37(2):267–71.
25. Ciolac EG, Bocchi EA, Bortolotto LA, Carvalho VO, Greve JM, Guimaraes GV. Effects of high-intensity aerobic interval training vs. moderate exercise on hemodynamic, metabolic and neuro-humoral abnormalities of young normotensive women at high familial risk for hypertension. Hypertens Res. 2010;33(8):836–43.
26. Maeda S, Tanabe T, Otsuki T, Sugawara J, Ajisaka R, Matsuda M. Acute exercise increases systemic arterial compliance after 6-month exercise training in older women. Hypertens Res. 2008;31(2):377–81.
27. Moreau KL, Donato AJ, Seals DR, DeSouza CA, Tanaka H. Regular exercise, hormone replacement therapy and the age-related decline in carotid arterial compliance in healthy women. Cardiovasc Res. 2003;57(3):861–8.

28. Hayashi K, Sugawara J, Komine H, Maeda S, Yokoi T. Effects of aerobic exercise training on the stiffness of central and peripheral arteries in middle-aged sedentary men. Jpn J Physiol. 2005;55(4):235–9.
29. Miyaki A, Maeda S, Choi Y, Akazawa N, Tanabe Y, Ajisaka R. Habitual aerobic exercise increases plasma pentraxin 3 levels in middle-aged and elderly women. Appl Physiol Nutr Metab. 2012;37(5):907–11.
30. Yoshizawa M, Maeda S, Miyaki A, Misono M, Choi Y, Shimojo N, et al. Additive beneficial effects of lactotripeptides and aerobic exercise on arterial compliance in postmenopausal women. Am J Physiol Heart Circ Physiol. 2009;297(5):H1899–903.
31. Sugawara J, Akazawa N, Miyaki A, Choi Y, Tanabe Y, Imai T, et al. Effect of endurance exercise training and curcumin intake on central arterial hemodynamics in postmenopausal women: pilot study. Am J Hypertens. 2012;25(6):651–6.
32. Joyner MJ, Green DJ. Exercise protects the cardiovascular system: effects beyond traditional risk factors. J Physiol. 2009;587(Pt 23):5551–8.
33. Kingwell BA, Sherrard B, Jennings GL, Dart AM. Four weeks of cycle training increases basal production of nitric oxide from the forearm. Am J Physiol. 1997;272(3 Pt 2):H1070–7.
34. Nualnim N, Parkhurst K, Dhindsa M, Tarumi T, Vavrek J, Tanaka H. Effects of swimming training on blood pressure and vascular function in adults >50 years of age. Am J Cardiol. 2012;109(7):1005–10.
35. Matsuda M, Nosaka T, Sato M, Ohshima N. Effects of physical exercise on the elasticity and elastic components of the rat aorta. Eur J Appl Physiol Occup Physiol. 1993;66(2):122–6.
36. Koutsis G, Kadi F, Vandewalle H, Lechat P, Hadjiisky P, Monod H. Effects of an endurance training programme on the passive and noradrenaline-activated compliances of rat aorta. Eur J Appl Physiol Occup Physiol. 1995;71(2–3):173–9.
37. Kingwell BA, Arnold PJ, Jennings GL, Dart AM. Spontaneous running increases aortic compliance in Wistar-Kyoto rats. Cardiovasc Res. 1997;35(1):132–7.
38. Kingwell BA, Arnold PJ, Jennings GL, Dart AM. The effects of voluntary running on cardiac mass and aortic compliance in Wistar-Kyoto and spontaneously hypertensive rats. J Hypertens. 1998;16(2):181–5.
39. Matsuda M, Nosaka T, Sato M, Iijima J, Ohshima N, Fukushima H. Effects of exercise training on biochemical and biomechanical properties of rat aorta. Angiology. 1989;40(1):51–8.
40. McEniery CM, Wilkinson IB, Avolio AP. Age, hypertension and arterial function. Clin Exp Pharmacol Physiol. 2007;34(7):665–71.
41. Shibata S, Levine BD. Biological aortic age derived from the arterial pressure waveform. J Appl Physiol. 2011;110(4):981–7.
42. Shibata S, Levine BD. Effect of exercise training on biologic vascular age in healthy seniors. Am J Physiol Heart Circ Physiol. 2012;302(6):H1340–6.
43. Cornelissen VA, Fagard RH. Effects of endurance training on blood pressure, blood pressure-regulating mechanisms, and cardiovascular risk factors. Hypertension. 2005;46(4):667–75.
44. Westhoff TH, Franke N, Schmidt S, Vallbracht-Israng K, Meissner R, Yildirim H, et al. Too old to benefit from sports? The cardiovascular effects of exercise training in elderly subjects treated for isolated systolic hypertension. Kidney Blood Press Res. 2007;30(4):240–7.
45. Guimaraes GV, Ciolac EG, Carvalho VO, D'Avila VM, Bortolotto LA, Bocchi EA. Effects of continuous vs. interval exercise training on blood pressure and arterial stiffness in treated hypertension. Hypertens Res. 2010;33(6):627–32.
46. Ferrier KE, Waddell TK, Gatzka CD, Cameron JD, Dart AM, Kingwell BA. Aerobic exercise training does not modify large-artery compliance in isolated systolic hypertension. Hypertension. 2001;38(2):222–6.
47. Seals DR, Tanaka H, Clevenger CM, Monahan KD, Reiling MJ, Hiatt WR, et al. Blood pressure reductions with exercise and sodium restriction in postmenopausal women with elevated systolic pressure: role of arterial stiffness. J Am Coll Cardiol. 2001;38(2):506–13.
48. Westhoff TH, Schmidt S, Gross V, Joppke M, Zidek W, van der Giet M, et al. The cardiovascular effects of upper-limb aerobic exercise in hypertensive patients. J Hypertens. 2008;26(7):1336–42.
49. Dimeo F, Pagonas N, Seibert F, Arndt R, Zidek W, Westhoff TH. Aerobic exercise reduces blood pressure in resistant hypertension. Hypertension. 2012;60(3):653–8.
50. Zebekakis PE, Nawrot T, Thijs L, Balkestein EJ, van der Heijden-Spek J, Van Bortel LM, et al. Obesity is associated with increased arterial stiffness from adolescence until old age. J Hypertens. 2005;23(10):1839–46.
51. Donnelly JE, Blair SN, Jakicic JM, Manore MM, Rankin JW, Smith BK. American College of Sports Medicine Position Stand. Appropriate physical activity intervention strategies for weight loss and prevention of weight regain for adults. Med Sci Sports Exerc. 2009;41(2):459–71.
52. Baynard T, Carhart Jr RL, Weinstock RS, Ploutz-Snyder LL, Kanaley JA. Short-term exercise training improves aerobic capacity with no change in arterial function in obesity. Eur J Appl Physiol. 2009;107(3):299–308.
53. Miyaki A, Maeda S, Yoshizawa M, Misono M, Saito Y, Sasai H, et al. Effect of habitual aerobic exercise on body weight and arterial function in overweight and obese men. Am J Cardiol. 2009;104(6):823–8.
54. Snowling NJ, Hopkins WG. Effects of different modes of exercise training on glucose control and risk factors for complications in type 2 diabetic patients: a meta-analysis. Diabetes Care. 2006;29(11):2518–27.
55. Yokoyama H, Emoto M, Fujiwara S, Motoyama K, Morioka T, Koyama H, et al. Short-term aerobic exercise improves arterial stiffness in type 2 diabetes. Diabetes Res Clin Pract. 2004;65(2):85–93.

56. Madden KM, Lockhart C, Cuff D, Potter TF, Meneilly GS. Short-term aerobic exercise reduces arterial stiffness in older adults with type 2 diabetes, hypertension, and hypercholesterolemia. Diabetes Care. 2009;32(8):1531–5.
57. Choi KM, Han KA, Ahn HJ, Hwang SY, Hong HC, Choi HY, et al. Effects of exercise on sRAGE levels and cardiometabolic risk factors in patients with type 2 diabetes: a randomized controlled trial. J Clin Endocrinol Metab. 2012;97(10):3751–8.
58. Briet M, Bozec E, Laurent S, Fassot C, London GM, Jacquot C, et al. Arterial stiffness and enlargement in mild-to-moderate chronic kidney disease. Kidney Int. 2006;69(2):350–7.
59. Blacher J, Guerin AP, Pannier B, Marchais SJ, Safar ME, London GM. Impact of aortic stiffness on survival in end-stage renal disease. Circulation. 1999;99(18):2434–9.
60. Mustata S, Chan C, Lai V, Miller JA. Impact of an exercise program on arterial stiffness and insulin resistance in hemodialysis patients. J Am Soc Nephrol. 2004;15(10):2713–8.
61. Toussaint ND, Polkinghorne KR, Kerr PG. Impact of intradialytic exercise on arterial compliance and B-type natriuretic peptide levels in hemodialysis patients. Hemodial Int. 2008;12(2):254–63.
62. Koh KP, Fassett RG, Sharman JE, Coombes JS, Williams AD. Effect of intradialytic versus home-based aerobic exercise training on physical function and vascular parameters in hemodialysis patients: a randomized pilot study. Am J Kidney Dis. 2010; 55(1):88–99.
63. Mustata S, Groeneveld S, Davidson W, Ford G, Kiland K, Manns B. Effects of exercise training on physical impairment, arterial stiffness and health-related quality of life in patients with chronic kidney disease: a pilot study. Int Urol Nephrol. 2011;43(4): 1133–41.
64. Bertovic DA, Waddell TK, Gatzka CD, Cameron JD, Dart AM, Kingwell BA. Muscular strength training is associated with low arterial compliance and high pulse pressure. Hypertension. 1999;33(6):1385–91.
65. Miyachi M. Effects of resistance training on arterial stiffness: a meta-analysis. Br J Sports Med. 2013;47(6): 393–6.
66. McCartney N. Acute responses to resistance training and safety. Med Sci Sports Exerc. 1999;31(1):31–7.
67. Williams MA, Haskell WL, Ades PA, Amsterdam EA, Bittner V, Franklin BA, et al. Resistance exercise in individuals with and without cardiovascular disease: 2007 update: a scientific statement from the American Heart Association Council on Clinical Cardiology and Council on Nutrition, Physical Activity, and Metabolism. Circulation. 2007;116(5): 572–84.
68. Okamoto T, Masuhara M, Ikuta K. Effect of low-intensity resistance training on arterial function. Eur J Appl Physiol. 2011;111(5):743–8.
69. Yang SJ, Hong HC, Choi HY, Yoo HJ, Cho GJ, Hwang TG, et al. Effects of a three-month combined exercise programme on fibroblast growth factor 21 and fetuin-A levels and arterial stiffness in obese women. Clin Endocrinol (Oxf). 2011;75(4):464–9.
70. Figueroa A, Park SY, Seo DY, Sanchez-Gonzalez MA, Baek YH. Combined resistance and endurance exercise training improves arterial stiffness, blood pressure, and muscle strength in postmenopausal women. Menopause. 2011;18(9):980–4.
71. Stewart KJ, Bacher AC, Turner KL, Fleg JL, Hees PS, Shapiro EP, et al. Effect of exercise on blood pressure in older persons: a randomized controlled trial. Arch Intern Med. 2005;165(7):756–62.
72. Spina RJ, Meyer TE, Peterson LR, Villareal DT, Rinder MR, Ehsani AA. Absence of left ventricular and arterial adaptations to exercise in octogenarians. J Appl Physiol. 2004;97(5):1654–9.

Index

M.E. Safar et al. (eds.), *Blood Pressure and Arterial Wall Mechanics in Cardiovascular Diseases*, DOI 10.1007/978-1-4471-5198-2, © Springer-Verlag London 2014

D

MIX
Papier aus verantwortungsvollen Quellen
Paper from responsible sources
FSC® C105338

If you have any concerns about our products,
you can contact us on
ProductSafety@springernature.com

In case Publisher is established outside the EU,
the EU authorized representative is:
Springer Nature Customer Service Center GmbH
Europaplatz 3, 69115 Heidelberg, Germany

Printed by Libri Plureos GmbH
in Hamburg, Germany